Pediatric Neoplasia
Morphology and Biology

Pediatric Neoplasia
Morphology and Biology

Editor

David M. Parham, M.D.

Chief
Department of Pediatric Pathology
Arkansas Children's Hospital
Vice-Chairman and Professor
Department of Pathology
University of Arkansas for Medical Sciences
Little Rock, Arkansas

Lippincott - Raven
PUBLISHERS
Philadelphia • New York

Lippincott-Raven Publishers, 227 East Washington Square, Philadelphia, Pennsylvania 19106

Made in the United States of America

Library of Congress Cataloging-in-Publication Data

Pediatric neoplasia: morphology and biology/edited by David M. Parham.
p. cm.
Includes bibliographical references and index.
ISBN 0-7817-0273-9
1. Tumors in children—Molecular aspects. 2. Tumors in children—Cytodiagnosis. 2. Pediatric pathology. I. Parham, David M.
[DNLM: 1. Neoplasms—in infancy & childhood. 2. Neoplasms—microbiology. 3. Neoplasms—pathology. QZ 275 P371 1996]
RC281.C4P326 1996
618.92'994—dc20
DNLM/DLC 95-42517
for Library of Congress

9 8 7 6 5 4 3 2 1

To the memory of my cousin,
William David Weatherly,
who died at St. Jude Children's Research Hospital on June 19, 1966,
of acute lymphoblastic leukemia, at the tender age of 15 years.

Contents

Color Figures

Chapter 6

Chapter 7

Chapter 8

Chapter 12

Chapter 13

Chapter 15

Chapter 16

Contributors

Richard A. Ashmun, Ph.D., *Associate Member, Department of Experimental Oncology, St. Jude Children's Research Hospital, 332 North Lauderdale Street, Memphis, Tennessee 38105*

Frederick G. Behm, M.D., *Associate Member, Department of Pathology and Laboratory Medicine, St. Jude Children's Research Hospital, 332 North Lauderdale Street, Memphis, Tennessee 38105*

M. Frederick Bugg, M.D., *Director, Rapid Service Laboratory and Staff Pathologist, Department of Pathology, MidSouth Pathology Group, Inc., Baptist Memorial Hospital, 899 Madison Avenue, Suite 270 Union East, Memphis, Tennessee 38146*

Andrew B. Cu-Unjieng, M.D., *Resident, Department of Ophthalmology and Visual Sciences, University of Louisville, Kentucky 40206*

Peter Dias, Ph.D., *Senior Scientist, Pharmingen, 10975 Torreyana Road, San Diego, California 92121*

Larry A. Donoso, M.D., Ph.D., *Director, Research Division, Wills Eye Hospital, 900 Walnut Street, Philadelphia, Pennsylvania 19107*

Gregory N. Fuller, M.D., Ph.D., *Assistant Professor of Pathology (Neuropathology), Department of Pathology, The University of Texas, M. D. Anderson Cancer Center, 1515 Holcombe Boulevard, Room G3.305, Houston, Texas 77030*

Glen S. Germain, B.S., M.S., *Associate Scientist, Department of Molecular Pharmacology, St. Jude Children's Research Hospital, 332 North Lauderdale Street, Memphis, Tennessee 38105*

Edith P. Hawkins, M.D., *Professor of Pathology and Associate Professor of Pediatrics, Department of Pathology, Texas Children's Hospital/Baylor College of Medicine, 6621 Fannin Street, Houston, Texas 77030*

David R. Head, M.D., *Member, Department of Pathology and Laboratory Medicine, St. Jude Children's Research Hospital, 332 North Lauderdale Street, Memphis, Tennessee 38105*

Peter J. Houghton, Ph.D., *Chairman, Department of Molecular Pharmacology, St. Jude Children's Research Hospital, 332 North Lauderdale Street, Memphis, Tennessee 38105*

Robert E. Hutchison, M.D., *Associate Professor of Pathology, Department of Pathology, State University of New York Health Science Center, 750 East Adams Street, Syracuse, New York 13210*

Jesse J. Jenkins III, M.D., *Associate Member, Department of Pathology and Laboratory Medicine, St. Jude Children's Research Hospital, 332 North Lauderdale Street, Memphis, Tennessee 38105*

Vijay V. Joshi, M.D., F.R.C.Path, *Professor of Pathology, Department of Pathology and Laboratory Medicine, East Carolina University School of Medicine, 200 Stantonsburg Road, Greenville, North Carolina 27858*

David R. Kelly, M.D., *Clinical Professor of Pathology, Department of Pathology, University of Alabama at Birmingham, Pathologist-in-Chief and Medical Director of Laboratories, The Children's Hospital of Alabama, 1600 Seventh Avenue South, Birmingham, Alabama 35233*

Geoffrey A. Machin, M.D., Ph.D., F.R.C.Path., F.R.C.P.(C), *Professor of Pediatric Pathology, Department of Pathology, University of Alberta Hospital, 8440 112th Street, Edmonton, Alberta T6G 2B7, Canada*

David Meyer, M.D., F.A.C.S., *Associate Clinical Professor, University of Tennessee, Memphis, Vitreoretinal Foundation, 825 Ridge Lake Boulevard, Memphis, Tennessee 38119*

David M. Parham, M.D., *Vice-Chairman and Professor, Department of Pathology, University of Arkansas for Medical Sciences, Chief, Department of Pediatric Pathology, Arkansas Children's Hospital, 800 Marshall Street, Little Rock, Arkansas 72202*

Kathleen Patterson, M.D., *Associate Professor, Department of Pathology, University of Washington/Children's Hospital, 4800 Sand Point Way, NE, Seattle, Washington 98105*

Elizabeth J. Perlman, M.D., *Director of Pediatric Pathology, Johns Hopkins Hospital, 600 North Wolfe Street, Baltimore, Maryland 21287*

Alfredo Pinto, M.D., *Assistant Professor, Department of Pathology, Faculty of Medicine, The University of Calgary/Alberta Children's Hospital, 1820 Richmond Road SW, Calgary, Alberta T2T 5C7, Canada*

Charles B. Pratt, M.D., *Professor of Pediatrics, University of Tennessee, Memphis, Member, Department of Hematology and Oncology, St. Jude Children's Research Hospital, 332 North Lauderdale Street, Memphis, Tennessee 38105*

Cynthia L. Trevenen, M.D., F.R.C.P.(C), *Associate Professor, Department of Pathology and Pediatrics, The University of Calgary/Alberta Children's Hospital, 1820 Richmond Road SW, Calgary, Alberta T2T 5C7, Canada*

Aysegul H. Uner, M.D., Ph.D., *Department of Pathology, State University of New York Health Science Center, 750 East Adams Street, Syracuse, New York 13210*

Ming X. Wang, M.D., Ph.D., *Assistant Professor of Ophthalmology, Research Division, Wills Eye Hospital, 900 Walnut Street, Philadelphia, Pennsylvania 19107*

Bruce L. Webber, M.B. B.Ch., F.F.Path. (S.A.), *Pathologist in Charge of Surgical Pathology, MidSouth Pathology Group, Inc., Baptist Memorial Hospital, 899 Madison Avenue, Memphis, Tennessee 38146*

Preface

The methods for diagnosing pediatric neoplasia have become so increasingly varied through the years that it has become imperative for pathologists, oncologists, radiologists, and tumor biologists to be keenly aware of other disciplines. Not only must we be updated of new findings but we must also learn to synthesize information from diverse fields.

Pediatric Neoplasia: Morphology and Biology is the first book to fully integrate both the morphologic and biologic studies on pediatric tumors. We believe that this integrated study will help us better understand and control the disease process. This volume will be of practical and scholarly use in studying all benign and malignant tumors of children through established and new data gathered from different sources. Classic observations of the gross, clinical, and microscopic features of pediatric tumors are reexamined in relation to new genetic and biologic findings relevant to tumor diagnosis.

Children can acquire not only pediatric tumors but also adult tumors of all types. Although we emphasize the more typical pediatric neoplasms, such as neuroblastoma, leukemia, and rhabdomyosarcoma, for tumors more commonly found in adults, we focus instead on the genetic and biologic factors that cause their unexpected development. We also describe the unique morphologic features of these malignant tumors in pediatric patients.

Pediatric Neoplasia: Morphology and Biology consolidates the latest study reports available and emphasizes ongoing research on diagnostic issues. It provides a solid framework for current reading and a strong reference guide for relevant topics under investigation.

With several illustrative anecdotes from veteran pediatric pathologists included for interest and informative viewpoints, this book will be helpful to a broad range of clinical and biological scientists, particularly those interested in the study and treatment of childhood tumors.

Acknowledgments

Any degree of success in the study of pediatric neoplasia I owe primarily to my co-workers and to the American Lebanese–Syrian Associated Charities (ALSAC, St. Jude's fund-raising organization) at the St. Jude Children's Research Hospital; the Pediatric Oncology Group; the Intergroup Rhabdomyosarcoma Study; and also to the collaborators and contributors who generously supplied me with materials.

My former chairman, Dr. Costan Berard, gave me advice, materials, time, and support for this project; and I thank him for these. Similarly, I thank my former colleague in anatomic pathology, Dr. Jesse Jenkins, for his magnanimity in giving me free time for writing. I also thank the staff of Lippincott-Raven Publishers, particularly Vickie Thaw and Jill Barnowski, for their patience, encouragement, and professional support.

At St. Jude's Children's Research Hospital, my co-workers in anatomic pathology have always supported my work in this project and in others with a professional attitude and high quality of workmanship. These esteemed colleagues include my secretaries, Trish McGhee, Vivian Turner, Hazel Beard, and Bobbye Allen; the Histology Laboratory, including Carolyn Beard, Inez Lewis, Nettie Turner, Charlene Henry, Alice Slusher, and the Reverend Darnell Johnson; Tumor Bank personnel, including Kent Williams, Fawn Learn, and the Immunopathology Laboratory Staff; and my most esteemed assistant in the Experimental Immunopathology Laboratory, Hallie Holt. I also thank my many colleagues in Hematology/Oncology, Surgery, and Diagnostic Imaging for their generosity in supplying illustrations and information. The employees of Biomedical Communications, particularly Jerry Luther, John Zacher, Klo Spelshouse, and Connie Coleman have been outstanding in their responsiveness to my needs and in their excellence at preparing the illustrations. I also thank Sharon Naron of Scientific Editing for her kind assistance in preparing the preface, and Teresa Springer and Helen Alexander, my assistants at Arkansas Children's Hospital, for helping me complete this project.

I gratefully acknowledge those who reviewed or helped with specific chapters, such as Drs. Sheila Shurtleff and Jesse Jenkins for Chapter 1; Drs. Susan Raimondi, Jim Downing, and Vivek Khare and Ms. Patsy Mardis for Chapter 2; Dr. Bob Castleberry for Chapter 6; Dr. Barry Fletcher for Chapters 8 and 9; and Dr. Costan Berard for Chapters 2 and 16. I am also grateful for the kind assistance of Mr. Ron Summer at the Health Science Library of the University of Tennessee, Memphis, for his help on research of Chapter 1. I thank The United States/Canadian Academy of Pathology and Drs. Bernard Wagner and Steven Vogel for giving me permission to reuse portions of the text from my article "Short course: pathology of selected pediatric embryonal neoplasms" in *Modern Pathology,* Vol. 7, 1994: 501–519.

Finally, I thank my family—Jean, Andrew, and Zack—for their patience, love, and forgiveness during the long hours I spent in preparing this book.

David M. Parham

Pediatric Neoplasia
Morphology and Biology

Pediatric Neoplasia: Morphology and Biology, edited by David M. Parham.
Lippincott-Raven Publishers, Philadelphia © 1996.

CHAPTER 1

History of the Pathologic Study of Pediatric Neoplasia

David M. Parham

INTRODUCTION

Perhaps no field in diagnostic pathology can boast the wide diversity of morphologic appearances or knowledge of biologic transformative events apparent in the study of pediatric neoplasia. These features are primarily due to the unquenched tendencies of these lesions to recapitulate embryonic events and structures in an often confusing nature divergent from their tissues of origin. As a result, one obtains skeletal muscle arising from the bladder, neural tissue arising from bone, and cartilage arising from the kidney. The degree to which these tumors differentiate also varies to an extreme degree, so that diagnosticians often grapple with uncommitted germinative neoplastic tissues or marvel at an interwoven array of neural, optic, and musculoskeletal caricatures. The oncogenesis of these lesions also holds extreme fascination for biologists, who relate these events to uncontrolled growth impulses normally functioning at such basic levels as the initial separation of tail and body segments in fly embryos.

Although childhood neoplasia is an uncommon event, it is nevertheless the second leading cause of death in pediatric medicine, following accidents (40). The extreme suffering and emotional torment that cancer causes has understandably propelled much investigation into its origins and cure in this age group. The results have also abetted our understanding of adult neoplasia, although in general the mechanisms of oncogenesis appear to differ from those of pediatrics (12). In addition, for peculiar reasons malignancies that usually occur in children may inexplicably arise in adults, so that a knowledge of these lesions is important to the general practice of pathology.

Finally, the results obtained with pediatric oncologic research have been stunning, with vastly improved survival figures obtained over a relatively short time (6). To some degree this phenomenon is a testament to the resiliency of children, but the methods and materials that have been used often have direct application for adult oncology (12). This improved survival is creating a burgeoning population of childhood cancer survivors whose surveillance will require knowledge of pediatric conditions by practitioners of adult oncology and surgical pathology (11). Also, the tools being developed for ancillary use in categorization of childhood tumors will also have application for general diagnosticians, so that a knowledge of their employment has become imperative.

D. M. Parham: Department of Pathology, Arkansas Children's Hospital, Little Rock, Arkansas 72202.

ANTIQUITIES THROUGH MEDIEVAL TIMES

According to Abt and Garrison (1), evidence that the ancients were familiar with childhood tumors is recorded in the Ebers Papyrus from 1500 B.C. However, interpretation of anatomic descriptions of tumors is severely hampered by the inclusion of infectious lesions and cysts as well as neoplasms into this general category. Thus, one can only speculate as to how many lymphoid malignancies compose the "scrofulous swellings, . . . growing chiefly in the neck, but also the armpits, groins, and sides," which are "slow to come to a head," as described by Celsus in his classic tome, *De Re Medicina*, which many consider to be the first systematic study of pathologic processes (24). Celsus also described splenomegaly that was externally palpable, but again many cases were doubtless (14) due to malaria. "Phymata," which later came to be known as "tubercles," were described; some of these may have been due to neoplasia as well as tuberculosis and other infections. One particularly intriguing passage of medical description regards abdominal tumors (hernias?) that were sometimes cancerous but that could be successfully treated surgically if the patient was between 7 and 14 years of age. Celsus, who was a historian as much as an observer, also refers to malignant nasal growths; according to Hajdu (16), angiofibromas were also known to Hippocrates. However, Celsus makes no direct reference to visceral cancers in either children or adults.

Following Celsus, the dominant medical writer was Galen, whose writings were considered to be the most authoritative texts until the Renaissance. Galen's knowledge of neoplasia was greatly hampered by his lack of experience at the gross dissection of patients, although he practiced often with pigs and baboons. He did, however, divide tumors into three groups: *tumores secundum naturum,* which were physiologic swellings such as the breast enlargement of thelarche; *tumores supra naturum,* which occurred after trauma, as with callus formation; and *tumores praeter naturum,* a broad group including inflammatory processes as well as true neoplasms (24). Galen was a great proponent of the humoral theory of disease advanced by Hippocrates, and he attributed all cancer to an overabundance of black bile (atra bilis) from the spleen. Unknowingly, of course, he was at least partially correct in some instances of leukemia and lymphoma. Regardless of his concept of the pathologic anatomy of cancer, Galen was quite familiar with the dire prognosis associated with its discovery. Galen used the term "fungus" to describe the fleshy swelling of sarcomas, both benign and malignant; this term persisted into the 19th century. Like Celsus, Galen had little knowledge of internal cancers.

RENAISSANCE THROUGH THE 18TH CENTURY

The advancement of medical knowledge during the Dark Ages was greatly stifled by a great reluctance to either perform postmortem dissections or to question the seemingly complete wisdom of Galen. Following the dissolution of the Roman Empire, the greatest practitioners of the medical arts were the Arabs, whose domain came to encompass the entire southern Mediterranean coast following the ascent of Islam. However, the Koran specifically prohibited the mutilation of dead bodies. The Catholic Church also took a dim view of autopsy procedures, largely because of the barbarous but common practice of cooking the flesh of dead Crusaders so that their bones could be transported to family cemeteries. Long (24) suggests that the use of anatomic dissection to teach medicine began in Bologna in 1260 under Taldeo di Alderotto.

In the latter part of the 15th century, Antonio Benivieni began making systematic postmortem examinations of his patients in order to deduce the cause of their infirmities. Thanks to his brother, Geronimo, his records were published under the title of *De Abditis Nonnullis ac Mirandis Morbundum et Sanationum Causis.* Included in this compendium are descriptions of 20 autopsies, including a description of a "callus" of the "mesaraic veins" obstructing the mesenteric circulation of an 8-year-old boy. This unfortunate child had suffered nausea and diarrhea which Benivieni ascribed to "a depraved appetite" with "eating of pebbles and rubbish," leading to a "state of lingering flesh." It is tempting for one with an interest in childhood neoplasia to classify this tumor as a retroperitoneal sarcoma, but infectious abdominal lymphadenitis cannot be excluded.

Another of Benivieni's patients was a 7-year-old girl with "elephantiasis" affecting the fibula. This untimely disorder led to "redness" of the overlying skin that "gradually began to change to blackness" with "great pain" and "no sign of pus." These alarming symptoms caused Benivieni to successfully perform a partial fibullectomy. The patient was "duly cured . . . and recovered," although we don't know the ultimate outcome. Again, it is tempting to consider this an osseous neoplasm, but osteomyelitis is also likely.

The most carefully detailed descriptions of gross pathology during the premodern era may be found in Giovanni Batista Morgagni's work, *De Sedibus et Causis Morbundi (The Seats and Causes of Disease).* The very first patient whom he describes is a 13-year-old boy with headaches and a pineal tumor. Accounts follow of a 20-year-old epileptic girl, whose autopsy uncovered hydrocephalus and multiple choroid plexus nodules, and an 18-year-old epileptic boy with an ill-defined tumor of the cerebrum. Other descriptions include bilateral renal enlargements in a virgin of unstated age, tumorous ascites in a 20-year-old girl with a large intrapelvic tumor, and a "growing exostosis" following trauma to the clavicle in a young man.

A number of previously recorded pediatric tumors are noted, including Hartmann's description of "a large tumour, in a girl of three years old, stretched out from the left spurious ribs, to the confines of the pubes." Morgagni also made numerous references to cystic ovarian teratomas, including one of "the magnitude of a goose's egg, full of oblong hairs and mucous material."

Morgagni's most classic description of childhood neoplasia is his account of lymphadenopathy in 15-year-old "noble youth," who had "prominent bodies, of the size of a pigeon's egg, resembling strumous glands, [in the] salivary [and] axillary [regions and] about the clavicles, . . . and abdominal integument." In an account eerily reminiscent of combination chemotherapy, Morgagni relates that "many remedies were made use of both internally and externally; and that in the beginning too, but still more in the progress of the disease, when the most powerful medicines were prescrib'd by the most skillful physicians in concert. But whether he made use of any, or none, the bulk of the tumours increas'd, and the disease had so rapid a course, that although it had begun only in the month of December, it finished its period in death about the end of May following." At autopsy, "the common integuments of the neck, breast, and abdomen, being cut into, it was found that those external tumours had their seats in the cells of the membrana adiposa [lymph nodes]; which was closely connected, in that part, to the subjected muscles. All of them were full of a whitish matter, which was in part somewhat fluid; but for the most part, solid and sebaceous." Morgagni's account continues with a description of massive abdominal and thoracic lymph node enlargement "to the size of a hen's egg." He concludes by mention of a similar case described by Meckel.

THE 19TH CENTURY AND THE BEGINNINGS OF HISTOPATHOLOGY

With the 19th century came the great leap of systematic cataloging of neoplasms according to their constituent cells. This great conceptual leap occurred largely by the efforts of Marie-François-Xavier Bichat, who first recognized the fundamental nature of tissues and their contribution as entities to human anatomy. In Germany, Johannes Müller established cells as the basic unit of neoplasms with his text, *On the Finer Structure and Form of Morbid Tumors*. It was during this period that the systematic study of childhood neoplasia truly began, as pathologists became more cognizant of the fleshy tumors that arise in children (Fig. 1). For example, Rudolph Virchow's landmark text, *Cellular Pathology*, contains the first description of leukemia as an entity composed of neoplastic leukocytes (Fig. 2) and the first usage of the term as we know it today. Virchow was quite familiar with the gross appearance of this disease and refers to an instance in which it created an abscesslike tumescence inside the heart. He also recognized two forms of the disease, one affecting primarily the spleen and the other the lymph nodes, thus engendering the categories of splenomyelogenous leukemia and lymphatic leukemia. The predilection of these patients to develop a hemorrhagic diathesis was also noted.

Virchow's basic theory, that human cells developed from other cells, had been previously elucidated by Theodor Schwann, but Virchow used this model to explain disease and to develop concepts of its pathogenesis. In doing so, he refuted the blastema theory of the day, which held that tumor cell formation proceeded from a

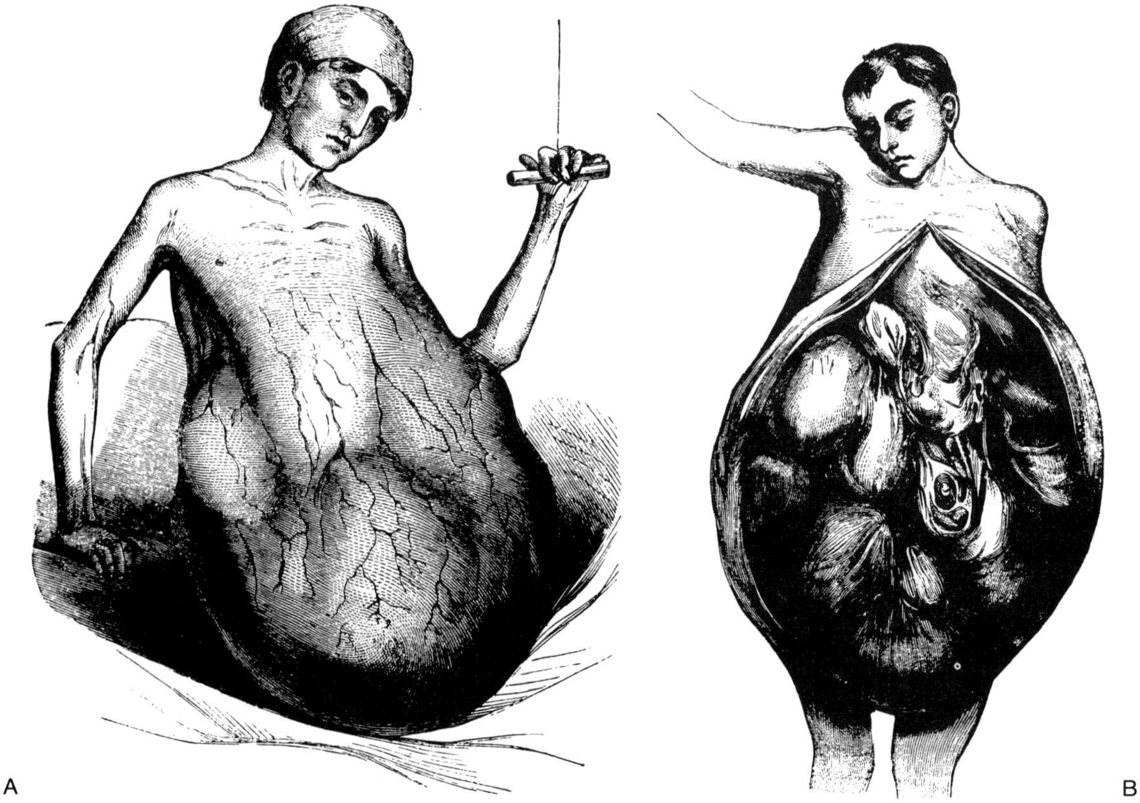

FIG. 1. Premortem **(A)** and postmortem **(B)** illustrations of fleshy intra-abdominal pediatric malignancy. (From Richard Bright's *Clinical Memoirs on Abdominal Tumors and Intumescence*, ref. 6a.)

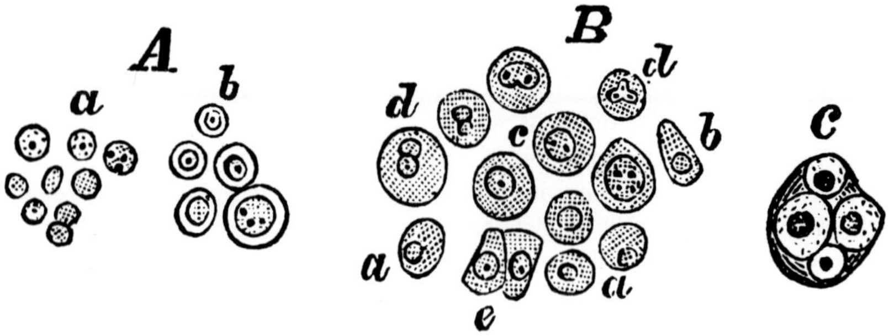

FIG. 2. Illustrations of leukocytes from Virchow's *Cellular Pathology* (ref. 8a).

formative fluid known as "blastema" or "cytoblastema." Virchow also disputed the "law of continuity," which held that all mesenchymal tissues developed from a common primordium and is a concept that we use today in explaining the differentiation of multipotential primitive mesenchyme. Instead he favored a doctrine of "histologic substitution" in which diseased tissues were replaced by a "histologic equivalent," similar to the squamous metaplasia that occurs in diseased bronchial epithelium. Virchow's basic criterion for determining the relative malignancy or benignancy of a tumor, as noted in *Cellular Pathology*, was the amount of fluid it contained, more succulent tumors being more clinically aggressive.

Shortly before Virchow's great work, the pathologist of the century was Carl Rokitansky, who published the standard four volume text, *Manual of Pathologic Anatomy*. This great text was divided into general pathology followed by systemic pathology, similar to the books we use today. Rokitansky seriously erred in his belief in the blastema theory to explain cell proliferation. However, he used the term "sarcoma" to refer to fleshy, benign, or malignant growths occurring primarily in children. Childhood neoplasms that he described arose in bone, muscle, nerve, eye, and kidney, but he did not characterize these lesions histologically. He also recognized the occurrence of brain tumors in children, but he described them as hyperplasias rather than neoplasms. Rokitansky recognized the limitations of the techniques available to him, stating that "to catalogue the species of these new-growths in a strictly philosophical order, is not feasible at this day." Rather, he divided lesions into categories based primarily on their gross structure, as with "gelatinous sarcoma," "albumino-fibrous tumour," or "albumen-like fibrous tumour."

A number of landmark articles on childhood neoplasms such as Wilms' tumor (Fig. 3) appeared during the 19th century. In his recounting of the history of Wilms' tumor, Gonzalez-Crussi (15) cites the description of a "fungus haematodes" in a 17-month-old infant by Thomas Rance in 1814; this tumor's relationship to Wilms' tumor is inferred by its rapid growth, bilaterality, and the patient's age. Eberth in 1872 provided a detailed histologic description of Wilms' tumor, including the appearance of striated muscle. The occurrence of muscle in these tumors was used to theorize their histogenesis, first as Wolffian by Eberth and later as myotomic by Cohnheim. With the advancement of surgery during the 1800s came the opportunity to examine renal tumors histologically, so that increasing numbers of reports appeared. As might be expected, the vast array of appearances that are part and parcel of childhood renal neoplasia gave rise to a confusion of diagnostic terminology and interpretations, which were unified into one nosologic entity by Birch-Hirschfeld. However, a subsequent monograph published by Max Wilms in 1899 also carefully described this tumor, so that ironically it is his name that we commonly use with these lesions today.

For an excellent historical account of the pathologic study of sarcomas, one must turn to the book by Hajdu (16). In it he credits Burns with the first account of a chloroma in 1811, Stafford with the first description of prostatic rhabdomyosarcoma in 1839, Odier with the coining of the term "neurom[a]" in 1806, Guersant with the first case report of botryoid rhabdomyosarcoma in 1854, We-

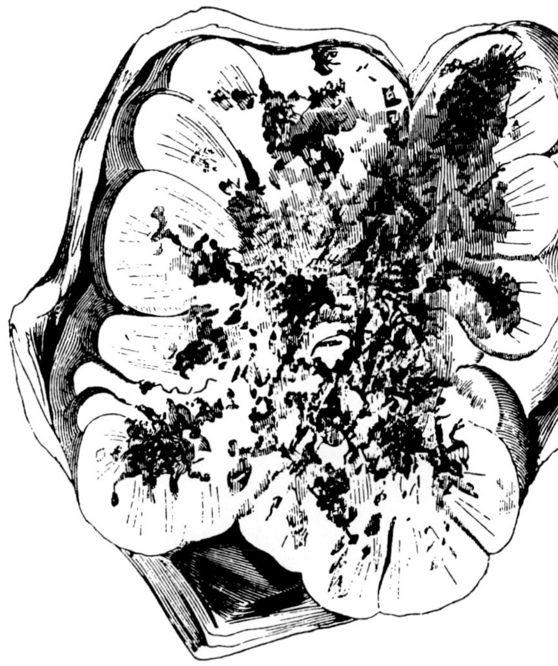

FIG. 3. Renal tumor illustrated in Samuel Gross's *Elements of Pathologic Anatomy* (ref. 15a, p. 646).

ber with the coining of the term "rhabdomyosarcoma" in his description of a tongue lesion, Malhéné with the first monograph on fibrous tumors in 1866, and Berard with the first association of rhabdomyosarcomas with embryonic striated muscle in coining the term "embryonal rhabdomyosarcoma" in 1899.

As noted by Hajdu (16), one of the most prescient 19th century authors in describing sarcomas was Samuel Gross of Philadelphia. His textbook, entitled *Elements of Pathologic Anatomy* and published in 1857, is replete with descriptions of pediatric tumors. Gross separated tumors into two broad groups: scirrhous and encephaloid. He begins his discourse on encephaloid by noting its occurrence "in various organs at every period of life," even "soon after birth" or "as an intrauterine affection" (Table 1). Of particular note to Gross was the more frequent occurrence of "encephaloid" of the eye in childhood (most likely retinoblastoma), and he personally saw a dozen cases (Fig. 4). Gross also noted the wide distribution of anatomic sites affected by encephaloid (Table 2). Other classic pathologic features of these tumors that he noted were their tendency to reappear after extirpation, to bleed profusely, to grow with "frightful rapidity," to ulcerate and discharge a "thin glairy fluid, resembling the white of an egg," and to "resemble a cauliflower." In these advanced stages, the patients would show a "rapid failure in strength, the flesh wastes, the appetite declines, the patient is harassed with a hectic fever, the countenance assumes a peculiar, yellowish hue, [and] the lymphatic ganglions in the neighborhood . . . become enlarged and converted into a substance resembling that of the original tumor." Among examples of pediatric encephaloid occurring in children described by Gross are ones found in lymphatic ganglions, bones (Fig. 5), brain, nerves, eye, peritoneum, and kidneys.

One glaring deficiency of Gross's text, considering the time in which it was written, is the minimal use of histology, although gross and clinical features of tumors are magnificently recorded. This deficiency is not present, however, in the writing of James Paget of London, who in 1854 published the first text on surgical pathology, *Lectures on Surgical Pathology Delivered at the Royal College of Surgeons of England.* This exquisite tome features extensive descriptions of pediatric cystic lesions occurring in the neck, scapular region, pubes, and other sites. Also noted are fibrocellular tumors of the scrotum, labia, vagina, and intermuscular spaces; these he describes as being "completely innocent." Possible examples of nodular fasciitis are described as "painful subcutaneous tumors . . . more frequent in women than men, not related to previous injury, [that] may resemble a scar." Recurring fibroid tumors, which may represent

TABLE 1. *Age groups affected by encephaloid, according to Gross*[a]

Age (yr)	No. of cases
1–3	8
3–7	4
7–14	5
14–21	9
21–30	20
30–40	14
40–50	18
50–60	7
60–70	4
70–75	9
Not specified	9

[a] Ref. 15a, p. 183.

TABLE 2. *Body sites affected by encephaloid, according to Gross*[a]

Site	No. of cases
Skull	3
Eye	10
Face	3
Neck	4
Shoulder	3
Interscapular region	1
Axilla	6
Forearm	5
Hand	1
Mammary gland	6
Chest	1
Abdomen	1
Groin	3
Thigh	8
Knee	8
Leg	4
Surface of the body	1
Fauces and larynx	1
Lungs and thoracic cavity	4
Liver and abdominal cavity	9
Uterus and pelvic cavity	3
Scrotum and testicle	14

[a] Ref. 15a, p. 183.

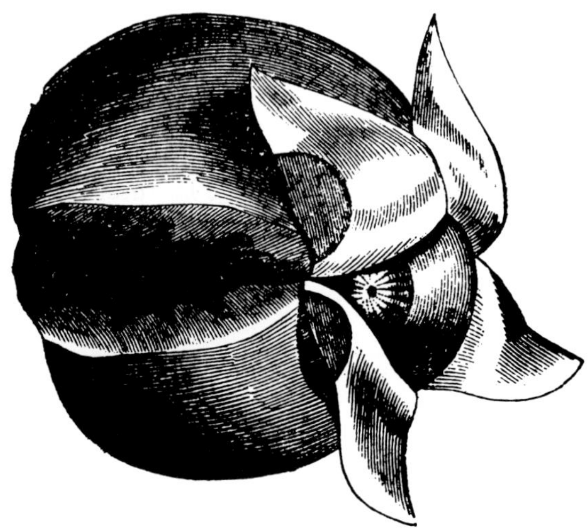

FIG. 4. Gross's illustration of an "encephaloid of the eye," with the sclera incised and everted anteriorly to display a large intraocular lesion. (From ref. 15a, p. 386.)

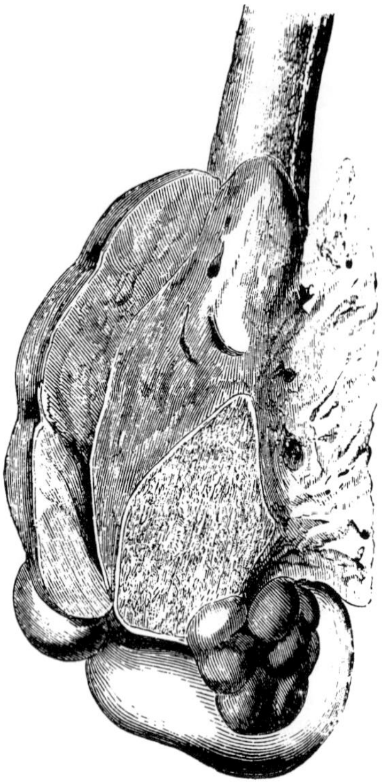

FIG. 5. Gross's illustration of "encephaloid of the bone." (From ref. 15a, p. 296.)

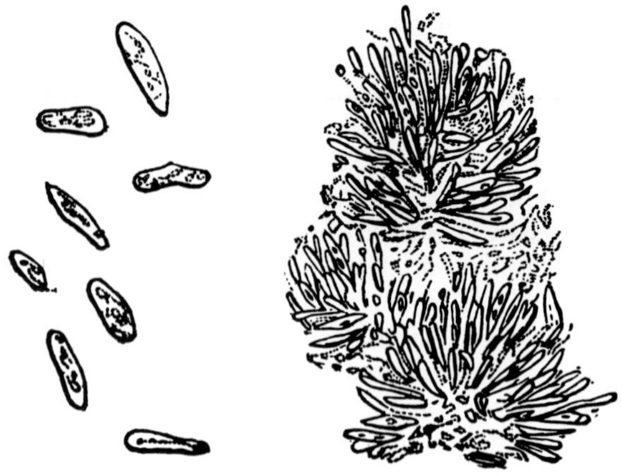

FIG. 6. Illustration of "fibronucleated tumor," from Paget's *Lectures on Surgical Pathology* (ref. 28a).

desmoids, are noted, as are "fibronucleated tumors" occurring in the soft tissues of children and young adults and microscopically consisting of "two materials: namely, nuclei, and sparing granular or molecular substance in which they are embedded." This description and the accompanying figure (Fig. 6) are reminiscent of synovial sarcoma. Pediatric bone tumors are also described in Paget's book.

Like Gross, Paget was cognizant of the unique properties of sarcomas, which he termed "medullary cancers," again noting their tendency to affect all ages and sites (Table 3). Paget noted that these tumors frequently followed a history of trauma, a frequently recorded observation to this day. Particularly prescient of Paget was his observation that a hereditary predisposition to cancer may occur that "is not cancer itself, but a tendency to the production of cancer at some time far future from the birth. . . . This tendency to cancerous disease is most commonly derived from a parent who is not yet manifestly cancerous; for, most commonly, the children are born before cancer is evident in the parent; so that, as we may say, that which is still future to the parent is transmitted potentially to the offspring. Nay, more: the tendency which exists in the parent may never become in him or her effective, although it may become effective in the offspring: for there are cases in which a grandparent has been cancerous, and although his or her children have not been so, the grandchildren have been." Another observation made by Paget that foretold 20th century research was his note that xenografts could be produced by the inoculation of "cancerous matter" into the subcutis of frogs. Unfortunately he was personally unable to verify this experiment, as his frogs "died soon thereafter."

20TH CENTURY HISTOLOGY

With the early 20th century came seminal discoveries on the nature of a number of childhood neoplasms. In 1918, James Ewing published his article on "endothelioma of bone," the sarcoma that bears his name today. This lesion elicited serious controversy, primarily by Sir Rubert Willis, who dismissed it as metastatic neuroblastoma. It was thus not until decades later that Lich-

TABLE 3. *Age groups and sites affected by medullary cancer, according to Paget*

Age	Breast	Soft parts	Lymph nodes	Bones	Eye, orbit	Testis	Total
<10	—	2	—	4	15	4	25
10–20	—	6	—	12	1	2	21
20–30	—	3	3	11	4	12	33
30–40	2	3	2	6	2	17	32
40–50	2	6	2	11	1	8	30
50–60	3	2	3	4	5	3	20
>60	—	1	—	6	3	—	10
Total	7	23	10	54	31	46	171

From ref. 28a.

tenstein and Jaffe reinstated it as a bona fide primary bone lesion and further characterized it as a unique clinicopathologic entity (10).

In spite of this error, Willis was a giant in the development of pediatric pathology, particularly as it relates to pediatric neoplasia. In his text *The Borderland of Pathology and Embryology* Willis built his experiences and those of his mentor, Dr. Nicholson, into a theoretical framework of pediatric neoplasia (19). Hamartomatous lesions were distinguished from true neoplasms and were considered to result from malformations in tissue development, resulting in abnormal overgrowths of excessive tissue indigenous to the site in which they arose. Although he did not consider these hamartomas to be neoplastic, he admitted that they had a potential for autonomous growth. Within this category he placed angiomatoses, enchondromatoses, fibrous dysplasias, lipoblastomas, neurofibromatoses, tuberous scleroses, melanocytic nevi, rhabdomyomas, sebaceous nevi, cylindromas, mesenchymal hamartomas, bronchial adenomas, and intestinal polyps. Willis recognized that genetic alterations in predisposed individuals were responsible for some lesions, which might not become apparent until years after birth.

Willis also introduced the term "embryonic tumour" to describe neoplasms arising from immature tissues. These he recognized as being fundamentally different from adult tumors and possessing a capacity for heterologous differentiation. Lesions in older children were considered to be a result of abnormal development of vestigial fetal tissues. Teratomas were included in this general category, although they differed from usual embryonic tumors in their lack of organ specificity. Besides teratomas, lesions discussed as embryonic tumors included neuroblastoma (Fig. 7), medulloblastoma, neuroepithelioma, retinoblastoma (Fig. 8), dictyoma, nephroblastoma, hepatoblastoma, and embryonic sarcomas, especially rhabdomyosarcoma. Willis hypothesized that these disturbances of organization and differentiation were not due to ordinary carcinogenic agents but rather to "excesses or deficiencies of particular mineral, nutritive, and maturation hormonal substances which are essential to normal growth and differentiation." However, Willis could see no evidence of a direct genetic etiology for any of these tumors except retinoblastoma and instead blamed them largely on intrauterine events.

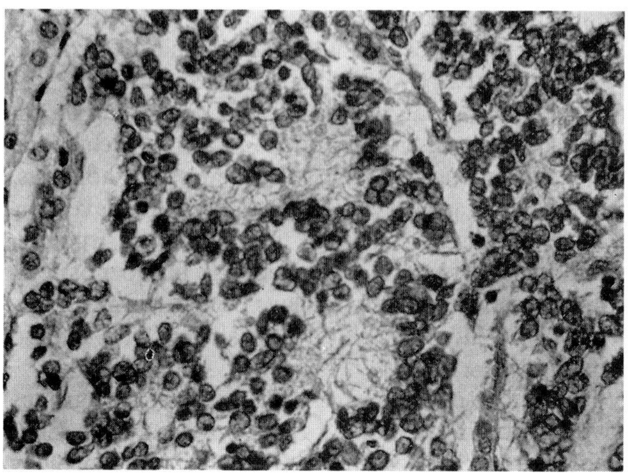

FIG. 7. Willis's photomicrograph of neuroblastoma, showing resemblance to fetal sympathetic ganglia, from *The Borderland of Pathology and Embryology* (ref. 39a).

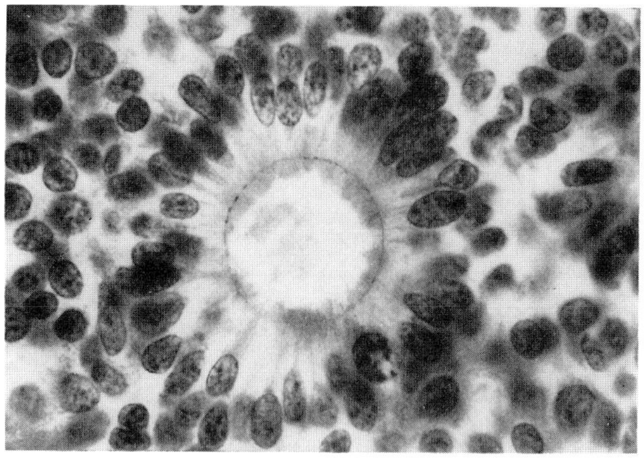

FIG. 8. Illustration of histology of retinoblastoma, from *The Borderland of Pathology and Embryology* (ref. 39a).

Another giant in pediatric tumor pathology during the 20th century was Arthur Purdy Stout. Dehner (9) has written an excellent account of Stout's work in the field of mesenchymal neoplasms. Stout was largely responsible for our modern classification of fibromatoses, which he categorized as desmoid fibromatosis, plantar and palmar fibromatoses, juvenile aponeurotic fibromatosis, keloid fibromatosis, diffuse muscular fibromatosis, differentiated fibrosarcoma, generalized fibromatosis, and fibromatosis, not otherwise specified. In particular, Stout recognized the nonmetastasizing nature of infantile fibrosarcoma.

Stout also developed the diagnostic concepts that we use with hemangiopericytoma and fibrous histiocytoma, both of which he recognized as being relatively benign tumors in young children. He also published reports on other pediatric soft tissue lesions, including synovial sarcoma, vascular tumors, lipomatous tumors, rhabdomyosarcomas, neurogenic tumors, and "mesenchymomas." One seminal contribution of Stout was the first description of a peripheral neuroepithelioma. With Margaret Murray, Stout also developed a method for in vitro study of tumor cells and made many original observations on this material (38).

Work by Drs. Cushing and Bailey must be considered the basis of our current knowledge of pediatric brain tumors. In their text, *A Classification of Tumors of the Glioma Group on a Histogenetic Basis with a Correlated*

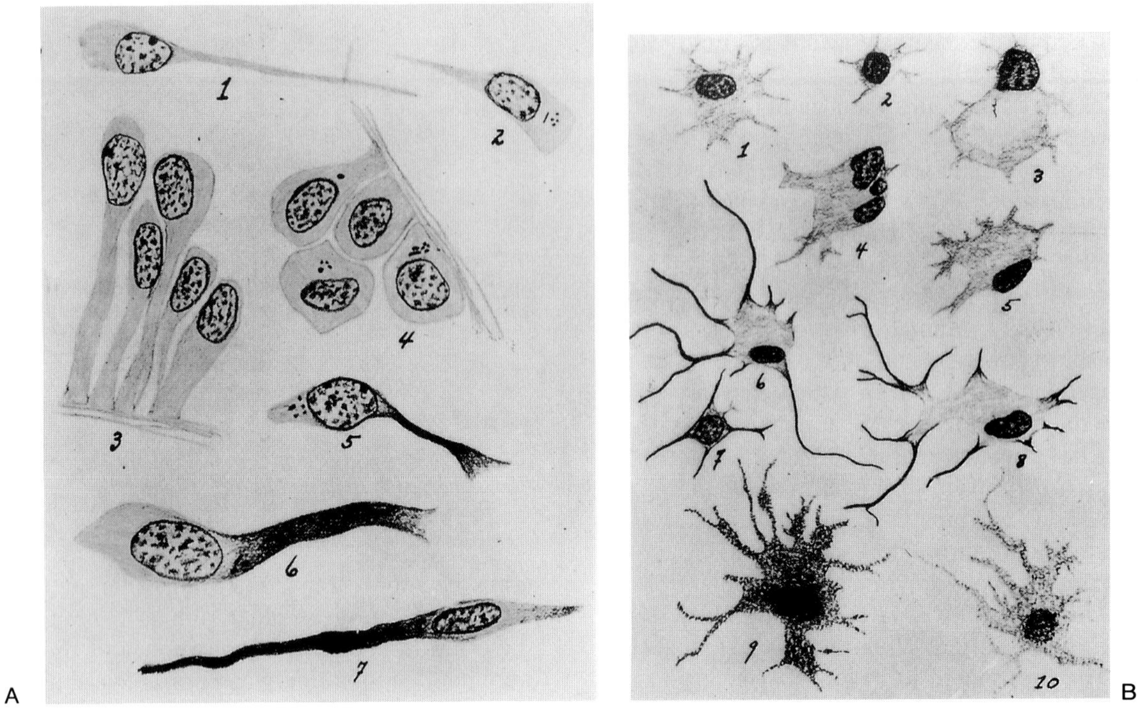

1. Ependymal spongioblast. (HE.)
2. Ependymal spongioblast. (NEVOG.)
3. Group of ependymal spongioblasts standing on a vessel. (HE.)
4. Group of eneddymal cells along a vessel. (NEVOG.)
5. 6, and 7. Ependymal spongioblasts. (PTAH.)

1. Typical protoplasmic astrocyte. (HE.)
2. Minute astrocyte. (HE.)
3. Astrocyte with hyalinized body. (HE.)
4. Multinucleated astrocyte. (HE.)
5. Astrocyte with eccentric nucleus. (HE.)
6. 7, and 8. Astrocytes of fibrillary type. (NEVOG.)
9 and 10. Protoplasmic astrocytes. (GS.)

FIG. 9. Bailey's illustrations of cells from ependymoma **(A)** and astrocytoma **(B)**. (From ref. 1a.)

Study of Prognosis, these investigators described many of the basic entities in pediatric neuropathology, and most are largely unchanged to this day (Fig. 9). As with leukemia, descriptions were abetted by the development of cytochemical stains, such as the silver stains developed by Ramon y Cajal (7). As for peripheral neural tumors, landmark events include Homer Wright's description of the neuroblastic rosette (41) (Fig. 7) and Flexner's description of the retinoblastic rosette (14) (Fig. 8).

Perhaps no writer in modern times has been more prolific in the description and delineation of pediatric lesions than Dr. Louis Dehner, author of *Pediatric Surgical Pathology* and countless publications in this field. Although Dehner's publications span the entire breadth of childhood neoplasia, his primary focus has remained on pediatric sarcomas. One of his major contributions in this field is a coherent classification of primitive neuroectodermal tumors (10).

INTERGROUP STUDIES

One of the major forces that have worked to produce the gratifying high survival rates and large knowledge base that we now associate with childhood neoplasia has been the formation of cooperative groups. These consortia combine the material of multiple pediatric hospitals in order to rapidly test experimental protocols and to pool tumor materials. One of the first groups to be formed was the Manchester University Children's Tumor Registry, instigated by Drs. Basil Marsden and James Steward (26). Using this material, Dr. Marsden made a number of seminal observations on childhood tumors, particularly renal neoplasms, which were enhanced by biologic investigations with Drs. William Lawler and Shant and Pat Kumar. Many of these observations were published in his text, *Tumours in Children.*

Dr. Marsden and colleagues have been highly instrumental in the pathologic investigations of another collaborative group, the Societé Internationale d'Oncologie Pédiatrique (SIOP), which has performed numerous prospective clinical trials and histopathologic studies on pediatric neoplasms. Similar European groups include the German Cooperative Group (CWS), whose pathologists, Drs. Dieter Harms and Dietmar Schmidt, have performed key investigations on the use of ultrastructure, immunohistochemistry, and ploidy in a number of pediatric cancers. Similar studies have been performed in Italy by Dr. Vito Ninfo and in Spain by Dr. Antonio Llombard-Bosch.

Two major collaborative pediatric oncology groups have formed in the United States; these are the Children's Cancer Study Group and the Pediatric Oncology Group. In three special circumstances, "intergroups" have been formed to address therapeutic and pathologic problems posed by specific childhood cancers. These comprise the National Wilms' Tumor Study (NWTS), the Intergroup Rhabdomyosarcoma Study (IRS), and the Intergroup Ewing's Sarcoma Study (IESS). The generous contributions of tumor tissue from numerous institutions and individuals has given great impetus to the pathobiologic study of these particular neoplasms.

The NTWS Pathology Center, formed in 1968, has been directed by Dr. Bruce Beckwith (Fig. 10). Using material from the NWTS-I study with Dr. Nigel Palmer, he formulated a new classification system for renal neoplasms (5). Dr. Beckwith and Dr. H. R. Wiedemann (3,39) independently described an unusual growth syndrome characterized by abnormal tissue development and tumor susceptibility. In 1990 (4), Beckwith published a landmark article on the definition and nature of nephrogenic rests of the kidney and their relationship to Wilms' tumor. He has made many other seminal observations and remains extremely active in this field.

The IRS Pathology Center was begun in 1972 under the direction of Dr. William Newton, Jr. Doctor Newton has made major contributions in the diagnosis and subclassification of rhabdomyosarcoma. To this end, he directed an international study of several classifications (Fig. 11) (see Chapter 5).

The IESS Pathology Committee, begun in 1972, was initially composed of Drs. John Kissane and Fred Askin. Doctor Kissane is also the author of the standard text on general pediatric pathology, *Pathology of Infancy and*

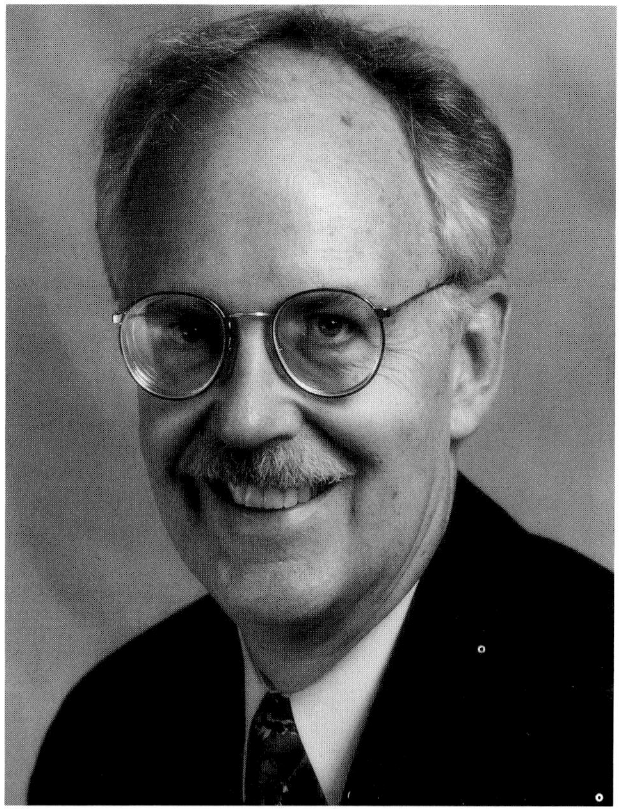

FIG. 10. J. Bruce Beckwith, Director of the NTWS Pathology Center. (Photograph courtesy of Dr. Beckwith.)

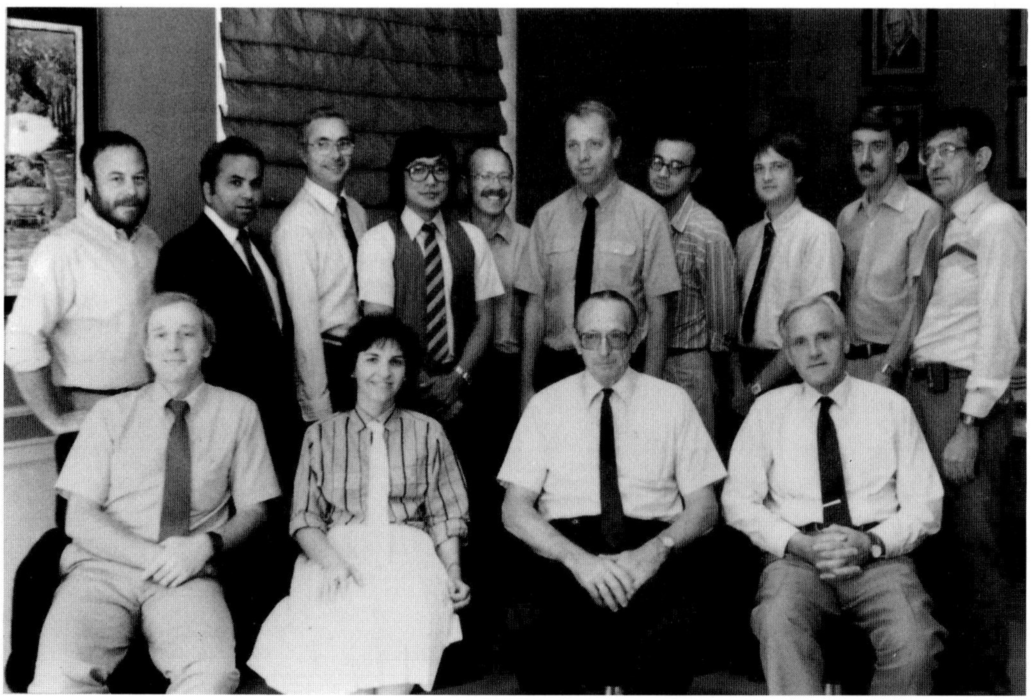

FIG. 11. Initial gathering of the working committee for the International Study of Rhabdomyosarcoma Classification. Top row (from left to right): Drs. Jean Cauillaud, Mohan Beltangady, Bruce Webber, Hiriyuko Shimada, Ambroglia Fascetti, Andrianne van Unnik, Andreas Cavazzana, David Parham, Nigel Palmer, and Ala Hamoudi; bottom row (from left to right): Drs. Tim Triche, Maria Tsokos, William Newton, and Basil Marsden. (Photograph courtesy of Dr. Newton.)

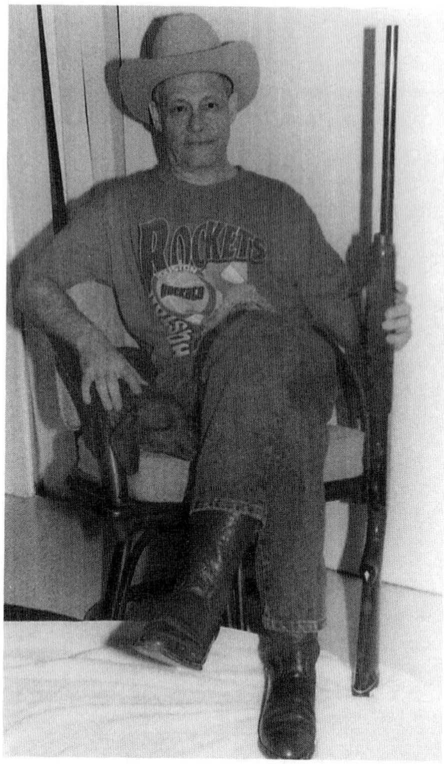

FIG. 12. Dr. Milton Finegold, in a casual mood. (Photograph courtesy of Dr. Finegold.)

Childhood. Dr. Askin is well known as the descriptor of the "Askin" tumor, or small cell tumor of the thoracopulmonary region, and has also devoted much time to the study of pediatric disease. With material from the IESS, Drs. Kissane and Askin analyzed the pathologic features of Ewing's sarcoma. Dr. Kissane's work has been updated by Drs. Dehner and Thomas Stocker with their multiauthored text, *Pediatric Pathology.*

PEDIATRIC SOCIETIES

The Society of Pediatric Pathology, founded in 1964 by Drs. George Fetterman and Frank Sherman as the Pediatric Pathology Club (18), has played a major role in the study and description of pediatric neoplasms. This Society owes a great debt to Drs. Benjamin Landing, Eugene Perrin, and Harvey Rosenberg, who were instrumental in the United States in the founding of pediatric pathology as an individual discipline of scientific study. This Society has encouraged the research of a number of investigators and has been the recipient of careful leadership by individuals such as Dr. Milton Finegold (Fig. 12). In 1986 Dr. Finegold published a major text devoted solely to pediatric neoplasia, *Pathology and Neoplasia in Children and Adolescents*, and he has also performed extensive work on hepatic tumors. The SPP has also supported young investigators in the field through grants and has disseminated information through two publications, *Pediatric Pathology* and *Perspectives in Pediatric Pathology.*

BIOLOGY OF CHILDHOOD NEOPLASIA

Biologic features of childhood tumors are without argument the aspect that holds the most fascination and promise in current research. One particular landmark occurred in 1911, when Dr. Peyton Rous discovered a chicken tumor virus that could produce tumors in healthy animals by inoculation of cell-free extracts. Similar discoveries followed with description of murine oncoviruses by Harvey and Abelson, frog oncovirus by Lucke, and feline oncovirus by McDonough, among others (32). Currently, a wide variety of these viruses are known (Table 4), and several, including herpesviruses, papillomaviruses, and retroviruses, are active in humans.

A great step forward was made in 1976 by Varmus and colleagues (36), who discovered that certain DNA sequences of oncoviruses, or oncogenes (designated v-gene name), were minimally altered variants of genes functioning in normal mammalian cells (designated c-gene name). These genes, called proto-oncogenes, have been

TABLE 4. *Some examples of retroviral oncogenes* *

Oncogene	Virus[a]	Host	Disease	Protein properties[b]	Protein location[c]
src	RSV	Chicken	Sarcoma	P-Tyr-K	PM
yes	Y73/ASV	Chicken	Sarcoma	P-Tyr-K	PM
fps	FuSV/FRCII	Chicken	Sarcoma	P-Tyr-K	PM
ros	UR2	Chicken	Sarcoma	P-Tyr-K	TM
crk	CT10	Chicken	Sarcoma	P-Tyr-K-Act	C
jun	ASV17	Chicken	Sarcoma	DB/TF	N
mil	MH2	Chicken	Sarcoma	P-Ser-Thr-K	C
*erb*B	AEV-H	Chicken	Sarcoma, erythroleukemia	P-Tyr-K-R	TM

* Reprinted with the kind permission of the author and publisher from Table 1 in Roussel MF. Oncogenes. In: Webster RG, Granoff A, eds. *Encyclopedia of Virology.* London: Academic Press; 1994:934–941.

[a] RSV, Rous sarcoma virus; Y73, Yamagushi 73 sarcoma virus; ASV, avian sarcoma virus; FuSV-Fujinami sarcoma virus; MH2, Mill Hill-2 virus; AEV, avian erthyroblastosis virus.

[b] P-Tyr-K, phosphotyrosine kinase; P-Try-K-Act, phosphotyrosine kinase activator; DB/TF, DNA-binding/transcription factor; P-Ser-Thr-K, phosphoserine-threonine kinase; P-Tyr-K-R, phosphotyrosine kinase receptor.

[c] PM, plasma membrane; TM, transmembrane; C, cytoplasmic; N, nuclear.

found to produce tumors in vivo and in vitro when critical mutations are introduced. A wide variety of protooncogenes are currently known to be present in the human genome. These genes function by producing critical growth-responsive proteins at various subcellular loci, ranging from the cell membrane to the nucleus.

Conversely, genetic sequences have been described that interact with DNA to prevent uncontrolled cell division and subsequent neoplasia. Alterations in these "antioncogenes," or tumor suppressor genes, are described in a number of syndromes that produce a heritable disposition to cancer. These include the Li–Fraumeni syndrome, hereditable retinoblastoma, the Wilms-aniridia syndrome, and others listed throughout this text. The initial work on anti-oncogenes proceeded from observations on bilateral retinoblastoma, leading to the discovery of the retinoblastoma gene. This phenomenon also led Drs. Knudson and Strong to propose a "two-hit" hypothesis of cancer formation in childhood (21), with the initial genetic event being either inherited, as with bilateral retinoblastoma, or somatic, as with unilateral retinoblastoma.

Using epidemiologic observations, Drs. Li and Fraumeni in 1969 described a cancer susceptibility syndrome associated with heritable rhabdomyosarcoma (23). The Li–Fraumeni syndrome was later associated with alterations in a gene, *p53*, whose protein product functions as a gateway to the S phase of the cell cycle. Similar observations have been made with neurofibromatosis 1, and more discoveries are certain to follow (20).

The discovery of these genes and the elucidation of their protein products have followed the development of methods used to demonstrate DNA, RNA, and protein sequences (described more fully in Chapter 2). The use of cytogenetics must be viewed as the premier technique for the discovery of gene sequences critical in cancer generation (34). The initial stains used to demonstrate the chromosomes seen in metaphase cells could only be used to determine their relative size and shape. Subsequent stains delineated chromosomal regions, or bands, and allowed further dissection of the genome. Chromosome banding was standardized by a series of conferences on cytogenetics held in the 1970s (31). Subsequently, a number of translocations, deletions, and other anomalies unique to specific pediatric neoplasms have been described (13).

While cytogenetic techniques were being developed, biochemists and microbiologists were generating technology for the analysis of DNA molecules, following the seminal description of this molecule by Drs. Watson and Crick in 1953. A number of microorganisms were found to produce DNases, or restriction enzymes, that recognize and cleave specific nucleotide sequences. Dr. Southern revolutionized this field in 1979 (35), when he described a method for separating and characterized cleaved DNA derived from whole cells. With this technique it became feasible to test for genetic mutations at the "molecular" level.

The sensitivity of molecular technology was markedly increased when polymerase chain reaction methodology was described by Saiki and colleagues in 1988 (33). By amplifying a genetic locus via repeated hybridization steps, it became possible to detect the presence of specific DNA sequences in a very few cells. This procedure thus has great potential for diagnostic use.

Another genetic technique used for diagnosis and prognosis is determination of DNA index, or ploidy. This determination requires quantitation of the amount of DNA present in tumor cells. It was initially developed using fluorimetric scanning of a stream of propidium iodine–stained cells using flow cytometry. This technique, invented by Walter Coulter in 1959 (30), was initially used to detect ploidy values of hematologic malignancies and adult tumors such as bladder cancer (28). Investigation of childhood neoplasms followed (25), and it became apparent that ploidy determination had prognostic significance in a number of these tumors. More recently, image analysis, which may be automated, has been used for ploidy determination.

Probably the most intriguing discoveries in childhood neoplasia in recent years have related them to molecular events that occur during embryogenesis. In these reports, genes characteristically disrupted in pediatric tumors have been found to exhibit homology to transcription family members. These transcription factors are DNA-binding proteins that regulate the transcription of DNA to RNA. They are encoded by genetic sequences known as homeobox genes (2,8,27), and they direct such basic blastomeric and gastrular events as determination of body axes and formation of viscera. The involvement of these genes in pediatric tumors may explain some of the confusing diversity of structure of these neoplasms.

Development of the newer biologic techniques and principles owes a large debt to the sacrifice of unwitting laboratory animals, particularly mice, which can be inbred or thymectomized to become recipients of human tumor tissue, or xenografts (17). Microinjection of foreign genes into embryo cells, followed by controlled breeding, can produce transgenic mice with an artificially altered genome. These animals permit "gene knockout" experiments in which selected genes are deleted or altered, becoming "null" or ineffective and thus allowing inference of gene function.

Another key development was the advent of cell culture techniques, which allow the perpetuation of tumor cells in vitro and their manipulation for biologic experimentation. Cell culture has been particularly important to cytogenetics and the study of growth factors. One particularly useful result of cell culture technique has been its use in the development of monoclonal antibodies during the 1970s (22). These immunologic reagents are produced by fusion of myeloma cells with sensitized lymphocytes using in vitro techniques. The resulting "hybridoma" can be propagated indefinitely and used to produce monoclonal antibodies having exquisite purity. These antibodies have had particular utility in immunohistochemistry, a method that has vastly improved the diagnostic capability and accuracy of surgical pathology.

Immunohistochemistry was initially practiced using fluorescent dye-tagged polyclonal antisera. Its applicability to routine diagnostic work was greatly enhanced in 1970, when Sternberger (37) published a staining method that offered visualization by bright field microscopy. A number of refinements to this basic technique have been forthcoming. With some caveats (29), these methods have had particular use in diagnosing pediatric small cell tumors that appear undifferentiated by routine light microscopy. As a consequence of their commonplace use, surgical pathologists have been obliged to add a broad working knowledge of cell biology to their morphology-based diagnostic skills. Currently, surgical pathology is indeed a practice of morphology and biology.

ACKNOWLEDGMENT

Supported by National Cancer Institute (NCI) Center Support Grant P30 CA217657 and American Lebanese Syrian Associated Charities (ALSAC).

REFERENCES

1. Abt AF, Garrison FH. *History of Pediatrics.* Philadelphia: WB Saunders; 1965.
1a. Bailey P. Cellular types in primary tumors of the brain. In: Penfield W, ed. *Cytology and Cellular Pathology of the Nervous System.* New York: Hafner; 1932:925(A), 931(B).
2. Beardsley T. Smart genes. *Sci Am* 1991;265:86–95.
3. Beckwith JB. Macroglossia, omphalocele, adrenal cytomegaly, gigantism, and hyperplastic visceromegaly. *Birth Defects* 1969;5: 188–196.
4. Beckwith JB, Kiviat NB, Bonadio JF. Nephrogenic rests, nephroblastomatosis, and the pathogenesis of Wilms' tumor. *Pediatr Pathol* 1990;10:1–36.
5. Beckwith JB, Palmer NF. Histopathology and prognosis of Wilms tumors: results from the First National Wilms' Tumor Study. *Cancer* 1978;41:1937–1948.
6. Bleyer WA. What can be learned about childhood cancer from "Cancer Statistics Review 1973–1988." *Cancer* 1993;71:3229–3236.
6a. Bright R. *Clinical Memoirs on Abdominal Tumors and Intumescence.* In: Barlow GH, Cantab MA, eds. New Sydenharm, London; 1860:32, 33.
7. Cajal WR. Quelques méthods simples pour la coloration de la névroglie. *Schwiez Arch Neurol Psychiatry* 1923;13:187–193.
8. De Robertis EM, Oliver G, Wright CV. Homeobox genes and the vertebrate body plan. *Sci Am* 1990;263:46–52.
9. Dehner LP. Mesenchymal neoplasms in childhood. Insights of Arthur Purdy Stout and where they have taken us. *Am J Surg Pathol* 1986;10 Suppl 1:32–42.
10. Dehner LP. Primitive neuroectodermal tumor and Ewing's sarcoma. *Am J Surg Pathol* 1993;17:1–13.
11. DeLaat CA, Lampkin BC. Long-term survivors of childhood cancer: evaluation and identification of sequelae of treatment. *CA Cancer J Clin* 1992;42:263–282.
12. Donaldson SS. Lessons from our children. *Int J Radiat Oncol Biol Phys* 1993;26:739–749.
13. Donner LR. Cytogenetics and molecular biology of small round-cell tumors and related neoplasms. Current status. *Cancer Genet Cytogenet* 1991;54:1–10.
14. Flexner S. A peculiar glioma (neuroepithelioma?) of the retina. *Johns Hopkins Hosp Bull* 1891;2:115–119.
15. Gonzalez-Crussi F. *Wilms' Tumor (Nephroblastoma) and Related Renal Neoplasms of Childhood.* Boca Raton: CRC Press; 1984.
15a. Gross SD. Elements of Pathological Anatomy. Philadelphia: Blanchard & Lea; 1887.
16. Hajdu SI. *Pathology of Soft Tissue Tumors.* Philadelphia: Lea and Febiger; 1979.
17. Houghton PJ, Shapiro DN, Houghton JA. Rhabdomyosarcoma: from the laboratory to the clinic. *Pediatr Clin North Am* 1991;38: 349–364.
18. Hubbard JD. George Fetterman, M.D. *Perspect Pediatr Pathol* 1984;8:98–100.
19. Kissane JM. Introduction. *Semin Diag Pathol* 1994;11:83–84.
20. Knudson AG. Antioncogenes and human cancer. *Proc Natl Acad Sci USA* 1993;90:10914–10921.
21. Knudson AG, Jr., Strong LC. Mutation and cancer: a model for Wilms' tumor of the kidney. *JNCI* 1972;48:313–324.
22. Krause M. The search for antibodies with molecular uniformity. *Adv Immunol* 1970;12:1–56.
23. Li FP, Fraumeni JF. Rhabdomyosarcoma in children: epidemiologic study and identification of a familial cancer syndrome. *JNCI* 1969;43:1365–1373.
24. Long ER. *A History of Pathology.* New York: Dover; 1965.
25. Look AT, Hayes FA, Nitschke R, McWilliams NB, Green AA. Cellular DNA content as a predictor of response to chemotherapy in infants with unresectable neuroblastoma. *N Engl J Med* 1984;311: 231–235.
26. Marsden HB. H.B. Marden. In: Taylor G, ed. *Pioneers in Pediatric Oncology.* Houston: The University of Texas M.D. Anderson Cancer Center; 1990:191–197.
27. Melton DA. Pattern formation during animal development. *Science* 1991;252:234–241.
28. Merkel DE, McGuire WL. Ploidy, proliferative activity and prognosis. DNA flow cytometry of solid tumors. *Cancer* 1990;65: 1194–1205.
28a. Paget J. *Lectures on Surgical Pathology.* Philadelphia: Lindsay & Blakiston; 1854:419.
29. Parham DM. Immunohistochemistry of childhood sarcomas: old and new markers. *Mod Pathol* 1993;6:133–138.
30. Patrick CW, Milson TJ, McFadden PW, Keller RH. Flow cytometry and cell sorting. *Lab Med* 1984;15:740–745.
31. Report of the Standing Committee on Human Cytogenetic Nomenclature. An international system for human cytogenetic nomenclature. *Cytogenet Cell Genet* 1978;21:309–404.
32. Roussel MF. Oncogenes. In: Webster RG, Granoff A, eds. *Encyclopedia of Virology.* London: Academic Press; 1994:934–941.
33. Saiki RK, Gelfand DH, Stoffel S, et al. Primer-directed enzymatic amplification of DNA with a thermostable DNA polymerase. *Science* 1988;239:487–491.
34. Sandberg AA. Cancer cytogenetics for clinicians. *CA Cancer J Clin* 1994;44:136–159.
35. Southern EM. Gel electrophoresis of restriction fragments. *Meth Enzymol* 1979;68:152–176.
36. Stehelin D, Varmus HE, Bishop JM, Vogt PK. DNA related to the transforming gene(s) of avian sarcoma viruses is present in normal avian DNA. *Nature* 1976;260:170–173.
37. Sternberger LA, Hardy PH, Cuculis JJ, Meyer HG. The unlabeled antibody enzyme method for immunohistochemistry. Preparation and properties of soluble antigen–antibody complex (horseradish peroxidase–antihorseradish peroxidase) and its use in the identification of spirochetes. *J Histochem Cytochem* 1970;18:315–333.
38. Stout AP, Murray MR. Neuroepithelioma of radial nerve with study of its behavior in vitro. *Rev Can Biol* 1942;1:651.
38a. Virchow R. *Cellular Pathology,* 2nd ed. Chance F (translator). Philadelphia: JB Lippincott; 1863:209.
39. Wiedemann HR. Complexe malformatif familial avec hernie ombilicale et macroglossie—un "syndrome noveau?" *J Génét Hum* 1995;13:223–232.
39a. Willis RA. The Borderland of Pathology and Embryology, 2nd ed. London: Butterworths; 1962:430.
40. Wingo PA, Tong T, Bolden S. Cancer statistics. *CA Cancer J Clin* 1995;45:8–30.
41. Wright JH. Neurocytoma or neuroblastoma, a kind of tumor not generally recognized. *J Exp Med* 1910;12:556–561.

Pediatric Neoplasia: Morphology and Biology, edited by David M. Parham.
Lippincott-Raven Publishers, Philadelphia © 1996.

CHAPTER 2

Diagnostic and Biologic Techniques

David M. Parham, David R. Head, Peter Dias, Richard A. Ashmun, Glen S. Germain, and Peter J. Houghton

ANATOMIC TECHNIQUES

David M. Parham

Introduction

In general, the techniques used for diagnosis of pediatric neoplasms are identical to those used in adult surgical pathology. However, unique clinical and biologic features of childhood tumors make careful consideration of specimen adequacy and handling imperative before beginning gross dissection. Excisional surgery may be delayed until after the patient is treated with a carefully defined protocol of radiation therapy and multiagent chemotherapy, so that the initial biopsy often assumes greater diagnostic significance than with the usual solid adult malignancy. Also, the recent discovery of unique biologic and karyotypic markers with prognostic and/or diagnostic significance dictates that thought be given to the adequacy and distribution of fresh biopsy material.

Gross Examination

The most critical step in the diagnosis of pediatric neoplasia is careful gross examination. This maxim applies equally to all areas of surgical pathology, but here it assumes particular importance because of the frequent heterogeneity of these lesions. Thus, one must learn to approach freshly excised childhood tumors with an acutely discriminating eye and a clear mind. It is particularly important to be acquainted with the intricacies of pathologic staging, the potential for invasion, and the array of microscopic appearances of a given lesion before undertaking a complicated dissection.

Of utmost importance in excisions is delineation of the contours of the surgical margins for subsequent microscopy. We accomplish this by the liberal application of India ink to the gross specimen before sectioning. Ink is often runny, particularly on fresh, wet tissue, so it is helpful to first dry the specimen with a towel and to apply Bouin's fixative to the surface after inking. The Bouin's solution acts as a mordant which dries the ink and is particularly helpful with small, immersible specimens. Specimens that have a large surface area present more of a problem, so usually the ink is dried with a hair blower before further dissection. If one is interested in obtaining sterile tumor tissue before detailed dissection, it is essential to remember to obtain this material before the inking step. In these instances, the author makes an effort to sterilely incise the specimen in a region with thick margins so as not to compromise critical thin areas. Following this maneuver, it is important to avoid inking of the subsequently exposed areas. Multiple colors of ink may be applied to differentiate various regions within the specimen.

Critical margins should be submitted before sectioning tumor, which frequently has a soft, runny consistency. Vascular, neural, soft tissue, cutaneous, and bony margins are thus obtained first. In tumors to be correlated with radiologic findings, it is critical to make sections in the plane of the presurgical radiographic images. Selection of the proper size of knife is also important, as jagged, irregular cuts detract from the aesthetic quality of subsequent photographs. It is generally advisable to use

D. M. Parham: Department of Pathology, Arkansas Children's Hospital, Little Rock, Arkansas 72202.
D. R. Head: Department of Pathology and Laboratory Medicine, St. Jude Children's Hospital, and Department of Pathology, University of Tennessee, Memphis, Tennessee 38105.
P. Dias, G. S. Germain, and P. J. Houghton: Department of Molecular Pharmacology, University of Tennessee, Memphis, Tennessee 38105.
R. A. Ashmun: Department of Experimental Oncology, University of Tennessee, Memphis, Tennessee 38105.

a knife larger than the specimen and not rely universally on a small surgical blade, except when cutting small, diagnostically critical areas such as close margins. Frequently the surgical margin is a thin rim of loose areolar tissue. It is thus helpful to fix surgical excisions in formalin overnight before dissection and after inking, so that the tissues are firmer and more amenable to sectioning. Formalin may be injected into hollow viscera such as the urinary bladder or intestine in order to facilitate fixation.

For bony specimens, the author performs sectioning with a band saw as used in butcher shops. Thin sections less than 5 mm in diameter must be obtained for histologic processing. Diamond-tipped saws as used with metal cutting give excellent results with small specimens. In general, hand-held vibrational saws as used with autopsies give less than satisfactory results with osseous dissections.

In selection of tissue for microscopic examination, viable tissue and potentially aggressive foci must be adequately sampled. Often large amounts of necrosis are present; this is more appropriately documented during gross dissection than microscopic examination, unless no other tissue is available or radiologic correlation is being performed. Viable embryonal tumor tissue has a pink, fleshy, mushy appearance reminiscent of the sea urchin roe served at sushi bars; these areas should be liberally sampled. In contrast, necrotic tissue has a granular, grayish yellow appearance (Fig. 1, see figure in color plate section). In addition, one must sample areas of nodularity or hemorrhage, which may yield focal choriocarcinoma or neuroblastoma. One must also look for areas of vascular and neural invasion. In tumors arising from peripheral nerves, longitudinal sections should include grossly normal nerve and its region of contact with the tumor. A list of sections noting their anatomic location should be submitted with the gross report.

One common question is the proper number of sections to be taken for histologic examination. The answer traditionally used in surgical pathology is to submit one section per centimeter of tumor as measured in the greatest dimension. This axiom functions well as a rough guide, but it is superseded by the rule that all heterogeneous areas should be examined. One must also remember the potentially focal nature of anaplasia or high-grade tumor in pediatric lesions, so that liberal sampling is important.

The use of multiple fixatives should be considered before total immersion of the specimen in formalin. A mixture of fixatives optimizes the potential for satisfactory immunohistochemistry (29), and glutaraldehyde fixation in particular is critically important for electron microscopy. Paraformaldehyde fixation is recommended for immunoelectron microscopy (see below). To avoid the artifacts that rapidly accrue with cellular degradation, sampling for electron microscopy should be performed as soon as possible after specimen removal. Finally, fresh tissue may be obtained for storage at −70°C in a tumor bank. This tissue is invaluable for subsequent biologic studies and is usually preferable to formalin-fixed, paraffin-embedded material. RNA is often tested in biologic assays and degrades quickly at room temperature. It is also wise to consider the possibility of infections as a cause of tumors, particularly with bone biopsies, so that sterile tissue should be obtained for microbiologic cultures if even the slightest indication is present.

Routine Microscopy

Foremost to successful light microscopic examination of human tissues is adequate histologic preparation (3). Of all critical procedural factors in histology, proper fixation is foremost. At St. Jude Children's Research Hospital we continue to use a phosphate-buffered 10% v/v formaldehyde solution as the standard fixative and prefer commercial reagents to in-house preparations. Tissue should be immersed in a sufficient volume of fixative, optimally a 1:10 ratio of tissue to solution. Formalin fixation should generally proceed for at least 8 hours for small biopsies and 12–18 hours for larger ones. Other fixatives, such as B5 or alcohol-based solutions, may require a different immersion time and should be monitored carefully.

Despite the great advances recently made in molecular biology and ancillary techniques, the most important component of tumor diagnosis remains the routinely stained histologic section. Routine stains vary from hospital to hospital, but in our laboratory we continue to use hematoxylin and eosin. A proper mixture of the two reagents are critical, as hematopathologists require crisp hematoxylin results to properly evaluate lymphoid lesions, and soft tissue pathologists prefer a good eosin stain for examination of sarcomas. It is possible to obtain a happy medium in a well-stained slide. Histochemical stains such as periodic acid–Schiff, reticulin, Grimelius, and others have assumed less diagnostic importance following the advent of immunohistochemistry, but they can still be fruitfully utilized in certain instances. Table 1 lists some specific examples.

Immunohistochemistry

The advent of immunohistochemistry has radically altered the profession of surgical pathology, not only by the diagnostic avenues which it has opened but by the increased knowledge of cell biology which its successful application requires. Thus, histopathologists can no longer be content to have familiarity only with tissue morphology but must be conversant in biochemistry and other heretofore foreign fields. Of particular use in assessment of these stains is knowledge of the normal cel-

TABLE 1. *Use of special stains in pediatric tumors*

Stain	To demonstrate
Reticulin	Reticulin fibers in hemangiopericytomas, fibrosarcomas
Trichrome	Collagen production in fibrous lesions
Fontana melanin	Melanin in melanoma, clear cell sarcoma of soft tissue
Grimelius	Argyrophilia in paragangliomas
Bielshowsky	Axonal fibers in neural lesions
PAS with and without diastase	Glycogen in Ewing's sarcoma, rhabdomyosarcoma, germ cell tumors
Alcian blue with and without hyaluronidase	Connective tissue mucin in soft tissue lesions
Best carmine	Mucin in signet ring carcinomas

TABLE 2. *Methods of immunohistochemistry*

Direct fluorescence
Indirect fluorescence
One-step (direct) immunoperoxidase
Two-step (indirect) immunoperoxidase
Peroxidase-antiperoxidase (three-step)
Simple avidin-biotin complex
Modified (labelled) avidin-biotin complex
Alkaline phosphatase-antialkaline phosphatase
Immunogold
Enhancement of antigenicity by:
Microwave oven-based retrieval
Pressure cooker–based retrieval
Enzymatic digestion

lular distribution of a given protein. Unusual antigen disposition may be a clue to artifactual staining. One must also be familiar with the array of both normal and neoplastic cell types that express a particular antigen. Finally, caution is advised in interpretations that modify impressions gained by routine light microscopy, as embryonal neoplasms are notorious in their capacity for pluripotent differentiation (30).

A partial list of techniques commonly used for immunohistochemical detection of cell markers is found in Table 2. The method used for immunohistochemistry must be modified according to the sensitivity of detection desired (47,57). When using purified monoclonal antibodies, it is possible to use very sensitive techniques such as the labeled avidin-biotin-peroxidase technique with relative impunity, but when working with relatively impure reagents such as polyclonal antisera, less sensitive techniques may avoid excessive background. In general, the sensitivity of a method is related to the number of signal moieties attached to the immunoglobulin sandwich (Fig. 2). Thus, one obtains minimal sensitivity with a one-step, direct method compared to the maximal sensitivity afforded by the labeled avidin-biotin-complex technique. These considerations are particularly important when working with novel antibodies with varying degrees of purity.

Of variables critical to successful immunohistochemistry, tissue fixation ranks as foremost. The addition of a formaldehyde solution to fresh tissues results in a dense fortress of molecular crosslinks that can render sites of antigenic recognition impervious to immunoglobulins (32). Alternatively, fixation may result in destruction of

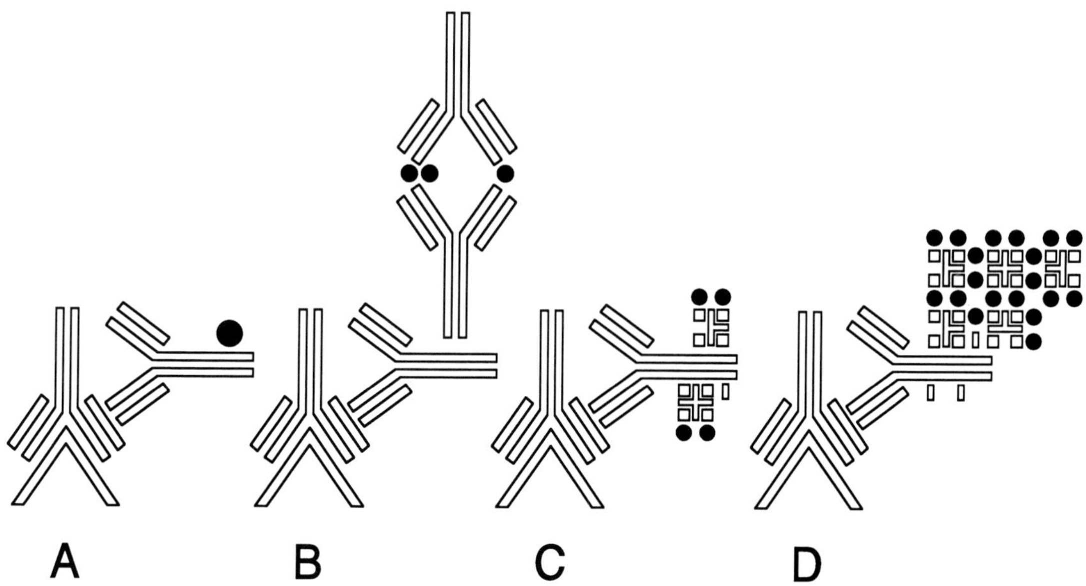

FIG. 2. Comparison of the number of signal moieties (*black dots*) attached in different immunohistochemical techniques. There is only one signal attached per antigen molecule with the indirect method (**A**) whereas the peroxidase–antiperoxidase (**B**), avidin–biotin complex (**C**), and labeled avidin–biotin complex (**D**) have progressively more. There is thus a hierarchy of sensitivities.

the epitope. Several strategies may thus be employed; first and foremost is to ensure a proper 10% v/v tissue-to-fixative balance and to avoid inadequate or prolonged fixation. A second helpful practice is to use a variety of fixatives if sufficient tissue is available. Variable results may be obtained with formalin, alcohol, Carnoy's solution, B5, or other fixatives (29,47,57).

The most recent advance in surmounting overfixation is the microwave antigen retrieval method. Antigen retrieval works by loosening the heavy bondage placed on epitopes by protein crosslinking, thus optimizing their presentation to permeating immunoglobulin molecules. The use of this technique is revolutionizing the ability of laboratories to obtain clean, standardized immunohistochemical results and promises a strategy to appease the jaundiced eyes of threatened governmental overseers (48). With antigen retrieval methods, tissue sections are heated in a special solution in a microwave oven before initiation of the immunostaining procedure. Initially, the solutions used contained heavy metals such as lead, creating potential problems with disposal and safe handling. Happily, nontoxic citrate buffers have been found to work equally well, so that the universal use of this method appears feasible. With few exceptions, this methodology appears to enhance the staining of most antigens and has been used to demonstrate highly comparable interlaboratory results (11).

Electron Microscopy

Immunohistochemistry has much to offer in terms of its ease and rapidity of examination and often stunning results. This has effected a decreased reliance on electron microscopy, with its cumbersome equipment, prolonged turnaround time, and sometimes equivocal interpretation. It is a grave error, however, to assume that ultrastructural examination no longer has a role in solving diagnostic problems. Because of their proclivity to coexpress diverse cell markers with a confusing array of immunohistochemical results, pediatric neoplasms frequently require electron microscopic examination for clarification of diagnostic uncertainty. Indeed, the two techniques should be considered synergistic rather than competitive in their capacity for divining tumor cell differentiation. As a result, one should be able to demonstrate intermediate filament arrays in tumors with vimentin positivity and neurosecretory granules in chromogranin-positive lesions. Electron microscopy has also been critical in the study of the structural biology of the cell. This book will thus describe ultrastructural appearances of pediatric neoplasms as part of their characterization as morphologic and biologic entities. A number of excellent texts and atlases that more thoroughly describe these features are available and are highly recommended (9).

As with the techniques listed above, the most critical step in electron microscopy is proper initial fixation. Promptness is critical, as hypoxia quickly dampens the membrane pumps separating the fragile cell interior from an osmotically hostile exterior. It is thus recommended that vials of glutaraldehyde be maintained in the surgery suite in order to promptly immerse excised tissues when pathologic consultation is requested. Glutaraldehyde is a relatively poor penetrant, so it is very important to submit *paper-thin* slices of tissue to allow adequate permeation. Otherwise, one will still observe subcellular hari-kari in spite of prompt specimen immersion.

Despite one's best efforts, cell degeneration not apparent with light microscopy may be painfully evident with ultrastructural examination. It is thus helpful to carefully evaluate the 1-μm-"thick" sections prepared for selection of blocks. If done carefully, this step optimizes the likelihood of finding well-preserved tumor cells. "Thick" sections also offer an opportunity to scan for areas of potential differentiation, as, for example, rosettes in a peripheral neuroepithelioma, strap cells in a rhabdomyosarcoma, or Langerhans cells in a histiocytic lesion.

Finally, one newer technique that is useful in evaluation of phenotypic markers and potentially even in diagnosis is immunoelectron microscopy. Using this method, one can detect the subcellular presence and locale of specific peptides. Although this method is attractive in principle, the vagaries of tissue processing and staining are amplified in practice. To be effective reagents, immunoglobulins must freely permeate an aqueous cellular milieu, which is not easily afforded by a polyacrylamide matrix. In addition, osmium cannot be used with this technique, with the unfortunate result that cellular detail is inferior. Special fixatives such as paraformaldehyde are also preferable to glutaraldehyde. Finally, the technician must exercise painstaking care to avoid excessive background. Various maneuvers have been used to overcome these difficulties (26). In our laboratory, we utilize a water-soluble resin for preparation of tissue blocks and immunogold particles for labeling. Others have used etching procedures to enhance the permeability of tissue blocks (26). If suitable results are obtained, this method may be used for diagnostic purposes such as distinguishing neurosecretory granules from lysosomes.

Cytology

Fine needle aspiration has great potential in diagnosis of pediatric neoplasms (51). Given the primitive nature of pediatric neoplasms with their often cryptic diagnostic features, a much different array of diagnostic questions are posed with childhood aspirates compared to the usual adult cancer. With adult neoplasms it is often not a problem to ascertain the presence of malignancy in a fine needle sample. Considering the range of neoplasms typically encountered, one can usually render a diagnostic opinion that is sufficient for further therapy, usually surgery. A different situation occurs with pediatric neoplasms in which standardized chemotherapy and radiotherapy are used before excision. Thus, it becomes critical to separate lesions such as peripheral neuroepithelioma and rhabdomyosarcoma, a feat that often requires extensive study on optimally preserved and quantitatively sufficient material. In spite of these caveats, the rapid turnaround time and low morbidity of fine needle aspiration hold great potential advantage over open biopsy (58). As may be surmised, this technique has become controversial among pediatric pathologists and has its share of adherents and detractors (25,44,49,52).

The author would caution readers that the requirement of *adequate* materials for a *reliable* diagnosis supersedes any other clinical consideration in desperately ill children. Also, I strongly urge careful apportionment of material before slide preparation and staining. In this vein, one must weigh the needs for electron microscopy, cytogenetics, molecular biology, and immunostaining against the requirement for material smeared on slides or spun with a cytocentrifuge. In addition, consideration should be given to the preparation of cell pellets for paraffin blocks, as one often obtains a "mini-biopsy" that can be profitably used for both routine stains and immunochemistry (20). There is no set rule for preparing aliquots for these various options; instead one must be guided by possible tumor diagnoses given the anatomic site, patient age, and radiographic findings.

Morphometry

Morphometry, or the measurement of anatomic structures, is a valuable research tool that has provided discrete numeric data to answer a number of embryological and anatomical questions in pediatric pathology (41). In surgical pathology, numeric measurement of prognostic and diagnostic variables has repeatedly been shown to produce significantly less variation than qualitative observation, even by panels of experts (28). In particular, morphometry is often applied to the grading of neoplasms, as this exercise requires assessment of semiquantitative features such as cellularity, amount of necrosis, mitotic index, and cellular pleomorphism. In the past, the amount of time necessary for careful, repeated measurement has limited the application of morphometry to research and precluded its use by busy hospital pathology services. However, technological advances in optics and computerization (55) have created a burgeoning market of instrumentation.

Foremost in the application of morphometry to the diagnosis and prognostication of pediatric neoplasms is assessment of mitotic index. This relatively simple procedure is based on morphometrically sound principles when performed in a standardized manner (2). Although it is theoretically a simple procedure, there are a number of caveats that necessitate some degree of caution and expertise in mitosis counting (2). Of particular importance is the correct recognition of a mitotic cell; one must be aware of cytologic mimicry and only count mitoses with the features listed in Table 3. Another consideration is the time between surgical excision and fixation, which may inversely affect the number of mitoses present at the time of examination (2). This could be a particularly critical feature of large tumors in which fixation is delayed. Finally, tumors may be heterogeneous in their growth, with emergence of aggressive clones in a background of low-grade activity. This can easily result in potential variability in counting if insufficient high-power fields are considered. One could circumvent this problem with the inclusion of only aggressive-appearing areas in a mitotic count, but this maneuver introduces an element of observer bias. Nevertheless, it is a maxim of surgical pathology that grade is determined by the most aggressive-appearing portion of the lesion.

More recently, morphometric assessment of other attributes such as mean nuclear and nucleolar size, circularity, and the standard deviation and coefficient of variation of these quantities have been used in tumor grading (10). In this manner, one obtains numeric values to assess hitherto semiquantitatively determined features of tumor cell pleomorphism. These values may be calculated very rapidly by computerized assessment of video images, and the images can be manipulated by the user for optimal data acquisition. In measurements of this sort, it is necessary to exclude variables such as adjoining or multinucleated cells by interaction with the video image. Another critical factor is the assessment of two-dimensional images, as oblique and tangential sections yield incorrect values for variables such as nuclear size. Mathematical computations and standardized section thicknesses may be employed to overcome this bias (34) or alternatively one may use whole cells or nuclei (46).

Another standard method in morphometry is point counting, wherein one assesses a variable such as number of tumor cells per square millimeter, thereby obtaining a mathematical value for cellularity. In its simplest form, this is performed using a standardized grid inserted into the eyepiece of a light microscope (Fig. 3); more sophisticated methods use electronic platens or image pixel points (23). Besides counting total numbers of cells, this

TABLE 3. *Features used for counting mitotic cells (2)*

Absence of a nuclear membrane
Absence of a central clear zone
Presence of hairy rather than triangular or spiky projections
Cytoplasmic basophilia rather than eosinophilia

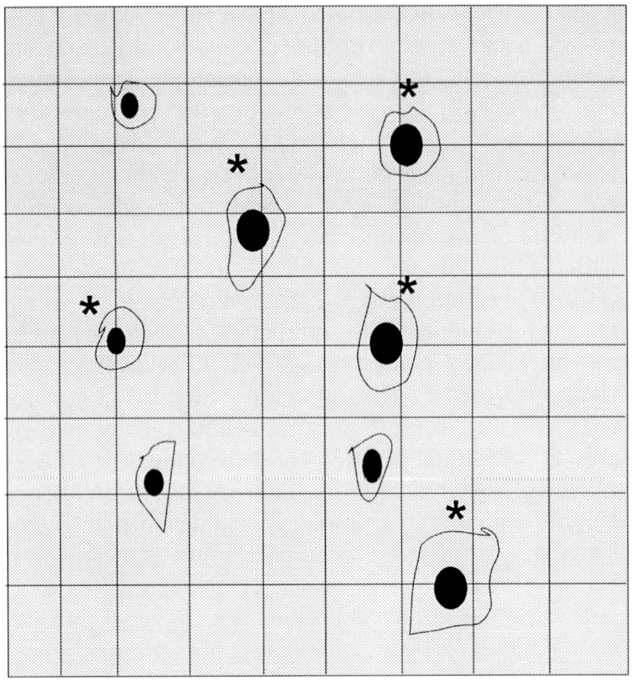

FIG. 3. Grid used for point counting. This is an overlap that in its simplest form is an etched glass lens inserted into a microscope eyepiece. Only the number of cells touching intersects are counted, thereby obtaining a discrete measurement of tumor cellularity.

method can be used to assess cells staining with a particular cell marker, yielding values of prognostic significance such as the proliferation index (16). The chief source of error in these counting methods is the inclusion of nontumor elements such as infiltrating macrophages or blood vessel cells into the total count, necessitating performance by operators experienced in cytologic and histologic examination.

One measurement that has generated numerous reports in the surgical pathology literature during the past decade is determination of the argyrophilic nucleolar organizer region (AgNOR) count. This morphometric technique is based on the presence of nuclear chromocenters, termed nucleolar organizing regions, which are best revealed by silver stains (24). At a molecular level, these sites represent areas of transcriptional activity (36). With this method, one counts the number of AgNORs in at least 200 cells and calculates the mean number per cell. In general, larger numbers of AgNORs has been associated with an increased propensity of tumors for recurrence and metastasis and decreased patient survival (24). In pediatrics, variable results have been obtained, with some tumors such as neuroblastoma showing a significant correlation of AgNOR count with survival (4), and others such as Wilms' tumor and Ewing's sarcoma showing no correlation (8,27).

Cytogenetics

Of all morphologic techniques, it is cytogenetics that most relates to current molecular biology and novel diagnostic approaches. This technique has formed the foundation of modern thought on the genesis and evolution of neoplasia. It is based on the observation that during mitosis and meiosis, DNA is bound into tightly strictured filaments, or chromosomes. These bodies are most apparent during metaphase, when they are normally aligned in a neat central row on the mitotic spindle apparatus. Cytogenetic abnormalities form the basis for neoplastic transformation of the cell and tend to be characteristic of specific types of pediatric neoplasms, thus forming the foundation of a new generation of diagnostic testing.

To observe metaphase cells, one must have a uniform slide preparation that contains evenly spread nuclei, so that the chromosomes of adjoining cells will not be mistaken for those of single isolated cells. Also, whole nuclei are required so that the entire genome can be observed. Finally, dividing cells must be present and can be found in the bone marrow of leukemia patients in a direct preparation or following propagation of tumor cells in a tissue culture medium. Tissue culture techniques are covered in a separate section of this chapter.

To increase the number of metaphases that one observes, colchicine may be added to the medium just before slide preparation. This drug paralyzes the mitotic spindle, freezing the cells in metaphase. The cells must then be hypotonically ruptured to release their nuclear contents and to allow observation of evenly spread chromosomes. The chromosomes may be altered to increase their length and enhance the visualization of their domains, or bands. Banding is performed by staining with Giemsa or quinacrine. Giemsa-stained bands, or G bands, are observable with routine bright field microscopy, whereas quinacrine-stained bands, or Q bands, are fluorescent and require fluorescence microscopy for their detection.

The technique of banding has been the primary step in mapping the human genome. In the study of pediatric neoplasia, banding has yielded clues to the basic biologic nature of a number of tumors, as recurring anomalies are present in malignancies such as alveolar rhabdomyosarcoma and acute lymphoblastic leukemia (31,42). These observations have begun to pay substantial dividends for both histogenetic theorists and diagnosticians, and newer molecular techniques are being developed and refined for their detection. This research will increase the availability of genetic testing, as routine cytogenetics suffers a relative insensitivity because of its requirement for in vitro tumor growth. Even with rapidly growing embryonal neoplasms, only 50% of attempted karyotypes are successful, even in the best of laboratories (56).

Turnaround time is also slowed by the need to first grow cells in vitro. Many neoplasms also have such marked distortion and duplication of chromosomes that detection of specific abnormalities via simple observation is difficult or impossible.

A number of abnormalities may be observed with cytogenetic study. Some of the more common are listed in Table 4. Understanding these anomalies requires knowledge of cytogenetic terminology and the normal karyotype (33,40). The normal diploid state, seen following mitotic division, consists of a 46,XX or 46,XY karyotype, corresponding to 46 autosomal chromosomes and 2 sex chromosomes. The haploid state, seen following meiosis, consists of a 23,X or 23,Y karyotype and is limited to germ cells. Chromosomes, as pictured in Figure 4, comprise two chromatids bound by a centromere; their distal regions are known as telomeres. The arms on either side of the centromere comprise the short, or p, arm and the long, or q, arm. The long and short arms are further divided into specific numeric regions based on their banding pattern.

Abnormalities such as translocations may link the long arm of one chromosome with the long arm of another chromosome, as in the 46,XX,t(11;22)(q24;q12) characteristic of Ewing's sarcoma. In this example, the tumor is composed of the diploid cells of a female, with a balanced translocation linking the 24 banding region of the long arm of chromosome 11 with the 12 region of chromosome 22. Examples of numeric abnormalities would include monosomy 7, listed as 45,XX,−7, or monosomy 22, listed as 45,XX,−22. These karyotypes lack a chromosome 7 (as seen with some forms of myeloid leukemia) or a chromosome 22 (as is characteristic of the atypical teratoid/rhabdoid tumor of the brain), respectively. Extra genetic material may also be obtained from duplications in which only a segment of a chromosome is added to the karyotype. This might be listed as 46,XX,dup(11)(p13→pter) if there was an extra segment of 11p stretching from the p13 band to the terminal end. These duplications may be direct or inverted (see below).

TABLE 4. *Cytogenetic abnormalities seen in pediatric neoplasms*

Numeric deletions (monosomy)
Numeric duplications (trisomy, etc.)
Translocations
Isochromosomes
Ring chromosomes
Marker chromosomes
Double minute chromosomes
Heterogeneous staining regions
Inverted chromosomes
Segmental deletions
Terminal
Interstitial
Dicentric chromosomes

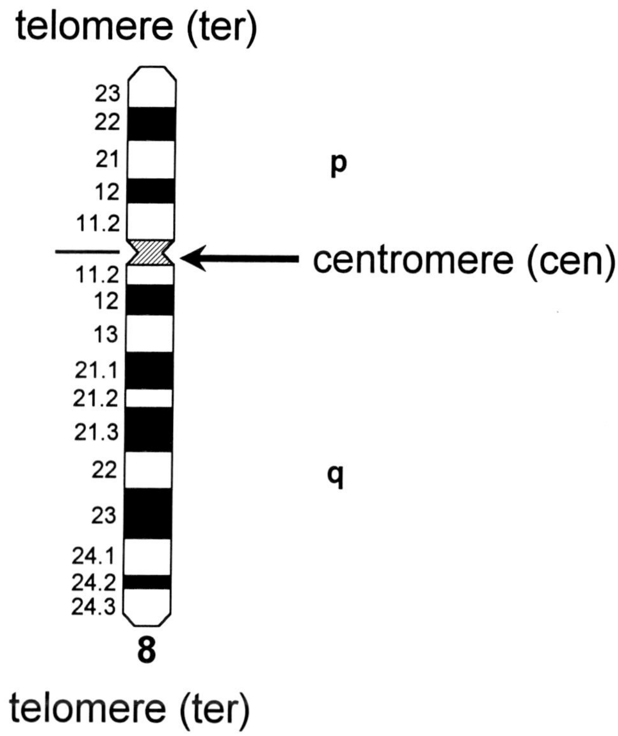

FIG. 4. Schematic diagram of one chromatid of chromosome 8. It is separated into p (short) and q (long) arms divided by a centromere and with distal telomeric ends. The chromosome is further subdivided into numeric regions as shown, based on the band pattern.

More complex cytogenetic abnormalities include ring, dicentric, and marker chromosomes, inversions, and isochromosomes. Ring chromosomes form a circle from fusion of telomeric ends, following breakage and deletion of their distal portions. This might be listed as 46,XY,r(2),(p21q31) if chromosome 2 forms a ring following deletional events at 2p21 and 2q31. Note that the result causes fusion of two normally separated genes. Dicentric chromosomes contain two centromeres rather than one. An example is 46,XY,dic(Y), in which the Y chromosome is dicentric. Marker chromosomes have such severe distortion that their identifying number cannot be reliably determined by visual observation alone. This might be listed as 47,XX,+mar, if a marker chromosome is present. Inverted chromosomes are somewhat analogous to translocated ones and are characterized by having segments that exhibit transposition within a single chromosome rather than between two. An example would be 46,XY,inv(1)(p12p23), in which there has been breakage at 1p12 and 1p23 followed by inversion and reunion. The net effect is still juxtaposition of normally separate genes. Isochromosomes are characterized by having identical long or short arms linked by a centromere. An example is the i(12p), typical of adolescent teratomas, in which there are short arms of 12 on both sides of the centromere.

Heterogeneous staining regions (HSRs) and double-minute chromosomes are related phenomena caused by genetic amplification. These amplified DNA segments produce an elongated, pale-staining region with HSRs and short isolated segments with double minutes. They are of particular note in neuroblastoma, where they represent amplification of the N-myc gene and are associated with aggressive clinical behavior.

Finally, a number of pediatric neoplasms show varying degrees of loss of genetic material. If the amount of genetic loss is severe enough, it is visually manifested as a segmental deletion. These deletions may cause loss of tumor suppressor genes that normally function to inhibit unbridled cell division. An example is the 11p− of the Wilms–aniridia syndrome, in which a portion or the short arm of chromosome 11 is lost, thus deleting the tumor suppressor gene *WT1*. Deletions may be terminal, with loss of the distal end, or interstitial, with loss of a midportion of the chromosome arm. Interstitial deletions of *WT1* occur in the Denys–Drash syndrome of Wilms' tumor, sexual ambiguity, and glomerulosclerosis, whereas terminal deletions of 11p are more common in the Wilms-aniridia syndrome (see Chapter 3).

FLOW CYTOMETRY AND CELL SORTING

Richard A. Ashmun

Flow cytometry is used to obtain rapid and reproducible measurements from large numbers of cells (43). These machines force single-cell suspensions under pressure into a fine fluid stream, which is then illuminated by a precisely aimed light source, usually a laser. Cells that have been labeled with specific fluorescent dyes or fluorescently tagged antibodies will fluoresce when illuminated by this source; the light emitted from these tags is collected by sensitive detectors and quantitated, together with measures of laser light that is physically scattered by the cells. The combination of measures of scattered light in the forward and side directions often permits an initial identification of cell subpopulations of interest; for example, lymphocytes, monocytes, and granulocytes can each be identified independently from a sample of peripheral blood leukocytes, using just light scatter measures. The information from all detectors is correlated for each individual cell at flow rates of up to thousands of cells per second; subsequent computer analysis of these data can be used to detect and characterize biologically important subpopulations of cells. The power of this technique lies in its ability to rapidly and reproducibly perform multiple quantitative measurements on individual cells, as opposed to single measurements from heterogeneous bulk populations of cells or measurements from far fewer cells by microscopic examination. Because flow cytometry requires analysis of single-cell suspensions, observations of cellular structure and cell-to-cell interaction are generally not possible with flow cytometry, whereas this information is routinely part of light microscopic examination of tissues. The intracellular localization of particular antigens of interest is similarly limited to microscopic examination. However, with flow cytometric analysis multiple measurements are possible from each cell, and the sensitivity of a flow cytometer's detectors exceeds that of the human eye in microscopic examination. Flow analysis also provides a good scheme of morphologic discrimination of cell subpopulations based on light scatter properties, and the flow machine can analyze hundreds of times more cells in an allotted time. Thus, these techniques of observation differ and are best used to complement each other.

Regardless of the application of this technique, proper machine preparation and documentation of performance are essential. While details vary with specific machines, proper preparation requires testing for proper alignment of the optical elements involved in the excitation laser beam and the detectors used to measure fluorescence emissions and scattered light. On some machines, this alignment is fixed and not subject to user adjustment, but on others detailed attention to alignment is required multiple times each day. Alignment usually requires the analysis of commercially available fluorescent standards, such as microbeads or fixed cells, which have fluorescence and light scatter properties that are documented and stable over time. Daily tests of the machine's performance will indicate any variation outside of prescribed limits; such discrepancies require corrective adjustments or else uninterpretable measurements will result. Typically, a flow cytometer can be tested quickly for both fluorescence sensitivity and linearity of response. Tests of sensitivity document the ability of the machine to detect a certain level of fluorescence above background; consistency in this test is essential to the daily interpretation of measures of cellular fluorescence. Linearity of response is especially important in the interpretation of measures of cellular DNA content and should also be tested daily.

One of the most common applications of flow cytometry is the measurement of cellular DNA content. DNA content abnormalities are common in malignant tumors; cytogenetics studies have shown that chromosomal abnormalities frequently involve a limited number of structural or numeric changes, which correlate with cell phenotype. DNA content analysis by flow cytometry remains the clinical flow cytometric procedure most widely used in oncology, and the quantitation of abnormal DNA content can often be a valuable determinant in the choice of therapy. The test is ideal for prognostic purposes, as it is rapidly and reproducibly performed in a semiautomated fashion using a relatively small number of cells.

The integrity of the sample is important in obtaining

good results. Pieces of fresh tissue or tumor must be disaggregated by careful mincing of the specimen, such as with scalpels in the presence of medium; the resulting cell suspension can be prefiltered to remove large clumps that remain. If tissue is minced too thoroughly, however, the cells of interest may actually be destroyed. Samples containing cells already in suspension, such as bone marrow or peripheral blood specimens, can be prepared using density-gradient centrifugation, which often suffices to produce clean single-cell suspensions. Samples containing a large number of red blood cells may require an extra step which lyses the red cells using an ammonium chloride buffer (or commercially available preparations for this purpose) while maintaining the integrity of nucleated cells present in the sample.

Nuclei from cells are stained with a DNA-specific dye and are analyzed for the amount of DNA present in each cell. Most commonly, cells are rapidly stained by suspending them in a hypotonic buffer containing the dye propidium iodide; in this buffer the cells lyse, exposing the bare nuclei to the dye. Propidium iodide, the dye of choice due to its fluorescent properties that are well suited to laser excitation, binds to both double-stranded DNA and double-stranded RNA. In order to eliminate any artificial broadening of the DNA histogram due to the presence of labeled RNA, samples should be treated with DNase-free RNase just before analysis for one-half hour at room temperature to digest the RNA. Just before analysis on the flow cytometer, samples should be filtered to eliminate any multicell aggregates or debris that could plug the fluidics system of the machine. During the analysis, the formation of the sample stream in the flow cytometer is partly dependent on the pressure applied to the sample, which in turn determines the flow rate. The best resolution of DNA content is obtained at these lower rates, although at the expense of longer analysis time.

The results of the analysis are plotted as a frequency histogram of DNA content versus cell number (Fig. 5). Under normal circumstances, nondividing cells should have the same amount of DNA, termed diploid (or referred to as 2N), and reside in the G0/G1 compartments of the cell cycle. DNA replication during S phase results in the cellular DNA amount increasing from 2N to 4N, while cells in the last part of S phase and during mitosis (M phase) have a DNA content of 4N. Upon division, a mitotic cell produces two daughter cells, each with a DNA content of 2N. In the real world, distributions exhibit some variation in DNA content of each compartment, due to variations in staining procedures, instrument performance, and possibly differences among cells. Samples of tumors or leukemic blood or bone marrow typically have some normal cells present in the sample; the DNA histogram of such a sample would be the composite of both the normal cells and the tumor cells. If the tumor cells have an aneuploid DNA content, the tumor population will be revealed by its own DNA distribution

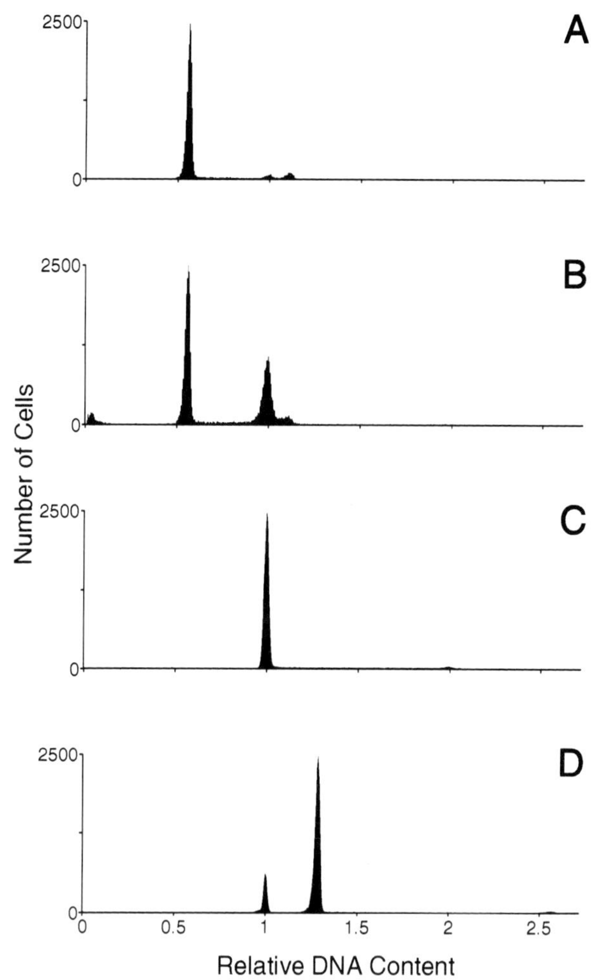

FIG. 5. Determination of DNA index (DI) in acute lymphoblastic leukemia. **A.** Case 1: near haploid tumor stemline (DI = 0.59), with some residual normal leukocytes (DI = 1.0). **B.** Case 1 mixed with normal leukocytes before staining. The histogram displays an increased diploid peak at DI = 1.0 as compared to Part A above. **C.** Case 2: diploid tumor stem line superimposed on normal leukocytes at DI = 1.0. **D.** Case 3: hyperdiploid tumor stem line (DI = 1.29), with some residual normal leukocytes (DI = 1.0).

at a different level of fluorescence proportional to the changed DNA content. The DNA content of tumor cells is expressed as a DNA index (DI), which is the ratio of the modal value of G0/G1 phase tumor cells to that of normal cells. In order to verify the ploidy of a tumor sample, a portion of the (unstained) sample is typically used to prepare a mix of tumor and normal cells (which can be normal lymphocytes or other cells with known DNA content); this mix is then stained with propidium iodide and run separately from the sample itself. The mix provides an internal reference point of a known DNA content; when the mix is analyzed, the sample DNA histogram will be modified by the added reference cells, providing a means of calculating the DI value for the sample. In cases where uncertainty or ambiguity exists, multiple mixes with samples of known DNA content may be required to be confident of the DI.

Flow cytometric analysis can also be performed on tissue that has been embedded in paraffin blocks (13). The success of such determinations varies widely, depending on the quality of the original sample, the method of recovering cells from the block, and the fixative used in the block preparation. Most commonly, relatively thick (50-μm) slices from blocks are rehydrated in a stepwise manner, followed by an enzymatic digestion chosen to help liberate cells from surrounding paraffin. Finally, recovered cells are stained with propidium iodide, filtered, and subjected to flow analysis. Standard mixing techniques to clearly identify cells with diploid DNA content do not work here due to inconsistent uptake of dye; the analysis must be accompanied by a microscopic analysis of a tissue slice from an adjacent section of the same block. The microscopic analysis is essential to estimate the percentage of tumor cells present in the entire sample, which is needed to interpret the identity of the cells comprising the DNA histogram. Despite the difficulties inherent in analyzing DNA content of paraffin-embedded material, the potential value of these measurements in studying archival material is frequently sufficient to make such efforts worthwhile.

In general, there is good agreement between flow cytometric assessment of ploidy and classical cytogenetic determination of chromosome number. As most flow cytometers cannot distinguish a change from diploidy of less than 3–4% (corresponding to a change of two chromosomes or less), the results from classical cytogenetics are especially informative in these cases. The advantages of the two techniques complement one another; whereas flow cytometry is rapid and accurately analyzes many cells, cytogenetic analysis is slower, analyzes far fewer cells, but is able to detect changes undetectable by flow (pseudodiploidy, translocations, etc.).

The flow cytometer is also routinely used for immunophenotyping tumor samples. This procedure has wide use in the characterization of cell lineage and levels of differentiation and can be extremely valuable in predicting prognosis. With the advent of monoclonal antibody (MAb) technique, a uniform nomenclature based on clusters of differentiation (or CD groups) has evolved based on reactivity of antibodies to cell surface antigens. Monoclonal antibodies to lymphocyte cell surface markers were among the very first to be characterized and remain the most frequently used reagents for flow phenotyping. For example, the lineage of acute leukemic blasts can be assigned based on the pattern of binding of a panel of monoclonal antibodies. The proper interpretation of results requires good controls; for a given immune reagent, the best control is an isotype-matched irrelevant antibody raised in the same species. The optimal titer for each reagent should be determined in controlled tests with known positive and negative cells as measured on the flow cytometer in order to guarantee saturation of binding to all available antigen sites. Frequently, the amount of MAb required for saturating binding conditions for flow cytometric studies is greater than the amount required for saturation on a light microscope–based assay.

Immunofluorescence staining may be either direct, whereby the MAb is conjugated to a fluorochrome and only a single staining step is required, or indirect, whereby the primary MAb is detectable only after a second fluorochrome-tagged reagent has been added. Indirect immunofluorescence has an advantage of amplifying the fluorescence level for a given number of antigen sites, at the expense of an additional step of staining. Each staining step is typically performed at 4°C for 20–30 minutes in a small volume (50–100 μL), followed by washes to remove unbound reagent. Samples should be filtered just before analysis to remove clumps or aggregates.

It is important to identify dying or dead cells within a sample that is otherwise viable; dead cells often bind nonspecifically to fluorescently labeled reagents, making these cells hard or impossible to distinguish from live cells that are specifically labeled by those reagents. Dead cells can often be distinguished from live ones by altered light scatter, but their detection is aided by counterstaining with a dye (such as propidium iodide) that does not penetrate the cellular plasma membrane of viable cells, but which can pass through the more porous membranes of dying or dead cells to stain nucleic acids. These stained dead cells can be electronically gated (or excluded) from the analysis, ensuring that the measurement of fluorescence is limited to viable cells. Stained samples can be fixed in 0.5–1% paraformadehyde, which stabilizes the labeling and permits storage at 4°C for analysis at a later time. The interpretation of immunofluorescence results usually includes an estimate of the percentage of cells that specifically bind a monoclonal antibody. The determination of this percentage remains somewhat of an art and involves computing the fraction of cells possessing fluorescence levels above a certain background threshold. The most important consideration is consistency and clarity of methodology.

Current flow cytometers can detect from three to five different fluorochromes if the order and wavelength specificity of the optical filters in the machine are chosen properly. The combination of several fluorochromes emitting at different wavelengths permits the simultaneous detection of binding of multiple monoclonal antibodies (Fig. 6). More complex flow cytometers may have two or three lasers for additional flexibility; recent availability of multiple fluorochromes that are excitable by the 48-nm light from a single argon-ion laser has enabled flow users to simultaneously label cells with up to four

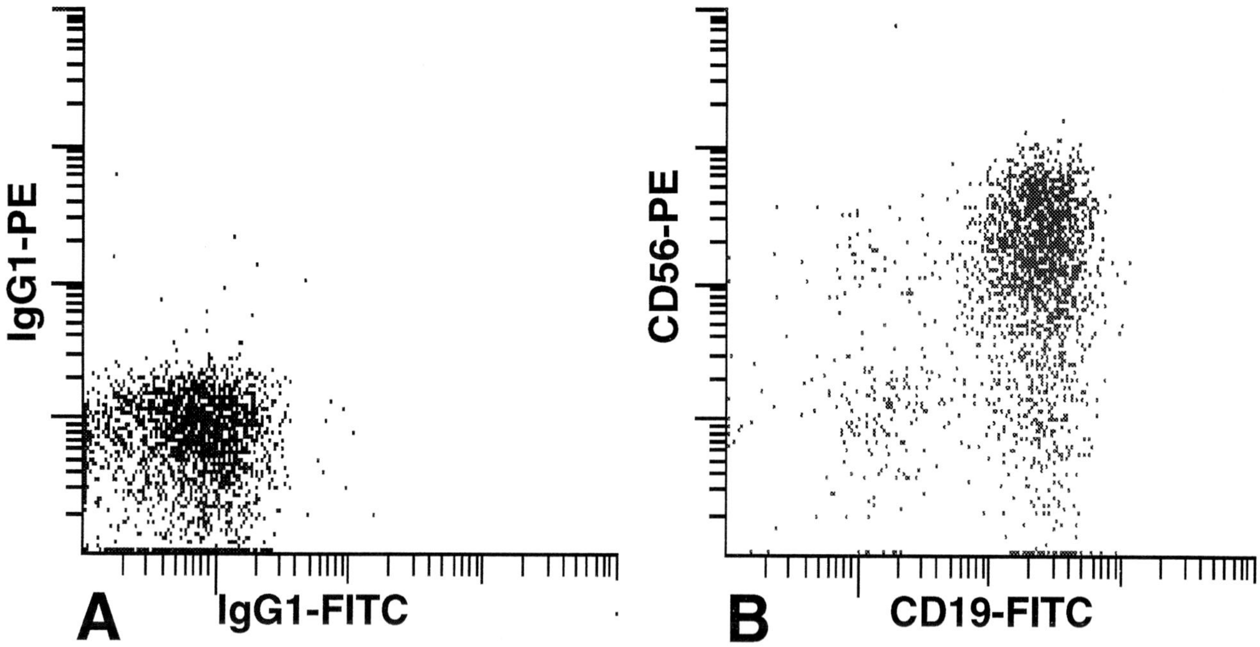

FIG. 6. Acute lymphoblastic leukemia tested with two-color flow cytometry. In panel **A**, testing for IgG1 with a phycoerythrin (PE) flourochrome, simultaneously with IgG1 conjugated to fluorescein isothiocyanate (FITC), reveals minimal staining. This result is used as a negative control. In panel **B**, testing for CD56, NK cell antigen, coupled to PE and for CD19, B-cell antigen, coupled to FITC, reveals a large positive population. This result indicates coexpression of both markers by the tumor cells. (Courtesy of Dr. Fred Behm, St. Jude Children's Research Hospital.)

tags, while exciting them all with only one laser. Commercial preparations are now available which combine two or three distinct antibodies, each with a unique fluorochrome, to simultaneously label a sample with multiple markers, including common combinations such as CD4 and CD8. Commercial cell stainers are also available that combine red cell lysis, staining, and fixation in a rapid series of semiautomated steps to facilitate routine staining. Additionally, certain flow cytometers can perform fluorescence-activated cell sorting (FACS), which can be used to physically separate cells possessing unique light scatter or fluorescence properties and contained in a mixed sample.

TISSUE CULTURE AND XENOGRAFTS

Peter Dias, Glen S. Germain, Peter J. Houghton

Diagnostic information may be gained from primary cell cultures, cell lines, and xenografts of tumors. Tumor-derived cell lines and xenografts also offer a means to propagate the tissue for studies on the biology of the tumors and their response to therapeutic agents.

The Knudson–Strong hypothesis (18) proposes that mutations of both alleles of a key growth-regulating gene are required for the uncontrolled proliferation resulting in neoplasia. The genes in question are often tumor suppressor genes, and it is now becoming clear that multiple changes involving the activation of oncogenes as well as inactivation of suppressor genes occur during malignant transformation (54). The transformed cells that have acquired these mutations have a selective growth advantage over the untransformed normal cells and increase in number, resulting in a clonal population. Because of this unregulated growth, transformed cells tend to accumulate further mutations in the process of tumor progression. If each mutation confers an aggressive growth property, then eventually highly malignant lines evolve that have minimal growth requirements. The understanding of malignant transformation is thus not only important in the study of cancer per se but also for the derivation and use of the tumor cell lines and xenografts.

Tissue Culture

Primary cell cultures, also referred to explant cultures, are by definition derived directly from normal, fetal, or diseased tissue, such as tumors. Such cultures are often used to examine for cytogenetic abnormalities and also sometimes for diagnosis of the derived cells by immunocytochemistry.

When a cell culture becomes confluent the cells are removed from the container, and a fraction, usually one half of the original cell number, is used to reseed a new flask of the same size. This process of subculturing is referred to as a passage. In culture, normal or nonneoplastic cells have a set number of cell divisions before they senesce. This is known as the Hayflick limit and was first conclusively demonstrated with diploid fibroblasts derived from embryonic lung (12). As a rough guide the number of cell divisions of a culture is determined by the number of its passages from the time it was derived from the tissue. Although the criteria tend to vary, a cell culture is regarded as a continuous cell line (simply referred to as cell line) after it has been passaged from 50 to 70 times or more, as these cells are immortal, or transformed, and do not have a Hayflick limit. If the cell line can form colonies on soft agar and also form tumors in immune-compromised animal models, then it is regarded as a malignant tumor cell line. It is important, however, to appreciate that not all immortal cell lines are malignant. Thus, just because a cell line does not have a Hayflick limit, it does not necessarily mean that it will grow on soft agar or form tumors in immune-compromised animals.

Obtaining and Processing Tumor Tissue at Biopsy/ Autopsy

In order to maintain viability in vitro it is important to obtain and process autopsy or biopsy specimens as rapidly as possible after excision, for these dissected tissues will not have a supply of oxygen and nutrients. The fresh tissue is obtained aseptically and placed in tissue culture medium containing at least 10% v/v fetal bovine serum for transportation and cell culturing. Tissue culture medium is an osmotically balanced salt solution usually containing all 20 amino acids, water-soluble vitamins, glucose, and a bicarbonate anion buffer. There are a number of commercially available tissue culture media, such as DMEM, medium 199, BME, MEM, and RPMI 1640. These media tend to have variations in the amounts of the constituents mentioned above.

It is important that the tissue not dry and be completely submerged in the tissue culture medium. Because there is a risk of microbial contamination, it is usually advisable to supplement the medium with a broad-spectrum antibiotic, such as gentamicin or a mixture of penicillin and streptomycin combined with an antifungal agent such as nystatin or amphotericin B. The specimen is immediately processed in a laminar flow tissue culture hood to maintain aseptic conditions. All equipment used in handling this material should be sterile. The tissue is rinsed in fresh medium containing the antimicrobial agents and cut into at least three representative samples, one for freezing viable samples of the original tumor tissue, one for deriving primary tumor cell cultures, and one for growth in immune-compromised rodents as xenografts.

Freezing Tissue

For freezing viable samples, the freshly obtained tumor is cut into 2-mm^3 pieces and immediately placed in a special medium for freezing tissue such as 90% v/v fetal calf serum with 10% v/v dimethyl sulfoxide (DMSO). The tissue suspension is then placed in cryovials and cooled at a controlled rate of 1°C per minute, until the temperature reaches at least below −40°C. The vials are then stored in liquid nitrogen until required. Control rate freezing is necessary to prevent intracytoplasmic ice crystal formation, which severely compromises cell viability.

Culture Derivation

Although the derivation of primary tumor cell cultures is technically simple, in practice success is not always guaranteed and depends on the degree of malignancy of the tumor being processed. The tumor tissue is placed in a petri dish (preferably glass) containing tissue culture medium and minced extensively with a pair of curved scissors. The best results are obtained when the tissue pieces are minced to smaller than 0.5 mm^3. Some investigators use enzymes such as collagenases in addition to the mincing process so as to obtain a single-cell suspension. The minced cell/tissue suspension is then carefully transferred to tissue culture flasks and placed in a temperature-controlled, humidified incubator maintained at 37°C and supplied with 5% carbon dioxide. The flasks are left undisturbed for several days to allow cells to grow out of the minced explant tissue and attach to the surface of the flasks. When the cells become confluent, they are released from the flask by treatment with trypsin. Samples of these cells are then frozen in liquid nitrogen for future reference, reseeded into fresh flasks for further propagation, and potentially used for characterization by techniques such as immunocytochemistry, cytogenetics, or DNA studies.

One of the biggest problems of deriving primary tumor cultures is growth of contaminating stromal cells, primarily fibroblasts. Fibroblasts tend to grow faster than tumor cells and if not suppressed will eventually outgrow the desired malignant cells, even though these stromal cells may not be immortal. Special techniques or media may be used that allow selective growth of tumor cells while keeping the fibroblast population suppressed. Some methods take advantage of the more rapid attachment of fibroblasts to tissue culture plastic to selectively deplete primary cultures of these stromal cells. Thus by placing the primary culture in flasks for a short time period such that only fibroblasts attach and then transferring the remaining cells to another flask, selective depletion has been achieved. Other studies report that tissue culture medium containing only the D-form of valine and no L-valine selectively inhibits fibroblast growth. Alternatively, enzymes can be used to break down the tissue to a homogeneous cell suspension, followed by incubation with an antibody to a cell surface lineage-specific marker that is specific for the desired cell type. After incubation with a fluorescent labeled secondary antibody, the primary antibody-tagged fluorescent labeled cells are then separated by the use of FACS. The labeled cells are then washed in tissue culture medium and seeded in tissue culture flasks.

Xenografts

A xenograft is a tissue from one animal species that is grafted in another animal species. In this context a human tumor xenograft is a human tumor that is grafted in immunocompromised animals of other species, generally rodents. Tumor xenografts retain most morphologic characteristics of the original tumor (Fig. 7). The changes that occur are exceptionally minor and undetectable even to skilled, experienced pathologists. Aside from the stromal component that is essentially of rodent origin, all the tumor cells are genetically human. Thus, in certain instances, use of xenografts has aided identification of characteristic cytogenetic abnormalities associated with particular tumor types. One advantage of using xenografts in this particular instance is that normal human stromal cells that might otherwise complicate cytogenetic assessment are absent because generally only tumor cells and not normal human cells will grow in immune-compromised rodents.

To grow human tumors as xenografts, immune-compromised mice such as NIH type II athymic nude mice (nu/nu) or rats such as the athymic PVG nude rats (rnu/rnu) may be used. However, for large xenograft studies it is cheaper to thymectomize, irradiate, and then reconstitute the marrow of genotypically normal mice. This will compromise their immune system sufficiently to allow transplantation of the human tumors. As in the derivation of cell lines from tumor tissue, the growth of human tumors in immune-compromised rodent models is technically simple but often difficult in practice. Not every human tumor transplanted into immune-compromised animals forms xenografts.

Xenografts may be formed by either subcutaneous injection of cells from a malignant cell line or by implantation of the original patient tumor. Approximately 5–10 million viable cells suspended in a small volume of saline (approximate volume of 0.2 cm^3) are used for subcutaneous injections. Alternatively, a piece of tumor tissue approximately 0.5 cm^3 in size or slightly larger is inserted subcutaneously through a small incision that is then briefly bathed in a solution of antibiotics and sealed by stapling or suturing. The implanted cells or tumor tissue may take between one to eight weeks to form xenograft tumors. The degree of malignancy of the patient tumor or the cell line will influence the rate of success of tumor take as well as the time to form xenografts. Most if not all highly malignant tumor cell lines form xenografts when a cell suspension is used for injection, although not all immortal cell lines form xenografts. Similarly, a specimen from a highly progressed tumor will take much more easily than a specimen from a tumor of low grade malignancy. It is also noted that clinically aggressive tumor subtypes such as alveolar rhabdomyosarcomas take more easily than do the less aggressive subtypes such as embryonal rhabdomyosarcomas (7). Furthermore, patients whose tumors form xenografts in immune-compromised rodents tend to have a poorer prognosis

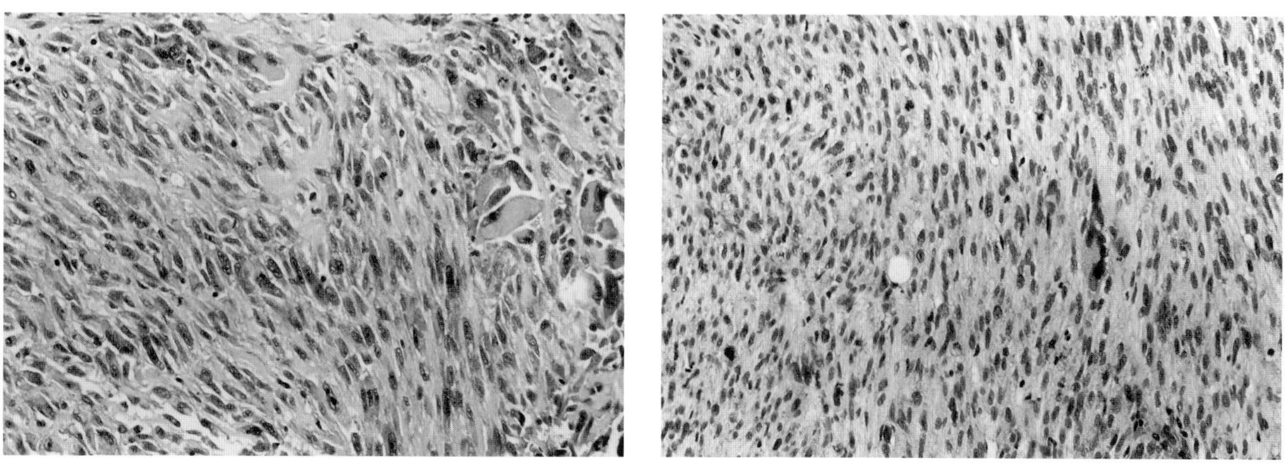

A B

FIG. 7. Sections of primary human osteosarcoma (**A**) and derived xenograft (**B**). Both tumors are similarly composed of pleomorphic spindle cells. (From Meyer WH et al. Development and characterization of pediatric osteosarcoma xenografts. *Cancer Res* 1990;50:2781–2785; courtesy of Dr. Meyer and the publisher.)

then those whose tumors do not grow as xenografts (35). However, such a relationship may depend on the tumor type.

When a xenograft has grown to approximately 2 cm^3, the tissue may be removed, cut into 2-mm^3 fragments, and reimplanted subcutaneously into other animals. It is good practice to freeze viable samples of xenograft tissues from each passage as reference material, as the tumor morphology may gradually change due to selection of highly aggressive, more rapidly growing clonal lines. It is also good practice to frequently examine xenograft histology, as rodent tumors have been reported to occur spontaneously (37) or grow at the site of implantation of the human tumor (14). It can be difficult to distinguish histologically between human and animal tumors. Thus, as long as the lineage of the tumor cells is known, the identity of the xenogeneic tumor may be determined by the use of antibodies to the lineage-specific marker. Antibodies to the major histocompatibility antigens of the host animal or human, or antibodies to human- or rodent-specific antigens may also be used to the differentiate between the two (7). Alternatively, the isoenzyme pattern for lactate dehydrogenase (14) or karyotyping can help to determine whether the tumor is of human or rodent origin.

MOLECULAR BIOLOGIC TECHNIQUES

David R. Head

Molecular biologic tests used for clinical evaluation and research of pediatric solid tumors include tests to analyze DNA (Southern blot, in situ hybridization [ISH], polymerase chain reaction [PCR]), RNA (northern blot, reverse transcriptase [RT]–PCR), and protein (western blot). Details of methodology and general uses will be discussed for these tests.

Southern Blot

To perform a Southern blot [after E. Southern (45)], genomic DNA is harvested from a cell sample and purified by differential extraction in organic solvents from protein, RNA, and other cellular constituents (5,53). Although DNA is a relatively resistant molecule containing billions of base pairs (bp), it is easily disrupted into small fragments. Since one aspect of testing consists of evaluation of the size of fragments of DNA, care must be taken to harvest the DNA as high molecular weight fragments. After harvest the DNA is digested with restriction endonucleases, which are bacterial enzymes apparently evolved for protection from viruses and which digest DNA at specific symmetric base sequences, typically 6 bp in length (1,21,53). For example, the commonly used restriction endonuclease EcoR1 cuts DNA at any locus that has the sequence GAATTC. This is exactly the same sequence when read in the opposite direction on the complementary strand, a characteristic of restriction endonuclease cut sites. This particular sequence also occurs irregularly at approximately 5000-bp intervals in eukaryotic DNA. Thus restriction endonucleases such as EcoR1 digest DNA reproducibly, creating variably sized fragments patterns of DNA with size based on the distribution of the DNA sequence recognized by the specific restriction endonuclease used. To perform a Southern blot, the digested DNA fragments are separated by size with electrophoresis, usually in an agarose or polyacrylamide gel, denatured to single-strand DNA, partially degraded to short fragments, blotted to a nitrocellulose or nylon membrane, permanently affixed to the membrane [eg, by ultraviolet (UV) crosslinking], and hybridized to a labeled DNA probe sequence specific for the DNA locus being studied. Sensitivity and specificity of the hybridization reaction are controlled by adjusting salt concentration, temperature, and the concentration of other agents such as formamide, all of which alter the hydrogen bonding forces between two complementary or near-complementary single strands of DNA. After hybridization is complete, the membrane is washed to remove nonspecifically bound probe, dried, exposed to photographic film (autoradiography), and the film developed to demonstrate the pattern of bands to which the probe adhered.

Southern blot analysis is used for multiple purposes, but most commonly for identification of gene amplifications, deletions, rearrangements, and abnormal restriction fragment length due to normally occurring polymorphisms, or restriction fragment length polymorphisms (RFLPs). Gene amplification is a common mechanism in the processes of transformation and genetic progression in neoplasia.

Southern blotting is also useful for analysis of DNA polymorphisms, which are genetic variations in DNA sequence that are usually unrelated to genes and alter either the length of a segment of DNA or a restriction endonuclease target site. One group of polymorphisms consist of short tandem repeats of nucleotides (STRs) or variable nucleotide tandem repeats (VNTRs), which are segments of DNA comprising short repeating sequences of DNA bases of unknown function; these are inherited DNA sequences that vary in length among individuals. In the analysis of tumors they have been used to identify the maternal or paternal source of reduplicated chromosomes, to recognize deletions of DNA, and to identify acquired defects of DNA mismatch repair (as in colon carcinoma). They can be visualized by Southern blot analysis or newer techniques as described below. RFLPs are likewise inherited from parents in a Mendelian fashion, and analyses of large numbers have been used to localize genetic mutations to specific chromosomal regions. RFLPs have been used as surrogate markers for the identification of neighboring defective genes, such as the neurofibromatosis genes; they can even be used before the defective genes themselves are cloned. A variation of restriction fragment length, or polymorphism, is manifested by a difference in the size of the reacting band on the Southern blot as compared to a standard length segment. This process of localizing genes based on their cosegregation with unrelated DNA markers is called linkage analysis.

Northern Blot

The northern blot (a play on words given the eponymic Southern blot for DNA analysis) is similar in many aspects to the Southern blot but uses RNA rather than DNA as its substrate (1,19,21,53). However, the northern blot procedure differs in several important aspects (5,39). RNA is more labile than DNA because of the ubiquity of RNases that degrade it, requiring care to avoid exposure of the sample to exogenous RNases and to inactivate endogenous RNases. The messenger RNA (mRNA) studied for diagnostic purposes is copied from DNA via transcription to pre-RNA and processed in the nucleus with excision of intronic sequences and addition of a polyadenine tail. mRNA is both the intermediary the cell uses to transfer the message to make a protein from nucleus to the cytoplasm and the template for making that protein sequence in ribosomes via translation. It is a relatively short single strand of nucleic acids, hundreds to thousands of bases in length. While DNA contains a large number of base sequences of unknown function unrelated to a coding gene sequence (on the order of 100:1), mRNA always contains as a major component the sequence of a gene encoding a protein. In addition it contains untranslated 5' and 3' regions that include elements that regulate the stability and the translation of the mRNA. Each mRNA species has a specific size that varies from one gene to the next and even within the same gene via alternative splicing and processing. To perform a northern blot analysis, mRNA is purified from a biologic sample, size-fractionated by electrophoresis in a gel, transferred to a nylon membrane, permanently affixed to the membrane by UV crosslinking, and visualized by probing with a labeled probe specific for the mRNA being studied. As with the Southern blot, sensitivity and specificity of the hybridization reaction are controlled by adjusting salt concentration, temperature, and the concentration of agents such as formamide, all of which alter the hydrogen bonding forces between two complementary or near-complementary strands of nucleic acids. After hybridization the membrane is dried, allowed to expose photographic film, and the film developed to demonstrate the electrophoretic size pattern of bands to which the probe adhered.

Northern blot analysis is primarily used to evaluate the level of expression of a particular gene in a tissue sample and the number and size of different (alternatively spliced) mRNA transcripts encoded by the given gene. It has been used to evaluate gene expression in both tumor and normal tissue, in tissue at varying stages of development (from embryologic to senescent), and in tissue from varying species. The northern blot has also been used for detection of specific chimeric gene products, e.g., mRNA from an abnormal gene formed by the fusion resulting from chromosomal translocation. The presence of chimeric genes may be suspected if the band labeling with a given probe indicates abnormal size, and it can confirmed by sequentially analyzing a northern blot by probes from each gene in question, observing whether a common band marks with both probes.

Western Blot

The western blot (a further play on words) consists of detection of a protein in tissue or fluid samples, after separation of the proteins by electrophoresis (50). To perform a western blot, proteins are extracted from a biologic sample, separated by electrophoresis in polyacrylamide, blotted to a nylon membrane, and then reacted with a specific antibody directed against the antigen in question (39). The presence of bound antibody is then detected by a radiolabeled or enzyme-labeled second antibody directed against the first, which is visualized by autoradiography or a colored reaction product. The sample to be studied can be tissue, serum or another body fluid, a cell suspension, or a tissue culture. The protein can be extracted by nonspecific methods or by specific procedures such as immunoprecipitation (IP). The latter technique may be followed by western blot analysis with another antibody in the so-called IP–western procedure.

Western blots are used to identify the presence of a protein in a biologic sample (1,21,53). The protein can be of any type for which an appropriate antibody is available, e.g., a normal product that is dysregulated in a given situation (over- or underexpressed), an abnormal chimeric protein created by a translocation, or a viral protein not present in uninfected individuals. The presence of a specific protein can be inferred by measuring the molecular weight of a band, as determined by comparing its migration pattern to that of a standard lane (Fig. 8). Western blots are also commonly used to confirm the specificity of immunologic reactions such as enzyme-linked immunosorbent assay (ELISA) tests or immunohistochemical stains. IP–western blot analysis can also be used to study the possible physical association of two proteins in biologic reactions.

Polymerase Chain Reaction

Polymerase chain reaction (PCR) is a technique that allows dramatic amplification of specific segments of

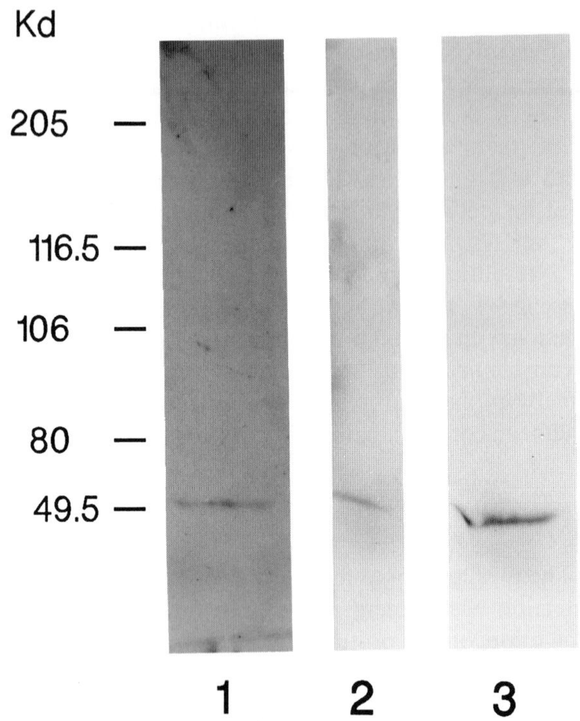

FIG. 8. Western blot of three tumor samples, testing for desmin. Lanes 1 and 2 are extracts of primary tumors and migrate similar to a rhabdomyosarcoma cell line extract in lane 3. The molecular weights are derived from a standard extract of purified substances with a known molecular weight. The distance traveled by all three bands corresponds to the molecular weight of desmin. (From Parham DM et al. Desmin positivity in primitive neuroectodermal tumors of childhood. *Am J Surg Pathol* 1992;16:483–492. Courtesy of Lippincott-Raven Publishers.)

DNA from minute amounts of starting material, providing at least some of the base sequence of the DNA region is known (38). Two critical elements are used in the procedure: template DNA for the reaction, and short (oligo-) nucleotide primers from each end of the specific segment of DNA to be amplified. Theoretically, only a single molecule of DNA is needed to serve as a template for the PCR reaction, and in practice a single drop of blood has sufficient nucleated cells to provide template DNA for multiple PCR reactions. Many other tissues have been used as starting material, including fresh and cryopreserved surgical specimens, buccal smears, and single hair follicles. The DNA sequence to be amplified in the reaction is determined by the choice of primers, which must be complementary to the 3' end of each chain of the DNA template (Fig. 9A); the region bracketed by the primers will be amplified if DNA from the appropriate region is present in the reaction mixture. For routine reactions the region to be amplified should be less than 1000 bases (1 kilobase or kb) in length; longer regions amplify poorly in the standard PCR reaction. In addition to template DNA and primers, the reaction requires buffer, nucleotide substrates, and the enzyme, DNA polymerase. DNA polymerase extends single-strand DNA from a double-stranded DNA nidus, adding complementary nucleotides in an upstream (5′) to downstream (3′) direction. To initiate PCR, a mixture of DNA, primers, substrates, and DNA polymerase is heated to 94°C to separate the double-strand DNA substrate into single strands. Next it is cooled to a predetermined temperature (usually around 50°C) to allow the primers to anneal to their targets, and finally heated to 72°C, the optimal temperature for the heat-resistant DNA polymerase used in the reaction (called *taq* polymerase). During this reaction both strands of the target serve as templates, resulting in doubling of the target sequence. This cycle is repeated 20–40 times in an automated thermal cycler, with a 10^3 increase of target for each 10 rounds of amplification (Fig. 9B). The amplified DNA can then be visualized by electrophoresis in agarose, with staining of the gel with a DNA-intercalating substance (ethidium bromide) that fluoresces under UV light (Fig. 9C). If the reaction is being used to detect a chimeric gene or a viral sequence (sequences not normally present), mere presence of an appropriately sized amplified product is sufficient for confirmation. A further degree of specificity can be obtained by Southern

FIG. 9. Polymerase chain reaction (PCR). **A.** Schematic outline of steps in a single cycle of PCR. From the top, the PCR reaction mixture (DNA, buffer, DNA nucleotide substrates, heat-resistant DNA polymerase [taq polymerase]) is heated to 94°C to denature double-stranded DNA to single strands, cooled to an appropriate temperature (usually 50–60°C) to allow primers to anneal to complementary single-strand DNA, and heated to 72°C to allow synthesis of new double-stranded DNA by DNA polymerase. This cycle is typically repeated 20–35 times. **B.** Schematic outline of 3 cycles of a PCR reaction. Each cycle of PCR leads to doubling of the amount of target DNA. Thus, 10 cycles of PCR theoretically result in an approximate 10^3-fold expansion of target DNA. **C.** Detection of PCR products. Analysis of PCR products typically consists of a single or two sequential procedures. First, reaction products are size-fractionated by electrophoresis in agarose gel and visualized by staining with the UV-fluorescent intercalating dye ethidium bromide. Second, for more specificity a Southern blot may be performed: the electrophoresed products are transferred to a nylon membrane, hybridized with a sequence-specific ^{32}P-labeled probe, and visualized by exposing X-ray film (autoradiogram). In the depicted gel and autoradiogram the negative control and pt.1 have no reaction product, while the positive control and pts.2 and 3 have reaction products of identical size; the top line in each lane is the application well in the gel, and the bottom line, where present, is the reaction product.

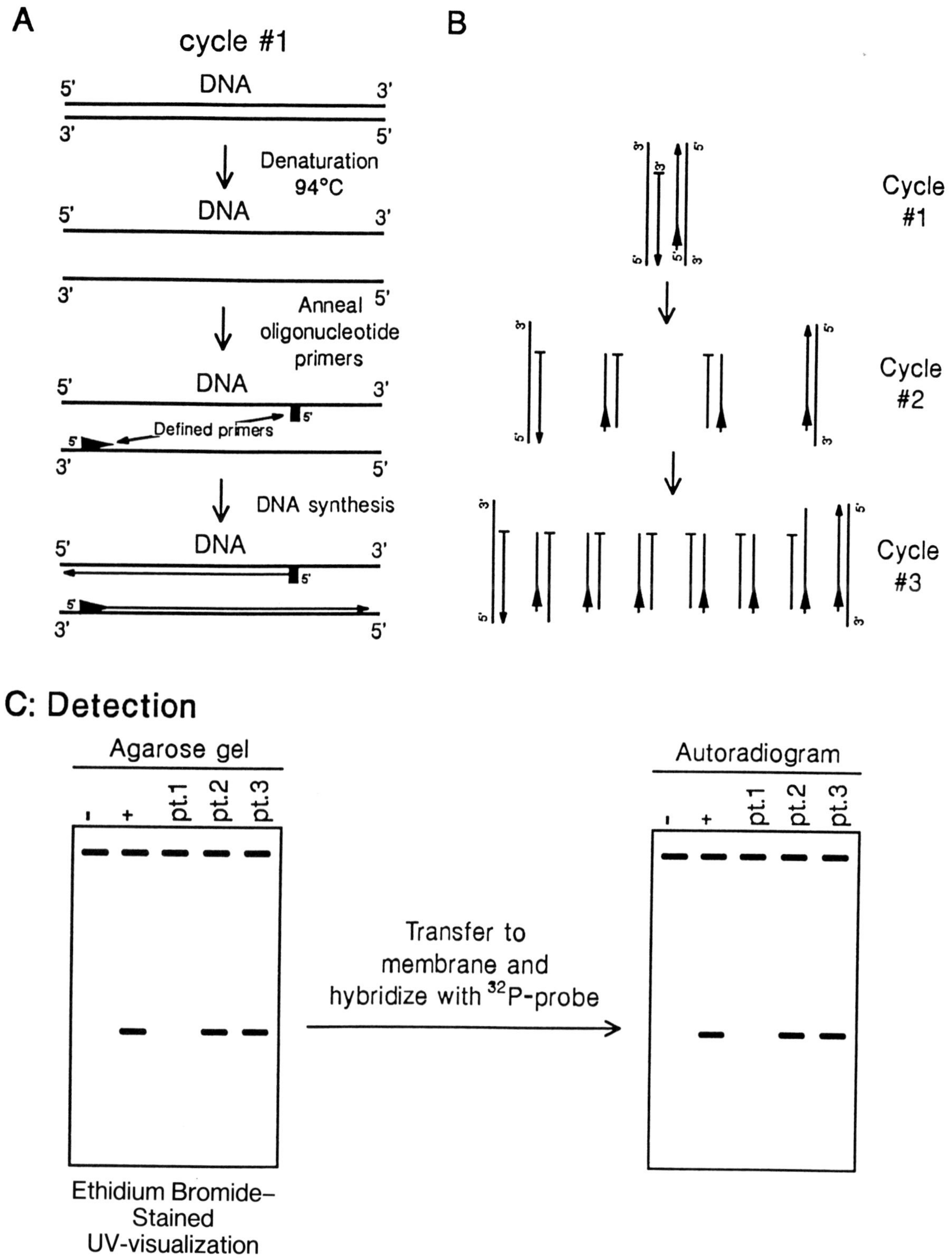
A
cycle #1
5' DNA 3'
3' 5'
Denaturation 94°C
5' DNA 3'
3' 5'
Anneal oligonucleotide primers
5' DNA 3'
Defined primers
3' 5'
DNA synthesis
5' DNA 3'
3' 5'
B
Cycle #1
Cycle #2
Cycle #3
C: Detection
Agarose gel
- + pt.1 pt.2 pt.3
Ethidium Bromide–Stained UV-visualization
Transfer to membrane and hybridize with 32P-probe
Autoradiogram
- + pt.1 pt.2 pt.3

blot hybridization of the product with a specific DNA probe, either blotting the electrophoretic gel or by direct blotting of the product to a membrane (slot blotting or dot blotting) (Fig. 9C). If mutations are suspected in the amplified DNA, the product can be analyzed by sequencing or by hybridization with oligonucleotide probes specific for the segment in question.

Applications of this technology are widespread. For example, DNA PCR can be used to amplify DNA for further analysis by another method, such as hybridization with a probe for a specific abnormality. Oncogenic activating point mutations of the signal transduction intermediary gene N-*ras* can be studied by PCR amplification of the gene, followed by blotting and hybridization with oligonucleotide probes specific for activating point mutations of the gene. The presence of hybridization indicates presence of the specific point mutation. PCR is used to demonstrate the presence of viral DNA sequence in a biologic specimen, although care is required in interpretation because the incredible amplification ability of the reaction imparts tremendous sensitivity. PCR is used to amplify HLA regions before hybridization analysis to determine whether molecular alleles are present in an individual. Because of its extreme sensitivity, the usefulness of PCR in studying tumors may be limited by contaminating normal tissue. This problem is obviated in cell lines, as there are no contaminating normal cells to confound analyses. For example, PCR amplification of marker segments of DNA located near two candidate tumor suppressor genes at 9p21, *P16/MTS1,* and *P15/MTS2,* was used to demonstrate deletion of both alleles of these genes in many tumor cell lines (15). Similar studies could not performed in tissue because of presence of normal connective tissue, blood vessels, and blood cells leads to normal results, even with malignancies shown by other methods to have biallelic deletion of this gene.

Reverse Transcriptase–PCR (RNA-Based PCR)

RNA-based PCR, or RT-PCR, is a very useful method for analyzing RNA in biologic specimens. To perform this reaction, RNA is converted to a double-stranded nucleic acid molecule using the retroviral enzyme, reverse transcriptase (RT), in a reaction buffer containing deoxynucleotides (5,39) (Fig. 9A). After completion of the RT reaction, routine PCR is performed (Fig. 9B, C). Uses of RT-PCR are several (1,21,53). It can be used to demonstrate inappropriate expression levels of a specific mRNA message or the expression of chimeric (or fusion) gene products resulting from chromosomal translocations. These are common in pediatric malignancies (6,17). The most reliable way to demonstrate gene fusion in a tumor is to detect the chimeric mRNA product of this gene by RT-PCR followed by electrophoresis or direct blotting to a nylon membrane and hybridization with an appropriately labeled probe.

In Situ Hybridization

In situ hybridization (ISH) refers to hybridization of a nucleic acid probe in an intact tissue section or cell preparation on a slide, rather than in a homogenized extracted specimen (39,53). The major benefit of this approach is that it allows visualization of the location of reaction positivity in individual cells in intact tissue. An appropriate probe must be selected to hybridize the nucleic acid sequence in question. In general, a large DNA probe is preferable to increase signal in the readout system. The reaction can be visualized using three different types of labels: a radioactive label that is developed by exposure to an overlaid photoactive gel; a fluorescent label that is interpreted with a fluorescent microscope (fluorescent ISH or FISH), and a histochemical label such as horseradish peroxidase or alkaline phosphatase that can be visualized by light microscopy. Since ISH allows visualization of genetic features in individual cells, it overcomes some limitations of DNA and RNA analysis in homogenates of patient samples. With modification ISH can be used to study either DNA or mRNA. It has been used to study the distribution pattern of mRNA expression by genes of unknown function in embryologic and adult tissues.

The most widespread uses to date of ISH, especially FISH, have been as a special stain for cytogenetics studies: to confirm ploidy for a given chromosome, to confirm the presence of a particular translocation by colocalization [or separation in different circumstances] of DNA sequences using two-color FISH, and to determine the chromosomal localization of newly isolated genes. Depending on probes used and purpose of study, the reaction may require metaphase nuclei with their condensed chromosomes. If probes are widely separated (millions of bases or megabases apart), condensed metaphase chromosomes may be necessary to demonstrate colocalization. If chromosomal localization of a gene is the issue, condensed and separated metaphase chromosomes will be required. Alternatively, some reactions can be interpreted in interphase nuclei, despite their markedly elongated chromosomes. Colocalization of closely linked probes separated by a megabase or less may be analyzed in interphase nuclei. Centromeric probes specific for a given chromosome can be interpreted in interphase nuclei by simply counting the number of fluorescing dots, corresponding to centromeres, in the nucleus with any given centromeric probe, with the normal complement for any centromere (except X or Y in a male) being 2 (see Chapter 4).

ADDITIONAL TECHNIQUES AND FUTURE DEVELOPMENTS

Dramatic advancements in the application of molecular biologic techniques to diagnostic pathology can be anticipated over the next several years. For example, from a technical standpoint we are already seeing the replacement of radioactive probes and gel-blot systems by semiautomated readout techniques and closed system approaches. Alternative labels have largely supplanted radionucleotides in ISH procedures. Multiplex RT-PCR systems currently under development will simplify screening tumor samples for the presence of multiple marker translocations. Automated systems for sequencing DNA are now available as a result of the human genome project. These systems greatly facilitate sequence analysis of new or abnormal genes.

The pace of identification of abnormal genes involved in both hereditary and acquired neoplasia has accelerated dramatically in the last several years, and as the genome project evolves it can be anticipated that the major genes involved in most hereditary and acquired diseases will be identified. Further study will be required to elaborate both normal function of these genes and exactly how they contribute to pathogenesis in disease states. This new information will undoubtedly create new diagnostic problems. For example, mutations of the tumor suppressor gene p53 have been implicated in the Li-Fraumeni syndrome of familial neoplasia (22). Mutations encompass many diverse areas of this large gene, creating a formidable problem in large-scale familial screening. Alternative techniques have been developed to address this problem. One is single-strand conformation polymorphism (SSCP). To perform SSCP, DNA from a target region is digested with a restriction endonuclease and then electrophoresed in a gel as single-rather than double-strand DNA under conditions that allow it to fold and partially hybridize with itself, thus altering its electrophoretic mobility. The majority of even single base substitutions alter mobility of the segment. Because many amino acid substitutions do not affect the function of a protein, in some instances it may be anticipated that functional assays of target proteins rather that genetic testing will be necessary for diagnosis.

Use of DNA markers such as with RFLP analysis will become obsolete as laboratories move to more direct analyses of defective genes and their protein products. Our knowledge of the molecular basis of the fundamental biologic properties of cells and their subversion in malignancy is progressing rapidly, revolutionizing our knowledge of both normal biology and disease states and leading to fundamental changes in treatment strategies for neoplasia. This progress will necessitate development of new diagnostic and monitoring strategies in the pathology laboratory, some of which are even now unanticipated. This is an exciting, revolutionary era in pathology, at which our predecessors would marvel with envy!

ACKNOWLEDGMENTS

Supported in part by Cancer Center Support CORE Grant P30 CA21765 and American Lebanese Syrian Associated Charities (ALSAC).

REFERENCES

1. Alberts B, Bray D, Lewis J, Raff M, Roberts K, Watson JD. *Molecular Biology of the Cell*. 2nd ed. New York: Garland; 1989.
2. Baak JP. Mitosis counting in tumors. *Hum Pathol* 1990;21:683–685.
3. Beard C, Nabers K, Bowling MC, Berard CW. Achieving technical excellence in lymph node specimens: an update. *Lab Med* 1985;16:468–475.
4. Brookes CN, Ooms BC, McGill F, England K, Hinchliffe SA, van Velzen D. Ploidy independence of Ag-NOR number in neuroblastoma. *Lab Invest* 1992;67:243–245.
5. Davis LG, Dibner MD, Battey JF. *Basic Methods in Molecular Biology*. New York: Elsevier; 1986.
6. Delattre O, Zucman J, Plougastel B, et al. Gene fusion with an ETS DNA-binding domain caused by chromosome translocation in human tumours. *Nature* 1992;359:162–165.
7. Dias P, Kumar P, Marsden HB, Kumar S. Induction of differentiation in human rhabdomyosarcoma. *Int J Oncol* 1992;1:243–251.
8. Egan M, Raafat F, Crocker J, Williams D. Prognostic importance of nucleolar organiser regions in Ewing's sarcoma of childhood (letter). *J Clin Pathol* 1988;41:232–236.
9. Erlandson RA. *Diagnostic Transmission Electron Microscopy of Tumors, with Clinicopathological, Immunohistochemical, and Cytogenetic Correlations*. New York: Raven Press; 1994.
10. Gamel JW, McLean IW, Greenberg RA, Zimmerman LE, Lichtenstein SJ. Computerized histologic assessment of malignant potential: a method for determining the prognosis of uveal melanomas. *Hum Pathol* 1982;13:893–897.
11. Gown AM, de Wever N, Battifora H. Microwave-based antigenic unmasking: a revolutionary new technique for routine immunohistochemistry. *App Immunohistochem* 1993;1:256–266.
12. Hayflick L, Moorhead PS. The serial cultivation of human diploid cell strains. *Exp Cell Res* 1961;25:585–621.
13. Hedley DW. DNA analysis from paraffin-embedded blocks. *Meth Cell Biol* 1990;33:139–147.
14. Houghton J, Houghton PJ. The suitability and use of human tumor xenografts. In: Kallman RF, ed. *Rodent Tumor Models in Experimental Cancer Therapy*, Oxford: Pergamon Press; 1987:199–204.
15. Kamb A, Gruis NA, Weaver-Feldhaus J, et al. A cell cycle regulator potentially involved in genesis of many tumor types. *Science* 1994;264:436–440.
16. Katz RL, Wojcik EM, El-Naggar AK, Ordonez NG, Johnston DA. Proliferation markers in non-Hodgkin's lymphoma: a comparative study between cytophotometric quantitation of Ki-67 and flow cytometric proliferation index on fine needle aspirates. *Anal Quant Cytol Histol* 1993;15:179–186.
17. Kawasaki ES, Clark SS, Coyne MY, Smith SD, Champlin R, Witte ON, McCormick FP. Diagnosis of chronic myeloid and acute lymphocytic leukemias by detection of leukemia-specific mRNA sequences amplified in vitro. *Proc Natl Acad Sci USA* 1988;85:5698–5702.
18. Knudson AG, Jr., Strong LC. Mutation and cancer: a model for Wilms' tumor of the kidney. *JNCI* 1972;48:313–324.
19. Lehrach H, Diamond D, Wozney JM, Boedtker H. RNA molecular weight determinations by gel electrophoresis under denaturing conditions, a critical reexamination. *Biochemistry* 1977;16:4743–4751.

20. Leung SW, Bedard YC. Simple miniblock technique for cytology. *Mod Pathol* 1993;6:630–632.
21. Lewin B. *Genes*. vol 4. New York: Oxford University Press; 1990.
22. Malkin D, Jolly KW, Barbier N, et al. Germline mutations of the p53 tumor-suppressor gene in children and young adults with second malignant neoplasms. *N Engl J Med* 1992;326:1309–1315.
23. Marchevsky AM, Gil J, Jeanty H. Computerized interactive morphometry in pathology: current instrumentation and methods. *Hum Pathol* 1987;18:320–331.
24. Martin H, Hufnagl P, Beil M, Wenzelides K, Gottschalk J, Rahn W. Nucleolar organizer region-associated proteins in cancer cells: quantitative investigations on gliomas, meningiomas, urinary bladder carcinomas and pleural lesions. *Anal Quant Cytol Histol* 1992;14:312–319.
25. McGahey BE, Moriarty AT, Nelson WA, Hull MT. Fine-needle aspiration biopsy of small round blue cell tumors of childhood. *Cancer* 1992;69:1067–1073.
26. Mount SL, Taatjes DJ, Von Turkovich M, Tindle BH, Trainer TD. Diagnostic immunoelectron microscopy in surgical pathology: assessment of various tissue fixation and processing protocols. *Ultrastruct Pathol* 1993;17:547 556.
27. Mourad WA, Lavallee-Grey M, Pappenhausen P, Essig YP, Rowlands DT, Jr. Argyrophilic nucleolar organizer regions in Wilms' tumors and related lesions: a histologic and chromosomal correlation. *Mod Pathol* 1991;4:247–252.
28. Ooms ECM, Kurver PHJ, Veldhuizen RW, Alons CL, Boon ME. Morphometric grading of bladder tumors in comparison with histologic grading by pathologists. *Hum Pathol* 1983;14:144–150.
29. Parham DM, Webber B, Holt H, Williams WK, Maurer HM. Immunohistochemical study of childhood rhabdomyosarcomas and related neoplasms: results of an Intergroup Rhabdomyosarcoma Study project. *Cancer* 1991;67:3072–3080.
30. Parham DM, Weeks DA, Beckwith JB. The clinicopathologic spectrum of putative extrarenal rhabdoid tumors: an analysis of 42 cases studies with immunohistochemistry and/or electron microscopy. *Am J Surg Pathol* 1994;18:1010–1029.
31. Parham DM. Small round cell tumors of childhood: importance of cytogenetics in prognosis and diagnosis. *Adv Pathol Lab Med* 1995;8:223–245.
32. Puchtler H, Meloan SN. On the chemistry of formaldehyde fixation and its effects on immunohistochemical reactions. *Histochemistry* 1985;82:201–204.
33. Report of the Standing Committee on Human Cytogenetic Nomenclature. An international system for human cytogenetic nomenclature. *Cytogenet Cell Genet* 1978;21:309–404.
34. Romppanen T. Practical approach to a morphometrical study. In: Collan Y and Romppanen T, eds. *Morphometry in Morphological Diagnosis*. Kuopio, Finland: Kuopio University Press; 1982:47–63.
35. Rousseau-Merck MF, Bigel P, Mouly H, Flamant F, Zucker JM, Wache AC, Nezelof C. Transplantability in nude mice of embryonic and other childhood tumours. *Br J Cancer* 1985;52:279–283.
36. Ruschoff J, Plate K, Bittinger A, Thomas C. Nucleolar organizer regions (NORs). Basic concepts and practical application in tumor pathology. *Pathol Res Pract* 1989;185:878–885.
37. Sadoff DA, Giddens WE, Jr., DiGiacomo RF, Vogel AM. Neoplasms in NIH type II athymic (nude) mice. *Lab Anim Sci* 1988;38:407–412.
38. Saiki RK, Gelfand DH, Stoffel S, et al. Primer-directed enzymatic amplification of DNA with a thermostable DNA polymerase. *Science* 1988;239:487–491.
39. Sambrook J, Fritsch EF, Maniatis T. *Molecular Cloning: A Laboratory Manual*. Cold Spring Harbor, NY: Cold Spring Harbor Laboratory Press; 1989.
40. Sandberg AA. Cancer cytogenetics for clinicians. *CA* 1994;44: 136–159.
41. Schmidt K, Pesce C. Quantitative methods in pediatric pathology. An overview with special consideration of developmental renal abnormalities. *Perspect Pediatr Pathol* 1992;16:134–159.
42. Schneider NR. Cytogenetic evaluation of childhood neoplasms. *Arch Pathol Lab Med* 1993;117:1220–1224.
43. Shapiro HM. *Practical Flow Cytometry*. 3rd ed. New York: Wiley-Liss; 1995.
44. Silverman JF, Gurley AM, Holbrook CT, Joshi VV. Pediatric fine-needle aspiration biopsy. *Am J Clin Pathol* 1991;95:653–659.
45. Southern EM. Detection of specific sequences among DNA fragments separated by gel electrophoresis. *J Mol Biol* 1975;98:503–517.
46. Stevens MW, Crowley KS, Fazzalari NL, Woods AE. Use of morphometry in cytological preparations for diagnosing follicular non-Hodgkin's lymphomas. *J Clin Pathol* 1988;41:370–377.
47. Taylor CR. *Immunomicroscopy: A Diagnostic Tool for the Surgical Pathologist*. Philadelphia: WB Saunders; 1986.
48. Taylor CR. An exaltation of experts: concerted efforts in the standardization of immunohistochemistry. *Hum Pathol* 1994;25:2–11.
49. Taylor SR, Nunez C. Fine-needle aspiration biopsy in a pediatric population. Report of 64 consecutive cases. *Cancer* 1984;54:1449–1453.
50. Towbin H, Staehelin T, Gordon J. Electrophoretic transfer of proteins from polyacrylamide gels to nitrocellulose sheets: procedure and some applications. *Proc Natl Acad Sci USA* 1976;76:4350–4354.
51. Vielh P, Howell LP. *Guides to Clinical Aspiration Biopsy: Pediatrics*. New York: Igaku-Shoin; 1993.
52. Wakely PE, Jr., Powers CN, Frable WJ. Metachronous soft-tissue masses in children and young adults with cancer: correlation of histology and aspiration cytology. *Hum Pathol* 1990;21:669–677.
53. Watson JD, Gilman M, Witkowski J, Zoller M. *Recombinant DNA*. New York: Scientific American Books; 1992.
54. Weinberg RA. Oncogenes and tumor suppressor genes. *CA* 1994;44:160–170.
55. Wells WA, Rainer RO, Memoli VA. Basic principles of image processing. *Am J Clin Pathol* 1992;98:493–501.
56. Whang-Peng J, Triche TJ, Knutsen T, Miser J, Kao-Shan S, Tsai S, Israel MA. Cytogenetic characterization of selected small round cell tumors of childhood. *Cancer Genet Cytogenet* 1986;21:185–208.
57. Wick MR, Siegal GP. *Monoclonal Antibodies in Diagnostic Immunohistochemistry*. New York: Marcel Dekker; 1988.
58. Zucker JM. The clinician's view. In: Vielh P, Howell LP, eds. *Pediatrics*. New York: Igaku-Shoin; 1995:229–236.

Pediatric Neoplasia: Morphology and Biology, edited by David M. Parham.
Lippincott-Raven Publishers, Philadelphia © 1996.

CHAPTER 3

Renal Neoplasms

David M. Parham

INTRODUCTION

Pediatric renal tumors constitute a diverse group of neoplasms (Table 1) with a wide range of appearances and clinical behaviors (68). By far the most common is Wilms' tumor, or nephroblastoma. The history of these lesions is one of the modern-day success stories in medicine. At the turn of the 19th century, the death rate of affected patients was over 90%. Thanks to improvements in surgery, chemotherapy, and radiotherapy, there is now an overall 4-year survival rate of 89% (41). Similarly, understanding of the pathology of nephroblastoma has improved considerably since publication of Max Wilms's scholarly monograph in 1899 (242). In the latter half of the 20th century, study of childhood renal neoplasms has resulted in a new histopathologic classification (13), discovery of relatively benign lesions (19), and the identification of genetic factors involved in tumorigenesis (36,88,219). Also newly described is the malignant rhabdoid tumor, for which remission is so unusual that it merits a case report (181). Discovery of novel pathologic entities and genetic factors continues unabated.

WILMS' TUMOR (NEPHROBLASTOMA)

Clinical Features

Wilms' tumors are relatively common neoplasms, composing 6.3% of pediatric cancers in the National Cancer Institute's Surveillance, Epidemiology, and End Results (SEER) program (134). As a result, renal neoplasms constitute an extremely important childhood tumor category and are sixth in frequency among pediatric cancers, respectively following leukemia, brain tumors, lymphomas, neuroblastic tumors, and soft tissue sarcomas (134). It is thus fortunate that we have attained the current high rate of success that we enjoy in treating these lesions, although the degree of this success is still dependent on stage and histologic grade (41).

Wilms' tumors are predominately lesions of young children; the vast majority are diagnosed before the age of 6 (142). Nevertheless, they are uncommon in neonates, who are more likely to have the most benign renal neoplasm, mesoblastic nephroma, or the most malignant one, rhabdoid tumor (124). Wilms' tumors are often first noted by attentive parents when bathing their child or by observant pediatricians during a routine physical examination. Hypertension is also a common clinical sign of this disease. Alternatively, intratumoral or peritumoral hemorrhage, often following blunt abdominal trauma, may lead to hematuria or the abrupt onset of abdominal pain. The finding of a renal mass is then confirmed by ultrasonography and computed tomography, which may also reveal tumor invasion into the renal vein (Fig. 1). Peripheral blood smears infrequently contain a characteristic precipitate resulting from circulating mucin (169), but this is an exceptionally rare phenomenon in the author's experience.

At surgery, the primary focus is to extirpate the affected kidney without rupturing the tumor or leaving behind residual gross disease. Because these lesions are soft and bulky, this task can be an onerous one, and if peritoneal spillage occurs, the patient will receive abdominal irradiation for high-stage (stage III) disease (41). Postirradiation complications include scoliosis, small bowel obstruction, and second malignancies (38,146). On the other hand, limited spillage does not affect survival (25), and tumor invading the renal vein and inferior vena cava may be excised, giving the patient an excellent outcome (25,146,178). Similarly, invasion of the liver is not necessarily cause for upstaging from stage II to stage

D. M. Parham: Department of Pathology, Arkansas Children's Hospital, Little Rock, Arkansas 72202.

TABLE 1. *Types of renal neoplasms occurring in the pediatric age group*

Wilms' tumor
Favorable histology
Anaplastic
Cystic
Rhabdomyomatous
Teratoid
Clear cell sarcoma of kidney
Congenital mesoblastic nephroma
Typical
Cellular
Malignant rhabdoid tumor
Renal cell carcinoma
Primitive neural tumors
Peripheral neuroepithelioma
Neuroblastoma
Neuroendocrine carcinoma
Juxtaglomerular cell tumor
Miscellaneous sarcomas and other soft tissue lesions
Hemangioma
Hematopoietic neoplasms
Renal medullary carcinoma
Nephrogenic adenofibroma

III (211). Besides the factors listed in the National Wilms' Tumor Study (NWTS) V Staging system (Table 2), age at diagnosis and weight of the excised specimen appear to independently affect clinical outcome, and the presence of microscopic disease at the margin of resection is predictive of aggressive tumor behavior in regional disease (25).

One therapy-related issue that affects surgical pathologists is whether to give preoperative chemotherapy, for this implies that histologic diagnosis will be made on the basis of a small-needle biopsy. Preoperative therapy is an attractive option because it appears to limit the incidence of intraoperative tumor rupture (74). On the other hand, it limits the amount of material available for diagnosis, so that questions have been raised regarding the adequacy of tumor grading following this procedure. Typically, there is severe modification of histology in treated Wilms' tumors (5,247). However, anaplasia is generally preserved (247). Because of the potential for tumor spread into the needle tract, preoperative biopsy was even omitted with a limited number of patients entering a Societé Internationale d'Oncologie Pediatrique (SIOP) trial (244), but this strategy incurred serious management problems.

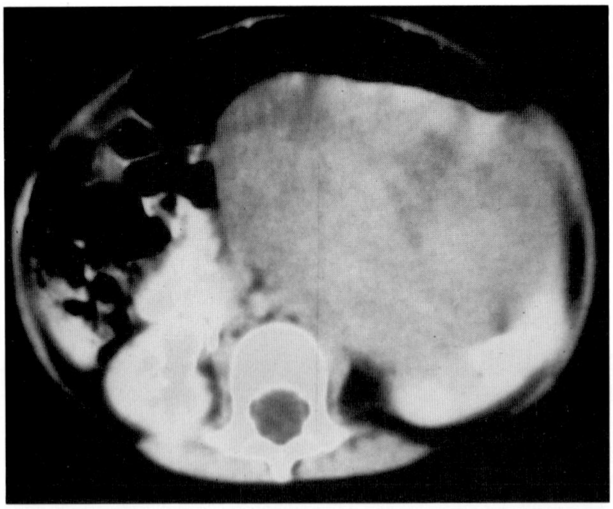

FIG. 1. Computed tomographic scan of abdomen in child with Wilms' tumor of left kidney. A large mass bulges from the kidney, fills the left abdomen, and crosses the midline. (Courtesy of Dr. Barry Fletcher, St. Jude Children's Research Hospital.)

TABLE 2. *NWTS V Clinicopathologic Staging System (74)*

Stage I
Tumor limited to kidney and completely excised. The surface of the renal capsule is intact.
Tumor was not ruptured before or during removal. There is no residual tumor apparent beyond the margins of resection.
Stage II
Tumor extends beyond the kidney but is completely removed. There is regional extension of the tumor, ie, penetration through the outer surface of the renal capsule into the perirenal soft tissues. Vessels outside the kidney substance are infiltrated or contain tumor thrombus. The tumor may have been biopsied or there has been local spillage of tumor confined to the flank. There is no residual tumor apparent or beyond the margins of excision.
Stage III
Residual nonhematogenous tumor confined to the abdomen. (1) Lymph nodes on biopsy are found to be involved in the hilus, the periaortic chains, or beyond. (2) There has been diffuse peritoneal contamination by tumor, such as spillage of tumor beyond the flank before or during surgery or by tumor growth that has penetrated through the peritoneal surface. (3) Implants are found on the peritoneal surface. (4) The tumor extends beyond the surgical margins either microscopically or grossly. (5) The tumor is not completely resectable because of local infiltration into vital structures.
Stage IV
Hematogenous metastases. Deposits beyond stage III, eg, lung, liver, bone, and/or brain.
Stage V
Bilateral renal involvement at diagnosis. An attempt should be made to stage each side according to the above criteria on the basis of the extent of disease before biopsy.

A number of epidemiologic studies have been performed to investigate the potential role of maternal and paternal factors in Wilms' tumorigenesis. Although a variety of maternal factors, such as consumption of cigarettes, coffee, tea, or oral contraceptives, have been speculated to cause a higher risk of Wilms' tumors, there was no verification of these hypotheses in a recent NWTS study (154). On the other hand, paternal occupation, particularly as a vehicle mechanic, auto body repairman, or welder, does increase the odds of occurrence of Wilms' tumor (153). These data are particularly provocative in light of the recent discovery of a parental imprinting mechanism in Wilms' tumor genetics (see below).

Gross Appearance

Grossly, Wilms' tumors are typically large bulging masses that markedly distort the renal contours. When the kidney is bivalved, the cut surface characteristically everts in an explosive fashion, necessitating care in sectioning to preserve the relation of the tumor to the renal capsule. There is often great heterogeneity in the cut surface of these lesions caused by alternating areas of viable tumor, hemorrhage, and necrosis (Fig. 2). Viable tumor tissue is opaque pale gray to yellow–gray with a soft, spongy consistency. Usually, the borders of Wilms' tumor are well defined, often by a fibrous pseudocapsule, in contrast to the infiltrating margins of mesoblastic nephroma. However, this is a deceptive feature because microscopic invasion of the adjacent kidney is common, particularly in higher stage lesions (227).

Determination of tumor stage and the corresponding therapy are intimately related to pathologic findings. As a result, Wilms' tumors present a critical challenge to the dissector, necessitating thoughtful, painstaking execution and deft specimen manipulation. A common problem is the artifactual presence of microscopic tumor fragments on the surface of the specimen or in vascular margins due to the mucinous consistency of these gelatinous, slimy tumors. It is thus important to section hilar margins before incising the tumor. A related problem is the tendency of the vessels to retract following their surgical division, misleading the pathologist into a false impression of marginal invasion (142).

Beckwith has devised a standard method of Wilms' tumor dissection (10). One particularly critical step is the inking of the external margins. To avoid artifactual leakage of tumor and contamination of the margins, Beckwith recommends fixation during overnight refrigeration prior to detailed dissection. Other important points are to *never* strip the renal capsule and to liberally sample the interface of the tumor with adjacent kidney and pseudocapsule.

One evolving issue in the staging of Wilms' tumors is the role of hilar invasion. Because the renal hilus is not normally encapsulated, hilar invasion has not been sufficient grounds for a stage II designation per se. However, extensive hilar invasion is associated with aggressive tumor behavior, and previous NTWS staging has been based on extension of tumor past the hilar plane, an anatomic landmark formed by the two medialmost

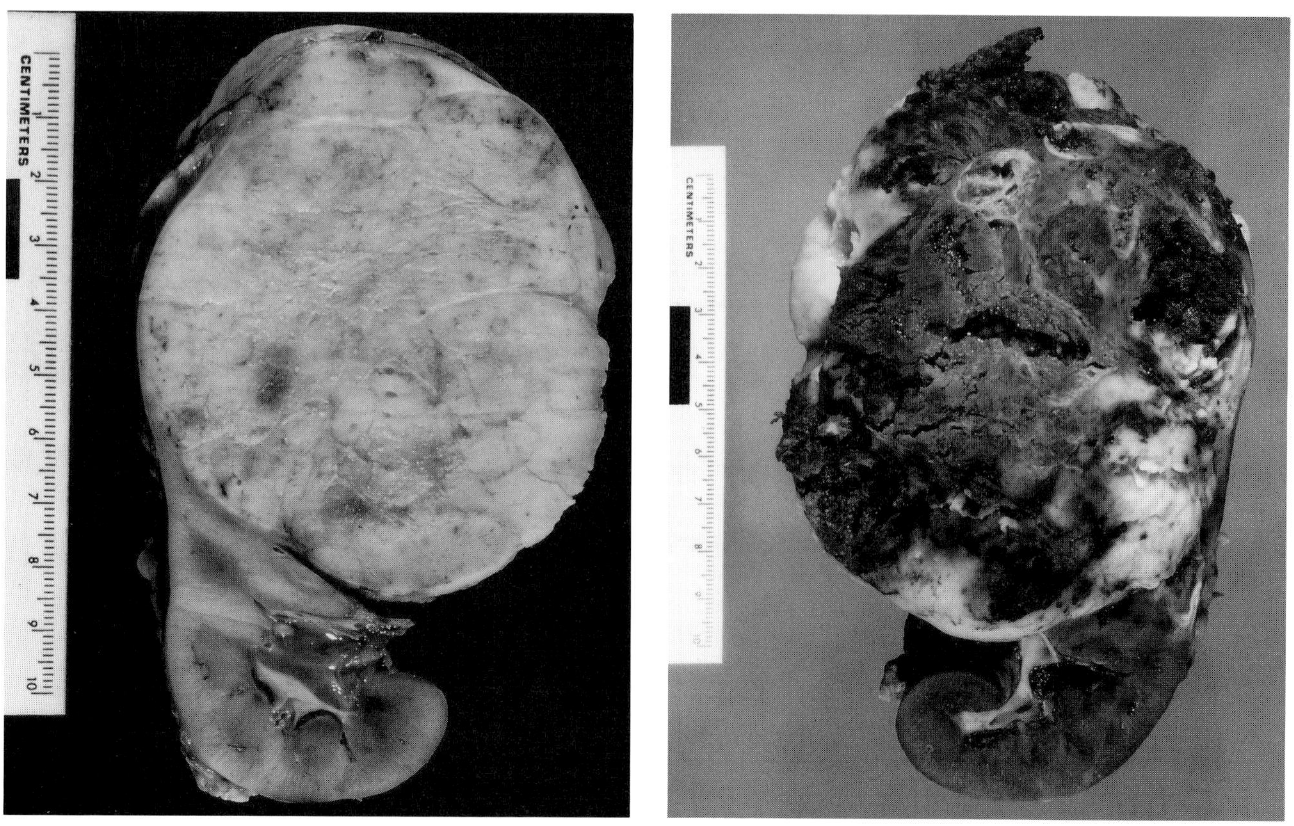

A B

FIG. 2. A. Gross photograph of bisected kidney with large, relatively homogeneous Wilms' tumor. **B.** Gross photograph of Wilms' tumor with extensive hemorrhage and necrosis.

limits of the bean-shaped kidney (228). Recent experience indicates that this landmark is difficult to assess in practice because of the anatomic distortion wrought by bulging tumors. Therefore, in the newest staging system (74) (Table 2), vascular invasion outside of the kidney substance is considered grounds for a stage II designation.

Another consideration in gross dissection is the adequacy of sampling to determine the presence of nephrogenic rests. Often these persistent embryonic foci are present adjacent to the tumor; hence, the emphasis on sectioning the tumor–kidney interface. Another frequent location in the subcapsular region. The strong possibility of finding these lesions necessitates careful sectioning of the normal-appearing kidney and sampling of any unusual or nodular foci. Even if nothing of note is found grossly, it is still helpful to submit several sections of uninvolved renal parenchyme because nephroblastomatosis may be microscopic and glomerulopathy also may be present on occasion.

Microscopic Appearance

Microscopically, Wilms' tumors are composed of three basic elements: blastema, stroma, and epithelium. The appearances produced by the mixture of these components tends to be so pronounced from case to case that, like snowflakes, no two Wilms' tumors are identical. The histologic features of Wilms' tumor closely recapitulates that of the developing kidney, which arises as a result of the interaction between the protruding ureteric bud and the abutting mesodermal blastema (Fig. 3). This inductive process proceeds through a series of well-characterized morphogenetic episodes to result in formation of the definitive nephron. These normal embryonic events are mimicked by Wilms' tumors to a remarkable degree, as described by Mierau et al. (133) in an excellent review. The resultant heterogeneity among these neoplasms derives from the wide variation in the stage, type, and degree of differentiation shown by their cellular constituents.

The blastemal elements of Wilms' tumors consist of undifferentiated small round cells that are analogous to the primitive mesenchyme forming the metanephric blastema of the developing embryo (Fig. 4A). From this primordium arises the epithelial elements of the tumor, predominantly in the form of abortive tubules (Fig. 4B). Glomerular structures are also commonly seen (Fig. 4C). The stromal element usually consists of a scaffolding of bland fibrous or myxoid tissue. Any of the three elements may be dominant in any given tumor. There is often a marked resemblance to fetal kidney (Fig. 5).

Poorly differentiated or blastemal-predominant Wilms' tumors (114) have been associated with poor prognosis in the older literature, but this factor showed no independent effect on outcome in the NWTS I–III studies (13,228). Blastemal-predominant tumors do tend to be higher stage lesions (227), thus possibly explaining the discrepant reports of the significance of this finding. Conversely, the predominance of epithelial differentiation in a Wilms' tumor has been associated with good prognosis (114), although again this feature loses its significance in multivariant analysis because of its association with low-stage tumors (227). Epithelial predominance tends to be more common in younger children (31,114). In one study (116), the diversity of epithelial differentiation was of more prognostic import than the abundance of epithelium.

Heterologous elements such as smooth muscle, striated muscle, adipose tissue, cartilage, bone, or even neu-

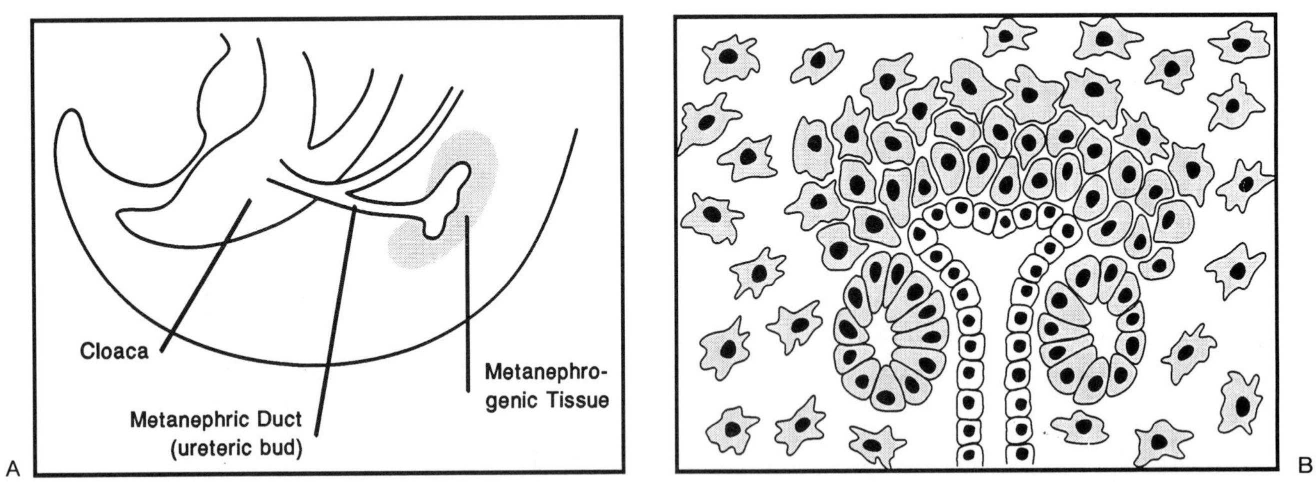

FIG. 3. A. Schematic diagram of nephrogenesis. The metanephric bud, which becomes the definitive ureter, arises from the mesonephros and extends into somatic mesoderm forming the metanephric blastema (*shaded area*). **B.** The cells lining the metanephric bud (*unshaded*) induce condensation of the metanephric blastema cells (*shaded*), with formation of primitive tubules.

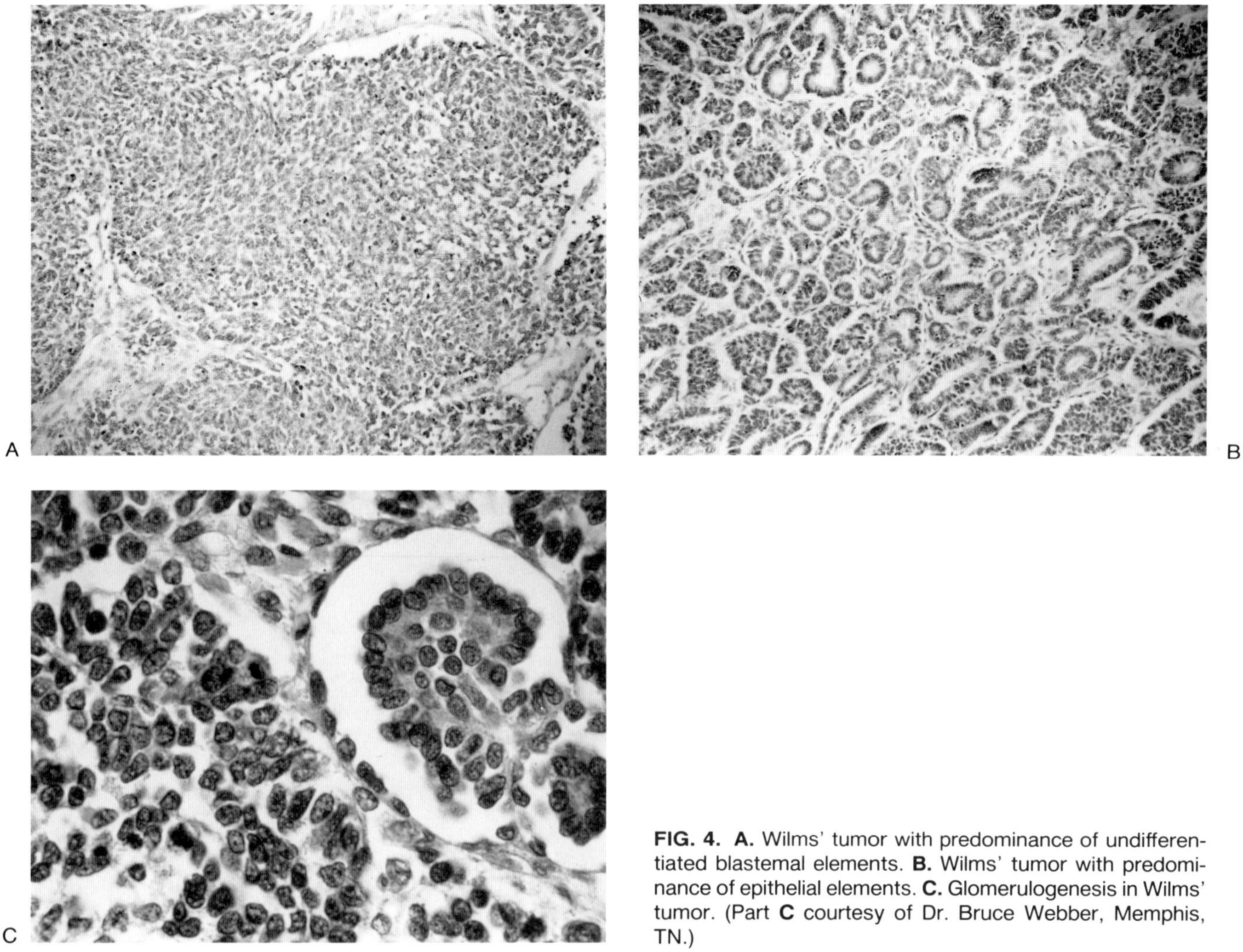

FIG. 4. **A.** Wilms' tumor with predominance of undifferentiated blastemal elements. **B.** Wilms' tumor with predominance of epithelial elements. **C.** Glomerulogenesis in Wilms' tumor. (Part **C** courtesy of Dr. Bruce Webber, Memphis, TN.)

roglial tissue are not unusual components of Wilms' tumors (Fig. 6). They may even predominate in a confusing array in lesions termed "teratoid" Wilms' tumors (56,220). The common occurrence of mesenchymal tissues such as muscle or bone in these tumors is a probable consequence of the mesodermal origin of the metanephrogenic blastema. However, the occasional presence of glial or neural tissues in Wilms' tumors (108) does not fit neatly into this supposition. Masson hypothesized that Wilms' tumors arose from neuroectoderm, and the persistent reports of neuroectodermally derived tissues in them provide continuous fuel for this argument. Others argue that these neoplasms are true "teratomas" not related to Wilms' tumors (56), and indeed it is difficult to draw a line of distinction in some cases. In fact, Wilms' tumorlike elements have been described in teratomatous lesions arising in extrarenal locations (37). Perhaps the most practical rule is to label teratomatous lesions of the kidney as teratoid Wilms' tumors only if they contain indisputable nephrogenic or blastemal elements.

One variant of the teratoid Wilms' tumor is the fetal rhabdomyomatous nephroblastoma, originally described by Wigger in 1976 (239). These tumors are distinguished by their large content of skeletal muscle, which has been described as composing at least 30% (71) and up to 99% (239) of the neoplasm (Fig. 6B). In some cases the amount of nephrogenic tissue is so miniscule that these tumors have been reported as "rhabdomyomas" (239). A perhaps related tumor is the "rhabdomyosarcoma" of the kidney (166), which contains primitive muscle more akin to that seen in the analogous soft tissue neoplasm. A close histogenetic relationship of embryonal rhabdomyosarcoma and Wilms' tumor may be inferred by their common genetic aberrations, so that the distinction may be more academic than biologic. To support this hypothesis, occasional reports of coexisting Wilms' tumors and vaginal rhabdomyosarcoma have appeared (144). Besides its striking abundance of skeletal muscle, fetal rhabdomyomatous nephroblastoma is a distinctive by virtue of its relatively benign behavior and tendency to occur bilaterally (239). In the author's expe-

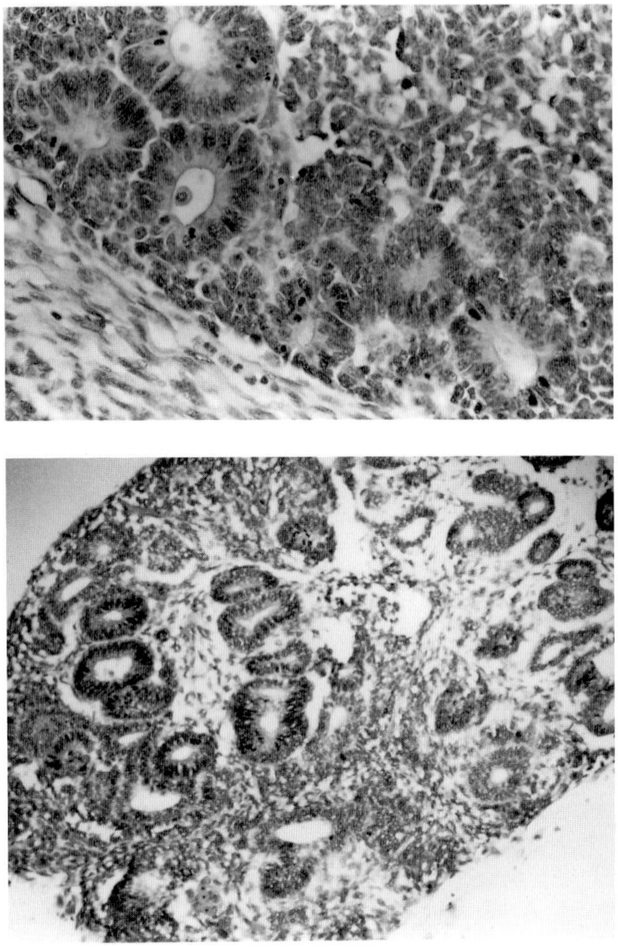

A

B

FIG. 5. There is often a marked similarity between Wilms' tumors (**A**) and fetal kidney (**B**).

rience, these tumors often contain other heterologous elements, such as cartilage or bone, so that their origin appears related to that of teratoid Wilms' tumor. Another recurring facet is the tendency of the myomatous elements to involve the medulla, usually with botryoid protrusion into the renal pelvis (121) (Fig. 7).

Classification of Wilms' Tumors

In their now classic histopathologic review of tumors accrued through the NTWS, Beckwith and Palmer separated Wilms' tumors into favorable and unfavorable subtypes (13). The favorable subtype consisted of the usual triphasic tumor as described above. The unfavorable subtypes were further subdivided into anaplastic Wilms' tumors and sarcomatous Wilms' tumors. The sarcomatous tumors, the clear cell sarcoma of the kidney and the malignant rhabdoid tumor, are now recognized as neoplasms distinct from Wilms' tumors and will be described separately.

The anaplastic subtype of Wilms' tumor is characterized by cells that are at least three times larger than adjacent cells of similar type and possess hyperchromatic nuclei. Enlarged, bizarre, multipolar mitotic figures (Fig. 8) are also essential to the diagnosis. These nuclear and mitotic irregularities correspond to hyperdiploidy and complex chromosomal rearrangements (Fig. 9) (49,77,194). Anaplasia may be focal or diffuse, so that adequate sampling of the tumor, generally one section per centimeter, is essential to confirm its absence, and a prolonged search may be necessary to find the required cells. Tumors are defined as having focal anaplasia if 10% or less of sections contain anaplastic cells and diffuse if greater than 10% contain anaplasia. A review of almost 1,200 patients entered on the first and second National Wilms' Study revealed that children with anaplastic tumors tended to be nonwhite, 1–2 years older at diagnosis than those with favorable histology, and have nodal metastases at diagnosis and decreased survival. However, modern chemotherapy appears to be improving the outlook in these patients (21). In a review of 58 unilateral anaplastic Wilms' tumors entered on NTWS-3, Zuppan and colleagues

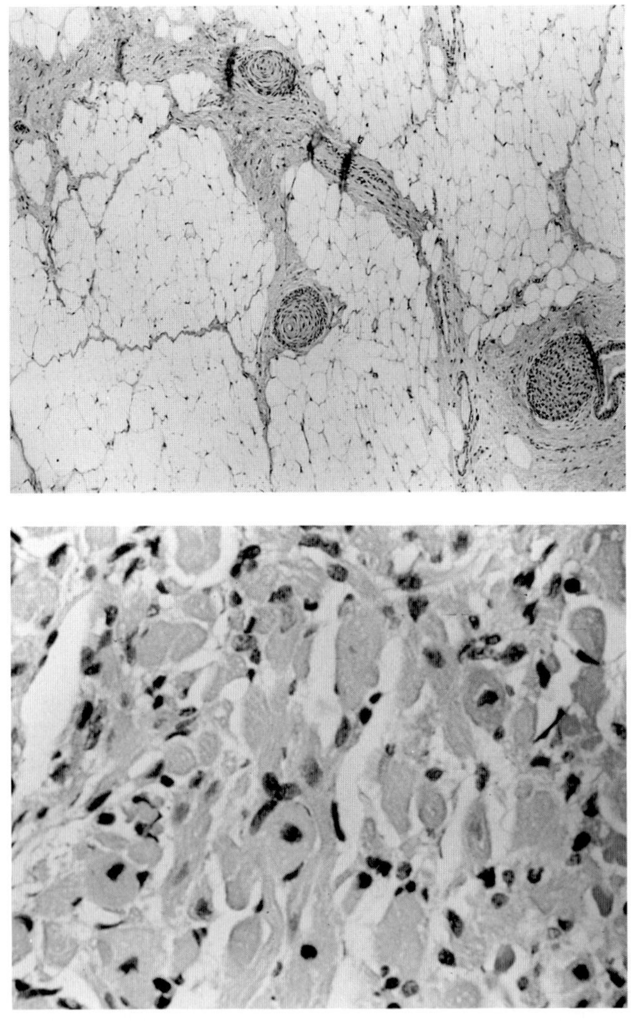

A

B

FIG. 6. Wilms' tumors may contain an abundance of heterologous elements such as squamous epithelium, fat (**A**), and skeletal muscle (**B**).

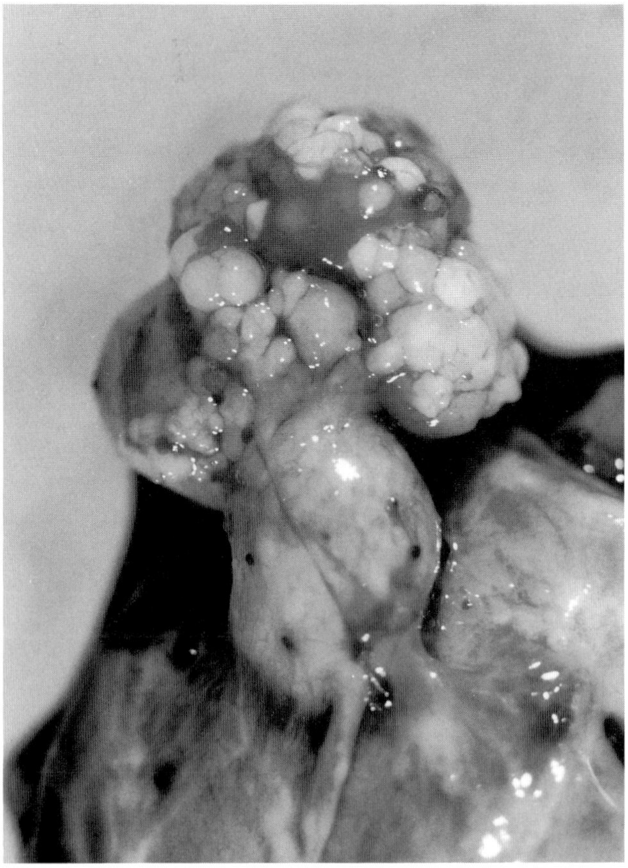

FIG. 7. Gross photograph of botryoid excrescence arising from the pelvic portion of a teratoid Wilms' tumor.

found that stage I tumors had a favorable outcome in spite of anaplasia. However, anaplasia associated with extrarenal occurrence or with predominantly blastemal tumors had a poor outcome (246).

Electron Microscopy and Immunohistochemistry

Diagnosis of Wilms' tumors is not difficult if one has abundant tissue, a renal primary, and obvious nephrogenesis. However, problems can arise with blastemal-predominant lesions, particularly on small percutaneous needle biopsies where the differential diagnosis may include the full spectrum of small round cell tumors of childhood. In these lesions, the primary diagnostic clue is given by the arrangement of the primitive tissues, which are often ordered into serpentine cords surrounded by a loose fibromyxoid stroma (142). Vague hints of epithelial differentiation, sometimes with rosette formation, may be present, particularly at the blastema–stroma interface. However, with fine needle aspirates undifferentiated blastemal cells may predominate and epithelial elements may be sparse or absent (172).

In these situations, one often resorts to immunohistochemistry and electron microscopy for additional hints at histogenesis. In this setting immunohistochemistry is often not helpful, as the blastemal tissues may be so primitive that even low molecular keratins are negative (3,4,48). Staining for WT1 protein may be of use in the future (141), but currently cytokeratin is the only widely available marker for Wilms' tumors. PAL-E, an endothelial marker (191), and desmoplakin, a desmosomal

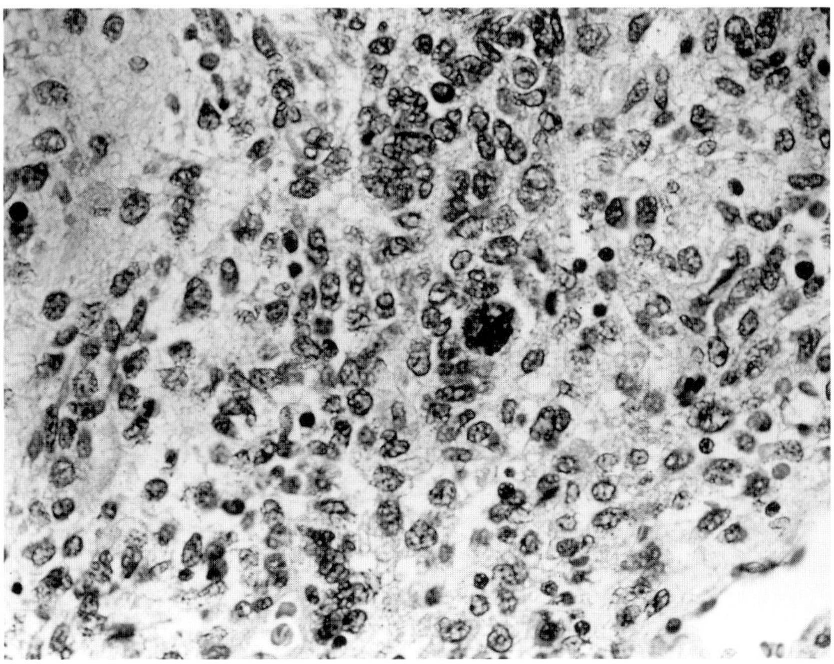

FIG. 8. Multipolar mitosis in anaplastic Wilms' tumor.

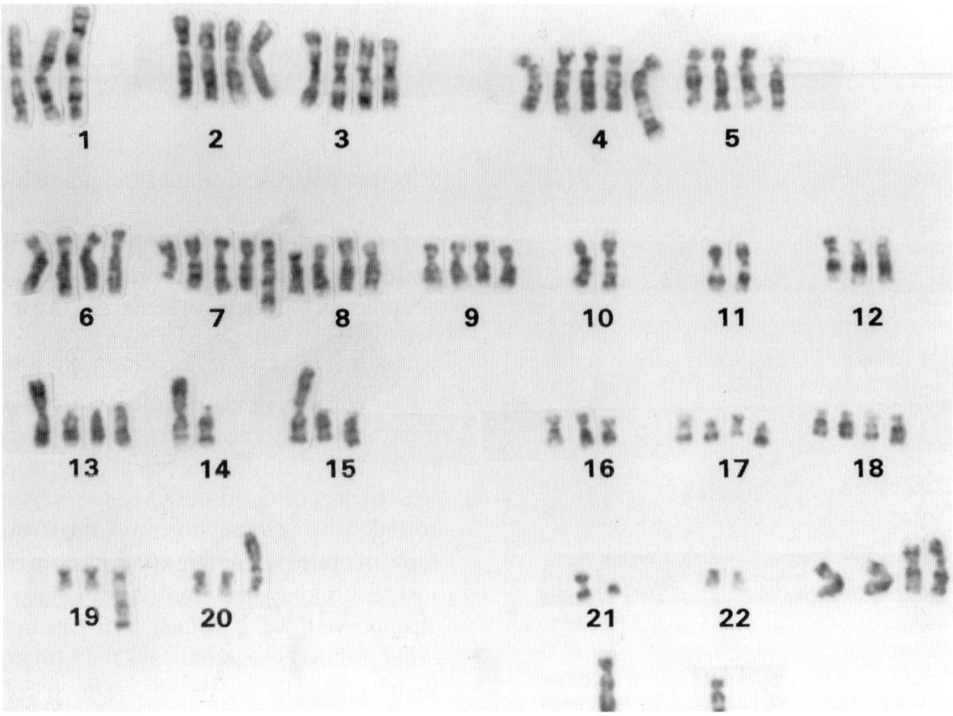

FIG. 9. Karyotype of anaplastic Wilms' tumor containing numerous chromosomal duplications. (Courtesy of Marc Valentine, St. Jude Children's Research Hospital.)

protein (48), may be found in cytokeratin-negative use but are not in wide diagnostic use.

On the other hand, the ultrastructural features of Wilms' tumors are well characterized and, like histology, closely recapitulate normal renal embryogenesis (90, 133). Thus, one observes condensation of cells with formation of lumens, microvilli, cilia, and basilar infoldings. Of particular note is the presence of a dense coat of basal lamina on the luminal surfaces of Wilms' tumor cells (Fig. 10) (133). This feature is due to the deposition of the neural cell adhesion molecule (NCAM) and is a characteristic feature even in primitive neoplasms (183). However, despite identification of ultrastructural features suggesting Wilms' tumor, fine needle aspiration cytology can be treacherous and misleading (149).

Microscopic Staging

Tantamount to the staging and clinical management of Wilms' tumor is the identification of spread through

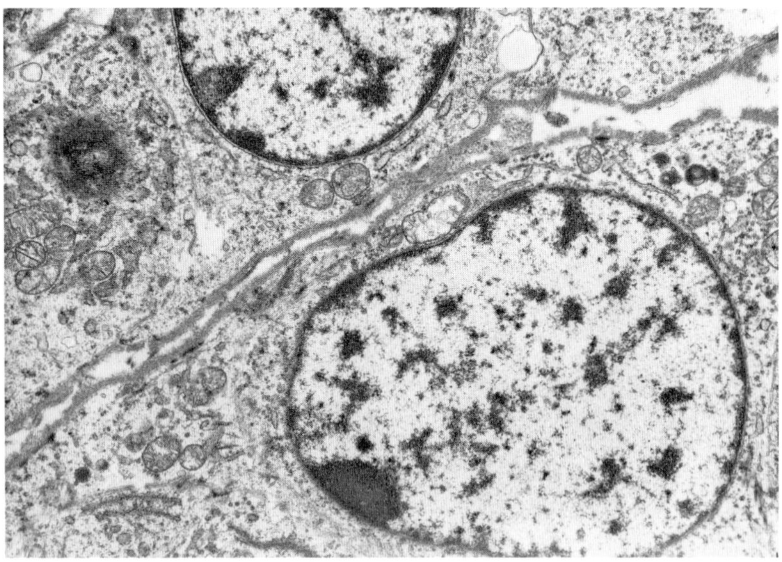

FIG. 10. Electron micrograph of Wilms' tumor containing a dense basal lamina lining the plasmalemma of tumor cells.

the renal capsule. This marker of tumor aggressiveness can mean the difference between no adjuvant treatment and a full course of potentially toxic chemotherapy. In practice, however, the microscopic identification of capsular invasion can be quite difficult because of the formation of a tumor-related pseudocapsule. The renal capsule is normally very thin and consists of only a few attenuated cells. This structure is damaged by the compressive effects of an adjacent neoplasm, leading to multiplication of fibroblasts and progressive collagenization. The result is a fibrous pseudocapsule of varying thickness that obscures the true stage of the tumor because of the obliteration of the defining boundary zone. To accurately assess the extent of tumor invasion in this circumstance, it is necessary to observe nonartifactual permeation of the lesion into fibroadipose tissue. To this end the best strategy is to liberally section areas that appear grossly suspicious or abut nonthickened capsule. Nevertheless, the presence of a fibrous pseudocapsule is an ominous sign (228).

Evaluation of pararenal lymph nodes can create other difficulties in microstaging because a number of nonmalignant lesions may superficially resemble metastatic Wilms' tumor (229). These entities include benign epithelial cells, reactive germinal centers, thickened endothelial cells, megakaryocytes, granulomas, and inspissated Tamm-Horsfall protein. The latter phenomenon is particularly common in my experience because the urinary obstruction caused by a bulging tumor frequently leads to leakage of this substance into the lymphatics. Damaged nephronic epithelium may accompany this extrusion.

Nephrogenic Rests

Critical to our understanding of Wilms' tumors is their association with persistent embryonal nephronic rests in the adjacent kidney (Fig. 11). These embryonal rests, termed "nephrogenic rests" ("nephroblastomatosis" if multiple or diffuse), have been demonstrated in 1% of neonatal autopsies (15) and in over one third of patients with Wilms' tumors (11,24). There is thus strong evidence that at least some Wilms' tumors develop according to the two-hit hypothesis of Knudson and Strong (99), with persistence of blastema representing the first mutational event and a postnatal stimulus on this blastemal tissue representing the second carcinogenic event.

Nephroblastomatosis was originally classified by Bove and McAdams (24) into pancortical, superficial diffuse, and multifocal variants. These were further subdivided into nodular renal blastema, which are small, well-circumscribed nodules of embryonal renal epithelium, sclerosing metanephric hamartomas, which are variably sized, collagenized nodules with an epithelial component, and incipient Wilms' tumors and Wilms' tumorlets, which are expansile nodules that respectively measure less than 1.0 cm or 3.5 cm. The sclerosing hamartomas appear to arise through progressive collagenization and atrophy of the blastemal elements, so that involution and eventual disappearance of these lesions probably occurs in many cases. Bove and McAdam also described other lesions, such as glomerulosclerosis, that were included in this complex.

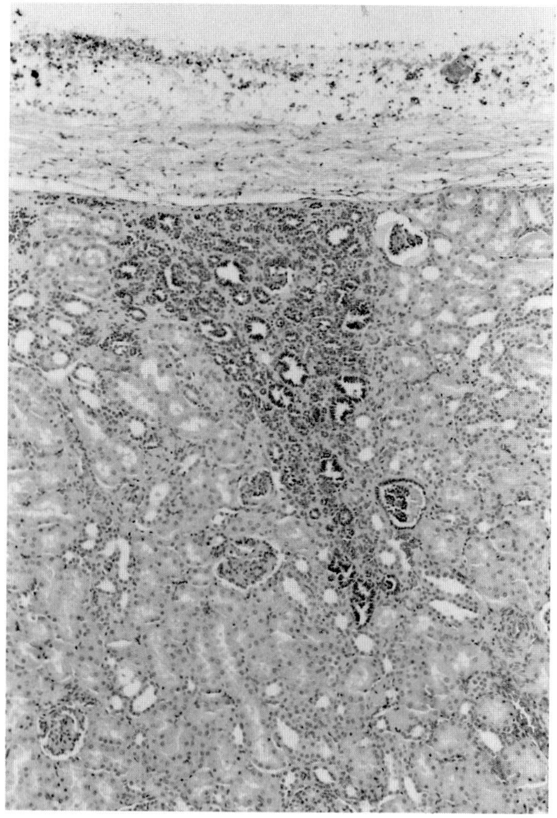

FIG. 11. Subcapsular nephrogenic rest, composed of persistent embryonic renal tissue.

More recently, Beckwith et al. (11) proposed another classification schema for nephrogenic rests, based on the location of the embryonal rests within the mature nephron. In this schema, the rests are subdivided into perilobar, intralobar, combined perilobar and intralobar, and panlobar nephroblastomatosis. The perilobar variant is located at the periphery of the renal lobe, whereas the intralobar variant is located within the inner portions of the cortex or medulla (Fig. 12) Intralobar rests may be noted at the periphery of Wilms' tumors (Fig. 13).

Mierau and colleagues (133) further proposed a correlation of nephrogenic rests with the pathologic features of the renal tumors that develop from these rests, further corresponding to the stage of embryonic development at which the error in nephrogenesis occurred (133). Perilobar rests are associated with synchronous bilateral Wilms' tumors with blastemal and epithelial predominance, and intralobar rests are associated with metachronous contralateral Wilms' tumors with stromal differ-

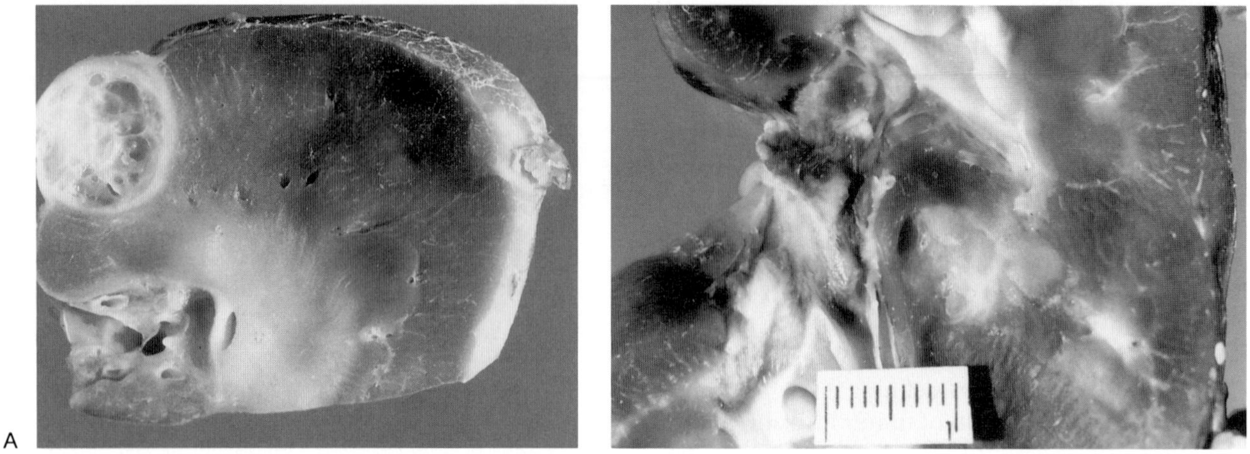

FIG. 12. Gross photographs of perilobar rest (**A**) and intralobar rest (**B**). The perilobar rest is cystic, sharply delimited, and situated at the periphery of the kidney, whereas the intralobar rest forms a poorly circumscribed pale focus in the center of the photograph, near the collecting system.

entiation. Thus, intralobar rests arise at a relatively early period of morphogenesis, thereby explaining their deeper location and greater tendency to contain heterologous elements. Recent observations at the molecular level appear to substantiate these distinctions (137).

By Beckwith's definition (11), nephrogenic rests can be hyperplastic or neoplastic. Hyperplastic rests are actively growing rests with mitotic activity, but a nonmalignant status is inferred by their configuration and spatial relationship to the adjacent kidney. This definition includes even massive infantile nephroblastomatosis, which is characterized by the presence of a thick melon-like rind of tissue enveloping both kidneys (Fig. 14) (44). On the other hand, neoplastic rests are globular or spherical lesions that arise from malignant clones (240). These tumors are more easily recognized by their configuration on CT scans than their histologic features, which may invite confusion if one relies solely on needle biopsy for diagnosis (236). Another lesion in Beckwith's classification is the adenomatous rest, which has the configuration of a neoplasm but with comparatively benign cytologic features. By use of Beckwith's system (11), terms such as "Wilms' tumorlet" and "incipient Wilms" are rendered obsolete, as neoplastic rests with the features of malignancy are technically Wilms' tumors regardless of their size.

Cystic Nephroma

Another common variation of Wilms' tumor is the cystic lesion. A large percentage of Wilms' tumors contain a variable number of cysts, probably caused by the dilatation of tubular components. The cystic component may be large, prominent, and filled with blood or clear fluid. At times the number of cysts may be quite remark-

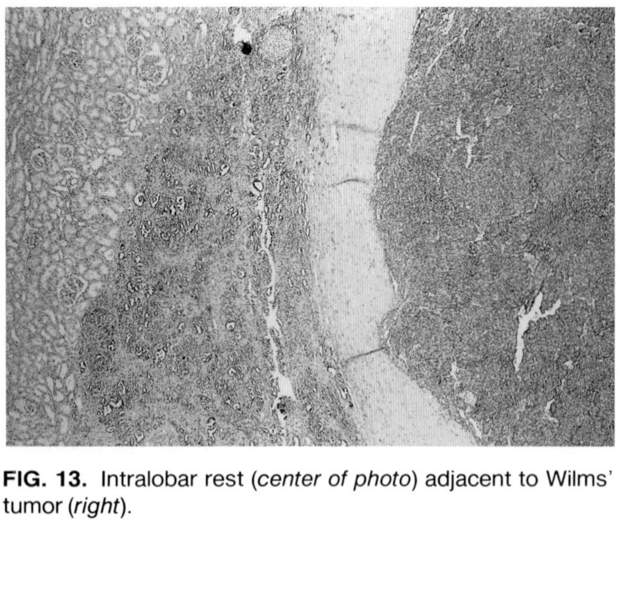

FIG. 13. Intralobar rest (*center of photo*) adjacent to Wilms' tumor (*right*).

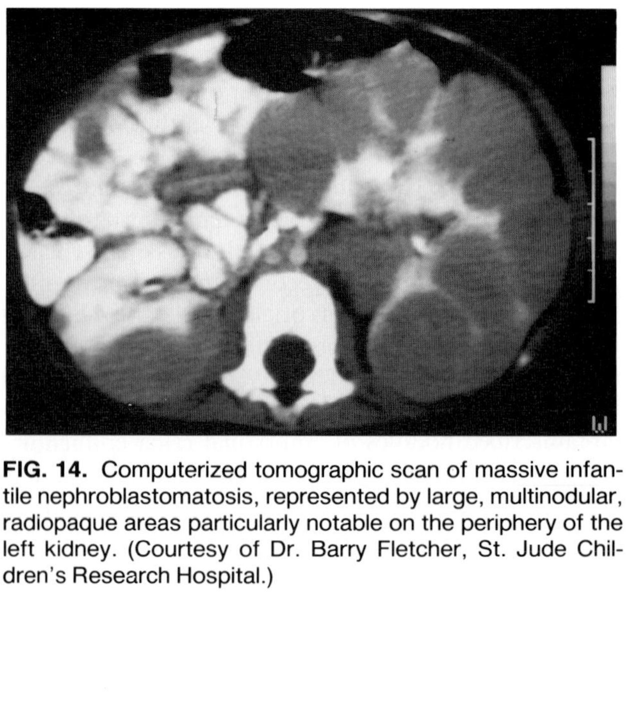

FIG. 14. Computerized tomographic scan of massive infantile nephroblastomatosis, represented by large, multinodular, radiopaque areas particularly notable on the periphery of the left kidney. (Courtesy of Dr. Barry Fletcher, St. Jude Children's Research Hospital.)

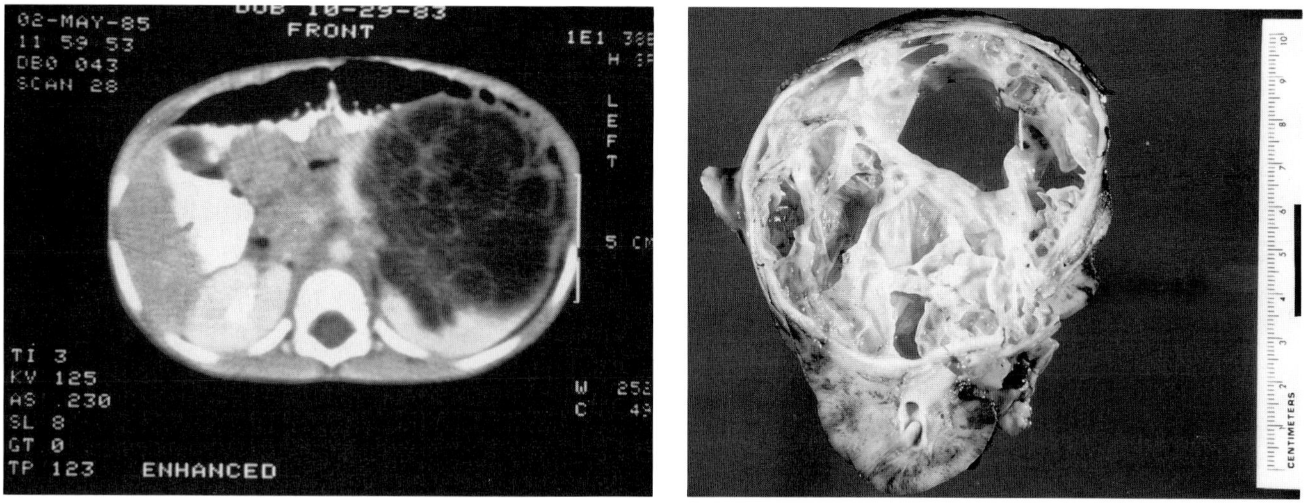

A B

FIG. 15. Computerized tomographic image (**A**) and gross photograph (**B**) of cystic nephromas. The lesions are composed of large, prominent cysts of varying sizes that form a striking radiographic image. (Part **A** courtesy of Dr. Barry Fletcher, St. Jude Children's Research Hospital; Part **B** from Webber BL et al.: Renal tumors in childhood. In Rosen PP, Fechner RE, eds. *Pathology Annual,* Vol. 27, Part 1, 1992: 191–232, courtesy of Appleton and Lange.)

able and call for the special designation of cystic partially differentiated nephroblastomas. These neoplasms, extensively studied by Joshi (93–95), will contain focal blastemal areas within the walls of the cysts and are thus technically Wilms' tumors. Like fetal rhabdomyomatous nephroblastomas, cystic partially differentiated nephroblastomas are characterized by a relatively benign clinical behavior and are usually low-stage lesions (142). A related lesion is the cystic nephroma, which is composed of variably sized cysts, often with a striking radiographic configuration (Fig. 15). The cystic nephroma, however, by definition should not contain any blastemal elements. It presumably arises from partially differentiated nephroblastoma by progressive maturation of the primitive elements and likewise exhibits a benign clinical behavior.

Molecular Biology and Cytogenetics

Recent studies into the molecular biology and cytogenetics of Wilms' tumors have proven particularly intriguing. These studies were prompted by the association of Wilms' tumors with certain congenital anomalies including aniridia, hemihypertrophy, and genitourinary malformations. Initial cytogenetic studies revealed that constitutional deletions of chromosome 11p13 (Fig. 16) were present in some patients with both aniridia and Wilms' tumor (177). Subsequent in vitro studies on Wilms' tumors removed from patients without aniridia revealed a similar deletion (201,202). Gene mapping, assisted by Southern blot analysis, revealed the presence of closely linked genetic loci termed the WAGR complex (W-Wilms', A-aniridia, G-genitourinary malformations, R-mental retardation) with variable expression depending on the length of the deleted segment (43). Loss of heterozygosity on chromosome 11 (Fig. 17) occurs more often in Wilms' tumors (122,123) and involves at least two distinct loci: a deletion in 11p13 that is associated with WAGR and aniridia, and a deletion in 11p15.5 that is associated with the Beckwith–Wiedemann syndrome (see below) (203,226).

Experiments on a putative Wilms' tumor cell line appeared to also substantiate the pivotal role of chromosome 11 in Wilms' tumor development by demonstrating loss of tumorigenicity when a normal chromosome 11 was inserted into the cells (235); however, this cell line was later shown to be derived from a rhabdoid tumor line (66). Of interest is the notorious resistance of Wilms'

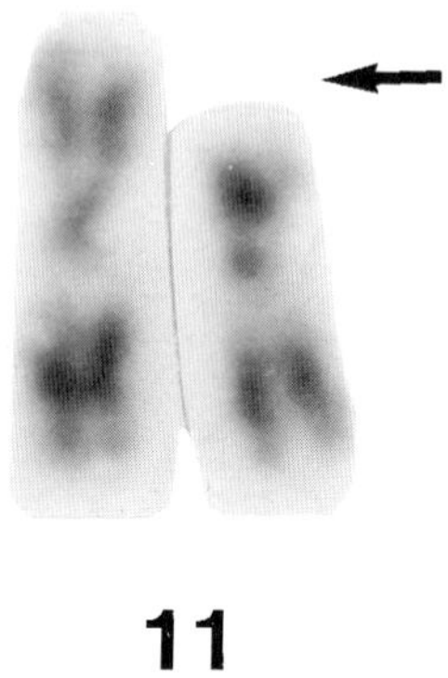

FIG. 16. Chromosomes 11 from constitutional karyotype of WAGR patient. There is a deletion of the distal portion of 11p in one chromosome (*arrow*). (Courtesy of Marc Valentine, St. Jude Children's Research Hospital.)

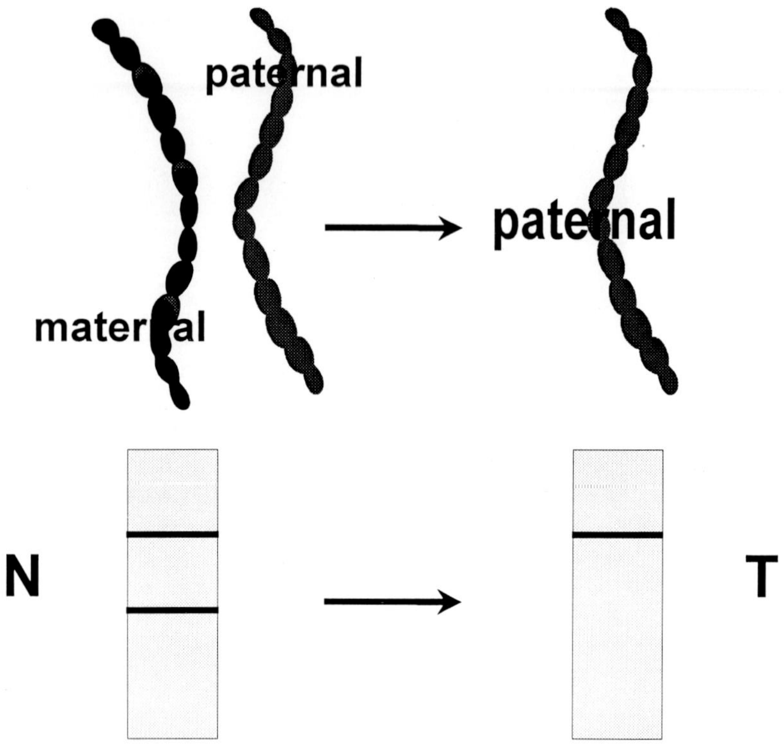

FIG. 17. Schematic illustration of genetic event causing loss of heterozygosity. There is a deletional event affecting one segment of DNA (*top*). This is manifested on a Southern blot by loss of a band on tumor tissue (T) as compared to normal tissue (N).

tumor cells to immortalization in cell lines (222), although they transiently exhibit vigorous growth in explants.

Other researchers demonstrated that the insulinlike growth factor–II (IGF-II) gene is located on chromosome band 11p14.1 and that IGF-II shows markedly elevated expression in Wilms' tumor (176,197). IGF-II is also found in the blastema of fetal kidneys, where its production appears to be inversely correlated with normal epithelial differentiation (157). Wilms' tumors also contain receptors for IGF-II, indicating an autocrine mechanism (Fig. 18) for tumor cell proliferation and abnormal differentiation (62). However, some have questioned the role of IGF-II in the tumorigenicity of Wilms' tumor

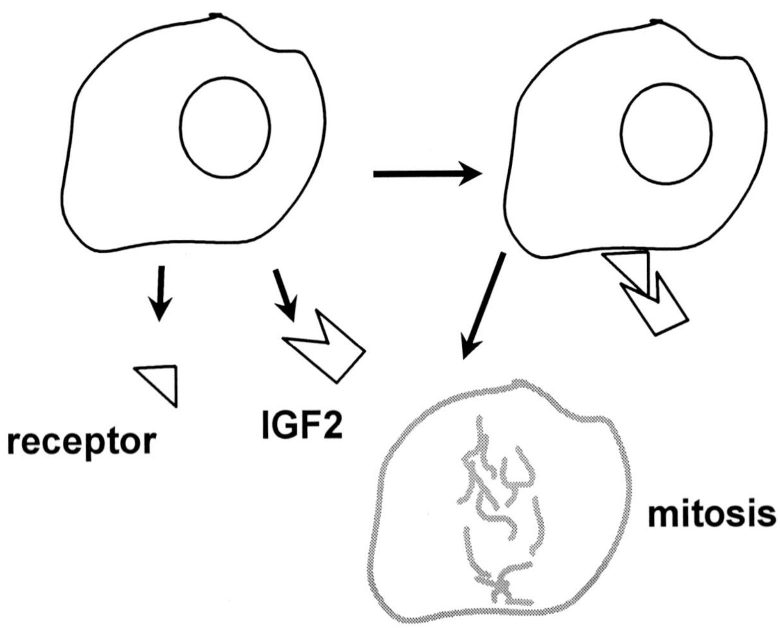

FIG. 18. Schematic illustration of autocrine secretion by Wilms' tumor cell. The cell produces both the IGF receptor and its ligand, leading to mitosis.

TABLE 3. *Genes associated with Wilms' tumor*

Name	Site	Association
WT1	11p13	WAGR, Denys–Drash
Wit1	11p13	?
WT2	11p15	Beckwith–Wiedemann
WT3	16p	Tumor progression
WT4?	?	Familial cases

(119). Nevertheless, antibodies directed against IGF-I inhibit the growth of Wilms' tumors in cell cultures and xenografts (63).

Recent publications have also detailed features of the putative Wilms' tumor gene (Table 3), *WT1*, which is located on chromosome 11p13 and appears to have a role in genitourinary embryogenesis (170,182). The protein encoded by this gene is a zinc finger peptide with significant homology to the early growth response–1 (or EGR-1) protein, a mitogen of mammalian cells (28,175). WT1 may affect cell growth by repressing the transcription of the *EGR-1* gene (120) and/or IGF-II (52). The mRNA produced by the *WT1* gene is expressed by a limited number of cell types, predominantly in the genitourinary tract (28), so it appears to be an organ-specific regulator of cell growth during embryogenesis. Limited expression is also seen in murine mesothelium and hindbrain (6). Defects in the *WT1* gene also cause defects other than renal neoplasia, including pseudohermaphrodism and glomerulonephritis (the Denys–Drash syndrome), juvenile granulosa cell tumors, hypospadias, and cryptorchidism (163,164), which is not surprising considering its expression in murine genitalia (165).

The *WT1* gene seems to normally function by genomic imprinting, with nonrandom inaction of paternal alleles (203). Genomic imprinting works by a non-Mendelian mechanism of action in which there is preferential gene function or loss of function by a parental allele (Fig. 19), as opposed to the random functioning predicted by Mendelian genetic theory. Preferential DNA methylation is one biochemical pathway by which this phenomenon occurs (207). A number of other pediatric neoplasms besides Wilms' tumor show dysfunction of this mechanism (97,102). As a consequence, loss of a preferentially expressed allele through a deletional event leads to a totally silent gene, as the other parental allele is normally not expressed anyway. Imprinting is thus important in tumor genes that show loss of heterozygosity. The evolutionary basis for imprinting is unknown, but its common presence in the animal kingdom (190) indicates that it is strongly conserved.

Another gene, *Wit1*, is closely linked to *WT1* and has a complementary nucleotide sequence (88). The function of this gene and its relationship to Wilms' tumor development are currently unknown.

Alterations in *WT1* with loss of gene expression occur in only 10% of Wilms' tumors, primarily those associated with intralobar nephrogenic rests and/or stromal predominance (88). Of interest is the observation that *WT1* gene function is also altered in nephrogenic rests (162), as might be predicted from Knudson and Strong's two-step hypothesis of tumorigenesis (99). Thus with WAGR and Denys–Drash patients, loss of *WT1* function appears to represent the primary molecular lesion in tumor development (80). Alteration of glomerular morphology occurs with Denys–Drash syndrome, with formation of mesangial nodules and malformed glomerular crescents. This pathology is due to the critical role that WT1 protein plays in glomerulogenesis (163). *WT1* is also altered in another neoplasm, the desmoplastic small

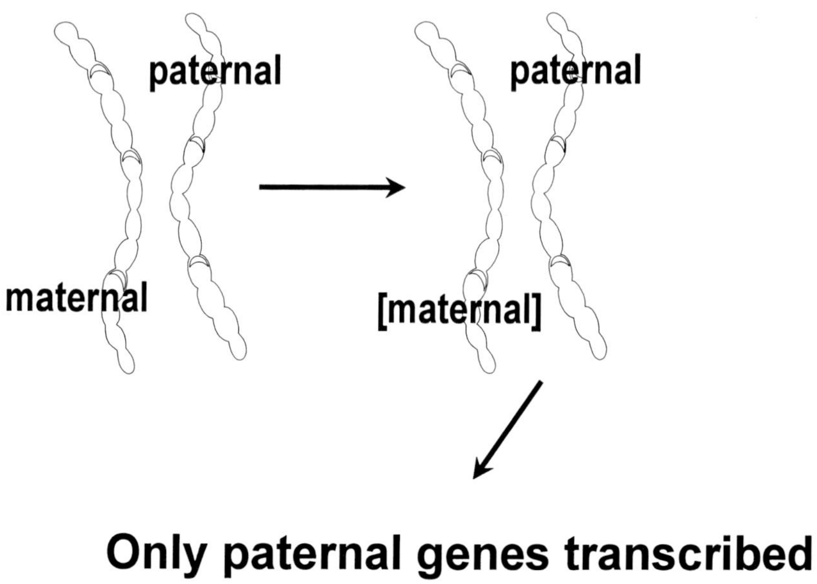

FIG. 19. Schematic illustration of imprinting. Although DNA segments from both parental alleles are present, only one allele functions in transcription, the other being functionally silent.

cell tumor, in which it is fused with *EWS* (110) (see Chapter 14).

Alterations in another Wilms' tumor gene *WT2*, located at 11p15.5, may also lead to neoplasia and hereditary Wilms' tumors without involvement of *WT1* (51,196). This gene also functions by an imprinting mechanism (27) and is involved in the development of other pediatric neoplasms, including embryonal rhabdomyosarcoma, adrenal cortical carcinoma, and hepatoblastoma (88,102). The *WT2* gene is either synonymous or closely linked to the *IGF-II* gene, which as noted above may be abnormally expressed in Wilms' tumors. Detection of deletions of this gene has proceeded from studies illustrating loss of heterozygosity of chromosome 11p (102,207), which indicate a variable loss of a portion of the 11p genome on one chromosome.

WT2 (or *BWS*) appears to be primarily responsible for the Beckwith–Wiedemann syndrome, which is associated with abnormal growth and development, a variety of embryonal tumors, and cytomorphologic lesions (205,233). Somatic defects seen in this syndrome include macroglossia, hepatosplenomegaly, and giantism (Fig. 20), due to abnormal organ growth, and omphalocele and umbilical hernias, due to abnormal abdominal wall development. A remarkable cytologic aberration occurs in the adrenal cortex, which is the site of adrenocortical cytomegaly. Embryonal rhabdomyosarcomas, adrenal cortical carcinomas, hepatoblastomas, and, rarely, neuroblastomas are also associated with this peculiar growth syndrome (205). It is noteworthy that these patients may show abnormal glucose tolerance, but the role of IGF-II in its production is unclear (245). As might be predicted, paternal imprinting plays a major role in familial cases of this syndrome (223).

A gene on 16q that does not act by genomic imprinting appears operative in at least some cases of Wilms' tumor (128). This gene may also be affected in hepatocellular carcinomas and is probably involved in tumor progression rather than initial tumorigenesis (36). Loss of heterozygosity of 16q is associated with aggressive clinical behavior independent of stage or histology (76).

Finally, studies of certain families with inherited Wilms' tumors have revealed no alterations in *WT1*, *WT2*, or the 16q gene. There thus appears to be even more genes, currently unidentified, that are associated with Wilms' tumor development (36).

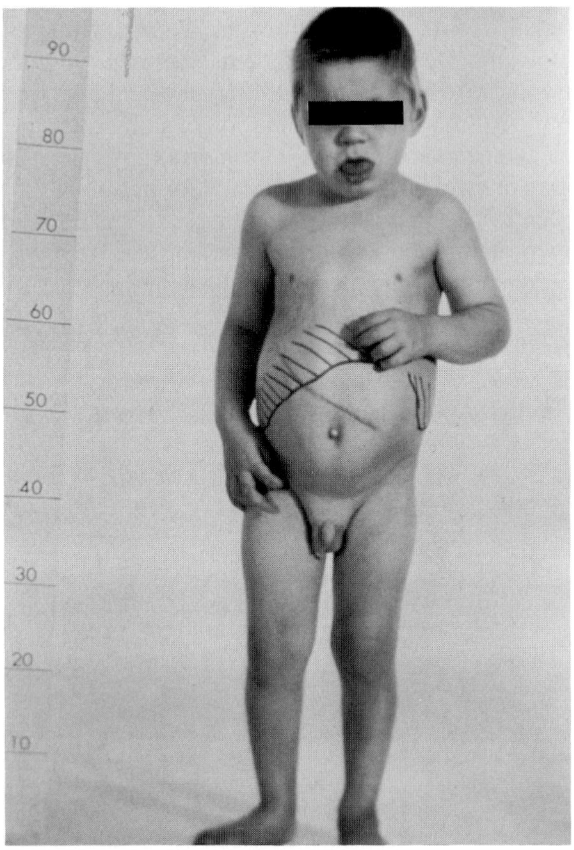

FIG. 20. Patient with Beckwith–Wiedemann syndrome, as evidenced by large overall size, macrocephaly, macroglossia, protuberant abdomen, and hepatosplenomegaly. (Courtesy of Dr. Judith Wilimas, St. Jude Children's Research Hospital.)

Ploidy

The association between abnormal ploidy in Wilms' tumors and prognosis has been controversial. There is a general consensus that hyperdiploidy is associated with the anaplastic variety of Wilms' tumors (49,77,107,136). This comes as no surprise, as the cytologic diagnosis is based on the presence of large, hyperchromatic nuclei and multipolar mitoses (Fig. 8). On the other hand, there are significant discrepancies between tumor aneuploidy and clinical outcome. To a large degree this appears to result from the cutoff level used to define a "bad" amount of DNA. In the study by Douglass et al. (49) using fresh tumor tissue, there was a discrete and striking difference in outcome between tumors with DNA indices above and below 1.3. Other studies claiming that aneuploidy has no effect on outcome have either included cases with DNA indices of <1.3 (77) or not stated the values included in the aneuploid population (107, 115,155). As evidenced by Douglass's studies (49), tumors with favorable histology can have minor aneuploid populations and a good outcome. This probably reflects the minor degrees of hyperchromatism and cellular enlargement sometimes present in favorable histology Wilms'. Reported instances of poor outcome in diploid tumors are more problematic. However, anaplastic Wilms' tumor cells may be diploid yet contain complex structural karyotypic abnormalities (Marc Valentine, personal communication). At any rate, as with other neoplasms, Wilms' tumor ploidy appear to reflect tumor progression with increasing loss of growth control and cell contact inhibition and a correspondingly more aggressive behavior as ploidy values increase.

Extrarenal Wilms' Tumors

Rare examples of Wilms' tumors occur outside of the kidney, particularly in the retroperitoneum and spermatic cord (55). Histologically, these tumors are defined by the presence of primitive nephrogenesis and should contain blastemal and tubular elements. Some reported cases may have been examples of the desmoplastic small cell tumor that occurs in the peritoneal cavity of adolescents and young adults (67). Extrarenal Wilms' tumors may also occur as a component of a teratoma (2).

MESOBLASTIC NEPHROMA

Mesoblastic nephroma is also known as congenital mesoblastic nephroma because of its strong predilection to occur in infants and newborns. Bolande et al. (20) reported this lesion in 1967 and presented evidence supporting its classification as a true neoplasm and a form of Wilms' tumor. It was further delineated as a clinical and pathologic entity in 1969 by Wigger (237), who considered it to be a fetal hamartoma unrelated to Wilms' tumor. More recent publications have focused on the delineation and diagnosis of aggressive forms of this tumor (8,168) and the molecular aberrations involved in its pathogenesis (106,195,212).

The most striking clinical feature of mesoblastic nephroma has been its almost exclusive occurrence in newborns and very young infants (54,82,189). In this age group, renal tumors are the third most commonly occurring abdominal tumor, respectively following neuroblastomas and germ cell neoplasms (82). Mesoblastic nephromas are usually reported to be the most frequent congenital renal neoplasm (82,237). The diagnosis of mesoblastic nephroma may be heralded by polyhydramnios (18,54,126), which may enhance the appearance of a renal mass on prenatal ultrasonography (18). Features of the Beckwith–Wiedemann syndrome, including microcephaly and hemihypertrophy, have been noted in one affected infant, and umbilical hernia and adrenal cytomegaly were noted in others (126). Hypercalcemia, related to tumor secretion of prostaglandin, a parathorminelike substance, or an intermediary (91,184,186), and hypertension related to hyperreninemia (35) have also been described.

Another salutory feature of mesoblastic nephroma is its generally benign behavior following nephrectomy (19,237). However, an aggressive form of this tumor may be associated with intra-abdominal and/or metastases and lead to the patient's demise (96). These aggressive tumors are more apt to occur in older patients and have even been reported in adults (213).

Grossly, mesoblastic nephroma has an appearance distinctly different from the usual Wilms' tumor. These features include a whorled fibrous-appearing cut surface likened to watered silk (237) and a firm consistency. In addition, the borders of mesoplastic nephromas typically show a lack of clear definition on gross inspection rather than the sharp margination usually present in Wilms' tumors. There is usually no gross evidence of necrosis, lobulation, or hemorrhage in mesoblastic nephromas (20), but cysts may be evident (19).

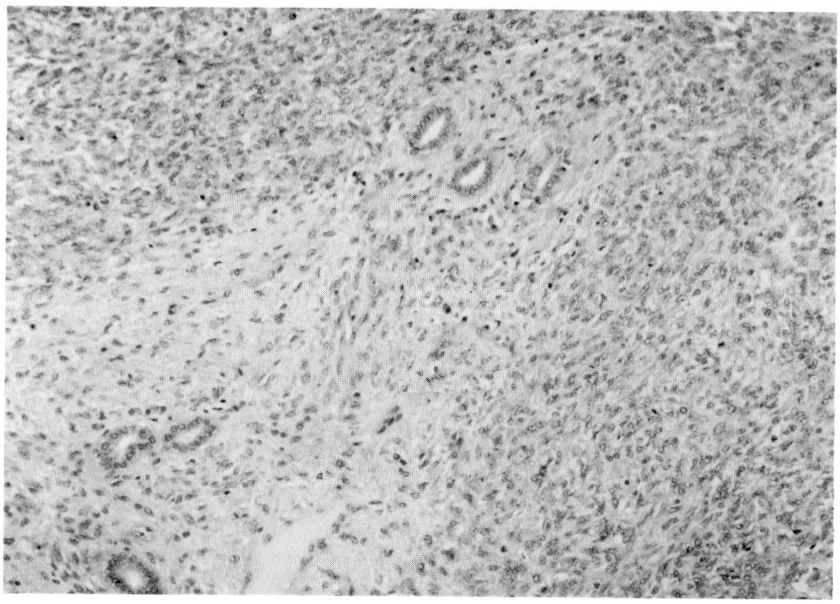

FIG. 21. Congenital mesoblastic nephroma arising from infant kidney and composed on bundles of bland myofibroblastic cells. There are interspersed tubules.

On routine light microscopy (Fig. 21), the fibromatous-appearing gross appearance of mesoblastic nephromas corresponds to a predominance of bland interlacing spindle cells likened to both smooth muscle (189,237) and fibroblasts (59). Varying amounts of collagenization are present, as well as a range of differentiation from immature fetal-type mesenchyme to fully developed myofibroblasts. Some tumors, particularly the more cellular forms, present a storiform fibrohistiocytic pattern. This variation in cellularity has been used to devise a subclassification system related to tumor behavior by some (189) but found to be of no significance by others (126,168), possibly because considerable overlap exists. Typically, recurrent lesions exhibit a higher degree of cellularity with less apparent differentiation (59,84).

In addition to the spindle cells that predominate in mesoblastic nephroma, heterologous elements may be interspersed. These tissues include cartilage and differentiated skeletal muscle with multinucleated giant cells (126). Islands of cornified squamous epithelium have also been described (126). Of particular note and engendering persistent debate among histogenetic theorists is the common appearance of scattered renal tubules and glomeruli within the body of the tumor (Fig. 21). Often, the tubular epithelial cells exhibit varying degrees of cytologic dysplasia. These elements were considered to be a integral part of the lesion by Bolande (19), who found this feature to be evidence of a relationship between mesoblastic nephroma and Wilms' tumor. On the other side of the coin, Wigger (237) believed that the epithelium represents entrapment of normally developing cells by a hamartomatous overgrowth of secondary renal mesenchyme. Of particular note in this regard is the tendency, admittedly not always the case, for the tubular elements to occur at the periphery of the lesion. Conversely, to date no epithelial elements have been in recurrences or metastases. However, the controversy has yet to be resolved (126).

Marsden and Newton (126), in their histologic study of a relatively large series of mesoblastic nephromas, took particular note of the renal tissue adjacent to the tumor, noting vacuolated and dysplastic tubules, cysts, and subcapsular renal tumorlets. The vacuolated tubules were likened to changes noted in the Denys–Drash syndrome. The description of subcapsular tumorlets is also intriguingly reminiscent of nephroblastomatosis, although Marsden and Newton disavowed this association.

Another striking pathologic feature of mesoblastic nephroma is its invasion of neighboring tissues. This may occur into the adjacent kidney, perirenal soft tissue, or renal pelvis (19). As a result, it behooves the surgical pathologist performing gross examination to pay particular attention to the surgical margins, as incomplete excision is predictive of recurrence (96).

Other features that portend aggressive tumor behavior include occurrence in patients older than 3 months of age (72), gross invasion of adjacent organs, and increased mitoses and cellularity (Fig. 22) (14,96). One or more of these features are usually present in lesions that recur or metastasize (72,96,118,189). However, the generally benign clinical behavior of mesoblastic nephromas has engendered doubt as to whether the aggressive tumors are truly forms of this lesion (142).

Electron microscopy of mesoblastic nephromas confirms the myofibroblastic character of the spindle cells, which typically contain cigar-shaped, tapered nuclei and abundant cisternae of rough endoplasmic reticulum that is often dilated by a granular procollagenous substance. Collagen fibrils of the usual type are commonly seen in the interstitium, and cells may be joined by zonulae ad-

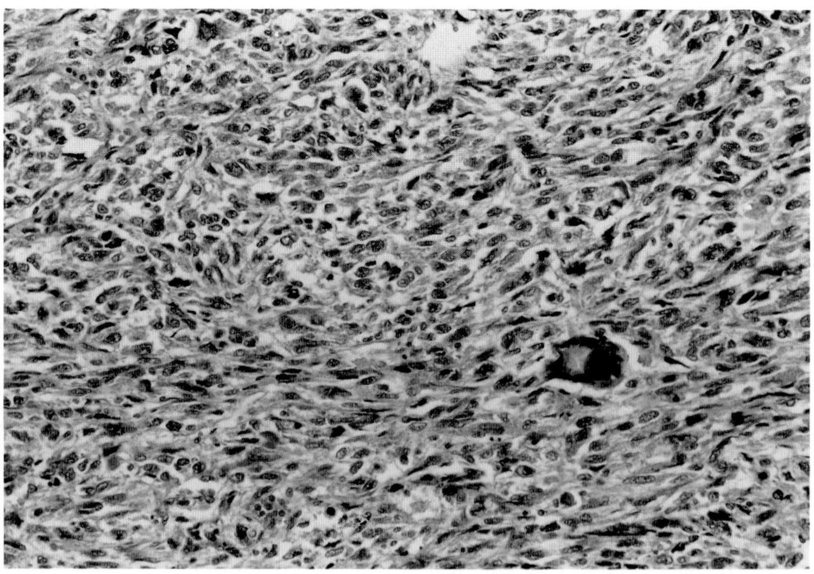

FIG. 22. Cellular mesoblastic nephroma arising from older patient. There is increased cellularity and focal atypia.

herens or zonulae occludens. Subplasmalemmal arrays of microfilaments with interspersed dense bodies, typical of smooth muscle, are also present in varying degrees; these cells may be invested by a basal lamina. Besides microfilaments, intracytoplasmic microtubules have been noted (54,59,168,238). Short filopodia, likened to microvilli, and an occasional cilium may be present (59,238). The myofibroblastic content of the lesion has been used to relate it to other visceral lesions of early childhood, such as the peribronchial myofibroblastic tumor (130). Cells with lesser differentiation, analogous to primitive mesenchymal cells, may be present in varying amounts and appear to predominate in recurrences and cellular forms (59,168).

Because of the distinctive histologic appearance of mesoblastic nephroma and the relatively nonspecific immunophenotype of its constituent cells, immunohistochemistry is not of great import in diagnosis. Reactivity with antibodies against vimentin, desmin, and actin supports the identity of the tumor cells as myofibroblasts (143,168). Cytokeratin positivity was observed in occasional spindle cells in one study (143) and was not observed in another (168). Kumar et al. (106) demonstrated the presence of intracellular and pericellular fibronectin and absence of stainable laminin in these tumors. They cited this result as indicative of origin from primitive nephrogenic mesenchyme, which has a similar phenotype, and against a histogenesis from secondary mesenchyme as proposed by Wigger (237). A similar conclusion regarding the origin of mesoblastic nephromas was given by their positivity for neural cell adhesion molecule-associated polysialic acid, which was observed in cellular areas (143). Nephronic segment-specific lectin staining was used to suggest that the intratumoral epithelial elements were primary distal tubules and collecting ducts, probably originating from the ureteric bud; origin from tumor cells was not entirely excluded, however (143). High levels of renin expression, the probable cause of associated hypertension, are found in blood vessels supplying the intratumoral epithelial cells (35).

Distinct karyotypic aberrations, primarily extra copies of chromosome 11, are present in mesoblastic nephroma. This genotype is typically found in the cellular forms of the lesion rather than the classic form. This aberration may be accompanied by nonrandom gains in chromosomes 8 and 17, as revealed by testing with fluorescence in situ hybridization using centromeric probes (195). These chromosome gains are associated with aneuploidy as detected by image analysis (195) or flow cytometry (168), but the clinical significance of this observation is unapparent at present (168). Chromosome losses have also been recorded (221). In contradistinction to Wilms' tumor, neither loss of heterozygosity on chromosome 11 nor N-myc expression was detected in two classic cases of mesoblastic nephroma (212), but marked expression of IGF-II was noted. More recently, a case with an 11p15 rearrangement has been reported (179), possibly furnishing a genetic link between mesoblastic nephroma and Wilms' tumor.

In vitro experiments have yielded interesting information on the differentiation potential of mesoblastic nephromas. Crocker and Vernier observed (39) that nephrogenesis with formation of tubular epithelium proceeded from organ culture. In their studies tumor tissue was incubated adjacent to fetal mouse brain, which presumably supplied needed differentiation factors; control experiments without brain failed to show differentiation. However, one cannot entirely exclude the possibility that "entrapped" epithelial elements within the tumor gave rise to the proliferating nephrogenic elements. This hurdle was cleared, however, by the demonstration of epithelial differentiation in tissue cultures of mesoblastic nephroma by Garvin et al. (65). In Garvin's experiment, epithelial cells formed islands that overlaid the spindle cell population.

Many of the features of mesoblastic nephroma, such as its occurrence in the kidneys of young children, entrapment of renal tubules, basic mesenchymal nature with apparent latent capacity for epithelial differentiation, and enigmatic derivation and relationship to Wilms' tumor, are reminiscent of the clear cell sarcoma of kidney (CCSK), a highly malignant renal neoplasm (see below). In fact, along with Wilms' tumor and malignant rhabdoid tumor of the kidney, CCSK must be considered in the differential diagnosis of these lesions (142). However, all efforts to date to construe CCSK as a malignant form of mesoblastic nephoma have been strictly conjectural.

CLEAR CELL SARCOMA OF THE KIDNEY

Clear cell sarcoma of the kidney is a relatively newly recognized renal tumor described during the latter half of the 20th century. Despite the name, it bears no relationship whatsoever to the clear cell sarcoma of tendons and aponeuroses (also known as melanoma of soft parts). Serendipitously, it was discovered almost simultaneously by three independent groups and published in the same journal in the same year, 1978 (13,125,138). Beckwith and Palmer bear the honor of its first description (13), which they initially published as a clinically aggressive or "sarcomatoid" variant of Wilms' tumor. The clear cell sarcomatoid Wilms' tumor formed one component of a group of three childhood renal tumors with distinctive histologic features and poor clinical outcome accrued through the National Wilms' Tumor Study (NWTS). The other two variants in the original description were the "rhabdomyosarcomatoid" Wilms' tumor, later to become the malignant rhabdoid tumor of the kidney (79), and the "hyalinizing" Wilms' tumor, later recognized as a morphologically peculiar form of either CCSK or rhabdoid tumor (9). In the initial NWTS report (13), these tumors had a strongly adverse prognosis.

Only a few months later, Marsden and colleagues (125) reported a peculiar lesion noted in their review of 231 pediatric renal tumors accrued through the first Medical Research Council Nephroblastoma Trial and the Manchester Children's Tumor Registry. These five tumors were distinguished clinically by their tendency to metastasize to bone, a property distinctly separate from the usual Wilms' tumor (113). They thus graced this tumor with the breathless sobriquet "bone metastasizing renal tumor of childhood." In the same journal issue, Morgan and Kidd (138) reported nine cases of an undifferentiated sarcoma of kidney, again recognizing an aggressive clinical behavior and tendency for bony metastases as well as a distinct histologic pattern. In retrospect, we recognize these tumors described by Marsden, Morgan, and their colleagues as being identical to the "clear cell sarcomatoid Wilms' tumor" described earlier by Beckwith and Palmer (13).

At the gross level, no distinction has been made between CCSK and Wilms' tumor, with both presenting as bulging, discretely outlined tan renal masses with varying degrees of necrosis and hemorrhage. Interesting clinical features have been noted, however, by Sotelo-Avila et al. (204), who reported a tendency of CCSK to be larger and diagnosed at an earlier age in boys than girls. Besides its aggressive behavior, CCSK is clinically noteworthy for its marked proclivity to skeletal metastasis, most often to the skull (Fig. 23) (204). One case (87) was associated with Cushing's syndrome due to elevated serum ACTH. This hormone could not be demonstrated in tumor cells by immunohistochemistry, so that the neoplasm was presumably secreting either a cortisol-releasing factor or bombesinlike substance.

CCSK has been found to present a variety of histologic patterns that may confuse and confound the unwary pathologist (12). Its basis component is an aggregate of seemingly undifferentiated tumor cells, usually presenting a clear or lightly staining appearance because of a finely distributed chromatin pattern and lucent cytoplasm (Fig. 24). However, despite the tumor's name, the tinctorial qualities of the cytoplasm are variable and may be scanty or even lightly eosinophilic. Common to all CCSK and essential to the diagnosis is a fine meshwork of small blood vessels that presents a pattern reminiscent of hemangiopericytoma or liposarcoma. The tumor cells produce variable amounts of a hyalinelike collagenizing ground substance that in greater quantities creates the "hyalinizing sarcoma" referred to by Beckwith in his original description of pediatric renal sarcomas (13). At

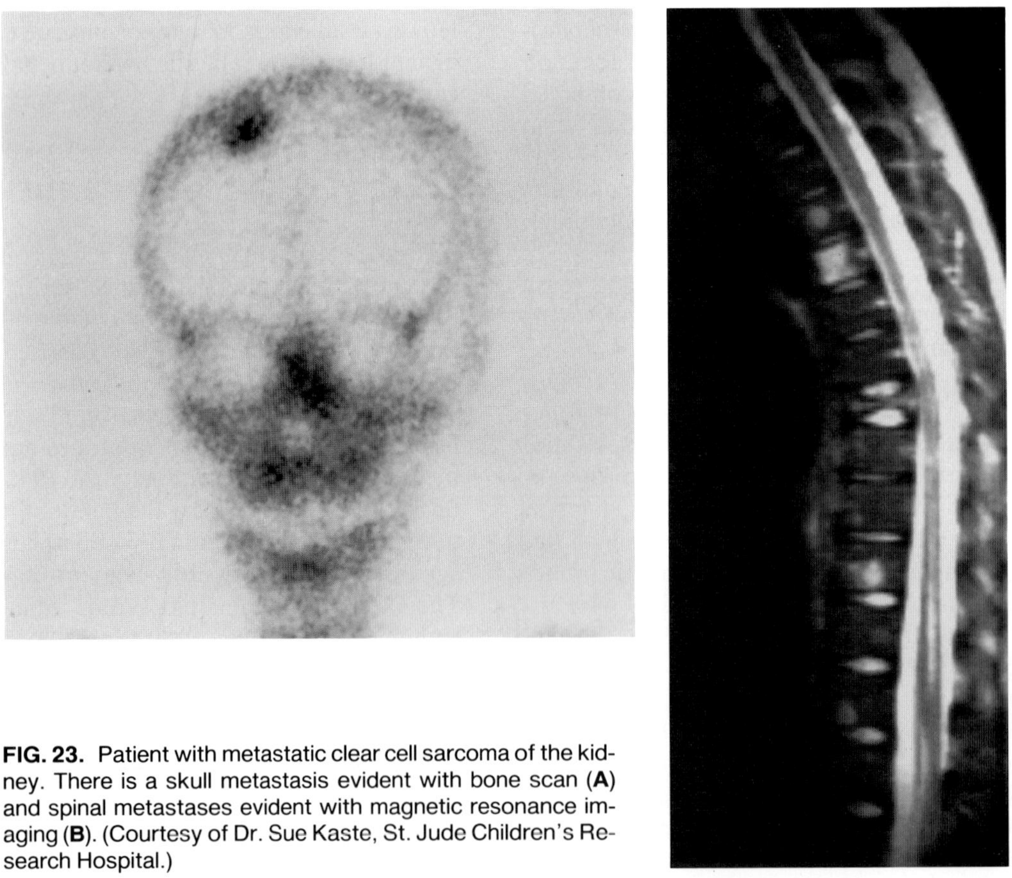

FIG. 23. Patient with metastatic clear cell sarcoma of the kidney. There is a skull metastasis evident with bone scan (**A**) and spinal metastases evident with magnetic resonance imaging (**B**). (Courtesy of Dr. Sue Kaste, St. Jude Children's Research Hospital.)

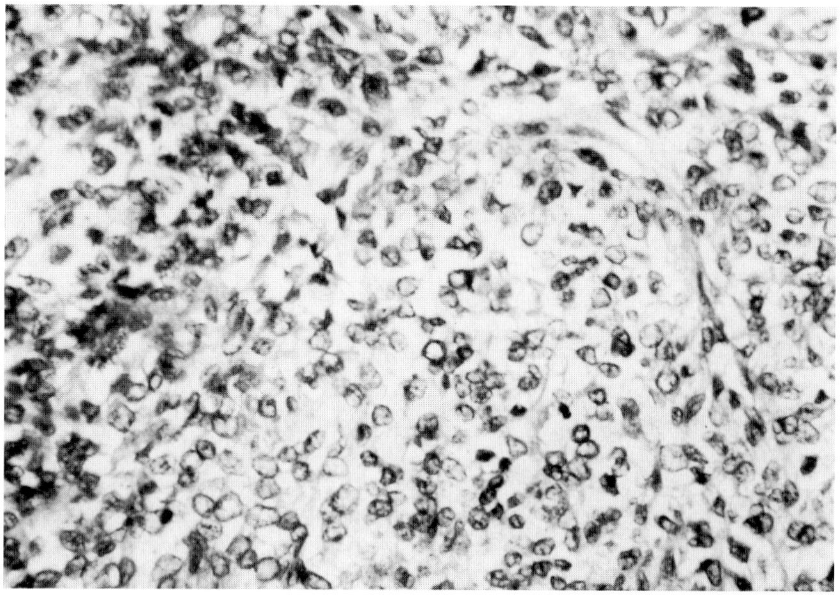

FIG. 24. Clear cell sarcoma of the kidney, composed of cells with clear cytoplasm and oval nuclei. Small arcuate vessels are apparent.

the extreme, this material may present an osteosarcomalike appearance (12). Alternatively, the tumor cells may secrete a mucoid substance producing myxoid or even cystic areas (Fig. 25).

Another histologic feature of the tumor cells of CCSK is their tendency to produce epithelioid aggregates (Fig. 26). Similar to mesoblastic nephroma, this feature has led to speculation about the relationship of the neoplasm to classical Wilms' tumor. To further develop this analogy, both tumors often contain tubular elements that are interpreted by most as entrapped normal structures. However, one case of CCSK with production of neoplastic epithelium has been reported (192). In this tumor, the epithelium was highly primitive and reminiscent of embryonal neuroectoderm. Other features of CCSK also have been cited as evidence of a capacity for epithelial differentiation (see below). Regardless of its interpretation, the formation of epithelioid aggregates of tumor cells nestled between a capillary meshwork may lead to a misleading histologic picture that must be correctly interpreted for proper prognostication and clinical management (12).

A

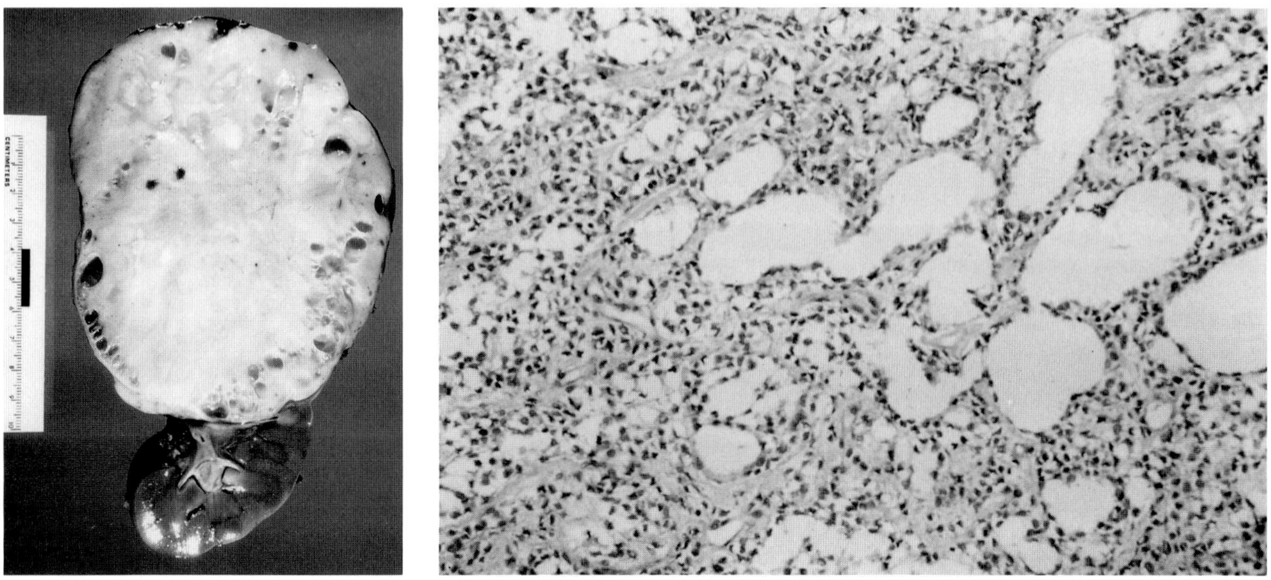

B

FIG. 25. Clear cell sarcoma of kidney containing prominent cystic component on gross (**A**) and microscopic (**B**) examination.

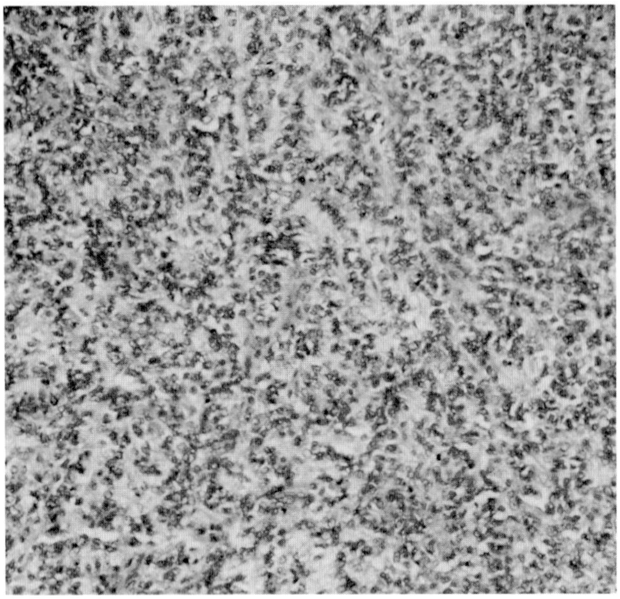

FIG. 26. Clear cell sarcoma of kidney with epithelioid aggregation of tumor cells.

Electron microscopy has been miserly to date in rewarding investigators with definitive evidence of the derivation of this neoplasm. Nevertheless, subtle clues have emerged, as several authors independently have noted cell clusters reminiscent of the primordial nephron, the metanephric blastemal cap (69,148,209). However, others contend that the ultrastructural features of CCSK are better deciphered as evidence of its origin from primitive undifferentiated mesenchyme (78). Regardless of the cryptic information it offers about the origin of CCSK, the electron microscopic features of these tumors comprise a distinctive motif of primitive cells, extracellular matrix, and small blood vessels. Particularly intriguing are the pools of extracellular matrix material, which may be partially enfolded by cytoplasmic processes (Fig. 27). This feature is at least partially responsible for the "clear cell" appearance of the tumor by light microscopy (78), so that the term "CCSK" is actually a misnomer. Tumor cell cytoplasm, on the other hand, may actually be dense, and as is typical of primitive cells, the most conspicuous cytoplasmic organelles are mitochondria, ergastoplasm, and Golgi complexes. Loose aggregates of intermediate filaments present in the cytoplasm should not be diagnostically misconstrued as evidence of rhabdoid tumor. Basal lamina is present at the tumor cell–capillary interfaces but not around individual cells. Fibroblasts and myofibroblasts accompany the vessels and are not tumoral in origin, as no transitional cells are apparent (78). Several authors have noted occasional cilia or similar structures on the apices of occasional tumor cells, but intercellular junctions do not attain the prominence usually seen in epithelium (69,148).

Similarly, anticytokeratin immunoreactivity is not found in CCSK except in entrapped tubular elements (151,209). Vimentin is usually present and probably constitutes the filaments seen with electron microscopy (151,209). Otherwise, CCSK lacks immunoexpression of a wide variety of cell-typic markers, including desmin, myoglobin, laminin, tissue polypeptide antigen, PNA-

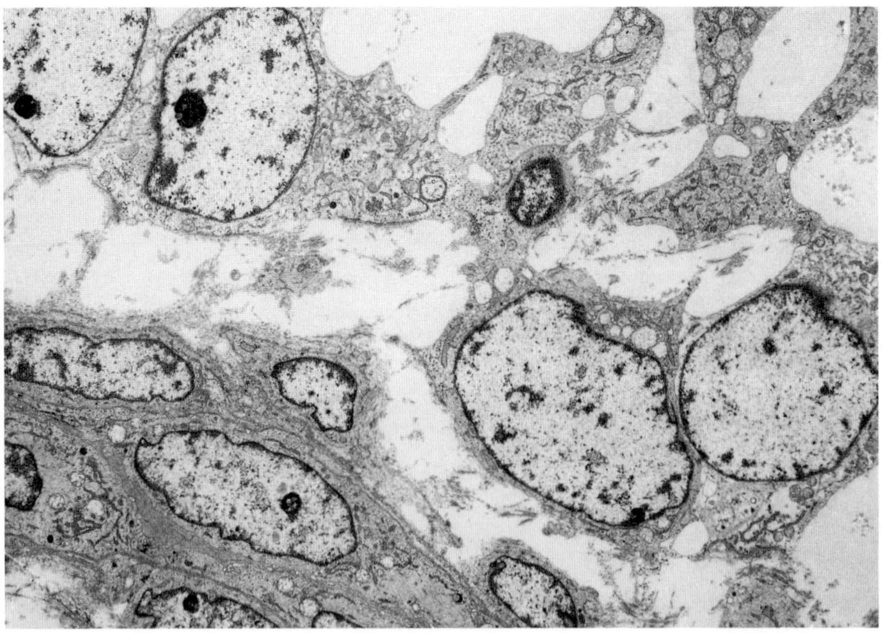

FIG. 27. Electron micrograph of clear cell sarcoma of kidney. Tumor cells enfold an abundant extracellular matrix containing scattered collagen fibrils. A blood vessel is at lower left.

lectin, and creatine kinase M (151,209). Even the epithelioid CCSK reported by Schmidt and colleagues (192) did not react with anticytokeratin.

On the other hand, cell lines derived from CCSK and capable of producing tumors in nude mice were found to be positive for cytokeratins 8 and 19 by immunoblotting and immunohistochemistry (89). This feature was accompanied by increased eosinophilic cytoplasm, mucin production, and the appearance of tonofilaments, microvilli, and intracellular lumina and was interpreted as evidence of a latent epithelial nature. Of interest is that the primary tumors showed typical CCSK features, including cytokeratin negativity. The authors of this study strongly favored these findings as indicating a relationship between CCSK and Wilms' tumor.

Contradictory evidence for this assumption comes from another recent cytogenetic study, which found a single case of CCSK to have a unique chromosomal aberration, a reciprocal translocation between chromosomes 10 and 17. This t(10;17)(q22;p13) has not been reported in any of the numerous cytogenetic studies on Wilms' tumors; neither did the reported case exhibit any of the aberrations such as 11p− typical of the latter lesion (171). Unfortunately, other cytogenetic reports of CCSK are not currently available.

Rare extrarenal instances of CCSK have been reported. These neoplasms have been found in the terminal ileum (98) and the pelvic soft tissues (232). CCSK-like tumors have also been reported in adults (135,150).

In summary, CCSK remains an enigmatic lesion to this date, distinguished by its histologic appearance and its tendency to produce bony metastases. Happily, modern therapy has improved the outlook of patients with this tumor, but success requires the correct recognition of the lesion by the surgical pathologist. CCSK appears to have a latent capacity for epithelial differentiation, but its exact relationship to Wilms' tumor is still controversial.

MALIGNANT RHABDOID TUMOR

Malignant Rhabdoid Tumor of the Kidney

The tremendous progress made with the favorable histology Wilms' tumors is unfortunately balanced by an appalling lack of understanding and effective therapy for the malignant rhabdoid tumor. Like CCSK, it was first recognized as a sarcomatous, unfavorable risk variant of Wilms' tumor, the rhabdomyosarcomatoid Wilms' tumor (13). At least one morphologically identical infantile tumor, originating in the thymus, was described just prior to this report (117). The tumor received its present name, malignant rhabdoid tumor, in the paper by Haas et al. (79), who established it as a distinct entity apart from Wilms' tumor and delineated its distinctive ultrastructural features.

Clinically, renal rhabdoid tumors generally present as abdominal masses in infants having a mean age of 11 months (230). Pathologically, they are distinctive tumors composed of noncohesive sheets of cells with abundant glassy eosinophilic cytoplasm and large eccentric nuclei with prominent central nucleoli (Fig. 28). The number of mitoses is variable from case to case and can be surprisingly low in view of the tumor's prognosis. One characteristic feature that is essential for the diagnosis is the presence of large oval cytoplasmic hyaline inclusions composed of 8- to 10-nm filaments by electron microscopy (Fig. 29) (79). Otherwise, Weeks et al. (230) encountered a wide range of histologic appearances in their series of 111 renal rhabdoid tumors. Morphologic patterns encountered included classical, epithelioid, sclerosing, lymphomatoid, histiocytoid, spindled, myxoid, palisaded, hemangiopericytomatous, organoid (paragangliomatous), pseudopapillary, and multicystic variants. However, no pattern had an independent effect on the clinical outcome, which was uniformly dismal (less than 20% survival for NTWS cases). Schmidt et al. (193) in their series of 16 cases also encountered the sclerosing and spindled patterns, as well as one they termed "pseudo-alveolar."

The diversity of phenotypic markers expressed by malignant rhabdoid tumors has been matched by a corresponding plethora of hypotheses concerning its histogenesis (70,105,185,187,209,214,224). Gonzalez-Crussi et al. (70) were some of the first investigators to use immunohistochemical techniques to study these tumors; their results indicated expression of histiocytic features. Given impetus by ultrastructural reports of cytoplasmic filaments, Vogel et al. (224) found coexpression of both cytokeratin (Fig. 30) and vimentin, the most common immunophenotype in subsequent publications. However, Tsokos et al. (214), Schmidt et al. (193), and Weeks et al. (230) found desmin positivity in some of their tumors, and Weeks et al. (230) even observed neurofilament positivity in some cases. In the Weeks series an impressive array of immunostains, including anti-leukocyte common antigen, stained the cytoplasmic inclusions, leading Weeks to conclude that the majority of stains were nonspecific. Additional evidence for an epithelial phenotype has come from Kumar et al. (105) and Higa et al. (86), who found epithelial membrane antigen positivity in their cases. Other authors have found myoglobin (230,243) and parathormone positivity (129), and Schmidt et al. (193) and Parham et al. (160) found neuron-specific enolase (NSE) positivity in a majority of cases.

One must be aware that not all renal tumors with a rhabdoid appearance are actually rhabdoid tumors. Weeks et al. (231) described 14 cases of these "pseudorhabdoid" tumors; they consisted of tumors lacking prominent nucleoli, cases with a serpentine growth pattern, cases with rhabdoid cells occurring in otherwise

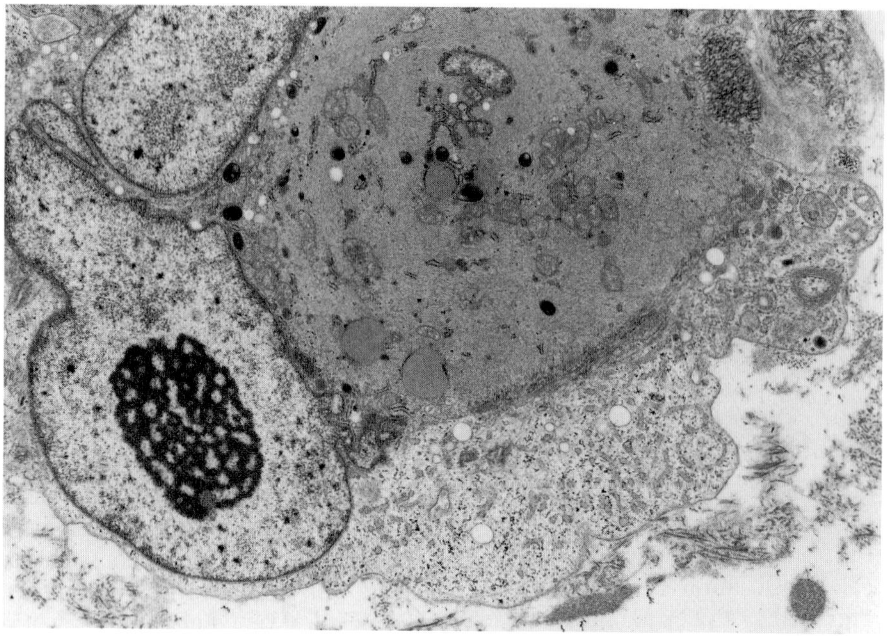

FIG. 29. Electron micrograph of malignant rhabdoid tumor. There is a large cytoplasmic inclusion composed of intermediate filaments and entrapped organelles.

typical Wilms' tumors, and, most importantly from a differential standpoint, cases of cellular congenital mesoblastic nephroma. The diagnostic boundary between malignant rhabdoid tumor and renal cell carcinoma also can be very fine. We have seen a renal tumor occurring in an adolescent patient and appearing to be composed of rhabdoid elements; however, consultants rendered opposing diagnoses of rhabdoid tumor and renal cell carcinoma. Another recent tumor in a 7-year-old boy had both rhabdoid cells and glandular elements, so that a diagnosis of renal cell carcinoma was rendered. However, the child unfortunately expired from his disease in a matter of a few months, an outcome quite reminiscent of rhabdoid tumors. Another rapidly fatal rhabdoidlike tumor occurring in an older child was discovered to be neuroendocrine in origin.

Extrarenal Rhabdoid Tumor

Even more controversial is the nature of the rhabdoid tumors described in extrarenal sites, such as the liver, prostate, heart, pelvis, paravertebral region, soft tissues, vulva, orbit, uterus, skin, and brain (161). Although reports of these extrarenal tumors keep appearing with a steady frequency, some authors are loathe to agree that they share any histogenetic relationship with the renal neoplasm, which appears to arise from primitive precursor cells in the renal medulla and sinus (230). Histologically, they are similar if not identical to renal rhabdoid tumors, being composed of cells with prominent nucleoli, abundant cytoplasm, and hyaline inclusions. The resemblance extends to their ultrastructural appearance, which shares a recurring motif of cytoplasmic whorls of intermediate filaments. When considering this diagnosis, one must be particularly mindful of unusual metastatic presentations of renal rhabdoid tumors (1).

Immunohistochemical findings in extrarenal rhabdoid tumors have been as diverse as those in renal tumors, but the most characteristic finding again appears to be vimentin and cytokeratin coexpression (53,161, 216). Although it is tempting to hypothesize that rhabdoid tumors are primitive carcinomas arising in organs such as kidney, liver and prostate, the origin of these lesions remains puzzling. The distinction of the soft tissue lesions from epithelioid sarcomas has been especially problematic, as they have similar morphologic and immunohistochemical features. However, putative extrarenal rhabdoid tumors should lack the multinodular, granulomalike pattern of epithelioid sarcomas and pursue a more aggressive biologic behavior (167). An intriguing observation is that of Tsuneyoshi et al., who observed areas of typical rhabdoid tumor in otherwise classified sarcomas (217). Similar features have been observed in epithelioid peripheral nerve sheath tumors (112), endometrial stromal sarcoma (57), a benign pelvic soft tissue neoplasm (145) and rhabdomyosarcomas submitted to the Intergroup Rhabdomyosarcoma Study (100), presenting a formidable diagnostic problem usually resolvable with electron microscopy, immunohistochemistry, and cytogenetic analysis (161).

Numerous carcinomas also contain cells similar to those of rhabdoid tumor. These include carcinomas of the thyroid, kidney, endometrium (131), colon (33), and

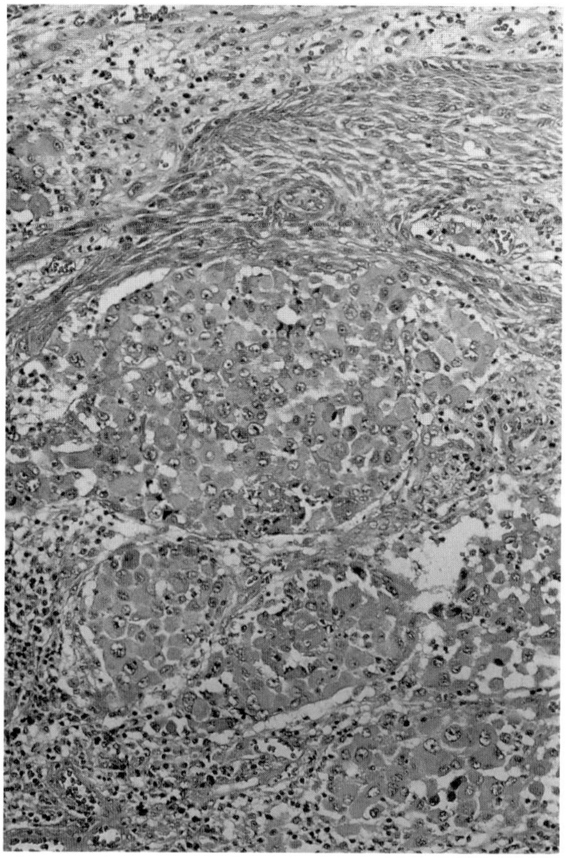

FIG. 31. Malignant melanoma containing rhabdoid cells.

urinary bladder (83). A metastatic melanoma with a rhabdoid phenotype (Fig. 31) has also been reported (17), as has a vulvar carcinoma (104), raising significant questions about many of the extrarenal rhabdoid tumors reported in the literature. In the review by Parham, Weeks, and Beckwith of 42 cases of extrarenal rhabdoid tumors gleaned from the files of St. Jude and NWTS (161), three major categories were apparent: tumors of diverse histologic types that contained rhabdoid cells, cases in which material was insufficient for detailed immunohistochemical and electron microscopic examination, and lesions of indeterminate histogenesis. It is this latter group that may constitute a unique entity, pending further analysis.

Cytogenetics of Rhabdoid Tumor

A number of cell lines and explants have been established from rhabdoid tumors and cytogenetic studies performed. Rhabdoid tumors of the brain characteristically have a monosomy 22 (16,50). A cell line derived from a paraspinal rhabdoid tumor, with immunostaining revealing positivity for vimentin, cytokeratin, actin, and desmin, had a karyotype with a t(18;22)(q21;p11.2). Culturing the cells in the presence of 1-β-D-arabinofuranosylcytosine induced neuronlike differentiation (81). In the renal rhabdoid cell line established by Gansler et al. (64), however, the differentiation-inducing agents TPA, nerve growth factor, and cAMP had no apparent effect on the microscopic features of the cells. Insulinlike growth factor–II was detected, analogous to Wilms' tumor, but *c-myc* rather that *N-myc* was expressed. In addition, the Wilms' tumor gene *WT1* was not detected (Garvin, personal communication). Somewhat paradoxically, the same investigators (64) more recently demonstrated that a cell line initially identified as Wilms' tumor, whose tumorigenicity was suppressed by insertion of a normal chromosome 11 (235), is actually a malignant rhabdoid tumor. The initial experiment was performed to demonstrate the integral function of chromosome 11 in Wilms' tumor development, but the conclusion now appears to apply to rhabdoid tumor.

In the St. Jude Hospital series of 10 rhabdoid tumor explants from a variety of sites, six cases had normal karyotypes, one case with an initially normal karyotype developed a del(13)(q14), a soft tissue tumor contained a t(8;15)(q12;p11), a liver tumor contained a del(3)(p21), and a single case of a brain tumor had monosomy 22 (50). These findings correlate well with the ploidy data of Schmidt et al., who found no aneuploid DNA stem lines as determined by flow cytometry (193). Recently, retroperitoneal and renal tumors which share an abnormality at chromosome 22q11.2 have been reported (156); the breakpoint on chromosome 22 is similar to that found in two brain tumors (16,50), suggesting that this group may be a unique entity. The *WT2* gene of Beckwith–Wiedemann syndrome appears to be involved in one rhabdoid tumor cell line, but *EWS* or *WT1* are not (147,188). More recently, involvement of chromosome 22 has been reported in a rhabdoid tumor of the kidney (199), indicating that some extrarenal and renal rhabdoid tumors are genetically related. However, there are contradictory data (58).

RENAL CELL CARCINOMA IN CHILDREN

Renal cell carcinoma (RCC) is typically a tumor of adulthood that rarely and often unexpectedly (244) occurs in children (23,26,29,46,109,158,173,227). The clinical features of RCC are protean (139,142) and will not be further discussed here. Suffice it to say that RCC is appropriately termed the "internists' tumor" because of the wide variety of manifestations caused by its local and paraneoplastic effects (142). Of particular note is the association of von Hippel–Lindau syndrome with RCC, as renal cell neoplasms often occur at a relatively young age in patients affected with this tumor complex (142). In children with bilateral RCC, this association is an even greater possibility (227).

Because they are unexpected causes of renal masses,

RCC may cause diagnostic confusion even at surgery. The author has personally encountered two neoplasms whose purulent-appearing liquefaction necrosis and discoloration grossly resembled a renal abscess. In both of these cases, the correct diagnosis was made only by close histologic examination of the necrotic areas, which contained ghosts of cells arranged in a papillary configuration. This propensity for mistaken identity is further caused by the relatively smaller size of pediatric RCC as compared to Wilms' tumor (227).

The cytohistologic features of RCC are well characterized (Fig. 32) (142,210) and have been related to prognosis in a number of adult series (60,208). This observation also holds in children, in whom well-differentiated clear cell tumors exhibit less aggressiveness than granular cell lesions (46). One caveat in this regard, however, is that granular RCC must be distinguished from renal oncocytomas, which are benign lesions (7,132). A diagnostically useful feature is the presence of cytokeratin-positive filamentous bodies in the cytoplasm of oncocytomas (22). Ironically, these filamentous bodies are reminiscent of rhabdoid tumor, so that the presence of a diffuse organoid pattern, absence of hemorrhage, necrosis, pleomorphism, ballooned cytoplasm, or clear cells, and characteristic tan gross appearance of oncocytoma must also be considered (7). Of particular note is the patient's age, as rhabdoid tumors are extremely rare outside of infancy, and oncocytomas are rare in children. Clear cell carcinomalike elements may also be encountered in Wilms' tumors (9).

A variety of cytogenetic aberrations have been described in RCC, and in fact genetic analysis has been proposed as a method for classification (103). In this system, nonpapillary RCC are characterized by 3p and 14q deletions and 5q rearrangements, papillary renal adenoma by trisomy 7 and 17 and loss of Y, papillary RCC by trisomy 16, 20, or 12, chromophobe RCC by diverse, exclusive allelic losses and rearrangements of mitochondrial DNA, and renal oncocytomas by normal or abnormal karyotypes with translocations and altered restriction of mitochondrial DNA. However, another study failed to find an association between RCC cytogenetics and stage, grade, or aggressiveness (73). A family with heritable RCC that occurred at an early age was notable for a balanced, reciprocal t(3;8)(p21;q24) in their constitutional genotype (34). Additional genetic events that appear to be associated with tumor progression also occur in this family (45).

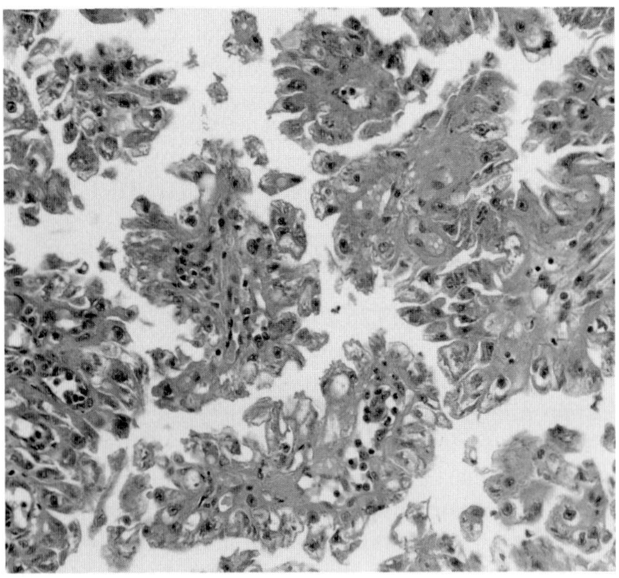

FIG. 32. Renal cell carcinoma arising in a pediatric patient. The tumor is composed of papillary clusters of tumor cells with clear cytoplasm.

The past decade has seen great strides in the molecular characterization of the genetic and molecular events responsible for cancer susceptibility. Pertinent to this chapter is the gene responsible for the von Hippel–Lindau syndrome. Beside RCC, von Hippel–Lindau syndrome is associated with pheochromocytoma, cerebellar hemangioblastoma, angiomas of the retina, cerebellum, and brain stem, cysts of the pancreas, liver, kidney, and epididymus, cystadenomas of the epididymus and ovarian adnexa, and an aggressive papillary tumor of the middle ear/temporal bone (61,111). As with the majority of cancer syndromes, von Hippel–Lindau syndrome is inherited in an autosomal dominant fashion. Cytogenetic analyses of the RCC occurring with this disease have revealed deletion of 3p as a primary alteration, with other secondary changes (92). Further genetic studies have isolated a tumor suppressor gene, *VHL,* that occurs at 3p25 and is deleted in sporadic RCC and those occurring in von Hippel–Lindau patients (40,200). Inactivation of both alleles of this gene appears necessary for tumorigenesis in either situation (40). Identification of this genetic alteration offers the opportunity for screening of potentially affected patients (111).

ANGIOMYOLIPOMA

Angiomyolipoma of the kidney is associated with another tumor susceptibility syndrome, tuberous sclerosis. In this clinical setting, angiomyolipoma is extremely common and often bilateral and multifocal (139). Renal neoplasms seen with tuberous sclerosis are usually discovered in childhood or adolescence and so have particular relevance to pediatric renal neoplasia. More often, however, angiomyolipomas occur in adults with no clinical evidence of this syndrome (139).

As implied for their name, angiomyolipomas are composed of a mixture of blood vessels, smooth muscle, and fat (Fig. 33) and are thus heterogeneous in gross and microscopic appearance. Fatty elements impart a yellow greasy element, myogenic elements a grey fleshy compo-

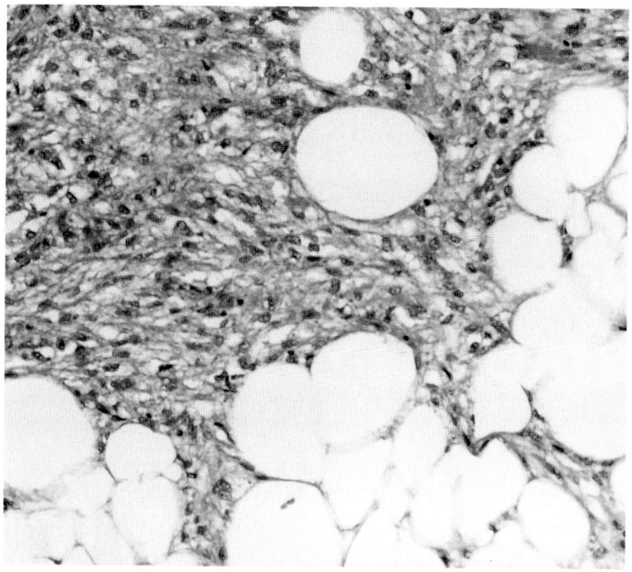

FIG. 33. Angiomyolipoma of kidney, containing fat cells and epithelioid smooth muscle cells. (Courtesy of Dr. Mahmoud El-Torky, University of Tennessee, Memphis.)

nent, and vascular elements a hemorrhagic portion. By light microscopy, the smooth muscle and vascular components are typically intertwined, with vessels occurring in tortuous bundles. The presence of nuclear pleomorphism and cytoplasmic vacuolization in the smooth muscle cells create features dissimilar to the cytology of normal smooth muscle, but mitoses are rare. The adipocytes may also appear atypical and exhibit anisocytosis and lipoblastoid features. The relative percentage of the three basic cytologic elements varies from case to case. Despite the benignancy of these lesions, degenerative phenomena such as hemorrhage, necrosis, and thrombosis are common (139).

One unexpected phenotypic feature of angiomyolipoma is its positivity for the melanoma-associated marker, HMB45 (30,215). Expression of this protein occurs in a perimembranous fashion in the epithelioid smooth muscle cells of this tumor. Not unexpectedly, these tumors also express desmin and muscle-specific actin (30). Another recently described feature of the epithelioid smooth muscle cells is their content of PAS-positive, diastase-resistant crystalloids that are not apparent with hematoxylin and eosin stains (140). Tumors associated with multiple hamartomas in the adjacent kidney, extending into adjacent renal parenchyma, or containing calcified spicules or tubular inclusions are more likely to be associated with tuberous sclerosis (218).

UNUSUAL PEDIATRIC RENAL NEOPLASMS

Ossifying Tumor of the Infantile Kidney

This tumor, described by Chatten in 1980 (32), is characterized by the abundant production of bone and osteoid (Fig. 34), which render the lesions stony-hard in consistency and brightly radiopaque with diagnostic imaging. They typically occur in the region of the renal pelvis of very young children, contain cytologically bland but invasive tumor cells, and have a benign clinical behavior (227).

Renal Medullary Carcinoma

Renal medullary carcinoma is a newly described entity that has been called the seventh sickle cell nephropathy because of its association with sickle cell trait or hemoglobin SC disease (42). Characteristically, this tumor occurs in adolescent and young adult black patients with gross hematuria or flank pain. As the name implies, these neoplasms occur in the medulla. Microscopically they have a reticular, yolk sac tumorlike, or adenoid cystic appearance, often with a dense fibroblastic stroma (Fig. 35). Of note is their frequent content of rhabdoid cells. The presence of sickled erythrocytes within blood vessels (Fig. 35, inset) offers an important clue to the diagnosis. Clinically, renal medullary carcinomas are highly malignant, with metastases usually evident at the time of clinical presentation. The mean duration of life after excision is 15 weeks, and no patients have survived to date.

Neural Tumors of the Kidney

Primitive neuroectodermal tumors (PNET) are embryonic neoplasms that arise from neural crest cells and are described in depth in Chapter 4. These tumors may rarely arise within the kidney (180,198), where their primitive histologic appearance can easily be confused

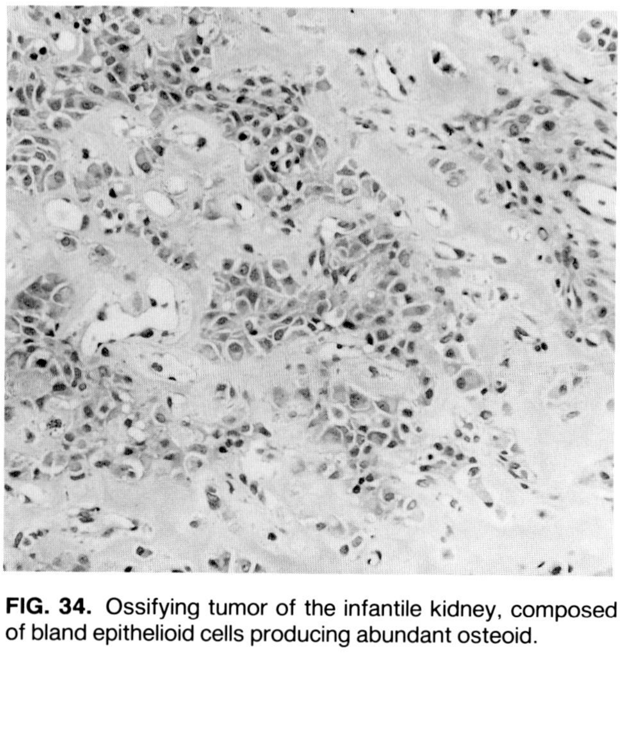

FIG. 34. Ossifying tumor of the infantile kidney, composed of bland epithelioid cells producing abundant osteoid.

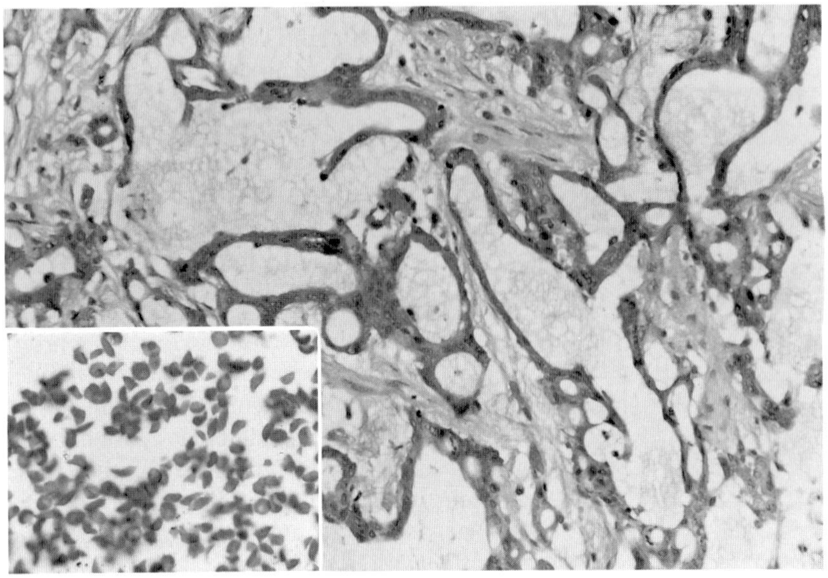

FIG. 35. Medullary carcinoma of the kidney, containing primitive glands in a yolk sac tumorlike arrangement, embedded in a fibrous stroma. Elsewhere, sickled erythrocytes were apparent (*inset*).

with that of blastemal Wilms' tumor. Aggravating this dilemma is the not-uncommon occurrence of rosettes, the histologic sine qua non of PNET, in Wilms' tumor. As noted above, the presence of neural elements within Wilms' tumors led to Masson's hypothesis that they are neuroectodermal in origin rather than mesoblastic (127). At any rate, PNET does occur in pure form as a renal neoplasm (Fig. 36) and may be responsible for some misdiagnoses of Wilms' tumor in adults (241). MIC2, the PNET/Ewing's sarcoma marker, may aid in identification of PNET of the kidney (180), as the blastemal component of Wilms' tumors is negative (234). Tubular elements, however, may stain positively (234). The distinction of renal PNET from Wilms' tumors is essential for proper patient management, as the therapy and prognosis of the two lesions is dramatically different. Besides PNET, carcinoid, paraganglioma, and neuroblastoma may occur within the kidney (159,174,180).

Juxtaglomerular Cell Tumor

Juxtaglomerular cell tumors are extremely rare neoplasms but cause dramatic clinical symptoms because of renin secretion. These symptoms are due to the hypertension, hyperaldosteronism, and hypokalemia resulting from the hyperreninemia and are eminently curable by surgical excision. Hyperreninemia may be seen with other pediatric neoplasms, such as mesoblastic nephroma, but is invariable with juxtaglomerular cell tumor (101). Juxtaglomerular cell tumors typically are small intrarenal lesions that occur in adolescents and

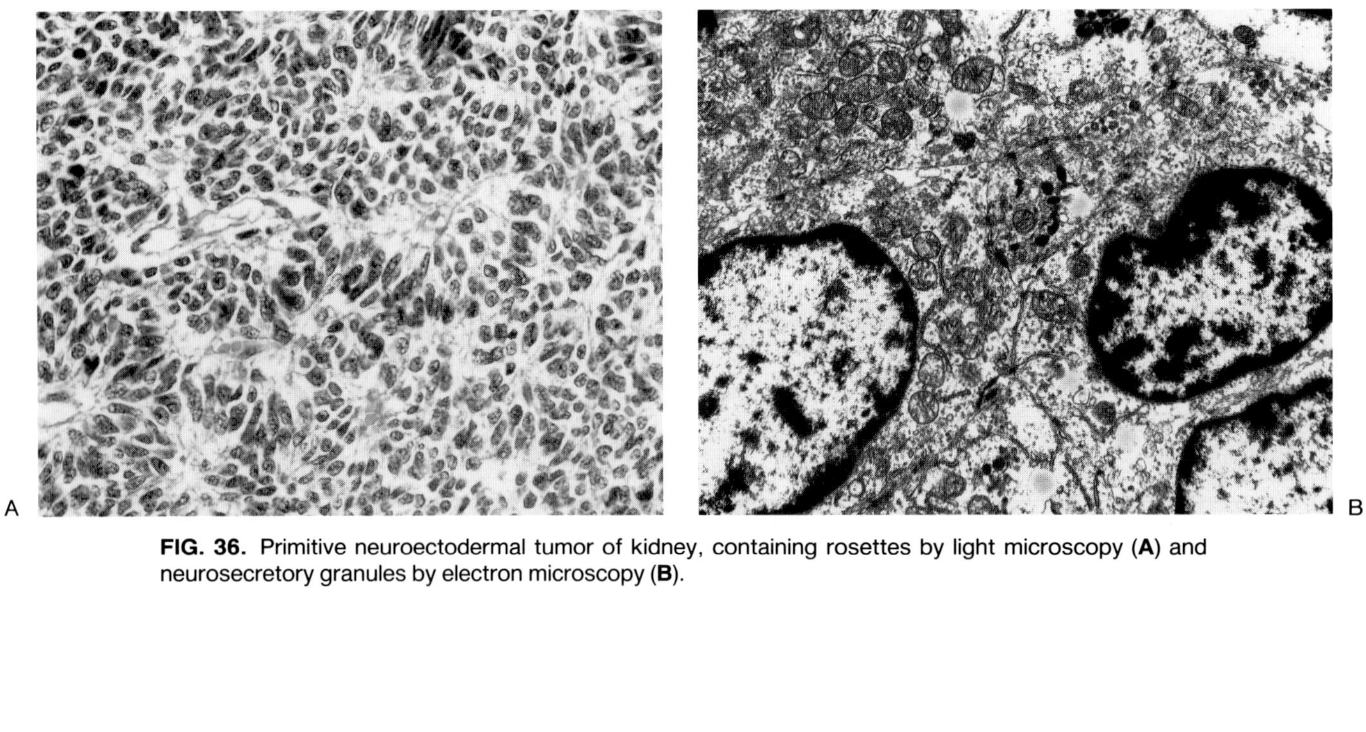

FIG. 36. Primitive neuroectodermal tumor of kidney, containing rosettes by light microscopy (**A**) and neurosecretory granules by electron microscopy (**B**).

young adults (101). A tumor cell line has been established (152).

Microscopically, juxtaglomerular cell tumors present a hemangiopericytomalike pattern of vascular sinusoids separated by cords of polygonal cells with clear cytoplasm, sometimes containing PAS-positive cytoplasmic granules. Mast cells may be prominent. Electron microscopy reveals a well-formed basal lamina, abundant Golgi complexes, and rhomboid and polygonal cytoplasmic granules, sometimes within Golgi cisternae (101,206). Immunohistochemical positivity can be demonstrated with antibodies against muscle-specific actin, smooth muscle actin, vimentin, and renin (101).

One important diagnostic consideration with juxtaglomerular cell tumor is to avoid confusion with clear cell sarcoma of the kidney (CCSK), which also has a hemangiopericytomalike appearance (see above). Besides the clinical features, clues to the diagnosis of juxtaglomerular cell tumor include the characteristic granules seen with PAS-staining and electron microscopy and the actin positivity, which is not a feature of CCSK. This is a highly important distinction because juxtaglomerular cell tumors are benign lesions, although they may be locally invasive (101,206).

Nephrogenic Adenofibroma

Nephrogenic adenofibroma is an extremely rare tumor described in 1992 by Hennigar and Beckwith (85), who reported a series of five patients culled from approximately 7,000 cases in the NWTS Pathology Center files. These lesions occur in young patients (mean age 13 years) and are not associated with metastatic disease or renal vein extension despite their lack of encapsulation. They have a distinctive histology (Fig. 37) composed of well-circumscribed nodules of embryonal epithelium with tubular, tubulopapillary, and papillary differentiation. Psammoma bodies are plentiful but mitoses and nuclear atypia are absent. These epithelial nodules are enmeshed in a mesoblastic nephromalike spindle cell stroma. They may contain foci of low grade collecting duct carcinoma near the renal pelvis. These tumors must be differentiated from Wilms' tumors with fibroadenomatous areas, which are otherwise typical Wilms' tumors (47,227), albeit with a good prognosis.

Miscellaneous Soft Tissue Neoplasms

As with adults (75,225), soft tissue sarcomas of various types may rarely be encountered in the kidneys of children.The author recently saw a pediatric renal fibroxanthosarcoma that contained xanthoma-type cells with a superficial resemblance of those of CCSK. They exhibited strong immunopositivity with antibodies against α_1-antichymotrypsin and CD56. Soft tissue neoplasms reported in adult kidneys include fibrosarcoma, malignant fibrous histiocytoma, myxoid liposarcoma, leiomyosarcomas, angiosarcomas, and hemangiopericytoma. These renal tumors are vanishingly rare in children in our experience.

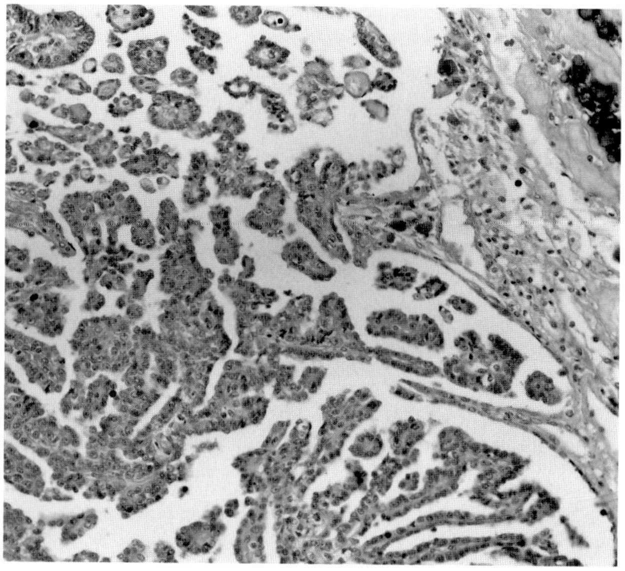

Fig. 37. Nephrogenic adenofibroma, composed of abundant, well-formed papillae lined by bland epithelium. Note the calcification in the upper right.

ACKNOWLEDGMENTS

Supported by National Cancer Institute (NCI) Center Support Grant P30 CA217657 and American Lebanese Syrian Associated Charities (ALSAC).

REFERENCES

1. Akhtar M, Ali MA, Sackey K, Bakry M, Johnson T. Malignant rhabdoid tumor of the kidney presenting as intraocular metastasis. *Pediatr Hematol Oncol* 1991;8:33–43.
2. Akhtar M, Kott E, Brooks B. Extrarenal Wilms' tumor: report of a case and review of the literature. *Cancer* 1977;40:3087–3091.
3. Albeda FW, Molenaar WM, De Leij L, Thijs-Ipema AH. Heterogeneity of Wilms' tumour blastema. An immunohistological study. *Virchows Arch A Histopathol Anat* 1989;414:263–271.
4. Altmannsberger M, Osborn M, Schafer H, Schauer A, Weber K. Distinction of nephroblastomas from other childhood tumors using antibodies to intermediate filaments. *Virchows Arch B Cell Pathol* 1984;45:113–124.
5. Bannayan GA, Huvos AG, D'Angio GJ. Effect of irradiation on the maturation of Wilms' tumor. *Cancer* 1971;27:812–818.
6. Bard JBL, Armstrong JF, Bickmore WA. WT1, a Wilms' tumour gene. *Exp Nephrol* 1993;1:218–223.
7. Barnes CA, Beckman EN. Renal oncocytoma and its congeners. *Am J Clin Pathol* 1983;79:312–318.
8. Beckwith JB. Mesenchymal renal neoplasms of infancy revisited. *J Pediatr Surg* 1974;9:803–805.
9. Beckwith JB. Wilms' tumors and other renal tumors of childhood. In: Finegold, M, ed. *Major Problems in Pathology. vol. 18. Pathology of Neoplasia in Children and Adolescents.* Philadelphia: WB Saunders; 1986:313–332.

10. Beckwith JB. Renal neoplasms of childhood. In: Sternberg, SS, ed. *Diagnostic Surgical Pathology*. New York: Raven Press; 1989: 1331–1353.
11. Beckwith JB, Kiviat NB, Bonadio JF. Nephrogenic rests, nephroblastomatosis, and the pathogenesis of Wilms' tumor. *Pediatr Pathol* 1990; 10:1–36.
12. Beckwith JB, Larson E. Case 7. Clear cell sarcoma of kidney. *Pediatr Pathol* 1989;9:211–218.
13. Beckwith JB, Palmer NF. Histopathology and prognosis of Wilms tumors: results from the First National Wilms' Tumor Study. *Cancer* 1978;41:1937–1948.
14. Beckwith JB, Weeks DA. Congenital mesoblastic nephroma: when should we worry? *Arch Pathol Lab Med* 1986; 110:98–99.
15. Bennington JL, Beckwith JB. *Atlas of Tumor Pathology. Second Series, Fascicle 12. Tumors of the Kidney, Renal Pelvis, and Ureter.* Washington, D.C.: Armed Forces Institute of Pathology; 1975.
16. Biegel JA, Rorke LB, Emanuel BS. Monosomy 22 in rhabdoid or atypical teratoid tumors of the brain. *N Engl J Med* 1989;321: 906.
17. Bittesini L, Dei Tos AP, Fletcher CDM. Metastatic malignant melanoma showing a rhabdoid phenotype: Further evidence of a non-specific histological pattern. *Histopathology* 1992;20:167–170.
18. Blank E, Neerhout RC, Burry KA. Congenital mesoblastic nephroma and polyhydramnios. *JAMA* 1978;240:1504–1505.
19. Bolande RP. Congenital mesoblastic nephroma of infancy. *Perspect Pediatr Pathol* 1973; 1:227–250.
20. Bolande RP, Brough AJ, Izant RJ, Jr. Congenital mesoblastic nephroma of infancy. A report of eight cases and the relationship to Wilms' tumor. *Pediatrics* 1967;40:272–278.
21. Bonadio JF, Storer B, Norkool P, Farewell VT, Beckwith JB, D'Angio GJ. Anaplastic Wilms' tumor: clinical and pathologic studies. *J Clin Oncol* 1985;3:513–520.
22. Bonsib SM, Bromley C, Lager DJ. Renal oncocytoma: diagnostic utility of cytokeratin-containing globular filamentous bodies. *Mod Pathol* 1991;4:16–23.
23. Booth CM. Renal parenchymal carcinoma in children. *Br J Surg* 1986;73:313–317.
24. Bove KE, McAdams AJ. The nephroblastomatosis complex and its relationship to Wilms' tumor: a clinicopathologic treatise. *Perspect Pediatr Pathol* 1976;3:185–223.
25. Breslow N, Sharples K, Beckwith JB, Takashima J, Kelalis PP, Green DM, D'Angio GJ. Prognostic factors in nonmetastatic, favorable histology Wilms' tumor: results of the Third National Wilms' Tumor Study. *Cancer* 1991;68:2345–2353.
26. Broecker B. Renal cell carcinoma in children. *Urology* 1991;38: 54–56.
27. Brown KW, Gardner A, Williams JC, Mott MG, McDermott A, Maitland NJ. Paternal origin of 11p15 duplications in the Beckwith–Wiedemann syndrome. A new case and review of the literature. *Cancer Genet Cytogenet* 1992;58:66–70.
28. Call KM, Glaser T, Ito CY, et al. Isolation and characterization of a zinc finger polypeptide gene at the human chromosome 11 Wilms' tumor locus. *Cell* 1990;60:509–520.
29. Chan HS, Daneman A, Gribbin M, Martin DJ. Renal cell carcinoma in the first two decades of life. *Pediatr Radiol* 1983; 13:324–328.
30. Chan JKC, Tsang WYW, Pau MY, Tang MC, Pang SW, Fletcher CDM. Lymphangiomyomatosis and angiomyolipoma: closely related entities characterized by hamartomatous proliferation of HMB-45-positive smooth muscle. *Histopathology* 1993;22:445–455.
31. Chatten J. Epithelial differentiation in Wilms' tumor: a clinicopathologic appraisal. *Perspect Pediatr Pathol* 1976;3:225–254.
32. Chatten J, Cromie WJ, Duckett JW. Ossifying tumor of infantile kidney: report of two cases. *Cancer* 1980;45:609–612.
33. Chetty R, Bhathal PS. Caecal adenocarcinoma with rhabdoid phenotype: an immunohistochemical and ultrastructural analysis. *Virchows Arch A Histopathol Anat* 1993;422:179–182.
34. Cohen AJ, Li FP, Berg S, Marchetto DJ, Tsai S, Jacobs SC, Brown RS. Hereditary renal-cell carcinoma associated with a chromosomal translocation. *N Engl J Med* 1979;301:592–595.
35. Cook HT, Taylor GM, Malone P, Risdon RA. Renin in mesoblastic nephroma: an immunohistochemical study. *Hum Pathol* 1988;19:1347–1351.
36. Coppes MJ, Williams BRG. The molecular genetics of Wilms tumor. *Cancer Invest* 1994; 12:57–65.
37. Coppes MJ, Wilson PCG, Weitzman S. Extrarenal Wilms' tumor: staging, treatment, and prognosis. *J Clin Oncol* 1991;9:167–174.
38. Cosentino CM, Raffensperger JG, Luck SR, Reynolds M, Sherman JO, Reyes-Mugica M. A 25-year experience with renal tumors of childhood. *J Pediatr Surg* 1993;28:1350–1355.
39. Crocker JF, Vernier RL. Congenital nephroma of infancy: induction of renal structures by organ culture. *J Pediatr* 1972;80:69–73.
40. Crossey PA, Foster K, Richards FM, et al. Molecular genetic investigations of the mechanism of tumourigenesis in von Hippel–Lindau disease: analysis of allele loss in VHL tumours. *Hum Genet* 1994;93:53–58.
41. D'Angio GJ, Breslow N, Beckwith JB, et al. Treatment of Wilms' tumor: results of the Third National Wilms' Tumor Study. *Cancer* 1989;64:349–360.
42. Davis CJ, Mostofi FK, Sesterhenn IA. Renal medullary carcinoma: the seventh sickle cell nephropathy. *Am J Surg Pathol* 1995;19:1–11.
43. Davis LM, Stallard R, Thomas GH, Couillin P, Junien C, Nowak NJ, Shows TB. Two anonymous DNA segments distinguish the Wilms' tumor and aniridia loci. *Science* 1988;241:840–842.
44. de Chadarevian JP, Fletcher BD, Chatten J, Rabinovitch HH. Massive infantile nephroblastomatosis: a clinical, radiological, and pathological analysis of four cases. *Cancer* 1977;39:2294–2305.
45. Decker H-JH, Wullich B, Whaley JM, et al. Cytogenetic and molecular studies of a familial renal cell carcinoma. *Cancer Genet Cytogenet* 1992;63:25–31.
46. Dehner LP, Leestma JE, Price EB, Jr. Renal cell carcinoma in children: a clinicopathologic study of 15 cases and review of the literature. *J Pediatr* 1970;76:358–368.
47. Delemarre JFM, Sandstedt B, Tournade MF. Nephroblastoma with fibroadenomatous-like structures. *Histopathology* 1984;8: 55–62.
48. Denk H, Weybora W, Ratschek M, Sohar R, Franke WW. Distribution of vimentin, cytokeratins, and desmosomal-plaque proteins in human nephroblastoma as revealed by specific antibodies: co-existence of cell groups of different degrees of epithelial differentiation. *Differentiation* 1985;29:88–97.
49. Douglass EC, Look AT, Webber B, Parham D, Wilimas JA, Green AA, Roberson PK. Hyperdiploidy and chromosomal rearrangements define the anaplastic variant of Wilms' tumor. *J Clin Oncol* 1986;4:975–981.
50. Douglass EC, Valentine M, Rowe ST, Parham DM, Wilimas JA, Sanders JM, Houghton PJ. Malignant rhabdoid tumor: a highly malignant childhood tumor with minimal karyotypic changes. *Genes Chrom. Cancer* 1990;2:210–216.
51. Dowdy SF, Fasching CL, Araujo D, Lai K-M, Livanos E, Weissman BE, Stanbridge EJ. Suppression of tumorigenicity in Wilms tumor by the p15.5-p14 region of chromosome 11. *Science* 1991;254:293–295.
52. Drummond IA, Madden SL, Rohwer-Nutter P, Bell GI, Sukhatme VP, Rauscher FJ, III. Repression of the insulin-like growth factor II gene by the Wilms tumor suppressor WT1. *Science* 1992;257:674–678.
53. Ekfors TO, Aho HJ, Kekomaki M. Malignant rhabdoid tumor of the prostatic region. Immunohistological and ultrastructural evidence for epithelial origin. *Virchows Arch A Histopathol Anat* 1985;406:381–388.
54. Favara BE, Johnson W, Ito J. Renal tumors in the neonatal period. *Cancer* 1968;22:845–855.
55. Fernandes ET, Kumar M, Douglass EC, Wilimas J, Parham DM, Rao BN. Extrarenal Wilms' tumor. *J Pediatr Surg* 1989;24:483–485.
56. Fernandes ET, Parham DM, Ribeiro RC, Douglass EC, Kumar AP, Wilimas J. Teratoid Wilms' tumor: the St Jude experience. *J Pediatr Surg* 1988;23:1131–1134.
57. Fitko R, Brainer J, Schink JC, August CZ. Endometrial stromal sarcoma with rhabdoid differentiation [letter]. *Int J Gynecol Pathol* 1990;9:379–382.

58. Fort DW, Tonk VS, Tomlinson GE, Timmons CF, Schneider NR. Rhabdoid tumor of the kidney with primitive neuroectodermal tumor of the central nervous system: associated tumors with different histologic, cytogenetic, and molecular findings. *Genes Chrom Cancer* 1994;11:146–152.
59. Fu Y, Kay S. Congenital mesoblastic nephroma and its recurrence. *Arch Pathol* 1973;96:66–70.
60. Fuhrman SA, Lasky LC, Limas C. Prognostic significance of morphologic parameters in renal cell carcinoma. *Am J Surg Pathol* 1982;6:655–663.
61. Gaffey MJ, Mills SE, Boyd JC. Aggressive papillary tumor of middle ear/temporal bone and adnexal papillary cystadenoma. Manifestations of von Hippel–Lindau disease. *Am J Surg Pathol* 1994;18:1254–1260.
62. Gansler T, Allen KD, Burant CF, et al. Detection of type 1 insulinlike growth factor (IGF) receptors in Wilms' tumors. *Am J Pathol* 1988;130:431–435.
63. Gansler T, Furlanetto R, Gramling TS, et al. Antibody to type I insulinlike growth factor receptor inhibits growth of Wilms' tumor in culture and in athymic mice. *Am J Pathol* 1989;135:961–966.
64. Gansler T, Gerald W, Anderson G, Gramling TS, Williams CH, Sens D, Garvin AJ. Characterization of a cell line derived from rhabdoid tumor of kidney. *Hum Pathol* 1991;22:259–266.
65. Garvin AJ, Hazen-Martin DJ, Sens DA. The in vitro differentiation of congenital mesoblastic nephroma (CMN) into epithelial cells. *Mod Pathol* 1991;4:108A (Abstract).
66. Garvin AJ, Re GG, Tarnowski BI, Hazen-Martin DJ, Sens DA. The G401 cell line, utilized for studies of chromosomal changes in Wilms' tumor, is derived from a rhabdoid tumor of the kidney. *Am J Pathol* 1993;142:375–380.
67. Gerald WL, Miller HK, Battifora H, Miettinen M, Silva EG, Rosai J. Intra-abdominal desmoplastic small round-cell tumor: report of 19 cases of a distinctive type of high-grade polyphenotypic malignancy affecting young individuals. *Am J Surg Pathol* 1991;15:499–513.
68. Gonzalez-Crussi F. *Wilms' Tumor (Nephroblastoma) and Related Renal Neoplasms of Childhood.* Boca Raton: CRC Press; 1984.
69. Gonzalez-Crussi F, Baum ES. Renal sarcomas of childhood. A clinicopathologic and ultrastructural study. *Cancer* 1983;51: 898–912.
70. Gonzalez-Crussi F, Goldschmidt RA, Hsueh W, Trujillo YP. Infantile sarcoma with intracytoplasmic filamentous inclusions: distinctive tumor of possible histiocytic origin. *Cancer* 1982;49: 2365–2375.
71. Gonzalez-Crussi F, Hsueh W, Ugarte N. Rhabdomyogenesis in renal neoplasia of childhood. *Am J Surg Pathol* 1981;5:525–531.
72. Gonzalez-Crussi F, Sotelo-Avila C, Kidd JM. Malignant mesenchymal nephroma of infancy: report of a case with pulmonary metastases. *Am J Surg Pathol* 1980;4:185–190.
73. Granata P, Portentoso P, Minelli E, et al. Clonal chromosome changes in renal carcinoma do not correlate with clinical stages and histopathologic grades. *Cancer Genet Cytogenet* 1992;64:30–34.
74. Green DM, Finklestein JZ, Breslow NE, Beckwith JB. Remaining problems in the treatment of patients with Wilms' tumor. *Pediatr Clin North Am* 1991;38:475–488.
75. Grignon DJ, Ayala AG, Ro JY, El-Naggar A, Papadopoulos NJ. Primary sarcomas of the kidney: A clinicopathologic and DNA flow cytometric study of 17 cases. *Cancer* 1990;65:1611–1618.
76. Grundy PE, Telzerow PE, Breslow N, Moksness J, Huff V, Paterson MC. Loss of heterozygosity for chromosomes 16q and 1p in Wilms' tumors predicts an adverse outcome. *Cancer Res* 1994;54:2331–2333.
77. Gururangan S, Dorman A, Ball R, Curran B, Leader M, Breatnach F, O'Meara A. DNA quantitation of Wilms' tumour (nephroblastoma) using flow cytometry and image analysis. *J Clin Pathol* 1992;45:498–501.
78. Haas JE, Bonadio JF, Beckwith JB. Clear cell sarcoma of the kidney with emphasis on ultrastructural studies. *Cancer* 1984;54: 2978–2987.
79. Haas JE, Palmer NF, Weinberg AG, Beckwith JB. Ultrastructure of malignant rhabdoid tumor of the kidney. A distinctive renal tumor of children. *Hum Pathol* 1981;12:646–657.
80. Haber DA, Housman DE. Role of the WT1 gene in Wilms' tumour. *Cancer Surv* 1992;12:105–117.
81. Handgretinger R, Kimmig A, Koscielnak E, et al. Establishment and characterization of a cell line (Wa-2) derived from an extrarenal rhabdoid tumor. *Cancer Res* 1990;50:2177–2182.
82. Harms D, Schmidt D, Leuschner I. Abdominal, retroperitoneal and sacrococcygeal tumours of the newborn and the very young infant. Report from the Kiel Paediatric Tumour Registry. *Eur J Pediatr* 1989;148:720–728.
83. Harris M, Eyden BP, Joglekar VM. Rhabdoid tumour of the bladder: a histological, ultrastructural and immunohistochemical study. *Histopathology* 1987;11:1083–1092.
84. Heidelberger KP, Ritchey ML, Dauser RC, McKeever PE, Beckwith JB. Congenital mesoblastic nephroma metastatic to the brain. *Cancer* 1993;72:2499–2502.
85. Hennigar RA, Beckwith JB. Nephrogenic adenofibroma: a novel kidney tumor of young people. *Am J Surg Pathol* 1992;16:325–334.
86. Higa TE, Mancer K, Thom H, Spicer P, Phillips MJ. Malignant rhabdoid tumor of infancy: an epithelial neoplasm. *Lab Invest* 1984;50:4P (Abstract).
87. Hsiao J-C, Yang C-P, Lin C-J, Chuen H. Ectopic ACTH syndrome due to clear cell sarcoma of the kidney. *Child Nephrol Urol* 1991;11:103–106.
88. Huff V, Saunders GF. Wilms tumor genes. *Biochim Biophys Acta Rev Cancer* 1993;1155:295–306.
89. Ishii E, Fujimoto J, Hara S, Tanaka S, Hata J. Human sarcomatous Wilms' tumor lines: evidence for epithelial differentiation in clear cell sarcoma of the kidney. *Cancer Res* 1989;49:5392–5399.
90. Ito J, Johnson WW. Ultrastructure of Wilms' tumor. I. Epithelial cell. *JNCI* 1969;42:77–99.
91. Jayabose S, Iqbal K, Newman L, San Filippo JA, Davidian MM, Noto R, Sagel I. Hypercalcemia in childhood renal tumors. *Cancer* 1988;61:788–791.
92. Jordan DK, Patil SR, Divelbiss JE, Vemuganti S, Headley C, Waziri MH, Gurll NJ. Cytogenetic abnormalities in tumors of patients with von Hippel–Lindau disease. *Cancer Genet Cytogenet* 1989;42:227–241.
93. Joshi VV, Banerjee AK, Yadav K, Pathak IC. Cystic partially differentiated nephroblastoma: a clinicopathologic entity in the spectrum of infantile renal neoplasia. *Cancer* 1977;40:789–795.
94. Joshi VV, Beckwith JB. Multilocular cyst of the kidney (cystic nephroma) and cystic, partially differentiated nephroblastoma: terminology and criteria for diagnosis. *Cancer* 1989;64:466–479.
95. Joshi VV, Beckwith JB. Pathologic delineation of the papillonodular type of cystic partially differentiated nephroblastoma: a review of 11 cases. *Cancer* 1990;66:1568–1577.
96. Joshi VV, Kasznica J, Walters TR. Atypical mesoblastic nephroma. Pathologic characterization of a potentially aggressive variant of conventional congenital mesoblastic nephroma. *Arch Pathol Lab Med* 1986;110:100–106.
97. Junien C. Beckwith–Wiedemann syndrome, tumourigenesis and imprinting. *Curr Opin Genet Dev* 1992;2:431–438.
98. Kataoka Y, Shimada H, Sugimoto T, et al. Congenital sarcoma in the terminal ileum histologically resembling clear cell sarcoma of the kidney: a case report with an immunohistochemical study. *Hum Pathol* 1993;24:1026–1030.
99. Knudson AG, Jr., Strong LC. Mutation and cancer: a model for Wilms' tumor of the kidney. *JNCI* 1972;48:313–324.
100. Kodet R, Newton WA, Jr., Hamoudi AB, Asmar L. Rhabdomyosarcomas with intermediate-filament inclusions and features of rhabdoid tumors: light microscopic and immunohistochemical study. *Am J Surg Pathol* 1991;15:257–267.
101. Kodet R, Taylor M, Vachalova H, Pycha K. Juxtaglomerular cell tumor. An immunohistochemical, electron-microscopic, and in situ hybridization study. *Am J Surg Pathol* 1994;18:837–842.
102. Koufos A, Hansen MF, Copeland NG, Jenkins NA, Lampkin BC, Cavenee WK. Loss of heterozygosity in three embryonal tumours suggests a common pathogenetic mechanism. *Nature* 1985;316:330–334.
103. Kovacs G. Molecular differential pathology of renal cell tumours. *Histopathology* 1993;22:1–8.
104. Kudo E, Hirose T, Fujii Y, Hasegawa T, Ino H, Hizawa K. Undifferentiated carcinoma of the vulva mimicking epithelioid sarcoma. *Am J Surg Pathol* 1991;15:990–1001.

105. Kumar S, Carr T, Marsden HB, Calabuig-Crespo MC. Study of childhood renal tumours using antisera to fibronectin, laminin, and epithelial membrane antigen. *J Clin Pathol* 1986;39:51–57.
106. Kumar S, Marsden HB, Carr T, Kodet R. Mesoblastic nephroma contains fibronectin but lacks laminin. *J Clin Pathol* 1985;38: 507–511.
107. Kumar S, Marsden HB, Cowan RA, Barnes JM. Prognostic relevance of DNA content in childhood renal tumours. *Br J Cancer* 1989;59:291–295.
108. Kuo TT. Observation of nervous tissue in a Wilms' tumor: its histogenetic significance. *Cancer* 1977;39:1105–1108.
109. Lack EE, Cassady JR, Sallan SE. Renal cell carcinoma in childhood and adolescence: a clinical and pathological study of 17 cases. *J Urol* 1985;133:822–828.
110. Ladanyi M, Gerald W. Fusion of the EWS and WT1 genes in the desmoplastic small round cell tumor. *Cancer Res* 1994;54:2837–2840.
111. Lamiell JM, Salazar FG, Hsia YE. von Hippel–Lindau disease affecting 43 members of a single kindred. *Medicine (Baltimore)* 1989;68:1–29.
112. Laskin WB, Weiss SW, Bratthauer GL. Epithelioid variant of malignant peripheral nerve sheath tumor (malignant epithelioid schwannoma). *Am J Surg* Pathol 1991;15:1136–1145.
113. Lawler W, Marsden HB. Bone metastases in children presenting with renal tumours. *J Clin Pathol* 1979;32:608–615.
114. Lawler W, Marsden HB, Palmer MK. Histopathological study of the first Medical Research Council Nephroblastoma Trial. *Cancer* 1977;40:1519–1525.
115. Layfield LJ, Ritchie AW, Ehrlich R. The relationship of deoxyribonucleic acid content to conventional prognostic factors in Wilms tumor. *J Urol* 1989;142:1040–1043.
116. Lemerle J, Tournade MF, Marchant RG, et al. Wilms' tumor: natural history and prognostic factors: a retrospective study of 248 cases treated at the Institut Gustave-Roussy 1952–1967. *Cancer* 1976;37:2557–2566.
117. Lemos LB, Hamoudi AB. Malignant thymic tumor in an infant (malignant histiocytoma). *Arch Pathol Lab Med* 1978;102:84–89.
118. Levin NP, Damjanov I, Depillis VJ. Mesoblastic nephroma in an adult patient: recurrence 21 years after removal of the primary lesion. *Cancer* 1982;49:573–577.
119. Little MH, Ablett G, Smith PJ. Enhanced expression of insulin-like growth factor II is not a necessary event in Wilms' tumour progression. *Carcinogenesis* 1987;8:865–868.
120. Madden SL, Cook DM, Morris JF, Gashler A, Sukhatme VP, Rauscher FJ III. Transcriptional repression mediated by the WT1 Wilms tumor gene product. *Science* 1991;253:1550–1553.
121. Mahoney JP, Saffos RO. Fetal rhabdomyomatous nephroblastoma with a renal pelvic mass simulating sarcoma botryoides. *Am J Surg Pathol* 1981;5:297–306.
122. Mannens M, Devilee P, Bliek J, et al. Loss of heterozygosity in Wilms' tumors, studied for six putative tumor suppressor regions, is limited to chromosome 11. *Cancer Res* 1990;50:3279–3283.
123. Mannens M, Slater RM, Heyting C, et al. Molecular nature of genetic changes resulting in loss of heterozygosity of chromosome 11 in Wilms' tumours. *Hum Genet* 1988;81:41–48.
124. Marsden HB, Lawler W. Primary renal tumours in the first year of life: a population based review. *Virchows Arch A Histopathol Anat* 1983;399:1–9.
125. Marsden HB, Lawler W, Kumar PM. Bone metastasizing renal tumor of childhood: morphological and clinical features, and differences from Wilms' tumor. *Cancer* 1978;42:1922–1928.
126. Marsden HB, Newton WA, Jr. New look at mesoblastic nephroma. *J Clin Pathol* 1986;39:508–513.
127. Masson P. The role of the neural crest in the embryonal adenosarcomas of the kidney. *Am J Cancer* 1938;33:1–32.
128. Maw MA, Grundy PE, Millow LJ, et al. A third Wilms' tumor locus on chromosome 16q. *Cancer Res* 1992;52:3094–3098.
129. Mayes LC, Kasselberg AG, Roloff JS, Lukens JN. Hypercalcemia associated with immunoreactive parathyroid hormone in a malignant rhabdoid tumor of the kidney (rhabdoid Wilms' tumor). *Cancer* 1984;54:882–884.
130. McGinnis M, Jacobs G, El-Naggar A, Redline RW. Congenital peribronchial myofibroblastic tumor (so-called "congenital leiomyosarcoma"). A distinct neonatal lung lesion associated with nonimmune hydrops fetalis. *Mod Pathol* 1993;6:487–492.
131. McNutt MA, Bolen JW, Gown AM, Hammar SP, Vogel AM. Coexpression of intermediate filaments in human epithelial neoplasms. *Ultrastruct Pathol* 1985;9:31–43.
132. Merino MJ, LiVolsi VA. Oncocytomas of the kidney. *Cancer* 1982;50:1852–1856.
133. Mierau GW, Beckwith JB, Weeks DA. Ultrastructure and histogenesis of the renal tumors of childhood: an overview. *Ultrastruct Pathol* 1987;11:313–333.
134. Miller RW, Young JL, Novakovic B. Childhood cancer. *Cancer* 1995;75:395–405.
135. Mishra VK, Krishnani N, Bhandari M. Clear cell sarcoma of kidney in an adult. *Br J Urol* 1993;72:118
136. Misra M, Rohatgi M, Mathur M, Sharma S. Flow cytometric analysis of DNA ploidy in 62 patients with Wilms' tumor. *Pediatr Surg Int* 1992;7:51–54.
137. Miwa H, Tomlinson GE, Timmons CF, Huff V, Cohn SL, Strong LC, Saunders GF. RNA expression of the WT1 gene in Wilms' tumors in relation to histology. *JNCI* 1992;84:181–187.
138. Morgan E, Kidd JM. Undifferentiated sarcoma of the kidney: a tumor of childhood with histopathologic and clinical characteristics distinct from Wilms' tumor. *Cancer* 1978;42:1916–1921.
139. Mostofi FK, Davis CJ, Jr. Tumors and tumor-like lesions of the kidney. *Curr Probl Cancer* 1986;10:53–114.
140. Mukai M, Torikata C, Iri H, et al. Crystalloids in angiomyolipoma. 1. A previously unnoticed phenomenon of renal angiomyolipoma occurring at a high frequency. *Am J Surg Pathol* 1992;16:1–10.
141. Mundlos S, Pelletier J, Darveau A, Bachmann M, Winterpacht A, Zabel B. Nuclear localization of the protein encoded by the Wilms' tumor gene WT1 in embryonic and adult tissues. *Development* 1993;119:1329–1341.
142. Murphy WM, Beckwith JB, Farrow GM. *Tumors of the Kidney, Bladder, and Related Urinary Structures.* Washington, D.C.: Armed Forces Institute of Pathology; 1994.
143. Nadasdy T, Roth J, Johnson DL, Bane BL, Weinberg A, Verani R, Silva FG. Congenital mesoblastic nephroma: an immunohistochemical and lectin study. *Hum Pathol* 1993;24:413–419.
144. Nakamura Y, Nakashima T, Nakashima H, Hashimoto T. Bilateral cystic nephroblastomas and botryoid sarcoma involving vagina and urinary bladder in a child with microcephaly, arhinencephaly, and bilateral cataracts. *Cancer* 1981;48:1012–1015.
145. Nakazato Y, Hirato J, Nakanishi Y, Tamaki O, Yazaki C. Immunohistochemical localization of five classes of intermediate filament in a benign pelvic soft tissue tumor of rhabdoid appearance. *Acta Pathol Jpn* 1991;41:65–72.
146. National Wilms' Tumor Study Committee. Wilms' tumor: status report, 1990. J *Clin Oncol* 1991;9:877–887.
147. Newsham I, Daub D, Besnard-Guerin C, Cavenee W. Molecular sublocalization and characterization of the 11;22 translocation breakpoint in a malignant rhabdoid tumor. *Genomics* 1994;19: 433–440.
148. Novak RW, Caces JN, Johnson WW. Sarcomatous renal tumor of childhood. An electron microscopic study. *Am J Clin Pathol* 1980;73:622–625.
149. Obers VJ, Phillips JI. Fine needle aspiration of pediatric abdominal masses: Cytologic and electron microscopic diagnosis. *Acta Cytol* 1991;35:165–170.
150. Oda H, Shiga J, Machinami R. Clear cell sarcoma of kidney. Two cases in adults. *Cancer* 1993;71:2286–2291.
151. Ogawa K, Nakashima Y, Yamabe H, Hamashima Y. Clear cell sarcoma of the kidney. An immunohistochemical study. *Acta Pathol Jpn* 1986;36:681–689.
152. Okumura A, Tanaka T, Mori H. Juxtaglomerular cell tumor cell line producing active renin and its precursors. *Virchows Arch B Cell Pathol* 1993;64:303–307.
153. Olshan AF, Breslow NE, Daling JR, et al. Wilms' tumor and paternal occupation. *Cancer Res* 1990;50:3212–3217.
154. Olshan AF, Breslow NE, Falletta JM, et al. Risk factors for Wilms tumor: Report from the National Wilms Tumor Study. *Cancer* 1993;72:938–944.
155. Oppedal BR, Glomstein A, Zetterberg A. Feulgen DNA values in Wilms' tumour in relation to prognosis. *Pathol Res Pract* 1988;183:756–760.
156. Ota S, Crabbe DCG, Tran TN, Triche TJ, Shimada H. Malignant rhabdoid tumor: a study with two established cell lines. *Cancer* 1993;71:2862–2872.

157. Paik S, Rosen N, Jung W, You JM, Lippman ME, Perdue JF, Yee D. Expression of insulin-like growth factor–II mRNA in fetal kidney and Wilms' tumor. An in situ hybridization study. *Lab Invest* 1989;61:522–526.
158. Palma LD, Kenny GM, Murphy GP. Childhood renal carcinoma. *Cancer* 1970;26:1321–1324.
159. Panuel M, Bourliere-Najean B, Gentet J-C, Scheiner C, Delarue A, Faure F, Devred P. Aggressive neuroblastoma with initial pulmonary metastases and kidney involvement simulating Wilms' tumor. *Eur J Radiol* 1992;14:201–203.
160. Parham DM, Jenkins JJ, Holt H, Callihan TR. Phenotypic diversity in pediatric rhabdoid tumors: a morphologic and immunohistochemical study. *Lab Invest* 1987;56:58A (Abstract).
161. Parham DM, Weeks DA, Beckwith JB. The clinicopathologic spectrum of putative extrarenal rhabdoid tumors: an analysis of 42 cases studies with immunohistochemistry and/or electron microscopy. *Am J Surg Pathol* 1994;18:1010–1029.
162. Park S, Bernard A, Bove KE, Sens DA, Hazen-Martin DJ, Garvin AJ, Haber DA. Inactivation of WT1 in nephrogenic rests, genetic precursors to Wilms' tumour. *Nature Genet* 1993;5:363–367.
163. Pelletier J, Bruening W, Kashtan CE, et al. Germline mutations in the Wilms' tumor suppressor gene are associated with abnormal urogenital development in Denys–Drash syndrome. *Cell* 1991;67:437–447.
164. Pelletier J, Bruening W, Li FP, Haber DA, Glaser T, Housman DE. WT1 mutations contribute to abnormal genital system development and hereditary Wilms' tumour. *Nature* 1991;353:431–434.
165. Pelletier J, Schalling M, Buckler AJ, Rogers A, Haber DA, Housman D. Expression of the Wilms' tumor gene WT1 in the murine urogenital system. *Genes Dev* 1991;5:1345–1356.
166. Penchansky L, Gallo G. Rhabdomyosarcoma of the kidney in children. *Cancer* 1979;44:285–292.
167. Perrone T, Swanson PE, Twiggs L, Ulbright TM, Dehner LP. Malignant rhabdoid tumor of the vulva: is distinction from epithelioid sarcoma possible? A pathologic and immunohistochemical study. *Am J Surg Pathol* 1989;13:848–858.
168. Pettinato G, Manivel JC, Wick MR, Dehner LP. Classical and cellular (atypical) congenital mesoblastic nephroma: a clinicopathologic, ultrastructural, immunohistochemical, and flow cytometric study. *Hum Pathol* 1989;20:682–690.
169. Powars DR, Allerton SE, Beierle J, Butler BB. Wilms' tumor clinical correlation with circulating mucin in three cases. *Cancer* 1972;29:1597–1605.
170. Pritchard-Jones K, Fleming S, Davidson D, et al. The candidate Wilms' tumour gene is involved in genitourinary development. *Nature* 1990;346:194–197.
171. Punnett HH, Halligan GE, Zaeri N, Karmazin N. Translocation 10;17 in clear cell sarcoma of the kidney: a first report. *Cancer Genet Cytogenet* 1989;41:123–128.
172. Quijano G, Drut R. Cytologic characteristics of Wilms' tumors in fine needle aspirates. A study of ten cases. *Acta Cytol* 1989;33:263–266.
173. Raney RB, Jr., Palmer N, Sutow WW, Baum E, Ayala A. Renal cell carcinoma in children. *Med Pediatr Oncol* 1983;11:91–98.
174. Raslan WF, Ro JY, Ordonez NG, Amin MB, Troncoso P, Sella A, Ayala AG. Primary carcinoid of the kidney. Immunohistochemical and ultrastructural studies of five patients. *Cancer* 1993;72:2660–2666.
175. Rauscher FJ, III, Morris JF, Tournay OE, Cook DM, Curran T. Binding of the Wilms' tumor locus zinc finger protein to the EGR-1 consensus sequence. *Science* 1990;250:1259–1262.
176. Reeve AE, Eccles MR, Wilkins RJ, Bell GI, Millow LJ. Expression of insulin-like growth factor–II transcripts in Wilms' tumour. *Nature* 1985;317:258–260.
177. Riccardi VM, Hittner HM, Francke U, Yunis JJ, Ledbetter D, Borges W. The aniridia–Wilms tumor association: the critical role of chromosome band 11p13. *Cancer Genet Cytogenet* 1980;2:131–137.
178. Ritchey ML, Kelalis PP, Breslow N, Offord KP, Shochat SJ, D'Angio GJ. Intracaval and atrial involvement with nephroblastoma: review of National Wilms Tumor Study-3. *J Urol* 1988;140:1113–1118.
179. Roberts P, Lockwood LR, Lewis IJ, Bailey CC, Batcup G, Williams J. Cytogenetic abnormalities in mesoblastic nephroma: a link to Wilms' tumour? *Med Pediatr Oncol* 1993;21:416–420.
180. Roloson GJ, Beckwith JB. Primary neuroepithelial tumors of the kidney in children and adults. A report from the NWTS Pathology Center. *Mod Pathol* 1993;6:67A (Abstract).
181. Roper M, Parmley RT, Crist WM, Kelly DR, Hyland CH, Salter M. Rhabdoid tumor of the kidney: complete remission induced by cis-platinum and adriamycin. *Med Pediatr Oncol* 1981;9:175–180.
182. Rose EA, Glaser T, Jones C, et al. Complete physical map of the WAGR region of 11p13 localizes a candidate Wilms' tumor gene. *Cell* 1990;60:495–508.
183. Roth J, Zuber C. Immunoelectron microscopic investigation of surface coat of Wilms tumor cells: dense lamina is composed of highly sialylated neural cell adhesion molecule. *Lab Invest* 1990;62:55–60.
184. Rousseau-Merck MF, de Keyzer Y, Bourdeau A, Cournot G, Mercier F, Nezelof C. PTH mRNA transcription analysis in infantile tumors associated with hypercalcemia. *Cancer* 1988;62:303–308.
185. Rousseau-Merck MF, Nogues C, Nezelof C, Marin-Cudraz B, Paulin D. Infantile renal tumors associated with hypercalcemia: characterization of intermediate-filament clusters. *Arch Pathol Lab Med* 1983;107:311–314.
186. Rousseau-Merck MF, Nogues C, Roth A, Nezelof C, Bourdeau A, Leblanc A, Trincard MD. Hypercalcemic infantile renal tumors: morphological, clinical, and biological heterogeneity. *Pediatr Pathol* 1985;3:155–164.
187. Rutledge J, Beckwith JB, Benjamin D, Haas JE. Absence of immunoperoxidase staining for myoglobin in the malignant rhabdoid tumor of the kidney. *Pediatr Pathol* 1983;1:93–98.
188. Sait SN, Nowak NJ, Singh-Kahlon P, Weksberg R, Squire J, Shows TB, Higgins MJ. Localization of Beckwith–Wiedemann and rhabdoid tumor chromosome rearrangements to a defined interval in chromosome band 11p15.5. *Genes Chrom Cancer* 1994;11:97–105.
189. Sandstedt B, Delemarre JF, Krul EJ, Tournade MF. Mesoblastic nephromas: a study of 29 tumours from the SIOP nephroblastoma file. *Histopathology* 1985;9:741–750.
190. Sapienza C. Genome imprinting and cancer genetics. *Semin Cancer Biol* 1992;3:151–158.
191. Sarawar SR, Schlingemann RO, Kelsey A, Fleming S, Kumar S. A monoclonal antibody stains blastemal but not tubular components of Wilms' tumour. *J Pathol* 1988;156:319–324.
192. Schmidt D, Harms D, Evers KG, Bliesener JA, Beckwith JB. Bone metastasizing renal tumor (clear cell sarcoma) of childhood with epithelioid elements. *Cancer* 1985;56:609–613.
193. Schmidt D, Leuschner I, Harms D, Sprenger E, Schäfer H-J. Malignant rhabdoid tumor: a morphological and flow cytometric study. *Pathol Res Pract* 1989;184:202–210.
194. Schmidt D, Wiedemann B, Keil W, Sprenger E, Harms D. Flow cytometric analysis of nephroblastomas and related neoplasms. *Cancer* 1986;58:2494–2500.
195. Schofield DE, Yunis EJ, Fletcher JA. Chromosome aberrations in mesoblastic nephroma. *Am J Pathol* 1993;143:714–724.
196. Schwartz CE, Haber DA, Stanton VP, Strong LC, Skolnick MH, Housman DE. Familial predisposition to Wilms tumor does not segregate with the WT1 gene. *Genomics* 1991;10:927–930.
197. Scott J, Cowell J, Robertson ME, et al. Insulin-like growth factor-II gene expression in Wilms' tumour and embryonic tissues. *Nature* 1985;317:260–262.
198. Seemayer TA, Thelmo WL, Bolande RP, Wiglesworth FW. Peripheral neuroectodermal tumors. *Perspect Pediatr Pathol* 1975;2:151–172.
199. Shashi V, Lovell MA, von Kap-herr C, Waldron P, Golden WL. Malignant rhabdoid tumor of the kidney: involvement of chromosome 22. *Genes Chrom Cancer* 1994;10:49–54.
200. Shuin T, Kondo K, Torigoe S, et al. Frequent somatic mutations and loss of heterozygosity of the von Hippel–Lindau tumor suppressor gene in primary human renal cell carcinomas. *Cancer Res* 1994;54:2852–2855.
201. Slater RM, De Kraker J. Chromosome number 11 and Wilms' tumor. *Cancer Genet Cytogenet* 1982;5:237–245.
202. Slater RM, De Kraker J, Voute PA, Delemarre JF. A cytogenetic study of Wilms' tumor. *Cancer Genet Cytogenet* 1985;14:95–109.
203. Slater RM, Mannens MMAM. Cytogenetics and molecular ge-

netics of Wilms' tumor of childhood. *Cancer Genet Cytogenet* 1992;61:111–121.
204. Sotelo-Avila C, Gonzalez-Crussi F, Sadowinski S, Gooch WM, Pena R. Clear cell sarcoma of the kidney: a clinicopathologic study of 21 patients with long-term follow-up evaluation. *Hum Pathol* 1985;16:1219–1230.
205. Sotelo-Avila C, Gooch WM. Neoplasms associated with the Beckwith–Wiedemann syndrome. *Perspect Pediatr Pathol* 1976;3:255–272.
206. Squires JP, Ulbright TM, DeSchryver-Kecskemeti K, Engleman W. Juxtaglomerular cell tumor of the kidney. *Cancer* 1984;53: 516–523.
207. Steenman MJC, Rainier S, Dobry CJ, Grundy P, Horon IL, Feinberg AP. Loss of imprinting of IGF2 is linked to reduced expression and abnormal methylation of H19 in Wilms' tumour. *Nature Genet* 1994;7:433–439.
208. Störkel S, Thoenes W, Jacobi GH, Engelmann U, Lippold R. Prognostic parameters of renal cell carcinoma. *Eur Urol* 1990;18 Suppl. 2:36–37.
209. Takagi M, Takakuwa T, Ushigome S, Nakata K, Fujioka T, Watanabe A. Sarcomatous variants of Wilms' tumor. Immunohistochemical and ultrastructural comparison with classical Wilms' tumor. *Cancer* 1987;59:963–971.
210. Thoenes W, Storkel S, Rumpelt HJ. Histopathology and classification of renal cell tumors (adenomas, oncocytomas and carcinomas). The basic cytological and histopathological elements and their use for diagnostics. *Pathol Res Pract* 1986;181:125–143.
211. Thomas PRM, Shochat SJ, Norkool P, Beckwith JB, Breslow NE, D'Angio GJ. Prognostic implications of hepatic adhesion, invasion, and metastases at diagnosis of Wilms' tumor. *Cancer* 1991;68:2486–2488.
212. Tomlinson GE, Argyle JC, Velasco S, Nisen PD. Molecular characterization of congenital mesoblastic nephroma and its distinction from Wilms tumor. *Cancer* 1992;70:2358–2361.
213. Trillo AA. Adult variant of congenital mesoblastic nephroma. *Arch Pathol Lab Med* 1990;114:533–535.
214. Tsokos M, Kouraklis G, Chandra RS, Bhagavan BS, Triche TJ. Malignant rhabdoid tumor of the kidney and soft tissues: evidence for a diverse morphological and immunocytochemical phenotype. *Arch Pathol Lab Med* 1989;113:115–120.
215. Tsui WMS, Yuen AKT, Ma KF, Tse CCH. Hepatic angiomyolipomas with a deceptive trabecular pattern and HMB-45 reactivity. *Histopathology* 1992;21:569–573.
216. Tsuneyoshi M, Daimaru Y, Hashimoto H, Enjoji M. Malignant soft tissue neoplasms with the histologic features of renal rhabdoid tumors: an ultrastructural and immunohistochemical study. *Hum Pathol* 1985;16:1235–1242.
217. Tsuneyoshi M, Daimaru Y, Hashimoto H, Enjoji M. The existence of rhabdoid cells in specified soft tissue sarcomas: histopathological, ultrastructural and immunohistochemical evidence. *Virchows Arch A Histopathol Anat* 1987;411:509–514.
218. van Baal JG, Becker AE, Fleury P, Brummelkamp WH. Renal angiomyolipomas: could the histology serve as a marker for tuberous sclerosis? *Histopathology* 1990;17:180–182.
219. Van Heyningen V, Hastie ND. Wilms' tumour: reconciling genetics and biology. *Trends Genet* 1992;8:16–21.
220. Variend S, Spicer RD, MacKinnon AE. Teratoid Wilms' tumor. *Cancer* 1984;53:1936–1942.
221. Varsa EW, McConnell TS, Dressler LG, Duncan M. Atypical congenital mesoblastic nephroma: report of a case with karyotypic and flow cytometric analysis. *Arch Pathol Lab Med* 1989;113:1078–1080.
222. Velasco S, D'Amico D, Schneider NR, Timmons C, Chappell E, Lee D, Nisen PD. Molecular and cellular heterogeneity of Wilms' tumor. *Int J Cancer* 1993;53:672–679.
223. Viljoen D, Ramesar R. Evidence for parental imprinting in familial Beckwith–Wiedemann syndrome. *J Med Genet* 1992;29:221–225.
224. Vogel AM, Gown AM, Caughlan J, Haas JE, Beckwith JB. Rhabdoid tumors of the kidney contain mesenchymal specific and epithelial specific intermediate filament proteins. *Lab Invest* 1984;50:232–238.
225. Vogelzang NJ, Fremgen AM, Guinan PD, Chmiel JS, Sylvester JL, Sener SF. Primary renal sarcoma in adults: a natural history and management study by the American Cancer Society, Illinois division. *Cancer* 1993;71:804–810.
226. Wadey RB, Pal N, Buckle B, Yeomans E, Pritchard J, Cowell JK. Loss of heterozygosity in Wilms' tumour involves two distinct regions of chromosome 11. *Oncogene* 1990;5:901–908.
227. Webber BL, Parham DM, Drake LG, Wilimas JA. Renal tumors in childhood. *Pathol Annu* 1992;27 Pt 1:191–232.
228. Weeks DA, Beckwith JB, Luckey DW. Relapse-associated variables in stage I favorable histology Wilms' tumor: a report of the National Wilms' Tumor Study. *Cancer* 1987;60:1204–1212.
229. Weeks DA, Beckwith JB, Mierau GW. Benign nodal lesions mimicking metastases from pediatric renal neoplasms: a report of the National Wilms' Tumor Study Pathology Center. *Hum Pathol* 1990;21:1239–1244.
230. Weeks DA, Beckwith JB, Mierau GW, Luckey DW. Rhabdoid tumor of kidney: a report of 111 cases from the National Wilms' Tumor Study Pathology Center. *Am J Surg Pathol* 1989;13:439–458.
231. Weeks DA, Beckwith JB, Mierau GW, Zuppan CW. Renal neoplasms mimicking rhabdoid tumor of kidney: a report from the National Wilms' Tumor Study Pathology Center. *Am J Surg Pathol* 1991;15:1042–1054.
232. Weeks DA, Malott RL, Zuppan C, Mierau GW, Beckwith JB. Primitive pelvic sarcoma resembling clear cell sarcoma of kidney. *Ultrastruct Pathol* 1991;15:403–408.
233. Wiedemann HR. Complexe malformatif familial avec hernie ombilicale et macroglossie - un "syndrome noveau"? *J Génét Hum* 1995;13:223–232.
234. Weidner N, Tjoe J. Immunohistochemical profile of monoclonal antibody O13: antibody that recognized glycoprotein p30/32^{MIC2} and is useful in diagnosing Ewing's sarcoma and peripheral neuroepithelioma. *Am J Surg Pathol* 1994;18:486–494.
235. Weissman BE, Saxon PJ, Pasquale SR, Jones GR, Geiser AG, Stanbridge EJ. Introduction of a normal human chromosome 11 into a Wilms' tumor cell line controls its tumorigenic expression. *Science* 1987;236:175–180.
236. White KS, Kirks DR, Bove KE. Imaging of nephroblastomatosis: an overview. *Radiology* 1992;182:1–5.
237. Wigger HJ. Fetal hamartoma of kidney. A benign, symptomatic, congenital tumor, not a form of Wilms' tumor. *Am J Clin Pathol* 1969;51:323–337.
238. Wigger HJ. Fetal mesenchymal hamartoma of kidney. A tumor of secondary mesenchyme. *Cancer* 1975;36:1002–1008.
239. Wigger HJ. Fetal rhabdomyomatous nephroblastoma–a variant of Wilms' tumor. *Hum Pathol* 1976;7:613–623.
240. Wilimas JA, Dow LW, Douglass EC, et al. Evidence for clonal development of Wilms' tumor. *Am J Pediatr Hematol Oncol* 1991;13:26–28.
241. Williams G, Colbeck RA, Gowing NFC. Adult Wilms' tumour: review of 14 patients. *Br J Urol* 1992;70:230–235.
242. Wilms M. *Die Mischgeschwülste.* Leipzig: Arthur Georgi; 1899.
243. Zanetti G, Giangaspero F. Rhabdomyoblastic nature of cytoplasmic inclusions in malignant rhabdoid tumor [letter]. *Hum Pathol* 1982;13:410
244. Zoeller G, Pekrun A, Lakomek M, Ringert R-H. Wilms tumor: the problem of diagnostic accuracy in children undergoing preoperative chemotherapy without histological tumor verification. *J Urol* 1994;151:169–171.
245. Zumkeller W, Schofield PN. The role of insulin-like growth factors and IGF-binding proteins in the physiological and pathological processes of the kidney. *Virchows Arch B Cell Pathol* 1992;62:207–220.
246. Zuppan CW, Beckwith JB, Luckey DW. Anaplasia in unilateral Wilms' tumor: A report from the National Wilms' Tumor Study Pathology Center. *Hum Pathol* 1988;19:1199–1209.
247. Zuppan CW, Beckwith JB, Weeks DA, Luckey DW, Pringle KC. The effect of preoperative therapy on the histologic features of Wilms' tumor: an analysis of cases from the third National Wilms' Tumor Study. *Cancer* 1991;68:385–394.

Pediatric Neoplasia: Morphology and Biology, edited by David M. Parham.
Lippincott-Raven Publishers, Philadelphia © 1996.

CHAPTER 4

Ewing's Sarcoma, Peripheral Neuroepithelioma, and Related Tumors

David M. Parham

EWING'S SARCOMA

Since 1921, when James Ewing first described the neoplasm he termed the "diffuse endothelioma of bone" (37), the sarcoma that bears Ewing's name has remained a source of mystery and intrigue for pathologists. Perhaps at no time since its recognition has the enthusiasm for probing the mysteries of this tumor been higher, what with the findings that Ewing's sarcomas and peripheral neuroepitheliomas share a unique chromosomal translocation (165), that a subgroup of small round cell tumors of bone expresses neural features in vivo (64), that tumors which are undifferentiated in vivo may express a neural phenotype in vitro (12), and that both tumors express a unique surface marker termed MIC2 (40). Recent work has focused on the molecular mechanisms of oncogenesis effected by the chromosomal translocation (26).

Ewing's insistence on the primary origin of the small cell neoplasm which he observed in bone was met with some derision by other pathologists. Noteworthy among them was Rupert Willis (168), who vehemently concluded that Ewing's sarcomas were metastases of neuroblastomas whose primary sites were undetected. The evidence for Willis's conclusion lay in his own autopsy observations of the frequency of metastatic neuroblastomas in skeletal sites; modern tools of diagnostic imaging were not available at that time, so that undetected primaries were relatively common. The fact that the giants of pathology of the time were confused pays great tribute to the enigmatic character of this lesion and to Ewing's recognition of it.

D. M. Parham: Department of Pathology, Arkansas Children's Hospital, Little Rock, Arkansas 72202.

Perhaps the most perceptive observation made at the time was that of Arthur Purdy Stout, who noted the not uncommon occurrence of rosettes in these neoplasms (140). Although this finding might have suggested that these tumors were of neuroectodermal origin, he wisely concluded that insufficient evidence was available for a histogenetic theory of Ewing's sarcoma.

The modern history of Ewing's sarcoma research is highlighted by the ability of the tumor to grow readily in cell culture, which in turn has led to the recognition of characteristic cytogenetic features (165), enzymatic and oncogenetic properties (150), and differentiation capacities (12) which in turn have given enhanced definition to an entity that can be considered the epitomy of the undifferentiated small round cell tumor.

Clinical Features

Ewing's sarcoma is primarily a tumor of the long bones of adolescents but it also affects the axial skeleton and ribs. Although typically these tumors occur in young adults, we have often seen examples in patients younger than 12 years of age, the youngest being 2.9 years (117). Nineteen patients under the age of 3 years were reported in the Intergroup Ewing's Sarcoma Study (IESS) series (89). The risk of development of these lesions appears to parallel periods of skeletal growth (30). In the IESS report (69), the mean age was 11 years, and the most commonly affected bones, in order of relative frequency, were the femur, ilium, fibula, tibia, and humerus. This tumor also has a distinctive racial distribution, as it virtually never occurs in black patients, who in our experience tend to have tumors with unusual histologic and/or clinical characteristics (109). Symptoms suggestive of osteomyelitis, such as fever, erythema, and increased

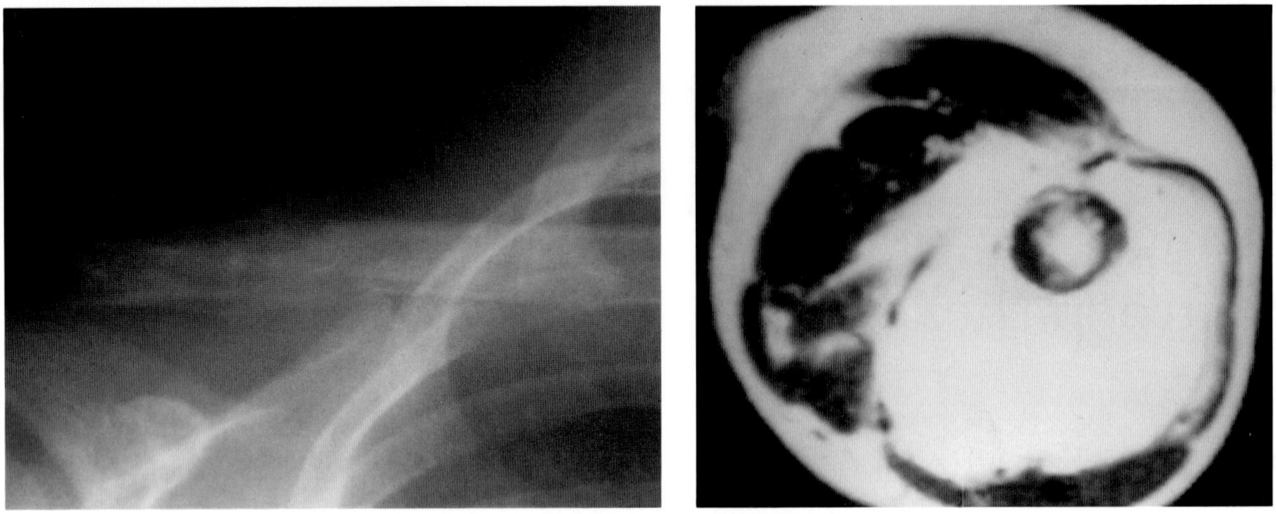

A B

FIG. 1. Radiographic studies of Ewing's sarcomas. **A.** Plain radiograph of a clavicular tumor demonstrating moth-eaten, lytic appearance with periosteal elevation. **B.** T2-weighted magnetic resonance image of a femoral tumor with a large, permeative area of soft tissue invasion. (Courtesy of Dr. Barry Fletcher, St. Jude Children's Research Hospital.)

erythrocyte sedimentation rate, may be present, often leading to delayed diagnosis. In addition, the tumor has been reported in siblings (62) and in clusters suggesting an infectious etiology (60).

On radiographic studies, Ewing's sarcomas are aggressive permeative lesions with extensive bone destruction and soft tissue invasion (Fig. 1). Frequently, the soft tissue component overshadows the osseous component, particularly in small bones. Periosteal expansion with reactive bone formation may create a sunburst effect. In contrast to osteosarcoma, which is usually a metaphyseal lesion, Ewing's sarcomas frequently involve the midshaft of the bone. Unfortunately, radiologic findings are still relatively nonspecific, even with newer techniques such as computed tomography scanning or magnetic resonance imaging. Relatively benign lesions such as Langerhans cell histiocytosis or even nonneoplastic lesions such as osteomyelitis often cannot be confidently excluded. Even osteosarcomas, which at times are predominately lytic, may present with similar radiographic features. As a result, biopsy is mandatory for diagnosis. Magnetic resonance imaging, however, can give an indication of the effectiveness of therapy, as replacement of the tumor-damaged marrow with loose, watery repair tissue gives a different signal from viable tumor (41).

Gross Features

Ewing's sarcomas are fleshy, gray–tan, expansile lesions with extensive destruction of the associated bone (Fig. 2). There is usually periosteal elevation and breakthrough, often with a large soft tissue component. However, these gross features are not commonly seen in modern-day practice, as resections are now usually performed after completion of combination chemotherapy. As a result, one more often encounters macroscopic evidence of repair, such as bony widening and sclerosis, hemorrhage, necrosis, and cystic degeneration, with no

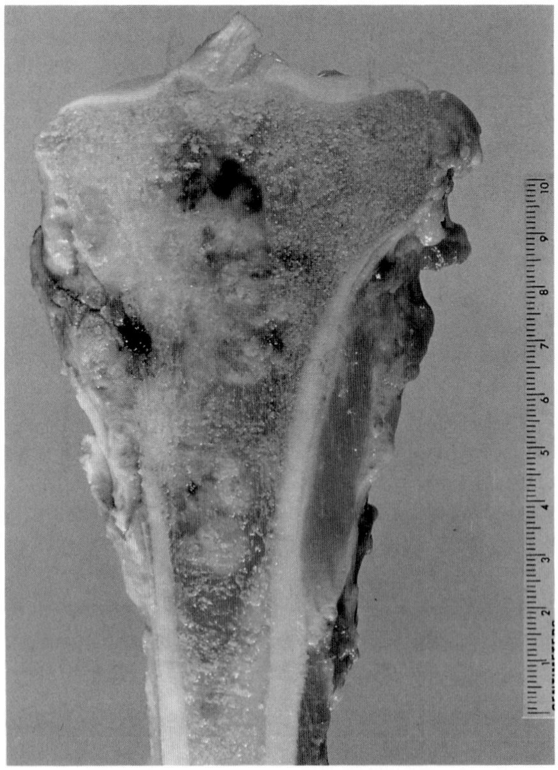

FIG. 2. Gross photograph of Ewing's sarcoma involving the proximal tibia. There is a poorly circumscribed, lytic lesion with cortical breakthrough and focal hemorrhage.

gross evidence of residual viable tumor. Microscopically, however, there are often scattered nests of tumor cells within a dense fibrous stroma.

Microscopic Features

Microscopically, Ewing's sarcoma is the prototypic small round cell tumor, composed of sheets of monotonous oval cells with primitive-appearing nuclei and modest amounts of clear to amphophilic cytoplasm (Fig. 3; see figure in color plate section). The nuclear characteristics of the prototypic Ewing's sarcoma are those of a primitive, uncommitted cell: an oval configuration with smooth contours, inconspicuous nucleoli, and finely distributed chromatin. These features have been likened to the appearance of the Thomsen variety of green grapes. The nuclei are generally centrally located and surrounded by a rim of clear cytoplasm. A high cell density is usually present with little intervening intercellular space, so that marked cell crowding is the rule. As a result, the diagnosis can often be suspected by gross visualization of the deep solid purple–blue color of hematoxylin and eosin stained sections. In spite of the high degree of cellularity, typical cases contain few mitoses.

Cytologically, these tumors are a mixture of lightly staining "primary" cells and darkly staining "secondary" cells (Fig. 3; see figure in color plate section). The difference in the relative intensity of staining is apparent in both nuclei and cytoplasm. The "secondary" cells are generally subtly intermingled with the "primary" cells with no discernible pattern formation. Although this feature is typical, it is nonspecific and may be noted in a variety of other small cell tumors.

"Atypical" or "large cell" Ewing's sarcoma is a variant tumor type having morphologic features departing from the classical cytology described above. In these tumors the cells are larger and more pleomorphic and have indented, irregular nuclear membranes and conspicuous nucleoli (Fig. 4). A higher mitotic rate may also be apparent. In spite of their ominous cytologic features, atypical Ewing's sarcomas do not generally have a different clinical outcome from "typical" lesions (98). These neoplasms appear to bridge a gap between the phenotypic extremes of typical Ewing's sarcoma and peripheral neuroepithelioma (9,155). However, one must be particularly cautious in diagnosis because atypical Ewing's sarcomas present cytologic features similar to those of non-Hodgkin's lymphoma of bone, an underrecognized and diagnostically difficult lesion with a diametrically opposed treatment regimen.

In point of fact, the undifferentiated microscopic features of Ewing's sarcoma often present a diagnostic dilemma. Table 1 lists the large group of pediatric tumors that must be considered in the differential diagnosis. Some of these lesions, such as desmoplastic small cell tumor (47), small cell mesothelioma (88), and acute megakaryocytic leukemia (3), are newly described sources of vexation, and others, such as the peripheral neuroepithelioma and Askin's tumor, appear to primarily be nosologic problems (23) which may be of more interest from a prognostic standpoint rather than a categorical one (see below). In cases such as small cell osteosarcoma and mesenchymal chondrosarcoma, the problem with diagnosis is related more to the limited amount of tissue available in a small biopsy. This factor necessitates that care be taken in obtaining and processing biopsy specimens so that optimal material is available for study. A great source of frustration in my own experience is the very fragile nature of primitive tumor cells, whose membranes are easily ruptured by rough handling, producing a mulligan stew of smeared DNA on histologic exam

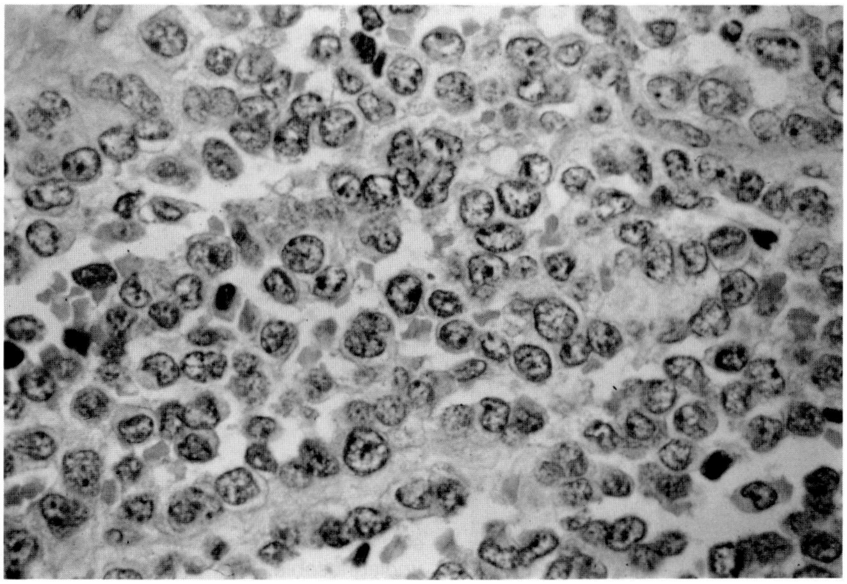

FIG. 4. Large cell, or "atypical," Ewing's sarcoma. Tumor cell nuclei are large and moderately irregular and contain conspicuous nucleoli.

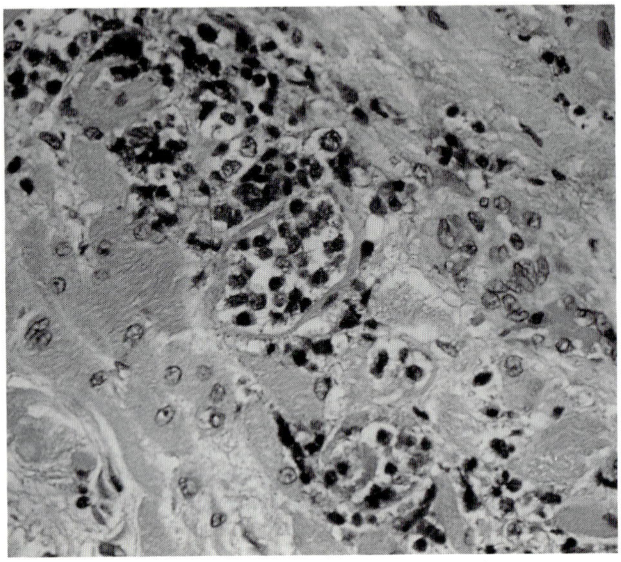

FIG. 7. Ewing's sarcoma with myofiber invasion.

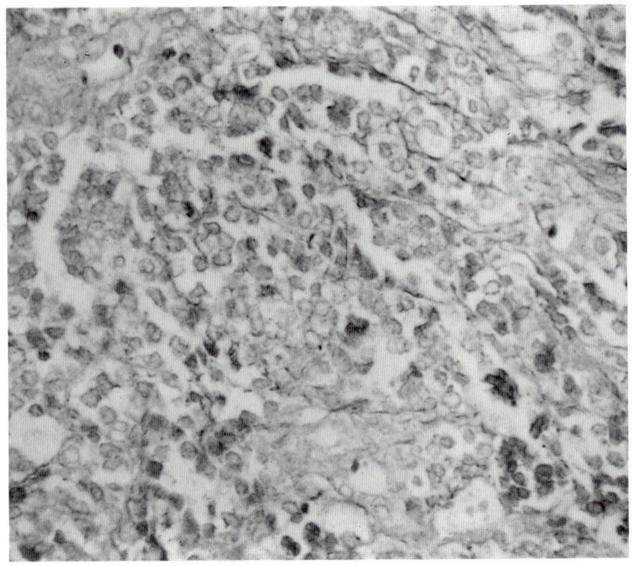

B

FIG. 8. Histochemical stains for Ewing's sarcoma, illustrating strong periodic acid–Schiff positivity **(A)** *(see color plate section)* and lack of reticulin fibers **(B)**.

such as alcohol fixation or tumor imprints, for optimal preservation. Newer diagnostic techniques, such as immunohistochemistry, have largely supplanted these procedures for routine diagnosis. Rhabdomyosarcomas and germ cell tumors in particular also contain an abundance of glycogen.

Electron Microscopy

Ultrastructural examination of Ewing's sarcoma typically reveals the same mixed population of light and dark cells noted on light microscopy. The most characteristic feature is the presence of cytoplasmic pools of glycogen, which at times may be quite prominent (Fig. 9). However, it must again be noted that cytoplasmic glycogen may be prominent in other embryonal tumors, such as rhabdomyosarcoma and neuroblastoma, so that it cannot be used as the sole diagnostic feature (153). In addition, a small percentage of Ewing's sarcomas (<10%) will not display glycogen even by electron microscopy (152). Perhaps the most reliable ultrastructural features of these

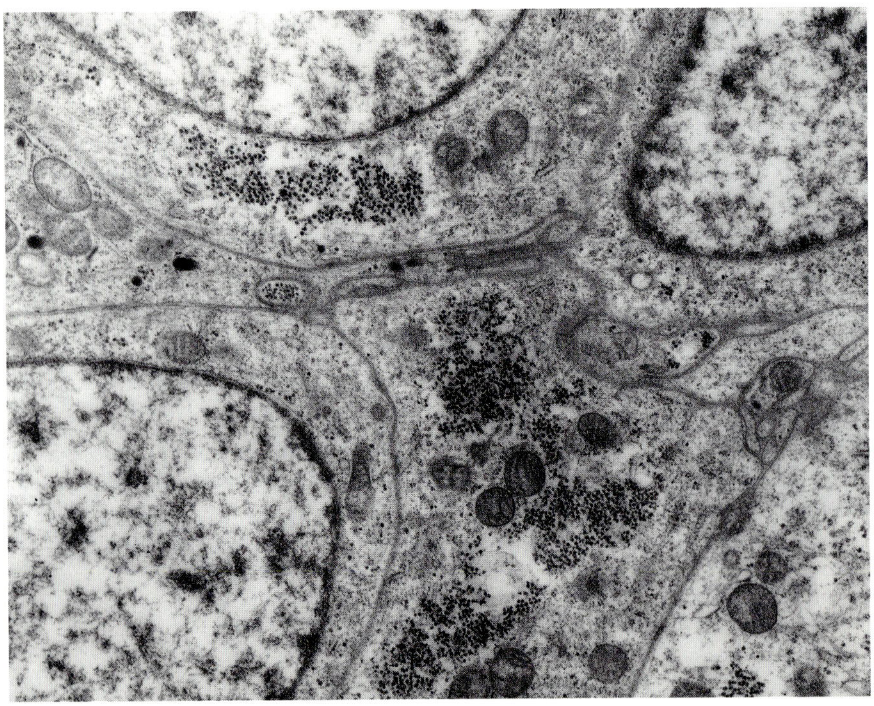

FIG. 9. Electron micrograph of Ewing's sarcoma, which contains cytoplasmic pools of glycogen.

tumors are an absence of a supporting stroma, lack of a cytoskeleton, relative paucity of organelles, and uniformity of nuclei and cell borders (152). Nevertheless, in Mierau's experience (personal communication), aggregates of β-rosette glycogen are characteristic of Ewing's sarcomas and distinguish them from other childhood tumors, which usually contain α-particulate glycogen. Ultrastructural evidence of neural (64,83,126,136,158) or endothelial (152) differentiation has also been noted in occasional cases of Ewing's sarcoma (Fig. 10). However, neural features have been used by Jaffe and colleagues (64) to define a separate entity, i.e., the primitive neuroectodermal tumor of bone. Whether these lesions represent a subset of Ewing's sarcoma or a unique lesion has been a source of much controversy.

Immunohistochemistry

A wide variety of immunohistochemical studies have been performed on Ewing's sarcoma. Vimentin, the intermediate filament that is contained in all mesenchymal cells, is commonly expressed and was the only marker initially found in these tumors (92,94). This apparent lack of cell marker specificity was disproven by the study of Moll and coworkers (94), who discovered that Ewing's sarcomas also contain desmoplakin, a desmosomal plaque protein, as well as cytokeratins found in simple epithelium (Fig. 11; see figure in color plate section). A minority of cases also contained dispersed or clustered cells which expressed neurofilaments. It thus became apparent that Ewing's sarcomas are derived from pluripotent cells capable of differentiating into a variety of cell types. Others have subsequently reported additional cytokeratin-positive cases (20,27,50). Ewing's sarcomas also commonly express neural proteins, such as neuron-specific enolase (NSE) synaptophysin, Leu 7, and E-26 (Fig. 12; see figure in color plate section) (64,67,83,136). The presence of these markers has been shown to be a bad prognostic sign by some (56), but other studies have failed to confirm this impression (20,116). At least for the time being, this confusion has been abated by the study by Schmidt et al. (125), which indicates that the presence of multiple neural markers and not neuron-specific enolase alone is predictive of a poor outcome. Markers for endothelial differentiation are usually negative (92), but even glial fibrillary acidic protein (GFAP) (Fig. 13; see figure in color plate section) may be expressed in some round cell tumors of bone (49,103,109).

Most recently, the cell surface marker MIC2 (or CD99) has been found to be relatively unique to Ewing's sarcomas and peripheral neuroepitheliomas (38,40,137). This molecule is a membrane-associated protein that is closely related to the murine THY-1 antigens, major cell

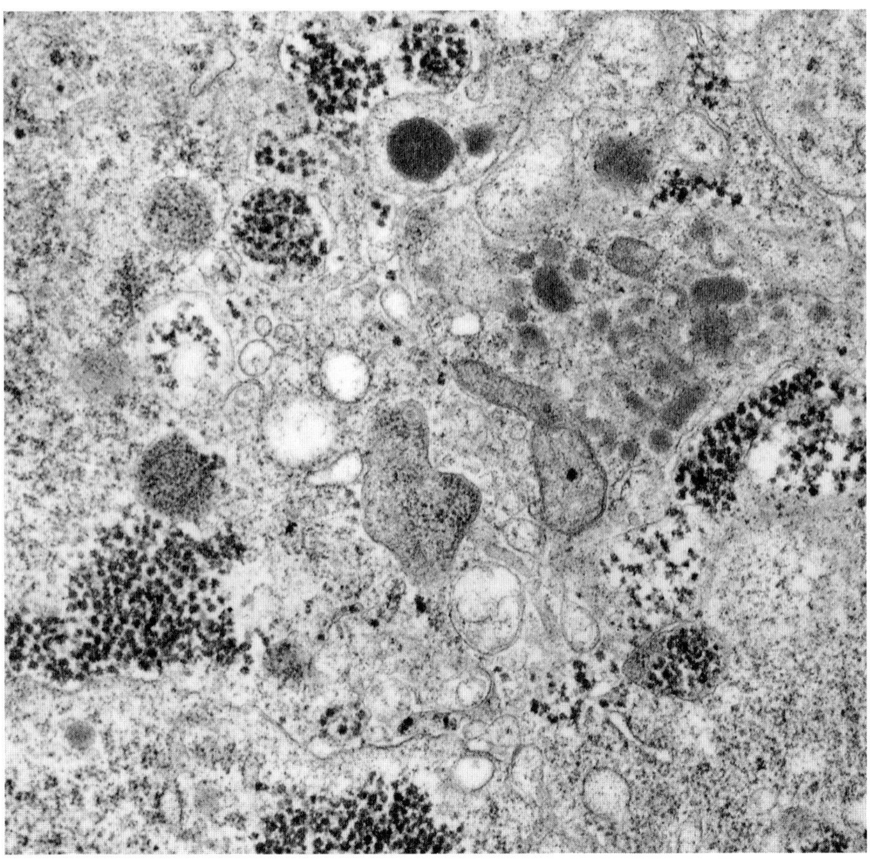

FIG. 10. Electron micrograph of tumor with histologic features of Ewing's sarcoma but containing processes with neurosecretory granules. Abundant glycogen is also present.

surface glycoproteins of murine brain and thymus cells (53). It is the product of the pseudoautosomal gene *MIC2*, found on the short arms of the X and Y chromosomes. Pseudoautosomal genes derive their name from the fact that they function in a manner more analogous to autosomal genes than sex chromosome–linked genes. Epitopes of the MIC2 antigen are recognized by the monoclonal antibodies HBA71, O13, and 12E7 (34,38,39,70,119,162), which were initially derived from studies of T-cell leukemia cell lines. In spite of this cross-reactivity with a subset of lymphoid cells, immunohistochemical studies of MIC2 have revealed a very high sensitivity (>90%) for this marker in Ewing's sarcomas and peripheral neuroepitheliomas (Fig. 14; see figure in color plate section). It is also relatively specific, staining only a few rhabdomyosarcomas, gliomas, Wilms' tumors, and neuroendocrine tumors (1,38,40,112,162). However, a recent large review (137) has documented staining in a wide variety of carcinomas and sarcomas. Its presence in lymphomas is particularly noteworthy (120), however, as they have a Ewing-like pattern of reactivity that could create diagnostic confusion in osseous neoplasms. The antigenicity of MIC2 is well preserved in formalin-fixed, paraffin-embedded tissue, which because of its higher specificity (40) is actually preferable to frozen tissue. MIC2 expression in Ewing's sarcomas does not appear to be related to expression of the t(11;22) fusion protein (see below) (34), but it may have an interactive function with insulinlike growth factors that function as potent autocrine growth stimulators in these neoplasms (54,159,170). At any rate, MIC2 appears to be the first discriminatory immunohistochemical marker for the diagnosis of Ewing's sarcoma, a tumor heretofore diagnosed often by exclusion, and offers additional evidence for its homology with peripheral neuroepithelioma, as discussed below.

Cytogenetics

Cytogenetically, Ewing's sarcoma is characterized by a balanced, reciprocal translocation, the t(11;22)(q24;q12) (Fig. 15) (32,157). Similar analyses have shown an identical translocation in cell lines of peripheral neuroepitheliomas (also known as peripheral primitive neuroectodermal tumors) and Askin's tumors (164,165), indicating a histogenetic relationship among these neoplasms. Although Ewing's sarcoma is generally not considered to be an inherited tumor, a similar constitutional translocation involving the same chromosome regions has been found in over 100 families. However, this constitutional t(11;22) is not associated with neoplasia, and by using in situ hydridization the constitutional and the tumor-associated translocations are found to involve different breakpoints (51). Other nonrandom cytogenetic abnormalities besides the t(11;22) have been reported in Ewing's sarcoma, including the der(16)t(1;16)(q21;q13) (31,97,169) and trisomy 8 (85,97). As is

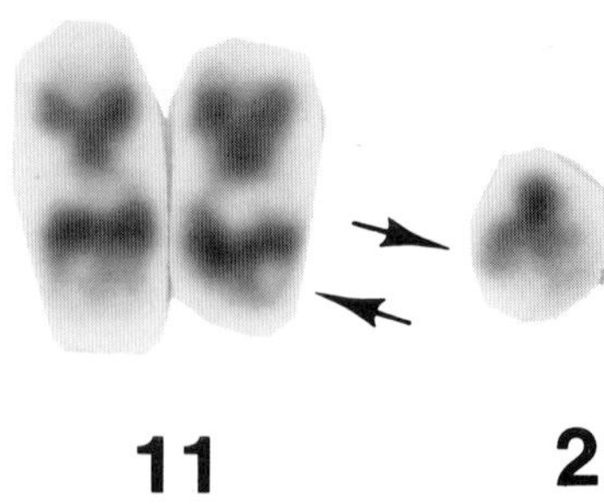

FIG. 15. t(11;22)(q24;q12) found in karyotype of case of Ewing's sarcoma. There is shortening of the long arm of chromosome 11 and lengthening of the long arm of chromosome 22. (Courtesy of Marc Valentine, St. Jude Children's Research Hospital.)

often the case with tumors possessing multiple karyotypic derangements, these additional anomalies may be evidence of malignant progression (161).

Ploidy studies in Ewing's sarcomas have yielded conflicting results. Dierick and colleagues (28) obtained evidence of aneuploidy in a sizable proportion of their patients and indicated that this feature portends a worse prognosis. However, different ploidy results were obtained depending on whether flow cytometry or image analysis was used. In our series (unpublished data) and that of Kowal-Vern et al. (71), aneuploidy is distinctly uncommon and not prognostically significant. Tetraploidy was not uncommon, but it also fails to show prognostic significance.

Cloning of the DNA sequences involved in the breakpoint of the t(11;22) has enabled identification of the genes affected by this characteristic aberration (Fig. 16). The translocation alters the open reading frame of the *EWS* gene on chromosome 22, by substituting the normal sequence that encodes a RNA binding domain with the DNA binding domain of the *Fli-1* gene of chromosome 11 (26). In mice, *Fli-1* is a retroviral integration site that is rearranged in erythroleukemia cell clones induced by the Friend murine leukemia virus (7,8). The presence of a similar alteration in the human homologue of this gene in Ewing's sarcoma suggests that its dysfunction as a DNA transcription factor leads to oncogenesis (87).

Besides the t(11;22), Ewing's sarcomas and peripheral neuroepitheliomas may contain an alternate translocation, t(21;22), in a minority of cases (133). In this translocation, the *ERG* gene on chromosome 21 fuses with the *EWS* gene on chromosome 22. The ERG protein belongs to the ETS family of transcription factors, similar to Fli-1, so that the fusion protein produced by the t(21;22) appears to have a tumorigenic effect similar to the t(11;22) and to result in histologically identical tumors (133). The *EWS* gene fuses not only with *Fli-1* and *ERG*, but also with several other genes in other types of tumors, such as the desmoplastic round cell tumor and

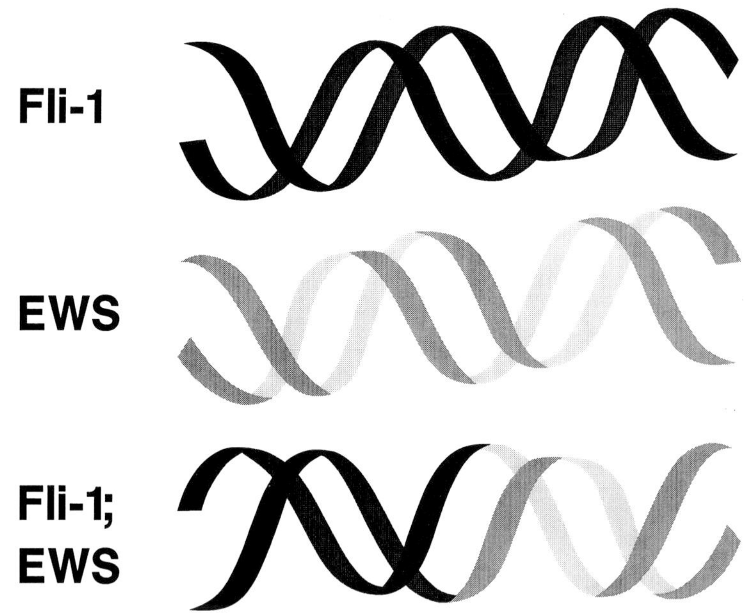

FIG. 16. Illustration of gene fusion occurring in t(11;22)(q24;q12) of Ewing's sarcoma. The *Fli-1* gene, located on chromosome 11 (black DNA, **top panel**) is fused to the *EWS* gene, located on chromosome 22 (gray DNA, **middle panel**), resulting in a *Fli-1;EWS* fusion gene (**lower panel**).

clear cell sarcoma of tendons and aponeuroses (73). Thus *EWS* appears to be a potent initiator of tumor formation in neoplasms with a variety of histologies.

Identification and cloning of the genetic sequence of the t(11;22) rearrangements have led to the creation of oligonucleotide primers that can be used as diagnostic reagents with the polymerase chain reaction (PCR) or fluorescence in situ hybridization (FISH) (33,147). To perform PCR, one uses reverse transcriptase to create a double-stranded cDNA template from the cellular RNA produced by the t(11;22) fusion. This template, which contains the translocation site derived from the fusion gene, then is subjected to the PCR reaction and amplified to create a visible signal (Fig. 17). The extreme sensitivity of this technique allows detection of very small amount of tumor RNA, and it can be enhanced by techniques such as the use of "nested" primers (33). RT-PCR can also be used to detect the alternate translocation of Ewing's sarcoma, the t(21;22) (25). The *Fli-1/EWS* gene fusion can also be directly detected using Southern blotting (74). Perhaps more attractive to the microscopist is the FISH technique, in which DNA primers containing the translocation are annealed to tumor DNA, producing a characteristic pattern of fluorescent dots on interphase nuclei (Fig. 18; see figure in color plate section) (48,147). However, with FISH whole nuclei must be tested in order to include the entire genome. Thus, because they include only a portion of the nucleus, 5-μm tissue sections are generally inadequate for reliable sampling.

Histogenesis

The undifferentiated cytologic nature of Ewing's sarcoma has intrigued pathologists since its inception as a diagnostic entity. As a result, a number of histogenetic

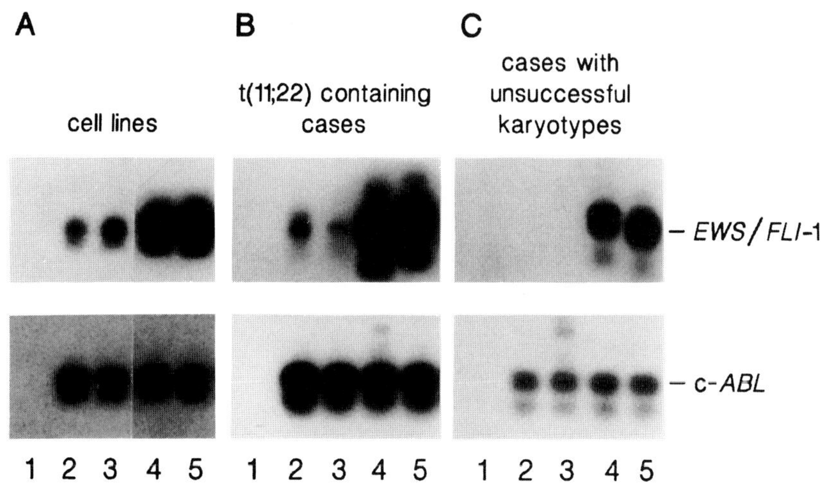

FIG. 17. Reverse transcriptase–polymerase chain reaction study of four Ewing's sarcoma cell lines **(A),** four frozen tumors demonstrated to contain the t(11;22)(q24;q12) by previous studies **(B),** and four cases with unsuccessful karyotypes **(C).** Lane 1 in each panel is a negative control, and the bottom panels are positive controls testing for the ubiquitously expressed gene *c-ABL.* The EWS/Fli-1 transcript is found in all cases previously verified to contain the t(11;22) and in two of four untested tumors. (From Downing JR et al. *Am J Pathol* 1993;143: 1294–1300, courtesy of the American Society of Investigative Pathology.)

theories have been postulated for this tumor; proposed candidates for the cell of origin include endothelial, pericytic, reticulum, myeloid, osteogenic, mesenchymal, and neuroectodermal cells (171). Currently, Ewing's sarcoma appears to most likely have a neuroectodermal origin, as evidenced by the finding of rosettes in some tumors, by the characteristic translocation which is identical to that found in peripheral neuroepitheliomas (164), and by seminal work performed by Cavazzana and colleagues (12), who tested five Ewing's sarcoma cell lines derived from tumors with typical histology and immunophenotype. The cells were treated in vitro with differentiating agents such as retinoic acid and nerve growth factors, which induced them to display neural features such as neurite production, neurosecretory granules, and NSE positivity. Others have confirmed this work either by similar in vitro induction of differentiation (81,105) or by noting the presence of neuroectodermal markers in untreated cell lines (80).

Clinical Behavior

Prior to the modern chemotherapy era, the prognosis for Ewing's sarcoma of bone was dismal, with a 5-year survival rate of 0–12% (135). Happily, recent advances in therapy have led to prolonged remissions in the majority of patients (99,115). In a St. Jude series, disease-free survival rates at 3 years were 82% for localized lesions <8 cm and 64% for localized lesions >8 cm (58). Fourteen of 18 patients with previously untreated metastatic disease were rendered grossly free of tumor by using chemotherapy and delayed surgery, and 10 patients were disease-free after a median of 47 months (59). There are a number of factors that affect these survival rates. In the Intergroup Ewing's Sarcoma Study (69), the site of the primary tumor ranked as the most important predictor of outcome in patients with localized tumors; patients with tumors in the pelvis had the poorest survival rate, whereas those with lesions in the distal extremities had a relatively good outcome. Predictably, metastatic disease at presentation, unfortunately a rather common occurrence, also has an adverse effect on survival (167). These metastases typically involve the lungs, pleura, bones, and regional lymph nodes (149). Other features reported to be of prognostic significance include tumor volume (66), amount of tumor necrosis (20,82), histologic (66) and clinical (106) response of tumor to chemotherapy, elevated erythrocyte sedimentation rate (167), and tumor extension into soft tissue (90).

Extraosseous Ewing's Sarcoma

In 1969 a group of four cases of paravertebral small cell tumors that did not involve bone but were histologically indistinguishable from Ewing's sarcoma was reported by Tefft and coworkers (148). A series of additional 39 cases of similar soft tissue sarcomas, called extraosseous Ewing's sarcoma, were later described by Angervall and Enzinger in 1975 (2). These tumors were subsequently included with tumors treated on the Intergroup Rhabdomyosarcoma Study (IRS) and were subdivided into types I and II, with type I corresponding to the conventional monomorphous small cell Ewing's sarcoma and type II to the large cell "atypical" Ewing's

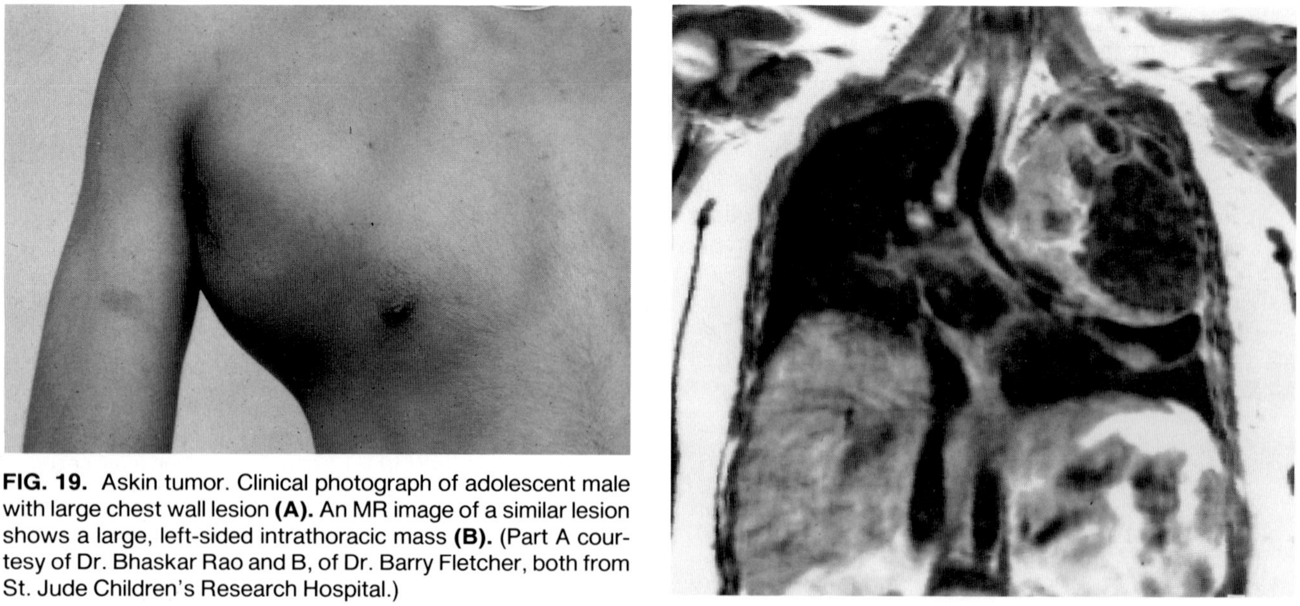

A B

FIG. 19. Askin tumor. Clinical photograph of adolescent male with large chest wall lesion **(A).** An MR image of a similar lesion shows a large, left-sided intrathoracic mass **(B).** (Part A courtesy of Dr. Bhaskar Rao and B, of Dr. Barry Fletcher, both from St. Jude Children's Research Hospital.)

sarcoma (134). IRS-I and II patients with these tumors had a response to therapy intermediate between botryoid and alveolar rhabdomyosarcomas and roughly corresponding to embryonal rhabdomyosarcomas (101). Retrospective pathologic analysis of the IRS extraosseous Ewing's sarcoma cases revealed that 13 of 14 exhibited single or multiple neural markers (neuron-specific enolase, S-100 protein, and/or neurosecretory granules) (130). Similar ultrastructural observations of primitive neural differentiation in extraosseous Ewing's sarcoma were made by Mierau (91). It has thus become apparent that there is a great deal of phenotypic overlap between extraosseous Ewing's sarcoma and peripheral neuroepithelioma (155). Diagnosis should not be attempted on these lesions without corroborative ancillary studies (155).

PERIPHERAL NEUROEPITHELIOMA (PERIPHERAL PRIMITIVE NEUROECTODERMAL TUMOR)

History

The first description of a peripheral neuroepithelioma was that of Stout (139), who in 1918 reported an ulnar nerve tumor composed of small round cells forming rosettes. After cells from a similar tumor grew axons in tissue culture, he postulated that this lesion bore a relationship to neuroblastoma (141). Sporadic but uncommon descriptions of similar neural tumors appeared thereafter (100), and it is now evident that this neoplasm was grossly underreported (17,124). This began to change in the 1970s, when Seemayer et al. (128) published a series of similar tumors that did not appear to involve nerves, Askin and coworkers (4) described a series of chest wall tumors (Fig. 19), and Liebermann (78) popularized the tumor in a series of lectures. The tumor described by Askin was termed the "malignant small round cell tumor of the thoracopulmonary region," but is better known as the Askin tumor. Askin's lesions are enigmatic in his original description, as they were PAS-negative and sometimes appeared to have neural features by electron microscopy, features not typical of Ewing's sarcoma (4). Later, Linnoila et al. (79) expanded this category of "Askin tumor" to include PAS-positive, diastase-sensitive neoplasms, all of which were also NSE-positive. More than anyone, Dehner has crystallized our concepts and understanding of these diverse, often baffling tumors through a series of enlightening editorials (21-23). As a result of a flurry of publications, peripheral neuroepitheliomas are now considered to be one of the most common pediatric soft tissue sarcomas (55).

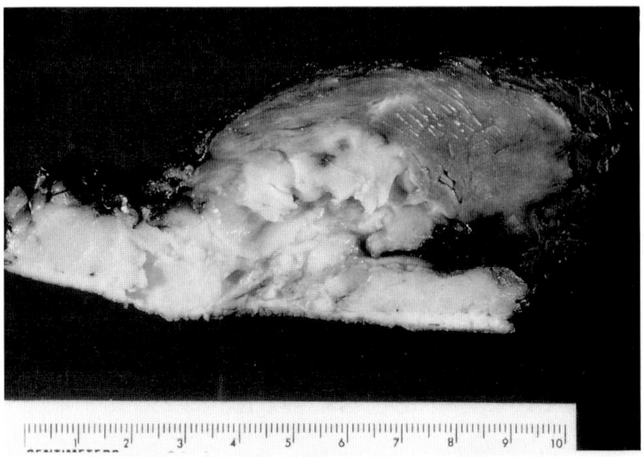

FIG. 20. Gross photograph of peripheral neuroepithelioma arising in the soft tissues and invading skeletal muscle.

Gross Features

Grossly, peripheral neuroepitheliomas are invasive, lobulated, gray–tan masses (Fig. 20) that may arise within or adjacent to a large nerve (65,86,100). In Enzinger and Weiss's series (36), the most common locations are buttock, upper thigh, shoulder, and upper arm. In the St. Jude series (86), pelvis and chest wall (Fig. 19) are also prominent. Other than the association with nerve, there are no particular gross features that would allow one to separate this lesion from rhabdomyosarcoma or other primitive tumors.

Microscopic Features

Microscopically, the most characteristic feature of peripheral neuroepithelioma is the Homer Wright rosette (Fig. 21; see figure in color plate section), which is quite reminiscent of those seen in neuroblastoma (see Chapter 6). Some have considered these structures mandatory for the diagnosis (84), but it is the opinion of the author and others (123) that immunohistochemistry, electron microscopy, and genetic analysis may identify peripheral neuroepitheliomas not having obvious rosettes. As with neuroblastoma, the rosettes have a central fibrillary core surrounded by a rim of primitive tumor cells with prominent nuclei, but they differ from neuroblastic tumors by often being poorly formed and difficult to recognize at first glance. At times these structures are scarce, and the tumor cells may be more sheetlike, corded, or trabecular, reminiscent of carcinoid tumors or small cell carcinomas. Spindle cell areas have been described (36). Flexner-type rosettes with a central lumen (Fig. 22; see figure in color plate section), as are characteristic of retinoblastoma, may be seen in some cases (57,86,123). Unlike neuroblastoma, ganglion cells and well-developed neuropil are vanishingly rare but have been reported (Fig. 23) (86,123,128).

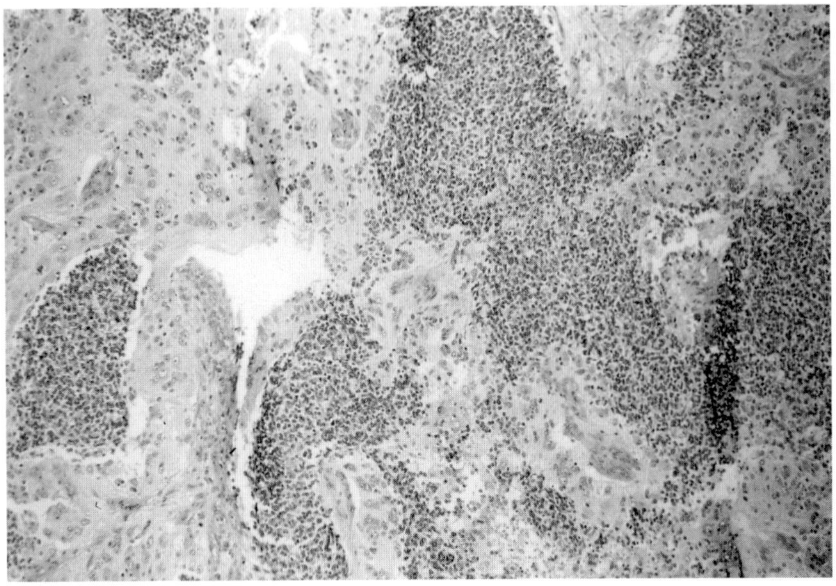

FIG. 23. Peripheral neuroepithelioma of chest wall of an infant. There are small cell foci admixed with areas of neural differentiation.

Electron Microscopy

The electron microscopic features of peripheral neuroepithelioma are also reminiscent of neuroblastoma, as both tumors characteristically include dendritic processes, microtubules, and dense core, neurosecretory-type granules (Fig. 24). The processes are best developed in the center of the rosettes (Fig. 25). Also conspicuous in these foci are the dense core granules, which may be also found in other areas of the tumor (36). However, one must be careful not to confuse neurosecretory dense core granules with primary lysosomes, which have a similar morphology and size range. Helpful features characteristic of primary lysosomes are their tendency to occur near Golgi structures and to be associated with phagolysosomes. Some cases contain a mixture of atypical neurosecretory granules and lysosomes (79). One must also beware of potential confusion with other cytoplasmic granules, such as the Weibel–Palade bodies of endothelial cells and the premelanosomes of melanocytes.

Although peripheral neuroepithelioma and neuroblastoma are similar tumors at an ultrastructural level,

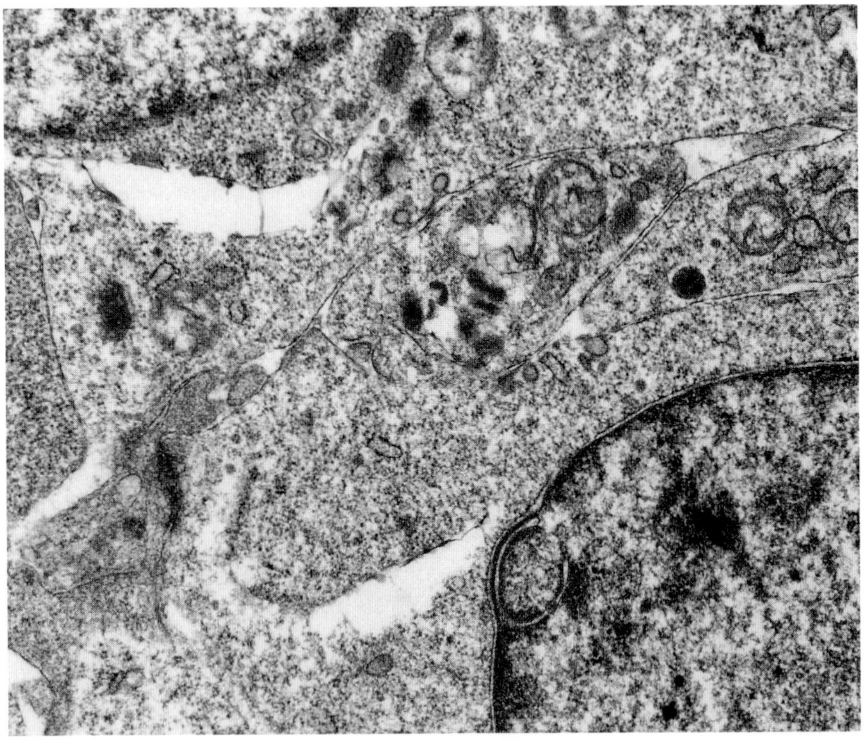

FIG. 24. Electron micrograph of peripheral neuroepithelioma containing dendritic processes with neurosecretory granules. Membrane-bound vesicles are also apparent.

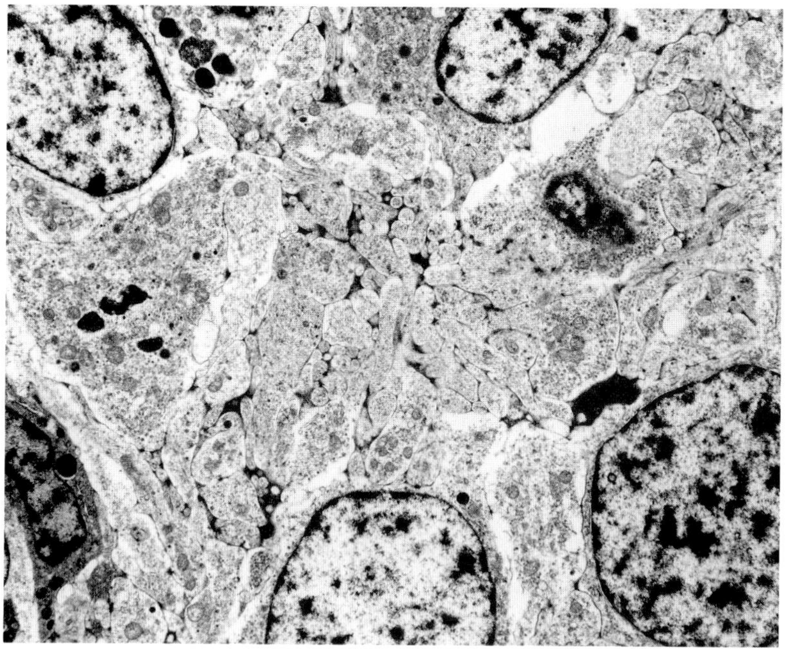

FIG. 25. Electron micrograph of central portion of a rosette seen in a peripheral neuroepithelioma. There are numerous interweaving processes in this region.

Mierau feels that they can usually be separated by the features of more advanced differentiation shown by neuroblastoma (personal communication). Peripheral neuroepitheliomas are poorly differentiated tumors, so that careful ultrastructural observation is required. Beside neural organelles, features of primitive epithelial differentiation may be found occasionally (Fig. 26). When observing processes, one must be aware of the possibility that formation of these structures is also a property of peripheral nerve sheath tumors, which are more commonly associated with large nerves. Thus, one must also search for structures such as basal lamina, pseudomesaxons, and long-spacing collagen (Luse bodies) (see Chapter 8).

Immunohistochemistry

Although helpful, electron microscopy can be misleading, so that correlation with immunohistochemistry is imperative. Immunohistochemical studies can be of great assistance in the diagnosis of peripheral neuroepithelioma (122), but it is also sometimes confusing, so that the author strongly recommends a full battery of

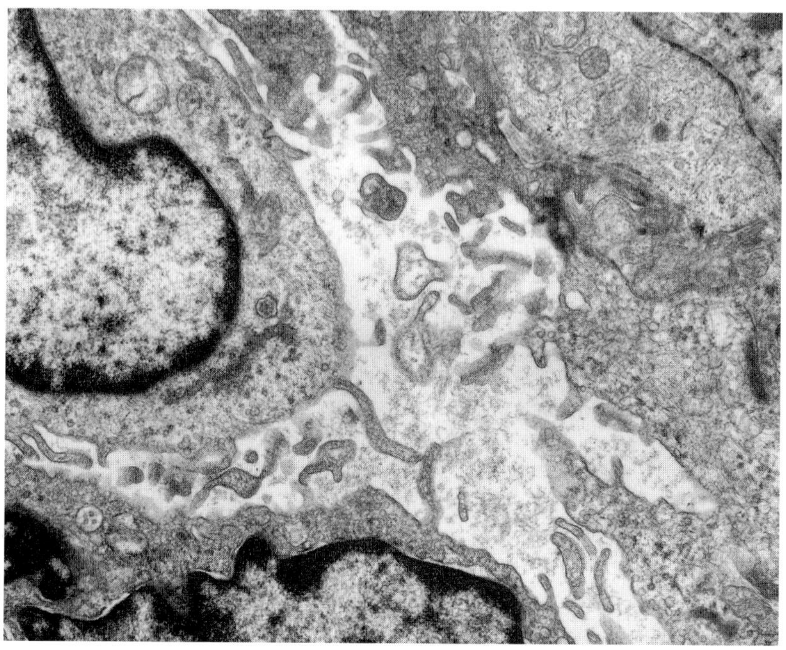

FIG. 26. Electron micrograph of peripheral neuroepithelioma with primitive epithelial differentiation. There is a central lumen lined by microvilli. Junctional complexes are seen in the juxtaluminal regions of the cells abutting the lumen. (From Parham DM et al. *Am J Clin Pathol* 1991;95:166–171, courtesy of American Society of Clinical Pathologists.)

testing in possible cases. Immunohistochemical study of peripheral neuroepithelioma may require a large battery of stains to exclude other diagnostic possibilities such as rhabdomyosarcoma or lymphoma and to determine the extent of neural differentiation. The stains that are employed in a typical panel are listed in Table 2. Immunohistochemical markers that have been reported as positive in peripheral neuroepithelioma are listed in Table 3. The most exhaustive immunohistochemical study has been that of Cavazzana et al. (13), who in a series of 42 cases of peripheral neuroepithelioma reported that NSE was positive in 95%, β_2-microglobulin in 77%, synaptophysin in 73%, S-100 protein in 67%, neurofilament triplet protein in 38%, and chromogranin in none. β_2-microglobulin is negative in neuroblastomas and can be used as a differential stain, just as chromogranin, which is positive in neuroendocrine tumors, might be used to distinguish poorly differentiated carcinoids and paragangliomas from peripheral neuroepithelioma. Cavazzana concluded that "NSE positivity plus beta-2-microglobulin positivity, preferably with positive synaptophysin and supportive electron microscopy, mandates a diagnosis of peripheral neuroepithelioma." Coffin and Dehner (17) were more exacting in their demand for neural differentiation, as in their series all peripheral neuroepitheliomas were positive for NSE, synaptophysin, and Leu 7.

Differentiation of peripheral neuroepithelioma from extraosseous Ewing's sarcoma can be quite perplexing and often seems arbitrary, as they can have similar immunohistochemical findings and even ultrastructural features (91,130). In fact, the histologic appearances of the two entities may merge in a given tumor (72). This distinction is generally made today by demonstration of positivity for two or more neural markers or by the presence of rosettes, such tumors being called peripheral neuroepithelioma (125). Distinction from rhabdomyosarcoma can generally be made by the use of electron microscopy and the muscle markers desmin and muscle-specific actin. However, we observed desmin- and actin-positive peripheral neuroepitheliomas (Fig. 27; see figure in color plate section) (108), which hypothetically are demonstrating the myogenic capability of neural crest cells (95). These lesions could be considered a form of

TABLE 2. *Initial immunohistochemical battery used at St. Jude for the diagnosis of peripheral neuroepithelioma*

MIC2
Neuron-specific enolase (NSE)
Synaptophysin
Leu 7
S100
Desmin
Muscle-specific actin
CD45 (leukocyte common antigen)

TABLE 3. *Immunohistochemical markers that may be positive with peripheral neuroepithelioma*

MIC2
Neuron-specific enolase
β_2-Microglobulin
Synaptophysin
S100
Neurofilaments
Desmin
Muscle-specific actin
Cytokeratin
Epithelial membrane antigen
Cholecystokinin
Carcinoembryonic antigen
Glial fibrillary acidic protein

primitive ectomesenchymoma (see below), multiphenotypic tumors with combined features of early neural and myogenic differentiation. Carcinoembryonic antigen, epithelial membrane antigen, and cytokeratin positivity (44,52,131) demonstrate the epithelial potential of neural crest development apparent in peripheral neuroepithelioma, glial fibrillary acidic protein (52,123) the potential for gliogenesis, and cholecystokinin production (127) the capacity for neuroendocrine differentiation.

As noted above, one of the most useful markers for peripheral neuroepithelioma is the recently described Ewing's sarcoma marker, MIC2, which is recognized by the monoclonal antibodies HBA71, 12E7, and O13 (1,40,137,162). One must note that this marker may also stain lymphomas (119,120) and occasional rhabdomyosarcomas (119). Although lymphomas are frequently MIC2-positive, rhabdomyosarcomas are usually MIC2-negative, usually only show staining in differentiated myoblasts, and typically exhibit diffuse cytoplasmic MIC2 positivity or nuclear positivity rather than the membranous pattern seen with peripheral neuroepithelioma (119,137).

Of particular diagnostic utility is the presence of MIC2 in the vast majority of peripheral neuroepitheliomas and its absence in poorly differentiated neuroblastomas (107). These two neoplasms may generate confusion because of their frequent occurrence in children in paraspinal or pelvic locations and their common neural features, but they have quite dissimilar treatment regimens. A similar distinction between neuroblastoma and neuroepithelioma may also be made with β_2-microglobulin and class I immunocompatibility antigens (29,45,75, 107,166). It must be noted in this regard that differentiating neuroblastic cells are β_2-microglobulin-positive (107). Conversely, neuroblastomas typically exhibit neural cell adhesion molecule (NCAM) and chromogranin positivity, contrasting with the absence of these markers in neuroepitheliomas (13,46). Neuroblastomas have also been distinguished from peripheral neuroepitheliomas by the use of morphometry (14).

Biology

Distinct differences also exist in the cytogenetics, proto-oncogene expression, and neurotransmitter production of peripheral neuroepithelioma and neuroblastoma. As noted above, peripheral neuroepithelioma is cytogenetically noted for the characteristic t(11;22) translocation, whereas neuroblastoma karyotypes tend to contain alterations in chromosome 1, double minutes, and homogeneously staining regions (see Chapter 6) (10,165). Double-minute chromosomes have been reported in two Askin tumors with a t(11;22) (129). Detection of the t(11;22) by FISH or PCR offers another potential means of tumor diagnosis, as noted above with Ewing's sarcoma (33,48,147). On the other hand, neuroblastomas can show *N-myc* amplification, elevated expression of N-*myc*, and decreased expression of C-*myc*, contrasting with the decreased expression of N-*myc* and the elevated expression of C-*myc* in peripheral neuroepitheliomas (151). There are also intriguing differences in neurotransmitter enzyme activities, as peripheral neuroepithelioma cell lines have high levels of cholinacetyltransferase, a key parasympathetic pathway enzyme, and neuroblastoma cell lines contain high levels of dopamine β-hydroxylase and tyrosine hydroxylase, sympathetic pathway enzymes (151). Peripheral neuroepitheliomas thus behave as tumors of the parasympathetic system, contrasting with the sympathetic differentiation of neuroblastoma. As a result, patients with peripheral neuroepithelioma typically have normal levels of urinary catecholamines (17), although exceptions have been reported (160).

Clinical Behavior

Patients with peripheral neuroepitheliomas have shown a poor survival rate. The patients in the series of chest wall tumors of Askin et al. (4) had a median survival of only 8 months. The St. Jude series (86) demonstrated a substantially shorter disease control interval than patients with Ewing's sarcoma of bone or neuroblastoma—10.5 months vs. 24 months. However, peripheral neuroepitheliomas show a definite response to chemotherapy, as patients treated at the National Cancer Institute showed an actuarial survival of 68% after a median follow-up of 18 months and an actuarial relapse-free survival rate of 56% at 12 months (93). An analysis of 42 patients in the German Society of Pediatric Oncology revealed a disease-free survival of 56% after 3 years for patients with localized tumors; however, 9 of 10 patients with metastatic tumors showed disease progression by this time (65). Peripheral neuroepithelioma characteristically metastases to the lungs, in contradistinction to neuroblastoma, which usually metastasizes to bone and liver and rarely spreads to lung (86).

ECTOMESENCHYMOMA

Ectomesenchymoma is a multiphenotypic tumor that typically contains elements of both skeletal muscle and nerve. In its most developed state, it is composed of well-differentiated rhabdomyosarcoma containing scattered ganglion cells (35). In the author's experience, these lesions are most apt to arise in paratesticular or inguinal

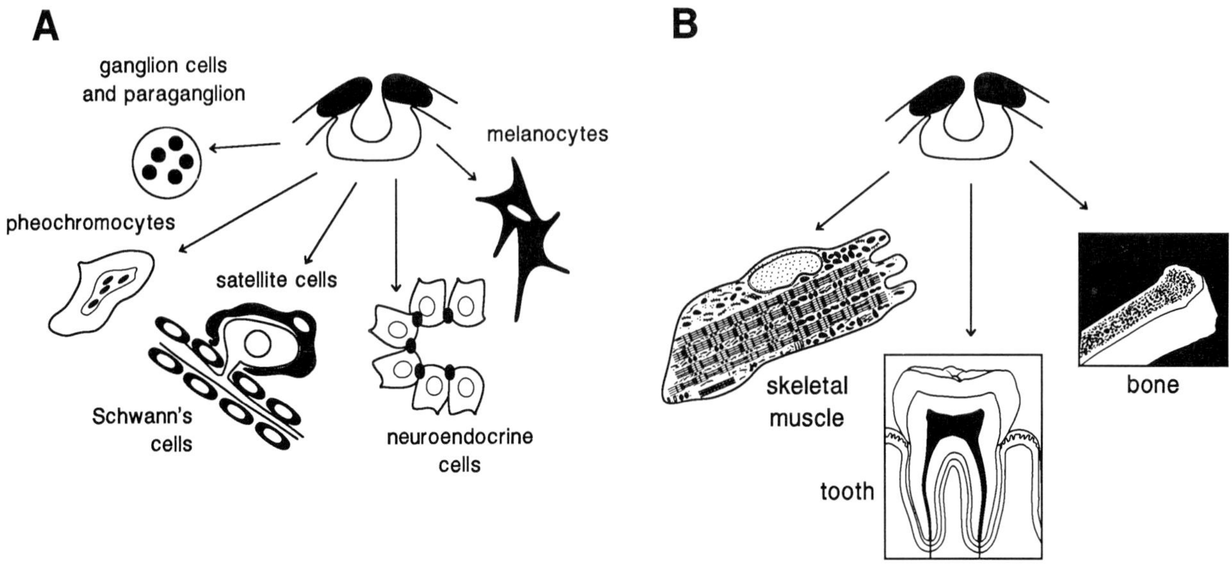

FIG. 29. Neural crest differentiation. Development of neuroectodermal tissues such as ganglion cells, pheochromocytes, Schwann cells, satellite cells, neuroendocrine cells, and melanocytes **(A)** is well known. However, neural crest cells in the developing head also differentiate into skeletal muscle, bone, and dental pulp **(B)**.

locations. Malignant, or primitive, ectomesenchymoma (68) is composed of less differentiated cells and may closely resemble peripheral neuroepithelioma in some areas and alveolar rhabdomyosarcoma in others. Immunohistochemical and ultrastructural examination should confirm the presence of both elements (Fig. 28; see figure in color plate section). Other cell types reported in these tumors include neuroglial cells, Schwann cells, lipoblasts, melanocytes, fibrohistiocytic cells, meningothelial cells, and chondrocytes (155).

Histogenetically, this occurrence should not occasion surprise, as the mesenchyme of the head is derived from neural crest elements (76). This phenomenon may explain why the head and neck are the most common sites of the primitive lesions (155). The wide diversity of tissues that originate from neuroectoderm (Fig. 29) is no doubt responsible for the plethora of cell types seen with its associated neoplasms. An ectomesenchymoma cell line with a t(11;22)(q24;q12) and translocation with a breakpoint involving chromosome 13q14, the site of the alveolar rhabdomyosarcoma t(2;13) disruption, has been reported (163). These two anomalies suggest that the cells have genotypic and as well as phenotypic features of both rhabdomyosarcoma and peripheral neuroepithelioma.

In a similar vein, the t(11;22) has been reported in small cell osteosarcoma (104) and mesenchymal chondrosarcoma (121), bone lesions that contain elements of Ewing's sarcoma as well as osteogenic and chondroid (see Chapter 9). These findings suggest that Ewing- type tumors are capable of other types of differentiation, as implied by the category of "primitive sarcoma of bone" defined by Tsokos and colleagues (156). These tumors are histologically similar to typical Ewing's sarcomas, but at the ultrastructural level they have features indicative of early mesenchymal differentiation. Another related tumor is the "polyhistioma," or "multipotential sarcoma of bone" (43,61,63), which contains a variety of phenotypes including small cell sarcoma.

MELANOTIC NEUROECTODERMAL TUMOR

Melanotic neuroectodermal tumor is a distinctive and relatively benign form of primitive neuroectodermal tumor, usually occurring in infants and very young children (24). It is also known by a number of other terms, foremost among them retinal anlage tumor and melanotic progonoma. These lesions typically arise in the facial region and jaw, but may occur in diverse locations such as the epididymis (18).

As the name implies, melanotic neuroectodermal tumors are composed of neuroepithelial cells with areas of melanin production (24). This pigment finely dusts nests of small embryonal cells having prominent nuclei and moderate amounts of cytoplasm. The tumor cells are dispersed as discrete cohesive nests surrounded by an abundant desmoplastic stroma, somewhat similar to the desmoplastic small cell tumor of the abdomen. Neuroblastlike small cells are typically intermingled with the pigmented cells (Fig. 30).

An array of phenotypic diversity is present in melanotic neuroectodermal tumors, as immunohistochemical stains demonstrate positivity for epithelial, mesenchymal, and neural markers as well as the melanocytic protein HMB45 (113,118,138). Conversely, S-100 protein, usually positive in melanoma, is negative in these tumors. However, muscle actin positivity can create a misleading impression of rhabdomyosarcomatous differentiation in small biopies (118). Electron microscopy reveals a mixture of cells with melanocytic and neuroblastic features (18,24,113).

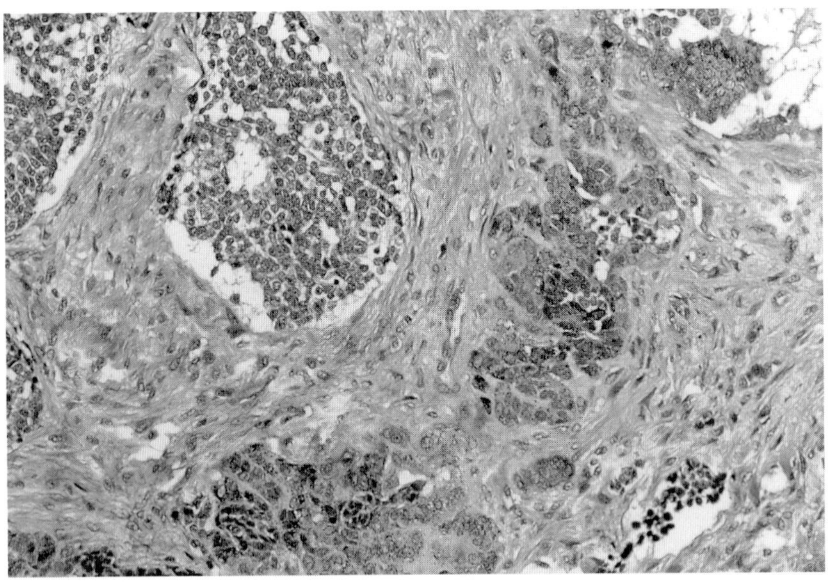

FIG. 30. Melanotic neuroectodermal tumor. There is a mixture of nests of primitive round cells **(upper left)** and pigment laden cells **(midright)** in a fibrous stroma.

Biologically, melanotic neuroectodermal tumors are akin to neuroblastoma, for they exhibit tyrosine hydroxylase activity (24). These lesions usually behave in a benign fashion, although malignancy has been reported (114). The benign behavior of this neoplasm and its histologic features suggest a choristomatous lesion, and an oropharyngeal case with simultaneous occurrence of brain heterotopia, indicating a neural tube defect, tends to corroborate this hypothesis (77).

ESTHESIONEUROBLASTOMA

Esthesioneuroblastoma is a primitive neuroectodermal tumor that arises from the neuroepithelium of the olfactory region of the nose (6,143). This typical location is useful for the clinical recognition of this region, for magnetic resonance (MR) scans reveal a distinctive but nondiagnostic picture with a destructive mass arising in the superior nasal cavity (Fig. 31). However, in the proper clinical setting, radiologic studies strongly suggest the diagnosis, which is often delayed because of an incorrect assumption that affected patients suffer from rhinitis or sinusitis.

Microscopically, esthesioneuroblastomas are invasive lesions composed of primitive small round cells that typically show no evidence of differentiation with routine stains. Rosettes and fibrillary material may be present, causing this tumor to be considered a neuroblastoma-type neoplasm until recently, when a Ewing-type t(11;22)(q24;q12) karyotypic anomaly was discovered (11). Thus, these malignancies appear to be more akin to peripheral neuroepithelioma than to neuroblastoma, although an EWS/Fli-1 transcript was not detected in a single case analyzed (110). Tyrosine hydroxylase activity in esthesioneuroblastoma cells (144) paradoxically would relate these neoplasms more to neuroblastomas than to peripheral neuroepitheliomas (150).

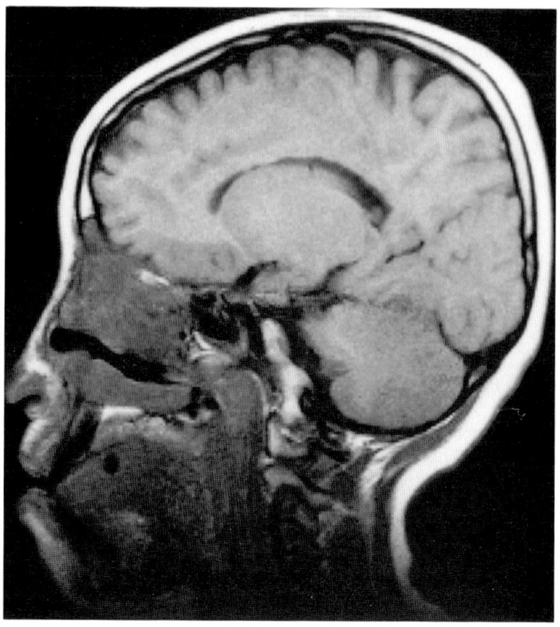

FIG. 31. Midsagittal magnetic resonance imaging scan of child with esthesioneuroblastoma. The tumor fills the upper nasal cavity and invades the superior-anterior portions of the overlying cranium. (Courtesy of Dr. James Langston, St. Jude Children's Research Hospital.)

Also unlike peripheral neuroepitheliomas, esthesioneuroblastomas are MIC2-negative (162). Positive immunohistochemical markers primarily include neural proteins such as synaptophysin, chromogranin, S-100, Leu 7, NSE, and neurofilaments (5,6,16,42,111,143, 145,154). As with peripheral neuroepitheliomas, markers such as cytokeratin, vimentin, and GFAP that are typical of other cell types may also be positive (6,16,42,143,145). Evidence of epithelial or myogenic differentiation may even be apparent with routine histology (102,132). Immunohistochemical studies may nevertheless be quite useful in distinguishing esthesioneuroblastoma from rhabdomyosarcomas, carcinomas, lymphomas, and gliomas that arise in the nasal cavity. Careful scrutiny of immunostains for neural markers will also reveal positivity in the neuroepithelial cells in the adjacent mucosa (Fig. 32; see figure in color plate section).

Electron microscopic studies of esthesioneuroblastomas are also often profitable for diagnosis, as neurosecretory granules, neuritic processes, synaptic vesicles, and microtubules may be found (15,143,145,146). Schwann cells are often seen by electron microscopy and resemble the sustentacular cells of the nasal epithelium (143,145); they correspond to S-100-positive cells found at the tumor–stroma interface (145).

Esthesioneuroblastomas are typically aggressive lesions that are therapeutically challenging and often locally recurrent. Metastases are not uncommon. Prognosis can be related to tumor grade (96).

ACKNOWLEDGMENT

Supported by National Cancer Institute (NCI) Center Support Grant P30 CA21765 and American Lebanese Syrian Associated Charities (ALSAC).

REFERENCES

1. Ambros IM, Ambros PF, Strehl S, Kovar H, Gadner H, Salzer-Kuntschik M. MIC2 is a specific marker for Ewing's sarcoma and peripheral primitive neuroectodermal tumors: evidence for a common histogenesis of Ewing's sarcoma and peripheral primitive neuroectodermal tumors from MIC2 expression and specific chromosome aberration. *Cancer* 1991;67:1886–1893.
2. Angervall L, Enzinger FM. Extraskeletal neoplasm resembling Ewing's sarcoma. *Cancer* 1975;36:240–251.
3. Ashfaq R, Weinberg AG, Argyle CA. Acute megakaryoblastic leukemia simulating carcinoma. *Am J Clin Pathol* 1992;98:55–60.
4. Askin FB, Rosai J, Sibley RK, Dehner LP, McAlister WH. Ma-

lignant small cell tumor of the thoracopulmonary region in childhood: a distinctive clinicopathologic entity of uncertain histogenesis. *Cancer* 1979;43:2438–2451.

5. Axe S, Kuhajda FP. Esthesioneuroblastoma: intermediate filaments, neuroendocrine, and tissue-specific antigens. *Am J Clin Pathol* 1987;88:139–145.
6. Banerjee AK, Sharma BS, Vashista RK, Kak VK. Intracranial olfactory neuroblastoma: evidence for olfactory epithelial origin. *J Clin Pathol* 1992;45:299–302.
7. Ben-David Y, Giddens EB, Bernstein A. Identification and mapping of a common proviral integration site Fli-1 in erythroleukemia cells induced by Friend murine leukemia virus. *Proc Natl Acad Sci USA* 1990;87:1332–1336.
8. Ben-David Y, Giddens EB, Letwin K, Bernstein A. Erythroleukemia induction by Friend murine leukemia virus: insertional activation of a new member of the ets gene family, Fli-1, closely linked to c-ets-1. *Genes Dev* 1991;5:908–918.
9. Berry J, Fairclough D, Parham D. Relationship between atypia, neuron-specific enolase (NSE) positivity, and nuclear morphometry in Ewing's sarcoma. *Mod Pathol* 1992;5:3A(Abstract).
10. Brodeur GM. Neuroblastoma: clinical significance of genetic abnormalities. *Cancer Surv* 1990;9:673–688.
11. Cavazzana AO, Navarro S, Noguera R, Reynolds PC, Triche TJ. Olfactory neuroblastoma is not a neuroblastoma but is related to primitive neuroectodermal tumor (PNET). In: Evans, AE, ed. *Advances in Neuroblastoma Research.* vol 2. Philadelphia: Alan R. Liss; 1988:463–473.
12. Cavazzana AO, Miser JS, Jefferson J, Triche TJ. Experimental evidence for a neural origin of Ewing's sarcoma of bone. *Am J Pathol* 1987;127:507–518.
13. Cavazzana AO, Ninfo V, Roberts J, Triche TJ. Peripheral neuroepithelioma: a light microscopic, immunocytochemistry, and ultrastructural study. *Mod Pathol* 1992;5:71–78.
14. Cavazzana AO, Santopietro R, Sforza V, et al. Morphometry and the differential diagnosis between peripheral neuroepithelioma and neuroblastoma. *Mod Pathol* 1991;4:615–620.
15. Chaudhry AP, Haar JG, Koul A, Nickerson PA. Olfactory neuroblastoma (esthesioneuroblastoma): a light and ultrastructural study of two cases. *Cancer* 1979;44:564–579.
16. Choi HS, Anderson PJ. Immunohistochemical diagnosis of olfactory neuroblastoma. *J Neuropathol Exp Neurol* 1985;44:18–31.
17. Coffin CM, Dehner LP. Peripheral neurogenic tumors of the soft tissues in children and adolescents: a clinicopathologic study of 139 cases. *Pediatr Pathol* 1989;9:387–407.
18. Cutler LS, Chaudhry AP, Topazian R. Melanotic neuroectodermal tumor of infancy: an ultrastructural study, literature review, and reevaluation. *Cancer* 1981;48:257–270.
19. Dahlin DC. *Bone Tumors: General Aspects and Data on 6,221 Cases.* 3rd ed. Springfield, IL: Charles C Thomas; 1978:274–287.
20. Daugaard S, Kamby C, Sunde LM, Myhre-Jensen O, Schiodt T. Ewing's sarcoma: a retrospective study of histological and immunohistochemical factors and their relation to prognosis. *Virchows Arch A Histolpathol Anat* 1989;414:243–251.
21. Dehner LP. Peripheral and central primitive neuroectodermal tumors. A nosologic concept seeking a consensus. *Arch Pathol Lab Med* 1986;110:997–1005.
22. Dehner LP. Whence the primitive neuroectodermal tumor? *Arch Pathol Lab Med* 1990;114:16–17.
23. Dehner LP. Primitive neuroectodermal tumor and Ewing's sarcoma. *Am J Surg Pathol* 1993;17:1–13.
24. Dehner LP, Sibley RK, Sauk JJ, Jr., et al. Malignant melanotic neuroectodermal tumor of infancy: a clinical, pathologic, ultrastructural and tissue culture study. *Cancer* 1979;43:1389–1410.
25. Delattre O, Zucman J, Melot T, et al. The Ewing family of tumors—A subgroup of small-round-cell tumors defined by specific chimeric transcripts. *N Engl J Med* 1994;331:294–299.
26. Delattre O, Zucman J, Plougastel B, et al. Gene fusion with an ETS DNA-binding domain caused by chromosome translocation in human tumours. *Nature* 1992;359:162–165.
27. Dellagi K, Lipinski M, Paulin D, Portier MM, Lenoir GM, Brouet JC. Characterization of intermediate filaments expressed by Ewing tumor cell lines. *Cancer Res* 1987;47:1170–1173.
28. Dierick AM, Langlois M, Van Oostveldt P, Roels H. The prognostic significance of the DNA content in Ewing's sarcoma: a retrospective cytophotometric and flow cytometric study. *Histopathology* 1993;23:333–339.
29. Donner L, Triche T, Israel MA. A panel of monoclonal antibodies which discriminate neuroblastoma from Ewing's sarcoma, rhabdomyosarcoma, neuroepithelioma and hemopoietic malignancies. In: Evans, AG, D'Angio, GJ and Seeger, RC, eds. *Advances in Neuroblastoma Research.* New York: Alan R. Liss; 1985:347–366.
30. Dos Santos Silva I, Swerdlow AJ. Sex differences in the risks of hormone-dependent cancers. *Am J Epidemiol* 1993;138:10–28.
31. Douglass EC, Rowe ST, Valentine M, Parham D, Meyer WH, Thompson EI. A second nonrandom translocation, der(16)t(1;16)(q21;q13), in Ewing sarcoma and peripheral neuroectodermal tumor. *Cytogenet Cell Genet* 1990;53:87–90.
32. Douglass EC, Valentine M, Green AA, Hayes FA, Thompson EI. t(11;22) and other chromosomal rearrangements in Ewing's sarcoma. JNCI 1986;77:1211–1215.
33. Downing JR, Head DR, Parham DM, et al. Detection of the (11;22)(q24;q12) translocation of Ewing's sarcoma and peripheral neuroectodermal tumor by reverse transcription polymerase chain reaction. *Am J Pathol* 1993;143:1294–1300.
34. Dworzak M, Stock C, Strehl S, Gadner H, Ambros PF. Ewing's tumor X mouse hybrids expressing the MIC2 antigen: analyses using fluorescence CDD-banding and non-isotopic ISH. *Hum Genet* 1992;88:273–278.
35. Enzinger FM, Weiss SW. *Soft Tissue Tumors.* 2nd ed. St. Louis: C.V. Mosby Company, 1988: 448–488.
36. Enzinger FM, Weiss SW. *Soft Tissue Tumors.* 2nd ed. St. Louis: C.V. Mosby, 1988: 806–810.
37. Ewing J. Diffuse endothelioma of bone. *Proc NY Pathol Soc* 1921;21:17–24.
38. Fellinger EJ, Garin-Chesa P, Glasser DB, Huvos AG, Rettig WJ. Comparison of cell surface antigen HBA71 (p30/32^{MIC2}), neuron-specific enolase, and vimentin in the immunohistochemical analysis of Ewing's sarcoma of bone. *Am J Surg Pathol* 1992;16:746–755.
39. Fellinger EJ, Garin-Chesa P, Su SL, DeAngelis P, Lane JM, Rettig WJ. Biochemical and genetic characterization of the HBA71 Ewing's sarcoma cell surface antigen. *Cancer Res* 1991;51:336–340.
40. Fellinger EJ, Garin-Chesa P, Triche TJ, Huvos AG, Rettig WJ. Immunohistochemical analysis of Ewing's sarcoma cell surface antigen p30/32^{MIC2}. *Am J Pathol* 1991;139:317–325.
41. Fletcher BD, Hanna SL, Fairclough DL, Gronemeyer SA. Pediatric musculoskeletal tumors: use of dynamic, contrast-enhanced MR imaging to monitor response to chemotherapy. *Radiology* 1992;184:243–248.
42. Frierson HF, Jr., Ross GW, Mills SE, Frankfurter A. Olfactory neuroblastoma: Additional immunohistochemical characterization. *Am J Clin Pathol* 1990;94:547–553.
43. Frydman CP, Klein MJ, Abdelwahab IF, Zwass A. Primitive multipotential primary sarcoma of bone: a case report and immunohistochemical study. *Mod Pathol* 1991;4:768–772.
44. Fujii Y, Hongo T, Nakagawa Y, et al. Cell culture of small round cell tumor originating in the thoracopulmonary region: evidence for derivation from a primitive pluripotent cell. *Cancer* 1989;64:43–51.
45. Funa K, Gazdar AF, Minna JD, Linnoila RI. Paucity of beta 2-microglobulin expression on small cell lung cancer, bronchial carcinoids and certain other neuroendocrine tumors. *Lab Invest* 1986;55:186–193.
46. Garin-Chesa P, Fellinger EJ, Huvos AG, Beresford HR, Melamed MR, Triche TJ, Rettig WJ. Immunohistochemical analysis of neural cell adhesion molecules: Differential expression in small round cell tumors of childhood and adolescence. *Am J Pathol* 1991;139:275–286.
47. Gerald WL, Miller HK, Battifora H, Miettinen M, Silva EG, Rosai J. Intra-abdominal desmoplastic small round-cell tumor: report of 19 cases of a distinctive type of high-grade polyphenotypic malignancy affecting young individuals. *Am J Surg Pathol* 1991;15:499–513.
48. Giovannini M, Selleri L, Biegel JA, Scotlandi K, Emanuel BS, Evans GA. Interphase cytogenetics for the detection of the t(11;22)(q24; q12) in small round cell tumors. *J Clin Invest* 1992;90:1911–1918.

49. Goji J, Sano K, Nakamura H, Ito H. Chondrocytic differentiation of peripheral neuroectodermal tumor cell line in nude mouse xenograft. *Cancer Res* 1992;52:4214–4220.
50. Greco MA, Steiner GC, Fazzini E. Ewing's sarcoma with epithelial differentiation: fine structural and immunocytochemical study. *Ultrastruct Pathol* 1988;12:317–325.
51. Griffin CA, McKeon C, Israel MA, et al. Comparison of constitutional and tumor-associated 11;22 translocations: nonidentical breakpoints on chromosomes 11 and 22. *Proc Natl Acad Sci USA* 1986;83:6122–6126.
52. Hachitanda Y, Tsuneyoshi M, Enjoji M, Nakagawara A, Ikeda K. Congenital primitive neuroectodermal tumor with epithelial and glial differentiation: an ultrastructural and immunohistochemical study. *Arch Pathol Lab Med* 1990;114:101–105.
53. Hamilton G, Havel M, Mallinger R. Expression of a new human THY-1 related antigen in Ewing's sarcoma and peripheral neuroectodermal tumors. *Immunol Lett* 1989;22:205–210.
54. Hamilton G, Mallinger R, Hofbauer S, Havel M. The monoclonal HBA-71 antibody modulates proliferation of thymocytes and Ewing's sarcoma cells by interfering with the action of insulin-like growth factor I. *Thymus* 1991;18:33–41.
55. Harms D, Schmidt D. Rare tumors in childhood: pathologic aspects. Experience of the Kiel Pediatric Tumor Registry. *Med Pediatr Oncol* 1993;21:239–248.
56. Hartman KR, Triche TJ, Kinsella TJ, Miser JS. Prognostic value of histopathology in Ewing's sarcoma: long-term follow-up of distal extremity primary tumors. *Cancer* 1991;67:163–171.
57. Hashimoto H, Enjoji M, Nakajima T, Kiryu H, Daimaru Y. Malignant neuroepithelioma (peripheral neuroblastoma): a clinicopathologic study of 15 cases. *Am J Surg Pathol* 1983;7:309–318.
58. Hayes FA, Thompson EI, Meyer WH, et al. Therapy for localized Ewing's sarcoma of bone. *J Clin Oncol* 1989;7:208–213.
59. Hayes FA, Thompson EI, Parvey L, Rao B, Kun L, Parham D, Hustu HO. Metastatic Ewing's sarcoma: remission induction and survival. *J Clin Oncol* 1987;5:1199–1204.
60. Holman CDJ, Reynolds PM, Byrne MJJ, Trotter JM, Armstrong BK. Possible infectious etiology of six cases of Ewing's sarcoma in Western Australia. *Cancer* 1983;52:1974–1976.
61. Hutter RVP, Foote FW, Francis KC, Sherman RS. Primitive multipotential primary sarcoma of bone. *Cancer* 1966;19:1–25.
62. Hutter RVP, Francis KD, Foote FW. Ewing's sarcoma in siblings: report of the second known occurence. *Am J Surg* 1964;4:598–603.
63. Jacobson SA. Polyhistioma: a malignant tumor of bone and extraskeletal tissues. *Cancer* 1977;40:2116–2130.
64. Jaffe R, Santamaria M, Yunis EJ, Tannery NH, Agostini RM, Medina J, Goodman M. The neuroectodermal tumor of bone. *Am J Surg Pathol* 1984;8:885–898.
65. Jürgens H, Bier V, Harms D, et al. Malignant peripheral neuroectodermal tumors. A retrospective analysis of 42 patients. *Cancer* 1988;61:349–357.
66. Jürgens H, Exner U, Gadner H, et al. Multidisciplinary treatment of primary Ewing's sarcoma of bone: a 6-year experience of a European cooperative trial. *Cancer* 1988;61:23–32.
67. Kawaguchi K, Koike M. Neuron-specific enolase and Leu-7 immunoreactive small round-cell neoplasm: the relationship to Ewing's sarcoma in bone and soft tissue. *Am J Clin Pathol* 1986;86:79–83.
68. Kawamoto EH, Weidner N, Agostini RM, Jaffe R. Malignant ectomesenchymoma of soft tissue: report of two cases and review of the literature. *Cancer* 1987;59:1791–1802.
69. Kissane JM, Askin FB, Foulkes M, Stratton LB, Shirley SF. Ewing's sarcoma of bone: clinicopathologic aspects of 303 cases from the Intergroup Ewing's Sarcoma Study. *Hum Pathol* 1983;14:773–779.
70. Kovar H, Dworzak M, Strehl S, Schnell E, Ambros IM, Ambros PF, Gadner H. Overexpression of the pseudoautosomal gene MIC2 in Ewing's sarcoma and peripheral primitive neuroectodermal tumor. *Oncogene* 1990;5:1067–1070.
71. Kowal-Vern A, Walloch J, Chou P, Gonzalez-Crussi F, Price J, Potocki D, Hermar . Flow and image cytometric DNA analysis in Ewing's sarcoma. *Mod Pathol* 1992;5:56–60.
72. Kudo M. Neuroectodermal differentiation in "extraskeletal Ewing's sarcoma." *Acta Pathol Jpn* 1989;39:795–802.
73. Ladanyi M, Gerald W. Fusion of the EWS and WT1 genes in the desmoplastic small round cell tumor. *Cancer Res* 1994;54:2837–2840.
74. Ladanyi M, Lewis R, Garin-Chesa P, Rettig WJ, Huvos AG, Healey JH, Jhanwar SC. EWS rearrangement in Ewing's sarcoma and peripheral neuroectodermal tumor. Molecular detection and correlation with cytogenetic analysis and MIC2 expression. *Diagn Mol Pathol* 1993;2:141–146.
75. Lampson LA, Fisher CA, Whelan JP. Striking paucity of HLA-A, B, C and beta 2-microglobulin on human neuroblastoma cell lines. *J Immunol* 1983;130:2471–2478.
76. Le Douarin NM, Ziller C. Plasticity in neural crest cell differentiation. *Curr Opin Cell Biol* 1993;5:1036–1043.
77. Lee SC, Henry MM, Gonzalez-Crussi F. Simultaneous occurrence of melanotic neuroectodermal tumor and brain heterotopia in the oropharynx. *Cancer* 1976;38:249–253.
78. Lieberman PH. Case twenty-one. Primitive neuroectodermal tumor. Proceedings of the Forty-fifth Annual Pathology Slide Seminar of the American Society of Clinical Pathologists 1979; Chicago:100–105.
79. Linnoila RI, Tsokos M, Triche TJ, Marangos PJ, Chandra RS. Evidence for neural origin and PAS-positive variants of the malignant small cell tumor of thoracopulmonary region ("Askin tumor"). *Am J Surg Pathol* 1986;10:124–133.
80. Lipinski M, Braham K, Philip I, et al. Phenotypic characterization of Ewing sarcoma cell lines with monoclonal antibodies. *J Cell Biochem* 1986;31:289–296.
81. Lizard-Nacol S, Volk C, Lizard G, Turc-Carel C. Abnormal expression of neurofilament proteins in Ewing's sarcoma cell cultures. *Tumor Biol* 1992;13:36–43.
82. Llombart-Bosch A, Contesso G, Henry-Amar M, et al. Histopathological predictive factors wwin Ewing's sarcoma of bone and clinicopathological correlations. A retrospective study of 261 cases. *Virchows Arch A Histopathol Anat* 1986;409:627–640.
83. Llombart-Bosch A, Lacombe MJ, Peydro-Olaya A, Perez-Bacete M, Contesso G. Malignant peripheral neuroectodermal tumours of bone other than Askin's neoplasm: characterization of 14 new cases with immunohistochemistry and electron microscopy. *Virchows Arch A Histopathol Anat* 1988;412:421–430.
84. Llombart-Bosch A, Terrier-Lacombe MJ, Peydro-Olaya A, Contesso G. Peripheral neuroectodermal sarcoma of soft tissue (peripheral neuroepithelioma): a pathologic study of ten cases with differential diagnosis regarding other small, round-cell sarcomas. *Hum Pathol* 1989;20:273–280.
85. Maletz N, McMorrow LE, Greco MA, Wolman SR. Ewing's sarcoma: pathology, tissue culture, and cytogenetics. *Cancer* 1986;58:252–257.
86. Marina NM, Etcubanas E, Parham DM, Bowman LC, Green A. Peripheral primitive neuroectodermal tumor (peripheral neuroepithelioma) in children: a review of the St. Jude experience and controversies in diagnosis and management. *Cancer* 1989;64:1952–1960.
87. May WA, Lessnick SL, Braun BS, et al. The Ewing's sarcoma EWS/FLI-1 fusion gene encodes a more potent transcriptional activator and is a more powerful transforming gene than FLI-1. *Mol Cell Biol* 1993;13:7393–7398.
88. Mayall FG, Gibbs AR. The histology and immunohistochemistry of small cell mesothelioma. *Histopathology* 1992;20:47–51.
89. Maygarden SJ, Askin FB, Siegal GP, et al. Ewing sarcoma of bone in infants and toddlers: a clinicopathologic report from the Intergroup Ewing's Study. *Cancer* 1993;71:2109–2118.
90. Mendenhall CM, Marcus RB, Enneking WF, Springfield DS, Thar TL, Million RR. The prognostic significance of soft tissue extension in Ewing's sarcoma. *Cancer* 1983;51:913–917.
91. Mierau GW. Extraskeletal Ewing's sarcoma (peripheral neuroepithelioma). *Ultrastruct Pathol* 1985;9:91–98.
92. Miettinen M, Lehto VP, Virtanen I. Histogenesis of Ewing's sarcoma. An evaluation of intermediate filaments and endothelial cell markers. *Virchows Arch B Cell Pathol* 1982;41:277–284.
93. Miser JS, Kinsella TJ, Triche TJ, et al. Treatment of peripheral neuroepithelioma in children and young adults. *J Clin Oncol* 1987;5:1752–1758.
94. Moll R, Lee I, Gould VE, Berndt R, Roessner A, Franke WW. Immunocytochemical analysis of Ewing's tumors: patterns of ex-

Pediatric Neoplasia: Morphology and Biology, edited by David M. Parham.
Lippincott-Raven Publishers, Philadelphia © 1996.

CHAPTER 5

Rhabdomyosarcomas and Related Tumors

David M. Parham

INTRODUCTION

Rhabdomyosarcomas are the most common soft tissue sarcomas encountered in children, constituting approximately 70% of mesenchymal malignancies and 15% of solid tumors treated at pediatric hospitals. They present a wide range of clinical and morphologic guises, ranging from deceptively innocuous-appearing lesions of the ear or vagina to widely metastatic lesions with bone marrow involvement that is easily misconstrued as leukemia. Their high relative incidence as soft tissue lesions in children markedly contrasts with their rarity in adults, who typically present with a different morphologic form of the disease. These tumors usually present as sporadic lesions with no evidence of clustering, although a tendency to develop them may be inherited as a component of the Li–Fraumeni syndrome, which is primarily caused by genetically transmitted alterations of the p53 tumor suppressor gene. The neoplasm tends to affect white children more than nonwhites and males more than females (78,113).

HISTORY

Recognition of rhabdomyosarcoma was necessarily preceded by histologic discovery of the myocyte. Identification of rhabdomyosarcoma was thus part of the great scientific leap taken by Virchow and his colleagues with the cellular theory of pathology and interest in histologic investigation. Rhabdomyosarcomas have been studied since 1854, when one was described in the tongue of a 21-year-old male patient (141); this lesion was remarkable for its strong resemblance to skeletal muscle. Since that report our understanding of these neoplasms has advanced concurrently with our knowledge of the biology of striated muscle. Recent gains in knowledge have proceeded largely as a result of cooperative groups such as the Intergroup Rhabdomyosarcoma Study (IRS), a large interinstitutional concern formed in 1972 (78).

Because of the often spectacular and enthralling microscopic appearance of neoplastic rhabdomyoblasts, numerous studies of rhabdomyosarcoma appeared soon after its discovery (see Chapter 1). To some degree, the well-defined cytology of highly developed examples has hindered the full recognition of rhabdomyosarcoma because well-differentiated cases are relatively uncommon. The strong diagnostic emphasis that pathologists initially gave to morphologic differentiation led to the common use of dyes that accentuate cross-striations, such as phosphotungstic acid-hematoxylin. These often led to prolonged, tiring microscopic searches for diagnostic cells. Needless to say, the threshold for recognizing cross-striations tended to be progressively lowered during laborious searches, as these structures are seen in only 40% of cases (4). According to Webber (personal communication), a premier midcentury surgical pathologist (who shall remain anonymous) lamented frequently that if he could have relived his existence, he wouldn't have searched for cross-striations!

The advent of electron microscopy led to some respite for the diagnostician, but histopathologists found that they were diverting their precious time from searches for cross-striations to searches for thick and thin filaments, which again may prove elusive. In recent years the use of immunohistochemistry has led to the seeming liberation of time-stressed microscopists, as even at low power magnification neoplastic cells with the antigenic features of muscle are usually easily identified. Unfortunately, there are still attendant problems and caveats that can lead to misdiagnoses.

In recent years our knowledge of the molecular genetics of rhabdomyosarcoma has expanded tremendously

D. M. Parham: Department of Pathology, Arkansas Children's Hospital, Little Rock, Arkansas 72202.

as a result of the discovery of two sets of genes: those that are key activators in the cascade of subcellular events leading to myogenesis and those whose fusion leads to production of unrestrained growth factors. The identification of these regulators of myogenic commitment and cell growth has profound implications for current understanding and diagnosis of rhabdomyosarcomas.

CLINICAL FEATURES

Rhabdomyosarcoma is primarily a tumor of childhood and arises in a wide diversity of organs, ranging from gallbladder to brain. It tends to occur primarily in the head and neck region (particularly the orbital soft tissues), the genitourinary region, the soft tissues of the extremities, and the paraspinal/parameningeal region. Age, primary site, and histology tend to be interrelated, with younger children having a predominance of embryonal tumors and genitourinary tract lesions and adolescents typically having alveolar rhabdomyosarcomas of the extremities.

A wide range of clinical symptoms may lead to presentation to the pediatrician, depending on the site of tumor origin. These clinical features are summarized in an excellent review by Ruymann (113). For example, lesions of the prostate and bladder neck (Fig. 1) may cause urinary incontinence, protruding lesions of the vagina (Fig. 2) may be externally visible, growing masses may appear in the extremities (Fig. 3), and orbital lesions (Fig. 4) may cause visual disturbances.

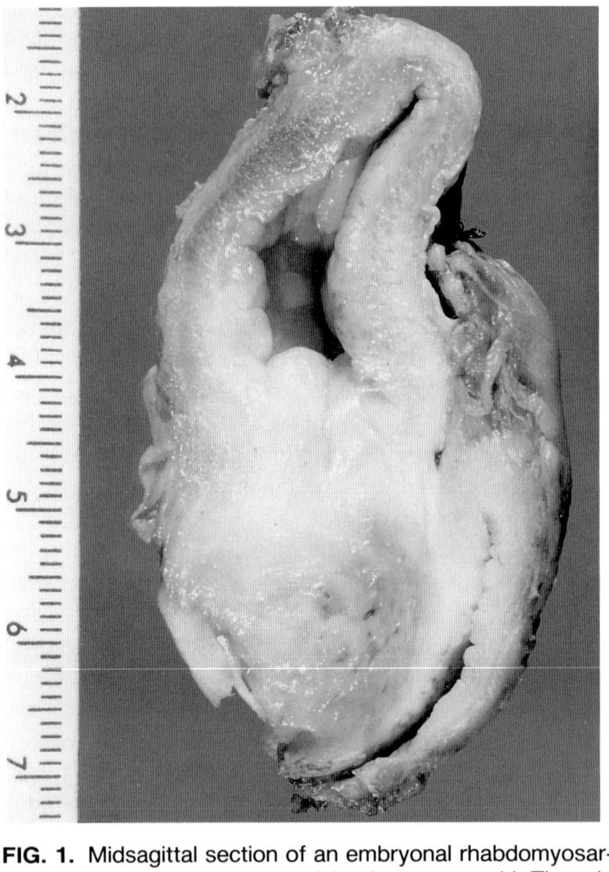

FIG. 1. Midsagittal section of an embryonal rhabdomyosarcoma of the urethral region, arising in a young girl. There is marked invasion of periurethral and anterovaginal tissues by a fleshy, poorly circumscribed tumor.

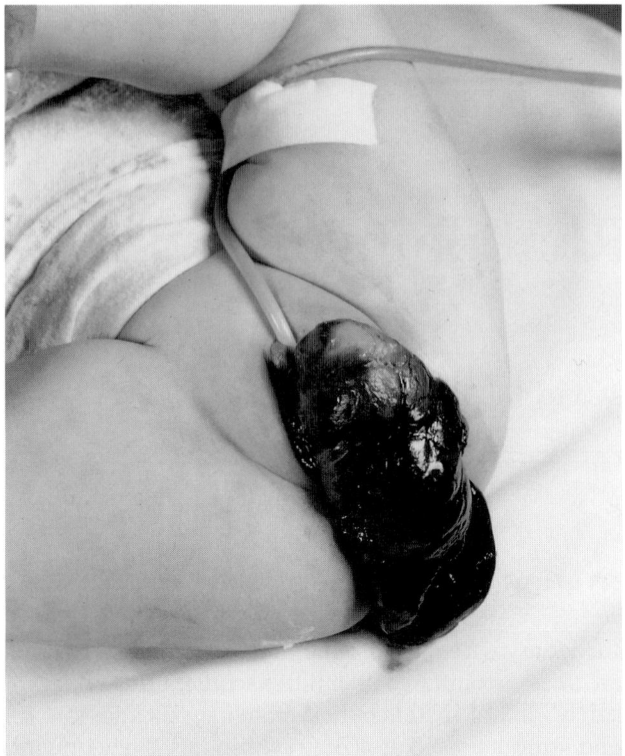

FIG. 2. Botryoid rhabdomyosarcoma protruding from vagina of an infant girl. (Courtesy of Dr. Charles Pratt, St. Jude Children's Research.)

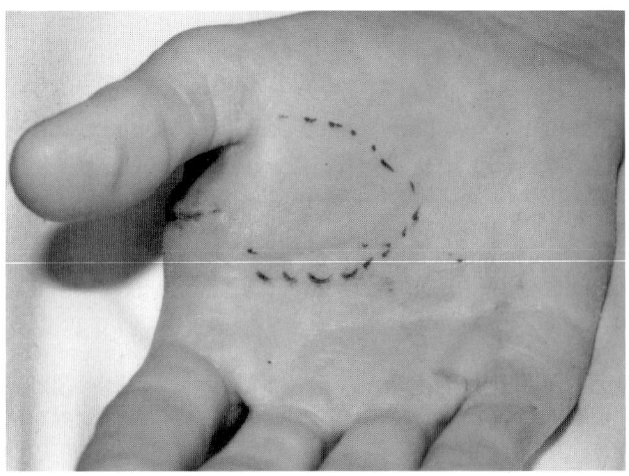

FIG. 3. Alveolar rhabdomyosarcoma causing a bulging mass in the thenar eminence of an adolescent boy.

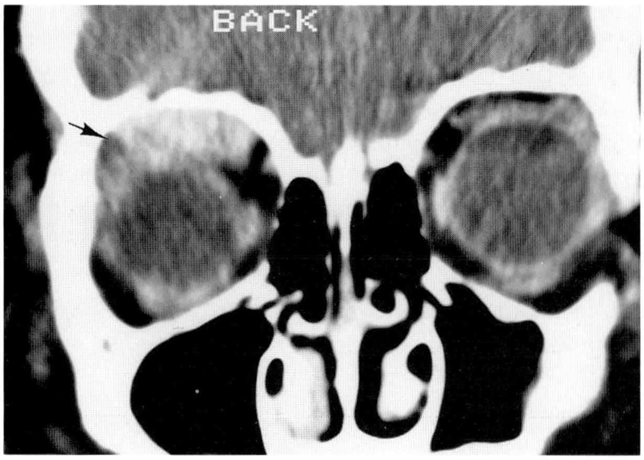

FIG. 4. Magnetic resonance image of orbital rhabdomyosarcoma *(arrow)*. (Courtesy of Dr. Barry Fletcher, St. Jude Children's Research Hospital.)

GROSS APPEARANCE

The gross appearance of rhabdomyosarcoma also varies widely, depending on histologic subtype. Perhaps the most familiar appearance is that of the botryoid rhabdomyosarcoma, or sarcoma botryoides, so named because of the resemblance of the tumor to a bunch of grapes (*botrus*, in ancient Greek). Botryoid tumors are polypoid masses that protrude from an epithelium-lined surface such as the vagina or urinary bladder (Fig. 5A; see figure in color plate section) and produce a characteristic appearance on computerized tomography or magnetic resonance imaging (Fig. 5B). Other varieties of rhabdomyosarcomas grossly present as fleshy gray–tan masses with poorly circumscribed margins. Consonant with their myxoid composition, embryonal and botryoid tumors are highly gelatinous with a glairy, semitranslucent cut surface. Other lesions are more fibrous, particularly following adjuvant therapy. Round cell lesions such as alveolar rhabdomyosarcomas have a pink–tan, fleshy, sea urchin roe–like appearance reminiscent of Wilms' tumors and may have areas of necrosis and hemorrhage. Except for botryoid tumors, rhabdomyosarcomas have no characteristic gross features that distinguish them from other sarcomas or embryonal neoplasms.

B

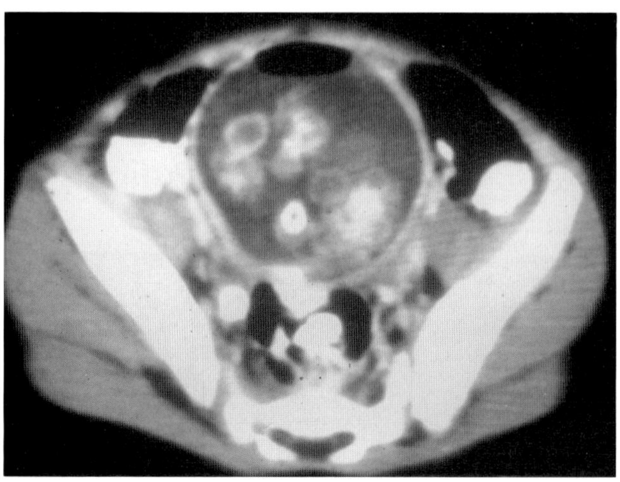

FIG. 5. Botryoid rhabdomyosarcomas of the urinary bladder, presenting as multiple, rounded polypoid lesions on gross examination **(A)** *(see color plate section)* or computerized tomography **(B)**.

MICROSCOPIC APPEARANCE

Rhabdomyosarcomas have a widely diverse set of microscopic appearances that range from highly cellular undifferentiated lesions to loosely textured myxoid tumors that may at first glance elicit a consideration of liposarcoma. To illustrate the diagnostic difficulties caused by the heterogeneity of these tumors, Table 1 depicts only part of the wide range of lesions that the author has seen misdiagnosed as rhabdomyosarcomas. To add to the potential for confusion, a wide variety of nonrhabdomyosarcomatous tumors, both benign and malignant, may exhibit myogenesis (Table 2). Thus, skeletal muscle differentiation alone does not perforce dictate a diagnosis of rhabdomyosarcoma.

Rhabdomyosarcomas are composed of cells analogous to fetal muscle at 10–12 weeks gestation (Fig. 6; see figure in color plate section). However, they commonly occur in areas such as the prostate or nasopharynx, which are devoid of skeletal muscle, indicating that they arise from mesenchymal precursor cells rather than myocytes. Thus, these neoplasms are not derived from muscle per se but from primitive mesenchyme having a myogenic tendency. In the so-called embryonal sarcoma, a subset of lesions included in the embryonal rhabdomyosarcoma category, a capacity for myogenesis is not histologically evident. In other tumors, there is pronounced myogenesis that leads to the consideration of a benign diagnosis (58). While these tumors resemble

TABLE 1. *Lesions misdiagnosed as rhabdomyosarcoma*

Extraosseous Ewing's sarcoma
Peripheral neuroepithelioma
Malignant lymphoma
Wilms' tumor
Langerhans' cell histiocytosis
Benign inflammatory pseudosarcomas
Malignant peripheral nerve sheath tumor
Synovial sarcoma
Pleuropulmonary blastoma
Extrarenal rhabdoid tumor
Intra-abdominal desmoplastic small cell tumor
Mesothelioma
Epithelioid angiosarcoma and hemangioendothelioma

TABLE 2. *Myogenic lesions in children and adolescents*

Malignant
Rhabdomyosarcoma
Wilms' tumor
Malignant triton tumor
Embryonal sarcoma of liver
Pleuropulmonary blastoma
Medulloblastoma
Hepatoblastoma
Immature teratoma
Ectomesenchymoma
Mesenchymal chondrosarcoma/polyhistioma
Meningeal sarcoma
Medulloepithelioma
Benign
Rhabdomyoma
Fetal
Adult
Genital
Mesenchymal hamartoma of skin
Leiomyoma
Benign triton tumor
Congenital mesoblastic nephroma
Mature teratoma
Localized hypertrophy
Supernumerary muscles

fully developed muscle, they are not innervated. This factor may be at least partially responsible for the high MyoD content of rhabdomyosarcomas (see below), as MyoD expression is inhibited by electrical impulses (101).

Because they are analogous to normally developing embryonal and fetal musculature, rhabdomyosarcoma cells closely recapitulate the stages of prenatal myogenesis (Fig. 7; *see figure in color plate section*). As such, one may encounter stellate primitive mesenchymal cells, myoblasts with abundant and somewhat elongated eosinophilic cytoplasm, myotubes with more abundant cytoplasm and more spindled contours, irregular myofiberlike cells resulting from the fusion of the myotubes and myoblasts, and elongated giant cells with nuclei arranged in tandem.

CLASSIFICATION

Because of their wide range of histologic appearances, rhabdomyosarcomas have been the subject of numerous studies relating morphology to prognosis. The best known and most widely used classification is that of Horn and Enterline (51), which subdivides rhabdomyosarcomas into embryonal, botryoid, alveolar, and pleomorphic types (Table 3).

Embryonal rhabdomyosarcomas are characterized by a mixture of dense spindle cell areas and loose myxoid foci (Fig. 6B), either of which may predominate in a given tumor. The essential ingredient for the diagnosis of these tumors is the rhabdomyoblast, a round to oval to elongated cell with an eccentric nucleus and abundant eosinophilic cytoplasm. These cells may have unusual shapes and appearances (Fig. 7), engendering the terms

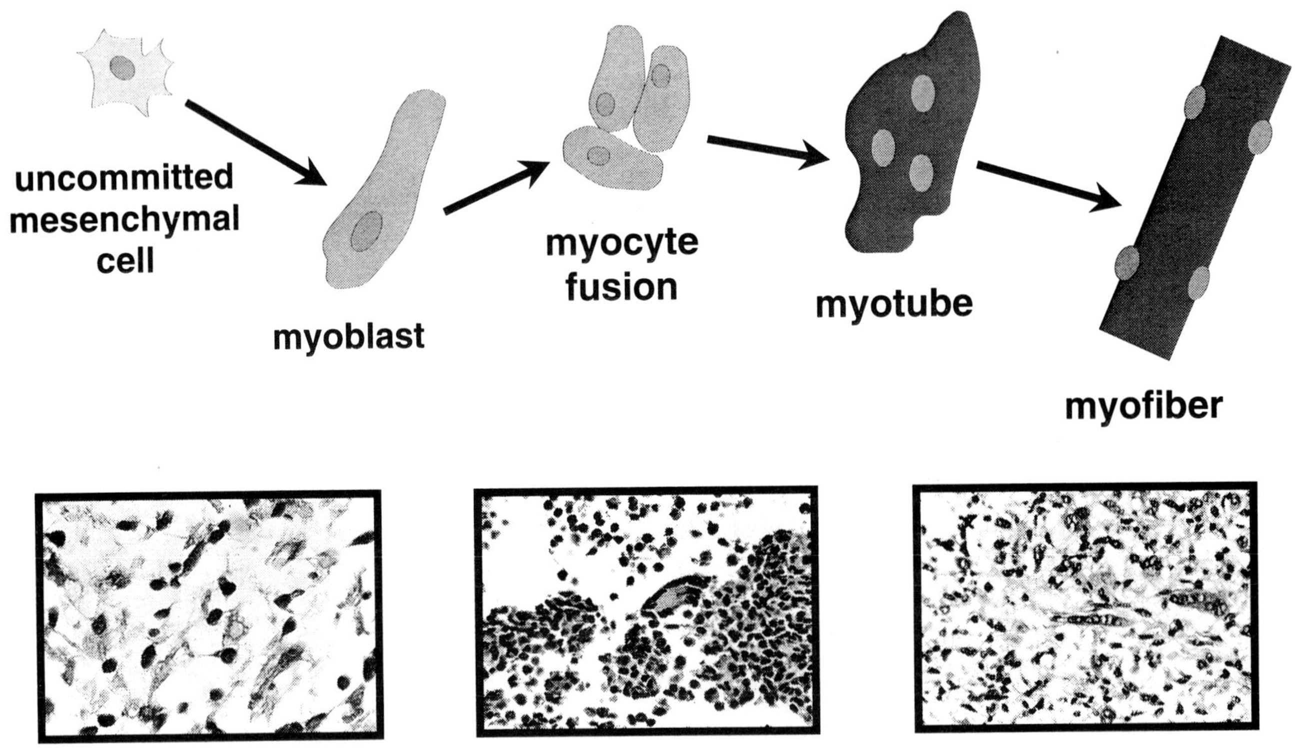

FIG. 7. Analogy of stages of myogenesis to cell types found in rhabdomyosarcoma. The flow diagram at the top illustrates the normal stages of embryonic myogenesis. The photomicrographs at the bottom illustrate compatible features in rhabdomyosarcoma, namely early myoblast formation **(left),** giant cells resulting from myocyte fusion **(middle),** and tandem cells similar to myofibers **(right).**

"racquet cell," "spider cell," or "tadpole cell." One may find further evidence of myogenesis in the form of strap cells with multiple tandem nuclei, and occasional cells may have cross-striations. Cross-striations are found in only a minority of cases (4).

The botryoid variant of rhabdomyosarcoma is typified by its gross appearance (Fig. 5) but also has a characteristic microscopic feature, the cambium layer. This histologic attribute (Fig. 8; see figure in color plate section) is derived from a dense subepithelial band of tumor cells that contrasts with the relatively hypocellular deeper portions of the tumor and resembles the outer or cambium growth zone of a tree. These tumors arise in hollow viscera such as the vagina, urinary bladder, pharynx, and biliary system.

The alveolar subtype of rhabdomyosarcoma also has a distinctive histologic appearance that is reminiscent of the pulmonary alveoli of fetal lung. It is characterized by the formation of fibrous septa from which individual myoblasts are suspended in a picket fence arrangement (Fig. 9, see figure in color plate section). These septa create a nested appearance and subtend groups of tumor cells which typically cluster in the center of the nests and lack cohesion at the edges, producing a clefted appearance. Another common feature is the presence of large multinucleated tumor giant cells that contain abundant eosinophilic cytoplasm (Fig. 7).

Alveolar tumors are largely composed of solid sheets of small round blue cells, so that differential diagnosis includes neuroblastoma, extraosseous Ewing's sarcoma, peripheral neuroepithelioma, lymphoma, and others (see Chapter 4). Tumors of this category may lack septa entirely (134). Conversely, even the presence of septa is not necessarily diagnostic, as similar structures may also be seen in primitive neural tumors (23), and focal desmoplasia can occur in embryonal rhabdomyosarcomas. Ancillary techniques such as electron microscopy, immunohistochemistry, and molecular genetics are usually of diagnostic assistance in these instances (114). To further confound matters, occasional rhabdomyosarcomas have a mixture of both embryonal and alveolar histology. Presently in the IRS-IV protocol, tumors with any component of alveolar histology are considered to be alveolar lesions.

Pleomorphic rhabdomyosarcoma is a highly cellular tumor composed of pleomorphic spindle cells with enlarged, hyperchromatic nuclei and bizarre mitoses (Fig. 10), arranged in a swirling pattern reminiscent of malignant fibrous histiocytoma or pleomorphic liposarcoma. It usually occurs in adults and is a distinctly uncommon tumor in children, as only 11 of 1,626 cases entered on IRS-I and IRS-II protocols were of this subtype, and of these 11 only 5 were "pure" (94). Usually in children this pattern is accompanied by embryonal-type histologic foci. The existence of this tumor in adults has been questioned (43), but recent data (128,144) confirm its status as a diagnostic and molecular entity.

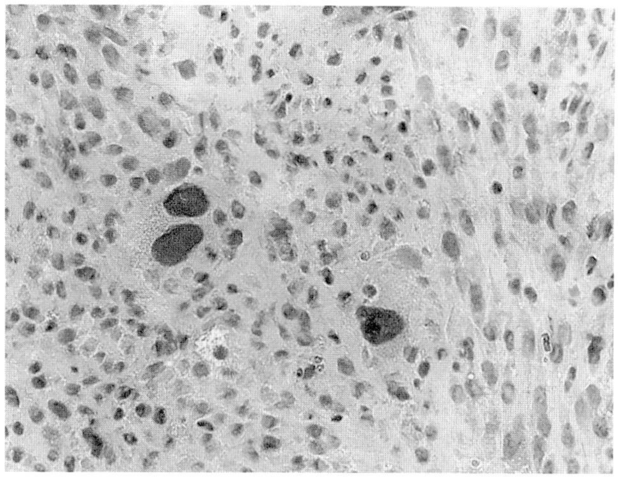

FIG. 10. Pleomorphic rhabdomyosarcoma. There is a mixture of spindle cells and large pleomorphic cells, reminiscent of malignant fibrous histiocytoma.

Although the Horn and Enterline classification of rhabdomyosarcomas correlates with clinical outcome in the majority of instances (94), some cases behave in an anomalous fashion. In St. Jude material, we have found that when the standard subtypes are matched for stage or primary site and compared with survival, there is no independently predictive value of histology (37). As a result of this factor and the marked histologic diversity, additional classification systems have been proposed in recent years.

Working with IRS-I and II cases, in 1983 Palmer (99) proposed a classification system based on the cytologic features of the tumor cells (Table 3). This study was conducted in a manner analogous to the work that Beckwith and he performed on pediatric renal tumors (6), in that he first carefully observed the range of cytologic features of a large number of specimens. These observations were used to catalog recurring cell types and to match them with subsequent tumor behavior in order to determine which cell types were predictive of poor patient outcome. In the cytohistologic system that Palmer subsequently devised (99), rhabdomyosarcomas were separated into anaplastic, monomorphous round cell, and mixed-histology types.

In Palmer's system, anaplastic tumors are characterized by the presence of enlarged, bizarre, multipolar mitotic figures (Fig. 11; see figure in color plate section), analogous to those found in anaplastic Wilms' tumors. Like Wilms' tumors, anaplastic rhabdomyosarcomas also typically contain variable numbers of nondividing pleomorphic cells, but these are not critical to the diagnosis. Monomorphous round cell tumors are characterized by sheets of round cells with uniform spherical nuclei (Fig. 12; see figure in color plate section). The nuclei contain a central nucleolus from which chromatin strands radiate into a thickened nuclear membrane. These nuclear features separate monomorphous round

TABLE 3. *Rhabdomyosarcoma classifications*

Horn and Enterline (51)
Embryonal
Alveolar
Botryoid
Pleomorphic
Palmer (99)
Anaplastic
Monomorphous round cell
Mixed
Type A
Societe Internationale d'Oncologie Pediatrique (SIOP) (11)
Embryonal sarcoma
Embryonal rhabdomyosarcoma
Loose botryoid
Loose nonbotryoid
Dense well differentiated
Dense poorly differentiated
Biphasic
Alveolar rhabdomyosarcoma
Myogenic
Round cell
Intermediate
Pleomorphic rhabdomyosarcoma
National Cancer Institute (134)
Embryonal rhabdomyosarcoma
Classic
Aggressive cytology
Pleomorphic
Leiomyomatous
Alveolar rhabdomyosarcoma
Pleomorphic
Ewing-like
Monomorphic
Solid
Pleomorphic rhabdomyosarcoma
International Classification (3)
Superior prognosis
Botryoid rhabdomyosarcoma
Spindle cell rhabdomyosarcoma
Intermediate prognosis
Embryonal rhabdomyosarcoma
Poor prognosis
Alveolar rhabdomyosarcoma
Undifferentiated

cell tumors from typical Ewing's sarcomas, which contain nuclei with finely divided chromatin and inconspicuous nucleoli. A primary emphasis is also placed on tumor cell uniformity. Mixed tumors are so named because they represent the conglomerate of the other cell types. The anaplastic and monomorphous round cell types comprise the unfavorable histologic variants and are associated with a marked decline in clinical outcome independent of stage or site (99).

Unfortunately, Palmer never published his work in article form, and others have failed to duplicate his results using a strict application of his definitions (3). However, subsequent publications have vindicated Palmer's system. The finding of a poor prognosis in anaplastic tumors was confirmed initially by the report of Hawkins and Camacho-Velasquez (47) and subsequently by a review of IRS material by Kodet and colleagues (59). However, less emphasis was placed on the finding of a single multipolar mitosis by these authors, who used a more traditional histologic approach. In Kodet's study (59), the distribution of the atypical cells appeared critical, as tumors that contained tight clusters of these cells were more aggressive than lesions with a few haphazardly dispersed pleomorphic cells. Palmer's monomorphic round cell lesions were probably comprised largely of typical and solid alveolar neoplasms, both types being aggressive tumors as in the study by Tsokos and colleagues (134).

In his original schema Palmer also identified a pattern with a good prognosis. He termed this tumor the "type A" variant and noted that it frequently was found in paratesticular lesions. Tumor cells with this histology exhibit a greater degree of differentiation than the usual embryonal rhabdomyosarcoma, a finding also evident with immunohistochemical studies (14). "Type A" tumors are arranged in tight fascicles composed of uniform elongate spindle cells that may be reminiscent of leiomyosarcoma, fibrous histiocytoma, or nerve sheath tumor (Fig. 13; see figure in color plate section). Palmer also noted that scattered, enlarged, oval cells were often embedded in this milieu. Pathologists have subsequently rediscovered this lesion, calling it a variety of terms that include "leiomyomatous embryonal rhabdomyosarcoma" (134) and "spindle cell rhabdomyosarcoma" (14,67). These reports also corroborate its association with a good clinical outcome and a paratesticular origin.

Tsokos and coworkers (134) subsequently devised a classification system (Table 3) in which the major deviation from the classical schema was the recognition of the "solid alveolar" variant. In this category are small round cell tumors with a solid, sheeted histologic pattern and no definite foci of cells hanging from fibrous septa (Fig. 12). These tumors would be classified as embryonal in the Horn–Enterline schema, although it must be remembered that the nested areas of the classic alveolar tumor may be focal. Although solid variant alveolar rhabdomyosarcomas lack the scaffolding of typical lesions, they possess similar karyotypic anomalies (105) and aggressive tendencies (134) that confirm their identity as "alveolar" tumors.

A third alternative schema for classifying rhabdomyosarcomas was devised by the pathologists of the Societé Internationale d'Oncologie Pédiatrique (SIOP) (11,146). In the SIOP schema embryonal tumors are subdivided according to their degree of differentiation and cellular density, and alveolar tumors are subcategorized based on the relative amount of differentiation (Table 3). As noted earlier, a key contribution of this system is the recognition of a primitive form of rhabdomyosarcoma termed the embryonal sarcoma. This term is also used to designate a mesenchymal tumor of the liver that has similar characteristics and relation to more differentiated forms of hepatic rhabdomyosarcoma (see Chapter 11) (103). The embryonal sarcoma of soft tissue, as envisioned by the SIOP pathologists, is a spindle cell lesion composed of primitive mesenchyme that does not exhibit definitive features of myogenesis, i.e., eosinophilic cytoplasmic tails (Fig. 14; see figure in color plate section). Because this definition is based primarily on cytohistologic features and not on the results of ancillary techniques such as electron microscopy or immunohistochemistry, there are doubtless a number of cases that would otherwise be classified as embryonal rhabdomyosarcoma by the standard schema. The embryonal sarcoma arises in relatively young children and generally behaves in a nonaggressive fashion (146).

These diverse systems have been the subject of a correlative study by the IRS that tested the ability of pathologists to consistently classify rhabdomyosarcomas and to predict their behavior (3). In this study an international panel of experts and proponents of the various classifications examined a large set of routinely stained tumors treated with IRS protocols. The results not unexpectedly indicate that use of a more familiar schema is easier and more reproducible, as the standard Horn-Enterline system gave better results than the Palmer system. As a consequence of the study, an international classification (Table 3) that combined clinically and histologically pertinent elements of the old and new systems was proposed and is currently being used in the IRS-IV protocol (3).

ELECTRON MICROSCOPY

Electron microscopy is often of great assistance in diagnosing problem cases of rhabdomyosarcoma. These are usually either small round cell tumors that only hint at myogenesis at the light microscopic level or spindle cell tumors that invite confusion with leiomyosarcoma, synovial sarcoma, fibrosarcoma, or malignant fibrous histiocytoma. The major finding of diagnostic importance is the association of myosin ("thick") and actin ("thin") filaments, which on cross section form hexagonal arrays (Fig. 15). Intermingled with these filaments are periodic densities representing primitive Z bands. In more differentiated tumors true sarcomeres with M and I bands are also formed.

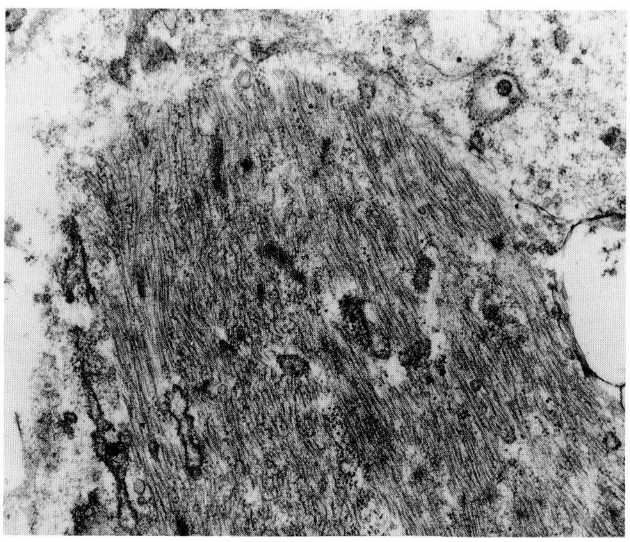

FIG. 15. Electron micrograph of rhabdomyosarcoma cell containing large numbers of alternating microfilaments and myosin filaments. Transverse sections appear as hexagonal arrays. The filaments are occasionally punctuated by primitive Z-band condensations.

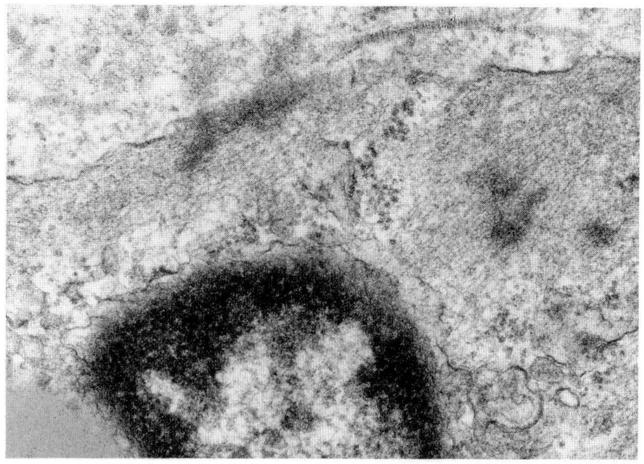

FIG. 16. Electron micrograph of rhabdomyosarcoma cell containing peripheral microfilaments with focal densities. These organelles are also features of smooth muscle cells.

Predictably, tumor cells that appear undifferentiated at the light microscopic level often exhibit similar features at the ultrastructural level, so that less restrictive criteria for ultrastructural diagnosis have been sought. In Lombardi and Pilotti's study (74), rudimentary sarcomeres could be identified in only one half of cases. According to Erlandson, "short, parallel bundles of rigid 15 nm myosin filaments with attached ribosomes arranged in single file" (myosin–ribosome complexes) represent the minimal ultrastructural criterion for diagnosis (36). These structures are also observed at the periphery of regenerating muscle (112) and represent nascent myofilament development. Erlandson (36) has also observed leptomeric fibrils, less common biostructural phenomena, in some rhabdomyosarcomas.

A even lesser degree of differentiation was accepted by Dickman and Triche in their studies of features separating primitive rhabdomyosarcomas from extraosseous Ewing's sarcomas. In their report (30), the ultrastructural characteristics that serve to distinguish rhabdomyosarcomas from extraosseous Ewing's sarcomas comprise the following: nuclear irregularity, 7-nm filaments, 10-nm filaments, focal densities, phagocytosed collagen, a collagen matrix, and basal lamina. However, these features are shared by a number of primitive sarcomas (16,39), so that their strict reliability for rhabdomyosarcoma diagnosis is controversial. Nevertheless, as Dickman and

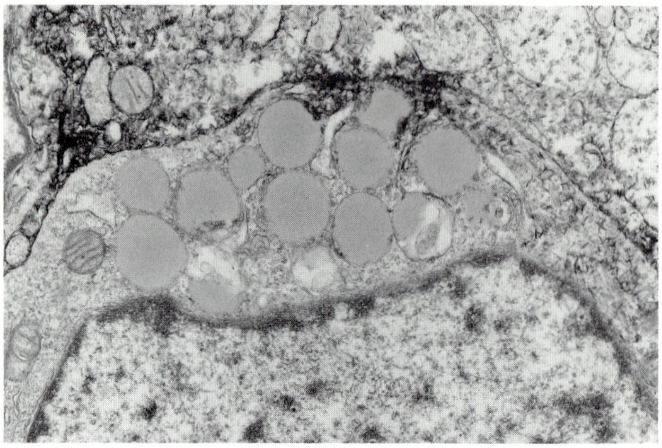

FIG. 17. Electron micrograph of rhabdomyosarcoma cell containing numerous cytoplasmic lipid droplets, characteristic of lipoblasts.

Triche stated, these submicroscopic aspects are not generally shared by Ewing's sarcoma, although the author has encountered intermediate filament bundles in occasional primitive neural tumor cells (102).

Prevailing evidence thus indicates that rhabdomyosarcomas exhibit a range of myogenesis and include embryonal sarcomas that contain only primitive mesenchymal cells. In this respect, Dickman and Triche (30) are correct in their definition of a category of primitive sarcoma that is allied with rhabdomyosarcoma, an observation reflected in the "embryonal sarcoma" category of the SIOP classification (11). For this reason, occasional tumors that demonstrate myogenic differentiation by immunohistochemistry may not show cytologic features of skeletal muscle by electron microscopy. As a result, immunohistochemistry appears to be more sensitive in the diagnosis of rhabdomyosarcoma than electron microscopy (29,41), but the specificity of most muscle markers is poorer than the ultrastructural demonstration of myogenesis. Conversely, by electron microscopy these primitive cells may show smooth muscle (Fig. 16) or lipoblastic (Fig. 17) differentiation (103,151).

IMMUNOHISTOCHEMISTRY

Striated muscle cells are largely composed of specialized structural and enzymatic proteins that are essential to mobility. As these proteins have been characterized, a scientific quest for the "holy grail" for primitive sarcoma diagnosis has unfolded. This search has been punctuated by reports of increasingly sensitive and/or specific antimuscle reagents. In the process immunohistochemistry has assumed an ascendant role in the diagnostic evaluation of rhabdomyosarcomas during the past decade (13,131). A list of some of the better characterized markers of muscle differentiation that have been investigated is presented in Table 4.

The potential utility of immunologic reagents in diagnosis of rhabdomyosarcoma was recognized at least a decade prior to the development of immunoperoxidase methods. In 1965 Johnson et al. (53) tested rhabdomyosarcomas for myosin by using indirect immunofluorescence and obtained impressive and prophetic results. Koh and colleagues (60) repeated this experiment in 1980, using the peroxidase–antiperoxidase technique, and again found great potential diagnostic utility for immunohistochemistry in pediatric tumor diagnosis.

Subsequent to the development and popularization of peroxidase-based immunohistochemistry, attention again turned to rhabdomyosarcoma with the development of antibodies against myoglobin (Fig. 18A; see figure in color plate section). Rosai and colleagues (90) demonstrated its usefulness in tumor categorization in a small series of cases, but soon after noted that anomalous staining of nonrhabdomyosarcoma tumor cells could be seen in neoplasms infiltrating skeletal muscle (Fig. 18B; see figure in color plate section) (38). One must also beware of misinterpreting myoglobin positivity in entrapped myofibers (Fig. 18C; see figure in color plate section). In spite of this caveat, other pathologists (10) have extolled the virtues of myoglobin immunohistochemistry in rhabdomyosarcoma diagnosis. In today's practice, it continues to be used as a definitive marker of skeletal muscle differentiation, but its sensitivity pales besides other markers such as desmin (66).

The next marker to be popularized for routine surgical pathology practice was desmin. Desmin is an intermediate filament, a class of structural proteins so-named because of their 8- to 10-nm width, which is intermediate between the widths of actin and myosin. In 1980, Lazarides (65) reported that desmin appeared only in muscle cells. Reports of desmin-positivity in neoplasms with muscle differentiation (81,82,97) (Fig. 19; see figure in color plate section) confirmed this association between desmin and myogenesis. Desmin initially appeared to be unreliable for routine use because its antigenicity wanes considerably following formalin fixation (106). This can be counteracted by using cryostat-frozen sections of fresh

TABLE 4. *Immunohistochemical markers of rhabdomyosarcoma*

Myoglobin
Creatine kinase M subunit
Desmin
Muscle-specific actin
Other forms of actin
Fetal myosin
Other forms of myosin
β-Enolase
Calsequestrin
Titin
Z protein
Myasthenia gravis serum
MyoD
Dystrophin

tissue or material fixed in alcohol solutions. However, hematoxylin and eosin stains of alcohol-fixed tissues tend to make even blasé cells as red as the most differentiated of rhabdomyoblasts. Happily, antigen retrieval methods and newer "supersensitive" immunohistochemical staining kits have increased the sensitivity of antidesmin antibodies in formalin-fixed tissues.

Desmin is a class-specific protein shared by smooth and cardiac muscle as well as striated muscle, so that it is also heavily expressed by leiomyosarcomas and tumors containing cells with a partial muscle phenotype (2,81,109,130). This factor diminishes its absolute specificity as a rhabdomyosarcoma marker, particularly with spindle cell lesions, but is less important with undifferentiated round cell tumors (Fig. 19). However, we have noted desmin positivity in primitive neural tumors (102), so that staining results must always be taken into context of light microscopic appearance and other studies (a good rule to follow with any marker!).

Contrasting with the loss of desmin sensitivity that follows routine fixation is the robustness of staining with muscle-specific actin (22,109,135). Found in practically all cell types, actin is ubiquitous, highly conserved, and essential for cell motility and intracytoplasmic trafficking. However, it exists in a variety of isoforms whose diversity rivals even cytokeratin (137). A number of these actin isotypes are cell type-specific; for example, the α isoform of smooth muscle actin may be used to demonstrate smooth muscle differentiation (see Chapter 8). However, α-smooth muscle actin is also transiently expressed in developing fetal muscle (149) and similarly in a subset of rhabdomyosarcomas (104). Antibodies unique to the striated muscle forms of actin have been used for rhabdomyosarcoma diagnosis (12).

Currently in wide use is HHF35, a monoclonal antibody that recognizes the entire group of cells with muscle differentiation (115,135,136). Like desmin, "muscle-specific" actin thus is present in leiomyosarcomas as well as rhabdomyosarcomas. It is extremely stable, so that low concentrations yield visually stunning results in routinely fixed tissue (Fig. 20; see figure in color plate section). As such the sensitivity of actin immunostaining with formalin-fixed lesions rivals that of desmin immunostaining with alcohol-fixed tissues (106). However, one must exert extra caution in interpretation, as pericytes are also strongly positive and are ubiquitous (Fig. 20) (117). Although the presence of these cells serves as an excellent internal control, they can lead to misinterpretation if tangentially-sectioned. A similar mistake can also occur in ultrastructural diagnosis.

Desmin and muscle-specific actin staining have been reported in desmoid tumors, malignant fibrous histiocytomas, glioblastomas, mesotheliomas, malignant peripheral nerve sheath tumors, and liposarcomas (48,80,109, 124), as well as primitive neural tumors (102,126), so that careful interpretation of the results is required. To further complicate matters, cytokeratin, S-100, and neuron-specific enolase staining has conversely been seen with rhabdomyosarcomas (17,83,106,133). Despite these caveats, immunohistochemistry can be of great value in the diagnosis of rhabdomyosarcoma when combined with careful light microscopic and ultrastructural observation.

MyoD AND RELATED GENES

In the past decade there has been isolation of a group of genes, called the *MyoD* family, that are capable of inducing muscle differentiation (64,70,143). The first gene to be studied, *MyoD1* (or myogenesis determination gene 1), was isolated subsequent to the observation that myogenesis followed gene demethylation (21,25). Its protein product was found to be a DNA transcription factor that binds to specific promoter sequences and leads to the production of mRNA that is translated into myogenic proteins such as desmin, myosin, and creatine kinase MM (70). The MyoD1 protein has a dimerized helix-loop-helix motif, a structural design characteristic of a number of growth and differentiating factors such as c-myc and the kappa chain promotor (92). When in vitro expression of *MyoD1* is induced in nonmyogenic cells such as fibroblasts or epithelial cells, they are transformed morphologically and biochemically into skeletal muscle. The DNA binding of *MyoD1* is regulated by dimerization with a variety of structurally similar molecules such as id or E1A, as well as by interaction with proto-oncogene products such as raf or jun and tumor suppressor molecules such as Rh1 (25,70,142).

Although this genetic scenario gives a seemingly complete version of the process of myogenesis, in real life it is too simplistic. For one thing, there are a number of MyoD-type genes besides *MyoD1,* including myogenin, *myf-3,* and *myf-4* (25). Also, in some myotomic regions of certain species, such as the forelimb of quail embryos, MyoD1 does not appear to function in myogenesis. Gene knockout experiments demonstrate that *MyoD1* alone is not essential to normal development of mice, but myogenin appears to be critical (25). On the other hand, either MyoD1 or Myf-5 is required for skeletal muscle formation (111).

Although MyoD1 function has a complexity not realized in initial experimentation, it has relatively straightforward diagnostic implications for rhabdomyosarcoma. In the initial report by Scrable et al. (118), expression of this gene was found in all rhabdomyosarcomas tested, regardless of subtype, and in no other tumors. Although the *MyoD1* gene is found in the distal portion of chromosome 11p, a possible site of rhabdomyosarcoma tumorigenesis, it does not appear to be the primary site of genetic alteration (119). When transfected into human rhabdomyosarcoma cells, the mouse *MyoD1* gene induces cytodifferentiation but does not decrease tumorigenicity (49). Immunohistochemical studies using antibodies against MyoD1 protein suggest that it is a more sensitive and specific marker of rhabdomyosarcoma than desmin (27,28), but additional investigations are warranted. With cryostat sections, MyoD1 staining in rhabdomyosarcoma shows strong nuclear positivity but may be heterogeneous and *granular* (Fig. 21; see figure in color plate section). By immunoelectron microscopy, this granular positivity appears to correlate with the binding of the protein to DNA transcription centers (27). Subsequent studies indicate that MyoD1 is present in adult pleomorphic rhabdomyosarcomas (128,144), alveolar soft part sarcomas (110,128), regenerating myocytes cells in primary myopathies, and atrophic myofibers in neuropathies (101).

The strong expression of MyoD1 in rhabdomyosarcomas appears to be due to an inability to degrade the protein or downregulate the gene (129). This may be similar to the MyoD1 expression seen in neurogenic atrophy, whose inappropriate MyoD1 accumulation is probably related to quenching of the inhibitory action of electrical stimulation (101). Rhabdomyosarcoma cells are also not innervated. At any rate, the biologic accident responsible for MyoD1 accumulation in rhabdomyosarcomas furnishes a unique diagnostic tool. In our studies frozen sections were necessary to demonstrate the presence of MyoD1, but paraffin sections may be adequate following microwave-based antigen retrieval (132). Additional experiments are needed for confirmation of this observation.

CYTOGENETICS AND MOLECULAR BIOLOGY

Cytogenetic studies indicate that a balanced, reciprocal translocation, t(2;13)(q35;q14) (Fig. 22), is specific for alveolar rhabdomyosarcoma (32). Variant chromosomal aberrations, all involving chromosome 13, have also been reported in this tumor (19,31,46,139). The t(2;13) fusion joins the *PAX3* gene sequence on chromosome 2q35 with the *FRKH* gene on chromosome 13 (Fig. 23) (5,122). *FRKH,* also reported as *ALV,* is a member of the forkhead family of transcription factors. *PAX* genes are characterized by a conserved DNA sequence, the paired box, and are important in organ development. The protein products of PAX act as DNA transcription factors (140) that bind to DNA in a site-specific manner to either or inhibit RNA sequencing. The *PAX3* gene is expressed in the mouse embryo in the developing nervous system and limbs (45). Forced expression of *PAX3* results in tumorigenesis in tissue culture cells and mice (77). The juxtaposition of *PAX3* with *FRKH,* which is also a transcription factor, apparently results in inappropriate gene function resulting in tumor growth. *PAX3* is also mutated in Waardenburg syndrome (5), which is

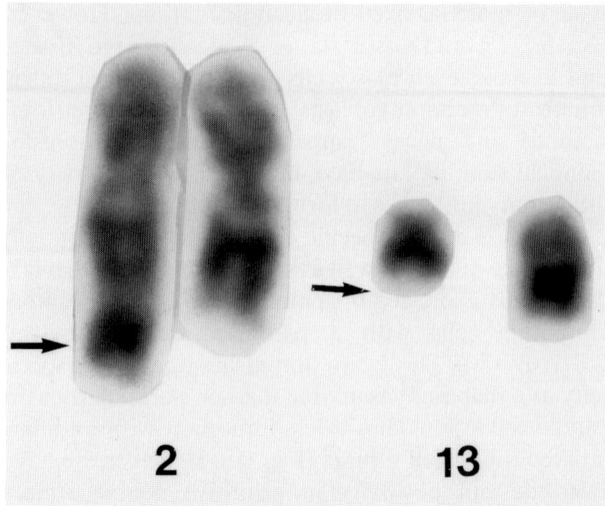

FIG. 22. t(2;13)(q35;q14) found in alveolar rhabdomyosarcoma. There is shortening of one chromosome 13q, with a corresponding lengthening of a 2q *(arrows).* Note that the normal 13q shows distal banding similar to that seen in the distal portion of the abnormally long 2q. (Courtesy of Marc Valentine, St. Jude Children's Research Hospital.)

characterized by deafness and pigmentary disturbances but not development of rhabdomyosarcoma.

Identification of the t(2;13) genetic abnormality can potentially be of great aid in diagnosis of alveolar rhabdomyosarcoma. Using cytogenetic analysis, we have demonstrated the presence of this karyotypic marker in solid variant tumors previously diagnosed as embryonal rhabdomyosarcoma (105). The solid alveolar rhabdomyosarcoma can be difficult to distinguish from embryonal rhabdomyosarcoma as a result of the lack of the prominent fibrous framework seen in more typical alveolar lesions. However, this distinction is important because of the aggressive behavior of the solid alveolar tumors compared to embryonal tumors (134).

Unfortunately, attempts at cytogenetic analysis are often unsuccessful and have a slow turnaround. However, Downing and colleagues (33) have demonstrated that the RNA fusion product of the t(2;13) may be identified by use of reverse transcriptase polymerase chain reaction (RT-PCR) technology (Fig. 24). This methodology has a rapid turnaround time and may be used in paraffin blocks in future studies. Combined with a t(11;22) transcript as a "multiplex" test (33), it has even greater potential for diagnosis of primitive round cell tumors. One of the most intriguing results of our experimentation with this methodology has been the identification of the t(2;13) fusion in mixed alveolar/embryonal rhabdomyosarcomas. One tumor arose as a paratesticular mass that is primarily composed of typical embryonal cells with a myxoid stroma. However, embedded within this prognostically favorable histology are scattered cellular foci that resemble a high-grade solid alveolar lesion (Fig. 25).

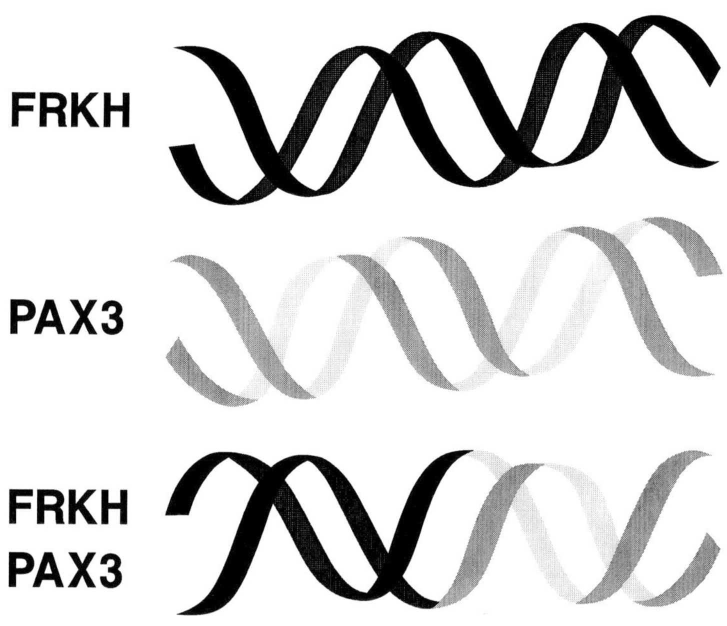

FIG. 23. Schematic of t(2;13)(q35;q14) gene fusion **(bottom).** DNA in the FRKH gene on chromosome 13 (black; **top)** is joined to the *PAX3* gene on chromosome 2 (gray; **middle).**

Presumably these foci are the source of the t(2;13) found with PCR examination and may represent sites of progressive neoplastic transformation.

Scrable and colleagues found that molecular testing also distinguishes embryonal rhabdomyosarcomas, which display loss of heterozygosity of chromosome 11p (118). Their later work on embryonal rhabdomyosarcoma has revealed two different growth suppressor genes, located on the short arm and long arm of chromosome 11 (71). One of these genetic loci, 11p15, may coincide with a major gene in the development of Wilms' tumor (52). Wilms' tumors frequently contain areas of myogenesis, and both rhabdomyosarcomas and Wilms' tumors arise in association with the Beckwith–Wiedemann syndrome (see Chapter 3), which apparently occurs as a result of an 11p15 aberration. Rhabdomyosarcomas also frequently arise in the genitourinary tract, the site where Wilms' tumor genes play key embryogenetic roles (91). Tumorigenesis of both Wilms' tumor and embryonal rhabdomyosarcoma may involve parental imprinting rather than strict Mendelian genetics (see Chapter 3) (55,150).

A major growth hormone, insulinlike growth factor–II (IGF-II), is produced by both Wilms' tumors and rhabdomyosarcomas and is encoded at the 11p15 locus (116). IGF-II causes both growth and motility in rhabdomyosarcoma cells (85,86). This is accomplished by interaction with two separate hormone receptors: the IGF-I re-

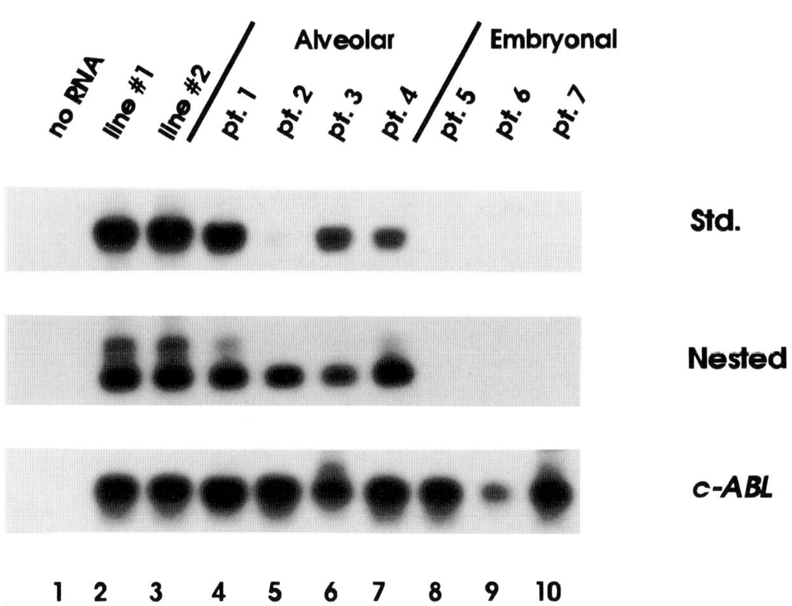

FIG. 24. Detection of t(2;13) fusion gene RNA by the reverse transcriptase–polymerase chain reaction (RT-PCR). Lane 1 in each panel represents a negative control, and the bottom panel depicts a series of positive controls detecting the RNA product of the ubiquitously expressed *c-ABL gene.* Using nested primers, the t(2;13) is detected in both alveolar rhabdomyosarcoma cell lines, in 4 of 4 tumors, and in no embryonal rhabdomyosarcomas. (From Downing et al. *Am J Pathol* 1995;146:626–634, courtesy of the American Society for Investigative Pathology.)

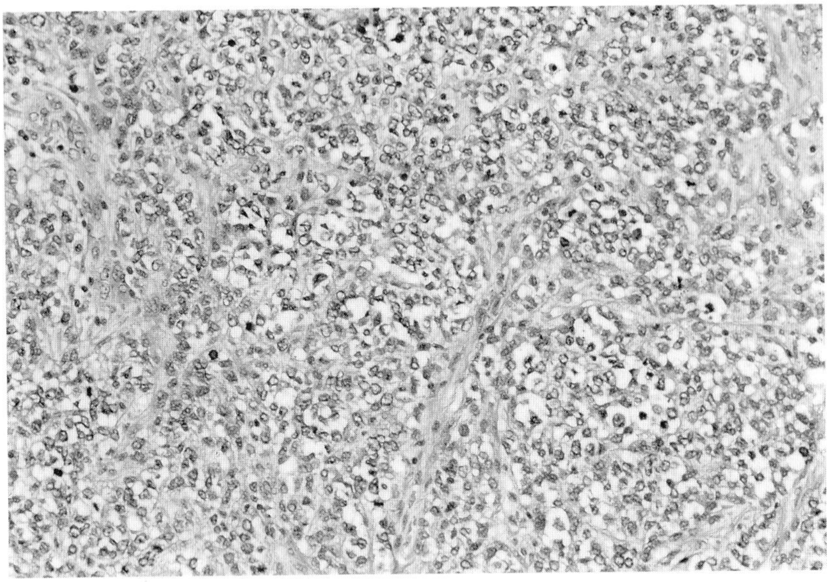

FIG. 25. High-grade-appearing, cellular focus in otherwise typical scrotal embryonal rhabdomyosarcoma that tested positive for the t(2;13) fusion gene RNA product by RT-PCR.

ceptor for an autocrine-type growth impulse and the IGF-II receptor for motility. Production of both receptors can be demonstrated in rhabdomyosarcoma cells (85). In this manner growth and motility of rhabdomyosarcoma occur in an independent fashion characteristic of neoplastic behavior and reminiscent of embryonal organ development.

p53

Knowledge of the p53 tumor suppressor gene, which has received a tremendous amount of attention in recent publications, began as a result of an epidemiologic study into heritable rhabdomyosarcomas (69). Thus Li and Fraumeni identified several families possessing a unique inheritable tendency to prematurely develop excessive numbers of epithelial, mesenchymal, hematopoietic, and glial malignancies. Later studies indicated there was disruption of a single DNA-binding gene that normally acts as a checkpoint for cells entering the S phase of the cell cycle (75). The gene was named p53 because gel electrophoresis of its derivative protein revealed a molecular weight of 53 kd. Further analyses showed that a number of benign polymorphs of the gene exist, but that if certain critical DNA sequences are mutated, cells are more susceptible to carcinogenesis (40,50,68). In many instances, there is deletion of a single nucleotide, causing a "frameshift" in the genetic signal. This aberrant signal can prematurely terminate transcription and result in a shortened, or "truncated," protein. Variable genetic penetrance of p53 mutations is indicated by the fact that some members of affected families do not develop tumors. Tragically, radiation and chemotherapy may render patients with p53 mutations more susceptible to a second malignancy (9,125). Immunohistochemical identification of cells with mutated p53 is made possible by their tendency to exhibit nuclear accumulation of the ineffectual protein product. However, the potential utility of this technique in distinguishing true sarcomas from lookalikes is currently controversial (24,57).

CYTODIFFERENTIATION

Recent morphologic observations of rhabdomyosarcoma reveal that tumor cells treated with combination chemotherapy may mature or terminally differentiate (Fig. 26; see figure in color plate section). This phenomenon occurs only in tumors that contain a population of moderately to well-differentiated cell prior to therapy. Thus, it appears that chemotherapy selectively eliminates undifferentiated tumor cells and induces partially differentiated cells to reach their full maturation potential (89). Cell lines derived from rhabdomyosarcoma may also undergo spontaneous terminal differentiation simulating myotube formation (42,120). This phenomenon, along with a diminution of proliferation, may be induced in rhabdomyosarcoma cell lines by deprivation of fetal calf serum or exposure to retinoic acid (44), nickel, Moloney murine sarcoma virus (93), various antineoplastic drugs (72), or X-irradiation (95,127). This differentiation process reduces the metastatic behavior of rhabdomyosarcoma cells injected into nude mice (73). Rhabdomyosarcoma cell maturation is also associated with production of extracellular matrix components such as laminin and fibronectin (63,138) and protooncogene proteins such as c-raf and c-fos, which transmit differentiation stimuli from the cell membrane to the nucleus (107,108).

Observation of cytodifferentiation in surgical pathology specimens has two important implications: it can cause difficulty in recognition of residual tumor cells in a seemingly benign resection specimen, and it may connote the effect of successful chemotherapy. Resection or mucosal biopsy of rhabdomyosarcomas may be attempted on lesions that demonstrate either stability or shrinkage following adjuvant chemotherapy. The resultant specimens typically comprise contain large amounts of an edematous fibrous stroma containing benign fibroblasts and vessels that show radiation- or chemotherapy-induced atypia. Scattered cells with brightly eosinophilic cytoplasm may pose a diagnostic dilemma of regenerating muscle vs. residual tumor vs. reactive stromal elements. In regions that normally lack skeletal muscle, such the urinary bladder, myoglobin positivity can be used to identify residual tumor (Fig. 18). The clinical significance of finding terminally differentiated tumor cells is uncertain at present.

CLINICAL BEHAVIOR

Clinical behavior of rhabdomyosarcomas is influenced by extent of disease (stage and clinical group), primary site, age, and histology (18,78). Of these factors, extent of disease (Table 5) is the most important. Primary site has also been repeatedly shown to be important in clinical outcome, with tumors of the orbit and genitourinary tract showing the best survival and those of the extremities, trunk, and retroperitoneum having worse outcomes. Younger age patients tend to do better than older ones, as they tend to have lower stage disease (78,79). Regarding histology, patients with botryoid tumors have the best survival, those with alveolar the worst, and those with embryonal neoplasms an intermediate outcome (94). Histology was the most important factor related to survival of Group I (low-stage) patients in IRS-I and II (18). In an autopsy survey, Shimada et al. (123) found that alveolar tumors tended to have more metastatic disease and that the most common sites of metastasis at death were the lungs, regional lymph nodes, bone, liver, and brain. Although metastatic alveolar rhabdomyosarcomas tend to recur rapidly, they ironically respond well to initial chemotherapy (61).

TABLE 5. *Clinical grouping system used for IRS I and II (18)*

Group I: Localized disease, completely resected
- A. Confined to organ or muscle of origin
- B. Infiltration outside organ or muscle of origin; regional nodes not involved

Group II: Compromised or regional resection including
- A. Grossly resected tumors with microscopic residual
- B. Regional disease, completely resected, in which nodes may be involved and/or tumor extends into an adjacent organ
- C. Regional disease with involved nodes, grossly resected, but with evidence of microscopic residual

Group III: Incomplete resection or biopsy with gross residual disease

Group IV: Distant metastases, present at onset

PLOIDY

A limited number of studies have been performed to determine the impact of ploidy on the clinical outcome of rhabdomyosarcomas. Molenaar et al. (88) and Boyce et al. (8) found that all rhabdomyosarcomas in two small series were aneuploid. In studies by Shapiro, Pappo, and colleagues on patients with unresectable Group III rhabdomyosarcomas (100,121), ploidy had a markedly significant impact on survival, with hyperdiploid values (DNA index >1.0) conferring the best prognosis and diploid values (DNA index $= 1.0$) the worst. Near tetraploidy (DNA index $+ 2.0$) was strongly associated with alveolar histology, and hyperdiploidy was exclusively associated with embryonal histology. Some investigators (54,96,145) have confirmed these observations, but others (26,62) have not. Ploidy studies at present appear most applicable to Group III unresectable, nonmetastatic tumors.

FETAL RHABDOMYOMA AND OTHER BENIGN MYOGENIC TUMORS

Fetal rhabdomyoma is a rare, highly differentiated myogenic neoplasm that, like embryonal rhabdomyosarcoma, tends to arise in young children (1,147). Because of morphologic overlap, this diagnosis should be kept in mind with well-differentiated myogenic lesions, particularly those that arise in the head and neck (56). The postauricular region is a distinctly common site of occurrence. Rarely this lesion appears to be capable of progression to rhabdomyosarcoma, as illustrated by the lingual case reported by Kodet and colleagues (58). Nevertheless, fetal rhabdomyoma should be considered to be a benign neoplasm in general and is curable with local excision (56).

Histologically, fetal rhabdomyoma is composed primarily of well-differentiated myotubes with peripheral nuclei and abundant cytoplasm. Characteristically the myotubes are embedded in a myxoid stroma containing primitive round or spindle cells with less cytoplasm. Cross-striations may be unexpectedly difficult to identify without special stains (35). More recently, Kapadia et al. (56) have called attention to a less common variety with smooth muscle features and a range of cellular maturation. Immunohistochemical staining of these "intermediate" fetal rhabdomyomas indicates both striated and smooth muscle characteristics, with smooth muscle actin positivity as well as desmin and muscle-specific actin staining (Fig. 27; *see figure in color plate section*).

Another form of rhabdomyoma, the adult rhabdomyoma, has a distinctive morphology and anatomic distribution unlike that of the fetal tumor. The neck is the most common location for the adult rhabdomyoma, and most patients are over 40 years of age (1,35,147). Histologically, the cells of the adult rhabdomyoma are rounded rather that spindly and vacuolated rather than eosinophilic. Ultrastructural examination reveals that this optical feature is due to abundant cytoplasmic glycogen.

Both forms of rhabdomyoma were considered to be hamartomatous lesions by Sir Rupert Willis (148), but are now considered neoplastic. Cardiac rhabdomyomas are occasionally encountered in children with hamartomatous syndromes (35) and more closely conform to this designation. Another hamartomatous lesion occurs in the skin of infants (35).

A rare but potentially devastating trap awaiting the surgical pathologist evaluating myogenous neoplasms is the occurrence of pseudosarcomatous lesions that occur in the female genital tract and strongly emulate embryonal rhabdomyosarcoma (15,98). These lesions, termed "genital rhabdomyomas" (35) or "pseudosarcoma botryoides" (34), typically occur in the vagina and cervix of young or middle-aged adult women, often during pregnancy (20,34,87). They may arise from atypical mesenchymal stem cells present in a narrow subepithelial zone of the entire vagina (15). Presumably these cells are capable of myogenous differentiation and react to hormonal stimuli such as those produced by pregnancy. No metastases have been reported to date.

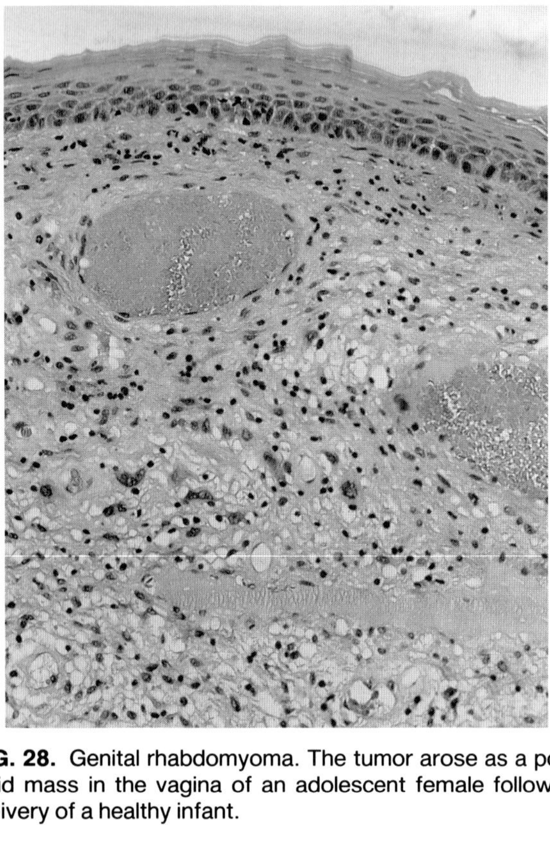

FIG. 28. Genital rhabdomyoma. The tumor arose as a polypoid mass in the vagina of an adolescent female following delivery of a healthy infant.

From the standpoint of differential diagnosis, genital rhabdomyomas do not exhibit the histologic features of botryoid rhabdomyomas (34). Instead, microscopic examination reveals a poorly circumscribed nodule composed of spindle cells of varying size and shapes (Fig. 28). The spindle cell nuclei may be enlarged and somewhat hyperchromatic, and mitotic activity may be present as well. Careful observation will disclose cross-striations in scattered cells (84). Immunohistochemistry and electron microscopy confirm the presence of skeletal muscle differentiation (35).

A number of other rare but benign lesions may exhibit myogenesis or bear a passing resemblance to rhabdomyosarcoma. At the most differentiated end of this spectrum, one may encounter unusual localized hypertrophy of isolated muscles in children. Pseudosarcomatous soft tissue lesions (see Chapter 8) may contain large eosinophilic cells superficially resembling muscle, and true myogenesis is encountered in a rare pediatric lesion of peripheral nerve, the benign triton tumor (also known as the neuromuscular hamartoma or neuromuscular choristoma) (7,76).

ACKNOWLEDGMENT

Supported in part by Cancer Center Support CORE Grant P30 CA21765 and American Lebanese Syrian Associated Charities (ALSAC).

REFERENCES

1. Agamanolis DP, Dasu S, Krill CE. Tumors of skeletal muscle. *Hum Pathol* 1986;17:778–795.
2. Angel CA, Gant LL, Parham DM, Rao BN, Douglass EC, Lobe T, Philippe PG. Leiomyosarcomas in children: clinical and pathologic characteristics. *Pediatr Surg Int* 1992;7:116–120.
3. Asmar L, Gehan EA, Newton WA, et al. Agreement among and within groups of pathologists in the classification of rhabdomyosarcoma and related childhood sarcomas: report of an international study of four pathology classifications. *Cancer* 1994;74: 2579–2588.
4. Bale PM, Parsons RE, Stevens MM. Pathology and behavior of juvenile rhabdomyosarcoma. In: Finegold M, ed. *Pathology of Neoplasia in Children and Adolescents. vol 18. Major Problems in Pathology*. Philadelphia: WB Saunders; 1986:196–222.
5. Barr FG, Galili N, Holick J, Biegel JA, Rovera G, Emmanuel BS. Rearrangement of the PAX3 paired box gene in the paediatric solid tumour alveolar rhabdomyosarcoma. *Nature Genet* 1993;3: 113–121.
6. Beckwith JB, Palmer NF. Histopathology and prognosis of Wilms tumors: results from the First National Wilms' Tumor Study. *Cancer* 1978;41:1937–1948.
7. Bonneau R, Brochu P. Neuromuscular choristoma: a clinicopathologic study of two cases. *Am J Surg Pathol* 1983;7:521–528.
8. Boyle ET, Jr., Reiman HM, Kramer SA, Kelalis PP, Rainwater LM, Lieber MM. Embryonal rhabdomyosarcoma of bladder and prostate: nuclear DNA patterns studied by flow cytometry. *J Urol* 1988;140:1119–1121.
9. Brachman DG, Hallahan DE, Beckett MA, Yandell DW, Weichselbaum RR. p53 gene mutations and abnormal retinoblastoma

protein in radiation-induced human sarcomas. *Cancer Res* 1991;51:6393–6396.

10. Brooks JJ. Immunohistochemistry of soft tissue tumors: myoglobin as a tumor marker for rhabdomyosarcoma. *Cancer* 1982;50: 1757–1763.
11. Caillaud JM, Gérard-Marchant R, Marsden HB, van Unnik AJM, Rodary C, Rey A, Flamant F. Histopathologic classification of childhood rhabdomyosarcoma: a report from the International Society of Pediatric Oncology Pathology Panel. *Med Pediatr Oncol* 1989;17:391–400.
12. Carter RL, Hall JM. A note on immunohistochemical staining for sarcomeric actin in rhabdomyosarcomas and other round cell tumours. *Histopathology* 1992;21:575–577.
13. Carter RL, McCarthy KP. Diagnosis of rhabdomyosarcomas with particular reference to immunohistochemical markers. *Prog Surg Pathol* 1992;12:251–267.
14. Cavazzana AO, Schmidt D, Ninfo V, et al. Spindle cell rhabdomyosarcoma: A prognostically favorable variant of rhabdomyosarcoma. *Am J Surg Pathol* 1992;16:229–235.
15. Chirayil SJ, Tobon H. Polyps of the vagina: a clinicopathologic study of 18 cases. *Cancer* 1981;47:2904–2907.
16. Churg AM, Kahn LB. Myofibroblasts and related cells in malignant fibrous and fibrohistiocytic tumors. *Hum Pathol* 1977;8: 205–218.
17. Coindre J, De Mascarel A, Trojani M, De Mascarel I, Pages A. Immunohistochemical study of rhabdomyosarcoma: unexpected staining with S100 protein and cytokeratin. *J Pathol* 1988;155: 127–132.
18. Crist WM, Garnsey L, Beltangady MS, et al. Prognosis in children with rhabdomyosarcoma: a report of the Intergroup Rhabdomyosarcoma Studies I and II. *J Clin Oncol* 1990;8:443–452.
19. Dal Cin P, Brock P, Sayed Aly M, Casteels-Van Daele M, De Wever I, Van Damme B, Van Den Berghe H. A variant (2;13) translocation in rhabdomyosarcoma. *Cancer Genet Cytogenet* 1991;55:191–195.
20. Davies SW, Makanje HH, Woodcock AS. Pseudo-sarcomatous polyps of the vagina in pregnancy. Case report. *Br J Obstet Gynaecol* 1981;88:566–568.
21. Davis RL, Weintraub H, Lassar AB. Expression of a single transfected cDNA converts fibroblasts to myoblasts. *Cell* 1987;51:987–1000.
22. de Jong ASH, van Kessel-van Vark M, Albus-Lutter CE, van Raamsdonk W, Voute PA. Skeletal muscle actin as tumor marker in the diagnosis of rhabdomyosarcoma in childhood. *Am J Surg Pathol* 1985;9:467–474.
23. Dehner LP. Primitive neuroectodermal tumor and Ewing's sarcoma. *Am J Surg Pathol* 1993;17:1–13.
24. Dei Tos AP, Doglioni C, Laurino L, Barbareschi M, Fletcher CDM. p53 protein expression in non-neoplastic lesions and benign and malignant neoplasms of soft tissue. *Histopathology* 1993;22:45–50.
25. Dias P, Dilling M, Houghton P. The molecular basis of skeletal muscle differentiation. *Semin Diag Pathol* 1994;11:3–14.
26. Dias P, Kumar P, Marsden HB, Gattamaneni HR, Kumar S. Prognostic relevance of DNA ploidy in rhabdomyosarcomas and other sarcomas of childhood. *Anticancer Res* 1992;12:1173–1178.
27. Dias P, Parham DM, Shapiro DN, Tapscott SJ, Houghton PJ. Monoclonal antibodies to the myogenic regulatory protein MyoD1: epitope mapping and diagnostic utility. *Cancer Res* 1992;52:6431–6439.
28. Dias P, Parham DM, Shapiro DN, Webber BL, Houghton PJ. Myogenic regulatory protein (MyoD1) expression in childhood solid tumors: diagnostic utility in rhabdomyosarcoma. *Am J Pathol* 1990;137:1283–1291.
29. Dickman PS, Bodner S, Salahi W, Parham D, Webber B, Gehan E, Maurer H. Electron microscopy (EM) and immunohistochemistry (IHC) of rhabdomyosarcoma: diagnosis and prognosis. *Mod Pathol* 1990;3:27A(Abstract).
30. Dickman PS, Triche TJ. Extraosseous Ewing's sarcoma versus primitive rhabdomyosarcoma: diagnostic criteria and clinical correlation. *Hum Pathol* 1986;17:881–893.
31. Douglass EC, Rowe ST, Valentine M, Parham DM, Berkow R, Bowman WP, Maurer HM. Variant translocations of chromosome 13 in alveolar rhabdomyosarcoma. *Genes Chrom Cancer* 1991;3:480–482.
32. Douglass EC, Valentine M, Etcubanas E, Parham D, Webber BL, Houghton PJ, Green AA. A specific chromosomal abnormality in rhabdomyosarcoma. *Cytogenet Cell Genet* 1987;45:148–155.
33. Downing JR, Khandekar A, Shurtleff SA, Head DR, Parham DM, Webber BL, Pappo AS, et al. Multiplex RT-PCR assay for the differential diagnosis of alveolar rhabdomyosarcoma and Ewing's sarcoma. *Am J Pathol* 1995;146:626–634.
34. Elliott GB, Elliott JD. Superficial stromal reactions of lower genital tract. *Arch Pathol* 1973;95:100–101.
35. Enzinger FM, Weiss SW. *Soft Tissue Tumors.* 3rd ed. St. Louis: CV Mosby; 1995:523–537.
36. Erlandson RA. The ultrastructural distinction between rhabdomyosarcoma and other undifferentiated "sarcomas." *Ultrastruct Pathol* 1987;11:83–101.
37. Etcubanas E, Parham D, Webber B, Dodge R, Pratt C, Husto O, Kun L, et al. An evaluation of histologic subtypes in the prognosis of childhood rhabdomyosarcomas (RMS) using conventional (CC) and Palmer classifications (PC). *Proc Annu Meet Am Soc Clin Oncol* 1987;6:215(Abstract).
38. Eusebi V, Bondi A, Rosai J. Immunohistochemical localization of myoglobin in nonmuscular cells. *Am J Surg Pathol* 1984;8:51–55.
39. Eyden BP, Christensen L. Leiomyosarcoma versus myofibrosarcoma: observations and terminology. *Ultrastruct Pathol* 1993;17: 231–239.
40. Felix CA, Chavez Kappel C, Mitsudomi T, et al. Frequency and diversity of p53 mutations in childhood rhabdomyosarcoma. *Cancer Res* 1992;52:2243–2247.
41. Fisher C. The value of electronmicroscopy and immunohistochemistry in the diagnosis of soft tissue sarcomas: a study of 200 cases. *Histopathology* 1990;16:441–454.
42. Gabbert HE, Gerharz C-D, Engers R, Müller-Klieser W, Moll R. Terminally differentiated postmitotic tumor cells in a rat rhabdomyosarcoma cell line. *Virchows Arch B Cell Pathol* 1988;55:255–261.
43. Gaffney EF, Dervan PA, Fletcher CDM. Pleomorphic rhabdomyosarcoma in adulthood: analysis of 11 cases with definition of diagnostic criteria. *Am J Surg Pathol* 1993;17:601–609.
44. Gerharz CD, Gabbert HE, Biesalski HK, Engers R, Luley C. Fetal calf serum and retinoic acid affect proliferation and terminal differentiation of a rat rhabdomyosarcoma cell line (BA-HAN-1C). *Br J Cancer* 1989;59:61–67.
45. Goulding MD, Chalepakis G, Deutsch U, Erselius JR, Gruss P. Pax-3, a novel murine DNA binding protein expressed during early neurogenesis. *EMBO J* 1991;10:1135–1147.
46. Harrison CJ, Johnson PRE, Yin JAL, Bhavnani M. Alveolar rhabdomyosarcoma with del(13q14). *Cancer Genet Cytogenet* 1991;55:257–259.
47. Hawkins HK, Camacho-Velasquez JV. Rhabdomyosarcoma in children. Correlation of form and prognosis in one institution's experience. *Am J Surg Pathol* 1987;11:531–542.
48. Hirose T, Kudo E, Hasegawa T, Abe J, Hizawa K. Expression of intermediate filaments in malignant fibrous histiocytomas. *Hum Pathol* 1989;20:871–877.
49. Hiti AL, Bogenmann E, Gonzales F, Jones PA. Expression of the MyoD1 muscle determination gene defines differentiation capability but not tumorigenicity of human rhabdomyosarcomas. *Mol Cell Biol* 1989;9:4722–4730.
50. Hollstein M, Sidransky D, Vogelstein B, Harris CC. p53 mutations in human cancers. *Science* 1991;253:49–53.
51. Horn RC, Enterline HT. Rhabdomyosarcoma: a clinicopathologic study of 39 cases. *Cancer* 1958;11:181-199.
52. Huff V, Saunders GF. Wilms tumor genes. *Biochim Biophys Acta Rev Cancer* 1993;1155:295–306.
53. Johnson W, Jurand J, Hiramoto R. Immunohistologic studies of tumors containing myosin. *Am J Pathol* 1965;47:1139–1155.
54. Jung WH, Jung SH, Yoo CJ, Kim YJ, Park C, Kim BS. Flow cytometric analysis of DNA ploidy in childhood rhabdomyosarcoma. *Yonsei Med J* 1994;35:34–42.
55. Junien C. Beckwith–Wiedemann syndrome, tumourigenesis and imprinting. *Curr Opin Genet Dev* 1992;2:431–438.
56. Kapadia SB, Meis JM, Frisman DM, Ellis GL, Heffner DK. Fetal

rhabdomyoma of the head and neck: a clinicopathologic and immunophenotypic study of 24 cases. *Hum Pathol* 1993;24:754–765.

57. Kawai A, Noguchi M, Beppu Y, et al. Nuclear immunoreaction of p53 protein in soft tissue sarcomas. A possible prognostic factor. *Cancer* 1994;73:2499–2505.
58. Kodet R, Fajstavr J, Kabelka Z, Koutecky J, Eckschlager T, Newton WA, Jr. Is fetal cellular rhabdomyoma an entity or a differentiated rhabdomyosarcoma? A study of patients with rhabdomyoma of the tongue and sarcoma of the tongue enrolled in the Intergroup Rhabdomyosarcoma Studies I, II, and III. *Cancer* 1991;67:2907–2913.
59. Kodet R, Newton WA, Jr., Hamoudi AB, Asmar L, Jacobs DL, Maurer HM. Childhood rhabdomyosarcoma with anaplastic (pleomorphic) features: a report of the Intergroup Rhabdomyosarcoma Study. *Am J Surg Pathol* 1993;17:443–453.
60. Koh S, Johnson WW. Antimyosin and antirhabdomyoblast sera: their use for the diagnosis of childhood rhabdomyosarcoma. *Arch Pathol Lab Med* 1980;104:118–122.
61. Koscielniak E, Rodary C, Flamant F, Carli M, Treuner J, Pinkerton CR, Grotto P. Metastatic rhabdomyosarcoma and histologically similar tumors in childhood: a retrospective European multi-center analysis. *Med Pediatr Oncol* 1992;20:209–214.
62. Kowal-Vern A, Gonzalez-Crussi F, Turner J, et al. Flow and image cytometric DNA analysis in rhabdomyosarcoma. *Cancer Res* 1990;50:6023–6027.
63. Langbein L, Kosmehl H, Katenkamp D, Neupert G, Stiller K-J. Experimentally induced murine rhabdomyosarcomas—correlation between cellular contacts, matrix formation and cellular differentiation. *Differentiation* 1990;44:185–196.
64. Lassar AB, Buskin JN, Lockshon D, Davis RL, Apone S, Hauschka SD, Weintraub H. MyoD is a sequence-specific DNA binding protein requiring a region of myc homology to bind to the muscle creatine kinase enhancer. *Cell* 1989;58:823–831.
65. Lazarides E. Intermediate filaments as mechanical integrators of cellular space. *Nature* 1980;283:249–256.
66. Leader M, Patel J, Collins M, Henry K. Myoglobin: an evaluation of its role as a marker of rhabdomyosarcomas. *Br J Cancer* 1989;59:106–109.
67. Leuschner I, Newton WA, Jr., Schmidt D, et al. Spindle cell variants of embryonal rhabdomyosarcoma in the paratesticular region: a report of the intergroup rhabdomyosarcoma study. *Am J Surg Pathol* 1993;17:221–230.
68. Levine AJ, Momand J, Finlay CA. The p53 tumour suppressor gene. *Nature* 1991;351:453–456.
69. Li FP, Fraumeni JF. Rhabdomyosarcoma in children: epidemiologic study and identification of a familial cancer syndrome. *JNCI* 1969;43:1365–1373.
70. Li L, Olson EN. Regulation of muscle cell growth and differentiation by the MyoD family of helix-loop-helix proteins. *Adv Cancer Res* 1992;58:95–120.
71. Loh WE, Jr., Scrable HJ, Livanos E, Arboleda MJ, Cavenee WK, Oshimura M, Weissman BE. Human chromosome 11 contains two different growth suppressor genes for embryonal rhabdomyosarcoma. *Proc Natl Acad Sci USA* 1992;89:1755–1759.
72. Lollini P-L, De Giovanni C, Del Re B, et al. Myogenic differentiation of human rhabdomyosarcoma cells induced in vitro by antineoplastic drugs. *Cancer Res* 1989;49:3631–3636.
73. Lollini P-L, De Giovanni C, Landuzzi L, Nicoletti G, Scotlandi K, Nanni P. Reduced metastatic ability of in vitro differentiated human rhabdomyosarcoma cells. *Invasion Metastasis* 1991;11:116–124.
74. Lombardi L, Pilotti S. Ultrastructural characterization of poorly differentiated rhabdomyosarcomas. *Ultrastruct Pathol* 1993;17:669–680.
75. Malkin D, Li FP, Strong LC, et al. Germ line p53 mutations in a familial syndrome of breast cancer, sarcomas, and other neoplasms. *Science* 1990;250:1233–1238.
76. Markel SF, Enzinger FM. Neuromuscular hamartoma: a benign "triton" tumor composed of mature neural and striated muscle elements. *Cancer* 1982;49:140–144.
77. Maulbecker CC, Gruss P. The oncogenic potential of Pax genes. *EMBO J* 1993;12:2361–2367.
78. Maurer HM, Beltangady M, Gehan EA, et al. The Intergroup Rhabdomyosarcoma Study I. A final report. *Cancer* 1988;61:209–220.
79. Maurer HM, Moon T, Donaldson M, et al. The Intergroup Rhabdomyosarcoma Study: A preliminary report. *Cancer* 1977;40:2015–2026.
80. Miettinen M. Antibody specific to muscle actins in the diagnosis and classification of soft tissue tumors. *Am J Pathol* 1988;130:205–215.
81. Miettinen M, Lehto VP, Badley RA, Virtanen I. Expression of intermediate filaments in soft-tissue sarcomas. *Int J Cancer* 1982;30:541–546.
82. Miettinen M, Lehto VP, Virtanen I. Antibodies to intermediate filament proteins in the diagnosis and classification of human tumors. *Ultrastruct Pathol* 1984;7:83–107.
83. Miettinen M, Rapola J. Immunohistochemical spectrum of rhabdomyosarcoma and rhabdomyosarcoma-like tumors: expression of cytokeratin and the 68-kD neurofilament protein. *Am J Surg Pathol* 1989;13:120–132.
84. Miettinen M, Wahlström T, Vesterinen E, Saksela E. Vaginal polyps with pseudosarcomatous features: a clinicopathologic study of seven cases. *Cancer* 1983;51:1148–1151.
85. Minniti CP, Kohn EC, Grubb JH, et al. The insulin-like growth factor II (IGF-II)/mannose 6-phosphate receptor mediates IGF-II-induced motility in human rhabdomyosarcoma cells. *J Biol Chem* 1992;267:9000–9004.
86. Minniti CP, Maggi M, Helman LJ. Suramin inhibits the growth of human rhabdomyosarcoma by interrupting the insulin-like growth factor II autocrine growth loop. *Cancer Res* 1992;52:1830–1835.
87. Mitchell M, Talerman A, Sholl JS, Okagaki T, Cibils LA. Pseudosarcoma botyroides in pregnancy: report of a case with ultrastructural observations. *Obstet Gynecol* 1987;70:522–526.
88. Molenaar WM, Dam-Meiring A, Kamps WA, Cornelisse CJ. DNA-aneuploidy in rhabdomyosarcomas as compared with other sarcomas of childhood and adolescence. *Hum Pathol* 1988;19:573–579.
89. Molenaar WM, Oosterhuis JW, Kamps WA. Cytologic "differentiation" in childhood rhabdomyosarcomas following polychemotherapy. *Hum Pathol* 1984;15:973–979.
90. Mukai K, Rosai J, Hallaway BE. Localization of myoglobin in normal and neoplastic human skeletal muscle cells using an immunoperoxidase method. *Am J Surg Pathol* 1979;3:373–376.
91. Mundlos S, Pelletier J, Darveau A, Bachmann M, Winterpacht A, Zabel B. Nuclear localization of the protein encoded by the Wilms' tumor gene WT1 in embryonic and adult tissues. *Development* 1993;119:1329–1341.
92. Murre C, McCaw PS, Vaessin H, et al. Interactions between heterologous helix-loop-helix proteins generate complexes that bind specifically to a common DNA sequence. *Cell* 1989;58:537–544.
93. Nanni P, Azzarello G, Tessarollo L, et al. In vitro differentiation of rhabdomyosarcomas induced by nickel or by Moloney murine sarcoma virus. *Br J Cancer* 1991;63:736–742.
94. Newton WA, Jr., Soule EH, Hamoudi AB, Reiman HM, Shimada H, Beltangady M, Maurer H. Histopathology of childhood sarcomas, Intergroup Rhabdomyosarcoma Studies I and II: clinicopathologic correlation. *J Clin Oncol* 1988;6:67–75.
95. Nicoletti G, De Giovanni C, Landuzzi L, Simone G, Rocchi P, Nanni P, Lollini P-L. Induction of myogenic differentiation in human rhabdomyosarcoma cells by ionising radiation, *N,N*-dimethylformamide and their combination. *Br J Cancer* 1992;65:519–522.
96. Niggli FK, Powell JE, Parkes SE, Ward K, Raafat F, Mann JR, Stevens MC. DNA ploidy and proliferative activity (S-phase) in childhood soft-tissue sarcomas: their value as prognostic indicators. *Br J Cancer* 1994;69:1106–1110.
97. Osborn M. Intermediate filaments as histologic markers: an overview. *J Invest Dermatol* 1983;81:104s–109s.
98. Ostor AG, Fortune DW, Riley CB. Fibroepithelial polyps with atypical stromal cells (pseudosarcoma botryoides) of vulva and vagina. A report of 13 cases. *Int J Gynecol Pathol* 1988;7:351–360.
99. Palmer NF, Foulkes M. Histopathology and prognosis in the second Intergroup Rhabdomyosarcoma Study (IRS II). *Proc Annu Meet Am Soc Clin Oncol* 1983;2:229(Abstract).

100. Pappo AS, Crist WM, Kuttesch J, et al. Tumor-cell DNA content predicts outcome in children and adolescents with clinical group III embryonal rhabdomyosarcoma. The Intergroup Rhabdomyosarcoma Study Committee of the Children's Cancer Group and the Pediatric Oncology Group. *J Clin Oncol* 1993;11:1901–1905.
101. Parham DM, Dias P, Bertorini T, von Wronski MA, Horner L, Houghton PJ. Immunohistochemical analysis of the distribution of MyoD1 in muscle biopsies of primary and neurogenic atrophy. *Acta Neuropathol (Berl)* 1994;87:605–611.
102. Parham DM, Dias P, Kelly DR, Rutledge JC, Houghton P. Desmin positivity in primitive neuroectodermal tumors of childhood. *Am J Surg Pathol* 1992;16:483–492.
103. Parham DM, Kelly DR, Donnelly WH, Douglass EC. Immunohistochemical and ultrastructural spectrum of hepatic sarcomas of childhood: evidence for a common histogenesis. *Mod Pathol* 1991;4:648–653.
104. Parham DM, Reynolds AB, Webber BL. Use of monoclonal antibody 1H1, anti-cortactin, to distinguish normal and neoplastic smooth muscle cells: comparison with anti-alpha-smooth muscle actin and anti-muscle specific actin. *Hum Pathol* 1995;26:776–783
105. Parham DM, Shapiro DN, Downing JR, Webber BL, Douglass EC. Solid alveolar rhabdomyosarcomas with the t(2;13): report of two cases with diagnostic implications. *Am J Surg Pathol* 1994;18:474–478.
106. Parham DM, Webber B, Holt H, Williams WK, Maurer HM. Immunohistochemical study of childhood rhabdomyosarcomas and related neoplasms: results of an Intergroup Rhabdomyosarcoma Study project. *Cancer* 1991;67:3072–3080.
107. Ramp U, Gerharz CD, Doehmer J, Oster O, Gabbert HE. Uniform response of c-raf expression to differentiation induction and inhibition of proliferation in a rat rhabdomyosarcoma cell line. *Virchows Arch B Cell Pathol* 1990;59:271–280.
108. Ramp U, Gerharz CD, Doehmer J, Oster O, Gabbert HE. Increase in proto-oncogene raf expression precedes differentiation induction in different clonal rhabdomyosarcoma subpopulations. *Anticancer Res* 1992;12:537–546.
109. Rangdaeng S, Truong LD. Comparative immunohistochemical staining for desmin and muscle-specific actin: a study of 576 cases. *Am J Clin Pathol* 1991;96:32–45.
110. Rosai J, Dias P, Parham DM, Shapiro DN, Houghton P. MyoD1 protein expression in alveolar soft part sarcoma as confirmatory evidence of its skeletal muscle nature. *Am J Surg Pathol* 1991;15:974–981.
111. Rudnicki MA, Schnegelsberg PNJ, Stead RH, Braun T, Arnold H-H, Jaenisch R. MyoD or Myf-5 is required for the formation of skeletal muscle. *Cell* 1993;75:1351–1359.
112. Russell B, Dix DJ, Haller DL, Jacobs-El J. Repair of injured skeletal muscle: a molecular approach. *Med Sci Sports Exerc* 1992;24:189–196.
113. Ruymann FB. Rhabdomyosarcoma in children and adolescents: a review. *Hematol Oncol Clin North Am* 1987;1:621–654.
114. Schmidt D, Harms D, Pilon VA. Small-cell pediatric tumors: histology, immunohistochemistry, and electron microscopy. *Clin Lab Med* 1987;7:63–89.
115. Schmidt RA, Cone R, Haas J, Gown AM. Diagnosis of rhabdomyosarcoma with HHF35, a monoclonal antibody directed against muscle actins. *Am J Pathol* 1988;131:19–28.
116. Schneid H, Seurin D, Vazquez MP, Gourmelen M, Cabrol S, Le Bouc Y. Parental allele specific methylation of the human insulin-like growth factor II gene and Beckwith–Wiedemann syndrome. *J Med Genet* 1993;30:353–362.
117. Schurch W, Skalli O, Lagace R, Seemayer TA, Gabbiani G. Intermediate filament proteins and actin isoforms as markers for soft-tissue tumor differentiation and origin. III. Hemangiopericytomas and glomus tumors. *Am J Pathol* 1990;136:771–786.
118. Scrable H, Witte D, Shimada H, et al. Molecular differential pathology in rhabdomyosarcoma. *Genes Chrom Cancer* 1989;1:23–35.
119. Scrable HJ, Johnson DK, Rinchik EM, Cavenee WK. Rhabdomyosarcoma-associated locus and MYOD1 are syntenic but separate loci on the short arm of human chromosome 11. *Proc Natl Acad Sci USA* 1990;87:2182–2186.
120. Shapiro DN, Houghton PJ, Hazelton BJ, Germain GS, Murti KG, Rahman A, Houghton JA. Morphological and molecular characterization of spontaneous myogenic differentiation in a human rhabdomyosarcoma cell line. *Cancer Res* 1990;50:6002–6009.
121. Shapiro DN, Parham DM, Douglass EC, et al. Relationship of tumor-cell ploidy to histologic subtype and treatment outcome in children and adolescents with unresectable rhabdomyosarcoma. *J Clin Oncol* 1991;9:159–166.
122. Shapiro DN, Sublett JE, Li B, Downing JR, Naeve CW. Fusion of PAX3 to a member of the forkhead family of transcription factors in human alveolar rhabdomyosarcoma. *Cancer Res* 1993;53:5108–5112.
123. Shimada H, Newton WA, Jr., Soule EH, Beltangady MS, Maurer HM. Pathology of fatal rhabdomyosarcoma. Report from Intergroup Rhabdomyosarcoma Study (IRS-I and IRS-II). *Cancer* 1987;59:459–465.
124. Skalli O, Schürch W, Seemayer T, Lagacé R, Montandon D, Pittet B, Gabbiani G. Myofibroblasts from diverse pathologic settings are heterogeneous in their content of actin isoforms and intermediate filament proteins. *Lab Invest* 1989;60:275–285.
125. Strong LC. Genetic implications for long-term survivors of childhood cancer. *Cancer* 1993;71 Suppl. 3435–3440.
126. Sugimoto T, Ueyama H, Hosoi H, et al. Alpha-smooth-muscle actin and desmin expressions in human neuroblastoma cell lines. *Int J Cancer* 1991;48:277–283.
127. Takizawa T, Matsui T, Maeda Y, et al. X-radiation-induced differentiation of xenotransplanted human undifferentiated rhabdomyosarcoma. *Lab Invest* 1989;60:22–29.
128. Tallini G, Parham DM, Dias P, Cordon-Cardo C, Houghton PJ, Rosai J. Myogenic regulatory protein expression in adult soft tissue sarcomas: a sensitive and specific marker of skeletal muscle differentiation. *Am J Pathol* 1994;144:693–701.
129. Tapscott SJ, Thayer MJ, Weintraub H. Deficiency in rhabdomyosarcomas of a factor required for MyoD activity and myogenesis. *Science* 1993;259:1450–1453.
130. Truong LD, Rangdaeng S, Cagle P, Ro JY, Hawkins H, Font RL. The diagnostic utility of desmin: a study of 584 cases and review of the literature. *Am J Clin* Pathol 1990;93:305–314.
131. Tsokos M. The role of immunocytochemistry in the diagnosis of rhabdomyosarcoma. *Arch Pathol Lab Med* 1986;110:776–778.
132. Tsokos M, Dias P, Jefferson J, Houghton PJ. Detection of the $MyoD_1$ gene product in paraffin sections of pediatric tumors. *Mod Pathol* 1994;7:148A(Abstract).
133. Tsokos M, Linnoila RI, Chandra RS, Triche TJ. Neuron-specific enolase in the diagnosis of neuroblastoma and other small, round-cell tumors in children. *Hum Pathol* 1984;15:575–584.
134. Tsokos M, Webber B, Parham D, et al. Rhabdomyosarcoma: a new classification scheme related to prognosis. *Arch Pathol Lab Med* 1992;116:847–855.
135. Tsukada T, McNutt MA, Ross R, Gown AM. HHF35, a muscle actin-specific monoclonal antibody. II. Reactivity in normal, reactive, and neoplastic human tissues. *Am J Pathol* 1987;127:389–402.
136. Tsukada T, Tippens D, Gordon D, Ross R, Gown AM. HHF35, a muscle-actin-specific monoclonal antibody. I. Immunocytochemical and biochemical characterization. *Am J Pathol* 1987;126:51–60.
137. Vandekerckhove J, Weber K. At least six different actins are expressed in a higher mammal: an analysis based on the amino acid sequence of the amino-terminal tryptic peptide. *J Mol Biol* 1978;126:783–802.
138. Vogel W, Kosmehl H, Katenkamp D, Langbein L. Differentiation dependent matrix formation (fibronectin and laminin) in an experimental murine rhabdomyosarcoma model. *Acta Histochem (Jena)* 1991;90:181–188.
139. Voullaire LE, Petrovic V, Sheffield LJ, Campbell P. Two forms of ring 13 in a child with rhabdomyosarcoma. *Am J Med Genet* 1991;39:285–287.
140. Walther C, Guenet JL, Simon D, et al. Pax: a murine multigene family of paired box-containing genes. *Genomics* 1991;11:424–434.
141. Weber CO. Anatomishche Untersuchung einer hypertrophische

Zunge nebst Bemerkunger uber die Neubildung quergestreifter Muskelfasern. *Virchows Arch A Histopathol Anat* 1854;7:115.
142. Weintraub H. The MyoD family and myogenesis: redundancy, networks, and thresholds. *Cell* 1993;75:1241–1244.
143. Weintraub H, Davis R, Tapscott S, et al. The myoD gene family: nodal point during specification of the muscle cell lineage. *Science* 1991;251:761–766.
144. Wesche WA, Fletcher CDM, Dias P, Houghton PJ, Parham DM. Immunohistochemistry of MyoD1 in adult pleomorphic soft tissue sarcomas. *Am J Surg Pathol* 1995;19:261–269.
145. Wijnaendts LC, van der Linden JC, van Diest P, van Unnik AJ, Delemarre JF, Voute PA, Meijer CJ. Prognostic importance of DNA flow cytometric variables in rhabdomyosarcomas. *J Clin Pathol* 1993;46:948–952.
146. Wijnaendts LCD, van der Linden JC, van Unnik AJM, Delemarre JFM, Voute PA, Meijer CJLM. Histologic classification of childhood rhabdomyosarcomas: relationship with clinical parameters and prognosis. *Hum Pathol* 1994;25:900–907.
147. Willis J, Abdul-Karim FW, di Sant'Agnese PA. Extracardiac rhabdomyomas. *Semin Diag Pathol* 1994;11:15–25.
148. Willis RA. *The Borderland of Embryology and Pathology*. 2nd ed. London: Butterworths; 1962.
149. Woodcock-Mitchell J, Mitchell JJ, Low RB, et al. Alpha-smooth muscle actin is transiently expressed in embryonic rat cardiac and skeletal muscles. *Differentiation* 1988;39:161–166.
150. Zhan S, Shapiro DN, Helman LJ. Activation of an imprinted allele of the insulin-like growth factor II gene implicated in rhabdomyosarcoma. *J Clin Invest* 1994;94:445–448.
151. Zuppan CW, Mierau GW, Weeks DA. Lipid-rich rhabdomyosarcoma—a potential source of diagnostic confusion. *Ultrastruct Pathol* 1991;15:353–359.

Pediatric Neoplasia: Morphology and Biology, edited by David M. Parham.
Lippincott-Raven Publishers, Philadelphia © 1996.

CHAPTER 6

Neuroblastoma and Related Tumors

David R. Kelly and Vijay V. Joshi

Neuroblastic tumors are derived from primordial neural crest cells, which ultimately populate the sympathetic ganglia, adrenal medulla, and other diverse sites. Variations in tumor site and degree of histopathologic differentiation result in tumors that display a wide range of clinical and biological characteristics and behavior (65). Neuroblastic tumors may show spontaneous and induced differentiation with maturation to benign neoplasms. They may also demonstrate spontaneous regression. The term "neuroblastic tumor" includes all tumors of the sympathetic nervous system of neuroblastic origin showing the presence or absence of differentiation along gangliocytic and Schwannian lineages, i.e., neuroblastoma, ganglioneuroblastoma, and ganglioneuroma. When the term "neuroblastoma" is used in the clinical context and in reference to the therapeutic protocols used by the national cooperative groups, it includes either or both neuroblastoma and ganglioneuroblastoma. When is used purely in a pathologic context, it includes only neuroblastoma.

In this chapter, we are concerned with peripheral neuroblastic tumors, i.e., classical neuroblastoma, ganglioneuroblastoma, and ganglioneuroma, and the embryologically related tumors, i.e., pheochromocytoma and paraganglioma. The following aspects are described in further detail: histogenesis; clinical features; biologic features; histologic, immunohistochemical, and ultrastructural characteristics; classification; and prognostic factors.

D. R. Kelly: Department of Pathology, University of Alabama at Birmingham, and the Children's Hospital of Alabama, Birmingham, Alabama 35233.

V. V. Joshi: Department of Pathology and Laboratory Medicine and Department of Pediatrics, East Carolina University School of Medicine, Brody Medical Sciences Building, Greenville, North Carolina 27858.

EPIDEMIOLOGY AND DEFINITION

Neuroblastoma is the fourth most common malignant tumor of childhood, being exceeded only by leukemia, malignant lymphoma, and brain tumors (289). It accounts for about 50% of malignancies in infants and 7–10% of all childhood neoplasms (111). The prevalence is about 1 case per 8,000 live births with an incidence of 7.0 per million per year in black children and 9.6 per million per year in white children. This incidence varies somewhat throughout the world; it is very low in much of Africa and parts of India and Puerto Rico (288). Boys are more commonly affected than girls; the male/female ratio is 1.2:1. The median age at diagnosis is 22 months. Thirty-six percent of patients are less than 1 year old at diagnosis, almost 85% are less than 4 years, and 97% are under 10 years old. Neuroblastoma has a biphasic age incidence with an initial peak before 1 year and a second peak between 2 and 4 years (65).

The question arises as to what a classical neuroblastoma actually is. Dehner (109,110,112) has given the following criteria: (a) It is an embryonal-appearing, small round cell tumor having a variable amount of neuropil and arising from neural crest precursors in the sympathetic nervous system, adrenal medulla, or sympathetic ganglia. Neuroblastic tumors can also occur in the central nervous system where they exhibit a different natural history. Examples include cerebral neuroblastoma (central primitive neuroectodermal tumor with neuroblastic-neuronal differentiation) and cerebellar ganglioneuroblastoma (gangliocytic medulloblastoma) (114). They can also arise from neural crest cells in primary, metastatic, or recurrent germ cell tumors (229). Olfactory neuroblastomas (esthioneuroblastomas), although morphologically similar to classical neuroblastoma, are more likely related to peripheral primitive neuroectodermal tumors (see Chapter 4) (78,110). (b) Catecholamines and/or their metabolites are elevated in patients with neuroblastoma. However, a minority of classical neuroblastomas are inactive with respect to catecholamine synthesis (437). Morphologic criteria, molecular biologic features, karyotype analysis, and site of origin can be used for the diagnosis of such tumors. (c) Neuroblastic tumors arise most commonly in children. Although neuroblastomas have been described in adults (12,13,292), it is likely that most of these cases represent peripheral primitive neuroectodermal tumors rather than neuroblastomas (109,110,417). Ganglioneuromas tend to occur more frequently in adults and in some instances represent maturation of a clinically silent neuroblastoma (402).

HISTORICAL ASPECTS

According to Willis (448), Virchow, in his clinical work on tumors (1863–1867), was the first to distinguish between tumors of nerve sheath origin and those of sympathetic origin when he proposed the existence of "neuroma gangliocellulare." A thoracic ganglion cell tumor was subsequently described in a 35-year-old woman by Loretz in 1870. Neuroblastic tumors were originally regarded as "round-celled sarcomas" or "lymphosarcomas" (448). Marchand (272) in 1891 correctly recognized the resemblance of these tumors to the developing sympathetic ganglia. Neuroblastic tumors were considered by Ribbert in 1904 as being of a glial nature (glioma). In 1905, Wiesel recognized the tumor cell rosettes of neuroblastic tumors as being similar to the embryonic adrenal medulla or sympathetic ganglia. James Homer Wright (453) described a group of tumors (particularly adrenal) in 1910 that he referred to as neuroblastoma (or neurocytoma). In 1912, Landau (246) drew attention to the diversity and extent of differentiation and its correspondence to the degree of malignancy. Wahl (439) in 1914 suggested a sequence of differentiation in neuroblastomas. Herxheimer in 1914 reviewed the histogenetic relationship of ganglioneuromas, neuroblastomas, and chromaffin tumors. Using the Bielschowsky method, he first demonstrated that the fibrils in neuroblastoma were fine nerve fibers and not nerve sheath cells (190). The term "ganglioneuroblastoma" was introduced by Robertson (356) in 1915. He described the combinations of, and transitions between, undifferentiated neuroblastomas and well-differentiated ganglioneuromas. Cushing and Wolbach (104) in 1927 described a patient whose paravertebral neuroblastoma spontaneously matured into a ganglioneuroma over time. Their report introduced tumor maturation as an important concept of cancer biology and stimulated early (but unsuccessful) efforts at chemotherapeutic induction of maturation (29). Bülbring in 1928 and Rinscheid in 1936 confirmed Herxheimer's earlier finding of argentophilic nerve fibers in neuroblastoma. Rinscheid stressed the variable degree of neuronal differentiation in neuroblastic tumors (448). In 1947 Murray and Stout (306) described formation of neuritic processes in tissue culture of neuroblastoma and, in 1948, the in vitro cultivation of a ganglioneuroma (307).

HISTOGENESIS OF PERIPHERAL NEUROBLASTIC TUMORS

Peripheral neuroblastic tumors arise from neuroectodermal cells originally derived from the neural crest (Fig. 1). With the development of the notochord, there is thickening of the overlying embryonic ectoderm to form the neural plate. The neural plate invaginates to form the neural groove by about the 18th day. By the end of the third week, the neural folds begin to fuse, converting the neural groove to the neural tube. As the neural tube develops, the neuroectodermal cells of the neural crest on each neural fold detach from the epidermis and the adjacent cells. Thus the neural tube becomes separated from the surface ectoderm. Neural crest cells move ventrolaterally on either side of the neural tube and form an irregular flattened mass between the neural tube and the over-

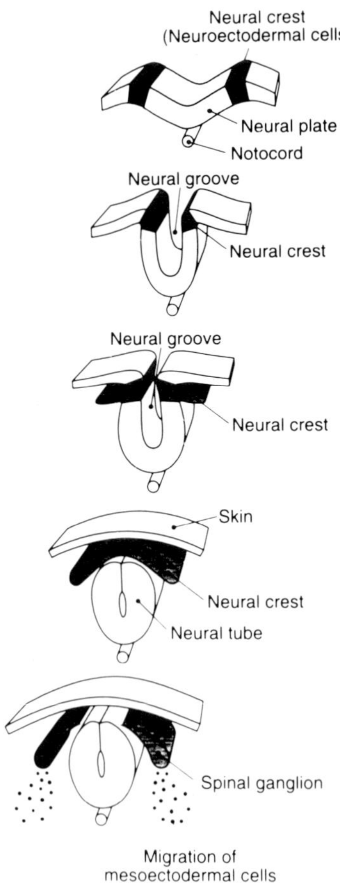

FIG. 1. Sequence of events in the development of the neural crest. (Adapted from Moore KL, ref. 298; used with permission.)

lying ectoderm. At this point, the neural crest divides into two lateral halves and the neural crest cells migrate (Fig. 1) and disperse in the body to give rise to different types of cells in different tissues (255) (Table 1).

The migrating neural crest cells on either side of the spinal column form the paravertebral sympathetic ganglia. The developing ganglia consist of neuroblasts, ganglion cells, and cells intermediate between the two. The neuroblasts may exhibit rosette formation. Neuritic processes arranged in a parallel manner and accompanied by Schwann cells emerge from the developing ganglion (Fig. 2).

The adrenal gland has a dual embryologic origin. The cortex is mesodermal and begins to form in the fifth week by aggregation of mesothelial cells located between the mesenteric root and the developing gonad on either side of the abdominal cavity (103). The cells that form the medulla are derived from the neural crest cells of the adjacent primitive sympathetic ganglion of the celiac plexus (255,298). They migrate to the center of the gland to form the adrenal medulla. Small clusters of dark-staining sympathochromaffin cells can be demonstrated in various sites in the cortex during this developmental stage (427) (Fig. 3A). These cells undergo differentiation to form pheochromoblasts and eventually pheochromocytes (Fig. 3B) during the fetal and neonatal period (189). A few ganglion cells similar to those found in sympathetic ganglia and other parts of the nervous system are present in the adrenal medulla. The adrenal neural crest cells that give rise to neuroblastoma may show a tendency to differentiate along the gangliocytic and Schwannian lineages seen in the sympathetic ganglia. Rarely, neoplastic transformation of the neural crest cells of the adrenal medulla is accompanied by a tendency to aberrant differentiation (or a change in the line of normal differentiation), giving rise to pheochromocytoma. The traditional pathways of differentiation and maturation are shown in Fig. 4, along with the various types of tumors that might be expected to occur.

TABLE 1. *Principal derivatives of the neural crest*

A. Cells
1. Neuronal cells of sensory ganglia [trigeminal (V), facial (VII), superior (IX), and jugulare (X) ganglia] and spinal dorsal root ganglia.
2. Neuronal cells of autonomic ganglia.
3. Schwann and sheath cells.
4. Glial and satellite cells of dorsal root ganglia and autonomic ganglia.
5. Glial and satellite cells of geniculate (VII), acoustic (VIII), petrosal (XI), and nodose (X) ganglia.
6. Melanocytes of dermis, epidermis, viscera; melanophores of iris.
7. Adrenal medullary cells and other adrenergic paraganglia.

B. Tissues
1. Bones and cartilages of facial and visceral skeleton.
2. Dermis of face and ventral neck.
3. Connective tissue of buccal and pharyngeal glands (salivary glands, thyroid, parathyroid and thymus).
4. Muscular and connective tissue wall of large arteries derived from aortic arches.

(Adapted from LeDouarin, ref. 255.)

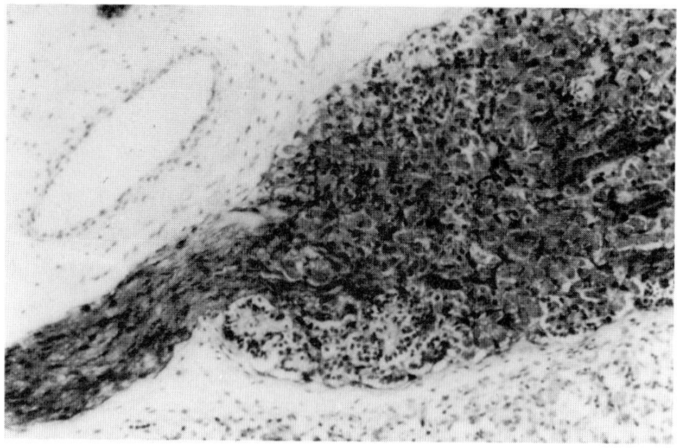

FIG. 2. Neuritic processes emerging from a developing ganglion in a fetus. (Used with permission, ref. 215.)

The histogenesis of stage 4S (S for special) neuroblastoma requires special consideration. This disease is characterized by infant onset of disseminated tumor with involvement of liver, skin, bone marrow, and/or ipsilateral lymph nodes, with generally favorable outcome (107,108). Although it is likely that the widespread involvement in stage 4S neuroblastoma is due to metastatic spread, the possibility of multicentric origin has been raised. It has been suggested that there may be heterotopic neural crest cells in the skin, liver, and bone marrow from which multicentric neuroblastoma arises, or there may be transdifferentiation of neural crest–derived cells normally present at some of these sites (melanoblasts or Schwann cells of nerves in the skin) (107,317). Similar histogenetic hypotheses can be applied to the primary neuroblastic tumors arising in the paraspinal region from the dorsal root ganglia of the spinal nerves (194,342) and from sites outside the sympathetic nervous system or adrenal medulla. These primary sites include kidney, urinary bladder, and spermatic cord (231,233). Alternatively, neuroblastic tumors can arise from the small sympathetic ganglia (some of which are of microscopic size) known to be present along the sympathetic nerves supplying various thoracic and abdominal viscera. Secondary involvement of these organs by neuroblastoma arising in an adjacent well-recognized primary site should be excluded before a diagnosis of primary neuroblastoma at an unusual site is made.

PRECURSOR LESIONS OF NEUROBLASTOMA

Theoretically, most malignant neoplasms in humans evolve through a morphologic phase that can be defined as in situ cancer (244). In that regard, Beckwith and Per-

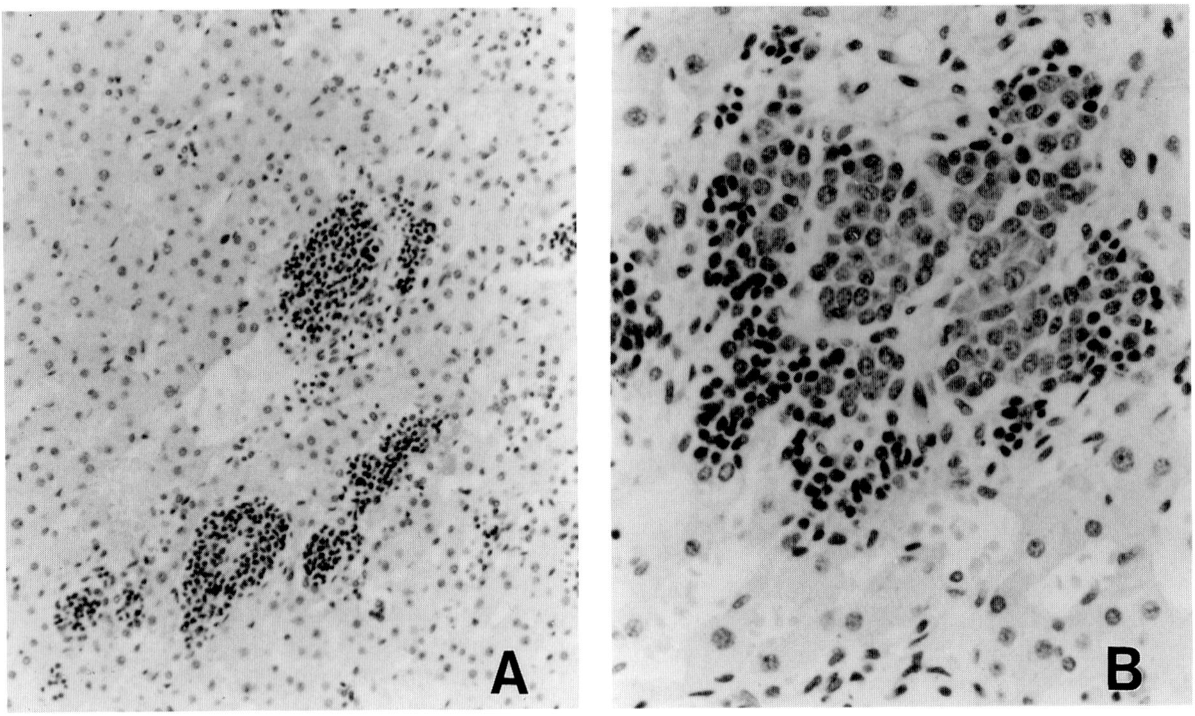

FIG. 3. A. Clusters of neuroblasts dispersed in the fetal adrenal cortex. **B.** Differentiation of neuroblasts to become adrenal medullary pheochromocytes. (Used with permission, ref. 215.)

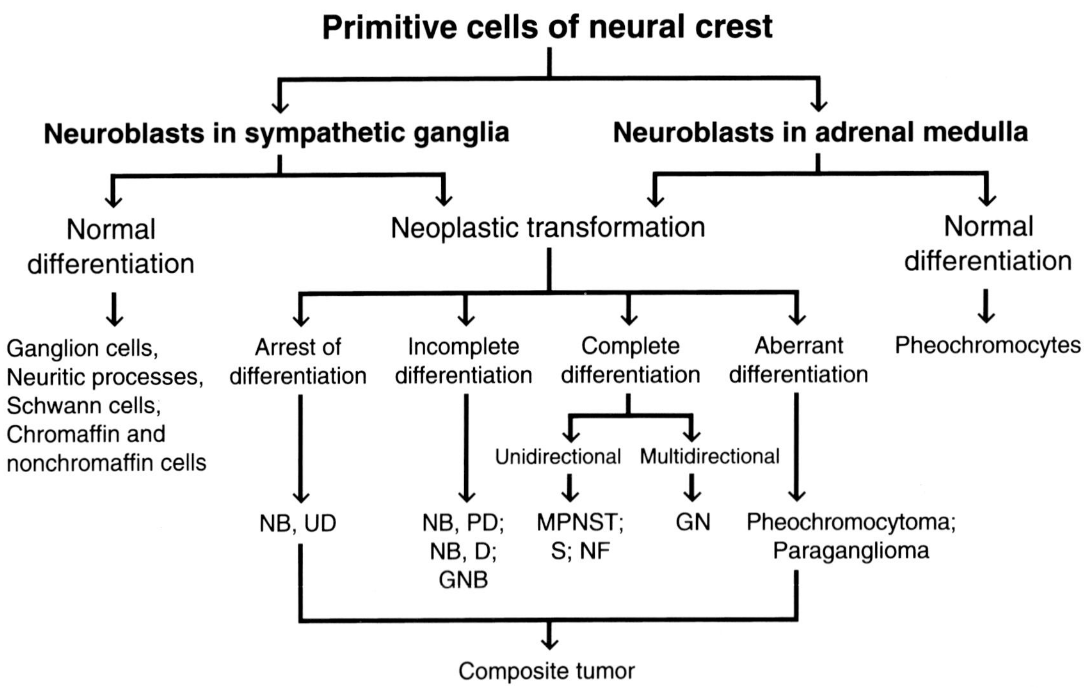

FIG. 4. The common embryogenesis of neuroblasts of the sympathetic ganglia and adrenal medulla from primitive cells of the neural crest. Neoplastic transformation and aberrant or divergent differentiation may result in a variety of tumors. NB, neuroblastoma; UD, undifferentiated; PD, poorly differentiated; D, differentiating; GNB, ganglioneuroblastoma; MPNST, malignant peripheral nerve sheath tumor; S, schwannoma; NF, neurofibroma; GN, ganglioneuroma. (Adapted from Joshi VV, Silverman JF, ref. 215; used with permission.)

rin (30) in 1963 described 13 cases of what they designated as neuroblastoma in situ. This was followed by a report of three similar cases by Shanklin and Sotello-Avila (382). All cases occurred in infants less than 3 months of age who died from other causes. The lesions varied from 0.7 to 9.5 mm in maximal dimension (Fig. 5) and histologically had the same features as a full-fledged neuroblastoma. Evidence of differentiation was present in only one case in which a small cluster of ganglion cells was found. There were no metastases to any organs in any of the cases. These findings were interpreted initially to indicate that neuroblastomas develop much more often than they are clinically detected. Beckwith and Perrin suggested that the majority of neuroblastomas in situ regress during early infancy and only rarely become full-fledged neuroblastomas.

Turkel and Itabashi (427) demonstrated microscopic clusters (nodules) of neuroblasts in the adrenal medulla of 92 fetuses of 17–20 weeks gestation. The neuroblasts in these "nodules" or clusters did not show any invasive features. They felt that the presence of neuroblastic "nodules" represents an essential event in the normal development of adrenal glands. However, the neuroblastic micronodules demonstrated by Turkel and Itabashi appear to be different from those of neuroblastoma in situ. The micronodules described by Beckwith and Perrin, measured in terms of millimeters (not micrometers), were unencapsulated, showed mitotic activity, and invaded the surrounding cortex and blood vessels (Fig. 6), whereas the neuroblastic "nodules" described by Turkel and Itabashi consisted merely of microscopic clusters of neuroblasts (Fig. 3) without any of the features of neuroblastoma in situ. Similar microscopic nodules (or clusters) of neuroblasts have been described by Ikeda et al. in the adrenal glands of fetuses from the seventh week of gestation (201). These authors found that larger mean nuclear diameter of neuroblasts was more characteristic of neuroblastoma in situ. Despite the controversial nature of neuroblastoma in situ, it remains an important concept. Knudsen and Meadows have suggested that in situ and stage 4S neuroblastomas may represent hyperplastic lesions lacking a "second hit" or "event" (29,232).

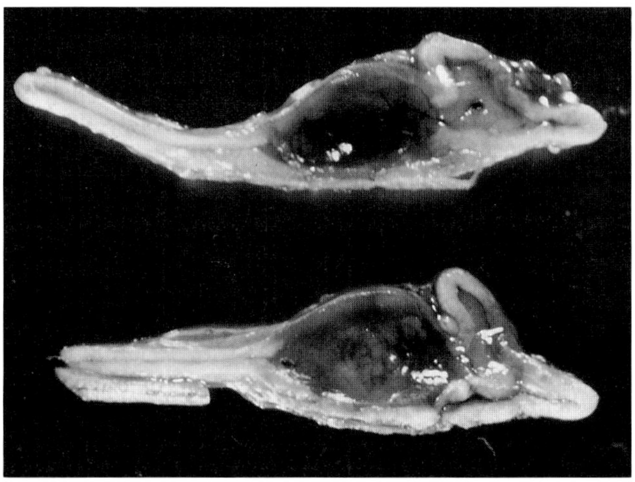

FIG. 5. Adrenal neuroblastoma in situ measuring 1.0 cm that was discovered in an infant who died with bronchopulmonary dysplasia.

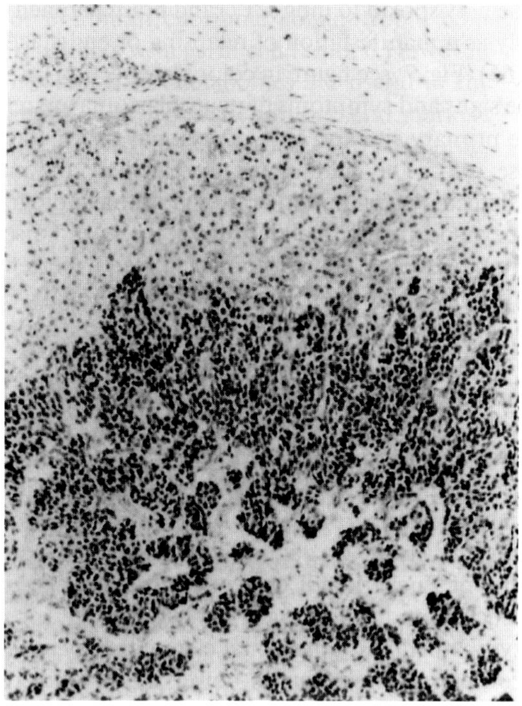

FIG. 6. Sheets of primitive cells invading adrenal cortex in neuroblastoma in situ.

CLINICAL FEATURES

The most common primary sites of neuroblastoma include adrenal gland (40%), abdominal sympathetic ganglia (25%), and sympathetic ganglia of the thorax (15%), neck (5%), and pelvis (5%). Infants have more thoracic and cervical primary tumors. Adrenal tumors are more common in children (40%) than in infants (25%). In about 1% of patients, a primary tumor cannot be found (65). Rare examples of multifocal primary neuroblastomas have been described (84,93,107,163,239). These tumors frequently occur in families and may present synchronously or metachronously. Unusual primary sites for neuroblastoma include orbit, kidney, lung, skin, ovary, spermatic cord, and urinary bladder (11,231,244). Metastatic extension of neuroblastoma occurs in two patterns: lymphatic and hematogenous. Regional lymph node metastases are noted in 35% of patients with apparently localized tumors. Spread of tumor to lymph nodes outside the cavity of origin is considered to be disseminated disease. Hematogenous spread occurs most frequently to bone marrow, bone, liver, and skin. Rarely,

TABLE 2. *Pediatric Oncology Group neuroblastoma staging system*

Stage	Features
A	Complete surgical excision of primary tumor, histologically negative or positive margins; nonadherent intracavitary lymph nodes histologically negative for tumor; liver negative for tumor in abdominal and pelvic primary tumor.
B	Incomplete surgical resection of primary tumor; lymph nodes and liver histologically negative for tumor as in stage A.
C	Complete or incomplete surgical resection of primary tumor; nonadherent intracavitary lymph nodes histologically positive for tumor; liver histologically negative for tumor.
D	Disseminated disease beyond intracavitary lymph nodes (i.e., bone marrow, bone, liver, skin, or lymph nodes beyond cavity containing primary tumor).
D-S[a]	Localized primary tumor with dissemination limited to liver, skin, and/or bone marrow (without evidence of bone metastasis).

(From Nitschke R et al., ref. 319; used with permission.)
[a] S, special.

lower for delayed or second-look procedures after tumor shrinkage by chemotherapy (35).

STAGING OF NEUROBLASTOMA

There are two staging systems used by the POG and CCG (130,183,319). A third staging system representing a combination of the two systems has been proposed by the International Conference on Neuroblastoma Staging and Response Criteria (62,64). These three staging systems are detailed in tables 2 through 4. It should be emphasized that the different stages in one system may not necessarily correspond to the respective stages in other systems. For example, stage A neuroblastoma according to the POG system will be considered as higher stages (II or III) according to the CCG system if the primary tumor shows involvement of adherent lymph nodes or extends beyond the midline. The revised International Staging System for Neuroblastoma (ISSN) is universally accepted and helps resolve the problems associated with the two earlier staging systems as well as furnish a unified basis for therapeutic and biologic studies.

TABLE 3. *Evans staging system for neuroblastoma used by Children's Cancer Group*

Stage	Features
I	Tumor confined to the primary site of origin
II	Tumor extending in continuity beyond the primary site of origin without crossing the midline. Regional lymph nodes on ipsilateral side may be involved.
III	Tumor extending in continuity beyond the primary site of origin and beyond the midline. Bilateral regional lymph node involvement may be present.
IV	Disease involving bone, viscera, soft tissues, distant lymph nodes, or bone marrow.
IV-S[a]	Disease involving one or more of the following sites: liver, skin, or marrow (without involvement of bone) in patients in whom the primary tumor would otherwise be considered as stage I or II.

(From Evans AE, et al., ref. 130, used with permission.)
[a] S, special.

TABLE 4. *Revised International staging system for neuroblastoma*

Stage	Features
1	Localized tumor with complete gross excision, with or without microscopic residual disease; representative ipsilateral lymph nodes are negative for tumor microscopically (lymph nodes adherent to and resected with the primary tumor may be positive).
2A	Localized tumor with incomplete gross excision; representative ipsilateral nonadherent lymph nodes are negative for tumor microscopically.
2B	Localized tumor with or without complete gross excision; ipsilateral nonadherent lymph nodes are positive for tumor; enlarged contralateral lymph nodes are negative for tumor on microscopic examination.
3	Unresectable tumor infiltrating across the midline defined as the vertebral column (i.e., tumors arising on one side must infiltrate to or beyond the opposite side of the vertebral column) with or without regional lymph node involvement; *or* midline tumor with bilateral extension by infiltration (unresectable) or by lymph node involvement.
4	Any primary tumor with dissemination to distant lymph nodes; bone, bone marrow, liver, skin, and/or other organs (except as defined in stage 4S).
4S	Localized primary tumor (as defined in stage 1, 2A, and 2B) with dissemination limited to skin, liver, and/or bone marrow (<10% of the total nucleated cells identified as malignant on bone marrow aspiration smear or biopsy); more extensive bone marrow involvement is considered as stage 4) (limited to infants <1 year of age).

(From Brodeur G et al., ref. 64; used with permission.)
Note: Multifocal primary tumors such as bilateral adrenal neuroblastomas should be staged according to the greatest extent of the disease; the stage is indicated by subscript "M."

PATHOLOGY OF NEUROBLASTIC TUMORS

Gross Features

Neuroblastoma typically presents as a circumscribed solid mass, especially when confined to the adrenal or located in the posterior mediastinum. Extra-adrenal, pelvic, retroperitoneal, or thoracoabdominal tumors may

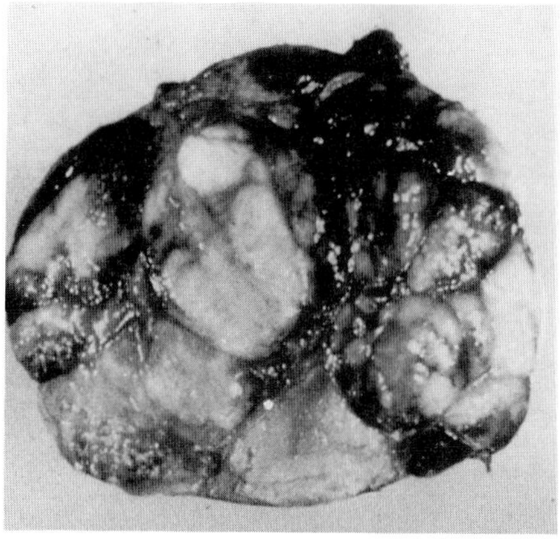

FIG. 9. Multinodular neuroblastoma from the abdomen.

be composed of several contiguous masses or consist of an ill-defined infiltrative mass within a dense bed of fibrous tissue (112). Most neuroblastomas measure from 1 to 10 cm. The compressed fibrous pseudocapsule of circumscribed tumors may have suspicious areas that represent penetration by tumor. Lymph nodes that may be adherent to the pseudocapsule should not be separated from it but included in the subsequent histologic sections of the adjacent pseudocapsule and tumor. On cut surface, neuroblastoma may consist of a multinodular tumor with variegated coloration, ranging from deep red to yellow–tan or glistening gray–tan (112) (Fig. 9). There may be diffuse hemorrhage. In rare cases, the tumor may be multicystic due to preoperative hemorrhage (19) (Fig. 10). Foci of necrosis and/or calcification may be grossly detectable. Typically, the calcification consists of dispersed fine punctate yellow granules or flecks. A variable rim of compressed adrenal tissue may be identified in some tumors that arise in the adrenal (112) (Fig. 11).

The gross appearance of ganglioneuroblastoma and ganglioneuroma is different from that of neuroblastoma. These tumors tend to have a firmer consistency and a tan–white color (Fig. 12). Ganglioneuroma and ganglioneuroblastoma of the intermixed and borderline subtypes also tend to be larger. In the nodular subtype of ganglioneuroblastoma, one or more grossly visible, usually encapsulated, neuroblastic nodules are present. These nodules have a softer consistency and gray–tan to red color (Fig. 13). Hemorrhage may be present in the nodule(s).

Basic Pathologic Components of Neuroblastic Tumors

Neuroblastoma is a tumor composed of neuroblasts and their derivatives, i.e., ganglion cells and Schwann cells that show progressive degrees of maturation and organization. There are three basic pathologic components: (a) neuroblastomatous, (b) intermediate, and (c) ganglioneuromatous.

The neuroblastomatous component is characterized by the presence of neuroblasts, i.e., undifferentiated small round cells with large nuclei containing a speckled or "salt-and-pepper" chromatin pattern (Fig. 14). Nucleoli, a thin rim of discernible cytoplasm, prominent mitotic activity, and foci of pleomorphism, are often present. The neuroblasts may be surrounded by "naked" neuropil (neuritic processes unaccompanied by Schwann cells) that appears as faintly eosinophilic fibrillary material in routinely stained sections (Fig. 15). The neuropil may be absent, minimal, or abundant. The neuroblasts are characteristically arranged in nests surrounded by variably developed fibrovascular septa (Fig. 16). Some neuroblastomas display Homer Wright rosettes characterized by a central tangle of neuropil surrounded by one or more layers of neuroblasts (Fig. 17; see figure in color plate section). These rosettes are

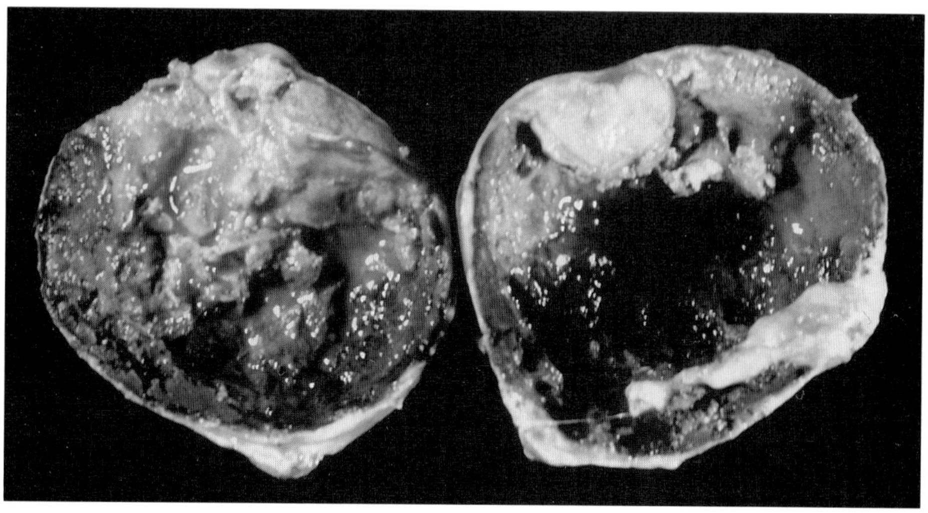

FIG. 10. Cystic adrenal neuroblastoma with a central hemorrhagic cavity.

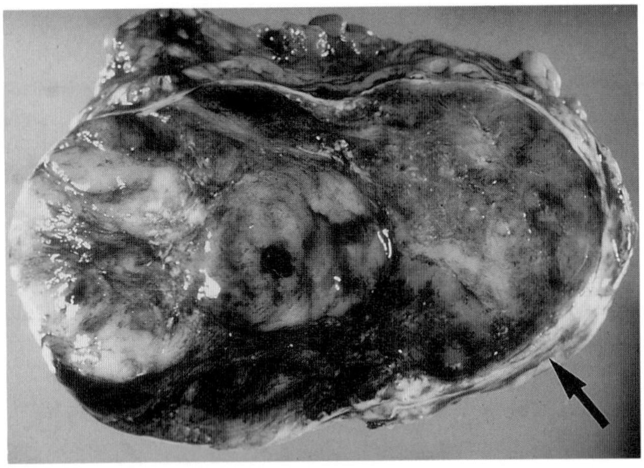

FIG. 11. A thin rim of adrenal cortical tissue *(arrow)* remains in this neuroblastoma.

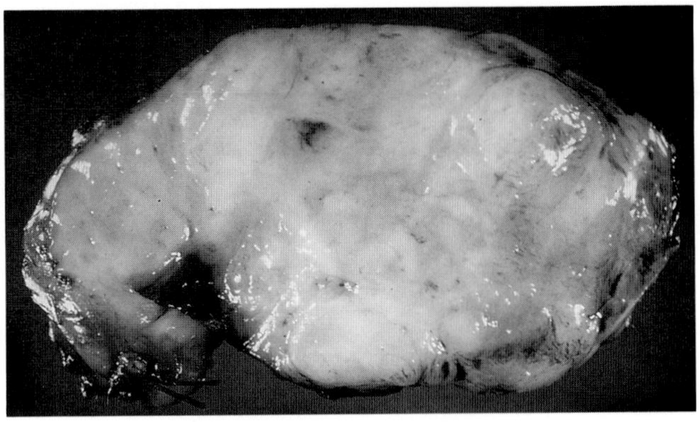

FIG. 12. Mediastinal ganglioneuroblastoma from a 2-year-old boy.

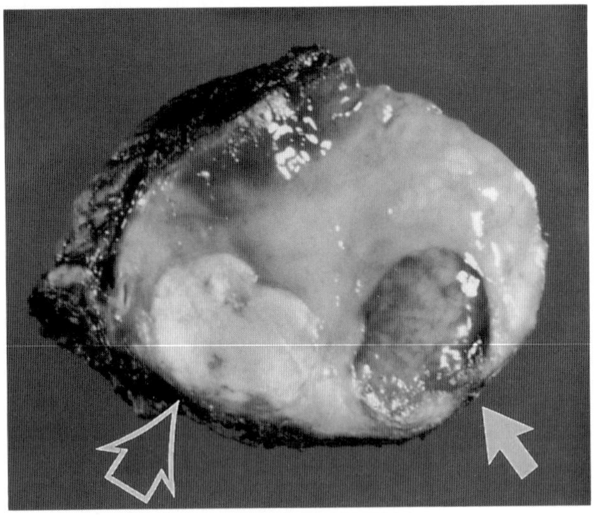

FIG. 13. Nodular ganglioneuroblastoma from the retroperitoneum in a 2-year-old boy. The neuroblastic nodule is well circumscribed *(arrow)*. A large area of coagulative necrosis *(open arrow)* is also present.

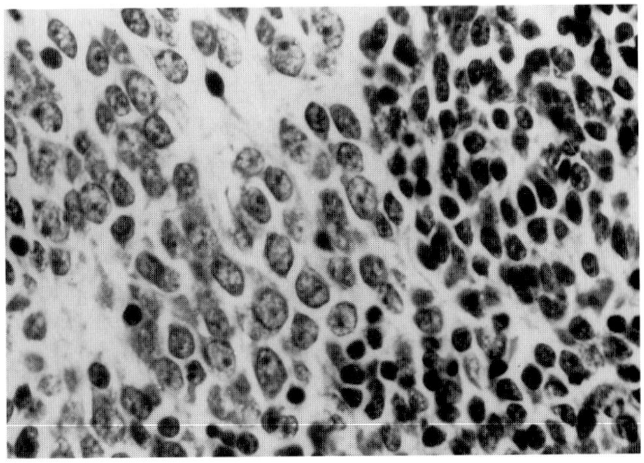

FIG. 14. Adrenal neuroblastoma showing an admixture of small hyperchromatic undifferentiated neuroblasts and larger differentiating neuroblasts. (Used with permission, ref. 211.)

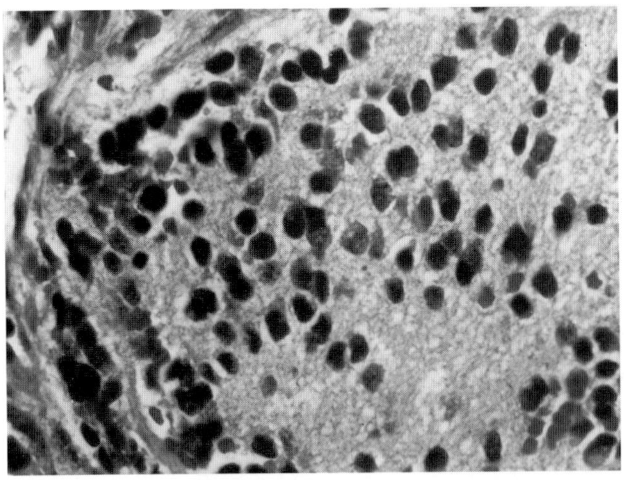

FIG. 15. Neuroblasts surrounded by "naked" neuropil in a retroperitoneal tumor.

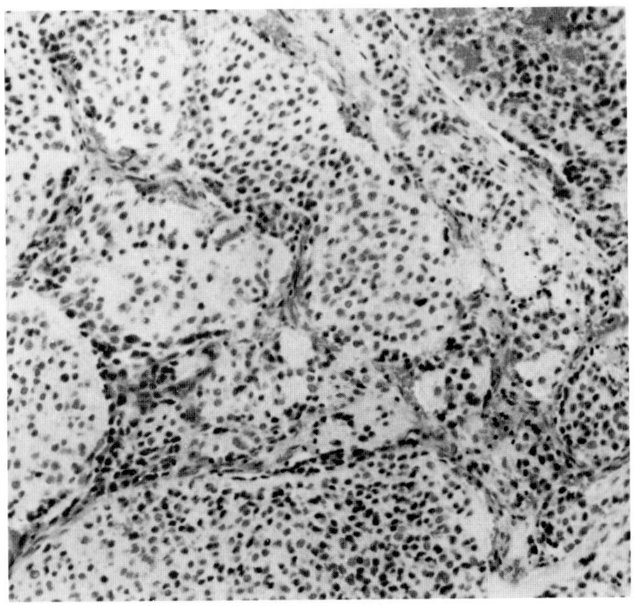

FIG. 16. Differentiating neuroblastoma with characteristic nesting pattern, abundant neuropil, and well-developed fibrovascular septa. (Used with permission, ref. 214.)

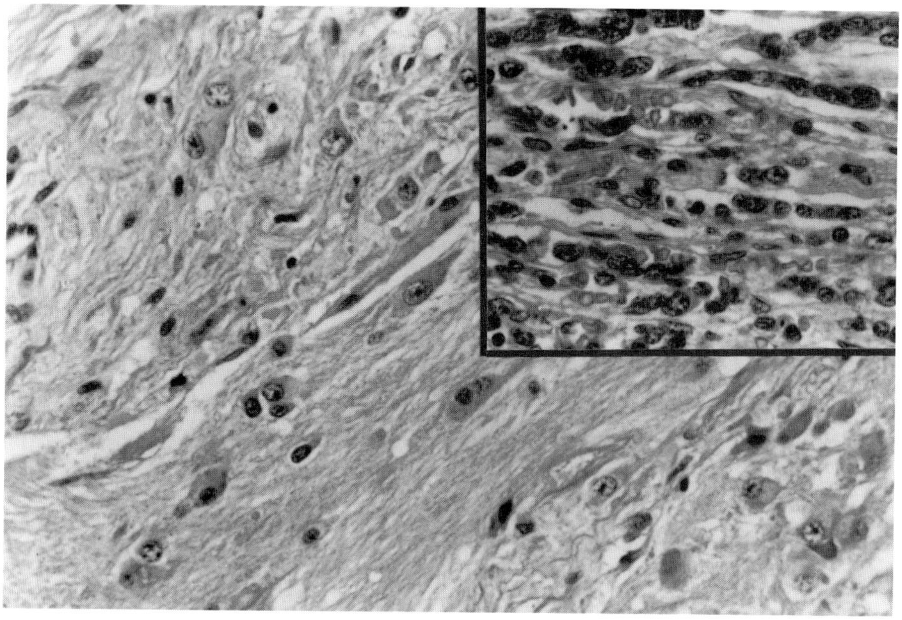

FIG. 19. Parallel ("streaming") arrangement of neuropil in the intermediate component. *Inset:* Single file rows of neuroblasts surrounded by compact neurofibrillary stroma. (Used with permission, ref. 215.)

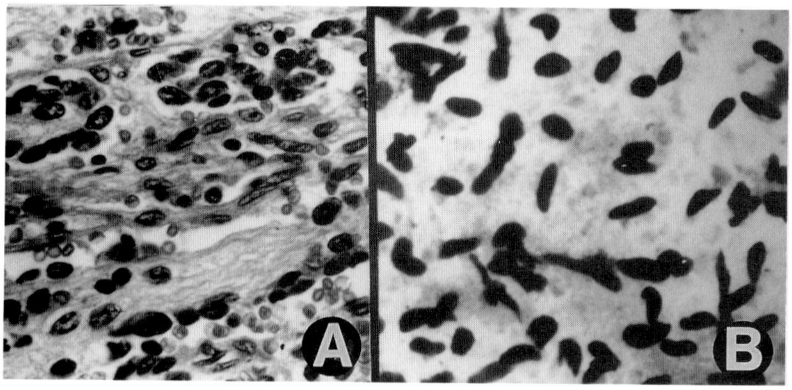

FIG. 20. A. Cells intermediate between neuroblasts and Schwann cells have oblong nuclei and are arranged along the parallel neuropil in a neuroblastoma. **B.** Intermediate cells in the fine needle aspiration specimen. (Used with permission, ref. 214.)

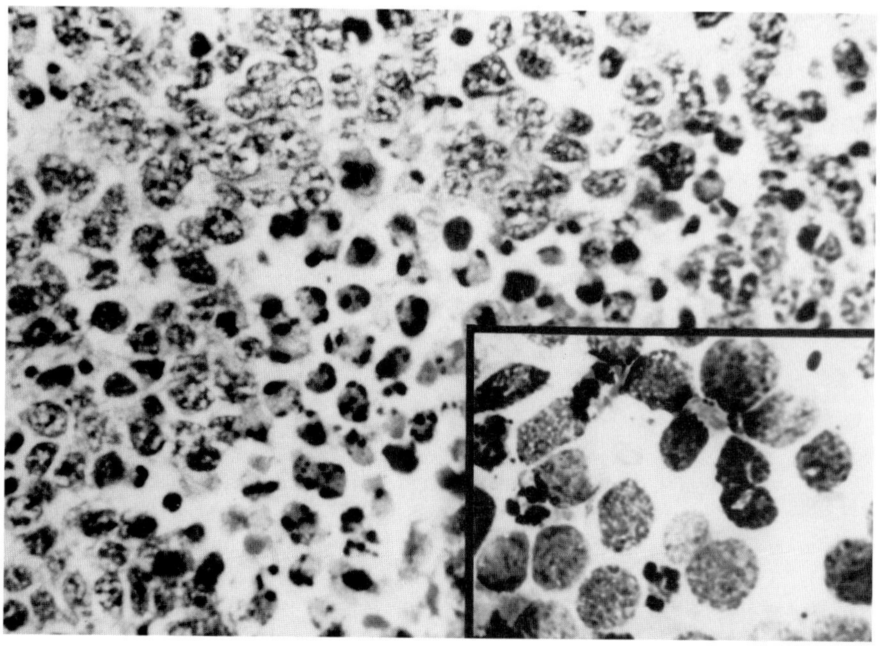

FIG. 21. Karyorrhectic cells of various types with punctate, neutrophillike, lymphocytelike, crescentic, and complex nuclear features. *Inset:* Fine needle aspiration cytologic features of karyorrhectic cells. (Used with permission, ref. 214.)

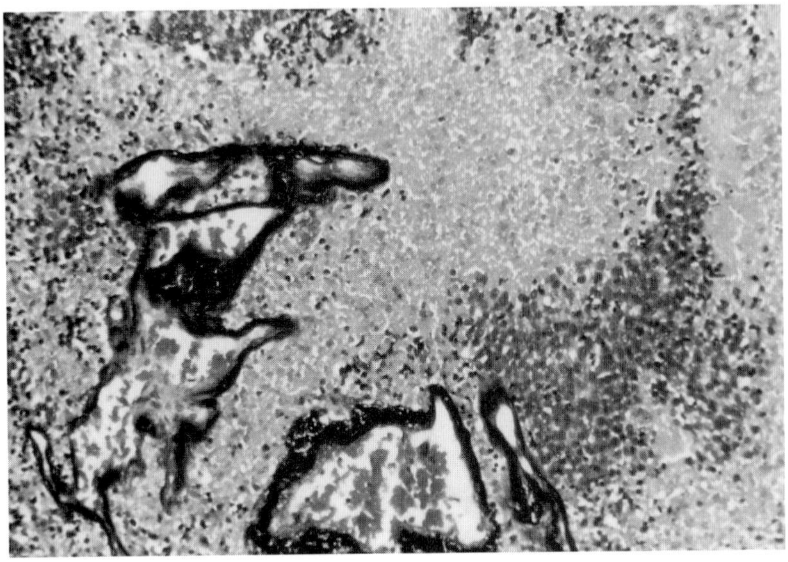

FIG. 22. Neuroblastoma showing an area of coagulative necrosis and a dense angiocentric deposit of basophilic material (the Azzopardi phenomenon).

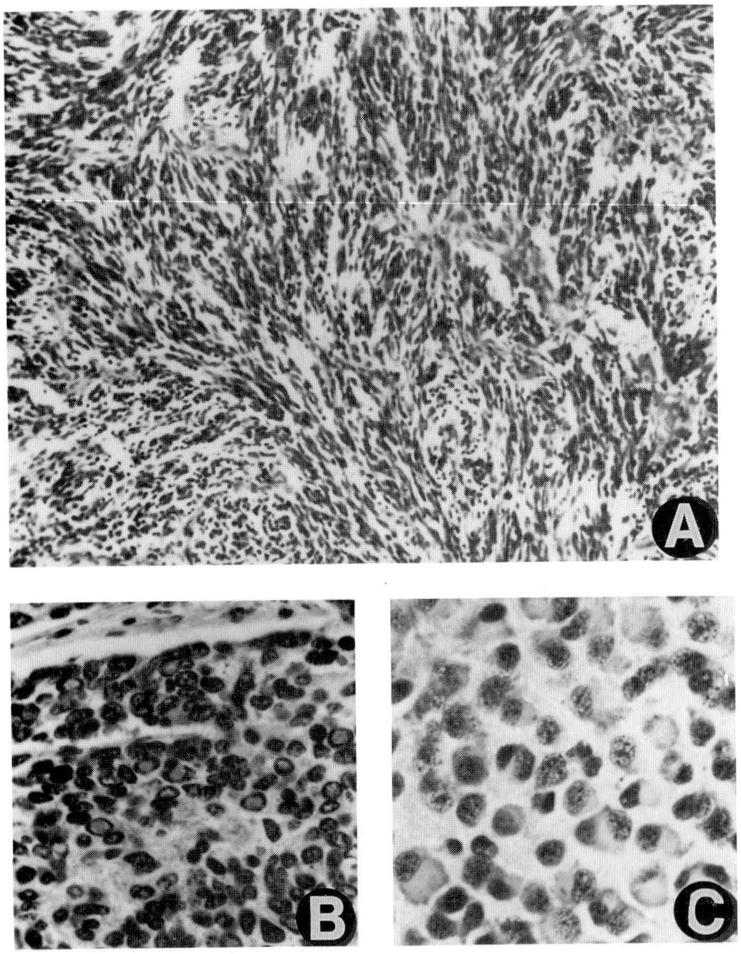

FIG. 23. Neuroblastomas with **(A)** spindle-shaped neuroblasts, **(B)** intranuclear cytoplasmic invaginations, and **(C)** pseudorhabdoid change. (Used with permission, ref. 214.)

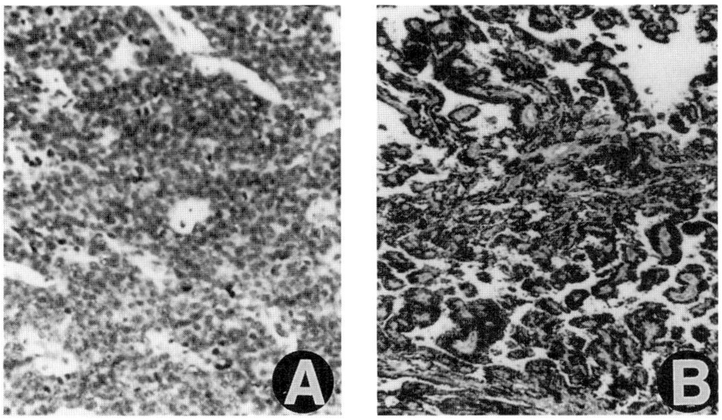

FIG. 24. "Starry sky" pattern **(A)** in undifferentiated neuroblastoma. A papillarylike pattern **(B)** results from degeneration, necrosis, and cell dropout from the central portions of the tumor cell nests. The residual mantle of tumor cells lining the fibrovascular septa resembles papillae. (Used with permission, ref. 214.)

characteristic but neither essential nor diagnostic for neuroblastoma.

The ganglioneuromatous component is characterized by an organized pattern of fascicles of neuritic processes accompanied by mature Schwann cells, mature ganglion cells, and fibrous tissue (Fig. 18; see figure in color plate section). The mere presence of ganglion cells in an area of a neuroblastic tumor does not constitute a ganglioneuromatous component. Schwann cells accompanied by neuritic processes arranged in an organized pattern must be present. The intermediate component shows various combinations of neuroblasts, maturing or atypical ganglion cells, parallel arrangement of neuropil, and fusiform or oblong cells that probably represent maturing Schwann cells (Figs. 19 and 20). Thus, the features are intermediate between the neuroblastomatous and ganglioneuromatous components. Gangliocytic differentiation of neuroblasts is characterized by cytoplasmic and nuclear enlargement, distinct cell borders, increased cytoplasmic eosinophilia, eccentrically located nuclei, peripherally condensed chromatin, a distinct nucleolus, and presence of Nissl substance in a granular or stippled rim at the periphery of the cytoplasm (244).

The neuroblastomatous component is present predominantly (more than 50%) or exclusively in neuroblastomas and focally in ganglioneuroblastomas. The ganglioneuromatous component is present predominantly in ganglioneuroblastomas, exclusively in ganglioneuromas, and may be present focally in neuroblastomas. The intermediate component may be seen in neuroblastomas and ganglioneuroblastomas but is not present in ganglioneuromas.

The basic morphology may be complicated by such secondary features (112,244) as karyorrhexis, necrosis, incrustation of blood vessel walls with DNA from necrotic tumor cells [the Azzopardi phenomenon (21)], hemorrhage, stippled or plaquelike dystrophic calcification, dense fibrosis, and lymphocytic infiltration (Figs. 21 and 22).

Joshi et al. (214) reported a number of previously undescribed features of neuroblastoma in 51 of 239 cases of neuroblastic tumors (Figs. 23–25). Some of the unusual features, such as rhabdoid or pseudorhabdoid change (330,441), large cells with eosinophilic cytoplasm, or pseudoalveolar, starry-sky, or papillarylike patterns, may be misleading if present in a small incisional or fine needle aspiration biopsy specimen. Some of the other unusual features may be related to the biology and natural history of neuroblastic tumors. Thus, the vascular proliferation seen in the septa may be related to elaboration of a tumor-derived angiogenesis factor (142). If hyalinization of the septa, a sclerosing pattern, and foci of dense lymphoplasmacytic infiltrates occur diffusely, they may be related to the phenomenon of spontaneous regression—an event that is not uncommon in the natural history of certain types of neuroblastoma (131).

There are several features of neuroblastic tumors that have not been sufficiently emphasized in the literature. Neuroblasts are usually "small" round cells measuring about 10 μM diameter. However, in 46% of the cases described by Joshi and colleagues (214), larger neuroblasts measuring up to 20 μM diameter were seen focally or diffusely. Large and small cells can also be recognized

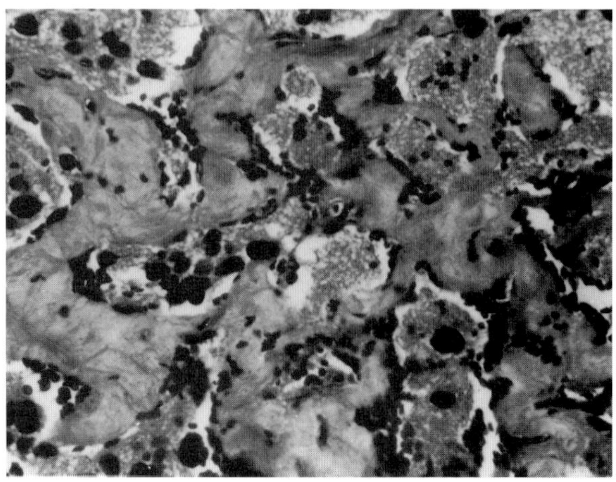

FIG. 25. Sclerosing pattern in neuroblastoma resulting from prominent collagenous fibrous stroma that obscures the typical nesting pattern. (Used with permission, ref. 214.)

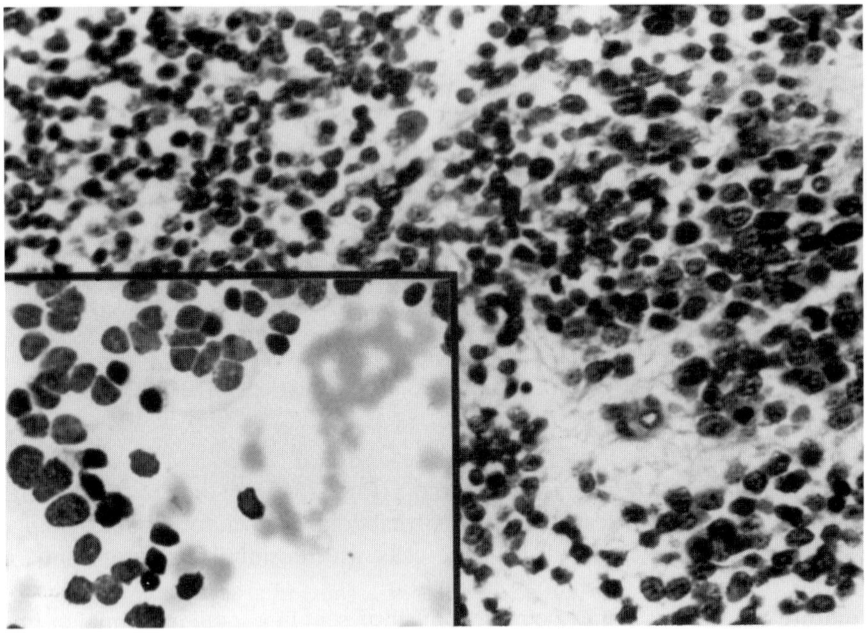

FIG. 26. Large and small neuroblasts from an undifferentiated adrenal neuroblastoma. *Inset:* Fine needle aspiration cytology specimen showing large and small neuroblasts. (Used with permission, ref. 214.)

in the fine needle aspiration biopsy (Fig. 26). A nesting pattern was seen in virtually all neuroblastomas in the series of Joshi et al. (215). In two cases, the nests were completely surrounded by fibrovascular septa, resulting in what is described as an organoid or paragangliomalike pattern (174). Fibrovascular septa can also be recognized in the fine needle aspiration biopsy. A nesting pattern is also frequently present in metastases. Various types of giant cells with single or multiple nuclei, with or without hyperchromasia, and regular or bizarre shapes are present in a high proportion of cases (Fig. 27). These tumor

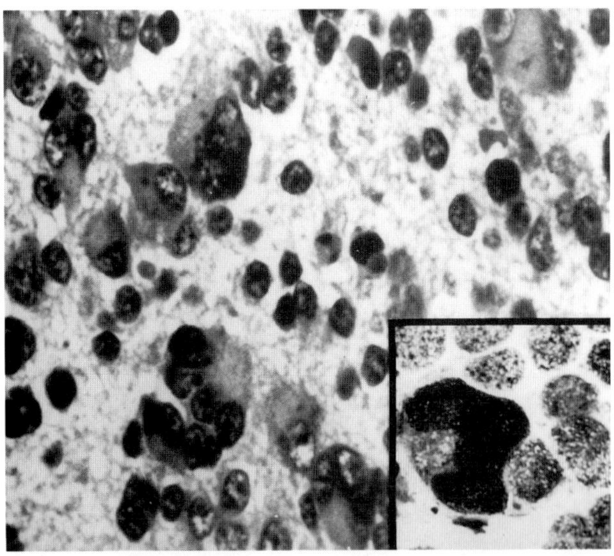

FIG. 27. Tumor giant cells in neuroblastoma. Some resemble ganglion cells; others have single or multiple enlarged nuclei, with or without hyperchromasia, and regular or bizarre shapes. *Inset:* Tumor giant cells in an fine needle aspiration specimen. (Used with permission, ref. 214.)

giant cells may resemble ganglion cells and in combination with nesting pattern may provide clues to the correct diagnosis in a small biopsy specimen, particularly in metastases. Nevertheless, a focal nesting pattern may be present in other small round cell tumors (primitive neuroectodermal tumor, Ewing's sarcoma, blastemal Wilms' tumor, etc.), so that it is a helpful but not necessarily diagnostic feature. Anaplasia as defined for Wilms' tumor (460) was seen in 19 cases. Only rarely are extreme degrees of nuclear pleomorphism and hyperchromasia present (100) (Fig. 28; see figure in color plate section). In contrast to Wilms' tumor, neuroblastomas showing anaplasia thus far have not been associated with statistically significant aggressive behavior (85).

CLASSIFICATION: NOMENCLATURE AND CRITERIA OF NEUROBLASTIC TUMORS

In the past 50 years most attempts at classification of neuroblastic tumors have been linked to histologic grading systems. Dehner (112) has reviewed the important contributions in this regard made by Stout (401), Poore et al. (343), Horn et al. (195), Beckwith and Martin (31), Mäkinen (271), Gitlow et al. (157), Hughes et al. (198), Meister et al. (282), and Sandstedt et al. (363). A review of these and other reports by various authors (3,48,167, 178,267,361,422,448) shows the following: (a) There is a lack of uniformity of terms and criteria for the various types of neuroblastic tumors, with a plethora of confusing and overlapping terms (Table 5). (b) In the descriptions of features of typical ganglioneuroblastoma, many authors neglect to mention the presence of neuritic processes and accompanying Schwann cells as an essential predominant component. (c) There are overlapping criteria for ganglioneuroblastoma and differentiating neuroblastoma. (d) Although the term "ganglioneuroma" is defined clearly by all authors, use of terms such as "immature ganglioneuroma" and "fully differentiated ganglioneuroma" creates confusion, leading to a tendency to diagnose some ganglioneuroblastomas as ganglioneuromas.

In 1984, Shimada et al. (386) introduced a new terminology and classification of neuroblastic tumors (see below). The amount of stroma, defined as Schwannian rather than other supportive elements, is the basis for classification of neuroblastic tumors into two broad groups: stroma-rich and stroma-poor. However, it appears that there has been reluctance on the part of pathologists to replace the widely used, deeply rooted, and time-honored conventional terms "neuroblastoma," "ganglioneuroblastoma," and "ganglioneuroma" with the Shimada terminology. Utilizing the conventional terminology in a review of over 200 cases of neuroblastic tumors, Joshi et al. (211) recommended the following pathologic criteria for various types of neuroblastic tumors (Table 6).

Neuroblastoma

There are three subtypes of neuroblastoma:

1. *Undifferentiated neuroblastoma.* Virtually all the tumor cells are undifferentiated neuroblasts. The neuropil is virtually absent to minimal (Fig. 29; see figure in color plate section). Immunoperoxidase stain for neuron-specific enolase (NSE) (425), electron microscopy for demonstration of characteristic neurosecretory granules and neuritic processes (422), and/or data on urinary catecholamines may be essential for a definitive diagnosis.
2. *Poorly differentiated neuroblastoma.* Less than 5% of the tumor cells show a tendency to gangliocytic differentiation. A variable amount of neuropil is clearly recognizable on routine stains. Rosettes may be present.
3. *Differentiating neuroblastoma.* In these tumors at least 5% of the neuroblasts show a tendency to differentiation (210) (Fig. 30; see figure in color plate section). The criteria for recognition of this tendency, described by Beckwith and Martin (31) and subsequently used by various authors (267,386), are as follows: nuclear enlargement, presence of a nucleolus, cytoplasmic eosinophilia and enlargement, development of a distinct cell border, and presence of cell processes.

Thus atypical, immature, and mature ganglion cells may be present along with undifferentiated neuroblasts and cells intermediate between the two (Fig. 19). Differentiating neuroblasts may be present focally or diffusely. Rare, occasional, or numerous ganglion cells may be present in a differentiating neuroblastoma, and a rare ganglion cell may be present in poorly differentiated neuroblastoma. Their presence is neither supportive nor contrary to the diagnosis of these two subtypes. Nests of undifferentiated neuroblasts may be present in variable amounts in poorly differentiated and differentiating neuroblastomas. Tumor giant cells resembling ganglion cells or with single large or multiple nuclei may also be seen in neuroblastomas (Fig. 27). Multipolar mitotic figures are observed in a few cases.

Ganglioneuroma

Ganglioneuroma is a tumor composed of mature elements that include ganglion cells, Schwann cells, and fi-

TABLE 5. *Conventional terminology for types and subtypes of neuroblastic tumors*

Type of neuroblastic tumor	Terms for subtypes	Reference
Neuroblastoma	Undifferentiated	31, 111, 178, 267, 361, 422, 448
	Predominantly undifferentiated	31
	Slightly differentiated	31
	Poorly differentiated	48
	Partially differentiated	48
	Differentiating	111, 267
	Predominantly differentiated	31
	Well differentiated	422
Ganglioneuroblastoma	Diffuse	3
	Imperfect	3, 361
	Complex	267
	Composite	48, 267, 361
	Immature	361
	Differentiated neuroblastoma	178
	Maturing neuroblastoma	167
Ganglioneuroma	Immature	178
	Fully differentiated	401

(Adapted from Joshi VV et al., ref. 21; used with permission.)

TABLE 6. *Recommended terminology and criteria for neuroblastic tumors*

Tumor type	Criteria	Comment
Neuroblastoma (NB), undifferentiated, poorly differentiated, or differentiating[a]	Neuroblasts and neuropil constitute the predominant (>50%) or exclusive component of the tumor. A small minority of NB contain small ganglioneuromatous focus or foci at the periphery or within the septa	The three subtypes are recognized on the basis of the proportion of differentiating neuroblasts (0, ≤5 and >5%, respectively)
Ganglioneuroma (GN)	The tumor is composed of mature ganglion cells, neurites accompanied by Schwann cells, and fibrous tissue	Mitotic figures should not be present
Ganglioneuroblastoma (GNB), nodular, intermixed, or borderline[a]	The tumor is composed of a predominant (>50%) ganglioneuromatous (Schwannian) component and a small neuroblastomatous component	The three subtypes are recognized on the basis of type of neuroblastomatous component. In almost all GNB, the GN component is far in excess of 50%. Nodular GNB has single or a few grossly demonstrable neuroblastomatous nodules; intermixed GNB has a few well-defined microscopic neuroblastomatous foci and borderline GNB has a few poorly defined neuroblastomatous foci
Neuroblastoma, not otherwise specified (NOS)	Clusters of neuroblastic cells or foci of NB are seen	This diagnosis should be made when the features are seen in a bone marrow aspirate, bone marrow biopsy, FNA, or incisional biopsy of primary or metastatic tumor or in a histologically inadequately sampled primary tumor resected before or after other modes of therapy. (There is a remote possibility that the FNA or incisional biopsy may sample only the neuroblastomatous nodule of nodular GNB.)
Mixed neuroblastic tumor, NOS	The tumor is composed of neuroblastomatous and ganglioneuromatous elements in unknown proportions	The diagnosis should be made when the features mentioned are seen in an incisional or FNA biopsy of primary or metastatic tumor or in a histologically inadequately sampled primary tumor resected before or after other modes of therapy

Abbreviation: FNA, fine-needle aspiration.
(Adapted from Joshi VV et al., ref. 214; used with permission.)
[a] The subtyping of NB and GNB should be done only on histologically adequately sampled primary tumors resected before other modes of therapy. Adequate histologic sampling is defined as one section for each centimeter of the longest dimension of the resected primary tumor.

brous tissue (Fig. 18; see figure in color plate section). Conceptually, immature elements such as neuroblasts, intermediate cells, and immature (atypical) ganglion cells are not part of ganglioneuroma. However, minor degrees of atypia are of no clinical or prognostic significance (386). Mitotic figures should not be seen in ganglioneuroma.

Ganglioneuroblastoma

Ganglioneuroblastoma consists of a ganglioneuromatous component which is predominant (greater than 50% of the tumor mass) and a minor neuroblastomatous component, the latter showing variable differentiation and distribution. In conventional terminology ganglioneuroblastoma is defined as a tumor containing greater than 5% mono- or multinucleated ganglion cells with or without cellular atypia (111). According to the recommended criteria as outlined above, a neuroblastic tumor containing ganglion cells without the predominant Schwann cell component accompanying the mature neurites is not considered ganglioneuroblastoma but differentiating neuroblastoma. Ganglioneuroblastoma is divided into the following three subtypes: nodular, intermixed, and borderline.

1. *Ganglioneuroblastoma, nodular.* The term "nodular" refers to the distribution of the neuroblastomatous component that is present in the form of one or a few discrete grossly demonstrable nodules of neuroblastoma embedded in a predominantly ganglioneu-

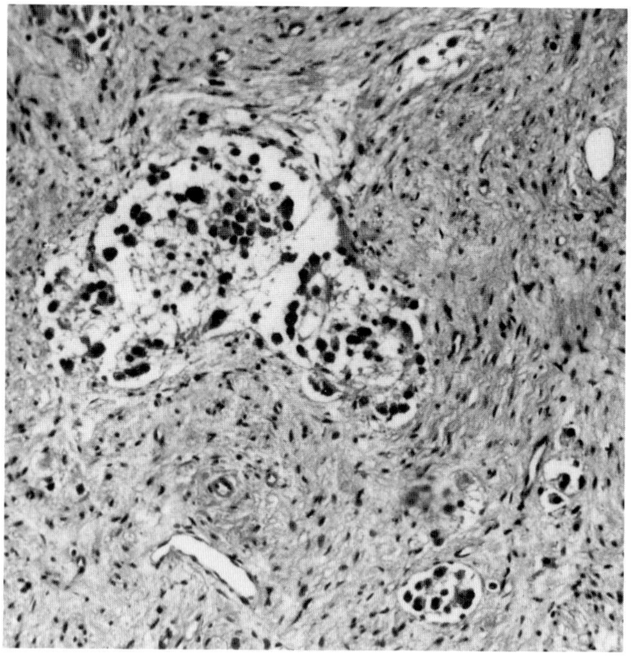

FIG. 31. Microscopic foci of neuroblastoma surrounded by fibrous Schwannian stroma in intermixed ganglioneuroblastoma. (Used with permission, ref. 215.)

romatous stroma (Fig. 13). The nodules may be encapsulated. There may be a few variably differentiated neuroblasts arranged in microscopic clusters or nests in the ganglioneuromatous component. In most cases, the neuroblastomatous nodule or nodules are much smaller than 50% of the area of the tumor. Rarely, the neuroblastomatous nodule may undergo marked expansion with the ganglioneuromatous component remaining as a thin rim at the periphery.

2. *Ganglioneuroblastoma, intermixed.* In this subtype the neuroblastomatous component is present in the form of variably sized, fairly well-defined but unencapsulated nests of neuroblasts and neuropil intermixed with the predominant ganglioneuromatous component (Fig. 31). These nests of neuroblasts can be recognized only on microscopic examination. A variable degree of differentiation with or without the presence of ganglion cells is exhibited by these neuroblasts.
3. *Ganglioneuroblastoma, borderline.* In this subtype the neuroblastomatous component is present in the form of a few scattered, evenly or unevenly distributed moderately differentiated neuroblasts and neuropil. In some cases only occasional neuroblastomatous foci may be present. Ganglion cells may be present in the neuroblastomatous component of both intermixed and borderline ganglioneuroblastoma. They tend to be more numerous in the latter.

"Neuroblastoma, not otherwise specified" is the designation used when clusters of neuroblasts are seen in smears of bone marrow aspirate or fine needle aspiration biopsy of a neuroblastic tumor or when only neuroblastomatous tumor is seen in a biopsy of bone marrow or incisional biopsy of primary or metastatic neuroblastic tumor. "Mixed neuroblastic tumor, not otherwise specified" is the designation for a neuroblastic tumor composed of neuroblastomatous and ganglioneuromatous elements in unknown proportions. This diagnosis is made when the features mentioned above are seen in an incisional or fine needle aspiration biopsy of primary or metastatic tumor or in a histologically inadequately sampled primary tumor. Although theoretically there may be transitional neuroblastic tumors that contain approximately equal proportions of neuroblastoma and ganglioneuroma, such tumors are rarely encountered in clinical practice (223). In some instances, a neuroblastic tumor with an adequate number of histologic slides may be unclassifiable according to the foregoing criteria for one or more of the following reasons: extensive necrosis,

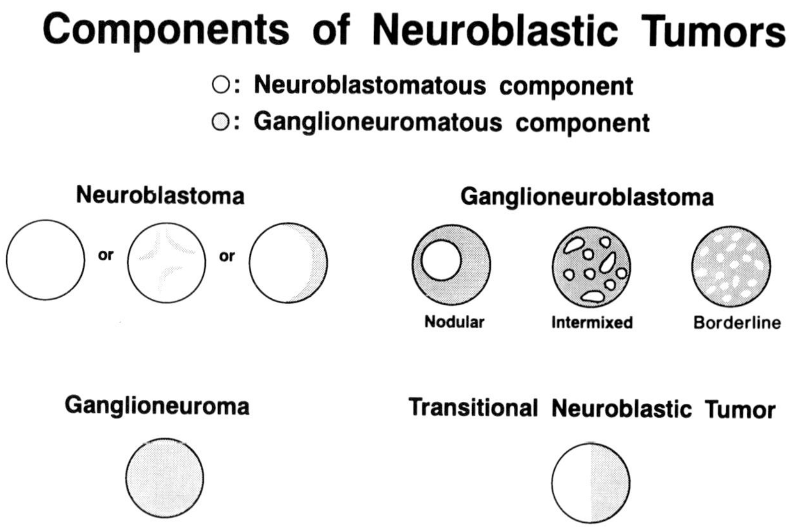

FIG. 32. Diagramatic representation of terminology in neuroblastic tumors. (Used with permission, ref. 212.)

TABLE 7. *Progressive differentiation, maturation, and organization in neuroblastic tumors*

Tumor type	Differentiation	Maturation	Organization	Behavior
Neuroblastoma, undifferentiated	None	None	Nesting pattern	Highly malignant
Neuroblastoma, poorly differentiated	<5% neuroblasts showing tendency to gangliocytic differentiation	Minimal	Nesting pattern, rosettes	Malignant
Neuroblastoma, differentiating	≥5% neuroblasts showing tendency to gangliocytic differentiation	Ganglion cells, cells intermediate between neuroblasts and Schwann cells may be present	Nesting pattern, foci of parallel arrangement of neuropil with alignment of immature Schwann cells, rosettes	Malignant
Ganglioneuroblastoma, nodular	Neuroblastoma area: variable, generally slight GN area (>50%): ganglion cells and Schwann cells	Neuroblastoma area: variable, generally slight GN area: complete (ganglion cells, Schwann cells)	Neuroblastoma area: nesting pattern GN area: neuritic processes accompanied by Schwann cells arranged in fascicles	Malignant
Ganglioneuroblastoma, intermixed	Neuroblastoma area: moderate GN area: same as in nodular GNB	Neuroblastoma area: moderate (ganglion cells may be present) GN area: same as in nodular GNB	Neuroblastoma area: nesting pattern may be present in relatively larger foci GN area: same as in nodular GNB but microscopically intermingled with neuroblastic foci	Borderline
Ganglioneuroblastoma, borderline	Neuroblastoma: moderate to good GN area: same as in nodular GNB	Neuroblastoma area: moderate to good (ganglion cells may be present) GN area: same as in nodular GNB	Neuroblastoma area: foci generally too small to show nesting pattern within themselves GN area: same as in nodular GNB but microscopically intermingled with neuroblastic foci	Borderline
Ganglioneuroma	Ganglion cells and Schwann cells	Complete	Same as in GN area of nodular GNB	Benign

(From Joshi VV et al., ref. 214; used with permission.)
Abbreviations: GN, ganglioneuroma; GNB, ganglioneuroblastoma.

TABLE 8. *Shimada Classification System*

Type of neuroblastic tumor	Favorable histology	Unfavorable histology
Neuroblastoma, stroma-rich (SR): age <5 years	Neuroblastoma, SR, well-differentiated subtype; intermixed subtype	Neuroblastoma, SR, nodular subtype (all ages)
Neuroblastoma, stroma-poor (SP): age ≤1.5 years	MKI <200	MKI >200
Neuroblastoma, SP: age 1.5–5 years	MKI <100 and differentiating	MKI >100 or undifferentiated
Neuroblastoma, SP: age >5 years	None	All

Abbreviation: MKI, mitosis-karyorrhexis index; SR, stroma-rich; SP, stroma-poor.

hemorrhage, calcification, crush artefact, severe cystic changes, or poor fixation and processing. Small sample size with or without the aforementioned changes also precludes definitive classification.

The major types of neuroblastic tumors are represented diagrammatically in Fig. 32. On the basis of progressive differentiation, maturation, and organization, neuroblastic tumors can be arranged in the following order: undifferentiated neuroblastoma, poorly differentiated neuroblastoma, differentiating neuroblastoma, nodular ganglioneuroblastoma, intermixed ganglioneuroblastoma, borderline ganglioneuroblastoma, and ganglioneuroma (Table 7).

Prognostic Significance of Pathologic Classification

Histopathologic characteristics such as degree of differentiation, maturation, lymphoid infiltration, calcification, anaplasia, necrosis, foam cells, mitotic activity, neuropil, and multinucleated cells have been evaluated by various authors in an attempt to distinguish neuroblastic tumors associated with better or worse prognosis (157,195,198,212,271,273,282,343,363,386,401). Two more recent schemes of prognostic categorization of neuroblastic tumors, based on detailed statistical analysis of morphologic features in two large series of cases, have been described by Shimada et al. (386) and Joshi et al. (212). Shimada and colleagues introduced a prognostic classification based on the integration of age with histologic features such as stromal (Schwannian) development, degree of differentiation along gangliocytic lineage, and mitosis-karyorrhexis index (MKI) (defined as the number of mitotic and karyorrhectic cells per 5,000 tumor cells in random fields). Shimada divided neuroblastic tumors into two broad groups according to stromal (Schwannian) development: (a) stroma-rich and (b) stroma-poor. In stroma-rich neuroblastoma there is a predominance of stroma, whereas in stroma-poor neuroblastoma, stromal development is minimal or absent. The stroma-rich group is subdivided into: (a) nodular type showing ganglioneuromatous tissue with the presence of one or more grossly discrete masses of stroma-poor neuroblastoma; (b) intermixed type showing ganglioneuromatous tissue studded with scattered nests of variably differentiated neuroblasts; and (c) well-differentiated type showing mature ganglioneuromatous tissue with only a few randomly distributed immature neuroblastic cells. Stroma-rich neuroblastomas of well-differentiated and intermixed types are considered as favorable histology types and stroma-rich neuroblastoma of nodular type as an unfavorable histology type (Table 8). The stroma-poor group is further subdivided by multifactorial analysis utilizing age at diagnosis (equal to or less than 1.5 years vs. greater than 1.5 years), extent of maturity determined by percentage of differ-

TABLE 9. *Survival in patients with neuroblastic tumors according to Shimada Classification*

Category	Favorable histology (survival)	Unfavorable histology (survival)
NB,[a] stroma-rich[a] at any age	Well differentiated[b] (100%) and intermixed subtypes (92%)	Nodular subtype (18%)
NB, stroma-poor at age <1.5 years	Any subtype with MKI < 200 (84%)	Any subtype with MKI > 200 (4.5%)
NB, stroma-poor at age 1.5 to 5 years	Differentiating subtype with MKI < 100 (84%)	Differentiating subtype with MKI > 100 *or* undifferentiated subtype with any MKI (4.5%)
NB, stroma-poor, at age >5 years	None	All subtypes (4.5%)

(Adapted from Joshi VV and Silverman JF, ref. 215; used with permission. Data from Shimada H et al., ref. 386.)
Abbreviations: NB, neuroblastoma; MKI, mitosis-karyorrhexis index.
[a] NB, stroma-rich category is designated as ganglioneuroblastoma in the modified conventional terminology.
[b] This subtype is designated as ganglioneuroblastoma of borderline subtype in modified conventional terminology.

TABLE 10. *Histologic grading system for neuroblastoma*[a c]

Grade	Criteria	Survival (%)[b]
1	Calcification *and* low mitotic rate[c]	90
2	Calcification *or* low mitotic rate	78
3	Absence of calcification *and* of low mitotic rate	34

(Data from Joshi VV et al., ref. 212.)
[a] Shimada classification is used for prognostic categorization of ganglioneuroblastomas.
[b] Survival at 5 years.
[c] Low mitotic rate = ≤10/10 high-power fields (hpf).

TABLE 11. *Risk groups of age-linked histologic grades of neuroblastoma*[a]

Risk group	Criteria	Survival (%)[b]
Low risk	All patients with grade 1 neuroblastoma and patients ≤1 year with grade 2 neuroblastoma	92
High risk	Patients >1 year of age with grade 2 neuroblastoma and all patients with grade 3 tumors	57

(Data from Joshi VV et al., ref. 212.)
[a] Adjusted for age and Pediatric Oncology Group stage.
[b] Survival at 5 years.

entiating tumor cells, and MKI. Immunohistochemical evaluation of proliferating cell nuclear antigen (MIB-1) (76,219) and the apoptosis oncoprotein *bcl-2* (74, 118,238) may further define the relationship of MKI to prognosis.

In the series reported by Shimada, analysis of the survival data, determined after a minimum 2-year follow-up, showed a striking difference between those patients with favorable histology and those with unfavorable histology (Table 9).

On the basis of a review of 211 cases of neuroblastoma enrolled into POG protocols, Joshi et al. (212) devised a histologic grading system of neuroblastoma related to prognosis. The criteria and survival at 5 years for the three histologic grades of neuroblastoma are given in Table 10. Survival differences in patients by histologic grades were statistically significant even after adjusting for groups according to age and POG stage ($p < 0.001$). Histologic grade was linked with two age groups (less than 1 year or greater than 1 year of age), in the manner of the Shimada classification, to develop two risk groups that showed statistically significant differences in survival (Table 11). However, in distinction from Shimada grouping, histologic grade can be used as a prognostic marker independent of age considerations.

The Shimada classification and histologic grading system should be done only on previously untreated primary tumors where an adequate number of histologic sections (a minimum of four sections, each at least 3 cm in perimeter) are available (212). According to the original criteria of Shimada et al. (386), a case of "pure" ganglioneuroma or ganglioneuroblastoma, intermixed or borderline type showing neuroblastomatous lymph node metastases, is classified as ganglioneuroblastoma, nodular type. Joshi et al. (211) do not use the histology of a metastasis to modify the classification of the primary tumor. It should be emphasized that histologic grades are applicable only to neuroblastomas and not ganglioneuroblastomas. The comparative designations for neuroblastic tumors in conventional, Shimada, and modified conventional terminology are given in Table 12.

FINE NEEDLE ASPIRATION BIOPSY OF NEUROBLASTIC TUMORS

The cytologic features of neuroblastic tumors revealed by fine needle aspiration biopsy have been described and illustrated above (Figs. 20, 21, 26, 27). Several investigators have shown that fine needle aspiration biopsy coupled with ancillary studies such as immunocytochemistry, electron microscopy, and cytogenetics is a reliable, rapid, and safe procedure that is extremely useful for primary diagnosis of inoperable neuroblastic tumors

TABLE 12. *Comparable designations of neuroblastic tumors*

Conventional	Shimada	Modified conventional
Classical NB	Neuroblastoma, SP, undifferentiated	Neuroblastoma, undifferentiated, poorly differentiated and differentiating subtypes
GNB	Neuroblastoma, SP, differentiating	Neuroblastoma, differentiating
Composite GNB	Neuroblastoma, SR, nodular	GNB, nodular
	Neuroblastoma, SR, intermixed	GNB, intermixed
	Neuroblastoma, SR, well differentiated	GNB, borderline[a]
GN	GN	GN

Abbreviations: NB, neuroblastoma; SP, stoma-poor; GNB, ganglioneuroblastoma; SR, stroma-rich; GN, ganglioneuroma.
[a] GNB, intermixed, and borderline may be labeled as GN in conventional terminology by some pathologists.

(8,9,393,394). Brodeur et al. (62,64) recommend that core needle biopsies of neuroblastic tumors be preferred to fine needle aspiration biopsies so that adequate tissue can be obtained for the biologic studies (N-*myc* copy number, DNA index, cytogenetics) that are helpful in diagnosis, prognostication, and therapy. These needle biopsies can be performed as closed biopsies under ultrasound guidance or, according to the preference and expertise available in a particular institution, as open biopsies (186). There is good correlation between the fine needle aspiration cytologic and histologic features of neuroblastic tumors. Fine needle aspiration biopsy is useful not only for the diagnosis of recurrence or metastasis but also for primary neuroblastic tumors. Immunocytochemical, flow cytometric, and ultrastructural studies can be done on fine needle aspiration biopsy material (215,216,393).

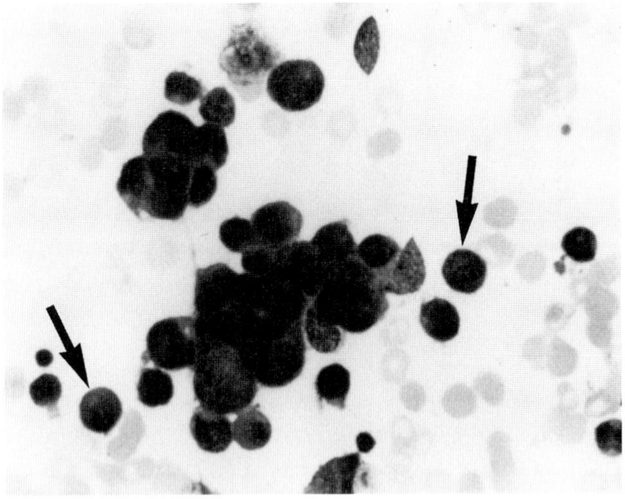

FIG. 34. Molded syncytial clumps of neuroblastoma cells with coarse chromatin and scant cytoplasm in a marrow aspirate. Discrete noncohesive tumor cells *(arrows)* are also present.

BONE MARROW ASPIRATION AND BIOPSY OF NEUROBLASTIC TUMORS

Bone marrow aspirates and/or biopsies are commonly submitted for diagnosis of neuroblastoma. A number of investigators have analyzed the type and amount of specimens to obtain. Franklin and Pritchard (148) found that bone marrow biopsy was more effective in detecting neuroblastoma cells in 20% of 154 paired samples whereas aspirate was more effective in 7%. They recommended that bilateral iliac crest marrow aspirates and trephine biopsies be obtained in children with neuroblastoma for initial staging as well as for subsequent monitoring of the disease. Bostrom et al. (45) also drew the conclusion that biopsy was superior to the aspirate. There is a trend toward obtaining bone marrow samples from two or more sites for diagnosis and monitoring. Bilateral aspirates and biopsies are recommended in the international criteria for diagnosis of bone marrow involvement (64). This will improve the reliability of initial staging and of subsequent monitoring. An adequate amount of bone marrow should be examined to exclude metastatic disease. Adequacy is defined as at least 1 cm of marrow (excluding cartilage) in a core biopsy (64) and the presence of particles in an aspirate smear. Involvement of tibial or sternal sites is not seen without involvement of the iliac crests. Imprints do not provide additional information (136). Cytocentrifuged preparations of bone marrow aspirates improve the detection rate of neuroblastoma cells (28). Adams and colleagues (5) have described a short-term tissue culture technique to detect minimal marrow involvement.

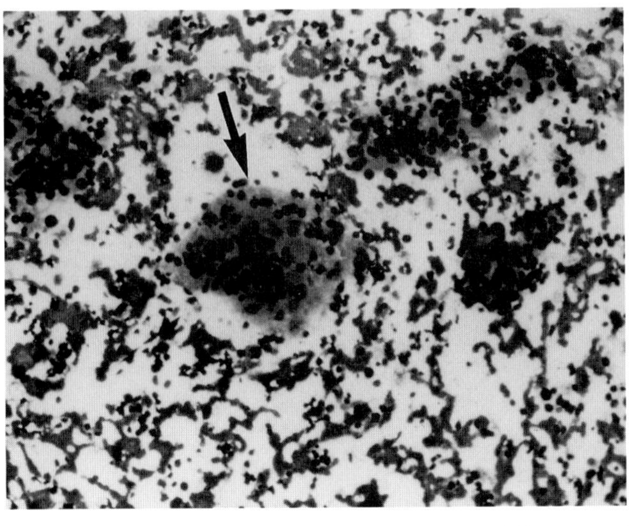

FIG. 33. Bone marrow aspirate in a child with ISSN stage 4 neuroblastoma shows several cohesive clusters of malignant cells with neuropil *(arrow)*.

Histopathology of Bone Marrow Aspirates and Biopsies in Neuroblastoma

There are no standardized and uniformly accepted criteria for the diagnosis of bone marrow involvement by neuroblastoma, which is surprising because neuroblastoma is the second most common cause of bone marrow involvement by a malignant process in children. Syncytial clusters of tumor cells showing nuclear molding, and in rare cases differentiating neuroblastoma cells with neuropil and/or rosettes, may be seen in positive smears (Figs. 33–35). Single neuroblastoma cells are difficult to identify with sufficient confidence by routine staining methods. Generally, tumor present or absent is the only grading used. However, the proportion of neuroblastoma cells among all nucleated cells in the bone marrow should be determined, particularly in cases suspected to be stage 4S, because according to the revised

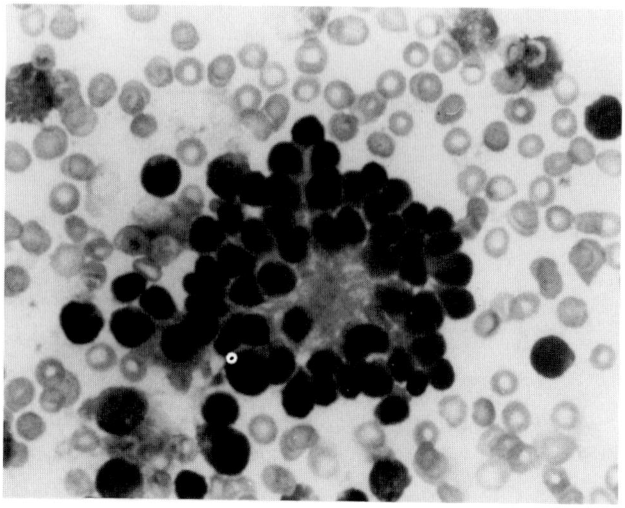

FIG. 35. Characteristic Homer Wright rosette of metastatic neuroblastoma in a marrow aspirate.

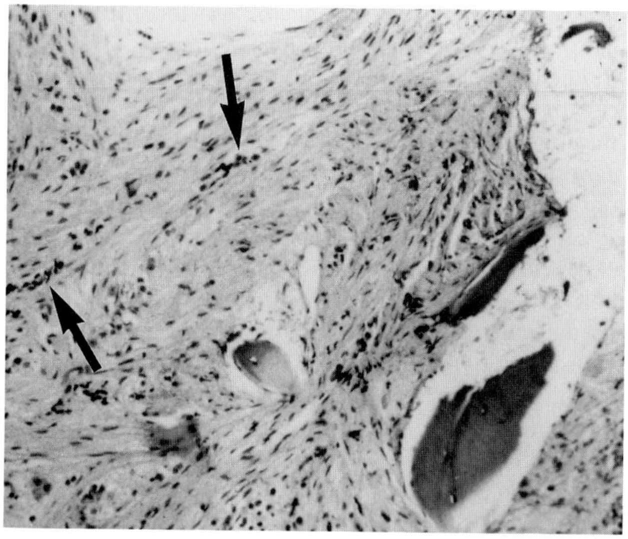

FIG. 36. Myelofibrotic pattern of bone marrow involvement by neuroblastoma. Distorted cords of relatively scanty small hyperchromatic metastatic tumor cells *(arrows)* are compressed by a surrounding desmoplastic reaction within the intertrabecular space.

guidelines for the International Neuroblastoma Staging System, greater than 10% of the total nucleated cells identified as neuroblastoma cells are considered stage 4 (64). For marrow biopsies, Reid and Hamilton (350) recommend routine performance of both hematoxylin-and-eosin and reticulin stains and a standardized description of the following features: cellularity of hematopoietic tissue (none, hypocellular, normal, or hypercellular), primitive cell infiltrate (none, slight, or extensive), fibrous stroma (none, slight, or extensive), and reticulin (none, slight, or extensive). Mills and Bird (290) found that marrow involvement by neuroblastoma is more common in patients with primary adrenal tumors and is often present at the time of presentation. They recognized several patterns of marrow involvement by neuroblastoma, noting a relatively high frequency of myelofibrosis (Fig. 36). Neuroblastoma is less easily identified in the marrow once treatment is begun. Reid and colleagues (351,428) found that distorted marrow architecture and persistent abnormal stromal reactions may be indicative of failure to eradicate tumor despite the absence of detectable primitive cells (Fig. 37). This abnormal fibrous stromal material was seen in previously biopsied as well as previously unbiopsied sites (Table 13). Immunostaining with monoclonal antibodies UJ13A and UJ127.11, which react with neuroblastoma cells in frozen sections (224), was seen in cells and stromal material in 8 of 12 staging procedures in which distorted architecture and fibrosis without obvious tumor were noted (351). The immunoreactivity of the stroma with neural markers in these bone marrow lesions suggests either a reaction to occult neuroblasts or Schwannian tumor differentiation (351). Tumor cells that cannot be morphologically appreciated in a fibrotic marrow may be demonstrable by cytogenetic studies (50).

Other immunohistochemical stains can be used to confirm the neuroblastic nature of the tumor cells and enhance the rate of recognition of positive bone marrows (301,326). A variety of immunologic reagents have been used to identify neuroblastoma cells, including NSE (68,101), synaptophysin, ganglioside G_{D2} (89), neural cell adhesion molecule (NCAM), neurofilament proteins, and chromogranin A (64). Decalcification may interfere with the demonstration of NSE (425). Alcohol fixation and immunohistologic stains on undecalcified bone marrow sections have been recommended by Oppedal et al. (326). In our experience, immunoperoxidase stains give consistent results even in the decalcified

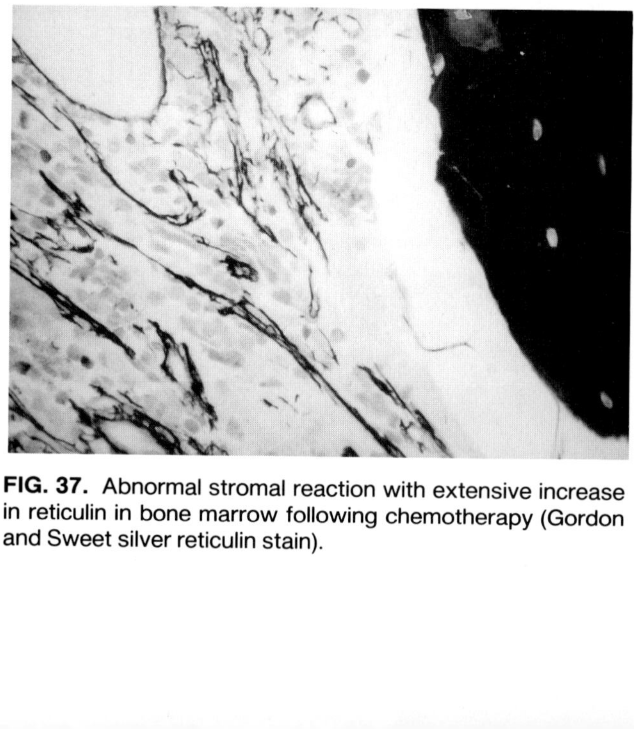

FIG. 37. Abnormal stromal reaction with extensive increase in reticulin in bone marrow following chemotherapy (Gordon and Sweet silver reticulin stain).

TABLE 13. *Histopathologic patterns seen in bone marrow biopsies in neuroblastoma*

Pattern	Additional features and comments
At diagnosis[a]	
Myelofibrotic	Desmoplastic reaction and marked increase in reticulin fibers around scanty tumor cells
Focal/multifocal	Islands of tumor cells with minimal or no increase in reticulin fibers
Interstitial	Sheets of tumor cells spread throughout the intertrabecular space not associated with increase in reticulin fibers
Mixed	Mixture of focal and interstitial pattern with patchy increase in reticulin fibers
After treatment[b]	
Normal marrow (grade 1)	Variable cellularity, normal architecture, no increased reticulin
Increased reticulin (grade 2)	Otherwise normal marrow
Distorted architecture containing fibrous stroma, no clearly identifiable tumor cells (grade 3)	Tumor cells may be demonstrable by immunostains
Marrow with readily identifiable tumor cells (grade 4)	Focal fibrosis may be present

(Adapted from [a]Mills AE and Bird AR, ref. 280, and [b] Reid MM and Hamilton PJ, ref. 350.)

bone marrow biopsy specimen (Fig. 38; see figure in color plate section). Alcohol or B5 fixation is recommended because either fixative preserves antigenicity of most cellular constituents better than crosslinking fixatives such as formalin. However, formalin fixation appears to give consistent results if excessive duration of fixation is avoided. Plastic or resin embedding (155) and/or microwave-based techniques for staining (43,234) and antigen retrieval in formalin-fixed tissues for immunohistochemical studies (165,257,384,403) provides superior results. It should be emphasized that the use of immunohistologic methods cannot replace a careful review of the hematoxylin and eosin–stained sections of the marrow biopsy (and also of the primary tumor).

IMMUNOHISTOCHEMISTRY OF NEUROBLASTOMA

Neuroblastoma morphologically resembles a number of malignant small blue cell tumors of infancy and childhood, including Ewing's sarcoma, peripheral primitive neuroectodermal tumor (PNET), malignant lymphoma, and rhabdomyosarcoma. Immunohistochemistry plays an important role in distinguishing these tumor types. Neuroblastoma can be diagnosed utilizing a variety of neural, neuroendocrine, supportive cell, intermediate filament, and cell surface antigen markers (Table 14). Unfortunately, many of these markers show inconsistent staining; display a wide spectrum of reactivity with other tumors; may be unreactive or poorly reactive in formalin-fixed, paraffin-embedded tissues; and/or fail to react with the most primitive tumors. NSE has been perhaps the most widely used marker for neuroblastoma despite the presence of reactivity in other tumors, e.g., PNET and rarely rhabdomyosarcoma (122,424,425). Consistent diffuse moderate to intense staining of tumor cells and neuropil is usually found, regardless of the degree of tumor cell differentiation (424) (Fig. 39; see figure in color plate section). S-100 protein antibody reliably demonstrates Schwann cells and their spindle-shaped precursor cells in the fibrovascular stroma of ganglioneuroblastoma and ganglioneuroma (Fig. 40; see figure in

TABLE 14. *Immunohistochemical markers in neuroblastic tumors*[a]

Marker
Neural markers
Neuron specific enolase (NSE)
Neurofilament triplet proteins 200, 160, 68 kd (NF)
Microtubule-associated proteins 1 and 2 (MAP1/MAP2)
β-tubulin (TU27, TUJ1)
τ protein
Dopamine-β-hydroxylase
Mab 5A7
NB84
Peripherin
Neuroendocrine markers
Chromogranin
Synaptophysin
Vasoactive intestinal peptide (VIP)
Protein gene product (PGP) 9.5
Supportive cell markers
S-100 protein
Glial fibrillary acidic protein (GFAP)
Myelin basic protein (MBP)
Cell surface markers
HNK-1 (Leu 7)
HSAN 1.2
KP-NAC8
UJ127.11
Neural cell adhesion molecule (NCAM, UJ13A)
UJ167.11
Ganglioside G_{D2}
Peanut agglutinin lectin (PNA)

[a] Refs. 16,18,68,89,101,136,140,173,193,216,224,283, 284,294,296,301,326,327,332,351,373,414,416,424,425, 445,446,450.

color plate section), providing a method for evaluation of differentiation and prognosis (16,294,387). Neurofilament proteins form part of the neuronal cytoskeleton. Commercial antibody preparations contain three proteins of approximately 200, 160, and 68 kd. The higher molecular weight antibodies are more readily detectable in the relatively mature neuroblastic tumors, and frozen sections are generally more suitable for demonstrating positive staining than is formalin-fixed paraffin-embedded tissue (296,327). Leu 7 (anti-CD57, HNK-1, human natural killer cell antigen) is a monoclonal antibody of the IgM class that has been found to recognize an epitope of myelin-associated glycoprotein and a glycoproteinaceous determinant in neurosecretory granule matrices (259), in addition to natural killer cells. Although it stains neuroblastoma, its usefulness is limited because other small blue cell tumors (Ewing's sarcoma, PNET, and Wilms' tumor) express this antigen (284). NB84 is another recently developed commercially available monoclonal antibody, raised against neuroblastoma tumor cells, that shows diffuse cytoplasmic staining in most formalin-fixed, paraffin-embedded neuroblastomas. However, some cases of Ewing's sarcoma and PNET also stain with this antibody (414). The monoclonal antibody HSAN 1.2 was raised against a human neuroblastoma cell line and directed against neuroectodermal cell surface antigenic determinants. It works well on frozen but not paraffin-embedded tissues and shows strong immunoreactivity in neuroblastoma and weak immunoreactivity in PNETs (424). Peripherin is an intermediate filament protein that displays cytoplasmic immunoreactivity with the entire spectrum of neuroblastic tumors, including undifferentiated and poorly differentiated neuroblastoma, ganglioneuroblastoma, and ganglioneuroma, but not other small blue cell tumors (140). Synaptophysin, a glycoprotein localized to the membrane of presynaptic vesicles, will stain well-differentiated neuroblasts and ganglion cells in optimally fixed (95% alcohol or Bouin's fixative, less consistently neutral buffered formalin) neuroblastomas (164,173, 296,446,450). Chromogranin A is an acidic water-soluble calcium-binding matrix protein of chromaffin granules that shows variable, weakly positive immunohistochemical staining of ganglion cells in about half of neuroblastomas (173,296,445,446). VIP also displays variable staining of ganglion cells in neuroblastic tumors (193,283,450). Exceptional cases may stain with antibodies directed against vimentin, glial fibrillary acidic protein (GFAP), desmin, or muscle-specific actin (296,424). A number of other recently characterized neural markers that recognize neuroblastoma have also been described. These include G_{D2}, microtubule-associated proteins (MAP-1 and MAP-2), peanut agglutinin lectin, and neural cell adhesion molecule (NCAM) (18,89,216,332,373).

Some antigens serve to distinguish neuroblastoma from other small blue cell tumors of childhood, particularly Ewing's sarcoma and PNET. Two of these antigens are β_2-microglobulin and MIC2, which is recognized by monoclonal antibodies HBA 71, 013, and 12E7. β_2-microglobulin is associated with class I histocompatibility molecules, while MIC2 is a cell surface glycoprotein closely related to the product of the pseudoautosomal gene MIC2 on the X and Y chromosomes. Antibodies against both markers react strongly with Ewing's sarcoma and PNET; neither reacts with neuroblastoma (329,424,442). Glyoxylic acid–induced catecholamine fluorescence has also been used as an ancillary technique for the diagnosis of neuroblastoma (352).

ULTRASTRUCTURAL APPEARANCES OF NEUROBLASTOMA

Ultrastructurally, the appearance of neuroblastic tumors varies with the degree of cytologic differentiation (293,359,411). The least differentiated cells may be difficult to distinguish from the primitive cells of other types of tumors (172). They have irregularly lobulated or indented nuclei, high nuclear-to-cytoplasmic ratio, and scant rims of cytoplasm with scarce organelles other than free ribosomes, a few mitochondria, and small numbers of heterogeneous osmiophilic granules measuring about 30–50 nm in diameter (293). More differentiated cells are recognized by larger cell size with increased amounts of cytoplasm (Fig. 41) and attenuated processes containing fine neurofilaments (8–12 nm) and microtubules (24 nm) (293,411) (Fig. 42). Variable numbers of dense core neurosecretory granules, measuring 50–200 nm in diameter, occur in small clusters in the elongated cell pro-

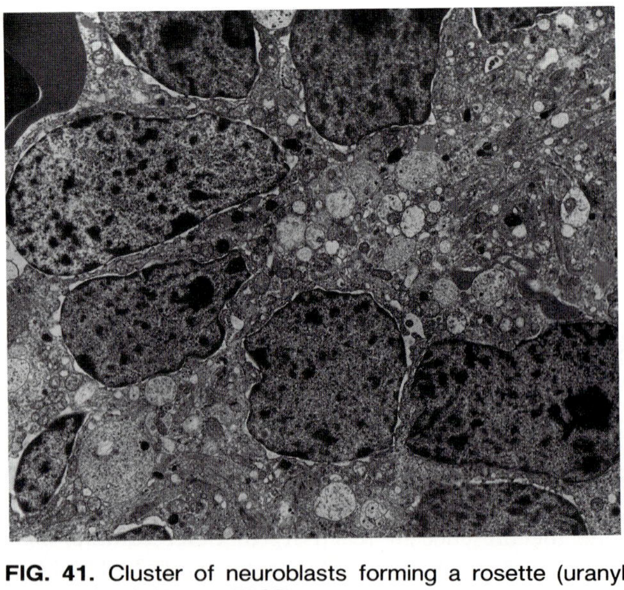

FIG. 41. Cluster of neuroblasts forming a rosette (uranyl acetate–lead citrate, x7560).

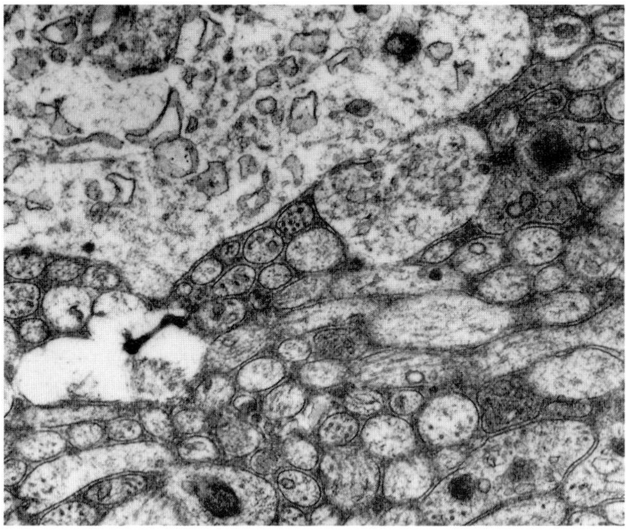

FIG. 42. Closely apposed cell processes in neuroblastoma contain a meshwork of fine neurofilaments and microtubules (uranyl acetate–lead citrate, x36,900).

cesses and less frequently in the perinuclear cytoplasm. The granules contain central dense cores surrounded by clear halos and delicate outer membranes (Fig. 43). Occasionally, smaller (25 nm) clear vesicles occurring mainly in synapselike structures are also noted. Glycogen is rarely conspicuous (235,421,456). Ganglionic differentiation is recognized by the large vesicular nucleus, prominent nucleolus, and abundant cytoplasm with a concomitant increase in mitochondria, smooth and granular endoplasmic reticulum, ribosomes, and perinuclear Golgi apparatuses. Small dense core granules are scattered throughout the cytoplasm, and larger heterogeneous granules containing myelin figures are present in significant numbers (293,411). In some cases the ganglion cells contain a proliferation of tightly packed 7- to 8-nm filaments that are arranged in whorled interlacing bundles to form one or more large intracytoplasmic inclusions (34). In addition to mature ganglion cells, ganglioneuromatous areas contain Schwann cells characterized by long tapered cytoplasmic processes invested with basal lamina and containing fine filaments, microtubules, and varying numbers of small and large granules. Occasional desmosomelike structures are found between cells, or between cells and processes, the latter occurring with collections of vesicles and granules simulating a synapse (411). Shimada (385) has described small round to spindle-shaped cells in ganglioneuroblastoma that contain 75- to 100-nm micropinocytotic vesicles near their plasma membranes. Irregular or complex infoldings of the cytoplasmic membrane and irregularly formed or multilayered basal lamina were present around the plasma membrane in some of these cells (Fig. 44). He suggested that these cells might be precursors of Schwann cells.

Although some neuroblastomas may have multiple classic well-formed dense core granules easily identified by routine electron microscopy, in others the granules may be sparse, pleomorphic, and difficult to recognize. Indeed, it may be difficult to differentiate the true dense core granules from lysosomal structures, degenerating mitochondria, or phagosomes in tumors that contain only a rare structure resembling a dense core neurosecretory granule (302). There are two techniques that can conclusively identify these structures as neurosecretory granules. The uranaffin reaction is a cytochemical stain that recognizes adenosine nucleotides in organelles rich in biogenic amines, such as the granules in platelets, adrenal medulla, sympathetic nerve terminals, and ganglion cells (334,354). Amine storage organelles of aldehyde-fixed tissues have a strong affinity for uranyl ions before their dehydration and appear highly electron-dense when examined by electron microscopy. The cytochemical reaction is the result of an interaction between uranyl ions and phosphate groups of 5′-phosphonucleotides. The dense cores (but not their membranes) of neurosecretory granules from both normal and neoplastic neuroendocrine cells exhibit a positive uranaffin reaction, whereas nonneuroendocrine electron-dense granules are negative (334). With immunoelectron microscopy, proteins such as chromogranin A can be used to identify neuroendocrine cells and their neoplasms (302,392). Utilizing immunocolloidal gold complexes (protein A–gold), chromogranin A can be localized ultrastructurally to membrane-bound dense core granules in neuroblastic tumors. Lysosomal granules and other nonneuroendocrine dense granules are nonreactive with this technique.

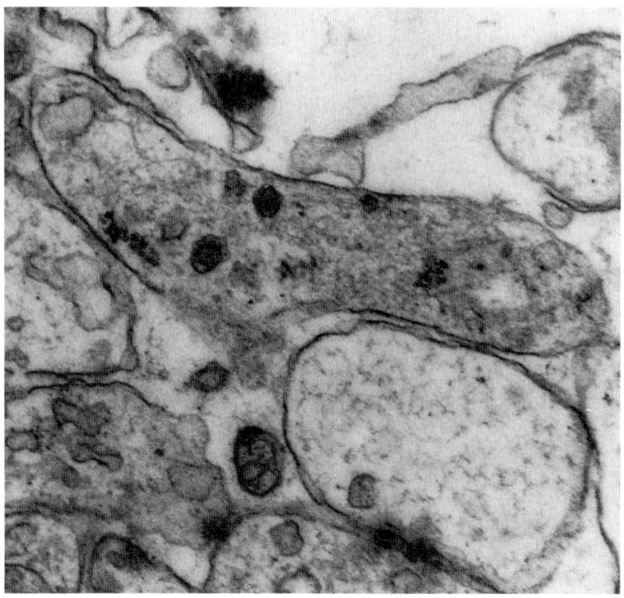

FIG. 43. Neuroblastoma with dense core granules in neuritic processes (uranyl acetate–lead citrate, x69,600).

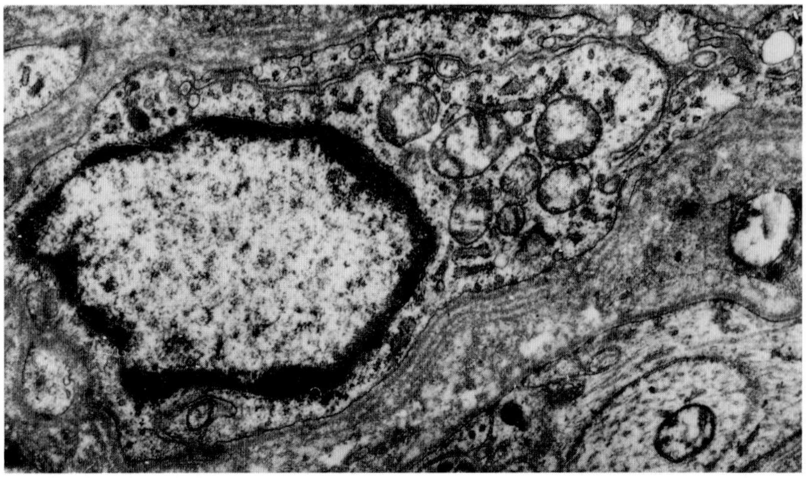

FIG. 44. Putative Schwannian precursor cell found in the perivascular area of an undifferentiated neuroblastoma (uranyl acetate and lead citrate, x18,000). (Courtesy of Dr. Hiroyuki Shimada, Children's Hospital of Los Angeles, Los Angeles, CA.)

SPECIAL CATEGORIES OF NEUROBLASTIC TUMORS

Congenital Neuroblastoma

Malignant congenital tumors are rare (22). In two series comprising 34 malignancies (102) and 110 cases of all types of tumors in the neonate (203), neuroblastoma was the commonest and third commonest lesion respectively. The abdomen (adrenals and retroperitoneum) was the most common primary site. Nine of the 14 neonatal neuroblastomas in the series reported by Isaacs (203) were stage IVS. Following therapy, eight of 14 patients had no evidence of tumor. Jennings et al. (209) and Dominici et al. (119) described the diagnosis of 5 and 32 cases, respectively, of fetal adrenal neuroblastoma by ultrasonography. The majority of prenatal neuroblastomas have a relatively favorable prognosis. Rare cases with unfavorable biological features do poorly despite early detection and treatment (119). A notable feature of fetal and congenital neuroblastomas is involvement of the placenta (300,337,396). In most cases the tumor cells are confined to the blood vessels of the villi. However, in the case reported by Perkins et al. (337), there was infiltration of the villous stroma by tumor cells that were identified definitively by electron microscopy. Fetal hydrops is common in infants with advanced stage congenital neuroblastoma and metastases (209).

Neuroblastoma in Adults

Over 100 cases of neuroblastoma have been reported in adults (12,13,32,161,220,269,292). The age range is 15–82 years (292) with a median of 34 years and an equal male/female distribution (13). The primary sites in 51 cases reviewed by Behr et al. (32) were abdomen (50%); head and neck (25%); thorax, pelvis, and lower extremities (25%). The survival rates are similar to those for INSS stages 3 and 4 childhood neuroblastoma (13). Many of these tumors are reported in sites that are unusual for classical neuroblastoma (parotid, kidney, gluteal soft tissues, lower extremity). Some may represent metastatic lesions associated with spontaneous regression and absence of the primary tumor (419). In most cases, however, adequate supportive evidence of classical neuroblastoma (catecholamine secretion, immunohistochemical studies, N-*myc* amplification, chromosomal abnormalities) is not available. There can be overlap between the morphologic features of neuroblastoma and peripheral primitive neuroectodermal tumor ("small blue round cell tumor" with or without Homer Wright rosettes, neuroendocrine granules, and/or neuritic processes) (180,372). With the application of immunohistochemistry for MIC2 and β_2-microglobulin (329) and karyotype analysis for the reciprocal translocation t(11;22)(q24;q12) (413,444) in these cases, it is likely that many would represent peripheral primitive neuroectodermal tumors (109,110,417,418).

Familial Neuroblastoma

Rare cases of neuroblastoma and ganglioneuroblastoma occur in related individuals such as siblings, monozygotic twins, half-siblings, cousins, and parent–child, suggesting an autosomal dominant inheritance (84,168, 239,335). In a review of 55 cases from 23 families, Kushner et al. (239) found that multiple primary sites, age less than 18 months, and diagnosis of tumor within 12 months in another family member are characteristic features of familial neuroblastoma. The median age at diagnosis is 9 months, which contrasts with a median age of 22 months for neuroblastoma in the general population. At least 20% of patients with familial neuroblastoma have bilateral adrenal or multifocal primary tumors

(64,93). The risk of neuroblastoma in siblings or offspring in the large majority of persons with neuroblastoma is less than 6% (239). Survival is comparable to that of unselected cases.

Pigmented Neuroblastic Tumors

Rare examples of pigmented or melanocytic neuroblastoma (304) and ganglioneuroblastoma (163,175, 322) have been reported. The pigment in these tumors may or may not be visible at the time of gross inspection. Microscopically, it is found in neuroblasts and ganglion cells and appears to be related to and histochemically indistinguishable from melanin (Fig. 45; see figure in color plate section). In most reports (163,304,322), the pigment is membrane-bound, coarsely granular, heterogeneous, and electron-dense with lipid residues, and has the ultrastructural features of neuromelanin, a waste product of catecholamine metabolism. An acquired defect of lysosomal function is the suggested mechanism of pigment storage in these cases. In the study by Hahn et al. (175), premelanosomes and melanosomes were observed ultrastructurally. This unusual feature of pigmentation is consistent with the phenotype of neuroblastoma cells in vitro, where the spectrum of neuronal, Schwannian, and melanocytic differentiation has been seen (426). The melaninlike pigment does not affect classification or prognosis.

SPONTANEOUS REGRESSION OF NEUROBLASTOMA

After renal carcinoma, neuroblastoma is the second most common human malignancy reported to undergo spontaneous regression (95). Regression occurs in 8% of all neuroblastomas and 87% of INSS stage 4S neuroblastomas (40). Evans et al. (131) reviewed 57 cases of neuroblastoma in which regression occurred following minimal, no, or unusual therapy. They found that the phenomenon occurs most frequently in stage II or stage IVS disease and that 65% of the patients whose tumors showed regression were less than 6 months of age at diagnosis. Spontaneous regression is characterized by total disappearance of the disease or maturation into ganglioneuroma or, rarely, a neurofibromatous mass (168). The total disappearance of the disease may be related to cytolysis resulting from an IgM antibody and complement-mediated immune response (41) or by cytotoxic lymphocytes (187). Hellstrom et al. (188) showed that lymphocytes from children with neuroblastoma are cytotoxic to neuroblastoma cells. They also demonstrated that the sera of children with neuroblastoma contain a factor that blocks the effect of cytotoxic lymphocytes. Cytolysis leads to a fibrous and calcified remnant or, in some cases, no trace of tumor at all.

The phenomenon of maturation has been documented morphologically in a number of cases (104, 123,146,171,278). It should be emphasized that the tumor at the end of the maturation must be sampled adequately before labeling it as ganglioneuroma. Spontaneous differentiation can also occur in metastatic sites (151). The mechanism in maturation is not known. It is not clear as to whether maturation is effected by certain hypothetical factors (primary and secondary organizers) found in the normal embryonic tissues that somehow are elaborated by an embryonal tumor such as neuroblastoma. It has been shown that highly malignant teratocarcinoma cells, when injected onto mouse blastocytes, become integrated into the blastocyst and follow normal pathways of differentiation (53). It is thus possible that the immediate environment of neuroblastoma in young infants may influence the subsequent differentiation and maturation of the tumor cells and that the incidence of this phenomenon is higher than reported.

Although neuroblastomas are known to undergo maturation in some cases, they also may remain dormant for long periods of time with late recurrences (5 or more years after initial diagnosis) (292,355). These cases are characterized by advanced disease at diagnosis with dissemination and a peculiar tendency for recurrence during the teenage years.

BIOLOGIC AND PROGNOSTIC FACTORS IN NEUROBLASTIC TUMORS

Prognostic factors in neuroblastoma include a number of clinical, biochemical, cytogenetic, molecular biologic, and morphologic variables (Table 15). Clinically, the age, stage, and site are related to prognosis. The outcome in infants less than 1 year of age is significantly better than in those who are older (52). However, in the series of 124 children with neuroblastoma from Children's Hospital of Philadelphia, the cutoff point for better survival was 2 years (133). The survival in patients with ISSN stages 1, 2, and 4S neuroblastoma is 80–90%. In contrast, the 2-year disease-free survival in stages 3 and 4 neuroblastoma patients is 20–30% (65). Neuroblastomas arising in the adrenal glands carry a worse prognosis than those arising in extra-adrenal sites, particularly the thorax (4,299).

The biochemical prognostic factors include serum NSE, ferritin, and lactate dehydrogenase (LDH), tumor ganglioside composition, tumor VIP and somatostatin concentration, and ratio of urine VMA to HVA. High serum NSE (>100 ng/mL), high serum ferritin (>150 ng/mL), high serum LDH (>1500 U/mL), and low urine VMA/HVA ratio (<1) are associated with worse prognosis (133,390,458). Neuroblastomas in patients who had ongoing disease or died of disease had more monosialogangliosides and fewer gangliotetraose gangliosides of B

TABLE 15. *Prognostic factors in neuroblastoma*

Factors	Favorable	Unfavorable
Tumor site	Extra-adrenal, particularly thorax	Adrenal
Age at diagnosis	≤1 year	>1 year
Stage	1, 2A, 2B, 4S	3, 4
Histopathology[a]	Favorable	Unfavorable
Histologic grade[b]	Grades 1 and 2	Grade 3
Lactate dehydrogenase	≤1500 U/mL	>1500 U/mL
VMA/HVA ratio	>1	<1
Ferritin	Normal	Elevated (≥142 ng/mL)
Neuron-specific enolase	≤100 ng/mL	>100 ng/mL
Ganglioside G_{D2}	Absent	Present
Vasoactive intestinal peptide (VIP)	Present	NA[c]
Somatostatin receptor expression	Present	Absent
DNA index (DI)	"hyperdiploid" (DI > 1)	"diploid" (DI = 1)
Chromosome 1p abnormalities	Absent	Present
Dmins, HSRs	Absent	Present
N-myc	Not amplified	Amplified
trk-A expression	Present	Absent
bcl-2 expression	Absent	Present
CD44 expression	Present	Absent
Hsp27 expression	Present	Absent

Abbreviations: VMA/HVA, vanillylmandelic acid/homovanillic acid; Dmins, extrachromosomal double-minute chromatin bodies; HSRs, chromosomally integrated homogeneously staining regions.

[a] Shimada classification (386).

[b] Joshi grading system (212).

[c] NA, not applicable. Lack of VIP secretion is not an unfavorable factor.

series than neuroblastomas in patients who were disease-free (371). High concentrations of tumor VIP (≥1.2 pg/μg DNA), as determined by radioimmunoassay, are correlated with cellular differentiation and favorable disease stage (347). Increased concentrations of somatostatin (>1.3 pg/μg DNA) are also found in neuroblastomas showing differentiation (347). Moertel et al. (295) found that somatostatin receptors, detected by autoradiographic techniques, were expressed more frequently in tumor tissue from patients with lower stages of disease, in those without N-*myc* amplification, and in patients with significantly longer survival.

Due to their unique biology and capacity for in vitro cell growth (Fig. 46), a relatively large number of neuroblastoma cell lines have been used to characterize the morphology, cell biology, biochemistry, and cytogenetics of neuroblastoma (96,344). Many of these tumor cell lines can be differentiated in vitro by treatment with a variety of biologic agents (retinoic acid, cyclic AMP, bromodeoxyuridine, VIP, nerve growth factor), thus providing excellent models for the study of the cytogenetic and molecular mechanisms that control cell growth and induce differentiation (56,207,344,374). The cytogenetic marker most often related to prognosis is the deletion of the short arm of chromosome 1 (Fig. 47). It is found in approximately 30% of primary tumors and 70–80% of cell lines that have been karyotyped. The region most commonly deleted is between 1p32 and 1pter (59). Neuroblastomas showing the deletion tend to have a poor prognosis (181). Historically, it has been suggested that this deletion represents the loss or inactivation of a putative neuroblastoma suppressor gene(s) (37). Lahti and colleagues (249,250) have recently demonstrated in neuroblastoma cell lines deletions or translocations affecting the p58 PITSLRE gene complex that is localized to 1p36.3. The group of protein kinase isoforms encoded by this gene complex is involved in apoptotic signaling. Lahti et al. suggest that the PITSLRE locus may harbor one or more tumor suppressor genes affected by chromosome 1p36 alterations in neuroblastoma.

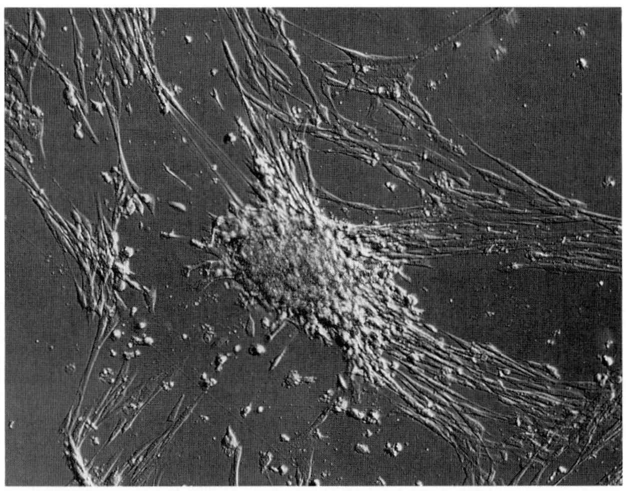

FIG. 46. Tissue culture of neuroblastoma, showing axonal outgrowths. (Courtesy of Dr. Thasia Leimig, St. Jude Children's Research Hospital, Memphis, TN.)

CYTOGENETIC ABNORMALITIES IN HUMAN NEUROBLASTOMAS

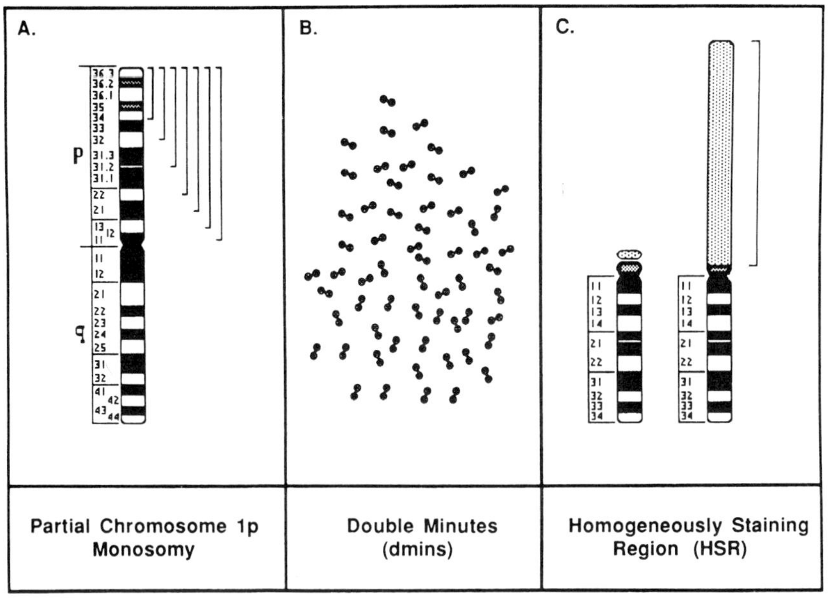

FIG. 47. Diagrammatic representations of the three most common cytogenetic abnormalities in neuroblastoma. **A.** Deletions of the short arm of chromosome 1. The brackets indicate that the region deleted in different tumors is variable in terms of its proximal breakpoint, but the distal short arm appears to be deleted in all cases, resulting in partial 1p monosomy. **B.** Extrachromosomal double-minute chromatin bodies (dmins). Dmins are seen in about 30% of primary neuroblastomas. **C.** Homogeneously staining region (HSR). A representative HSR on the short arm of chromosome 13 is shown in this example. (Used with permission (55).)

The molecular biological marker most related to prognosis in neuroblastic tumors is N-*myc* amplification (375). N-*myc* is a proto-oncogene found on the distal short arm of chromosome 2 (2p23-24). Myc functions as a transcription regulator of other genes apparently involved in the control of cell proliferation. The effects of *myc* on both gene expression and cell growth are differentially regulated by other recently described basic region helix-loop-helix leucine zipper DNA binding transcription factors known as Max and Mad. These proteins can either cooperate or compete with myc for sequence-specific DNA binding. Overexpression of *myc* appears to block differentiation and drive cells into proliferation (236,281). The phenomenon of N-*myc* amplification was discovered during investigations of double-minute chromatin bodies and chromosomally integrated homogeneously staining regions in neuroblastoma cell lines (23,36,58,59) (Fig. 47). Amplification of a large region of chromosome 2, which includes the N-*myc* locus, occurs initially as many double-minute chromosomes, separate from the normal 46 chromosomes. In a small percentage of primary tumors and about half of established neuroblastoma cell lines, the amplified DNA becomes linearly integrated into a chromosome in the form of tandem repeats as a homogeneously staining region (56,279) (Fig. 47). Seeger et al. (379) determined the number of copies of the N-*myc* oncogene in 89 neuroblastomas by Southern blot and densitometric analysis. Genomic amplification (3–300 copies) was associated with rapid progression and poor prognosis. Up to 40% of advanced stage neuroblastomas showed amplification. The progression-free survival at 18 months was 70%, 30%, and 5% in patients whose tumors had 1, 3–10, and greater than 10 N-*myc* copies. N-*myc* amplification occurs in about 25–30% of primary neuroblastomas from untreated patients (65), and in about 90% of established cell lines (56), suggesting a critical role in autocrine growth necessary for in vitro propagation. Although N-*myc* amplification is found predominantly in advanced stages of neuroblastomas (INSS stages 3 and 4) (60), it may also occur in stages 1 and 2 disease, where it is not necessarily associated with poor outcome (94). This suggests that other prognostic factors can modify the deleterious effects of N-*myc* amplification. N-*myc* amplification only rarely occurs with INSS stage 4S, a stage known to undergo spontaneous regression. It is consistently found in association with chromosome 1p deletions. The proliferation advantage offered by increased N-*myc* expression in neuroblastoma may require that an apoptotic pathway be blocked by deletion or inactivation of one or more of the PITSLRE kinases (249,250). N-*myc* copy number is consistent in multiple samples from the same specimen and in consecutive specimens from the same patient (61), and amplification is almost always present at the time of diagnosis if it is going to occur (63). It is usually the paternal allele of N-*myc* that is amplified, possibly demonstrating an example of genomic imprinting in tumors (see Chapter 3) (86). Virtually all tumors with amplified N-*myc* also have increased N-*myc* expression at the mRNA and the protein levels, and in the absence of N-*myc* amplification, increased N-*myc* mRNA expression is not necessarily associated with poor outcome (376,380). Recently, polymerase chain reaction (PCR) (39) and fluorescence in situ hybridization (FISH) (258) have been used with routine histologic sections, tumor imprints and bone marrow smears (412), and tumor cell suspensions (383) for quantitative estimation of the N-*myc* copy number and detection of deletions of chromosome 1p (258,412) in neuroblastoma (Fig. 48; see figure in color plate section).

The *trk* family of proto-oncogenes encodes tyrosine kinase neurotrophic receptors that are important in regulating growth and differentiation in normal and neoplastic nerve cells. *trk*-A is a transmembrane glycoprotein that encodes the primary component of nerve growth factor receptor, a protein that is selectively expressed in the developing nervous system and in many neuroblastomas. Nerve growth factor promotes survival and induces terminal neuronal differentiation in developing sympathetic neuroblasts. *trk*-A expression is inversely related to N-*myc* amplification, high levels of expression of the *trk*-A gene being associated with favorable outcome in neuroblastoma (311). Nakagawara and colleagues (311) have shown that tumors with high *trk* proto-oncogene expression may be more likely to differentiate, regress spontaneously, or respond well to therapy. Conversely, aggressive neuroblastomas, especially those with N-*myc* amplification, express little or no *trk*-A, and many cell lines have a defective nerve growth factor receptor signaling pathway (57,312). A considerable number of *trk*-A-expressing neuroblastomas remain histologically undifferentiated. Peters and colleagues (338) have shown that those patients older than 1.5 years whose tumors express less of the neuronal isoform of *trk*-A (*trk*-A II) have a poor outcome. *trk*-B encodes a receptor for brain-derived neurotrophic factor (BDNF). BDNF appears to promote cell survival and neurite outgrowth. Truncated *trk*-B appears to be preferentially expressed in more differentiated tumors (ganglioneuromas and ganglioneuroblastomas), whereas full-length *trk*-B is expressed in immature neuroblastomas with N-*myc* amplification. The BDNF/*trk*-B pathway may be particularly important for growth and differentiation of neuroblastomas with N-*myc* amplification (313).

Since N-*myc* expression is greatest in advanced stage tumors with poorly differentiated histology, which tend to be most refractory to drug treatment, it has been suggested that this oncogene may regulate the transcription of critical drug resistance genes (33). P-glycoprotein, the product of the *mdr*-1 gene, is a 170-kd plasma membrane protein that is implicated in cross-resistance to anticancer drugs that are not structurally related. The mechanism of this effect may be related to the function of P-glycoprotein as an ATP-dependent drug efflux pump (80,81). Increased concentrations of P-glycoprotein are thought to confer multiple drug resistance by decreasing net intracellular accumulation of cytotoxic drugs. There is some controversy with regard to P-glycoprotein expression in childhood solid tumors (420), with authors variously claiming no expression (323), positive association (81,82), or inconclusive results (27,97). In neuroblastoma, the relationship between *mdr*-1 gene expression and amplification/overexpression of N-*myc* is also unclear. *mdr*-1 expression has been reported to be unrelated to (46,82,162) or inversely correlated with N-*myc* amplification/overexpression (98,310). The expression of the *mdr*-1 gene in neuroblastoma has been shown to increase concomitantly with retinoic acid–induced morphologic differentiation (26,44), suggesting that increased *mdr*-1 gene expression may be specifically related to the degree of differentiation rather than contributing to drug resistance in this disease (310). A membrane-bound glycoprotein that does appear to regulate multidrug resistance in neuroblastoma is encoded by the *MRP* gene, the expression of which correlates with amplification and overexpression of N-*myc* (44).

Determination of the DNA index (DI) of neuroblastoma from infants can also provide important information that can be predictive of response to particular chemotherapeutic regimens as well as outcome. Tumors with a "hyperdiploid" DNA content (DI > 1) are more likely to have lower stages of disease and to respond to cyclophosphamide and doxorubicin. Those with a "diploid" DNA content (DI = 1) are more likely to have advanced stages of disease and do not respond to this combination (262,263).

Other genetic and cell biologic features currently under investigation that will likely provide further insight into the biologic heterogeneity of neuroblastoma include loss of heterozygosity of chromosome 14 (144,399,404, 409), abnormalities of chromosome 17 (435), activity of the ribonucleoprotein enzyme telomerase (225), expression of oncogenes *smg* p25A (365), c-*src* (38,275), *bcl-2* (74,118,238), and c-Ha-*ras* p21 (297,410), protooncogenes HER-2/*neu* (c-erbB-2, ERBB2) (254) and *ret* (206,407), tumor suppressor gene p53 (196,254), tumor metastasis suppressor protein p19/*nm*23 (176,256), heat shock protein Hsp27 (431), cell adhesion molecule CD44 (138,169), the transmembrane-spanning cell adhesion receptor family of integrins (137,158,280), and the microtubule-associated proteins MAP-1, MAP-2, and tau (121,264).

Correlations Between Various Prognostic Markers

Correlations between histologic grade and N-*myc* copy number, DNA index, and serum LDH value and between Shimada classification and N-*myc* copy number have been demonstrated (213,388). In a study by Joshi and colleagues, the low histologic grades 1 and 2 were associated with N-*myc* copy number per haploid genome of 1, DNA index of >1, and serum LDH of >1,500 U/mL, whereas histologic grade 3 was associated with N-*myc* copy number per haploid genome of >1, DNA index of 1, and serum LDH of >1,500 U/mL (213). Shimada et al. (388) have demonstrated the association of high MKI in stroma-poor neuroblastomas with N-*myc* gene amplification.

In a series of 91 cases of neuroblastoma in which a second-look surgery specimen was available, lymphocytic infiltration of the remnant tumor was found to be associated with serum LDH of ≤1,500 U/mL, N-*myc* gene copy number of 1 in samples of tumor obtained before therapy, and better eventual outcome (223) (Fig. 49; see figure in color plate section).

Qualman et al. (347) found correlation between high concentrations of tumor tissue VIP and degree of tumor differentiation. Strong association was observed between age, stage, serum NSE, and serum ferritin by Evans et al. (133). Fong et al. (143) have described correlation between N-*myc* amplification and loss of heterozygosity for chromosome 1p. George and colleagues (153) have demonstrated that successful engraftment of human neuroblastoma in the nude mouse is associated with patient age greater than 2 years, stage III–IV disease, abdominal primary site, patient tumor aneuploidy, high incidence of chromosome 1p abnormalities, unfavorable Shimada histologic pattern, and poor prognosis (5% 3-year patient survival).

Based on the correlation between various prognostic markers, a number of investigators have attempted to divide neuroblastomas into prognostic groups. The German Neuroblastoma Study Group has recognized four risk groups based on stage and N-*myc* amplification: A—localized, almost completely resectable (90–100% survival); B—localized, usually incomplete resection (65–80% survival); C—metastatic, including all N-*myc*-amplified tumors (20–30% survival); and D—stage IVS tumors (75–80% survival) (374). Evans and colleagues (133) have proposed three groups as follows: group 1—normal serum ferritin concentration, age less than 2 years (93% 2-year survival); group 2—normal serum ferritin concentration and age equal to or greater than 2 years (58% 2-year survival); and group 3—high serum ferritin concentration and age greater than 2 years (19% 2-year survival). Silber and colleagues (391) described the correlations between age, Evans stage, serum ferritin, and histopathology. The survival curves derived from the model incorporating all four variables identified three risk groups: low (greater than 90% survival), intermediate (30–70% survival), and high (less than 10% survival). Brodeur and colleagues (63,65) have proposed three biologic subtypes of neuroblastoma with good (greater than 95% survival), intermediate (25–50% survival) and bad (less than 5% survival) outcome based on the combination of the following features: ploidy, loss of heterozygosity for chromosome 1p, N-*myc* copy number, *trk*-A expression, age, and stage. Castleberry (75) has proposed prognostic strata for neuroblastoma therapy based on age, INSS stage, N-*myc* copy number, and DNA index (Table 16).

Therapy and Prognosis of Neuroblastic Tumors

Unfortunately, the majority of patients (60–80%) have advanced stage 3 or 4 disease at the time of diagnosis and only 20–40% of patients have stage 1, 2, or 4S disease. Aggressive measures are required for the management of advanced disease. Cisplatin, teniposide (VM-26), etoposide (VP16), cyclophosphamide, doxorubicin (Adriamycin), carboplatin, ifosfamide, and topotecan are among the chemotherapeutic agents used to treat neuroblastoma. Primary resection of the tumor can be done in stage 1 and 2 disease, but in advanced stages only a biopsy or partial resection may be feasible and the remnant tumor must be resected at second-look surgery. Intraoperative detection of radiolabeled octreotide, a somatostatin analog, may facilitate the staging of neuroblastoma and the detection of disseminated occult disease, resulting in more effective surgical reduction of tumor burden (348). In stage 1 disease no chemotherapy is given after complete gross surgical resection. Radiation therapy may be used in the multimodality management of residual neuroblastoma, bulky unresectable tumors, and disseminated disease. The response to therapy is graded as complete response, very good partial response, partial response, mixed response, no response, and progressive disease, depending on the disappearance of or reduction in size of the primary tumor, metastases, and normal uri-

TABLE 16. *Prognostic strata for neuroblastoma*

Risk category	Age (yr)	INSS stage	N-*myc* copy number	DNA index	Survival
Low	<1	1, 2A, 2B, 3, 4, 4S	1	>1	>90%
	≥1	1, 2A	1	NA	
Intermediate	<1	2B, 3, 4, 4S	1	1	30–50%
	≥1	2B, 3	1	NA	
High	<1	2B, 3, 4, 4S	>1	1 or >1	<20%
	≥1	2B, 3, 4	>1	NA	
	≥1	4	>1	NA	
Unclear	<1	1, 2A	>1	and/or 1	
	≥1	1, 2A	>1	NA	

(Adapted from Castleberry RP, ref. 75; used with permission.)
NA, not applicable.

nary catecholamines (62,64). Other modes of therapy include autologous bone marrow transplantation (134), monoclonal anti-G_{D2} antibody, ^{131}I-MIBG (*meta*-iodobenzylguanidine) therapy (276), immunotherapy with tumor-infiltrating lymphocytes (360), and differentiation therapy with nerve growth factor, retinoic acid, and cyclic nucleotides (378).

The disease-free survival at 2 years in patients with stage 1, 2, 3, 4, and 4S disease is 75–95%, 60–90%, 35–80%, 5–10%, and 75–90%, respectively. Despite dissemination, the prognosis in stage 4S disease is relatively good. Therapy is controversial because there is spontaneous regression of disseminated disease following resection of the primary tumor in about 30% of patients (132). In the report by Haas et al. (171), there was maturation from a poorly differentiated neuroblastoma to ganglioneuroma in serial biopsies of subcutaneous nodules over a period of 76 months without any cytotoxic therapy. Based on the review of 212 cases of stage 4S disease in the literature, Haas found that 13% show progression of the disease and fatal outcome. Therefore, the question of whether stage 4S is a heterogeneous disease has been raised (449). N-*myc* gene copy number and DNA index have been determined in a few cases of stage 4S disease (47,309). Bourhis et al. (47) reported that nine patients with stage 4S disease in whom the tumors showed aneuploidy (DNA index >1) and absence of N-*myc* amplification were free of disease at the end of the follow-up period (1–41 months with a mean of 20 months). In contrast, in three cases with N-*myc* amplification and/or diploidy there was a rapid progression with fatal outcome. Histologic grading has been reported in 18 cases of stage 4S neuroblastoma. Eight tumors were Joshi grade 1 and the remaining cases were grade 2 (210).

NEUROBLASTOMA SCREENING STUDIES

Mass screening programs for neuroblastoma have been performed in Japan for over 20 years (368) and for the past several years in parts of Canada and England (452). Infants have usually been screened at 6 months of age using a qualitative VMA spot test. These studies have yielded a marked increase in the detection of patients with neuroblastoma who were under 1 year of age and had low-stage disease, increased tumor resectability, favorable DNA index, and absence of N-*myc* amplification (65). There are persistent concerns with regard to false-negative screens, however, because the prevalence of neuroblastoma in patients over 1 year of age has not changed (204,318). These findings suggest that mass screening is identifying a substantial number of tumors that would have regressed or matured without therapy (65,305). Recently, the Japanese National Ministry of Health recommended screening by quantitative measurement of VMA, HVA, and creatinine using high-performance liquid chromatography, and a regional protocol for second screening for 18-month-old children has been instituted to rescue false-negative cases (182). Further studies are necessary to determine whether early detection, especially of patients whose tumors have poor prognostic biologic features, will result in a decline in population-based mortality for neuroblastoma (65,452).

PHEOCHROMOCYTOMA

Pheochromocytoma is a neural crest–derived neoplasm originating from the adrenal medulla (Fig. 4). The term was introduced by Pick (341) in 1912 to describe an adrenal medullary tumor that darkened upon exposure to chromate-containing fixatives. The chromaffin reaction is dependent on the oxidation of epinephrine and norepinephrine to adrenochrome pigments. However, the method is relatively insensitive, and many morphologically and functionally indistinguishable tumors of the adrenal medulla and paraganglia show a negative reaction (129,242).

Pheochromocytoma is rare in childhood, as only about 10% of these tumors occur in the pediatric age group (5 months to 19 years). About one third of patients have multiple primary tumors, almost a quarter have bilateral tumors, and 15% have extra-adrenal tumors (or paragangliomas) (77,199,400,432). Overproduction of norepinephrine and epinephrine by the tumor is responsible for most of the characteristic clinical signs and symptoms (438,443), and elevated concentrations of these two hormones in plasma and urine, together with normetanephrine, metanephrine, and VMA in the urine, are diagnostic (145,207,432). In children these neoplasms often secrete more norepinephrine than epinephrine, unlike those in adults (438). Paroxysmal or sustained hypertension and headaches are present in virtually all patients (221). Rarely, patients present without hypertension and are found to have pheochromocytomas that predominantly or exclusively secrete dopamine (227,345). Nausea, vomiting, diaphoresis, palpitations with and without tachycardia, tremors, weakness, fatigue, anxiety, chest and abdominal pain, and visual disturbances are also common clinical manifestations. Weight loss, hypermetabolism, fasting hyperglycemia, and glucosuria also occur. Serious and occasionally fatal complications of untreated pheochromocytomas include myocardial arrhythmias and infarction, cerebral hemorrhage, nephrosclerosis, and retinopathy (51,170, 328,438). Pheochromocytomas may also be associated with polycythemia, increased platelet aggregation, and thrombotic complications. Catecholamine overproduction may result in a distinctive type of cardiomyopathy (202,369). Rarely, these tumors may secrete other hormones in quantities sufficient to produce other neuroendocrine syndromes. Cases of ACTH and VIP overproduction resulting in Cushing's syndrome and watery diarrhea syndrome, respectively, have been reported (241,251,398). On occasion, pheochromocytomas may also secrete *leu-* and *met*-enkephalin, endorphins, somatostatin, prostaglandins, and calcitonin (117,184, 241,266). Plasma chromogranin A concentrations are elevated in patients with pheochromocytoma and provide a sensitive and specific method for detecting both familial and sporadic tumors (197). Pheochromocytomas may uncommonly present with no clinical hormonal syndromes (170). Computed tomography (77, 185,362,432), magnetic resonance imaging (120,139, 221), and ^{131}I-MIBG scintigraphy (77,226,340) can be used to detect occult as well as overt tumors.

Familial pheochromocytoma has, in most cases, an autosomal dominant inheritance pattern with variable penetrance and expressivity (242). Patients with familial tumors tend to be younger at onset than those with nonfamilial tumors and are more apt to have bilateral and multifocal tumors (241). Pheochromocytomas and multiple paragangliomas are described in families (331), and there is a relationship between congenital heart disease and familial pheochromocytoma (115). Pheochromocytoma occurs as part of the multiple endocrine neoplasia (MEN) 2 syndromes (66,67,166,241,328,357, 436,438) (Table 17). In the type 2a variant, pheochromocytomas are associated with medullary thyroid carcinoma and parathyroid hyperplasia or adenomas. In type 2b, they are also associated with medullary thyroid carcinoma and mucosal ganglioneuromas, particularly of the lips and tongue, intestinal ganglioneuromatosis, and a marfanoid habitus (72,73). Diffuse or nodular adrenal medullary hyperplasia is thought to precede the development of pheochromocytoma in the MEN 2 syndromes (71,243). Criteria for the diagnosis of medullary hyperplasia include the demonstration of increased medullary volume as determined morphometrically and extension of the medulla into the tail and alar regions of the gland (71,241,243,328). Adrenal medullary hyperplasia and the presence of S-100 protein–positive sustentacular cells are unique morphologic features of familial or hereditary pheochromocytomas (260) and may be used to differentiate them from sporadic lesions (349).

Recently, the genes responsible for MEN 2a and 2b have been localized to chromosome 10q11.2 by genetic and physical mapping (245,277,321,395). The affected DNA segment encompasses the *ret* proto-oncogene (*RE*arranged during *T*ransfection), a transmembrane receptor tyrosine kinase gene that is expressed in neuroblastoma, medullary thyroid carcinoma, and pheochromocytoma (314,366). Dominantly acting point mutations in the gene cause neoplasia in endocrine organs (128,192,303,367) and are associated with the aganglionosis of Hirschsprung's disease (274). The gene for MEN 1 has also been localized, in this instance by tumor deletion mapping and family linkage studies, to chromosome 11q13 (247). Like the putative neuroblastoma gene, this gene most likely acts as a tumor suppressor gene, the allelic loss of which may initiate tumor development (248). There is also an increased incidence of pheochromocytomas in neurofibromatosis type 1, tuberous sclerosis, ataxiatelangiectasia, and von

TABLE 17. *Multiple Endocrine Neoplasia (MEN) syndromes*

Feature	MEN 1	MEN 2a	MEN 2b
Pituitary hyperplasia or adenoma with acromegaly, hyperprolactinemia, or hypopituitarism	+	−	−
Parathyroid hyperplasia, adenoma, multiple adenomas, or carcinoma with hyperparathyroidism	++	+	−
Pancreatic hyperplasia, adenoma, or carcinoma, with hypersecretion of insulin, glucagon, gastrin, somatostatin, vasoactive intestinal peptide, or pancreatic polypeptide	+	−	−
Thyroid adenoma, carcinoma, thyrotoxicosis, colloid goiter, thyroiditis	±	−	−
Bronchial, thymic, and intestinal carcinoid tumors	±	−	−
Multiple lipomas	±	−	−
Adrenal cortical adenoma	±	−	−
Schwannoma	±	−	−
Pineal parenchymal tumors	±	−	−
Colonic aganglionosis (Hirschsprung's disease)	−	±	−
Cutaneous lichen amyloidosis	−	+	−
Thyroid C-cell hyperplasia/medullary carcinoma	−	++	++
Adrenal medullary hyperplasia/pheochromocytoma	−	++	++
Extra-adrenal paraganglioma	−	+	+
Mucosal ganglioneuromas of lips, tongue, and eyelids	−	−	+
Gastrointestinal ganglioneuromatosis	−	−	+
Marfanoid habitus	−	−	+

Hippel–Lindau disease (cerebelloretinal hemangioblastomatosis) (20,208,243,308,316,328).

Loss of heterozygosity for chromosome 1p is universally present in pheochromocytomas from MEN 2a and MEN 2b patients, but is less common in sporadic pheochromocytomas (455). The common breakpoint is 1p32. Loss of heterozygosity has also been reported with significant frequency for chromosomes 3, 17, and 22. These three chromosomes harbor the genes for von Hippel–Lindau disease, neurofibromatosis type 1, and hereditary acoustic neuroma (neurofibromatosis type 2), respectively. Pheochromocytomas have not been reported in patients with neurofibromatosis type 2 (315).

Compound adrenal medullary tumor (composite pheochromocytoma) is an unusual neoplasm in which there are components of pheochromocytoma, neuroblastoma, ganglioneuroblastoma, and/or ganglioneuroma (7,24,88,215,237,241,243,416). Although quite rare, these tumors should not be unexpected, given the common neural crest origin of ganglion cells of the sympathetic ganglia and pheochromocytes of the adrenal medulla (96) (Fig. 4). Such tumors are typically discovered in middle-aged individuals, sometimes in association with neurophakomatosis syndromes (237), with symptoms related to excess catecholamine secretion (7,241,416), or with watery diarrhea syndrome (423). However, three examples in children have been described. Wahl and Robinson (440) reported a mediastinal tumor with neuroblastic and pheochromocytic foci and neuroblastic cervical lymph node metastases in a 4-year-old boy. The second case was a young girl with a large cystic adrenal mass that showed a spectrum of medullary differentiation (111). A third such tumor has been reported in a 14-year-old girl with neurofibromatosis who had bilateral adrenal involvement and widespread metastases (308). Composite pheochromocytoma and malignant peripheral nerve sheath tumors have been reported in adults (286,291).

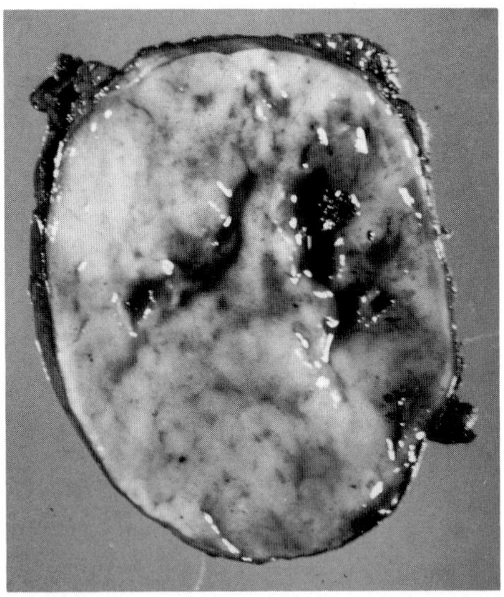

FIG. 50. Right adrenal pheochromocytoma (6 cm, 31 g) from a 9-year-old male with a 1-year history of night sweats, intermittent hypertension, and skin rash. An adrenal pheochromocytoma was surgically excised from the child's father at age 17 years.

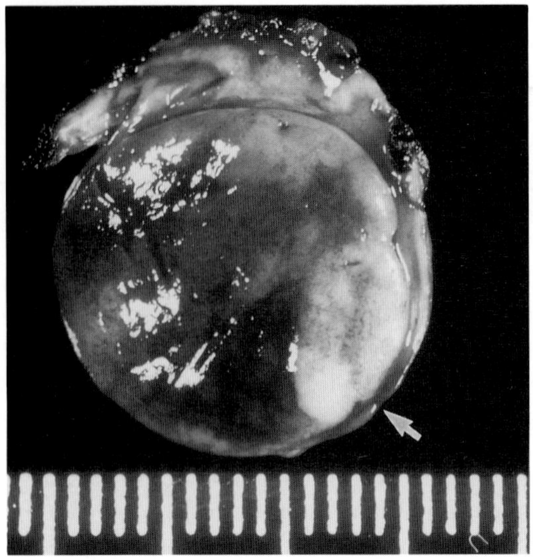

FIG. 51. Left adrenal pheochromocytoma (1.5 cm, 7.5 g) removed from the same patient 2 years later. Note the narrow rim of residual adrenal cortex *(arrow)*.

Most pheochromocytomas are round, apparently encapsulated masses that are 3–5 cm in diameter and weigh less than 100 g (328) (Fig. 50). They usually arise in the head or body area of the adrenal and may be single or multiple. The right adrenal is more often involved with tumor than the left. Cut surfaces have a gray–pink to tan color and soft consistency. As in neuroblastoma, a rim of bright yellow adrenal cortex may be seen at the periphery (Fig. 51). Hemorrhage, myxoid change, necrosis, calcification, and cyst formation are frequent in large tumors (170). The characteristic microscopic pattern is one of solid round cell aggregates (zellballen), trabeculae, or ribbons separated by a reticulin-rich fibrovascular stroma (243) (Fig. 52). Elongated sustentacular cells may surround the tumor cell aggregates. The tumor cells are polyhedral with round to oval vesicular nuclei, coarsely clumped chromatin, and a single nucleolus. The cytoplasm is granular, rarely vacuolated, and eosinophilic or basophilic (Fig. 53). Nuclear pseudoinclusions of invaginated cytoplasm are found in some cells. Other tumor cells display PAS-positive cytoplasmic inclusions. Excessive intracytoplasmic lipid accumulation may simulate an adrenocortical tumor (349). Pigmented pheochromocytomas have also been described (87,252).

The methods for demonstrating catecholamines in tissues include glyoxylic acid– and formaldehyde-induced fluorescence and immunohistochemical techniques

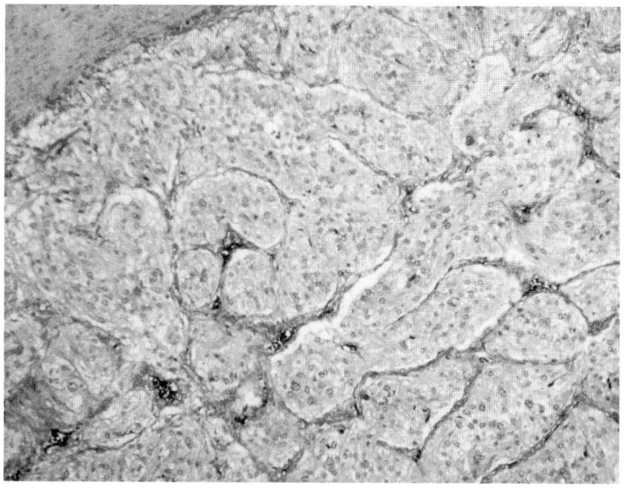

FIG. 52. Characteristic nesting pattern (zellballen) of pheochromocytoma.

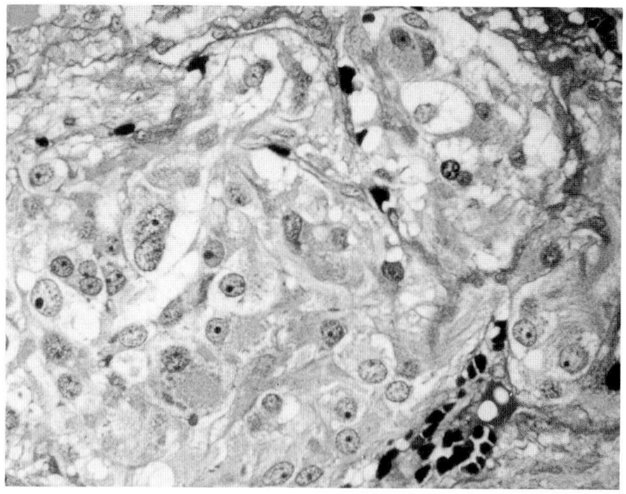

FIG. 53. Clusters of polyhedral tumor cells with granular cytoplasm and single prominent nucleolus in pheochromocytoma.

(116,135,227,261). Most pheochromocytomas show immunoreactivity with antibodies to NSE, chromogranin A, synaptophysin, Leu 7, and neurofilaments (147,164, 243,260,285). Neuropeptides including calcitonin, VIP, ACTH, bombesin, somatostatin, and some catecholamine-synthesizing enzymes may also be detected immunohistochemically, regardless of clinical manifestations (129,184,227,241,266). Insulinlike growth factor (IGF)–II immunoreactivity is expressed in normal (adrenal and retroperitoneal) and neoplastic (adrenal and extra-adrenal) paraganglionic tissues (405). Pheochromocytes express high concentrations of tumoral (but not plasma) IGF-II and both type I and type II receptors, suggesting that IGF-II may act through both receptors to alter tumor growth (152). The Schwann-like sustentacular cells express vimentin and S-100 protein (129,170,241).

Ultrastructurally, abundant neurosecretory granules ranging from 330 to 550 nm are seen. Norepinephrine-storing granules tend to predominate. They have highly electron-dense granules with eccentric cores and crescent-shaped halos (Fig. 54). The smaller epinephrine-storing granules (165 nm) have less dense, finely granular matrix and no circumferential lucent zones. Pleomorphic rod- or comma-shaped granules of variable size (110 x 360 nm) and density, consistent with storage of other materials, are also prominent in most tumors. Inconspicuous desmosomelike junctions, interdigitating contiguous cell membranes, arrays of microtubules, and intranuclear cytoplasmic extensions are also encountered. Spindle-shaped, Schwann-like sustentacular cells devoid of neurosecretory granules and axons are rarely identified (129).

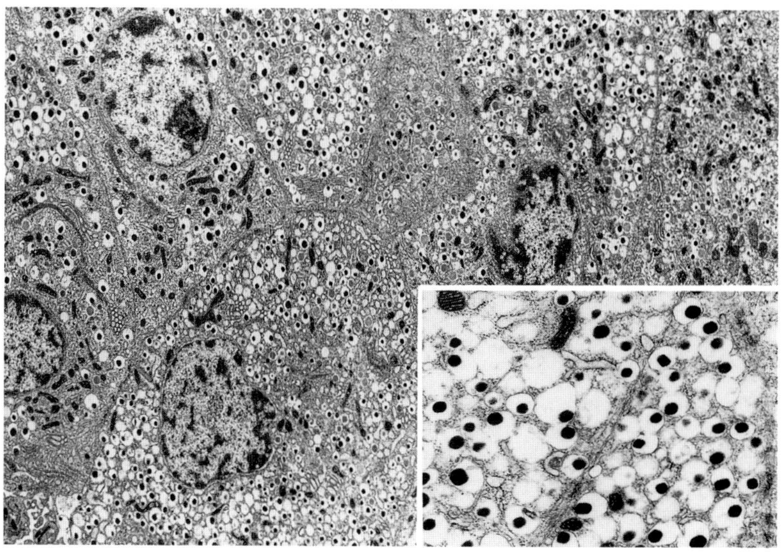

FIG. 54. Pheochromocytoma shows interdigitating cell processes and numerous "norepinephrine-type" granules with a prominent eccentric electron-dense core, crescent-shaped lucent space, and limiting membrane. (Uranyl acetate and lead citrate, x1910; inset: x11,000.) (Courtesy of Dr. Guillermo Herrera, University of Alabama at Birmingham, Birmingham, AL.)

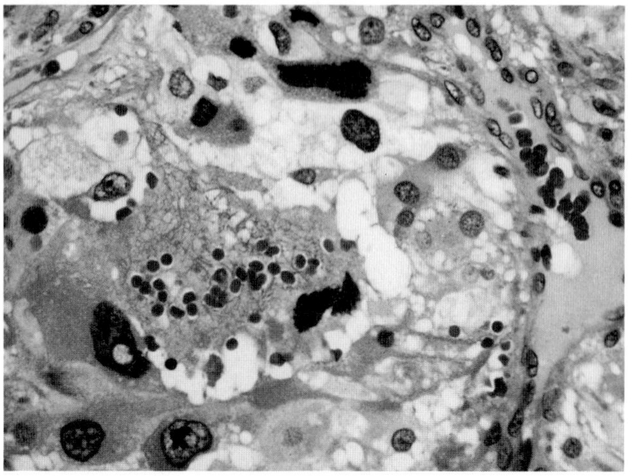

FIG. 55. Nuclear pleomorphism in a nonmetastasizing pheochromocytoma.

Recurrences, distant metastases, and development of pheochromocytoma in the remaining adrenal are more frequent in patients with a family history of this or related tumors (226,433). Malignant pheochromocytomas, however, are very rare in children (124,270). In sporadic cases, malignant potential is more likely to be associated with the large tumor size than with cellular pleomorphism or capsular invasion. Nuclear pleomorphism and atypia may be considerable (Fig. 55), and focal vascular invasion or rare mitoses may be encountered; but none of these features are predictive of malignant behavior (170). Helpful but not absolute features include extensive necrosis, small tumor cell size, and abundant mitoses (270,328). Pathologic demonstration of tumor in an area where chromaffin tissue does not normally exist or a clinical course characterized by recurrence or metastases of the tumor are the only

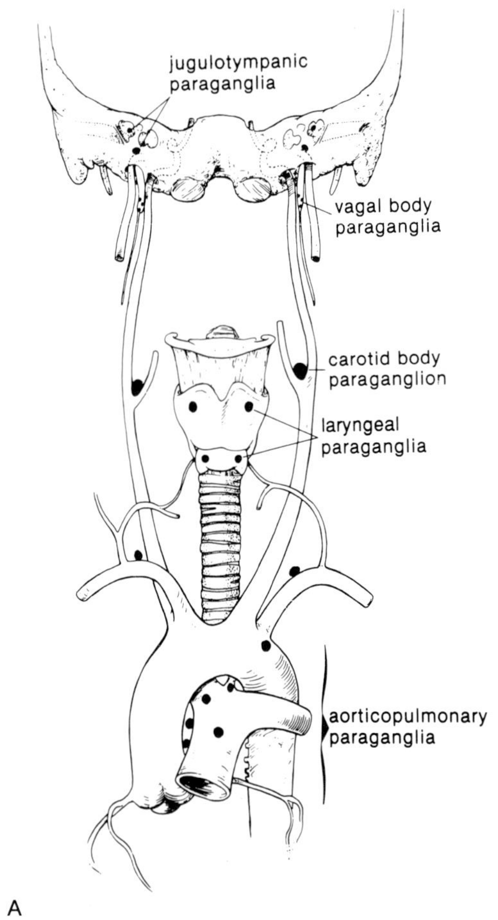

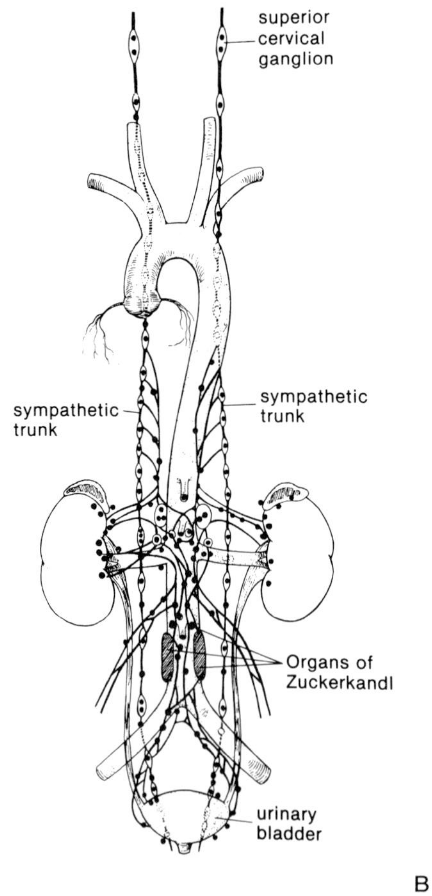

FIG. 56. A. Anatomic distribution of paraganglia in the head and neck region including base of the heart. Carotid bodies are the largest compact collection of paraganglia. (Used with permission (242).) **B.** Anatomic distribution of sympathoadrenal neuroendocrine system with adrenal medullae representing the largest compact collections of paraganglia in adults. Multiple extra-adrenal paraganglia along the lower part of the aorta represent organs of Zuckerkandl. (Adapted from Coupland RE. (99), used with permission.)

certain means of establishing malignancy (270). Bone, liver, lymph nodes, lung, pleura, and brain are the usual metastatic sites (328). Dense infiltration of tumors by HLA-DR (Ia)–antigen-positive dendritic cells in patients who have high urinary or serum catecholamine concentrations has been suggested as a favorable prognostic feature (149).

The treatment of pheochromocytoma is surgical, with careful intraoperative management to avoid cardiac arrhythmias and blood pressure instability (10,125, 126,362,429). Lifelong follow-up of all patients is mandatory (433).

PARAGANGLIOMA

While tumors arising from adrenal medullary pheochromocytes are designated as "pheochromocytomas," similar neoplasms originating from the extra-adrenal paraganglia are called "paragangliomas." Functional paraganglionic tumors are uncommon and are often called "extra-adrenal pheochromocytomas." Extra-adrenal paraganglia originate from cells of the neural crest and are classified into four main groups, emphasizing their anatomic distribution (Fig. 56). The branchiomeric paraganglia consist of carotid bodies, jugulotympanic paraganglia, and other cranial, cervical, and mediastinal paraganglia. Intravagal paraganglia (vagal body) are situated below the perineurium along the vagus nerve. Aorticosympathetic paraganglia extend from the aortic arch to the bladder and include the superior cervical paraganglion, abdominal preaortic paraganglia, and the organ(s) of Zuckerkandl. Visceral-autonomic paraganglia consist of poorly definedvisceral-associated paraganglia (e.g., bladder, duodenum, gallbladder, thyroid, etc.) (129,159,242,243).

The incidence of extra-adrenal sites of origin in pheochromocytoma/paraganglioma is approximately 10% in

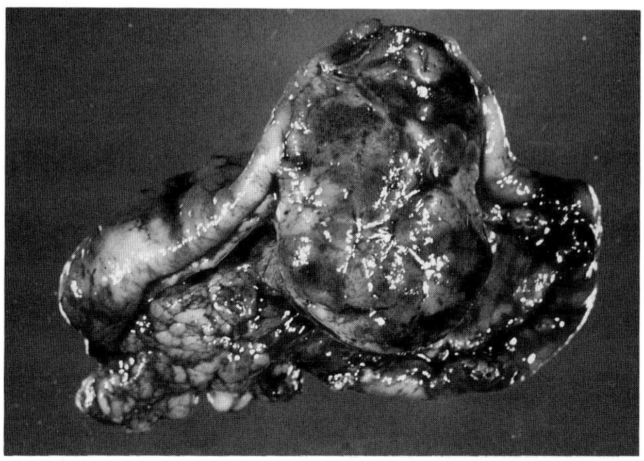

FIG. 57. Gastric paraganglioma (3 cm) in a 12-year-old female who presented with gastrointestinal bleeding and anemia.

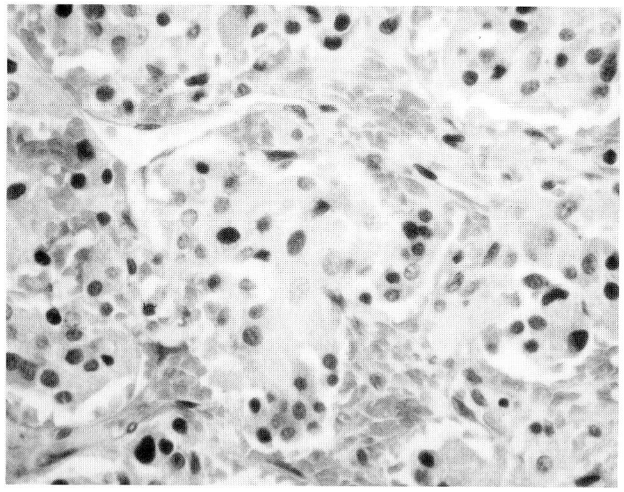

FIG. 58. Small nests of rounded tumor cells surrounded by hemorrhage in gastric paraganglioma.

adults and 25% in children (340). While 90–95% of these tumors in children arise in the retroperitoneum and abdominal cavity, they may occur anywhere from the base of the skull to the bladder (179,432) (Fig. 57). Paragangliomas in children are more often multicentric and familial (7–9% of cases) than those occurring in adults (160,325). Multiple paragangliomas are one manifestation of Carney's triad (1,17,70) (gastric epithelioid leiomyosarcoma, pulmonary chondroma, paraganglioma), which is found primarily in young girls.

Most tumors appear well circumscribed but poorly encapsulated. They have a tan to red–brown color and measure from 1–3 cm in greatest dimension. The average diameter is dependent to some extent on the primary site. Polygonal to ovoid chief cells with clear to granular cytoplasm and smaller, less conspicuous sustentacular cells are arranged in anastomosing cell cords, sheets, or spindle cell or organoid nests (zellballen) (242,243) (Fig. 58). There may be considerable variation in nuclear size and shape with marked pleomorphism. A conspicuously hemorrhagic stroma is present in some tumors, occasionally to such a degree that the underlying pathology may be obscured.

Ultrastructurally, neurosecretory granules are less conspicuous in extra-adrenal paragangliomas than in pheochromocytomas. They are distributed diffusely throughout the cytoplasm of the chief cells, located in the ectoplasm or clustered in cytoplasmic processes. Virtually all of the dense core granules have a distinct but narrow halo and a diameter of 100–400 nm (average 140 nm) (Fig. 59). Synapses are frequent between chief cells and axons. Large atypical mitochondria are common and often abundant. Rudimentary cell junctions, long cytoplasmic processes that envelope adjacent chief cells, and thin basal lamina are other ultrastructural features (129,230).

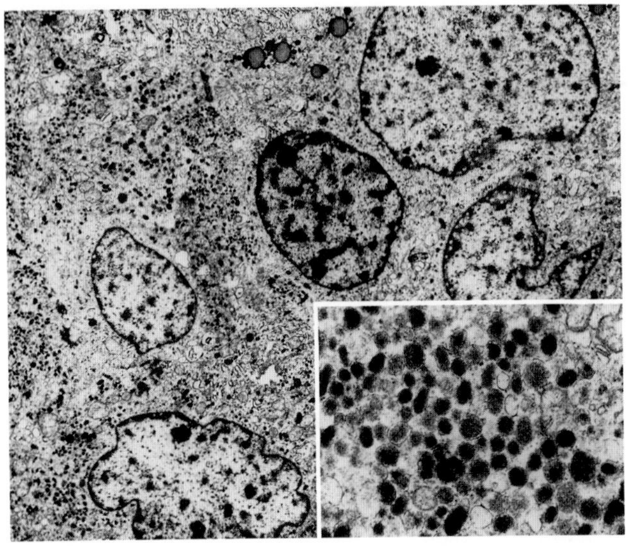

FIG. 59. Paraganglioma demonstrates abundant "epinephrine-type" granules (uranyl acetate and lead citrate, x4400; inset: x12,900). (Courtesy of Dr. Guillermo Herrera, University of Alabama at Birmingham, Birmingham, AL.)

Paragangliomas are immunoreactive for NSE, serotonin, chromogranin, synaptophysin, and S-100 protein, and occasionally for GFAP, bombesin, *leu-* and *met*-enkephalins, VIP, somatostatin, protein gene product (PGP) 9.5, and catecholamine-synthesizing enzymes (2,129,227,230,243) (Fig. 60; see figure in color plate section).

The prognosis is excellent in most instances, but local recurrences develop in 5–10% of cases (340). Malignant behavior is uncommon (228), especially among the familial paragangliomas (160), but as with pheochromocytomas, is impossible to predict. Although surgical excision of paraganglioma is the treatment of choice, radiotherapy may be indicated in patients with locally advanced or surgically inaccessible disease.

COMMENT

There is a wide spectrum of childhood neural crest-derived neoplasms. Many are hormonally active and produce unique signs and symptoms that facilitate diagnosis. Pheochromocytomas and paragangliomas are uncommon, and most are, fortunately, benign. Of all the pediatric malignancies, neuroblastoma poses the greatest challenge in terms achieving a high cure rate, due largely to the high frequency of dissemination of the disease at presentation. In recent years, great advances have been made in understanding the biology of neuroblastoma. The development of more effective modes of therapy, utilizing novel agents, e.g., differentiation therapy, autologous bone marrow transplantation, cytokines (360), and viral therapy (265), remains one of the most important avenues of research. Brodeur and Castleberry (65) have suggested that improvements in the management of patients with neuroblastoma will also come from the development of mass screening strategies for the early detection of high-risk patients, identification of individuals with genetic predisposition to develop disease, and the discovery of better morphologic, biologic, and immunologic markers that can be related to prognosis.

REFERENCES

1. Acha T, Picazo B, Garcia-Martin FJ, Urda A, Campos J. Carney's triad: apropos of a new case. *Med Pediatr Oncol* 1994;22:216–220.
2. Achilles E, Padberg BC, Holl K, Kloppel G, Schroder S. Immunocytochemistry of paragangliomas—value of staining for S-100 protein and glial fibrillary acidic protein in diagnosis and prognosis. *Histopathology* 1991;18:453–458.
3. Adam A, Hochholzer L. Ganglioneuroblastoma of the posterior mediastinum: a clinicopathologic review of 80 cases. *Cancer* 1981;47:373–381.
4. Adams GA, Shochat SJ, Smith EI, et al. Thoracic neuroblastoma: a Pediatric Oncology Group study. *J Pediatr Surg* 1993;28:372–376.
5. Adams JA, Kelsey AM, Carr TF, Stevens RF, Morris-Jones P. Detection of bone marrow metastases in neuroblastoma using a short term tissue culture technique. *J Clin Pathol* 1992;45:424–426.
6. Aguirre P, Scully RE. Testosterone-secreting adrenal ganglioneuroma containing Leydig cells. *Am J Surg Pathol* 1983;7:699–705.
7. Aiba M, Hirayama A, Ito Y, et al. A compound adrenal medullary tumor (pheochromocytoma and ganglioneuroma) and a cortical adenoma in the ipsilateral adrenal gland. A case report with enzyme histochemical and immunohistochemical studies. *Am J Surg Pathol* 1988;12:559–566.
8. Akhtar M, Ali MA, Sabbah RS, Bakry M, Sackey K, Nash EJ. Aspiration cytology of neuroblastoma. Light and electron microscopic correlations. *Cancer* 1986;57:797–803.
9. Akhtar M, Ali MA, Sackey K, et al. Aspiration cytology of neuroblastoma. Light microscopy with transmission and scanning electron microscopic correlations. *Diagn Cytopathol* 1988;4:323–327.
10. Albanese CT, Wiener ES. Routine total bilateral adrenalectomy is not warranted in childhood familial pheochromocytoma. *J Pediatr Surg* 1993;28:1248–1252.
11. Albregts AE, Cohen MD, Galliani CA. Neuroblastoma invading the kidney. *J Pediatr Surg* 1994;29:930–933.
12. Aleshire SL, Glick AD, Cruz VE, Bradley CA, Parl FF. Neuroblastoma in adults. Pathologic findings and clinical outcome. *Arch Pathol Lab Med* 1985;109:352–356.
13. Allan SG, Cornbleet MA, Carmichael J, Arnott SJ, Smyth JF. Adult neuroblastoma. Report of three cases and review of the literature. *Cancer* 1986;57:2419–2421.
14. Altman AJ, Baehner RL. Favorable prognosis for survival in children with coincident opso-myoclonus and neuroblastoma. *Cancer* 1976;37:846–852.
15. Ando S. Gangliosides in the nervous system. *Neurochem Int* 1983;5:507–537.
16. Aoyama C, Qualman SJ, Regan M, Shimada H. Histopathologic features of composite ganglioneuroblastoma. Immunohistochemical distinction of the stromal component is related to prognosis. *Cancer* 1990;65:255–264.
17. Argos MD, Ruiz A, Sanchez F, Garcia C, Gaztambide J. Gastric leiomyoblastoma associated with extraadrenal paraganglioma and pulmonary chrondroma: a new case of Carney's triad. *J Pediatr Surg* 1993;28:1545–1549.
18. Artlieb U, Krepler R, Wiche G. Expression of microtubule-associated proteins, Map-1 and Map-2, in human neuroblasto-

mas and differential diagnosis of immature neuroblasts. *Lab Invest* 1985;53:684–691.
19. Atkinson GO Jr, Zaatari GS, Lorenzo RL, Gay BB Jr, Garvin AJ. Cystic neuroblastoma in infants: radiographic and pathologic features. *AJR* 1986;146:113–117.
20. Atuk NO, McDonald T, Wood T, et al. Familial pheochromocytoma, hypercalcemia, and von Hippel-Lindau disease. A ten year study of a large family. *Medicine (Baltimore)* 1979;58:209–218.
21. Azzopardi JG. Oat cell carcinoma of the bronchus. *J Pathol Bacteriol* 1959;78:513–519.
22. Bader JL, Miller RW. US cancer incidence and mortality in the first year of life. *Am J Dis Child* 1979:133:157–159.
23. Balaban-Malenbaum G, Gilbert F. Relationship between homogeneously staining regions and double minute chromosomes in human neuroblastoma cell lines. *Prog Cancer Res Ther* 1980;12: 97–107.
24. Balázs M. Mixed pheochromocytoma and ganglioneuroma of the adrenal medulla: a case report with electron microscopic examination. *Hum Pathol* 1988;19:1352–1355.
25. Banks E, Yum M, Brodhecker C, Goheen M. A malignant peripheral nerve sheath tumor in association with a paratesticular ganglioneuroma. *Cancer* 1989;64:1738–1742.
26. Bates SE, Mickley LA, Chen Y-N, et al. Expression of a drug resistance gene in human neuroblastoma cell lines: modulation by retinoic acid-induced differentiation. *Mol Cell Biol* 1989;9:4337–4344.
27. Bates SE, Shieh CY, Tsokos M. Expression of *mdr*-1/P-glycoprotein in human neuroblastoma. *Am J Pathol* 1991;139:305–315.
28. Bayle C, Allard T, Rodary C, Vanderplancke J, Hartman O, Lemerle J. Detection of bone marrow involvement by neuroblastoma: comparison of two cytological methods. *Eur Pediatr Hematol Oncol* 1985;2:123–128.
29. Beckwith JB. Neuroblastoma and related tumors. In: Henson DE, Albores-Saavedra J, eds. *Pathology of incipient neoplasia.* 2nd ed. Philadelphia: WB Saunders; 1993:435–441.
30. Beckwith JB, Perrin EV. In situ neuroblastomas: a contribution to the natural history of neural crest tumors. *Am J Pathol* 1963;43:1089–1104.
31. Beckwith JB, Martin RF. Observations on the histopathology of neuroblastomas. *J Pediatr Surg* 1968;3:106–110.
32. Behr A, Uijs RR, Phillips JI. Neuroblastoma in adults. A report of 3 cases. *S Afr Med J* 1989;75:333–335.
33. Benard J, Bourhis J, de Vathaire, et al. Prognostic value of *MDR1* gene expression in neuroblastoma: results of multivariate analysis. In: Evans AE, Biedler JL, Brodeur GM, D'Angio GJ, Nakagawara A, eds. *Advances in Neuroblastoma Research.* New York: Wiley-Liss; 1994:4:111–116.
34. Bender BL, Ghatak NR. Light and electron microscopic observations on a ganglioneuroma. *Acta Neuropathol (Berl)* 1978;42:7–10.
35. Berthold F, Utsch S, Holschneider AM. The impact of preoperative chemotherapy on resectability of primary tumor and complication rate in metastatic neuroblastoma. *Z Kinderchir* 1989;44: 21–24.
36. Biedler JL, Ross RA, Shanske S, Spengler BA. Human neuroblastoma cytogenetics: search for significance of homogeneously staining regions and double minute chromosomes. *Prog Cancer Res Ther* 1980;12:81–96.
37. Biegel JA, White PS, Marshall HN, et al. Constitutional 1p36 deletion in a child with neuroblastoma. *Am J Hum Genet* 1993;52: 176–182.
38. Bjelfman C, Hedborg F, Johansson I, Nordenskjold M, Pahlmans S. Expression of the neuronal form of pp60c-*src* in neuroblastoma in relation to clinical stage and prognosis. *Cancer Res* 1990;50:6908–6914.
39. Boerner S, Squire J, Thorner P, McKenna G, Zielenska M. Assessment of *MYCN* amplification in neuroblastoma biopsies by differential polymerase chain reaction. *Pediatr Pathol* 1994;14: 823–832.
40. Bolande RP. Spontaneous regression and cytodifferentiation of cancer in early life: the oncogenic grace period. *Surv Synth Pathol Res* 1985;44:296–311.
41. Bolande RP. A natural immune system in pregnancy serum lethal to human neuroblastoma cells: a possible mechanism of spontaneous regression. In: Garvin AJ, O'Leary TJ, Bernstein J, Rosenberg HS, eds. *Pediatric molecular pathology: quantitation and applications. Perspect Pediatr Pathol* 1992;16:120–133.
42. Bolande RP, Towler WF. A possible relationship of neuroblastoma and von Recklinghausen's disease. *Cancer* 1970;26: 162–175.
43. Boon ME, Kok LP, Moorlag HE, Gerrits PO, Suurmeijer AJH. Microwave-stimulated staining of plastic embedded bone marrow sections with the Romanowsky–Giemsa stain: improved staining patterns. *Stain Technol* 1987;62:257–264.
44. Bordow SB, Haber M, Madafiglio J, Cheung B, Marshall GM, Norris MD. Expression of the multidrug resistance-associated protein (*MRP*) gene correlates with amplification and overexpression of the N-*myc* oncogene in childhood neuroblastoma. *Cancer Res* 1994;54:5036–5040.
45. Bostrom B, Nesbit ME, Brunning RD. The value of bone marrow trephine biopsy in the dignosis of metastatic neuroblastoma. *Am J Pediatr Hematol Oncol* 1985;7:303–305.
46. Bourhis J, Benard J, Hartmann O, Boccon-Gibod L, Lemerle J, Riou G. Correlation of *MDR1* gene expression with chemotherapy in neuroblastoma. *JNCI* 1989;81:1401–1405.
47. Bourhis J, Dominici C, McDowell H, et al. N-*myc* genomic content and DNA ploidy in stage IV-S neuroblastoma. *J Clin Oncol* 1991;9:1371–1375.
48. Bove KE, McAdams AJ. Composite ganglioneuroblastoma. An assessment of the significance of histological maturation in neuroblastoma diagnosed beyond infancy. *Arch Pathol Lab Med* 1981;105:325–330.
49. Bower RJ, Adkins JC. Ondine's curse and neurocristopathy. *Clin Pediatr* 1980;19:665–668.
50. Bown N, Reid MM, Pearson ADJ, Davison EV, Malcolm AJ, Craft AW. Cytogenetic investigations in the assessment of response to treatment in neuroblastoma. *J Clin Pathol* 1987;40: 1334–1336.
51. Bravo EL, Gifford RW. Pheochromocytoma: diagnosis, localization, and management. *N Engl J Med* 1984;311:1984.
52. Breslow N, McCann B. Statistical estimation of prognosis for children with neuroblastoma. *Cancer Res* 1971;31:2098–2103.
53. Brinster RL. The effect of cells transferred into the mouse blastocyst on subsequent development. *J Exp Med* 1974;140:1049–1056.
54. Brock CE, Ricketts RR. Hemoperitoneum from spontaneous rupture of neonatal neuroblastoma. *Am J Dis Child* 1982;136: 370–371.
55. Brodeur GM. Neuroblastoma—clinical applications of molecular parameters. *Brain Pathol* 1990;1:47–54.
56. Brodeur G. Molecular biology and genetics of human neuroblastoma. In: Pochedly C, ed. *Neuroblastoma: Tumor Biology and Therapy.* Boca Raton, FL: CRC Press; 1990:31–50.
57. Brodeur GM. *trk*-A expression in neuroblastomas: a new prognostic marker with biological and clinical significance. *JNCI* 3;85:344–345.
58. Brodeur GM, Sekhon GS, Goldstein MN. Chromosomal aberrations in human neuroblastomas. *Cancer* 1977;40:2256–2263.
59. Brodeur GM, Green AA, Hayes FA, Williams KJ, Williams DL, Tsiatis AA. Cytogenetic features of human neuroblastomas and cell lines. *Cancer Res* 1981;41:4678–4686.
60. Brodeur GM, Seeger RC, Schwab M, Varmus HE, Bishop JM. Amplification of N-*myc* in untreated human neuroblastomas correlates with advanced disease stage. *Science* 1984;224:1121–1124.
61. Brodeur GM, Hayes FA, Green AA, et al. Consistent N-*myc* copy number in simultaneous or consecutive neuroblastoma samples from 60 individual patients. *Cancer Res* 1987;47:4248–4253.
62. Brodeur GM, Seeger RC, Barrett A, et al. International criteria for diagnosis, staging and response to treatment in patients with neuroblastoma. *J Clin Oncol* 1988;6:1874–1881.
63. Brodeur GM, Azar C, Brother M, et al. Neuroblastoma. Effect of genetic factors on prognosis and treatment. *Cancer* 1992;70: 1685–1694.
64. Brodeur GM, Pritchard J, Berthold F, et al. Revisions of the international criteria for neuroblastoma diagnosis, staging, and response to treatment. *J Clin Oncol* 1993;11:1466–1477.
65. Brodeur GM, Castleberry RP. Neuroblastoma. In: Pizzo PA,

regulation of $\alpha v\beta 5$ as neuroblastoma cells differentiate in vivo. *Am J Pathol*; in press.
159. Glenner GG, Grimley PM. *Tumors of the Extra-adrenal Paraganglion System (Including Chemoreceptors): Atlas of Tumor Pathology.* Second Series, Fascicle 9. Washington, DC: Armed Forces Institute of Pathology; 1974.
160. Glowniak JV, Shapiro B, Sisson JC, et al. Familial extra-adrenal pheochromocytoma. A new syndrome. *Arch Intern Med* 1985;145:257–261.
161. Gohji K, Nakanishi T, Hara I, Hamami G, Kamidono S. Two cases of primary neuroblastoma of the kidney in adults. *J Urol* 1987;137:966–968.
162. Goldstein LJ, Fojo AT, Ueda K, et al. Expression of the multidrug resistance, MDR1, gene in neuroblastoma. *J Clin Oncol* 1990;8: 128–136.
163. Gonzalez-Crussi F, Hsueh W. Bilateral adrenal ganglioneuroblastoma with neuromelanin. Clinical and pathologic observations. *Cancer* 1988;61:1159–1166.
164. Gould VE, Lee I, Weidenmann B, Moll R, Chejfec G, Franke WW. Synaptophysin: a novel marker for neurons, certain neuroendocrine cells, and their neoplasms. *Hum Pathol* 1986;17:979–983.
165. Gown AM, de Wever N, Battifora H. Microwave–based antigenic unmasking. A revolutionary new technique for routine immunohistochemistry. *Appl Immunohistochem* 1993;1:256–266.
166. Granner DK, Lee FJ. The multiple endocrine neoplasia syndromes. In: Moosa AR, Robson MC, Schimpff SC, eds. *Comprehensive Textbook of Oncology.* Baltimore: Williams & Wilkins; 1986:815–825.
167. Greenfield LJ, Shelley WM. The spectrum of neurogenic tumours of the sympathetic nervous system: maturation and adrenergic function. *JNCI* 1965;35:215–226.
168. Griffin ME, Bolande RP. Familial neuroblastoma with regression and maturation to ganglioneurofibroma. *Pediatrics* 1969;43: 377–382.
169. Gross N, Beretta C, Peruisseau G, Jackson D, Simmons D, Beck D. CD44H expression by human neuroblastoma cells: relation to MYN amplification and lineage differentiation. *Cancer Res* 1994;54:4238–4242.
170. Gruhn JG, Gould VE. The adrenal glands. In: Kissane JM, ed. *Anderson's Pathology.* 9th ed. St. Louis: CV Mosby; 1990:1608–1611.
171. Haas D, Ablin AR, Miller C, Zoger S, Matthay KK. Complete pathologic maturation and regression of stage IVS neuroblastoma without treatment. *Cancer* 1988;62:818–825.
172. Hachitanda Y, Tsuneyoshi M, Enjoji M. An ultrastructural and immunohistochemical evaluation of cytodifferentiation in neuroblastic tumors. *Mod Pathol* 1989;2:13–19.
173. Hachitanda Y, Tsuneyoshi M, Enjoji M. Expression of panneuroendocrine proteins in 53 neuroblastic tumors. An immunohistochemical study with neuron-specific enolase, chromogranin, and synaptophysin. *Arch Pathol Lab Med* 1989;113:381–384.
174. Hachitanda Y, Tsuneyoshi M. Neuroblastoma with a distinct organoid pattern: a clinicopathologic, immunohistochemical, and ultrastructural study. *Hum Pathol* 1994;25:67–72.
175. Hahn JF, Netsky MG, Butler AB, Sperber EE. Pigmented ganglioneuroblastoma: relation of melanin and lipofuscin to schwannomas and other tumors of neural crest origin. *J Neuropathol Exp Neurol* 1976;35:393–403.
176. Hailat N, Keim DR, Melham RF, et al. High levels of p19/*nm*23 protein in neuroblastoma are associated with advanced stage disease and with N-myc gene amplification. *J Clin Invest* 1991;88: 341–345.
177. Hann H-WL, Levy HM, Evans AE. Serum ferritin as a guide to therapy in neuroblastoma. *Cancer Res* 1980;40:1411–1413.
178. Harkin JC, Reed RJ. *Tumors of the Peripheral Nervous System: Atlas of Tumor Pathology.* Second Series, Fascicle 3. Washington, DC: Armed Forces Institute of Pathology; 1969:137–149.
179. Hartman GE, Hintz R, Northway W Jr, Mihm FG. Extra-adrenal pheochromocytoma: an unusual location. *J Pediatr Surg* 1988;11:045–1047.
180. Hashimoto H, Enjoji M, Nakajima T, Kiryu H, Daimaru Y. Malignant neuroepithelioma (peripheral neuroblastoma). A clinicopathologic study of 15 cases. *Am J Surg Pathol* 1983;7:309–318.
181. Hayashi Y, Kanda N, Inaba T, et al. Cytogenetic findings and prognosis in neuroblastoma with emphasis on marker chromosome 1. *Cancer* 1989;63:126–132.
182. Hayashi Y, Ohi R, Yaoita S, et al. Problems of neuroblastoma screening for 6 month olds and results of second screening for 18 month olds. *J Pediatr Surg* 1995;30:467–470.
183. Hayes FA, Green A, Hustu O, Kumar M. Surgicopathologic staging of neuroblastoma: prognostic significance of regional lymph node metastases. *J Pediatr* 1983;102:59–62.
184. Heath H III, Edis AJ. Pheochromocytoma associated with hypercalcemia and ectopic secretion of calcitonin. *Ann Intern Med* 1979;91:208–210.
185. Hecht ST, Brasch RC, Styne DM. CT localization of occult secretory tumors in children. *Pediatr Radiol* 1982;12:67–71.
186. Hedborg F, Lindgren PG, Johansson I, et al. N-myc gene amplification in neuroblastoma: a clinical approach using ultrasound guided cutting needle biopsies collected at diagnosis. *Med Pediatr Oncol* 1992;20:292–300.
187. Hellstrom I, Hellstrom KE, Bill AH, Pierce GE, Yang JPS. Studies on cellular immunity to human neuroblastoma cells. *Int J Cancer* 1970;6:172–188.
188. Hellstrom I, Sjogren HO, Warner G, Hellstrom KE. Blocking of cell-mediated tumor immunity by sera from patients with growing neoplasms. *Int J Cancer* 1971;7:226–237.
189. Hervonen A. Development of catecholamine storing cells in human fetal paraganglia and adrenal medulla. A histochemical and electron microscopic study. *Acta Physiol Scand Suppl* 1971;368: 1–94.
190. Herxheimer G. Ueber Tumoren des Nebennierenmarkes, insbesondere das Neuroblastoma sympathicum. *Beitr Pathol Anat* 1914;57:112–117.
191. Hiyama E, Yokoyama T, Ichikawa T, et al. Poor outcome in patients with advanced stage neuroblastoma and coincident opsomyoclonus syndrome. *Cancer* 1994;74:1821–1826.
192. Hofstra RM, Landsvater RM, Ceccherini I, et al. A mutation in the ret proto-oncogene associated with multiple endocrine neoplasia type 2B and sporadic medullary thyroid carcinoma. *Nature* 1994;367:375–376.
193. Hokfelt T, Schultzbert M, Lundberg JM, et al. Distribution of vasoactive intestinal polypeptide in the central and peripheral nervous systems as revealed by immunocytochemistry. In: Said SI, ed. *Vasoactive Intestinal Peptide.* New York: Raven Press; 1982:5–89.
194. Holgersen LO, Santulli TV, Schullinger JN, Berdon WE. Neuroblastoma with intraspinal (dumbbell) extension. *J Pediatr Surg* 1983;18:406–411.
195. Horn RC Jr, Koop CE, Kiesewetter WB. Neuroblastoma in childhood. Clinicopathologic study of forty-four cases. *Lab Invest* 1956;5:106–119.
196. Hosoi G, Hara J, Okamura T, et al. Low frequency of the p53 gene mutations in neuroblastoma. *Cancer* 1994;73:3087–3093.
197. Hsiao RJ, Neumann HP, Parmer RJ, Barbosa JA, O'Connor DT. Chromogranin A in familial pheochromocytoma: diagnostic screening value, prediction of tumor mass, and post-resection kinetics indicating two-compartment distribution. *Am J Med* 1990;86:607–613.
198. Hughes M, Marsden HB, Palmer MK. Histologic patterns of neuroblastoma related to prognosis and clinical staging. *Cancer* 1974;34:1706–1711.
199. Hume DM. Pheochromocytoma in the adult and in the child. *Am J Surg* 1960;99:458–496.
200. Iancu TC, Shiloh H, Kedar A. Neuroblastomas contain iron-rich ferritin. *Cancer* 1988;61:2497–2502.
201. Ikeda Y, Lister J, Bouton JM, Buyukpamukcu M. Congenital neuroblastoma, neuroblastoma in situ, and the normal fetal development of the adrenal. *J Pediatr Surg* 1981;16:636–644.
202. Imperato-McGinley J, Gautier T, Ehlers K, Zullo MA, Goldstein DS, Vaughan ED Jr. Reversibility of catecholamine-induced cardiomyopathy in a child with a pheochromocytoma. *N Engl J Med* 1987;316:793–797.
203. Isaacs H Jr. Perinatal (congenital and neonatal) neoplasms: a report of 110 cases. *Pediatr Pathol* 1985;3:165–216.
204. Ishimoto K, Kiyokawa N, Fujita H, et al. Problems of mass

screening for neuroblastoma: analysis of false-negative cases. *J Pediatr Surg* 1990;25:398–401.
205. Israel MA. The evolution of clinical molecular genetics. Neuroblastoma as amodel tumor. *Am J Pediatr Hem Oncol* 1986;8: 163–172.
206. Itoh F, Ishizaka Y, Tahira T, et al. Identification and analysis of the ret proto-oncogene promoter region in neuroblastoma cell lines and medullary thyroid carcinomas from MEN 2A patients. *Oncogene* 1992;7:1201–1206.
207. Itoh T, Omori K. Biosynthesis and storage of catecholamines in pheochromocytoma and neuroblastoma cells. *J Lab Clin Med* 1973;81:889–896.
208. Jansson S, Dahlstrom A, Hansson G, Tisell LE, Ahlman H. Concomitant occurrence of an adrenal ganglioneuroma and a contralateral pheochromocytoma in a patient with von Recklinghausen's neurofibromatosis. An immunohistochemical study. *Cancer* 1989;63:324–329.
209. Jennings RW, LaQuaglia MP, Leong K, Hendren WH, Adzick NS. Fetal neuroblastoma: prenatal diagnosis and natural history. *J Pediatr Surg* 1993;28:1168–1174.
210. Joshi VV, Chatten J, Sather H, Shimada H. Evaluation of the Shimada classification in advanced neuroblastoma with a special reference to the mitosis-karyorrhexis index: a report from the Childrens Cancer Study Group. *Mod Pathol* 1991;4:139–147.
211. Joshi VV, Cantor AB, Altshuler G, et al. Recommendations for modification of terminology of neuroblastic tumors and prognostic significance of Shimada classification. A clinicopathologic study of 213 cases from the Pediatric Oncology Group. *Cancer* 1992;69:2183–2196.
212. Joshi VV, Cantor AB, Altshuler G, et al. Age-linked prognostic categorization based on a new histologic grading system of neuroblastomas. A clinicopathologic study of 211 cases from the Pediatric Oncology Group. *Cancer* 1992;69:2197–2211.
213. Joshi VV, Cantor AB, Brodeur GM, et al. Correlation between morphologic and other prognostic markers of neuroblastoma. A study of histologic grade, DNA index, N-myc gene copy number, and lactic dehydrogenase in patients in the Pediatric Oncology Group. *Cancer* 1993;71:3173–3181.
214. Joshi VV, Silverman JF, Altshuler G, et al. Systematization of primary histopathologic and fine needle aspiration cytologic features and description of unusual histopathologic features of neuroblastic tumors: a report from the Pediatric Oncology Group. *Hum Pathol* 1993;24:493–504.
215. Joshi VV, Silverman JF. Pathology of neuroblastic tumors. *Sem Diagn Pathol* 1994;11:107–117.
216. Kahn HJ, Baumal R, Thorner PS, Chan H. Binding of peanut agglutinin to neuroblastomas and ganglioneuroblastomas: a marker for differentiation of neuroblasts into ganglion cells. *Pediatr Pathol* 1988;8:83–93.
217. Kalra R, Zoger S, Kosovich MS, Matthay KK. Miliary pulmonary neuroblastoma. *Arch Pediatr Adolesc Med* 1995;149:195–196.
218. Kaplan SJ, Holbrook CT, McDaniel HG, Buntain WL, Crist WM. Vasoactive intestinal peptide secreting tumors of childhood. *Am J Dis Child* 1980;134:121–124.
219. Karamitopoulou E, Perentes E, Diamantis I, Maraziotis T. Ki-67 immunoreactivity in human central nervous system tumors: a study with MIB 1 monoclonal antibody on archival material. *Acta Neuropathol* 1994;87:47–54.
220. Kaye JA, Warhol MJ, Kretschmar C, Landsberg L, Frei E III. Neuroblastoma in adults. Three case reports and a review of the literature. *Cancer* 1986;58:1149–1157.
221. Keiser HR, Doppman JL, Robertson CN, Linehan WM, Averbach SD. Diagnosis, localization, and managment of pheochromocytoma. In: Lack EE, ed. *Pathology of the Adrenal Glands*. New York: Churchill Livingstone;1990;237–255.
222. Keller SM, Papazoglou S, McKeever P, Baker A, Roth JA. Late occurrence of malignancy in a ganglioneuroma 19 years following radiation therapy to a neuroblastoma. *J Surg Oncol* 1984;25: 227–231.
223. Kelly DR, Joshi VV, Cantor AB, et al. Prognostic significance of histopathologic features of neuroblastic tumors resected at second look surgery. A Pediatric Oncology Group pilot study. *J Pediatr Surg;* in press.
224. Kemshead JT, Clayton J, Patel K. Monoclonal antibodies used for the diagnosis of the small round cell tumors of childhood. In: Kemshead JT, ed. *Pediatric Tumors: Immunological and Molecular Markers*. Boca Raton, FL: CRC Press; 1989:31–45.
225. Kim NW, Piatyszek MA, Prowse KR, et al. Specific association of human telomerase activity with immortal cells and cancer. *Science* 1994;266:2011–2015.
226. Khafagi FA, Shapiro B, Fischer M, Sisson JC, Hutchinson R, Beierwaltes WH. Phaeochromocytoma and functioning paraganglioma in childhood and adolescence: role of iodine 131 metaiodobenzylguanidine. *Eur J Nucl Med* 1991;18:191–198.
227. Kimura N, Miura Y, Nagatsu I, Nagura H. Catecholamine synthesizing enzymes in 70 cases of functioning and non-functioning phaeochromocytoma and extra-adrenal paraganglioma. *Virchows Arch A Histopathol Anat* 1992;421:25–32.
228. Kitahara M, Mori T, Seki H, et al. Malignant paraganglioma presenting as Cushing syndrome with virilism in childhood. Production of cortisol, androgens, and adrenocorticotrophic hormone by the tumor. *Cancer* 1993;72:3340–3345.
229. Kleinman GM, Young RH, Scully RE. Primary neuroectodermal tumors of the ovary. A report of 35 cases. *Am J Surg Pathol* 1993;17:764–778.
230. Kliewer KE, Wen D-R, Cancilla PA, Cochran AJ. Paragangliomas: assessment of prognosis by histologic, immunohistochemical and ultrastructural techniques. *Hum Pathol* 1989;20:29–39.
231. Knoedler CJ, Kay R, Knoedler JP Sr, Wiig TH. Pelvic neuroblastoma. *J Urol* 1989;141:905–907.
232. Knudsen AG Jr, Meadows AT. Regression of neuroblastoma IV-S: a genetic hypothesis. *N Engl J Med* 1980;302:1254–1256.
233. Kogut MD, Donnell GN. Cushing's syndrome in association with renal ganglioneuroblastoma. *Pediatrics* 1961;28:566–577.
234. Kok LP, Boon ME. *Microwave Cookbook for Microscopists. Art and Science of Visualization*. 3rd ed. Leiden, The Netherlands: Coulomb Press; 1992.
235. Koppersmith DL, Powers JM, Hennigar GR. Angiomatoid neuroblastoma with cytoplasmic glycogen. A case report and histogenetic considerations. *Cancer* 1980;40:553–560.
236. Koskinen PJ, Makela TP, Vastrik I, Aitalo K. Myc amplification: regulation of myc function. *Clin Chim Acta* 1993;217:57–62.
237. Kragel PJ, Johnston CA. Pheochromocytoma-ganglioneuroma of the adrenal. *Arch Pathol Lab Med* 1985;109:470–472.
238. Krajewski S, Chatten J, Hanada M, Reed JC. Immunohistochemical analysis of the Bcl-2 oncoprotein in human neuroblastomas. Comparisons with tumor cell differentiation and N-myc protein. *Lab Invest* 1995;71:42–54.
239. Kushner BH, Gilbert F, Helson L. Familial neuroblastoma. Case reports, literature review and etiologic considerations. *Cancer* 1986;57:1887–1893.
240. Lacey SR, Gribble TJ, Kosloske AM. Favorable prognosis of vasoactive intestinal peptide-secreting ganglioneuroblastoma. *Pediatr Surg Int* 1989;4:217–219.
241. Lack EE. Adrenal medullary hyperplasia and pheochromocytoma. In: Lack EE, ed. *Pathology of the Adrenal Glands*. New York: Churchill Livingstone, 1990;173–235.
242. Lack EE. Paragangliomas. In: Sternberg SS, ed. *Diagnostic Surgical Pathology*. 2nd ed. New York: Raven Press, 1994;599–621.
243. Lack EE. *Pathology of Adrenal and Extra-adrenal Paraganglia*. Philadelphia: WB Saunders; 1994.
244. Lack EE, Kozakewich HPW. Adrenal neuroblastoma, ganglioneuroblastoma, and related tumors. In: Lack EE, ed. *Pathology of the Adrenal Glands*. New York: Churchill Livingstone; 1990: 277–309.
245. Lairmore TC, Howe JR, Korte JA, et al. Familial medullary thyroid carcinoma and multiple endocrine neoplasia type 2B map to the same region of chromosome 10 as multiple endocrine neoplasia type 2A. *Genomics* 1991;9:181–192.
246. Landau M. Die malignen Neuroblastome des Sympathikus. *Frankf Z Pathol* 1912;11:26–77.
247. Larsson C, Skogseid B, Öberg K, Nakamura Y, Nordenskjold M. Multiple endocrine neoplasia type 1 gene maps to chromosome 11 and is lost in insulinoma. *Nature* 1988;332:85–87.
248. Larsson C, Friedman E. Localization and identification of the multiple endocrine neoplasia type 1 disease gene. *Endocrinol Metab Clin North Am* 1994;23:67–79.

249. Lahti JM, Valentine M, Xiang J, et al. Alterations in the PITSLRE protein kinase gene complex on chromosome 1p36 in childhood neuroblastoma. *Nat Genet* 1994;7:370–375.
250. Lahti JM, Xiang J, Heath LS, Campana D, Kidd VJ. PITSLRE protein kinase activity is associated with apoptosis. *Mol Cell Biol* 1995;15:1–11.
251. Lamovec J, Memoli VA, Terzakis JA, Sommers SC, Gould VE. Pheochromocytoma producing ACTH with Cushing's syndrome. *Ultrastruct Pathol* 1984;7:41–48.
252. Landas SK, Leigh C, Bonsib SM, Layne K. Occurrence of melanin in pheochromocytoma. *Mod Pathol* 1993;6:175–178.
253. Laug WE, Siegel SE, Shaw KNF, Landing B, Baptista J, Gutenstein M. Initial urinary catecholamine metabolite concentrations and prognosis in neuroblastoma. *Pediatrics* 1978;62:77–83.
254. Layfield LJ, Thompson JK, Kerns BJ. Prognostic indicators for neuroblastoma; stage, grade, DNA ploidy, MIB-1-proliferation index, p53, HER-2/*neu*, and EGFr: a survival study. *Lab Invest* 1995;72:144A.
255. LeDouarin N. Migration and differentiation of neural crest cells. *Curr Top Dev Biol* 1980;16:31–85.
256. Leone A, Seeger RC, Hong CM, et al. Evidence for *nm*23 RNA overexpression, DNA amplification and mutation in aggressive childhood neuroblastomas. *Oncogene* 1993;8:855–865.
257. Leong AS-Y, Milios J. An assessment of the efficacy of the microwave antigen-retrieval procedure on a range of tissue antigens. *Appl Immunohistochem* 1993;1:267–274.
258. Leong PK, Thorner P, Yeger H, Ng K, Zhang A, Squire J. Detection of mycN gene amplification and deletions of chromosome 1p in neuroblastoma by in situ hybridization using routine histologic sections. *Lab Invest* 1993;69:43–50.
259. Lipinski M, Braham K, Caillaud J-M, Carlu C, Tursz T. HNK-1 antibody detects an antigen expressed on neuroectodermal cells. *J Exp Med* 1983;158:1775–1780.
260. Lloyd RV, Blaivas M, Wilson BS. Distribution of chromogranin and S100 protein in normal and abnormal adrenal medullary tissues. *Arch Pathol Lab Med* 1985;109:633–635.
261. Lloyd RV, Sisson JC, Shapiro B, Verhofstad AAJ. Immunohistochemical localization of epinephrine, norepinephrine, catecholamine synthesizing enzymes and chromogranin in neuroendocrine cells and tumors. *Am J Pathol* 1986;125:45–54.
262. Look AT, Hayes FA, Nitschke R, McWilliams NB, Green AA. Cellular DNA content as a predictor of response to chemotherapy in infants with unresectable neuroblastoma. *N Engl J Med* 1984;311:231–235.
263. Look AT, Hayes FA, Shuster JJ, et al. Clinical relevance of tumor cell ploidy and N-myc gene amplification in childhood neuroblastoma: a Pediatric Oncology Group study. *J Clin Oncol* 1991;9:581–591.
264. Loomis PA, Howard TH, Castleberry RP, Binder LI. Identification of nuclear τ isoforms in human neurblastoma cells. *Proc Natl Acad Sci USA* 1990;87:8422–8426.
265. Lorence RM, Reichard KW, Katubig BB, et al. Complete regression of human neuroblastoma xenografts in athymic mice after local Newcastle disease virus therapy. *JNCI* 1994;86:1228–1233.
266. Lundberg JM, Hamberger B, Schultzberg M, et al. Enkephalin- and somatostatin-like immunoreactivities in human adrenal medulla and pheochromocytoma. *Proc Natl Acad Sci USA* 1979;76: 4079–4083.
267. Machin GA. Histogenesis and histopathology of neuroblastoma. In: Pochedly C, ed. *Neuroblastoma, Clinical and Biological Manifestations.* New York: Elsevier Biomedical, 1982;195–231.
268. Mack E, Sarto GE, Crummy AB, Carlson IH, Curet LB, Wu J. Virilizing adrenal ganglioneuroma. *JAMA* 1978;239:2273–2275.
269. Mackay B, Luna MA, Butler JJ. Adult neuroblastoma. Electron microscopic observations in nine cases. *Cancer* 1976;37:1334–1351.
270. Mahoney EM, Harrison JH. Malignant pheochromocytoma: clinical course and treatment. *J Urol* 1977;118:225–229.
271. Ma¨kinen J. Microscopic patterns as a guide to prognosis of neuroblastoma in childhood. *Cancer* 1972;29:1637–1646.
272. Marchand F. Beitraege zur kenntnis der normalen und pathologischen anatomie der glandula carotica an der nebennieren. *Int Beitr Wiss Med Festschr Berlin: Vershow* 1891;1:535–581.
273. Martin RF, Beckwith JB. Lymphoid infiltrates in neuroblastomas: their occurrence and prognostic significance. *J Pediatr Surg* 1968;3:161–163.
274. Martucciello G, Favre A, Takahashi M, Jasonni V. Immunohistochemical localization of RET protein in Hirschsprung's disease. *J Pediatr Surg* 1995;30:433–436.
275. Matsunaga T, Takahashi H, Ohnuma N, et al. Expression of N-myc and c-*src* protooncogenes correlating to the undifferentiated phenotype and prognosis of primary neuroblastomas. *Cancer Res* 1991;51:3148–1352.
276. Matthay KK, Huberty JP, Hattner RS, et al. Efficacy and safety of ^{131}I-metaidobenzylguanidine therapy for patients with refractory neuroblastoma. *J Nucl Biol Med* 1991;35:244–247.
277. Matthew CGP, Chin KS, Easton DF, et al. A linked genetic marker for multiple endocrine neoplasia type 2A on chromosome 10. *Nature* 1987;328:527–528.
278. McLaughlin JE, Urich H. Maturing neuroblastoma and ganglioneuroblastoma: a study of four cases with long survival. *J Pathol* 1977;121:19–26.
279. McRobert TL, Rudduck C, Kees UR, Garson OM. Detection of *MYCN* amplification in three neuroblastoma cell lines by nonradioactive chromosomal *in situ* hybridization. *Cancer Genet Cytogenet* 1992;59:128–134.
280. Mechtersheimer G, Barth T, Quentmeier A, Moller P. Differential expression of β_1, β_3 and β_4 integrin subunits in nonneoplastic neural cells of the peripheral and autonomic nervous system and in tumors derived from these cells. *Lab Invest* 1994;70:740-752.
281. Meichle A, Philipp A, Eilers M. The function of Myc proteins. *Biochim Biophys Acta* 1992;1114:129–146.
282. Meister P, Middeke M, Selbmann H-K. Nephroblastoma and neuroblastoma—histology and prognosis. *Z Krebsforsch* 1978; 92:315–326.
283. Mendelsohn G, Eggleston JC, Olson JL, Said SI, Baylin SB. Vasoactive intestinal peptide and its relationship to ganglion cell differentiation in neuroblastic tumors. *Lab Invest* 1979;41:144–149.
284. Michels S, Swanson PE, Robb JA, Wick MR. Leu-7 in small cell neoplasms. An immunohistochemical study with ultrastructural correlations. *Cancer* 1987;60:2958–2964.
285. Miettinen M, Lehto V-P, Virtanen I. Immunofluorescence microscopic evaluation of the intermediate filament expression of the adrenal cortex and medulla and their tumors. *Am J Pathol* 1985;118:360–366.
286. Miettinen M, Saari A. Pheochromocytoma combined with malignant schwannoma: unusual neoplasm of the adrenal medulla. *Ultrastruct Pathol* 1988;12:513–527.
287. Miller DR, Patel K, Allen JC, Horten B. Neuroblastoma, tuberous sclerosis, and subependymal giant cell astrocytoma. *Am J Pediatr Hematol Oncol* 1983;5:213–218.
288. Miller RW. Ethnic differences in cancer ocurrence: genetic and environmental differences with particular reference to neuroblastoma. In: Mulvihill J, Miller R, Fraumeni J, eds. *Genetics of Human Cancer.* New York: Raven Press; 1977:1–14.
289. Miller RW, Young Jr JL, Novakovic B. Childhood cancer. *Cancer* 1995;75:395–405.
290. Mills AE, Bird AR. Bone marrow changes in neuroblastoma. *Pediatr Pathol* 1986;5:225–234.
291. Min K-W, Clemens A, Bell J, Dick H. Malignant peripheral nerve sheath tumor and pheochromocytoma. A composite tumor of the adrenal. *Arch Pathol Lab Med* 1988;112:266–270.
292. Mir R, Phillips SL, Schwartz G, Mathur R, Khan A, Kahn LB. Metastatic neuroblastoma after 52 years of dormancy. *Cancer* 1987;60:2510–2514.
293. Misugi K, Misugi N, Newton WA Jr. Fine structural study of neuroblastoma, ganglioneuroblastoma, and pheochromocytoma. *Arch Pathol* 1968;86:160–170.
294. Misugi K, Aoki I, Kikyo S, Sasaki Y, Tsunod A, Nakajima T. Immunohistochemical study of neuroblastoma and related tumors with anti-S-100 protein antibody. *Pediatr Pathol* 1985;3: 217–226.
295. Moertel CL, Reubi J-C, Scheithauer BS, Schaid DJ, Kvols LK. Expression of somatostatin receptors in childhood neuroblastoma. *Am J Clin Pathol* 1994;102:752–756.
296. Molenaar WM, Baker DL, Pleasure D, Lee VM-Y, Trojanowski JQ. The neuroendocrine and neural profiles of neuroblastomas,

ganglioneuroblastomas, and ganglioneuromas. *Am J Pathol* 1990;136:375–382.

297. Moley JF, Brother MB, Wells SA, Spengler BA, Biedler JL, Brodeur GM. Low frequency of *ras* gene mutations in neuroblastomas, pheochromocytomas, and medullary thyroid carcinoma. *Cancer Res* 1991;51:1596–1599.
298. Moore KL. *The Developing Human. Clinically Oriented Embryology.* 4th ed. Philadelphia: WB Saunders; 1988.
299. Morris JA, Shochat SJ, Smith EI, et al. Biological variables in thoracic neuroblastoma: a Pediatric Oncology Group study. *J Pediatr Surg* 1995;30:296–303.
300. Moss TJ, Kaplan L. Association of hydrops fetalis with congenital neuroblastoma. *Am J Obstet Gynecol* 1978;132:905–906.
301. Moss TJ, Reynolds CP, Sather HN, Romansky SG, Hammond GD, Seeger RC. Prognostic value of immunocytologic detection of bone marrow metastases in neuroblastoma. *N Engl J Med* 1991;324:219–226.
302. Mount SL, Taatjes DJ, von Turkovich M, Tindle BH, Trainer TD. Diagnostic immunoelectron microscopy in surgical pathology: assessment of various tisue fixation and processing protocols. *Ultrastruct Pathol* 1993;17:547–556.
303. Mulligan LM, Kwok JBJ, Healey CS, et al. Germ-line mutations of the RET proto-oncogene in multiple endocrine neoplasia type 2A. *Nature* 1993;363:458–460.
304. Mullins JD. A pigmented differentiating neuroblastoma. A light and ultrastructural study. *Cancer* 1980;46:522–528.
305. Murphy SB, Cohn SL, Craft AW, et al. Do children benefit from mass screening for neuroblastoma? Consensus statement from the American Cancer Society Workshop on Neuroblastoma Screening. *Lancet* 1991;1:344–346.
306. Murray MR, Stout AP. Distinctive characteristics of the sympathicoblastoma cultivated in vitro. *Am J Pathol* 1947;23:429–441.
307. Murray MR, Stout AP. A sympathetic ganglioneuroma cultivated in vitro. *Cancer* 1948;1:242–247.
308. Nakagawara A, Ikeda K, Tsuneyoshi M, Daimaru Y, Enjoji M. Malignant pheochromocytoma with ganglioneuroblastomatous elements in a patient with von Recklinghausen's disease. *Cancer* 1985;55:2794–2798.
309. Nakagawara A, Sasazuki T, Akiyama H, et al. N-*myc* oncogene and stage IV-S neuroblastoma. Preliminary observations on ten cases. *Cancer* 1990;65:1960–1967.
310. Nakagawara A, Kadomatsu K, Sato S, et al. Inverse correlation between expression of multidrug resistance gene and N-*myc* oncogene in human neuroblastomas. *Cancer Res* 1990;50:3043–3047.
311. Nakagawara A, Arima M, Azar CG, Scavarda N, Brodeur GM. Inverse relationship between *trk* expression and N-*myc* amplification in human neuroblastomas. *Cancer Res* 1992;52:1364–1368.
312. Nakagawara A, Arima-Nakagawara M, Scavarda NJ, Azar CG, Cantor AB, Brodeur GM. Association between high levels of expression of the *trk* gene and favorable outcome in human neuroblastoma. *N Engl J Med* 1993;328:847–854.
313. Nakagawara A, Azar CG, Scavarda NJ, Brodeur GM. Expression and function of *trk*-B and BDNF in human neuroblastomas. *Mol Cell Biol* 1994;14:759–767.
314. Nakamura T, Ishizaka Y, Nagao M, Hara M, Ishikawa T. Expression of the *ret* proto-oncogene product in human normal and neoplastic tissues of neural crest origin. *J Pathol* 1994;172:255–260.
315. Nelkin BD, Ball DW, Baylin SB. Molecular abnormalities in tumors associated with multiple endocrine neoplasia type 2. *Endocrinol Metab Clin North Am* 1994;23:187–213.
316. Neumann HP, Berger DP, Sigmund G, et al. Pheochromocytomas, multiple endocrine neoplasia type 2, and von Hippel-Lindau disease. *N Engl J Med* 1993;329:1531–1538.
317. Nguyen AV, Argenyi ZB. Cutaneous neuroblastoma. Peripheral neuroblastomas. *Am J Dermatopathol* 1993;15:7–14.
318. Nishi M, Miyake H, Takeda T, et al. Cases of neuroblastoma missed by the mass screening programs. *Pediatr Res* 1989;26:603–607.
319. Nitschke R, Smith EI, Shochat S, et al. Localized neuroblastoma treated by surgery: a Pediatric Oncology Group Study. *J Clin Oncol* 1988;6:1271–1279.
320. Normann T, Havnen J, Mjolnerod O. Cushing's syndrome in an infant associated with neuroblastoma in two ectopic adrenal glands. *J Pediatr Surg* 1971;6:169–175.
321. Norum RA, Lafreniere RG, O'Neal LW, et al. Linkage of the multiple endocrine neoplasia type 2B gene (MEN2B) to chromosome 10 markers linked to MEN2A. *Genomics* 1990;8:313–317.
322. O'Dowd GM, Gaffney EF. Pigmented ganglioneuroblastoma: a tumour cell "storage disease"? *Histopathology* 1993;22:591–593.
323. O'Meara A, Imamura A, Johnson P, et al. Reactivity of P-glycoprotein monoclonal antibodies in childhood cancers. *Oncology* 1992;49:203–208.
324. Omenn GS. Ectopic hormone syndromes associated with tumors in childhood. *Pediatrics* 1971;47:613–622.
325. Ophir D. Familial multicentric paragangliomas in a child. *J Laryngol Otol* 1991;105:376–380.
326. Oppedal BR, Storm-Mathisen I, Kemshead JT, Brandtzaeg P. Bone marrow examination in neuroblastoma patients: a morphologic, immunocytochemical, and immunohistochemical study. *Hum Pathol* 1989;20:800–805.
327. Osborn M, Dirk T, Kaser H, Weber K, Altmannsberger M. Immunohistochemical localization of neurofilaments and neuron specific enolase in 29 cases of neuroblastoma. *Am J Pathol* 1986;122:433–442.
328. Page DL, DeLellis RA, Hough AJ Jr. *Tumors of the Adrenal: Atlas of Tumor Pathology.* Second Series, Fascicle 23, Washington, DC: Armed Forces Institute of Pathology; 1986.
329. Pappo AS, Douglass EC, Meyer WH, Marina N, Parham DM. Use of HBA 71 and anti-β_2-microglobulin to distinguish peripheral neuroepithelioma from neuroblastoma. *Hum Pathol* 1993;24:880–885.
330. Parham DM, Weeks DA, Beckwith JB. The clinicopathologic spectrum of putative extrarenal rhabdoid tumors. An analysis of 42 cases studied with immunohistochemistry or electon microscopy. *Am J Surg Pathol* 1994;18:1010–1029.
331. Parkin JL. Familial multiple glomus tumors and pheochromocytomas. *Ann Otol* 1981;90:60–63.
332. Patel K, Moore SE, Dickson G, et al. Neural cell adhesion molecule (NCAM) is the antigen recognized by monoclonal antibodies of similar specificity in small cell lung carcinoma and neuroblastoma. *Int J Cancer* 1989;44:573–578.
333. Patrone PM, Chatten J, Weinberg P. Neuroblastoma and DiGeorge anomaly. *Pediatr Pathol* 1990;10:425–430.
334. Payne CM. Use of the uranaffin reaction in the identification of neuroendocrine granules. *Ultrastruct Pathol* 1993;17:49–82.
335. Pegelow CH, Ebbin AJ, Powars D, Towner JW. Familial neuroblastoma. *J Pediatr* 1975;87:763–765.
336. Pendergrass TW, Hanson JW. Fetal hydantoin syndrome and neuroblastoma. *Lancet* 1976;2:150.
337. Perkins DG, Kopp CM, Haust MD. Placental infiltration in congenital neuroblastoma: a case study with ultrastructure. *Histopathology* 1980;4:383–389.
338. Peters J, Miyake N, Seeger RC, et al. Splicing pattern of the high affinity nerve growth factor receptor (*trk*A) transcript in neuroblastomas: correlation with histopathology and clinical outcome. *Lab Invest* 1995;72:144A.
339. Pham BN, Villanueva RP. Ganglioneuromatous proliferation associated with juvenile polyposis coli. *Arch Pathol Lab Med* 1989;113:91–94.
340. Phillips AF, McMurtry RJ, Taubman J. Malignant pheochromocytoma in childhood. *Am J Dis Child* 1976;130:1252–1255.
341. Pick L. Das ganglioma embryonale sympathicum (Sympathoma embryonale); eine typische bo¨sartige Geschwulstform des sympathischen Nervensystems. *Berl Klin Wochenschr* 1912;49:16–22.
342. Plantaz D, Hartmann O, Kalifa C, Sainte-Rose C, Lemoine G, Lemerle J. Localized dumbbell neuroblastoma: a study of 25 cases treated between 1982 and 1987 using the same protocol. *Med Pediatr Oncol* 1993;21:249–253.
343. Poore TN, Dockerty MB, Kennedy RLJ, Walters W. Abdominal neuroblastomas. *Surg Clin North Am* 1951;31:1121–141.
344. Prasad KN. Differentiation of neuroblastoma cells: a useful

model for neurobiology and cancer. *Biol Rev Camb Philos Soc* 1991;66:431–451.

345. Proye C, Fossati P, Fontaine P, et al. Dopamine-secreting pheochromocytoma: an unrecognized entity? Classification of pheochromocytomas according to their type of secretion. *Surgery* 1986;100:1154–1162.
346. Punt J, Pritchard J, Pincott JR, Till K. Neuroblastoma: a review of 21 cases presenting with spinal cord compression. *Cancer* 1980;45:3095–3101.
347. Qualman SJ, O'Dorisio MS, Fleshman DJ, Shimada H, O'Dorisio TM. Neuroblastoma: correlation of neuropeptide expression in tumor tissue with other prognostic factors. *Cancer* 1992;70: 2005–2012.
348. Qualman SJ, Martinez D, O'Dorisio MS, Robinson A, Hanson RP, O'Dorisio TM. In vitro/in vivo imaging of human neuroblastoma (NB) via somatostatin receptor (SSR) binding. *Lab Invest* 1995;72:144A.
349. Ramsey JA, Asa SL, van Nostrand AWP, Hassaram ST, de Harven E. Lipid degeneration in pheochromocytomas mimicking adrenal cortical tumors. *Am J Surg Pathol* 1987;11:480–486.
350. Reid MM, Hamilton PJ. Histology of neuroblastoma involving bone marrow: the problem of detecting residual tumor after initiation of chemotherapy. *Br J Haematol* 1988;69:487–490.
351. Reid MM, Wallis JP, McGuckin AG, Pearson AD, Malcolm AJ. Routine histological compared with immunohistological examination of bone marrow trephine biopsy specimens in disseminated neuroblastoma. *J Clin Pathol* 1991;44:483–486.
352. Reynolds CP, Smith RG, Frenkel EP. The diagnostic dilemma of the "small round cell neoplasm": catecholamine fluorescence and tissue culture morphology as markers for neuroblastoma. *Cancer* 1981;48:2088–2094.
353. Ricci A Jr, Parham DM, Woodruff JM, Callihan TA, Green A, Erlandson RA. Malignant peripheral nerve sheath tumors arising from ganglioneuromas. *Am J Surg Pathol* 1984;8:19–29.
354. Richards JG, Da Prada M. Uranaffin reaction: a new cytochemical technique for the localization of adenine nucleotides in organelles storing biogenic amines. *J Histochem Cytochem* 1977;25: 1322–1326.
355. Richards MJS, Joo P, Gilbert EF. The rare problem of late recurrence in neuroblastoma. *Cancer* 1976;38:1847–1852.
356. Robertson HE. Das Ganglioneuroblastom ein besonderer Typus im system der Neurome. *Virchows Arch Pathol Anat Physiol Klin Med* 1915;220:147–168.
357. Robinson MF, Furst EJ, Nunziata V, et al. Characterization of the clinical features of five families with hereditary primary cutaneous lichen amyloidosis and multiple endocrine neoplasia type 2. *Henry Ford Hosp Med J* 1992;40:249–252.
358. Robinson MJ, Howard RN. Neuroblastoma, presenting as myasthenia gravis in a child aged 3 years. *Pediatrics* 1969;43:111–113.
359. Romansky SG, Crocker DW, Shaw KNF. Ultrastructural studies on neuroblastoma. Evaluation of cytodifferentiation and correlation of morphology and biochemical and survival data. *Cancer* 1978;42:2392–2398.
360. Rossi AR, Pericle F, Rashleigh S, Janiec J, Djeu JY. Lysis of neuroblastoma cell lines by human natural killer cells activated by interleukin-2 and interleukin-12. *Blood* 1994;83:1323–1328.
361. Russell DS, Rubinstein LJ. *Pathology of Tumors of the Nervous System*. 4th ed. Baltimore: Williams & Wilkins; 1977:402–436.
362. Samaan NA, Hickey RC, Shutts PE. Diagnosis, localization, and management of pheochromocytoma. Pitfalls and follow-up in 41 patients. *Cancer* 1988;62:2451–2460.
363. Sandstedt B, Jereb B, Eklund G. Prognostic factors in neuroblastomas. *Acta Pathol Microbiol Immunol Scand A*;1983:91: 365–371.
364. Sanger WG, Howe J, Fordyce R, Purtilo DT. Inherited partial trisomy #15 complicated by neuroblastoma. *Cancer Genet Cytogenet* 1984;11:153–159.
365. Sano K, Nakamura H, Mabuchi S, Tanaka T, Nakagawara A, Takai Y. Expression of the *smg* p25A (a *ras* p21-like GTP-binding protein) gene in human neuroblastoma cell lines and tumor tissues. *Cancer Res* 1990;50:7242–7245.
366. Santoro M, Rosati R, Grieco M, et al. The *ret* proto-oncogene is consistently expressed in human pheochromocytomas and thyroid medullary carcinomas. *Oncogene* 1990;5:1595–1598.
367. Santoro M, Carlomagno F, Romano A, et al. Activation of *RET* as a dominant transforming gene by germline mutations of MEN2A and MEN2B. *Science* 1995;267:381–383.
368. Sawada T. Past and future of neuroblastoma screening in Japan. *Am J Pediatr Hematol Oncol* 1992;14:320–326.
369. Schaffer MS, Zuberbuhler P, Wilson G, Rose V, Duncan WJ, Rowe RD. Catecholamine cardiomyopathy: an unusual presentation of pheochromocytoma in children. *J Pediatr* 1981;99:276–279.
370. Scheibel E, Rechnitzer C, Fahrenkrug J, Hertz H. Vasoactive intestinal peptide (VIP) in children with neural crest tumours. *Acta Paediatr Scand* 1982;71:721–725.
371. Schengrund C-L, Repman MA, Schochat SJ. Ganglioside composition of human neuroblastomas. Correlation with prognosis. A Pediatric Oncology Group study. *Cancer* 1985;56:2640–2646.
372. Schmidt D, Harms D, Burdach S. Malignant peripheral neuroectodermal tumours of childhood and adolescence. *Virchows Arch A Histopathol Anat* 31985;406:351–365.
373. Schulz G, Cheresh DA, Varki NM, Yu A, Staffileno LK, Reisfeld RA. Detection of ganglioside G_{D2} in tumor tissues and sera of neuroblastoma patients. *Cancer Res* 1984;44:5914–5920.
374. Schwab M. Molecular cytogenetics of human neuroblastoma. *Biochim Biophys Acta* 1992;1114:43–50.
375. Schwab M. Amplification of N-*myc* as a prognostic marker for patients with neuroblastoma. *Semin Cancer Biol* 1993;4:13–18.
376. Schwab M, Ellison J, Busch M, Rosenau W, Varmus HE, Bishop JM. Enhanced expression of the human gene N-*myc* consequent to amplification of DNA may contribute to malignant progression of neuroblastoma. *Proc Natl Acad Sci USA* 1984;81:4940–4944.
377. Scully RE, Cohen RB. Ganglioneuroma of adrenal medulla containing cells morphologically identical to hilus cells (extraparenchymal Leydig cells). *Cancer* 1961;16:421–425.
378. Seeger RC, Siegel SE, Sidell N. Neuroblastoma: clinical perspectives, monoclonal antibodies, and retinoic acid. *Ann Intern Med* 1982;97:873–884.
379. Seeger RC, Brodeur GM, Sather H, et al. Association of multiple copies of the N-*myc* oncogene with rapid progression of neuroblastomas. *N Engl J Med* 1985;313:1111–1116.
380. Seeger RC, Wada R, Brodeur GM, et al. Expression of N-*myc* by neuroblastomas with one or multiple copies of the oncogene. *Prog Clin Biol Res* 1988;271:41–49.
381. Seeler RA, Israel JN, Royal JE, Kaye CI, Rao S, Abuladan M. Ganglioneuroblastoma and fetal hydantoin–alcohol syndromes. *Pediatrics* 1979;63:524–527.
382. Shanklin DR, Sotello-Avila C. In situ tumors in fetuses, newborns and young infants. *Biol Neonate* 1969;14:286–316.
383. Shapiro DN, Valentine MB, Rowe ST, et al. Detection of N-*myc* gene amplification by fluorescence *in situ* hybridization. Diagnostic utility for neuroblastoma. *Am J Pathol* 1993;142:1339–1346.
384. Shi S-R, Key ME, Kalra KL. Antigen retrieval in formalin-fixed, paraffin-embedded tissues: an enhancement method for immunohistochemical staining based on microwave oven heating of tissue sections. *J Histochem Cytochem* 1991;39:741–748.
385. Shimada H: Transmission and scanning electron microscopic studies on tumors of neuroblastoma group. *Acta Pathol Jpn* 1982;32:415–426.
386. Shimada H, Chatten J, Newton WA Jr, et al. Histopathologic prognostic factors in neuroblastic tumors: definition of subtypes of ganglioneuroblastoma and an age-linked classification of neuroblastomas. *JNCI* 1984;73:405–416.
387. Shimada H, Aoyama C, Chiba T, Newton WA Jr. Pathologic subgroups for undifferentiated neuroblastoma. Immunohistochemical study with anti-S-100 protein antibody. *Hum Pathol* 1985;16: 471–476.
388. Shimada H, Stram D, Chatten J, et al. Histopathology and N-*myc* gene in neuroblastoma. A report from the Children's Cancer Study Group. *Lab Invest* 1992;66:10P.
389. Shown TE, Durfee MF. Blueberry muffin baby: neonatal neuroblastoma with subcutaneous metastases. *J Urol* 1970;104:193–195.
390. Shuster JJ, McWilliams NB, Castleberry RP, et al. Serum lactate dehydrogenase in childhood neuroblastoma: a Pediatric Oncol-

ogy Group recursive partitioning study. *Am J Clin Oncol* 1992;15:295–303.
391. Silber JH, Evans AE, Fridman M. Models to predict outcome from childhood neuroblastoma: the role of serum ferritin and tumor histology. *Cancer Res* 1991;51:1426–1433.
392. Silver MM, Lines LD, Hearn SS. Immunogold detection of chromogranin A in the neuroendocrine tumor. *Ultrastruct Pathol* 1993;17:83–92.
393. Silverman JF, Dabbs DJ, Ganick DJ, Holbrook CT, Geisinger KR. Fine-needle aspiration cytology of neuroblastoma, including peripheral neuroectodermal tumor with immunocytochemical and ultrastructural confirmation. *Acta Cytol* 1988;32:367–376.
394. Silverman JF, Berns LA, Holbrook CT, Neill JSA, Joshi VV. Fine-needle aspiration cytology of primitive neuroectodermal tumors. A report of three cases. *Acta Cytol* 1992;36:541–550.
395. Simpson NE, Kidd KK, Goodfellow PJ, et al. Assignment of multiple endocrine neoplasia 2A to chromosome 10 by genetic linkage. *Nature* 1987;328:528–530.
396. Smith CR, Chan HS, DeSa DJ. Placental involvement in congenital neuroblastoma. *J Clin Pathol* 1981;34:785–789.
397. Smith IE, Castleberry RP. Neuroblastoma. In: Wells SA Jr, ed. *Current Problems in Pediatric Surgery*. St. Louis: C.V. Mosby 1990;27:577–620.
398. Spark RK, Connolly PB, Gluckin DS, White R, Sacks B, Lansberg L. ACTH secretion from a functioning pheochromocytoma. *N Engl J Med* 1979;301:416–418.
399. Srivatsan ES, Murali V, Seeger RC. Loss of heterozygosity for alleles on chromosomes 11q and 14q in neuroblastoma. *Prog Clin Biol Res* 1991;366:91–98.
400. Stackpole RH, Melicow MM, Uson AC. Pheochromocytoma in children. Report of 9 cases and review of the first 100 published cases with follow-up studies. *J Pediatr* 1963;63:315–330.
401. Stout AP. Ganglioneuroma of the sympathetic nervous system. *Surg Gynecol Obstet* 1947;84:101–110.
402. Stowens D. Neuroblastoma and related tumors. *Arch Pathol* 1957;63:451–458.
403. Suurmeijer AJH, Boon ME. Notes on the application of microwaves for antigen retrieval in paraffin and plastic tissue sections. *Eur J Morphol* 1993;31:144–150.
404. Suzuki T, Mugishima H, Fujisawa T, et al. Loss of heterozygosity on chromosome 14 in neuroblastoma. *Prog Clin Biol Res* 1991;366:135–145.
405. Suzuki T, Watanabek K, Sugino T, Tanigawa T, Satoh S. Immunocytochemical demonstration of IGF-II immunoreactivity in human phaeochromocytoma and extra-adrenal abdominal paraganglioma. *J Pathol* 1992;167:199–203.
406. Swenson SJ, Brown ML, Sheps SG, et al. Use of ^{131}I-MIBG scintigraphy in the evaluation of suspected pheochromocytoma. *Mayo Clin Proc* 1985;60:299–304.
407. Tahira T, Ishizaka Y, Itoh F, Nakayasu M, Sugimura T, Nagao M. Expression of the *ret* proto-oncogene in human neuroblastoma cell lines and its increase during neuronal differentiation induced by retinoic acid. *Oncogene* 1991;6:2333–2338.
408. Takahashi H, Yoshizaki K, Kato H, et al. A gonadotrophin-responsive virilizing adrenal tumor identified as a mixed ganglioneuroma and adrenocortical tumor. *Acta Endocrinol* 1978;89: 701–709.
409. Takayama H, Suzuki T, Mugishima H, et al. Deletion mapping of chromosomes 14q and 1p in human neuroblastoma. *Oncogene* 1992;7:1185–1189.
410. Tanaka T, Slamon DJ, Shimada H, et al. A significant association of Ha-*ras* p21 in neuroblastoma cells with patient prognosis. *Cancer* 1991;68:1296–1302.
411. Taxy JB. Electron microscopy in the diagnosis of neuroblastoma. *Arch Pathol Lab Med* 1980;104:355–360.
412. Taylor CPF, McGuckin AG, Boen NP, et al. Rapid detection of prognostic genetic factors in neuroblastoma using fluorescence *in situ* hybridization on tumour imprints and bone marrow smears. *Br J Cancer* 1994;69:445–451.
413. Thiele CJ, McKeon C, Triche TJ, Ross RA, Reynolds CP, Israel MA. Differential protooncogene expression characterizes histopathologically indistinguishable tumors of the peripheral nervous system. *J Clin Invest* 1987;80:804–811.
414. Thomas JO, Nijjar J, Turley H, Micklem K, Gatter KC. NB84: a new monoclonal antibody for the recognition of neuroblastoma in routinely processed material. *J Pathol* 1991;163:69–75.
415. Tiedemann K, Pritchard J, Long R, Bloom SR. Intractable diarrhea in a patient with vasoactive intestinal peptide-secreting neuroblastoma. Attempted control by somatostatin. *Eur J Pediatr* 1981;137:217–219.
416. Tischler AS, Dayal Y, Balogh K, Cohen RB, Connolly JL, Tallberg K. The distribution of immunoreactive chromogranins, S-100 protein, and vasoactive intestinal peptide in compound tumors of the adrenal medulla. *Hum Pathol* 1987;18:909–917.
417. Triche TJ. Neuroblastoma—biology confronts nosology. *Arch Pathol Lab Med* 1986;110:994–996.
418. Triche TJ. Differential diagnosis of neuroblastoma and related tumors. In: Lack EE, ed. *Pathology of the Adrenal Glands*. New York: Churchill Livingstone; 1990:323–350.
419. Triche TJ. Neuroblastoma and other childhood neural tumors: a review. *Pediatr Pathol* 1990;10:175–193.
420. Triche TJ. Multiple drug resistance in Ewing's sarcoma and peripheral primitive neuroectodermal tumors. *Am J Clin Pathol* 1994;102:1–2.
421. Triche TJ, Ross WE. Glycogen-containing neuroblastoma with clinical and histopathologic features of Ewing's sarcoma. *Cancer* 1978;41:1425–1432.
422. Triche TJ, Askin FB. Neuroblastoma and the differential diagnosis of small round blue cell tumors. *Hum Pathol* 1983;14:569–595.
423. Trump DL, Livingston JN, Baylin SB. Watery diarrhea syndrome in an adult with ganglioneuroma-pheochromocytoma. Identification of vasoactive intestinal peptide, calcitonin, and catecholamines and assessment of their biologic activity. *Cancer* 1977;40:1526–1532.
424. Tsokos M. Peripheral primitive neuroectodermal tumors. Diagnosis, classification, and prognosis. In: Garvin AJ, O'Leary TJ, Bernstein J, Rosenberg HS, eds. *Pediatric Molecular Pathology: Quantitation and Applications. Perspectives in Pediatric Pathology*. Basel: Karger; 1992:16:27–98.
425. Tsokos M, Linnoila RI, Chandra RS, Triche TJ. Neuron-specific enolase in the diagnosis of neuroblastoma and other small, round-cell tumors in children. *Hum Pathol* 1984;15:575–584.
426. Tsokos M, Scarpa S, Ross RA , Triche TJ. Differentiation of human neuroblastoma recapitulates neural crest development. Study of morphology, neurotransmitter enzymes and extracellular matrix proteins. *Am J Pathol* 1987;128:484–496.
427. Turkel SB, Itabashi HH. The natural history of neuroblastic cells in the fetal adrenal gland. *Am J Pathol* 1974;76:225–244.
428. Turner GE, Reid MM. What is marrow fibrosis after treatment of neuroblastoma? *J Clin Pathol* 1993;46:61–63.
429. Turner MC, Lieberman E, DeQuattro V. The perioperative management of pheochromocytoma in children. *Clin Pediatr* 1992;31:583–589.
430. Uderzo C, Rajnoldi AC, Schiro R, et al. Neuroblastoma during acute lymphoblastic leukemia in remission. *Cancer* 1988;62: 1359–1363.
431. Ungar DR, Hailat N, Strahler JR. Hsp27 expression in neuroblastoma: correlation with disease stage. *JNCI* 1994;86:780–784.
432. Van Heerden JA, Sheps SG, Hamberger B, Sheedy PF II, Poston JG, ReMine WH. Pheochromocytoma: current status and changing trends. *Surgery* 1982;91:367–373.
433. Van Heerden JA, Roland CF, Carney JA, Sheps SG, Grant CS. Long-term evaluation following resection of apparently benign pheochromocytoma(s)/paraganglioma(s). *World J Surg* 1990;14: 325–329.
434. Vanier MT, Holm M, Ohman R, Svennerholm L. Developmental profiles of gangliosides in human and rat brain. *J Neurochem* 1971;18:581–592.
435. Van Roy N, Laureys G, Cheng NC, et al. 1;17 translocations and other chromosome 17 rearrangements in human primary neuroblastoma tumors and cell lines. *Genes Chrom Cancer* 1994;10: 103–114.
436. Vasen HF, van der Feltz M, Raue R, et al. The natural course of multiple endocrine neoplasia type IIb. A study of 18 cases. *Arch Intern Med* 1992;152:1250–1252.
437. Voorhess ML. Neuroblastoma with normal urinary catecholamine excretion. *J Pediatr* 1971;78:680–683.

438. Voorhess ML. Disorders of the adrenal medulla and multiple endocrine adenomatoses. *Pediatr Clin North Am* 1979;26:209–222.
439. Wahl HR. Neuroblastomata: with a study of a case illustrating the three types that arise from the sympathetic system. *J Med Res* 1914;30:205–260
440. Wahl HR, Robinson D. Neuroblastoma of the mediastinum with pheochromoblastomatous elements. *Arch Pathol* 1943;35:571–578.
441. Weeks DA, Beckwith JB, Mierau GW, Luckey DW. Rhabdoid tumor of kidney. A report of 111 cases from the National Wilms' Tumor Study Pathology Center. *Am J Surg Pathol* 1989;13:439–458.
442. Weidner N, Tjoe J. Immunohistochemical profile of monoclonal antibody 013: antibody that recognizes glycoprotein p30/32^{MIC2} and is useful in diagnosing Ewing's sarcoma and peripheral neuroepithelioma. *Am J Surg Pathol* 1994:18;486–494.
443. Weinblatt ME, Heisel MA, Siegel SE. Hypertension in children with neurogenic tumors. *Pediatrics* 1983;71:947–957.
444. Whang-Peng J, Triche TJ, Knutsen T, Miser J, Douglass EC, Israel MA. Chromosome translocation in peripheral neuroepithelioma. *N Engl J Med* 1984;311:584–585.
445. Wick MR. Monoclonal antibodies to chromogranin: characterization and comparison with other "neuroendocrine" markers. In: Wick MR, Siegal GP, eds. *Monoclonal Antibodies in Diagnostic Immunohistochemistry.* New York: Marcel Dekker; 1988:521–537.
446. Wiedenmann B, Huttner WB. Synaptophysin and chromogranins/secretogranins. Widespread constituents of distinct types of neuroendocrine vesicles and new tools in tumor diagnosis. *Virchows Arch B* 1989;58:95–121.
447. Williams TH, House RF Jr, Burgert EO, Lynn HB. Unusual manifestations of neuroblastoma: chronic diarrhea, polymyoclonia-opsoclonus, and erythrocyte abnormalities. *Cancer* 1972;29:475–480.
448. Willis RA. Neuroblastoma and ganglioneuroma. In: *Pathology of tumours.* London: Butterworths, 1967;857–885.
449. Wilson PCG, Coppes MJ, Solh H, et al. Neuroblastoma stage IV-S: a heterogeneous disease. *Med Pediatr Oncol* 1991;19:467–472.
450. Wirnsberger GH, Becker H, Ziervogel K, Höfler H. Diagnostic immunohistochemistry of neuroblastic tumors. *Am J Surg Pathol* 1992;16:49–57.
451. Witzleben CL, Landy RA. Disseminated neuroblastoma in a child with von Recklinghausen's disease. *Cancer* 1974;34:786–790.
452. Woods WG, Lemieux B, Tuchman M. Neuroblastoma represents distinct clinical-biologic entities: a review and perspective from the Quebec Neuroblastoma Screening Project. *Pediatrics* 1992;89:114–118.
453. Wright JH. Neurocytoma or neuroblastoma, a kind of tumor not generally recognized. *J Exp Med* 1910;12:556.
454. Yamaguchi K, Abe K, Otsubo K, et al. The WDHA syndrome: clinical and laboratory data in 28 Japanese cases. *Peptides* 1984;5:415–421.
455. Yang KP, Nguyen CV, Castillo SG, Samaan NA. Deletion mapping on the distal third region of chromosome 1p in multiple endocrine neoplasia type IIA. *Anticancer Res* 1990;10:527–533.
456. Yunis EJ, Agostini RM Jr, Walpusk JA, Hubbard JD. Glycogen in neuroblastomas. A light- and electron-microscope study of 40 cases. *Am J Surg Pathol* 1979;3:313–323.
457. Zeltzer P, Schneider S, Bell R, Marangos PJ. Neuronal enolase and BB isoenzyme of creatine kinase are biological markers for neuroectodermal tumors. *Clin Res* 1982;30:139A.
458. Zeltzer PM, Marangos PJ, Parma AM. Raised neuron-specific enolase in serum in children with metastatic neuroblastoma. A report from Children's Cancer Study Group. *Lancet* 1983;2:361–363.
459. Zheng HL, Maruyama T, Matsuda S, Satomura K. Neuroblastoma presenting with the nephrotic syndrome. *J Pediatr Surg* 1979;14:414–419.
460. Zuppan C, Beckwith JB, Luckey DW. Anaplasia in unilateral Wilms' tumor. A report from the National Wilms' Tumor Pathology Center. *Hum Pathol* 1988;19:1199–1209.

Pediatric Neoplasia: Morphology and Biology, edited by David M. Parham.
Lippincott-Raven Publishers, Philadelphia © 1996.

CHAPTER 7

Central Nervous System Tumors

Gregory N. Fuller

INTRODUCTION

Tumors of the central nervous system rank second only to leukemia in frequency and as a cause of mortality among childhood malignancies, and they constitute the single largest class of solid tumors in the pediatric age group. Approximately 1,500–2,000 new cases occur annually in the United States (298) and an estimated 40,000 worldwide (43).

The central nervous system is composed of a diverse array of cellular constituents (114). This remarkable diversity is reflected in the wide range of primary neoplasms arising from the nervous system and its investing meninges. Over 120 categories and subtypes are listed in the most recent revision of the World Health Organization (WHO) classification of tumors of the central nervous system (199). However, approximately 80% of pediatric brain tumors are encompassed by only five histologic categories: medulloblastoma, juvenile pilocytic astrocytoma, the diffuse astrocytomas, ependymoma, and craniopharyngioma (Table 1). Each of the remaining disparate entities constitutes only a small fraction of the total.

Much has been made in general texts of the distribution of pediatric brain tumors, particularly with respect to an infratentorial (posterior fossa) predominance in childhood compared to the supratentorial predominance seen in adult patients. This is a gross and misleading oversimplification of the data. In a recent survey by the Childhood Brain Tumor Consortium (CTBC) of 3,291 children with biopsied brain tumors, only a slight overall infratentorial predominance was seen (43.2% infratentorial, 40.9% supratentorial, 4.9% spinal cord, 11% involving multiple compartments) (70). A more meaningful evaluation is provided by analyzing the distribution of brain tumors as a function of age, in which three phases can be distinguished (70,250). Initially, from birth through the first year of life, supratentorial tumors predominate and are more common than posterior fossa tumors. This is due to the comparatively high incidence of teratomas and choroid plexus papillomas in these very young patients. Teratomas, while occurring throughout the neuraxis during childhood, arise predominantly supratentorially in this age group, as do pediatric choroid plexus papillomas. From age 1 through 8–10, infratentorial tumors predominate, primarily because of the high incidence of cerebellar medulloblastomas and juvenile pilocytic astrocytomas during this middle period of childhood (70,250). Finally, from about age 10 through adolescence supratentorial tumors once again predominate, as the distribution merges with that of young adults.

Only 5% of pediatric intrathecal (intradural) tumors arise in the spinal cord. The three most common histologic types in this location observed in the CBTC study were pilocytic astrocytoma (13.0%), myxopapillary ependymoma (10%), and schwannoma (9.6%) (70).

Concepts of the classification, biology, and treatment of pediatric brain tumors are changing rapidly in response to an ever-increasing infusion of data from clinical and basic research. This chapter is intended to provide a summary of the morphologic and biologic diversity of childhood brain tumors with an emphasis on current research trends.

ASTROCYTIC NEOPLASMS

Astrocytic tumors as a group comprise about 40% of all pediatric brain tumors (70) and based on clinicopathologic features can be divided into two major categories: (**a**) the diffusely infiltrating fibrillary astrocytomas ("ordinary" astrocytomas) and (**b**) a heterogeneous group comprising juvenile pilocytic astrocytoma (JPA), pleo-

G. N. Fuller: Department of Pathology, University of Texas M. D. Anderson Cancer Center, Houston, Texas 77030.

TABLE 1. *Histologic subtypes of childhood brain tumors*

Neoplasm	Approximate percentage of all pediatric brain tumors
Medulloblastoma/PNET (95% infratentorial)	20
Juvenile pilocytic astrocytoma (75% infratentorial)	20
Low-grade astrocytoma	15
High-grade astrocytoma	7
Ependymoma (70% infratentorial)	7
Craniopharyngioma	7
Unclassified primary tumors	7
Choroid plexus tumors (75% supratentorial)	2
Germ cell tumors	2
Oligodendroglioma	1–2
Meningioma	1–2
Metastatic tumors	1
Ganglion cell tumors	1
Pineal parenchymal tumors	1
Schwannoma	<1
Teratoma	<1
Pituitary adenoma	<1

PNET, primitive neuroectodermal tumors.

morphic xanthoastrocytoma (PXA), desmoplastic cerebral astrocytoma of infancy (DCAI), and subependymal giant cell astrocytoma (SGCA). These latter four entities are mutually distinctive but share several characteristics: (**a**) occurrence at an early age, (2) very limited infiltration of surrounding brain parenchyma, (**c**) a tendency to spread into the overlying leptomeninges, (**d**) little tendency for anaplastic progression, and (**e**) a relatively favorable prognosis compared to the fibrillary astrocytomas. Because these tumors do not exhibit a spectrum of anaplasia, they do not require stratification by grade (in contrast to the fibrillary astrocytomas).

Juvenile Pilocytic Astrocytoma

Discussion of astrocytic brain tumors conventionally begins with fibrillary astrocytomas, largely because they are the most common astrocytic neoplasms of adulthood. In contrast, the most common astrocytic tumor of childhood is the juvenile pilocytic astrocytoma (JPA), which comprises about 20% of all childhood brain tumors (Table 1) (70).

JPAs constitute a unique group of astrocytic tumors with favored neuroanatomic locations, distinctive histologic features, very little tendency for malignant progression, and a significantly more favorable clinical outlook than is associated with the fibrillary astrocytomas. The three classic locations are cerebellum, hypothalamic/third ventricular region, and optic nerves (at which site they are commonly referred to as "optic gliomas"). By far the most common site is the cerebellum, where around 75% of juvenile pilocytic astrocytomas arise (70). This site also carries the most favorable prognosis, due in large part to the potential for complete surgical resection. In contrast, hypothalamic lesions are not amenable to gross total excision. Optic nerve pilocytic astrocytomas are intermediate in outlook. Those distal to the chiasm may be resected (with sacrifice of the nerve), but involvement of the chiasm and more proximal structures poses the same impediment to surgical extirpation as encountered with hypothalamic lesions. Approximately 20% of children with neurofibromatosis type 1 have an optic glioma (225,232). Conversely, in one study 12.5% of pediatric patients with an optic glioma had NF1(243).

JPAs also occur at other sites within the central nervous system, including the cerebrum (105), brain stem ("dorsally exophytic" tumors) (196), and spinal cord (327). Those of the midbrain tectum and periaqueductal region are sometimes referred to as "pencil gliomas" (399). Among low grade astrocytomas of the cerebral hemispheres, JPAs are slightly more frequent than low grade fibrillary astrocytomas (70,299).

JPAs, particularly in the cerebellum, often present with a classic neuroradiologic appearance composed of a contrast-enhancing nodule in the wall of a large cyst. Other patterns, including solid tumors and tumors with multiple intrinsic cysts, are also recognized (25). Contrast enhancement is a typical feature of these low-grade tumors and does not carry the same caveats as when found in association with fibrillary astrocytomas (110).

By light microscopy, pilocytic astrocytomas exhibit a distinctive biphasic appearance, with bundles of dense fibrillary tissue separated by loose, spongy, microcystic areas (Fig. 1). The compact areas exhibit fascicles of elongated, spindle-shaped astrocytes (pilocytes) and often contain prominent Rosenthal fibers (Fig. 2A; see figure in color plate section). Rosenthal fibers are compacted masses of glial filaments that distend and irregularly distort astrocytic processes (Fig. 2B). Although typical of the JPA, it must be kept in mind that Rosenthal fiber formation is a very common astrocytic response to chronic compressive conditions and may be seen in neuropil adjacent to a wide variety of neoplastic and nonneoplastic lesions, including craniopharyngiomas, hemangioblastomas, syringomyelia, vascular malformations, and incidental pineal cysts.

The microcystic areas of JPAs contain loosely arranged stellate astrocytes and often eosinophilic granular bodies. The latter structures are most commonly seen in slowly growing, low-grade neoplasms such as JPA, pleomorphic xanthoastrocytoma, and ganglioglioma (157) (see Fig. 5B). Microvascular proliferation is often a prominent component of JPA (Fig. 3) and constitutes the presumed morphologic basis for the contrast enhancement seen on neuroimaging studies. Cells with enlarged, pleomorphic, hyperchromatic nuclei are also frequently seen (Fig. 3). The latter are presumed to

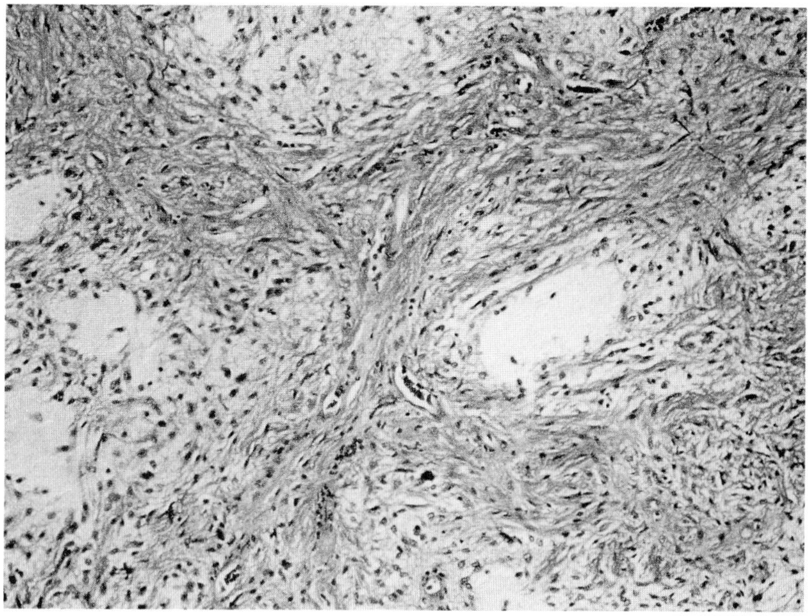

FIG. 1. Juvenile pilocytic astrocytoma (JPA). JPAs characteristically exhibit a biphasic architectural pattern consisting of dense bands of elongated glial cells ("pilocytes") separated by hypocellular, microcystic areas.

represent "degenerative atypia" and, as with vascular proliferation and contrast enhancement, do not have the adverse prognostic significance as when seen in fibrillary astrocytomas. Notably, mitotic figures are generally inconspicuous or absent, and tumor necrosis is rare. Invasion of the overlying leptomeninges is quite common and, as with other low-grade glial tumors that exhibit this propensity (pleomorphic xanthoastrocytoma, desmoplastic infantile ganglioglioma), does not constitute a negative prognostic indicator (Fig. 4). Juvenile pilocytic astrocytomas occasionally disseminate widely throughout the neuraxis via the ventricular and subarachnoid space cerebrospinal fluid pathways (118,298). With appropriate use of adjuvant therapy, such "metastatic" spread is not incompatible with extended survival (118, 298). Very rarely, JPA may undergo anaplastic progression (55).

It should be noted that fibrillary astrocytomas, including rare glioblastomas, may also be seen in the cerebellum (144). Although high-grade neoplasms usually do

B

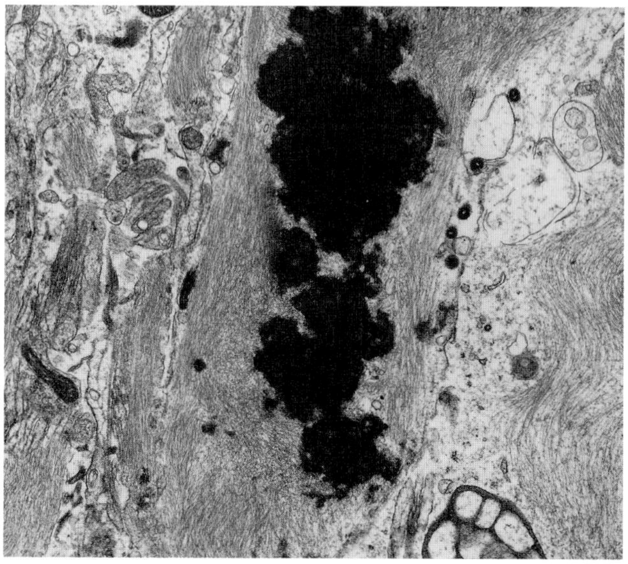

FIG. 2. Juvenile pilocytic astrocytoma. Rosenthal fibers **(A)** *(see color plate section)* are a prominent feature of most JPAs. Ultrastructural examination **(B)** shows amorphous aggregates of electron-dense material. Note the close association of the Rosenthal fiber material with glial intermediate filaments.

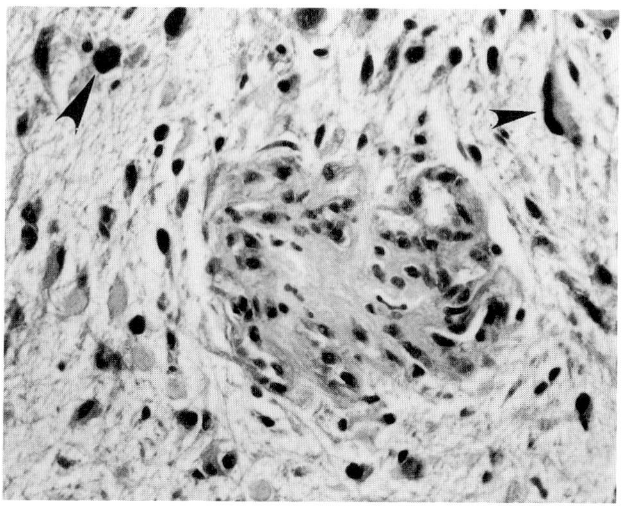

FIG. 3. Juvenile pilocytic astrocytoma. Two common features of JPAs that may lead to overgrading are microvascular proliferation, which may assume the florid "glomeruloid" proportions seen in the center of the field, and atypical hyperchromatic nuclei *(arrowheads)*.

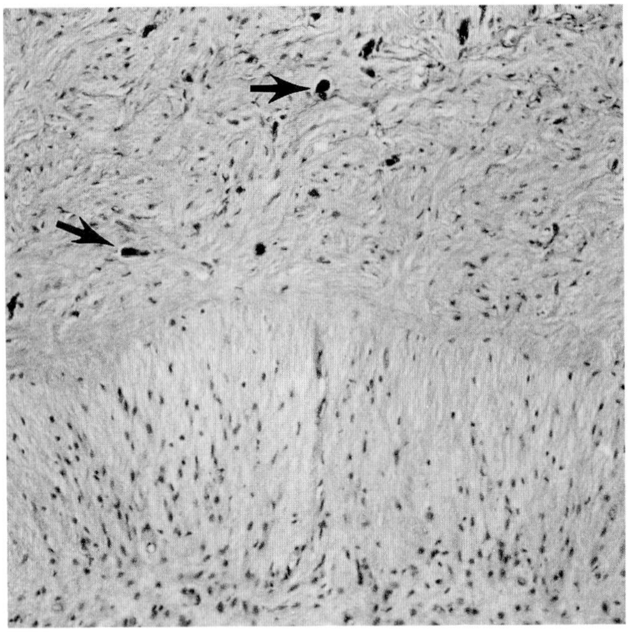

FIG. 4. Juvenile pilocytic astrocytoma. Invasion of the leptomeninges, as illustrated above, is frequent in JPAs and, like microvascular proliferation, is devoid of prognostic significance. The dark structures *(arrows)* are Rosenthal fibers.

not pose diagnostic difficulty, low-grade tumors may be difficult to distinguish from peripheral areas of JPA if only limited biopsy tissue is available for examination. JPAs are, however, much more common in the cerebellum than are low-grade diffuse astrocytomas, outnumbering them in this location by almost 4:1 (70).

Preliminary molecular studies of JPA have shown marked differences as compared to the fibrillary astrocytomas, including a lack of *p53* mutation, absence of allelic losses on chromosomes 10 and 19q, and lack of amplification of the epidermal growth factor receptor (EGFR) gene (226,394–396). In contrast, deletion of 17q has been reported in 20% of pilocytic astrocytomas in one study, suggesting possible involvement of a tumor suppressor gene (394).

Pleomorphic Xanthoastrocytoma

The pleomorphic xanthoastrocytoma (PXA) is a unique astrocytic neoplasm of late childhood and adolescence that occurs most frequently in the cerebral hemispheres, particularly the temporal lobe (192,193). Vigorous debate over the progenitor cell of this highly pleomorphic tumor has now largely been resolved in favor of an astrocytic origin, primarily because of tumor cell immunoreactivity for glial fibrillary acidic protein (GFAP).

PXAs characteristically exhibit robust infiltration of the overlying leptomeninges but quite limited infiltration of surrounding brain parenchyma. Striking cellular pleomorphism is typically accompanied by the presence of multinucleated giant cells and numerous eosinophilic granular bodies (Fig. 5). Other features include lipidized tumor cells and perivascular infiltrates of chronic inflammatory cells. Most importantly, mitotic figures are very rare, and no necrosis or microvascular proliferation is seen.

Ultrastructural examination of these tumors has revealed the presence of basal lamina associated with the neoplastic astrocytes. Given the superficial location of PXAs and the fact that subpial astrocytes are known to possess a basement membrane, it has been hypothesized that PXAs originate from this specialized astrocyte. A similar argument can be made for the desmoplastic cerebral astrocytoma of infancy (discussed below).

The prognosis for patients with PXA is very good compared to the fibrillary astrocytomas, and the possibility of surgical cure exists. However, residual tumor will recur and well-documented cases of recurrence with progression to anaplastic astrocytoma or glioblastoma have been reported (11,124,191). Given the fact that the existence of PXA has only been recognized for 15 years and that a majority of these patients will experience extended survival, the late sequelae of PXA and therapy used to treat it are only now becoming manifest.

Desmoplastic Cerebral Astrocytoma of Infancy (Superficial Cerebral Astrocytoma)

Desmoplastic cerebral astrocytoma of infancy (DCAI) is typically a very large astrocytic neoplasm of the cerebral hemispheres that occurs during in the first 2 years of life (231,373,387). Despite their enormous size, these tumors have a comparably favorable prognosis. There are shared similarities with the desmoplastic infantile ganglioglioma (discussed under "Neoplasms of Mixed Neuronal/Glial Phenotype").

Microscopically, DCAIs are composed of highly spindled cells interspersed with collagen (Fig. 6A). This histologic appearance, along with the characteristic invasion of the overlying leptomeninges (Fig. 6B), gives the neoplasm a strong resemblance to sarcoma. Confirmation of the glial nature is provided by immunoreactivity of the neoplastic cells for GFAP.

Preliminary molecular genetic analysis suggests that tumor suppressor genes on chromosomes 10 and 17p (including the p53 gene) are not involved in the genesis of at least some of these tumors (231). These data are consistent with accumulating evidence that p53 gene mutation lacks a significant role in several types of astrocytic tumors in the pediatric population and provide another example of the fundamental differences between adult and pediatric tumors of the same histogenetic lineage (226). Further studies on additional tumors are clearly needed.

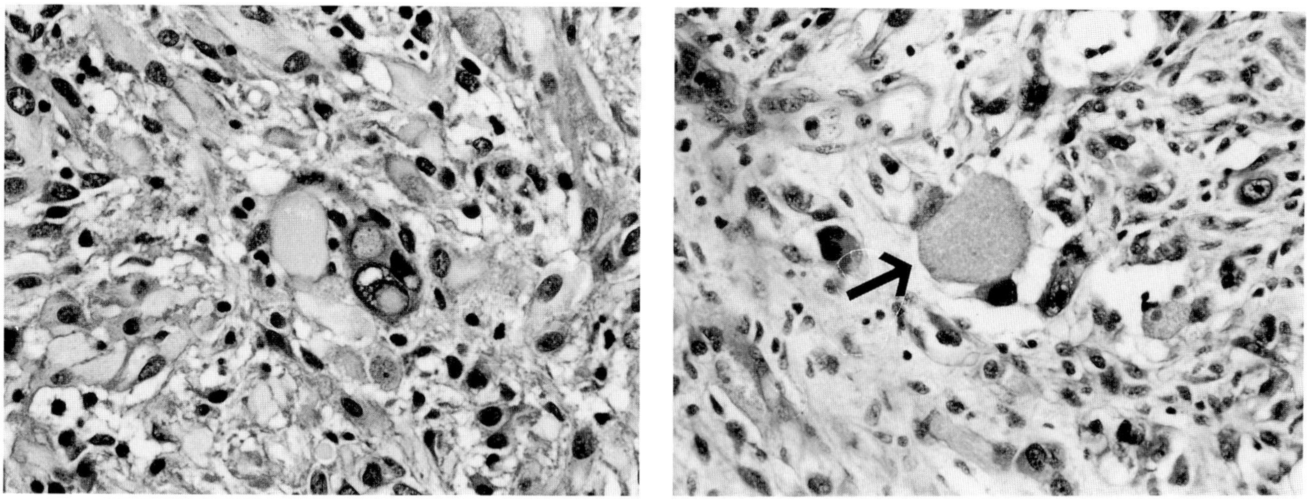

A B

FIG. 5. Pleomorphic xanthoastrocytoma (PXA). PXA is typified by strikingly pleomorphic cellular constituents **(A)**. Eosinophilic granular bodies (*arrow,* **B**) are numerous in most PXAs. Mitotic figures are rare and necrosis and microvascular proliferation are absent.

On the biologic level, an interesting hypothesis that relates the striking desmoplasia to the indolent growth of these tumors has been proposed (231). In brief, it is known from ultrastructural studies that the neoplastic astrocytes of desmoplastic cerebral astrocytomas are associated with basal laminae, hence the postulated origin from subpial astrocytes. Cell culture studies have demonstrated the ability of extracellular matrix proteins to inhibit glioma growth (336,337). Louis et al. (231) have therefore speculated that indolent behavior in this class of tumors may be in part related to an autocrine type of inhibition of growth by glia-elaborated basal lamina components. A similar growth control mechanism could be postulated for other superficial astrocytic neoplasms (e.g., pleomorphic xanthoastrocytoma) that possess basal laminae and are hypothesized to originate from subpial astrocytes.

Subependymal Giant Cell Astrocytoma

The subependymal giant cell astrocytoma (SGCA) is traditionally included with the astrocytic neoplasms, even though the cells of this low-grade tumor exhibit variable immunoreactivity for both glial and neuronal

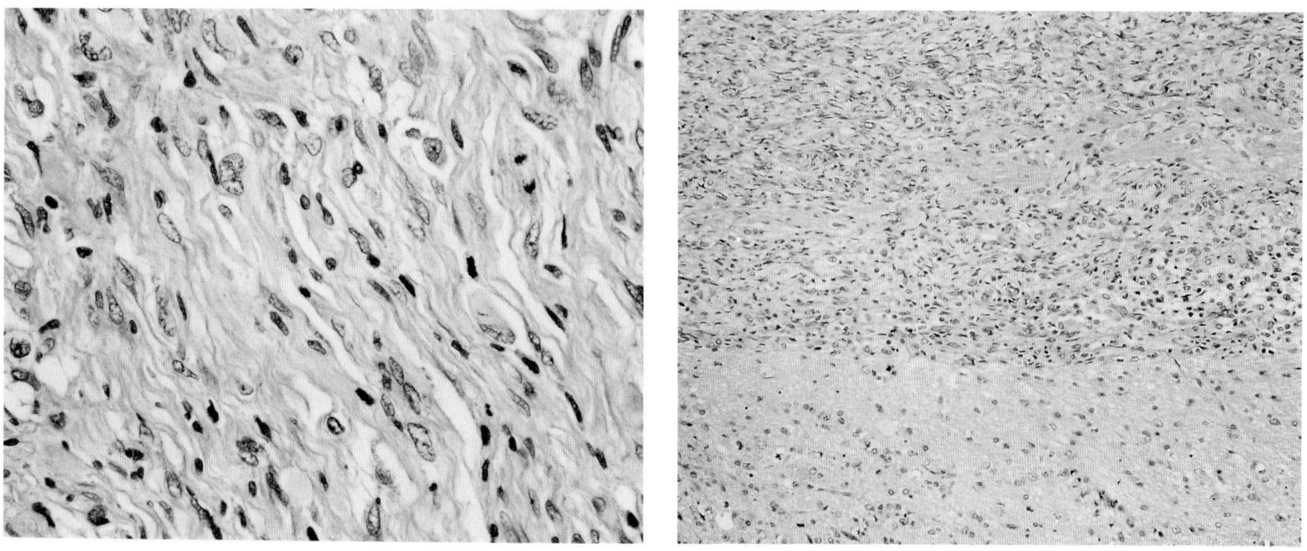

A B

FIG. 6. Desmoplastic cerebral astrocytoma of infancy. These typically enormous tumors are composed of highly spindled cells **(A)** that are immunopositive for glial fibrillary acid protein (GFAP) (not shown). Invasion of the overlying subarachnoid space **(B)** is common and does not adversely affect the prognosis.

markers. The lineage remains a subject of spirited debate (54,55).

Subependymal giant cell astrocytomas constitute one of the classic lesions associated with tuberous sclerosis and often present in that context in childhood, occasionally as early as the neonatal period (46,278,362). In some cases, hydrocephalus secondary to the tumor precipitates the initial clinical presentation, and a history of tuberous sclerosis is therefore not available to the surgical pathologist at the time of intraoperative consultation. Moreover, in a minority of cases, additional stigmata of tuberous sclerosis are not found when specifically searched for (362). Thus, a high index of suspicion is required, based on the neuroimaging data and a familiarity with the variable morphologic features of this unique tumor.

As the name implies, SGCAs originate in a subependymal location and grow in an exophytic fashion into the lateral ventricle. Symptoms usually relate to hydrocephalus produced by obstruction of the foramen of Monro. Histologically, SGCAs exhibit large cells with abundant cytoplasm and sometimes cacifications. These cells may closely resemble gemistocytic astrocytes (Fig. 7A) or, less commonly, ganglion cells. A fibrillary pattern may also be seen (Fig. 7B). As already mentioned, the cells exhibit variable reactivity for glial and neuronal markers. Given this ambiguity, use of the less restrictive term "subependymal giant cell tumor" has been recommended.

Fibrillary Astrocytoma

Fibrillary astrocytomas occur less frequently in children than pilocytic astrocytomas. The most common location in children is the brainstem, but supratentorial and spinal cord tumors occur as well. Brainstem tumors will be discussed under a separate heading below.

Fibrillary astrocytomas differ from the four special categories of astrocytic neoplasms just described by exhibiting diffuse infiltration of neural parenchyma and a tendency for anaplastic progression over time. Grading of this class of tumors has a long and complicated history. To provide an overview and facilitate comparison, seven systems that figure prominently in the current and historical literature are illustrated in Table 2. Approximate equivalencies relative to the three traditional categories consisting of astrocytoma, anaplastic astrocytoma, and glioblastoma multiforme are indicated along with the grades as assigned in the original publications, including faithful adherence to the use of either Arabic or Roman numerals as chosen by the respective authors. It is readily apparent from perusal of Table 2 that failure to specify the system used for numeric grading may lead to ambiguity. For example, a grade 3 astrocytoma in the St. Anne–Mayo system is equivalent to an anaplastic astrocytoma but would be a glioblastoma in the Kernohan system. The WHO system employs Roman numerals for grades, but this convention is often ignored. For these reasons, it is strongly recommended that if a diagnosis is rendered using a numeric grading system, the particular system should be specified.

The individual grading systems warrant brief comment. The historic, original classification of Bailey and Cushing (18) was devised as a histogenetic scheme based on the morphologic resemblance of tumor cells to contemporaneously recognized stages of normal astrocytic differentiation. This system thus fundamentally differs from contemporary schemes, which represent attempts

A

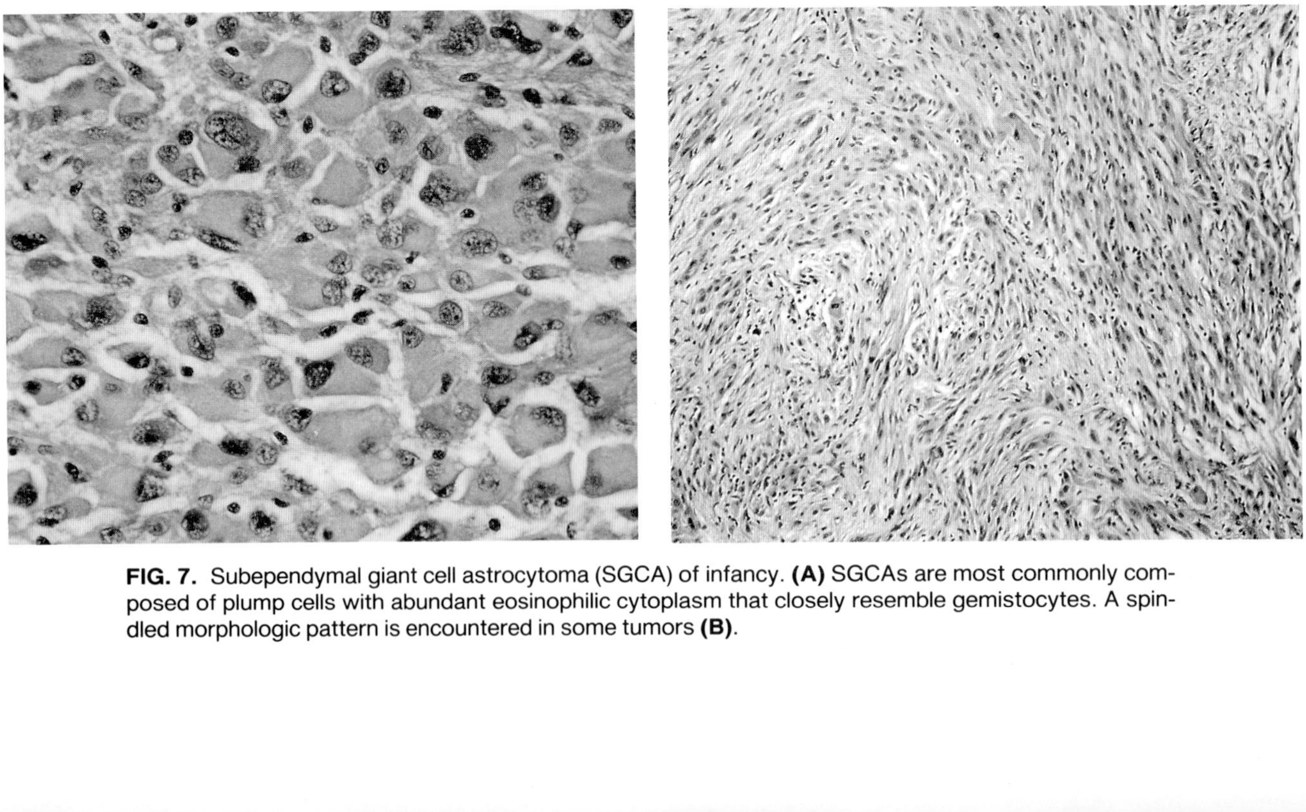

B

FIG. 7. Subependymal giant cell astrocytoma (SGCA) of infancy. **(A)** SGCAs are most commonly composed of plump cells with abundant eosinophilic cytoplasm that closely resemble gemistocytes. A spindled morphologic pattern is encountered in some tumors **(B)**.

TABLE 2. *Fibrillary astrocytoma grading systems*

Bailey & Cushing (1926)	Kernohan (1949)	Ringertz (1950)	Univ. California-San Francisco	Modified Ringertz	St. Anne-Mayo (1988)	WHO (1993)
	Astrocytoma grade 1		Mildly anaplastic astrocytoma		Astrocytoma grade 1	
Astrocytoma		Astrocytoma		Astrocytoma		Astrocytoma (grade II)
			Moderately anaplastic astrocytoma		Astrocytoma grade 2	
	Astrocytoma grade 2					
Astroblastoma		Intermediate type	Highly anaplastic astrocytoma	Anaplastic astrocytoma	Astrocytoma grade 3	Anaplastic astrocytoma (grade III)
	Astrocytoma grade 3					
Spongioblastoma multiforme		Glioblastoma multiforme	Glioblastoma multiforme	Glioblastoma multiforme	Astrocytoma grade 4	Glioblastoma multiforme (grade IV)
	Astrocytoma grade 4					

Modified from Fuller and Burger, Ref. 115.

to generate prognostically meaningful stratification of astrocytomas based on their degree of anaplasia. Typical anaplastic features assessed in the various schemes include nuclear pleomorphism and hyperchromasia, cellular pleomorphism, mitotic activity, microvascular proliferation, and tumor necrosis. The earliest grading system of this type was introduced by Kernohan et al. in 1949 (194) and segregated the astrocytomas into four tiers (Table 2). However, the last two tiers (grades 3 and 4) were simply subdivisions of glioblastoma, and the status of grade 2 tumors was ambiguous. Although grade 2 lesions were regarded by the author as rapidly growing tumors akin to the "astroblastoma" of Bailey and Cushing, the histologic criteria specifically stated that mitotic figures were absent. As indicated in Table 2, only two prognostically significant categories result from rigorous application of the Kernohan criteria, i.e., low grade and high grade (84).

Ringertz introduced a three-tiered system (319) that with some modification has been widely adopted by numerous investigators (55,259,335). A major feature of the modified Ringertz systems is the use of tumor necrosis, with or without surrounding pseudopalisading of tumor cells, to separate glioblastomas from anaplastic astrocytomas. A four-tiered system with a unique nomenclature has been extensively employed at the University of California at San Francisco (86).

The two most recently introduced systems are the St. Anne–Mayo (84) and the revised WHO (199). In the St. Anne–Mayo system, tumor grading is accomplished by simply tabulating the presence or absence of four morphologic features: (a) nuclear atypia, (b) mitotic figures, (c) microvascular proliferation, and (d) necrosis. Tumors exhibiting none of these features (i.e., very low-grade tumors characterized only by increased cellularity and perhaps distortion of native parenchymal architecture) are classified as grade 1; those with only one feature (usually nuclear pleomorphism) are grade 2; those with two features (usually nuclear pleomorphism and mitotic figures) are grade 3; and tumors exhibiting three or four features are classified together as grade 4. Grade 1 tumors are extremely uncommon and, as indicated in Table 2, may be grouped with the grade 2 tumors for purposes of comparison to other systems. The original WHO classification published in 1979 (418) did not recognize the glioblastoma as an astrocytic neoplasm. Instead, these tumors were relegated to a rubric termed "poorly differentiated and embryonal tumors." In contrast, the 1993 revised WHO system (199) adopts a more conventional three-tiered stratification similar to that of the modified Ringertz systems (Table 2). However, similar to the St. Anne–Mayo system, the presence of necrosis is not an absolute requirement for a diagnosis of a grade IV (glioblastoma) tumor. Rather, the criteria state: "Essential for the diagnosis is the presence of vascular proliferation and/or necrosis."

As seen in Table 2, by convention all of the three-tiered systems use descriptive terms rather than numerical designations, whereas the four-tiered systems use either Arabic numerals (St. Anne–Mayo; Kernohan) or Roman numerals (revised WHO). However, these conventions are often flouted. For example, some investigators have appropriated Arabic or Roman numeral designators for the three tiers of modified Ringertz systems.

A 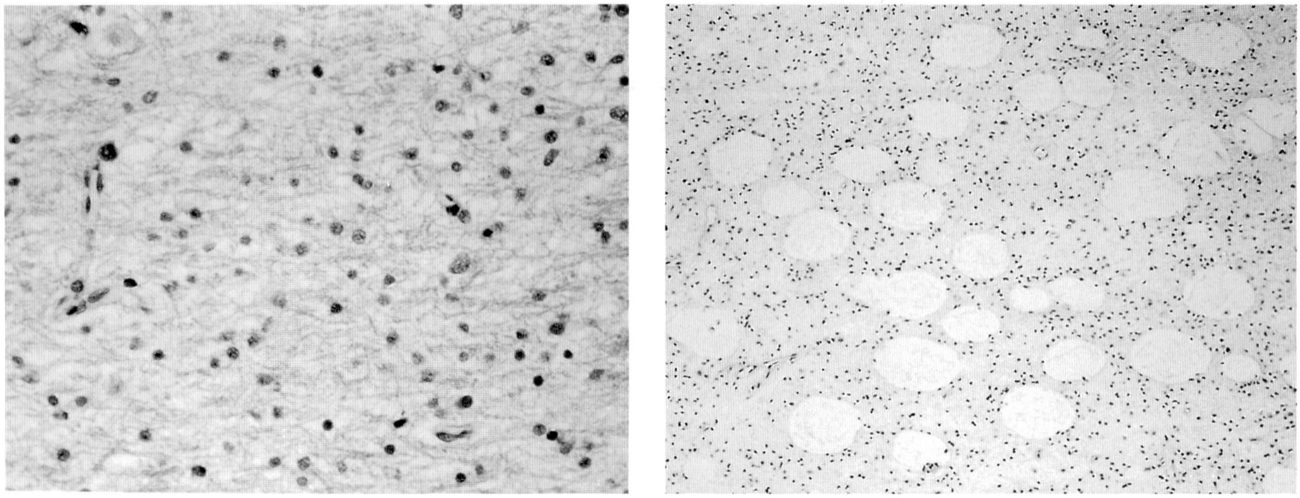 B

FIG. 8. Low-grade fibrillary astrocytoma. Low-grade astrocytomas show mild to moderately increased cellularity **(A)**. Mitotic figures and microvascular proliferation are not present. In some cases, the normal architecture of the neural parenchyma is disrupted by microcyst formation **(B)**.

Once again, to avoid confusion or ambiguity, the particular system or criteria employed should be specified.

As a final comment on the various classification and grading systems, it should be noted that the Kernohan system has now largely passed into desuetude. Its continued use is thus to be discouraged, not only because the criteria fail to stratify patients into more than two prognostically meaningful groups, but also because of the potential problems arising from confusion between its numeric terminology and that of more contemporary systems. The modified Ringertz, St. Anne–Mayo, and revised WHO systems are all currently employed worldwide.

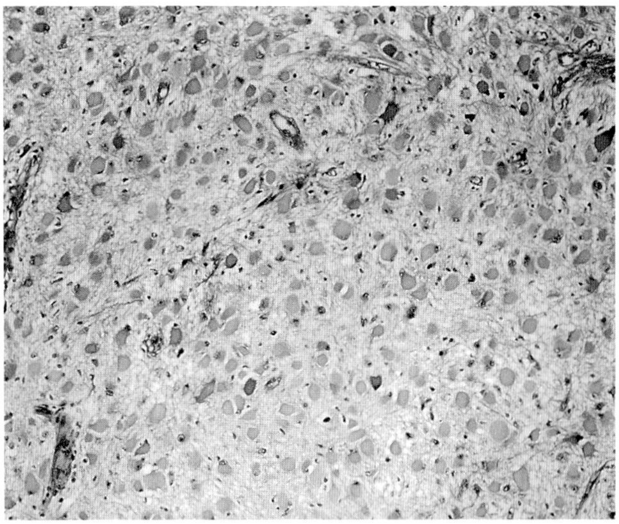

FIG. 9. Gemistocytic astrocytoma. The cells exhibit eccentric nuclei and abundant, globular cytoplasm.

Astrocytoma (Low-Grade)

Low-grade fibrillary astrocytomas exhibit mild to moderately increased cellularity over that found in normal brain parenchyma (Fig. 8A). The rounded to oval nuclei resemble normal astrocytic nuclei with a delicate chromatin pattern but may be mildly pleomorphic. Microcysts may also be present (Fig. 8B). Mitotic figures, however, are absent, as are microvascular proliferation and necrosis.

Brief comment is warranted concerning the gemistocytic astrocytoma (Fig. 9). Although these tumors have traditionally been considered variants of low-grade astrocytomas and are maintained in that position in the revised WHO classification (199), recent studies have shown that they exhibit a tendency for rapid anaplastic progression and should be considered anaplastic astrocytomas (214).

Neuroimaging studies of low-grade astrocytomas usually show lack of tumor enhancement following contrast agent administration. The presence of enhancement should strongly suggest the presence of either a higher grade fibrillary astrocytoma or one of the special low-grade categories of brain tumor (e.g., juvenile pilocytic astrocytoma, pleomorphic xanthoastrocytoma, ganglion cell tumor).

Data suggest that gross total resection, when possible, offers the best opportunity for long-term progression-free survival in these patients (299).

Anaplastic Astrocytoma

Anaplastic astrocytomas exhibit increased cellularity and nuclear and cellular pleomorphism compared to

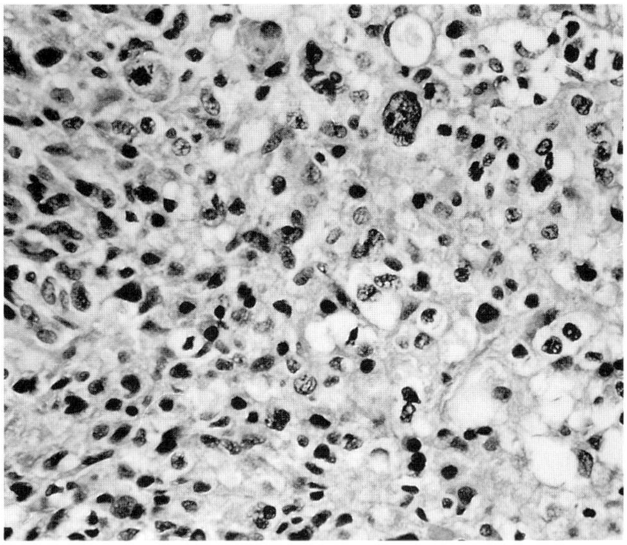

FIG. 10. Anaplastic astrocytoma. The tumor exhibits increased cellularity and pleomorphism compared with low-grade tumors.

low-grade astrocytomas (Fig. 10). Mitotic figures are usually present but may be difficult to identify in some cases, particularly if only limited tissue is available for examination, such as with stereotactic biopsy. Microvascular proliferation may also be seen, but the presence of tumor necrosis warrants raising the grade from anaplastic astrocytoma to glioblastoma (56,259).

A majority of anaplastic astrocytomas exhibit contrast enhancement, but absence of enhancement does not exclude an anaplastic neoplasm. Such lack of enhancement in a minority of malignant astrocytomas has been well documented in adult patients (67,204) and can also be seen with childhood fibrillary astrocytomas (personal observations).

Glioblastoma Multiforme

The term "glioblastoma multiforme" is derived from "spongioblastoma multiforme," an appellation previously used by Globus and Strauss (126), in which the modifier "multiforme" reflects the great cellular heterogeneity seen in these tumors. Glioblastomas generally exhibit dense cellularity, mitotic figures, microvascular proliferation, and foci of tumor necrosis (Fig. 11). Mitotic figures are actually quite variable from case to case and may be difficult to find in some instances. Although most glioblastomas are at least focally positive for GFAP, some cases are so poorly differentiated as to lack significant immunoreactivity. Proliferation of small vessels is a common accompaniment of malignant astrocytomas and reaches its zenith in large nodular tangles termed "glomeruloid vascular proliferation" (Fig. 12). Endothelium was formerly considered to be the sole proliferative element as reflected in the common term "vascular endothelial proliferation." Recent immunohistochemical and immunoelectron microscopic studies have demonstrated that activated pericytes and/or vascular smooth muscle cells also contribute to this process both in the florid glomeruloid-type structures as well as in the early proliferative stages (132,402,403). Use of the term "microvascular proliferation" or simply "vascular proliferation" is therefore recommended as a more accurate characterization of the process.

Brainstem Astrocytomas

Brainstem astrocytomas are common tumors of childhood, variously estimated to comprise 6–15% of all pediatric brain tumors (298). Rare gangliogliomas also occur in the brainstem.

Brainstem astrocytomas are separable into two pri-

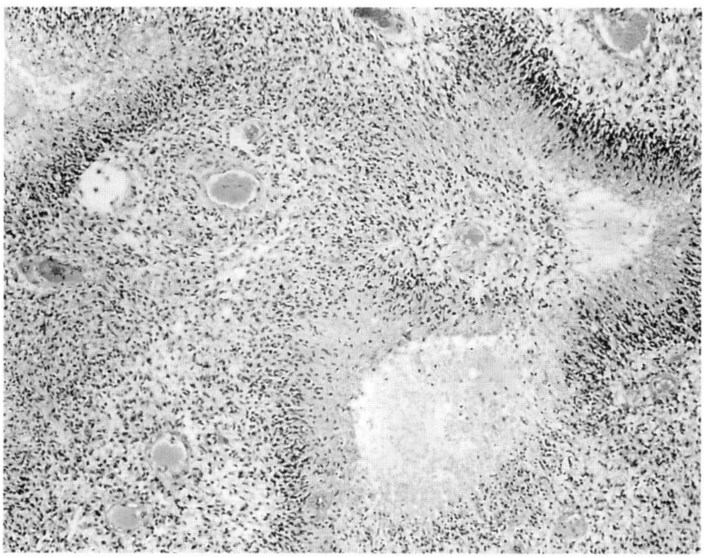

FIG. 11. Glioblastoma multiforme. The cellular constituents of glioblastomas are quite heterogeneous both within and between tumors. Many grading systems require the presence of tumor necrosis for the diagnosis. Pseudopalisading of tumor cells around zones of necrosis, as seen in this case, is a typical finding but need not be present.

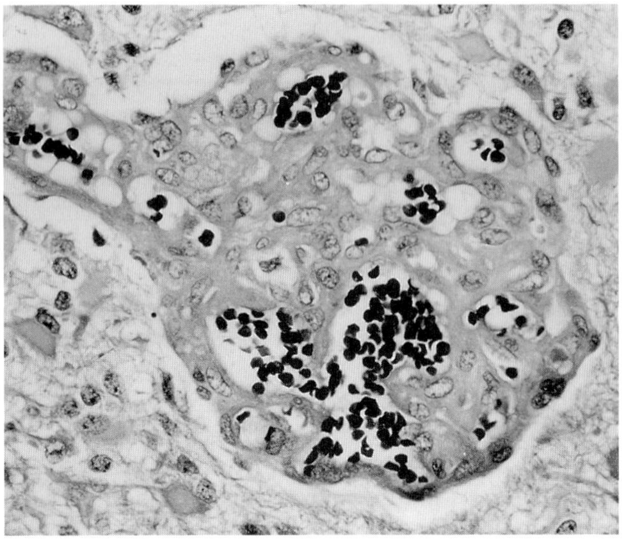

FIG. 12. Glioblastoma multiforme. Microvascular proliferation is commonly seen in glioblastomas.

mary categories. The larger group, unfortunately, is typified by the classical pontine astrocytoma—a highly infiltrative, fibrillary astrocytoma that diffusely expands the pons and often surrounds and engulfs the basilar artery. Like adult fibrillary astrocytomas, these tumors exhibit a tendency for malignant progression over time and have a uniformly dismal prognosis. The median survival is only about 10 months. The second group of brainstem astrocytomas are so-called focal gliomas, including a "dorsally exophytic" subgroup, which are relatively circumscribed neoplasms that exhibit morphologic features of either low-grade astrocytoma or juvenile pilocytic astrocytoma and have an expansive, rather than infiltrative, growth pattern (98,196,319). In contrast to those with diffuse brainstem astrocytomas, these patients generally experience extended survival, often with only subtotal resection (296,300,388).

Molecular Biology of Pediatric Fibrillary Astrocytomas

Several factors have hindered the molecular biologic characterization of fibrillary astrocytomas in children. As previously noted, the most common location for this class of tumors in the pediatric age range is the brainstem. Because of the vital functions concentrated in this region of the neuraxis, tumors that exhibit characteristic neuroimaging features of brainstem astrocytoma are commonly treated without biopsy confirmation (8). When biopsy is performed, the amount of tissue removed is generally quite small and often limited to stereotactic needle biopsy cores. Although tissue obtained at postmortem examination can be used for some types of genetic analysis, it is frequently of suboptimal quality and also has usually been subjected to the alterations produced by therapeutic irradiation and/or chemotherapy. In addition, the absolute numbers of diffuse astrocytomas in the pediatric age group are also far less than those in the adult population. Thus, there is in general a significant paucity of suitable research material. However, recent technical advances, particularly in the burgeoning number of polymerase chain reaction (PCR)–based methods, are permitting more to be done with less (229).

Preliminary data on pediatric brainstem gliomas suggest a high incidence of p53 gene mutation, allelic loss of chromosome 17p, and allelic loss of the long arm of chromosome 10 (229, 415). These tumor suppressor gene—related alterations are similar to those found in hemispheric glioblastomas occurring in young adults (398). Alternatively, another preliminary study found no p53 gene mutations in a series of 18 pediatric fibrillary astrocytomas that included 4 diffuse low-grade astrocytomas, 12 anaplastic astrocytomas, and 2 glioblastomas (226). Although individual sites of origin were not specified for this series of tumors, a comparison of these results with those from the brainstem series suggests that fibrillary astrocytomas arising in different parts of the pediatric neuraxis may occur via different oncogenic mechanisms.

A role for bcl-2 in suppressing apoptosis in adult gliomas that express wild-type p53 has recently been suggested (10). The possible relevancy of this finding to pediatric fibrillary astrocytomas awaits further investigation. With respect to oncogenes, amplification of the epidermal growth factor receptor (EGFR) gene, which is a major oncogene alteration found in approximately one third of adult glioblastomas (112), does not appear to have a role in the pediatric tumors (229).

Among the many unanswered questions regarding this class of tumors, no explanation currently exists for the high incidence of pediatric fibrillary astrocytomas in the brainstem.

Gliomatosis Cerebri

Gliomatosis cerebri is the extensive, diffuse involvement of the central nervous system by a malignant glioma (260). Gliomatosis is a controversial issue whose precise definition, pathophysiology, and nosologic position with respect to less extensive infiltrative gliomas are the subject of spirited debate. Most authors would agree on the following points: (a) neoplastic infiltration seen in gliomatosis is remarkably extensive, often involving an entire hemisphere and sometimes both hemispheres as well as the brainstem; (b) infiltrating tumor cells diffusely expand large regions of the nervous system without destroying native tissue architecture; (c) compact epicenters of tumor with foci of necrosis are not a part of the early stages of tumor evolution; and (d) the individual tumor cells are either frankly astrocytic (immunopositive for GFAP) or undifferentiated ("naked nuclei"). Rare cases of oligodendroglial gliomatosis have been described (21). There are a few reported cases of gliomatosis with extended survival, but most pursue a relentlessly aggressive course.

Gliomatosis cerebri should not be confused with the term "leptomeningeal gliomatosis," which refers to invasion and spread through the subarachnoid space. Most such cases arise from an intra-axial malignant astrocytoma that subsequently breaches the pia and spreads secondarily through the leptomeninges ("secondary leptomeningeal gliomatosis"). Very rare cases have apparently arisen directly from extra-axial heterotopic glial rests in the leptomeninges ("primary leptomeningeal gliomatosis"). It is stressed that leptomeningeal invasion is also a characteristic feature innate to the biology of several well-differentiated childhood astrocytic neoplasms, including juvenile pilocytic astrocytoma, pleomorphic xanthroastrocytoma, and desmoplastic cerebral astrocytoma of infancy. In none of these special categories does leptomeningeal invasion signify a worse prognosis.

Astroblastoma

The question of whether astroblastoma exists as a legitimate clinicopathologic entity is controversial and unresolved. The entity is described as a very rare astrocytic tumor arising primarily in the cerebral hemispheres during the first three decades of life (335,166). Characteristic features include prominent gliovascular pseudorosettes and immunopositivity for GFAP. A possible cytogenetic relationship to the tanycyte has been postulated (332). Besides a few sporadic case reports, only one recent series, consisting of only 23 tumors, has been described (48). In that series, approximately half of the cases were indolent, well-differentiated tumors and the remainder were malignant neoplasms, one of which progressed to glioblastoma and another to gliosarcoma. Astroblastoma-like morphologic features occur focally within several other types of gliomas, including malignant astrocytomas and ependymomas. Examples of "pure" astroblastoma are exceptionally rare. No cases were reported in the Childhood Brain Tumor Consortium review of 3,291 childhood brain tumors, which included contributions from ten different medical centers (70). Molecular biologic data are not available, and cytogenetic studies are limited to case reports (172).

OLIGODENDROGLIOMAS

Oligodendrogliomas are comparatively rare tumors of childhood and constitute only about 1–2% of tumors of the pediatric central nervous system. They occur primarily in the cerebrum, followed by the spinal cord, and are least common in the posterior fossa (70). The supratentorial tumors are located primarily in the cerebral hemispheres. A large majority of so-called intraventricular oligodendrogliomas are now known to be central neurocytomas (discussed below). Oligodendrogliomas are infiltrating gliomas that, like the fibrillary astrocytomas, exhibit a spectrum of anaplasia ranging from well-differentiated to anaplastic. Rare examples may progress to glioblastoma.

Typical low-grade oligodendrogliomas are composed of small, uniform cells with rounded nuclei that, in formalin-fixed permanent sections, are surrounded by prominent cleared cytoplasmic spaces termed perinuclear halos (Fig. 13A, B). The perinuclear halo is a useful artefact of delayed fixation that results from hydropic swelling of oligodendroglial cytoplasm. This change is not seen in cryostat sections prepared for intraoperative frozen section diagnosis (Fig. 13C).

Anaplastic oligodendrogliomas exhibit increased cellularity, nuclear pleomorphism, and mitotic figures and may also have foci of vascular proliferation and necrosis (Fig. 14). The presence of the latter feature raises the issue of differentiating high-grade oligodendroglioma from glioblastoma. Making this distinction may be difficult, but tumors that retain recognizable oligodendroglial features such as prominent perinuclear halos and a branching vascular pattern should not be reclassified as glioblastomas based solely on the focal presence of necrosis for two reasons. First, even the most anaplastic oligodendrogliomas can be expected to have a better prognosis than glioblastoma (12); second, the recently recognized sensitivity of anaplastic oligodendrogliomas to chemotherapy may provide an additional therapeutic option for malignant tumors of this lineage (60,61).

Several different systems have been used for grading oligodendrogliomas. Smith et al. (364) devised a four-tiered system that distinguishes three prognostically significant groups (grade A, grades B + C, and grade D). The Kernohan criteria (194) and the St. Anne–Mayo criteria for fibrillary astrocytomas (84) have also been applied to the grading of oligodendrogliomas (359). Both systems yielded two statistically significant survival curves: low-grade tumors comprising grades 1 and 2, and high-grade tumors comprising grades 3 and 4. Because the majority of patients in these studies were adults, applicability of the systems to childhood tumors is uncertain. Nevertheless, many authors employ a simple two-tiered system, stratifying oligodendrogliomas as either low-grade or anaplastic (115,116,199).

Oligodendrogliomas are infiltrative tumors that usually originate in white matter and secondarily invade the cortex, where they tend to cluster around neuronal cell bodies and blood vessels. This process is termed neoplastic satellitosis. Such clustered formations reflect intrinsic affinities of the oligodendroglial cell (Fig. 15) and are the most frequently encountered examples of so-called secondary structures of Scherer. In his classic paper, Scherer (351) described the various morphologic patterns produced by infiltrating gliomas. Those patterns that the tumor was capable of producing out of its own innate bio-

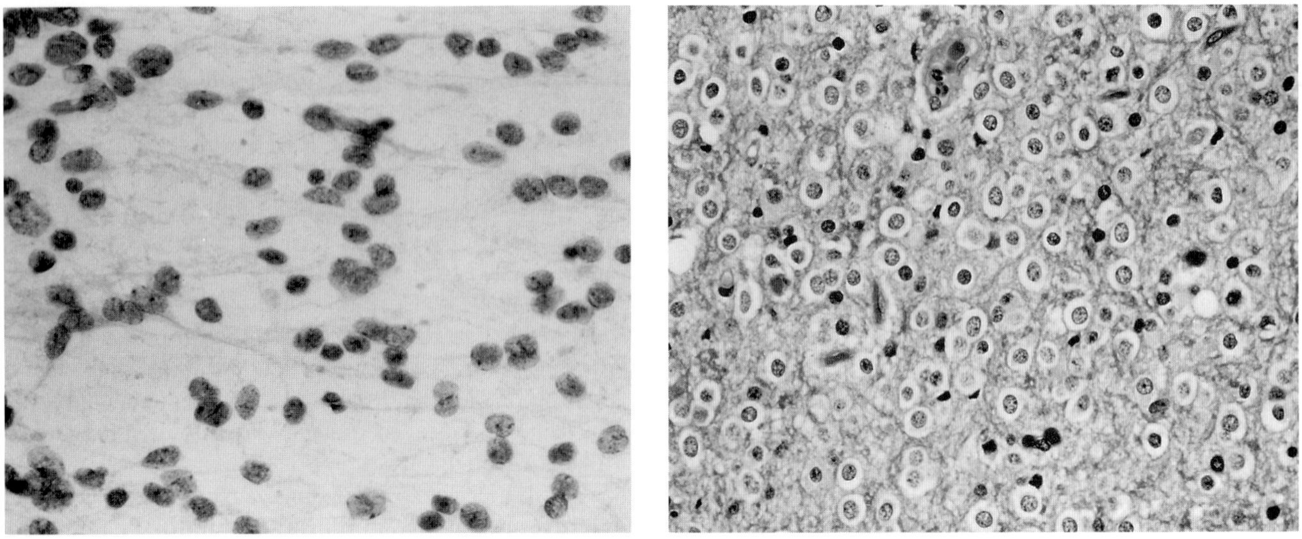

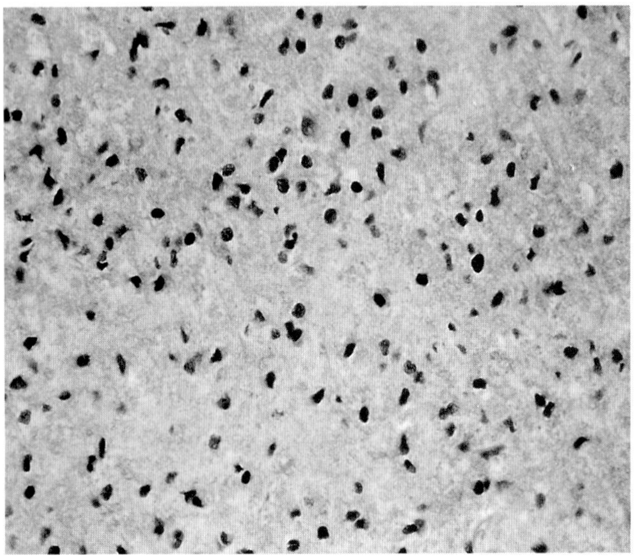

FIG. 13. Oligodendroglioma. The cells of oligodendrogliomas are typically rounded with very little cytoplasm as seen in smear preparations performed at the time of intraoperative frozen section **(A)**. Permanent sections reveal the classic "fried egg" appearance **(B)**. The perinuclear halos are useful artefacts of delayed fixation and are not observed in rapidly frozen tissue **(C)**. Also note the considerable distortion of nuclear architecture produced by freezing **(C)**, which can lead the unwary to render a frozen section diagnosis of high-grade astrocytoma.

logic potential, such as rosettes and palisades, were termed proper (primary) structures. Those morphologic arrangements that were dependent on preexisting host structures, such as perineuronal and perivascular satellitosis, he termed secondary structures. Additional examples of secondary structures include subpial accumulation of tumor cells and the patterns produced by tumor cell infiltration between or within dense fiber tracts (inter- and intrafascicular spread). Lastly, Scherer employed the term "tertiary structure" for the various interactions of tumor cells with proliferating mesenchymal connective tissue, such as that seen when gliomas invade the leptomeninges (desmoplastic response) or when organization of necrotic tumor by blood vessel–derived fibroblasts occurs.

In addition to cortical infiltration with satellitosis, oligodendrogliomas may exhibit a variety of other growth patterns, including nodular aggregates, clusters, and palisades (Fig. 16). Oligodendrogliomas generally show strong nuclear immunopositivity for S-100 protein (as do astrocytomas). In addition, several special cell types may be reactive for GFAP (discussed below in section on mixed gliomas).

Several studies from independent laboratories have found evidence implicating a role for possible tumor suppressor genes located on chromosomes 1 and 19 in the genesis of oligodendrogliomas (30,209,311,315,396). Preferential allelic losses occur on 1p and 19q in a significant percentage of both low-grade and high-grade (anaplastic) oligodendrogliomas.

MIXED GLIOMAS

Given the common embryologic heritage of the three types of glial cells (astrocytes, oligodendroglia, and ependymocytes), it is not surprising that focal areas of heterologous glial differentiation may be seen in an otherwise "pure" glioma. The presence of such differentiation is in

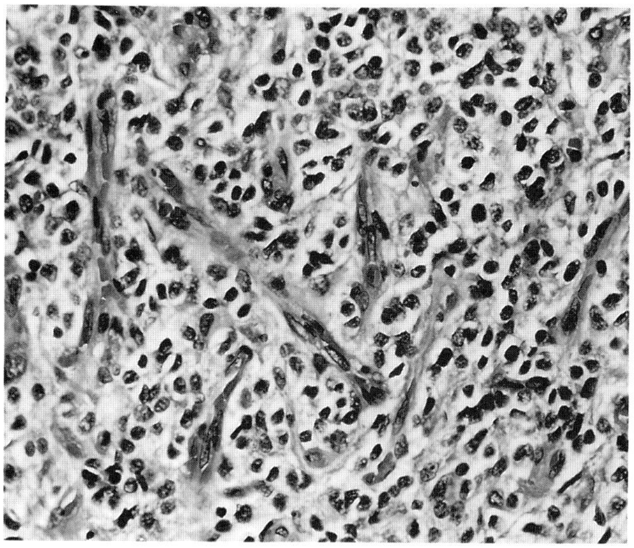

FIG. 14. Anaplastic oligodendroglioma. Increased cellularity, pleomorphism, and mitotic activity are evident.

fact a very common occurrence, and its presence in limited foci does not, per se, warrant a diagnosis of mixed glioma. However, when two or more glial lines each constitute a significant proportion of the neoplasm, a diagnosis of mixed glioma is appropriate. Unfortunately, the threshold for determining what percentage constitutes a "significant proportion" is subjective, as no specific, objective, universally accepted criteria exist.

In principle, a mixed glioma may be composed of any combination of two or three glial cell types, and all of the possible permutations are allowed for in most classification systems (199,322). In practice, however, only the oligoastrocytoma occurs in significant numbers (140). In the pediatric population, mixed oligoastrocytoma accounts for less than 1% of brain tumors; most of these occur in the cerebral hemispheres (70). A diagnosis of mixed oligoastrocytoma requires the unequivocal identification of both a neoplastic astrocytic and a neoplastic oligodendroglial component. These may be present as separate, discrete areas ("compact" type) or as closely intermingled components ("diffuse" type) (140).

There are two additional factors that require comment with respect to the differential diagnosis between oligodendroglioma and mixed oligoastrocytoma. First, oligodendrogliomas often elicit a prominent reactive astrocytosis. These cells tend to be quite eye catching and must be recognized as reactive in nature (Fig. 17A). Second, two types of GFAP-positive neoplastic cell types are now recognized to occur as integral components of some otherwise typical oligodendrogliomas: gliofibrillary oligodendrocytes and miniature gemistocytes (minigemistocytes, microgemistocytes) (152,211). Gliofibrillary oligodendrocytes exhibit a ring of GFAP-immunoreactive cytoplasm encircling the nucleus and minigemistocytes display a small, eccentric cytoplasmic mass that is similarly GFAP-immunoreactive (Fig. 17B,C). These cell types are considered closely related and are postulated to be transitional forms between oligodendrocytes and astrocytes. Current data suggest that their presence does not influence biologic behavior and accordingly should not alter the diagnosis. In contrast, however, it should be noted that the presence of large, clearly astrocytic gemistocytes is a negative prognostic indicator (212).

The diagnosis of mixed glioma is based on recognition of the classical morphologic features of the three glioma subtypes in routine hematoxylin and eosin–stained tissue sections, i.e., prominent eosinophilic cytoplasmic processes for astrocytoma, clustered nuclei with surrounding prominent perinuclear halos for oligodendro-

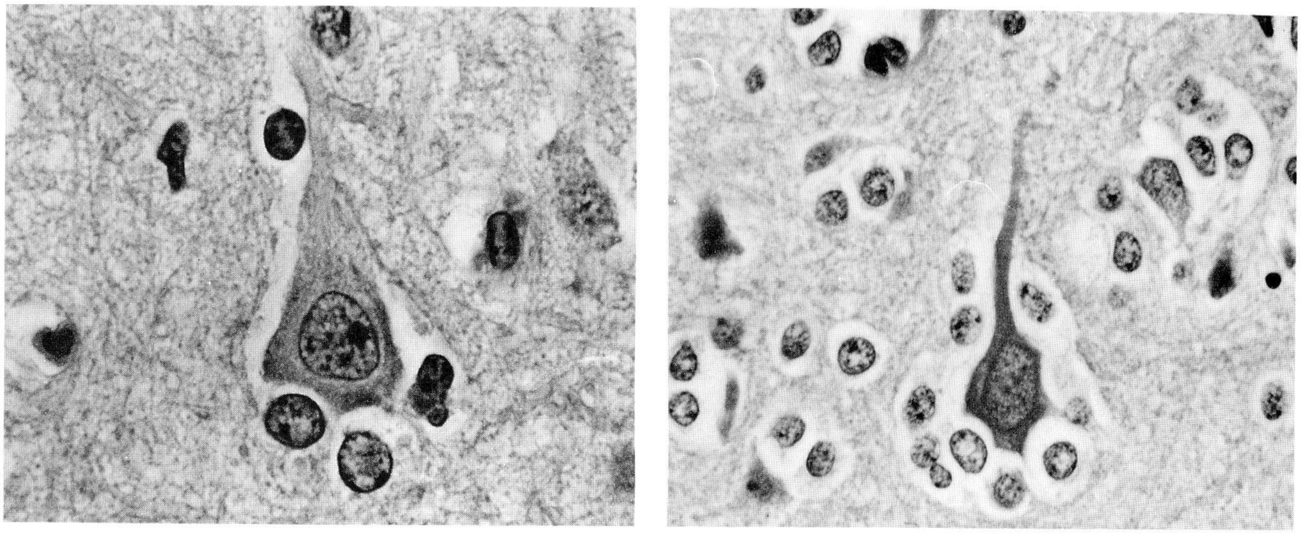

A B

FIG. 15. Oligodendroglioma. Oligodendroglia, astrocytes, and microglia are normally found in close apposition to neuronal perikarya ("satellite cells") **(A)**. Neoplastic satellitosis is a reflection of this affinity that is seen in both oligodendrogliomas **(B)** and astrocytomas.

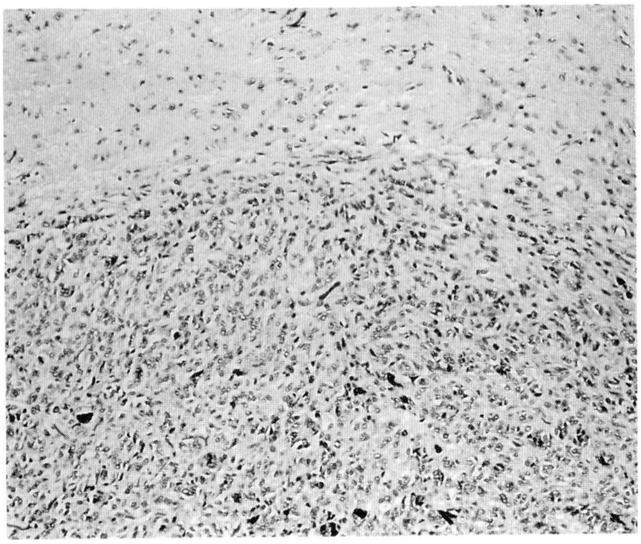
A

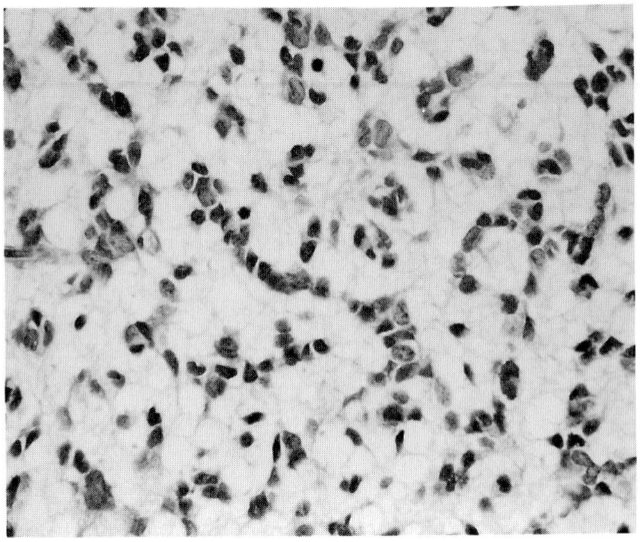
B

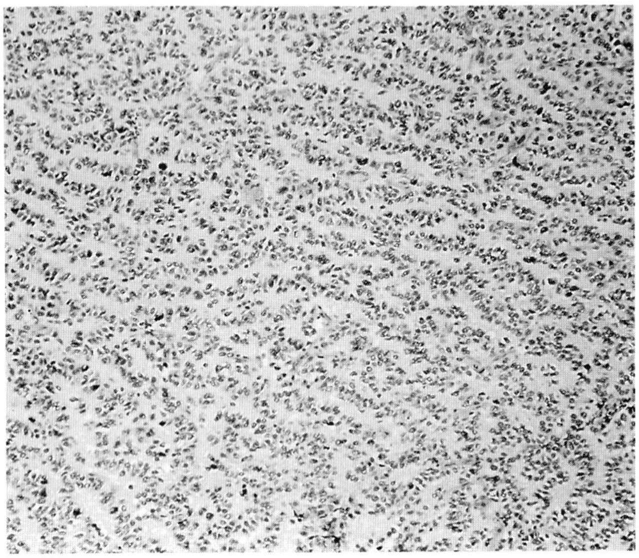
C

FIG. 16. Oligodendroglioma. Several growth patterns may be seen in oligodendrogliomas in addition to satellitosis, including the commonly observed nodular growth **(A)**, clusters and short cords **(B)**, and palisading (enfilades) **(C)**.

glioma, and perivascular pseudorosettes for ependymoma. However, rapid advances in molecular biology described throughout this chapter are beginning to impact this area of neuropathology as well. The allelic losses of chromosomes 1p and 19q that are frequently found in oligodendrogliomas are also seen in mixed oligoastrocytoma (30,209,315,396,397). Kraus et al. (209) used a PCR-based technique to separately assay small areas of relatively pure astrocytoma and relative pure oligodendroglioma from three mixed oligoastrocytomas. The results for all three cases showed loss of heterozygosity for both 1p and 19q in both the astrocytic and oligodendroglial domains of the tumors, suggesting in each case a monoclonal origin of the two components. Thus it would appear from these studies that not only are the two cellular components of classical mixed oligoastrocytoma very closely related but also that oligoastrocytomas in general are more akin to oligodendrogliomas than to astrocytomas. This line of research also serves to illustrate the ever-increasing impact of molecular approaches in addressing long-standing issues of brain tumor classification and biology.

CHOROID PLEXUS NEOPLASMS

The choroid plexus is formed by an invagination of the leptomeninges through the neural mantle into the ventricular cavity during development. The structure of choroid plexus reflects its mode of genesis and consists of papillary tufts of vascular connective tissue (derived from the leptomeninges) covered with modified ependyma (choroid plexus epithelium). The embryologic origin of the fibrovascular stroma from the pia-arachnoid membrane explains the incidental presence of scattered nests of arachnoid cells (meningothelial cells) in normal choroid plexus (see Fig. 42). Such nests constitute the

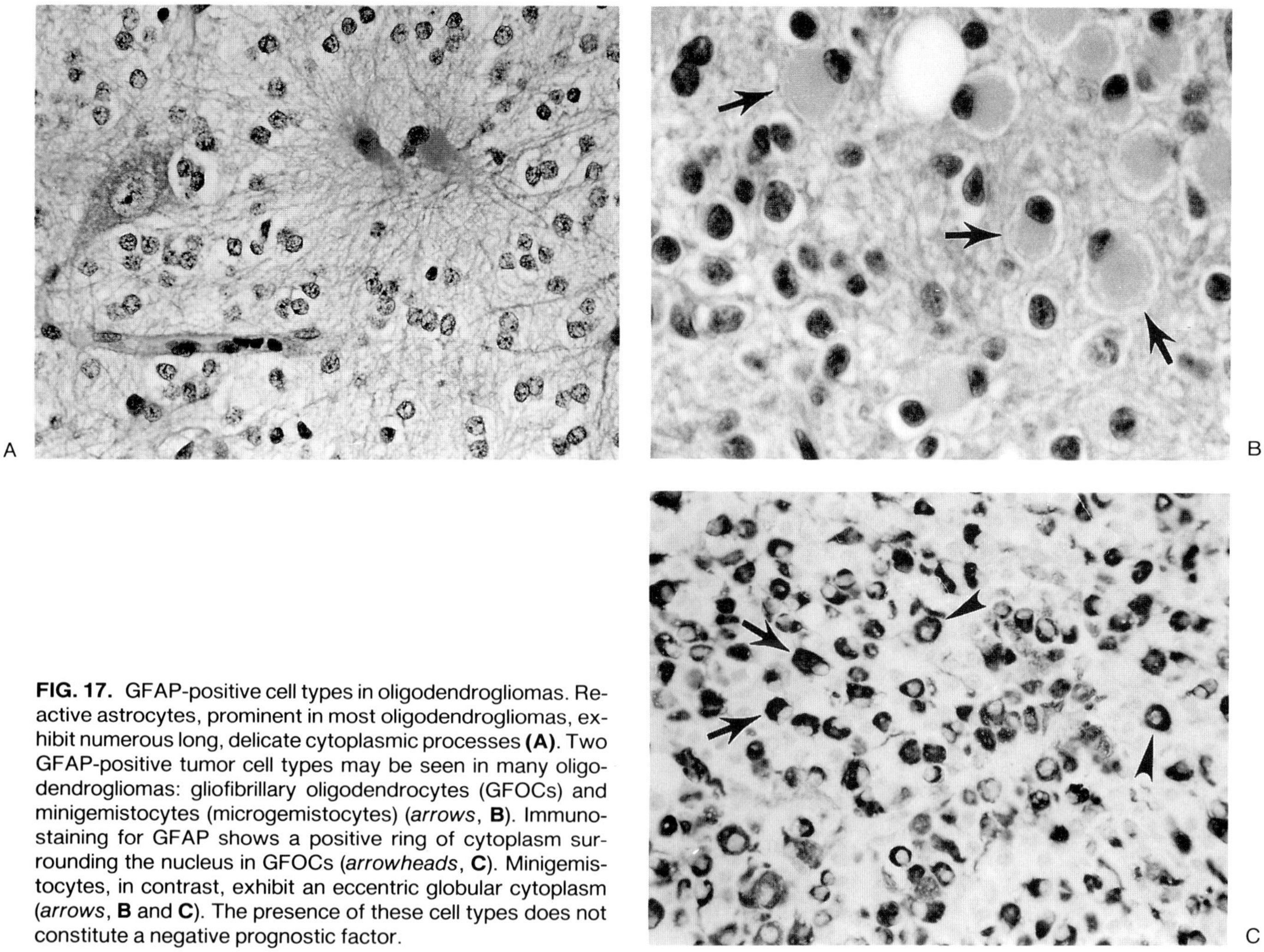

FIG. 17. GFAP-positive cell types in oligodendrogliomas. Reactive astrocytes, prominent in most oligodendrogliomas, exhibit numerous long, delicate cytoplasmic processes **(A)**. Two GFAP-positive tumor cell types may be seen in many oligodendrogliomas: gliofibrillary oligodendrocytes (GFOCs) and minigemistocytes (microgemistocytes) (*arrows*, **B**). Immunostaining for GFAP shows a positive ring of cytoplasm surrounding the nucleus in GFOCs (*arrowheads*, **C**). Minigemistocytes, in contrast, exhibit an eccentric globular cytoplasm (*arrows*, **B** and **C**). The presence of these cell types does not constitute a negative prognostic factor.

presumed site of origin for intraventricular meningiomas, which, although rare, comprise a comparatively greater percentage of meningiomas occurring in children than in adults (101,342).

Neoplasms of the choroid plexus epithelium occur as both low-grade tumors (choroid plexus papillomas) and high-grade tumors (anaplastic choroid plexus papillomas and choroid plexus carcinomas). The latter entity is most confidently diagnosed in childhood, as the vast majority of carcinomas presenting in the choroid plexus of adult patients are metastatic rather than primary in origin.

Choroid plexus papillomas compose approximately 2% of childhood brain tumors. Most (75%) occur supratentorially in the lateral ventricles (70). In contrast, the majority of choroid plexus tumors in adults occur in the fourth ventricle. High-grade choroid plexus neoplasms also present primarily in the lateral ventricles of children but compose less than 0.5% of pediatric brain tumors. Within the lateral ventricle, the favored location for all choroid plexus tumor types (including meningioma) is the atrium (the site of convergence of the body, temporal horn, and lateral horn of the ventricle). This finding is explained in part by the fact that although choroid plexus is found in all four ventricles, the largest masses (termed glomera choroidea) are located in the atria of the lateral ventricles (114).

Choroid plexus papillomas recapitulate the papillary architecture of normal choroid plexus with high fidelity, differing mainly in the denser packing of often more columnar cells (Fig. 18). Anaplastic choroid plexus papillomas and choroid plexus carcinomas display increasingly more atypical features, including pleomorphism, increased mitotic rate, foci of necrosis, and progressive effacement of the papillary architecture (Fig. 18).

Choroid plexus papillomas are strongly immunopositive for cytokeratins and S-100 protein. Focal positivity for GFAP is sometimes present and reflects glial or ependymal differentiation. However, the strong, widespread immunopositivity for GFAP like that present diffusely in

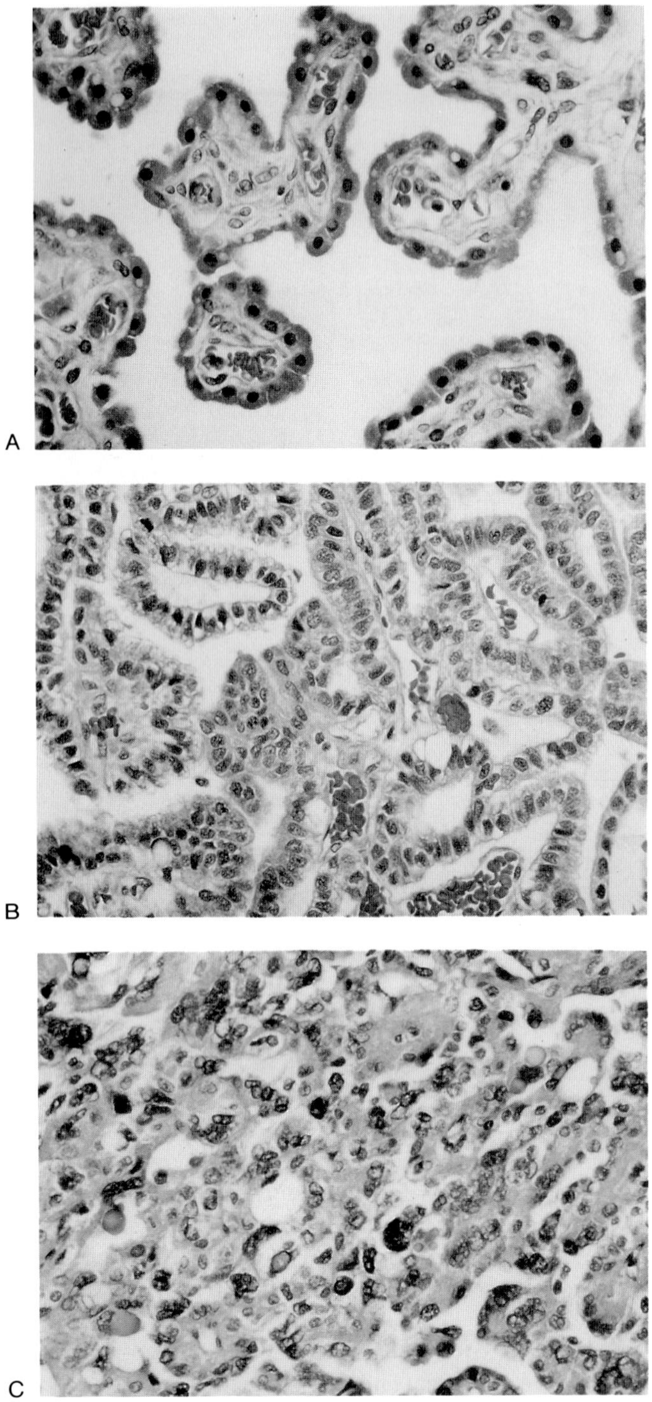

FIG. 18. Choroid plexus neoplasms. Choroid plexus papillomas **(B)** mimic the papillary architecture of normal choroid plexus **(A)** but are more cellular and the closely packed eithelium is frequently more columnar rather than cuboidal. Choroid plexus carcinomas **(C)** exhibit more pleomorphism and usually focal loss of papillary architecture. Necrosis is also frequently present.

astrocytomas and in the perivascular pseudorosettes of ependymomas is typically not seen. An additional marker of some utility is transthyretin (prealbumin), for which normal choroid plexus and some papillomas are strongly positive. However, most choroid plexus carcinomas are only focally positive at best and often weakly so, thus limiting the usefulness of this marker (7). Ultrastructurally, choroid plexus neoplasms reflect an epithelial origin with the apical surfaces of papillary fronds exhibiting abundant microvilli and occasional cilia (Fig. 19).

Little is known about the origin of choroid plexus neoplasms. A recent provocative report noted the presence of a segment of the simian virus 40 (SV40) T-antigen gene in half of choroid plexus tumors examined (10 of 20) and in 10 of 11 ependymomas (32), suggesting a possible etiologic role for this or a closely related virus. Further investigation is necessary. Only a few reported cytogenetic studies of choroid plexus tumors have been published to date (308).

EPENDYMAL NEOPLASMS

There are four types of neoplasms derived from the ependymal lining of the ventricular system: (a) classical ependymoma, of which there are a number of histological variants, (b) ependymoblastoma, a malignant primitive neuroectodermal tumor, (c) myxopapillary ependymoma of the filum terminale, and (d) subependymoma. Of these, classical ependymoma is by far the most common in childhood and accounts for up to 10% of intracranial pediatric tumors in some series. Examples of the other ependyma-derived tumor types are much rarer in the pediatric population.

Ependymoma

A majority of ependymomas in children arise in the posterior fossa (approximately 70% of cases), although cerebral examples occur as well (about 25% of cases) and infrequent examples present as spinal cord tumors (less than 5% of cases). The infratentorial lesions are typically diagnosed before the age of 5 years and grow exophytically into the fourth ventricle. Some tumors fill the lateral recesses of the fourth ventricle and extend out into the subarachnoid space to surround the brainstem ("plastic ependymomas") (79). A rare neoplasm arises directly from the ependyma-lined glial sleeve at the foramen of Luschka and proliferates as a primary tumor of the cerebellopontine angle cistern. In contrast to posterior fossa ependymomas, which favor an intraventricular growth pattern, approximately 70% of supratentorial tumors occur as intraparenchymal hemispheric masses without a ventricular component (281). For reasons that are not understood, ependymomas arising from the third ventricle are quite rare in both children and adults; only isolated pediatric cases have been reported in this location (270,281). The male/female incidence of pediatric ependymomas is approximately equal.

The most commonly encountered and diagnostically important morphologic feature of ependymomas is the perivascular pseudorosette (sometimes referred to as

A 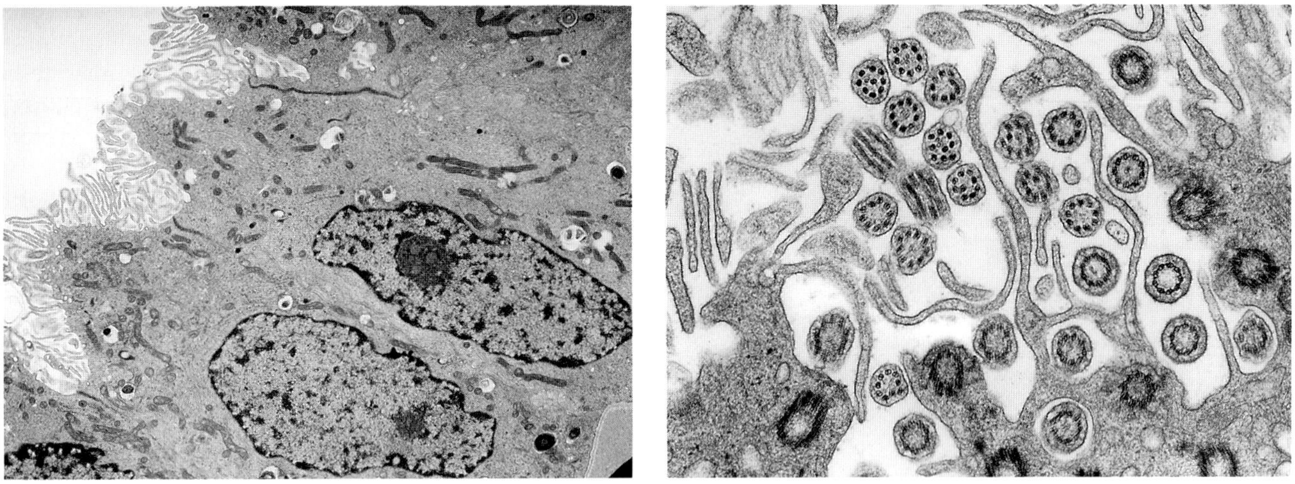 B

FIG. 19. Choroid plexus neoplasms. Ultrastructural examination reveals epithelial properties with columnar cells resting on a basement membrane **(A)**. The apical surface displays microvilli, and some cells may also have cilia **(B)**.

"gliovascular rosettes"). Perivascular pseudorosettes are eosinophilic, nucleus-free zones that surround blood vessels. Recognition of these structures is a critical clue to the correct diagnosis at the time of intraoperative frozen section (Fig. 20A). In permanent sections, the delicate, radiating fibrillary processes of ependymal tumor cells that form the anuclear perithelial collars are often visible (Fig. 20B) and constitute the primary site of immunopositivity for GFAP in ependymomas. GFAP immunoreactivity is a useful diagnostic feature and reflects the glial lineage of these tumors.

Although of glial lineage, the ependyma also serves an epithelial function as the lining membrane of the ventricular system in the brain and central canal of the spinal cord. It is therefore not surprising that this biologic potential is sometimes expressed by neoplastic ependymal cells in the form of so-called true ependymal rosettes (Fig. 21A) or as more extensive tubules and prominent epithelial surfaces (Fig. 21B). It must be emphasized, however, that these morphologically aesthetic manifestations of the epithelial capabilities of ependymal cells are far less frequently seen than are the perivascular pseudorosettes that reflect the cells' glial heritage and more often facilitate correct diagnosis.

There are several histologic variants of ependymoma that do not have prognostic significance but are important because of their potential to confuse or mislead the pathologist. The most often mentioned is papillary epen-

A 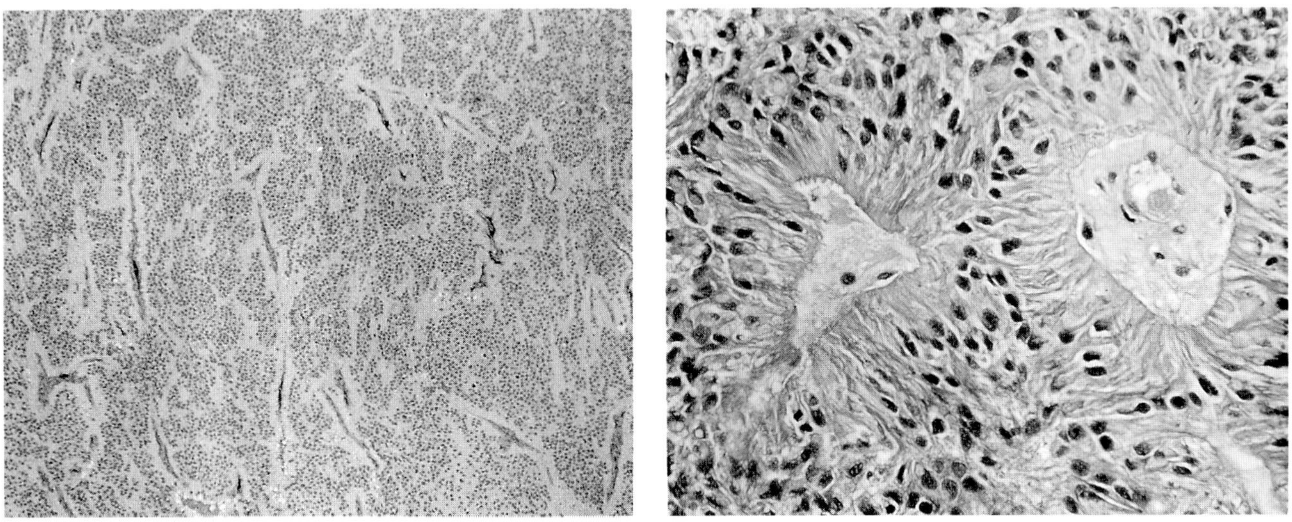 B

FIG. 20. Ependymoma. The most characteristic feature of ependymomas are perivascular nucleus-free zones (perivascular pseudorosettes) that are very helpful diagnostic features at the time of frozen section **(A)**. Permanent sections sometimes show the delicate elongated fibrillary cell processes that form the perivascular anuclear cuffs **(B)**.

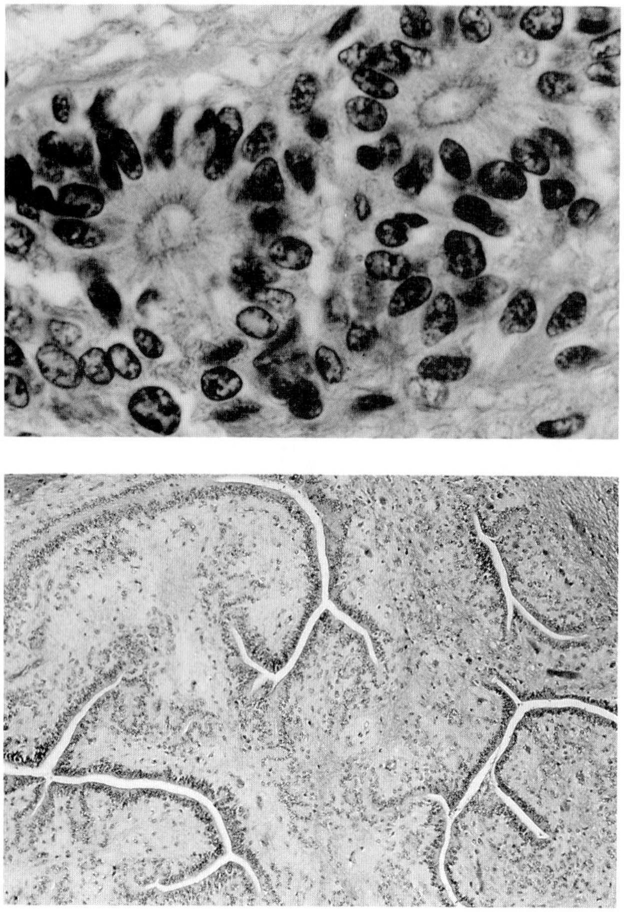

A

B

FIG. 21. Ependymoma. "True" ependymal rosettes, which consist of a ring of tumor cells surrounding a central lumen, are seen in some ependymomas **(A)**. Less commonly encountered are long branching tubules **(B)**.

dymoma, in which the neoplastic cells assume a papillary or pseudopapillary configuration. Most textbooks allude to the potential difficulty in distinguishing between papillary ependymoma and choroid plexus papilloma, emphasizing the importance of identifying the glial papillary cores of the former tumor as opposed to the fibrovascular cores of the latter. However, in practice papillary ependymomas are in fact quite rare compared to choroid plexus papillomas, and for those ependymomas that do exhibit papillary features, close inspection of the tumor generally permits at least focal identification of the characteristic perivascular pseudorosettes. Another variant is so-called clear cell ependymoma, which is composed of neoplastic cells with rounded nuclei surrounded by cleared cytoplasm ("perinuclear halos"), features that mimic oligodendroglioma and central neurocytoma (Fig. 22). In approaching this differential diagnosis, it should be kept in mind that the fourth ventricle is not a site of origin for central neurocytoma and immunopositivity for synaptophysin in central neurocytomas readily resolves the issue for tumors originating in the lateral ventricle. As for the other mimic, oligodendrogliomas exclusively confined to the ventricular space are exceedingly rare (most examples of so-called "intraventricular oligodendroglioma" have been shown to be central neurocytomas) and, as with papillary ependymomas, careful search of the tissue usually uncovers perivascular pseudorosettes even in ependymomas with predominant clear cell morphology. A potential fourth entity in the differential diagnosis, intraventricular meningioma with clear cell features, is a technical possibility but would be exceptional. Some investigators consider ependymomas with focal or extensive clear cell features as mixed oligoependymomas, but convincing data to justify this distinction are generally lacking, and the majority of such tumors can be expected to behave as ependymomas and should be treated accordingly.

The final variant that warrants brief mention is tanycytic ependymoma. These rare tumors are characterized by fascicles of highly spindled cells that may resemble schwannoma (Fig. 23). Confirmation of the diagnosis is dependent on finding typical areas with perivascular pseudorosettes, demonstration of immunopositivity for GFAP, or identification of characteristic ependymal ultrastructural features by electron microscopy (discussed below).

Grading of ependymomas is a subject frought with controversy. Virtually all authors acknowledge the existence of an anaplastic category of ependymoma, and the results of survival studies attest to the significantly worse prognosis for this group (206,215,329). The difficulty arises from a lack of specific, reliable criteria for grading. Clearly, the criteria applied for grading fibrillary astrocytomas are not valid for ependymomas. For example, the presence of small foci of necrosis and focal nuclear atypia

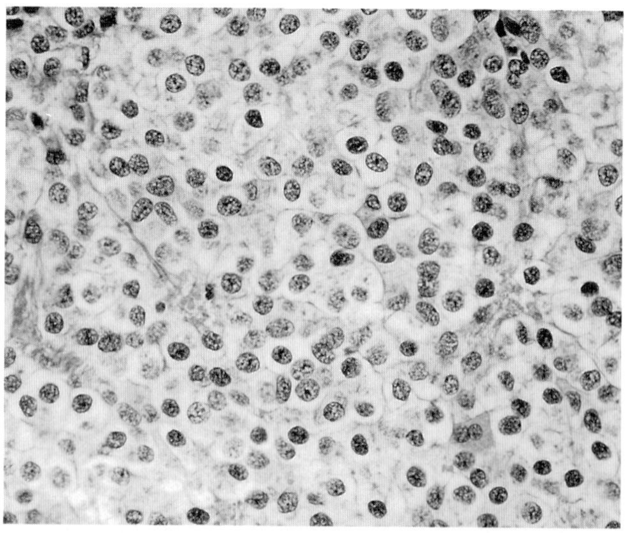

FIG. 22. Clear cell ependymoma. The morphologic features of this variant of ependymoma mimic other tumors such as oligodendroglioma. If sufficient tissue is available for examination, however, the characteristic perivascular pseudorosettes can usually be found (not shown).

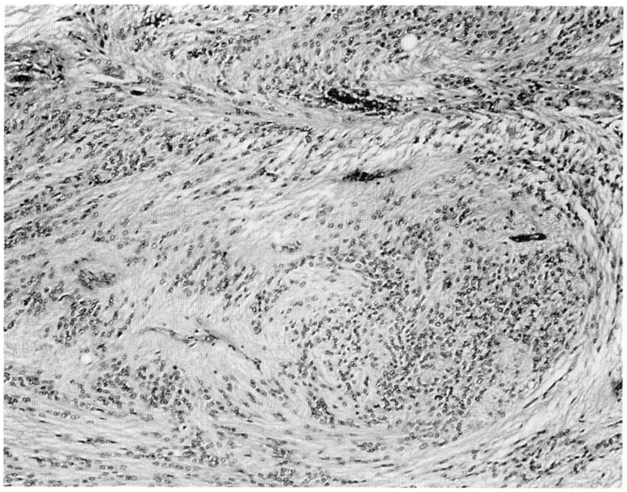

FIG. 23. Tanycytic ependymoma. This distinctive variant of ependymoma exhibits elongated cell processes.

do not, per se, mandate a diagnosis of high-grade tumor, as these features may be seen in many otherwise typical low-grade ependymomas. Cases in which the predominant portion of the neoplasm exhibits a clearly malignant morphology, including hypercellularity with numerous readily identifiable mitotic figures, large areas of tumor necrosis, and microvascular proliferation, are not the subject of debate. The problem concerns the significant number of tumors that exhibit focal areas of hypercellularity with an increased mitotic rate. Whether or not the presence and extent of such foci in an otherwise low-grade ependymoma constitute clinically significant negative prognostic indicators is currently unresolved and is one of many important issues in pediatric neuro-oncology that requires further investigation. The 5-year survival of ependymoma patients has improved significantly with radiation therapy and falls in the range of 40–70%, although the long-term prognosis remains guarded (71,177,206,215,329).

Ependymomas are immunopositive for S-100 protein and at least focally for GFAP. As mentioned previously, GFAP immunoreactivity is usually most prominent around blood vessels in the cell processes that form perivascular pseudorosettes. While GFAP immunopositivity reflects the glial nature of ependymomas, ultrastructural examination reveals the epithelial qualities, ie, lumina filled with microvilli and occasional cilia surrounded by cells firmly attached to each other by elongated tight junctions (343) (Fig. 24).

Spinal cord ependymomas are one of the well-known associated lesions of neurofibromatosis type 2 (NF2). Rare instances of familial ependymoma without the presence of NF2 have also been reported (263). Cytogenetic analyses of sporadic ependymomas have revealed a wide range of chromosomal abberations (320,346).

Ependymoblastoma

Ependymoblastoma is a rare, malignant primitive neuroectodermal tumor that typically arises in very young children and exhibits only glial and ependymal differentiation. The most characteristic morphologic feature is the presence of prominent ependymal rosettes often having elongated slit-like lumens (termed ependymoblastomatous rosettes). There is a predilection for leptomeningeal dissemination (251,361). Mitotic figures are numerous in these malignant neoplasms, but microvascular proliferation and tumor necrosis with pseudopalisading are typically scant or absent. The histologic features of ependymoblastomas thus differ from those of

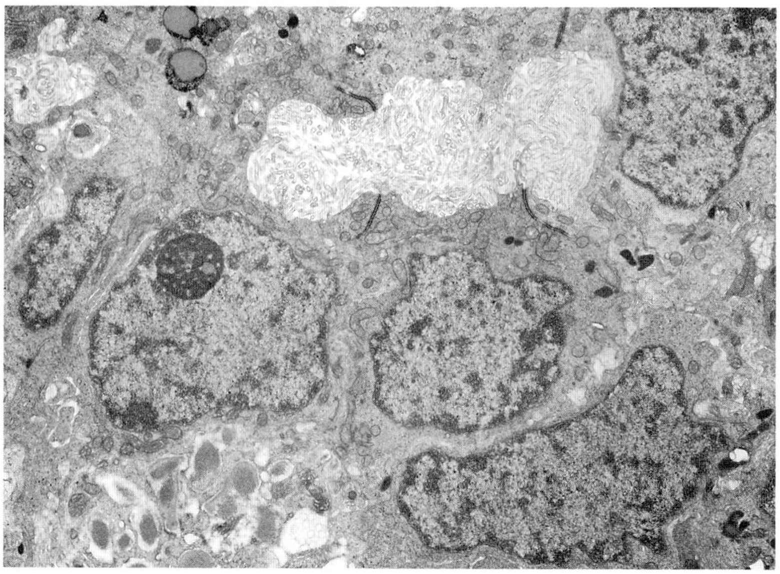

FIG. 24. Ependymoma. Ultrastructural examination can be very helpful in the diagnosis of ependymoma in cases in which routine H&E-stained tissue sections are not definitive or are very limited in amount. The salient feature is the presence of intercellular lumens filled with microvilli. Long intercellular junctions are visible. These structures are often identified by electron microscopy even when no hint of rosette formation can be discerned by light microscopic examination.

high-grade (anaplastic) ependymomas, so that distinction is drawn between them (54,81,199,220,251,335).

Myxopapillary Ependymoma

Myxopapillary ependymoma is an ependyma-derived neoplasm that occurs almost exclusively in the filum terminale and conus medullaris of the spinal cord. The morphologic features are unique and quite unlike those of ependymomas that arise elswhere in the nervous system. The distinctive morphologic features of the human filum terminale probably contribute to this exceptional histologic appearance. The filum is composed primarily of collagen, with a few blood vessels, small peripheral nerve fascicles, and, most significant from an oncologic perspective, an ependymal remnant of the central canal of the spinal cord (114). It is the latter structure that provides the presumptive cell of origin for the myxopapillary ependymoma. In addition, asymptomatic ependymal rests are a common finding in the subcutaneous tissues of the sacrococcygeal region (20,74,306) and constitute the source of extraspinal myxopapillary ependymomas in this region. These rare tumors occur predominantly in children and may arise as early as infancy (74,148).

The most distinctive feature of the myxopapillary ependymoma is the accumulation of mucin in small cystic spaces and in collars surrounding blood vessel walls (Fig. 25A). The tumor cells themselves range from stellate to markedly elongated. The latter appearance may be quite similar to that of the pilocytes of pilocytic astrocytoma (Fig. 25B; compare with Fig. 1). Myxopapillary ependymoma is a uniformly low-grade neoplasm with no demonstrated potential for malignant progression and therefore does not require histologic grading. Those rare tumors arising from subcutaneous sacrococcygeal rests, however, do have the potential for lymph node and pulmonary metastasis (130,148,408).

Subependymoma

Subependymomas are derived from the cellular constituents of the ependymal lining and subependymal plate. The latter structure consists of a hypocellular zone of glial processes with scattered nests of ependymal cells and astrocytes—the so-called subependymal glia. The precise histogenetic origin of subependymomas has been extensively debated, with different camps adducing various ultrastructural and immunohistochemical findings to buttress arguments favoring either an ependymal, astrocytic, or combined cellular origin.

Subependymomas are most frequently encountered incidentally in older adults at autopsy as small growths arising from the floor of the fourth ventricle. They also occur in the lateral ventricles. A much rarer but well-documented location is the spinal cord. Similar to ependymomas, the occurrence of subependymomas as primary tumors of the third ventricle is exceedingly rare; most of the few reported cases represent extension of a lateral ventricle subependymoma through the intraventricular foramen of Monro into the third ventricle. If appropriately situated, subependymomas of either the fourth or lateral ventricle may attain sufficient size to cause obstructive hydrocephalus. Rare cases of symp-

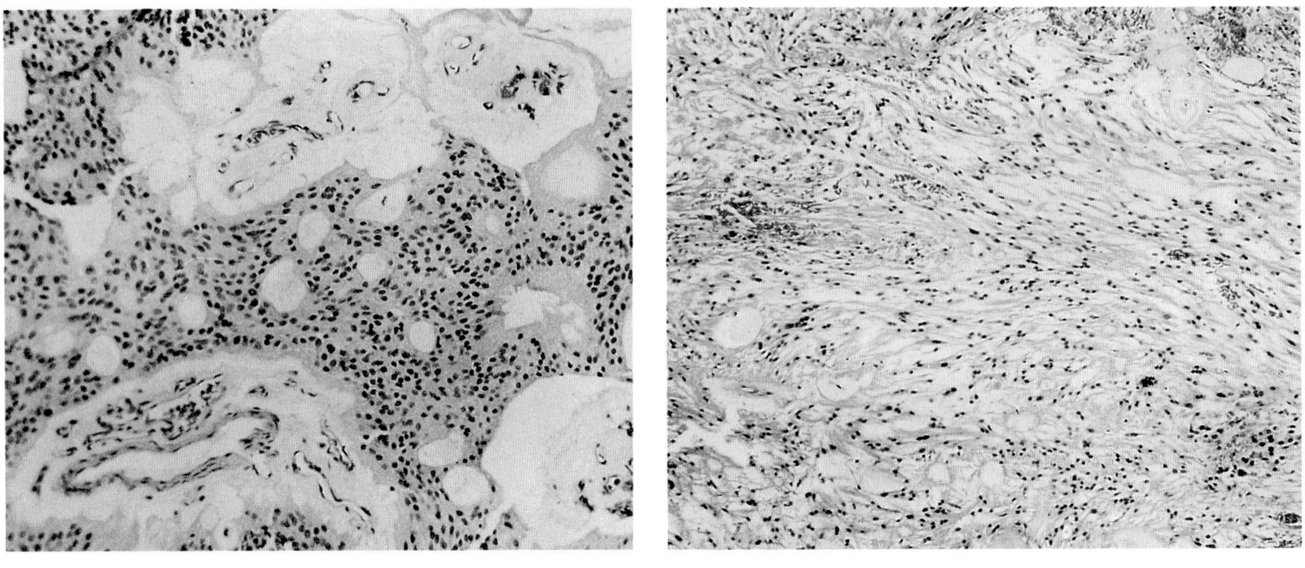

A B

FIG. 25. Myxopapillary ependymoma. This tumor arises almost exclusively from the conus medullaris and filum terminale of the spinal cord. The most distinctive feature is the presence of mucin that is found in collars around blood vessels and in microcysts **(A)**. Focal areas of highly spindled tumor cells, very similar to those of juvenile pilocytic astrocytoma, are often observed **(B)**.

tomatic subependymomas of the lateral and fourth ventricles have been reported in children (281,313,350).

The histologic pattern of subependymoma is quite distinctive and consists of small clustered nests of bland nuclei embedded in a fibrillary matrix; hence the older appelation "subependymal glomerate astrocytoma" (Fig. 26A). Tumors occurring in the lateral ventricles may show a strikingly vacuolated appearance, but upon close inspection the clustered arrangement of the constituent nuclei can be appreciated (Fig. 26B). Classical subependymomas are benign, low-grade tumors for which anaplastic transformation is unknown; however, surgical morbidity and mortality, particularly for those lesions arising from the floor of the fourth ventricle, has been significant. Progress in surgical technique has decreased the operative risk.

Rare instances of familial subependymoma have been described (69,160,340). The molecular genetic characterization of these tumors as well as the much more common sporadic subependymomas awaits further investigation.

Brief mention should be made of mixed tumors, most common in the first two decades of life, that exhibit areas of both subependymoma and ependymoma (sometimes referred to as "mixed ependymoma-subependymoma"). Clinical data indicate that these tumors will express the more aggressive biologic behavior associated with ependymoma and should be treated accordingly.

NEURONAL NEOPLASMS

Central nervous system tumors composed exclusively of neuronal elements are quite rare compared to glial neoplasms. There are only three principal entities: (a) cerebral neuroblastoma, (b) gangliocytoma, and (c) central neurocytoma. A questionable fourth entity is primitive polar spongioblastoma (discussed below). Gangliocytomas, tumors composed exclusively of large, mature ganglion cells without evidence of a glial component, occupy one end of the spectrum of ganglion cell tumors and are discussed under that rubric.

Cerebral Neuroblastoma

Cerebral neuroblastoma is a rare embryonal neoplasm that typically presents in the cerebral hemispheres of young children during the first decade. These tumors are composed of dense sheets of small cells with a high nuclear/cytoplasmic ratio. Intervening anuclear zones display dense fibrillarity produced by neuritic processes emanating from the tumor cells. These areas are typically immunopositive for neuronal markers such as synaptophysin. Focal ganglionic differentiation is not uncommon, but fully developed ganglioneuroblastoma, such as is seen outside the central nervous system, is rare. The presence of elongated GFAP-positive cytoplasmic processes of entrapped reactive astrocytes is expected, but the unequivocal presence of GFAP immunopositivity in a subset of tumor cells suggests a primitive neuroectodermal tumor with neuronal and glial differentiation. The prognosis is not as sanguine as for posterior fossa medulloblastomas. One recent series observed an overall survival of 34% at 5 years (9).

Central Neurocytoma

Prior to the discovery of central neurocytoma by Hassoun et al. in 1982 (142,143), the only known tumors of

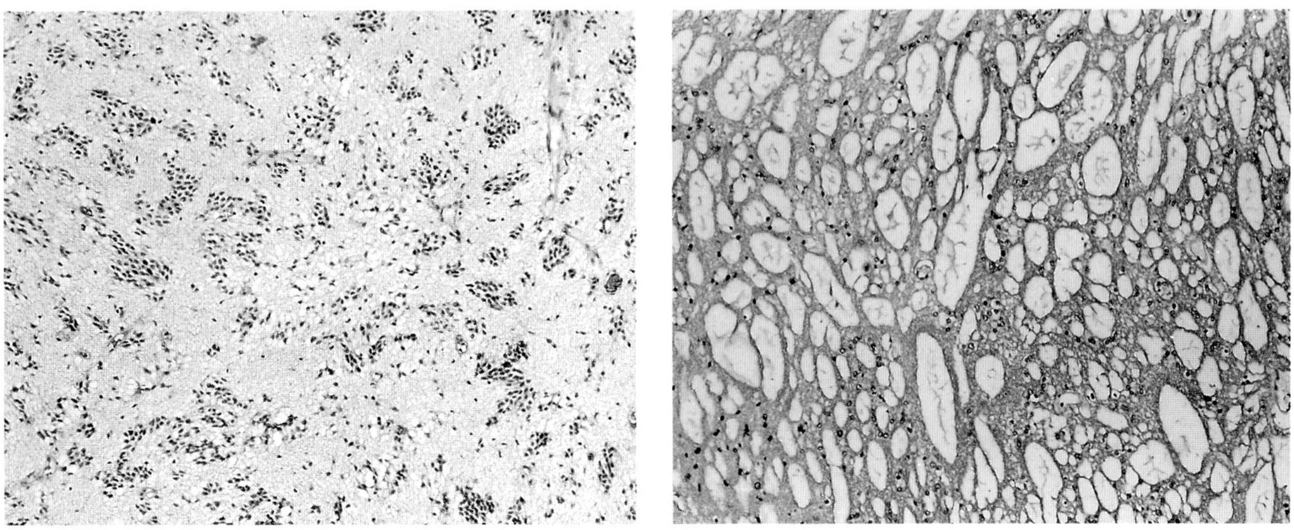

A B

FIG. 26. Subependymoma. Subependymomas are composed of clusters of benign-appearing glial nuclei distributed in a finely fibrillar matrix **(A)**. In some examples, particularly those arising in the lateral ventricles, prominent microcyst formation may dominate the morphologic appearance **(B)**.

the central nervous system that exhibited relatively pure neuronal differentiation were either primitive small cell embryonal neoplasms (neuroblastoma) or well-differentiated tumors composed of large, mature-appearing ganglion cells (gangliocytoma). In contrast to these extremes, the central neurocytoma is composed of small tumor cells that are roughly the size of those seen in neuroblastoma but are more differentiated, like those of gangliocytoma. In contrast to ganglion cell tumors, however, the neoplastic cells of central neurocytoma differentiate along the lines of small, mature neurons similar to those found in the granular cell layer of the cerebellum or hippocampal formation (Fig. 27).

The true identity of this class of tumors escaped detection for decades due to their close morphologic resemblance to oligodendroglioma (compare Fig. 27A and B with Fig. 13A and B). Both tumors are composed of small cells with regular, rounded nuclei and scant cytoplasm that often exhibits prominent artefactual clearing (perinuclear halos) in formalin-fixed tissue. Both neoplasms may also display a delicate, branching vascular pattern and scattered microcalcifications. Thus, prior to the seminal report by Hassoun et al. (142), these tumors were regularly misdiagnosed as intraventricular oligodendrogliomas. The initial discovery of the neuronal nature of central neurocytoma came through the application of electron microscopy, which revealed the presence of synaptic structures and cell processes with neuritic features (142) (Fig. 28A). Immunopositivity for the neuronal marker synaptophysin was subsequently demonstrated (24,393) and has become the mainstay of diagnosis (Fig. 28B; see figure in color plate section).

Although central neurocytomas occur primarily in young adults (mean age 29 years), a significant number present in older children during the second decade of life (143). The sex distribution is approximately equal. An overwhelming majority of these tumors arise in the lateral ventricles. In a review of 127 cases published in the literature, one or both lateral ventricles were involved in 95% (121 of 127) of patients; only six tumors were restricted to the third ventricle (143). No cases arising primarily in the fourth ventricle have been reported. An ex-

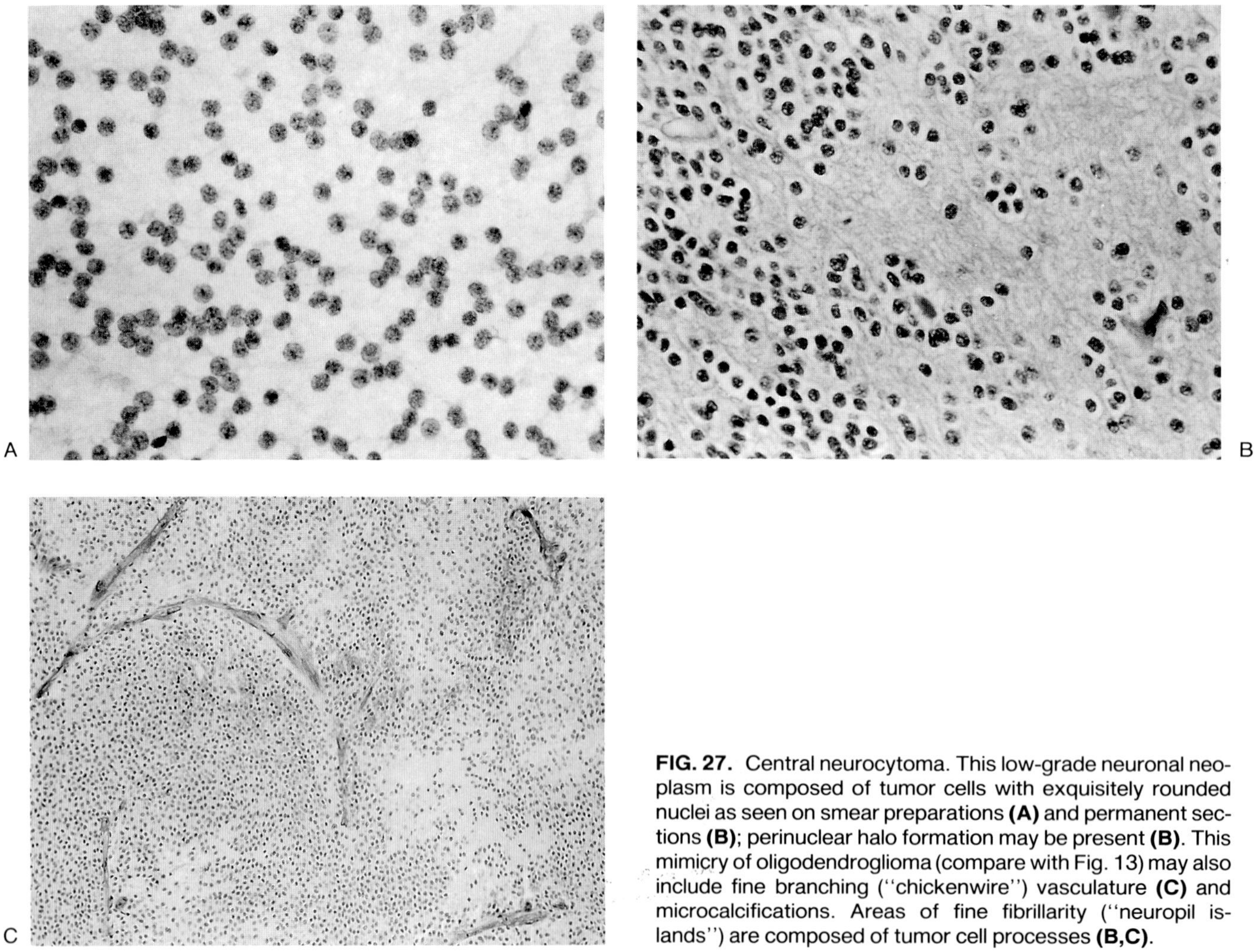

FIG. 27. Central neurocytoma. This low-grade neuronal neoplasm is composed of tumor cells with exquisitely rounded nuclei as seen on smear preparations **(A)** and permanent sections **(B)**; perinuclear halo formation may be present **(B)**. This mimicry of oligodendroglioma (compare with Fig. 13) may also include fine branching ("chickenwire") vasculature **(C)** and microcalcifications. Areas of fine fibrillarity ("neuropil islands") are composed of tumor cell processes **(B,C)**.

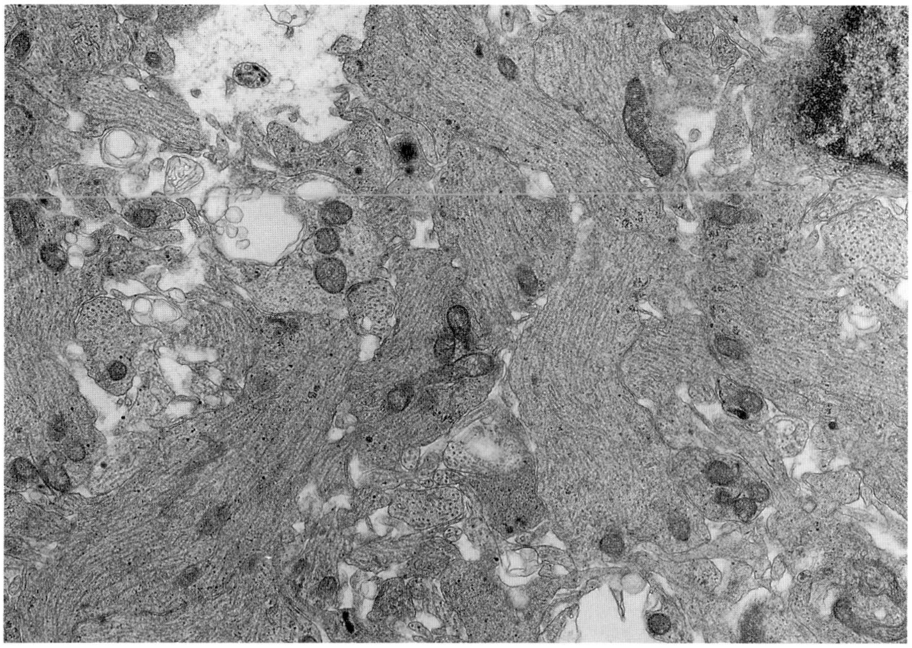

A

FIG. 28. Central neurocytoma. Ultrastructural examination shows neuronal features such as neuritic processes containing parallel arrays of microtubules and occasional dense core granules **(A)**. Central neurocytomas are strongly immunopositive for the neural marker synaptophysin **(B)** *(see color plate section)*.

ceptional case of a massive tumor with extension throughout the entire ventricular system, including the fourth ventricle, was noted by Yasargil et al. (412). Most central neurocytomas arise from the septum pellucidum or lateral wall of the ventricle and grow by exophytic expansion into the ventricular cavity. The subsequent production of mechanical obstruction of the interventricular foramen of Monro causes the patient to come to clinical attention with symptoms of increased intracranial pressure.

Central neurocytomas are well-differentiated neuronal tumors that have a favorable prognosis, often with surgical resection alone. Tumor recurrence, however, is recognized and may contribute to morbidity in some patients. Several issues await further clarification (50), including the role of radiation therapy and the possible existence of an anaplastic variant characterized by a high mitotic rate, foci of necrosis, and microvascular proliferation (104,412).

Primitive Polar Spongioblastoma

This tumor shares with astroblastoma the distinction of being a controversial entity defined primarily by a histologic pattern that is often seen focally in many other central nervous system neoplasms. In the case of primitive polar spongioblastoma, the morphologic pattern is that of palisading cells with elongated bipolar cytoplasmic processes—an architectural motif that has been described for a number of other tumors, including ependymomas, juvenile pilocytic astrocytomas, oligodendrogliomas, medulloblastomas, and cerebral neuroblastomas (221,269,353). Examples of "pure" polar spongioblastoma are very rare. No cases of this entity were reported among the 3,291 pediatric brain tumors of the Childhood Brain Tumor Consortium (70).

Although earlier reports described these tumors as glial in nature, more recent studies have stressed the presence of neuronal features, such as immunoreactivity for synaptophysin and the ultrastructural finding of dense core (neurosecretory-type) vesicles, and noted a lack of immunoreactivity for GFAP (171,261). Similar to astroblastoma, the validity of primitive polar spongioblastoma as a distinct clinicopathologic entity has been questioned (353).

It should be noted that the terms "polar spongioblastoma" and "spongioblastoma polare" have also been used in the past by some authors as synonyms for juvenile pilocytic astrocytoma.

NEOPLASMS OF MIXED NEURONAL/GLIAL PHENOTYPE

A variety of central nervous system tumors exhibit a mixed glial-neuronal lineage with highly variable representation of the two components. The principal members of this group are the ganglion cell tumors (gangliocytoma and ganglioglioma), the desmoplastic neuroepithelial tumors of infancy (superficial cerebral astrocytoma of infancy and desmoplastic infantile ganglioglioma), and dysembryoplastic neuroepithelial tumor.

Ganglion Cell Tumors

Ganglion cell tumors constitute a spectrum that ranges from gangliocytoma to anaplastic ganglioglioma. A majority of these tumors occur in the first two decades of life and are located in the cerebral hemispheres, especially the temporal lobe. A significant number also arise in the spinal cord and brainstem. As might be expected, the supratentorial lesions most commonly present with a history of seizures that often have been treated medically for years with poor response.

Gangliocytoma

Gangliocytomas are tumors composed exclusively of well-differentiated neurons ("ganglion cells"). These neoplasms are very rare and occur significantly less frequently than tumors of mixed neuronal and glial differentiation (gangliogliomas). They merge on the nosologic continuum with tumors of the ganglioglioma series. In some cases it may not be possible to determine whether or not a neoplastic glial component is present, and resort is taken to the general term "ganglion cell tumor." Microscopically, gangliocytomas contain clusters of variably sized ganglion cells surrounded by a highly fibrillar matrix composed of neuritic processes arising from the tumor cells (Fig. 29). Mitotic figures are usually not observed but may occasionally be identified.

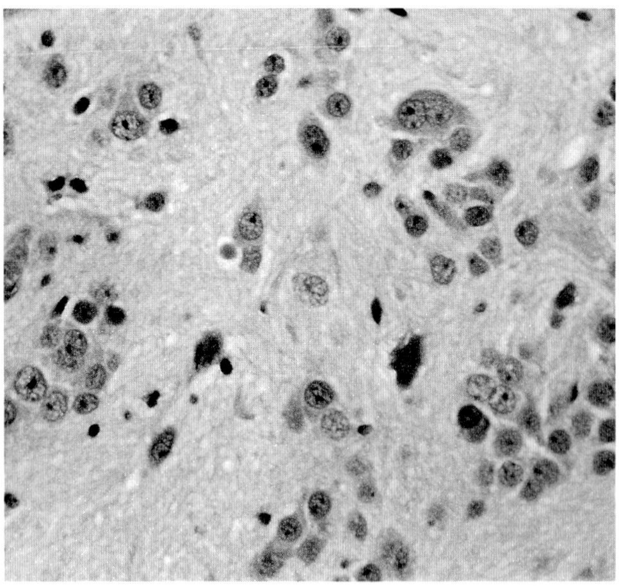

FIG. 29. Gangliocytoma. This very low-grade neuronal tumor is composed exclusively of large, mature-appearing ganglion cells. No glial component is present.

Dysplastic Gangliocytoma of the Cerebellum (Lhermitte–Duclos Disease)

Dysplastic gangliocytoma of the cerebellum (Lhermitte–Duclos disease), although bearing the descriptor "gangliocytoma," is a unique quasi-hamartomatous clinicopathologic entity that is unrelated to the other ganglion cell tumors under discussion. Numerous cases of dysplastic cerebellar gangliocytoma have been reported in association with multiple hamartoma syndrome (Cowden's disease) (392), including some that presented in infancy and childhood (91,401). The pathogenesis of this unusual lesion remains to be defined.

Another central nervous system lesion, hypothalamic hamartoma (which is notable as a rare cause of precocious puberty), is also occasionally referred to as hypothalamic "gangliocytoma." However, it arises as a developmental dysplasia and, like dysplastic cerebellar gangliocytoma, is distinct from other pediatric gangliocytomas.

Ganglioglioma

Gangliogliomas are far more common than gangliocytomas. Although the term "ganglioglioma" leaves open the possibility of participation by any glioma subtype, in practice the glial element in the overwhelming majority of cases is astrocytoma. Only in an exceptional case is oligodendroglioma found. The astrocytic component is generally diffusely distributed within the neoplasm, with ganglion cells often assuming a clustered arrangement (Fig. 30A).

Desmoplasia with collagen deposition is common in ganglion cell tumors and should raise the index of suspicion. The astrocytic component is usually low grade but can be higher (213,249). An exceptional case of malignant transformation of the neuronal component as well as the astrocytic component of a ganglioglioma has been reported (174).

Neoplastic ganglion cells often exhibit characteristic light microscopic features such as large nuclei with single prominent nucleoli and large amounts of cytoplasmic Nissl substance (Fig. 30B). However, Nissl substance may not be evident, and neoplastic astrocytes may also have large nuclei with prominent nucleoli. Binucleate or multinucleate forms may or may not be present. Immunohistochemistry, although rarely needed for the typically well-differentiated tumors, is useful for questionable cases and reveals strong reactivity for synaptophysin (249). Eosinophilic granular bodies are often prominent in gangliogliomas, a feature shared with juvenile pilocytic astrocytomas and pleomorphic xanthoastrocytomas (Fig. 30C).

One diagnostic caveat is worthy of emphasis. The presence of prominent tumor cell perineuronal satellitosis is

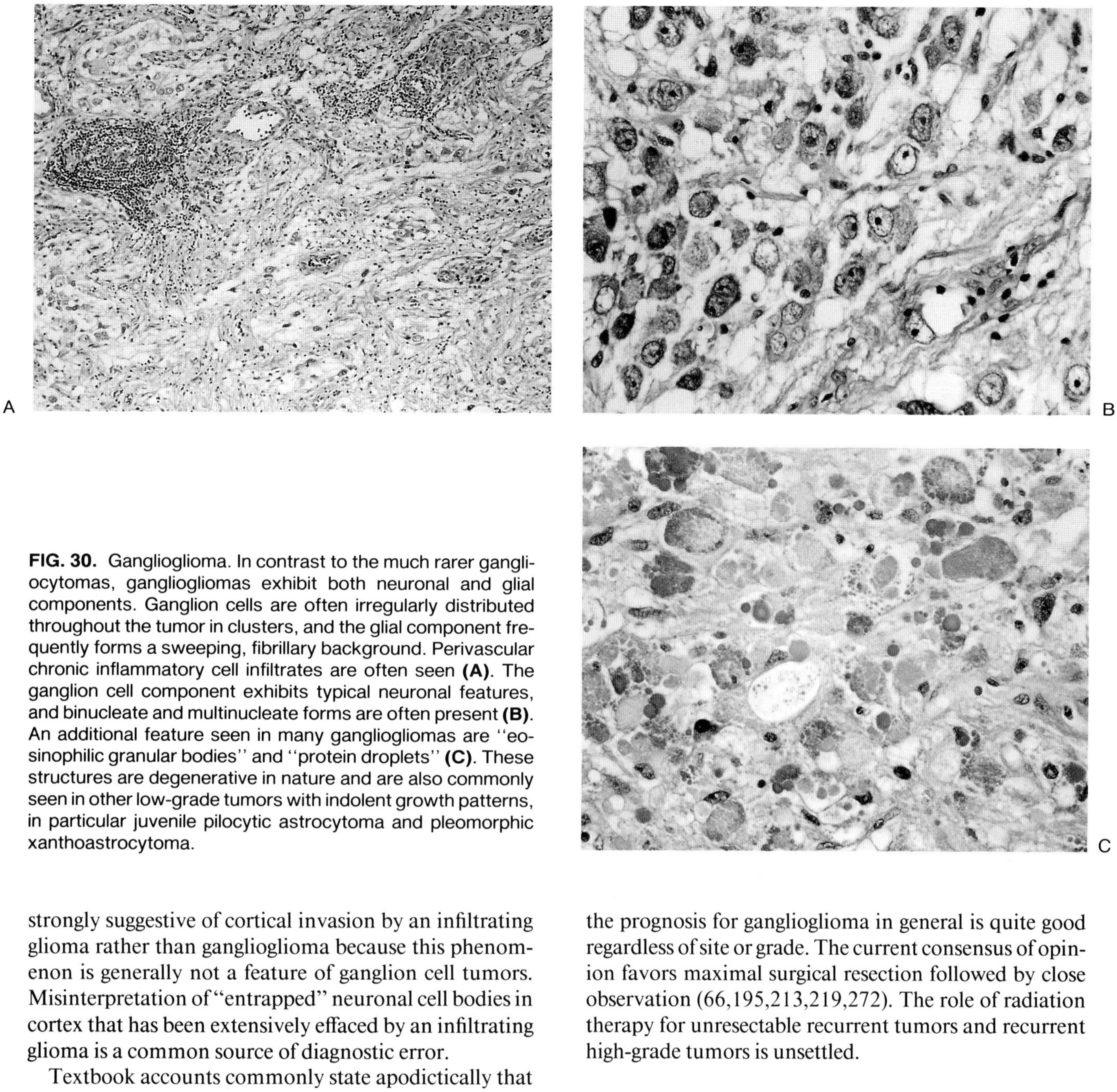

FIG. 30. Ganglioglioma. In contrast to the much rarer gangliocytomas, gangliogliomas exhibit both neuronal and glial components. Ganglion cells are often irregularly distributed throughout the tumor in clusters, and the glial component frequently forms a sweeping, fibrillary background. Perivascular chronic inflammatory cell infiltrates are often seen **(A)**. The ganglion cell component exhibits typical neuronal features, and binucleate and multinucleate forms are often present **(B)**. An additional feature seen in many gangliogliomas are "eosinophilic granular bodies" and "protein droplets" **(C)**. These structures are degenerative in nature and are also commonly seen in other low-grade tumors with indolent growth patterns, in particular juvenile pilocytic astrocytoma and pleomorphic xanthoastrocytoma.

strongly suggestive of cortical invasion by an infiltrating glioma rather than ganglioglioma because this phenomenon is generally not a feature of ganglion cell tumors. Misinterpretation of "entrapped" neuronal cell bodies in cortex that has been extensively effaced by an infiltrating glioma is a common source of diagnostic error.

Textbook accounts commonly state apodictically that prognosis for gangliogliomas is dependent on the grade of the astrocytic component. Such conclusions, however, appear to be largely based on scattered case reports. In contrast, both older and more recent series suggest that prognosis is less dependent on grade than on completeness of surgical excision (178,195,213,219). When gross total resection is possible (as with many supratentorial hemispheric lesions), it is often curative. For brainstem lesions, complete resection is not possible in a majority of cases and the recurrence rate is therefore higher. Spinal cord tumors also have an increased risk of recurrence and less favorable prognosis, most likely due to residual microscopic tumor (219). Malignant progression of some unresectable cases has been reported. Nevertheless, the prognosis for ganglioglioma in general is quite good regardless of site or grade. The current consensus of opinion favors maximal surgical resection followed by close observation (66,195,213,219,272). The role of radiation therapy for unresectable recurrent tumors and recurrent high-grade tumors is unsettled.

Desmoplastic Infantile Ganglioglioma

Desmoplastic infantile gangliogliomas (DIGs) share many clinicopathologic features with desmoplastic (or superficial) cerebral astrocytoma of infancy (discussed separately in section on astrocytic neoplasms), including a comparatively sanguine prognosis. It has been suggested that these two tumors are in fact variants of a single entity for which the designation "desmoplastic neuroepithelial tumor of infancy" has been proposed (288,334,386). The unique clinicopathologic features exhibited by desmoplastic infantile gangliogliomas, including predominant occurrence in the first 2 years of life, massive size, and exclusively supratentorial location, differ from those of the other pediatric gangliogliomas discussed above and warrant separation of DIGs from them.

The presence of a neuronal component may be obvious on hematoxylin and eosin—stained sections or require immunostaining for synaptophysin for confirmation. Important from a diagnostic perspective is the frequent presence of anaplastic-appearing, hypercellular areas of mitotically active, undifferentiated tumor cells (Fig. 31). In conjunction with the typically enormous tumor size and marked desmoplasia, such foci have resulted in misdiagnoses that invariably overgrade the lesion. In a review of one series, DIGs were initially mistaken for malignant neoplasms such as leptomeningeal fibrosarcoma, high-grade astrocytoma, malignant meningioma, and gliosarcoma (94).

The importance of correctly diagnosing this tumor lies in its far more favorable prognosis compared to the aforementioned mimics and in its extended progression-free survival, often following surgical resection alone. For cases in which progression occurs and further resection is not feasible, chemotherapy appears to be a suitable form of treatment (94). Given the extremely young age at diagnosis, irradiation is generally not an acceptable therapeutic option.

Dysembryoplastic Neuroepithelial Tumor

Dysembryoplastic neuroepithelial tumor (DNET) is a recently recognized entity that characteristically presents in children with medically intractable complex partial seizures, often of many years duration (82,83,374). Over 80 cases have been reported, including clinical series from four institutions (83,312,374). A review of the literature shows that all reported lesions are supratentorial and most involve the temporal lobe. Smaller numbers are located in the frontal lobe, and only rare cases arise primarily in the occipital or parietal lobes. The male/female ratio is approximately 3:2. Surgery is virtually always curative, and seizure control is often achieved even with partial resection. Recurrence and malignant progression do not occur.

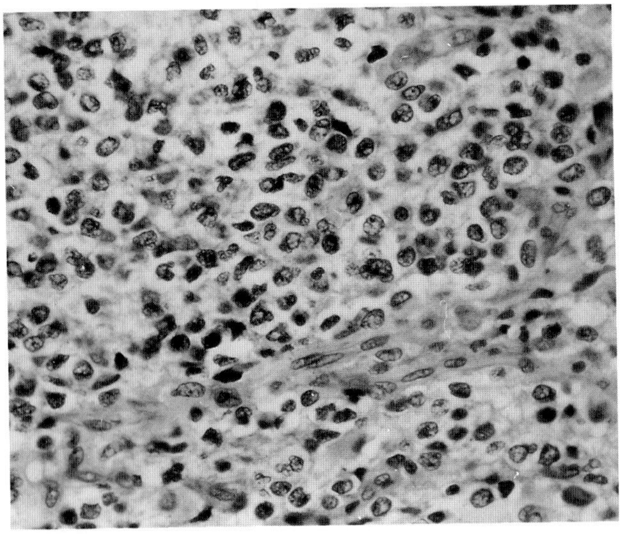

FIG. 31. Desmoplastic infantile ganglioglioma. This tumor is closely related clinically and biologically to the desmoplastic cerebral astrocytoma of infancy, differing mainly by the presence of a neuronal component identified by either the presence of typical ganglion cell features or synaptophysin immunopositivity. Focal mitotically active hypercellular areas, as seen in this illustration, may be present but do not alter the diagnosis or prognosis.

Major architectural properties of DNET include (a) an intracortical location, (b) multinodular composition, and (c) mixed glial and neuronal elements (82,83) (Fig. 32A). When sufficient tissue is available for examination, the lesion is often found to be encompassed by regions of cortical dysplasia. The most characteristic histologic feature of the lesion is the so-called specific glioneuronal element, composed of oligodendroglia-like cells and astrocytes, and neurons lying in a variably mucin-rich extracellular matrix (Fig. 32B). The nodular component often has a similar composition but exhibits greater morphologic variability. Occasional nodules are composed primarily of astrocytes. The lesion resembles oligodendroglioma or mixed oligoastrocytoma, particularly in limited tissue samples in which the characteristic architectural features cannot be fully appreciated. In contrast to oligodendroglioma and oligoastrocytoma, however, perineuronal satellitosis is virtually absent or extremely minimal.

The predominant cell type in both the "specific element" and the nodules is a monotonous population of small cells with rounded nuclei and very scant cytoplasm (Fig. 32B). These cells closely resemble oligodendroglia and have been referred to as "oligodendroglia-like cells (OLC)" (156). The majority are strongly immunopositive for S-100 protein. Occasional reactivity for GFAP and rare positivity for neuronal markers are seen (156). Ultrastructural studies likewise show a predominance of features consistent with oligodendroglial differentiation, with a smaller population exhibiting astrocytic or neuronal characteristics (82,156).

The hamartomatous vs. neoplastic nature of this interesting lesion has been debated (82,374). Regardless of classification, the indolent nature of DNET is unequivocally demonstrated by the absence of recurrence even following partial resection and the uniformly excellent prognosis with no reported examples of anaplastic progression. It is emphasized that treatment for this lesion is exclusively surgical; the use of adjunctive radiation therapy or chemotherapy is not warranted.

EMBRYONAL NEOPLASMS (PRIMITIVE NEUROECTODERMAL TUMORS)

Neoplasms composed of primitive neuroectodermal constituents compose a significant percentage of pediatric brain tumors, up to 25% in some series (298). Much

A 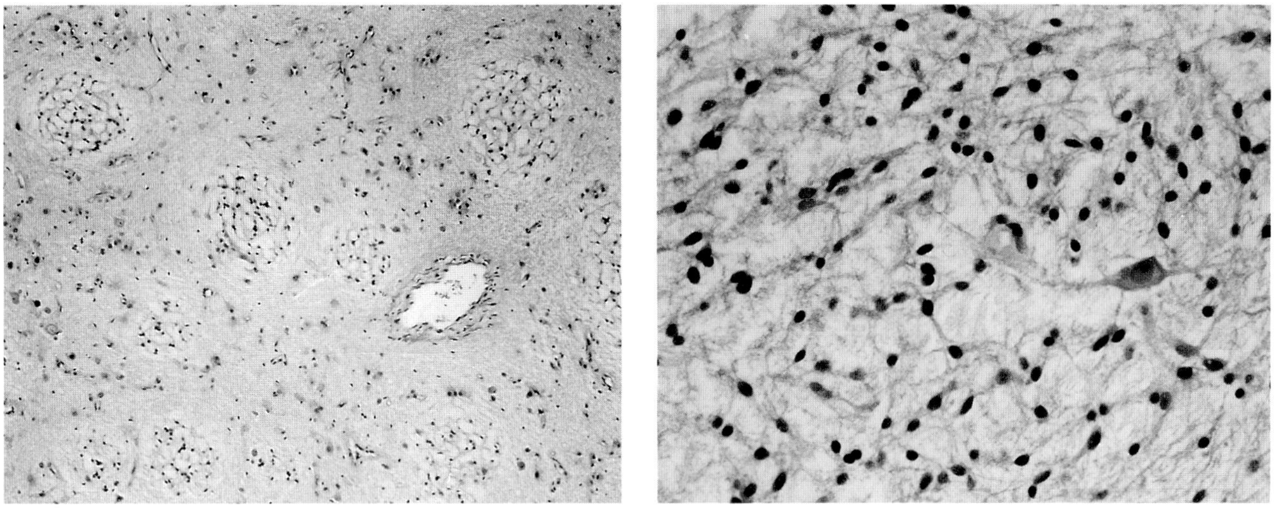 B

FIG. 32. Dysembryoplastic neuroepithelial tumor. A principal feature of this lesion is an intracortical location with nodular architecture **(A)**. Histologically, the "specific glioneuronal element" consists of oligodendrocyte-like cells **(B)**.

energy has been expended in an ongoing debate concerning the appropriate nomenclature for this class of tumors, with some arguing for retention of traditional categories (medulloblastoma, pineoblastoma, cerebral neuroblastoma, etc.) and others championing the more recently proposed unifying concept of the primitive neuroectodermal tumor (PNET). Both camps have presented cogent, detailed apologias, and the reader is urged to consult those publications for a fully nuanced explication of the issues (27,29,53,55,247,322–325,330, 331,335). Examples of the principal systems in current use are listed in Table 3 and include a traditional classification scheme (55), PNET classification (324), and the recently revised hybrid classification of the World Health Organization (199). The latter has appropriated the term "primitive neuroectodermal tumour" but otherwise retains traditional rubrics.

Part of the problem with classification of embryonal neoplasms stems from a lack of comparative data concerning the oncogenetic mechanisms operative in these tumors. Although molecular dissection of cerebellar medulloblastomas is progressing (discussed below), information accrual has been slow and sporadic for other PNET subtypes, due in large part to their relatively lower frequency of occurrence. It is hoped that molecular biologic studies will ultimately provide a firmer foundation for classification than that based upon morphologic patterns, immunohistochemical detection of differentiation antigens, and speculative theories of cytogenesis. To this end, technical advances such as PCR-based methodologies for analysis of minute tissue samples and collaborative efforts between well-established consortia for pooling and sharing of rarer tumor subtypes offer promising avenues for surmounting these limitations.

One terminologic footnote: the phrase "primitive neuroectodermal tumor" is also applied to malignant small

TABLE 3. *Classification systems for primitive small cell neoplasms of the central nervous system*

Burger and Scheithauer (1994)	Rorke (1993)	World Health Organization (1993)
Pineoblastoma[a]	Primitive neuroectodermal tumor, not otherwise specified	Pineoblastoma[a]
Mixed pineocytoma/pineoblastoma	Primitive neuroectodermal tumor with glial differentiation	Mixed pineocytoma/pineoblastoma
Pineal parenchymal neoplasms of intermediate differentiation	Primitive neuroectodermal tumor with ependymal differentiation	
Embryonal tumors:	Primitive neuroectodermal tumor with neuronal differentiation	*Embryonal tumors:*
Medulloepithelioma	Primitive neuroectodermal tumor with multipotential or bipotential differentiation (including muscle or melanocytic)	Medulloepithelioma
Neuroblastoma		Neuroblastoma
Ganglioneuroblastoma		Ganglioneuroblastoma
Ependymoblastoma		Ependymoblastoma
		Primitive neuroectodermal tumours
Medulloblastoma		Medulloblastoma
		Desmoplastic medulloblastoma
Medullomyoblastoma		Medullomyoblastoma
Melanotic medulloblastoma		Melanotic medulloblastoma
Other embryonal tumors		

[a]Classified with the pineal parenchymal tumors.

cell neuroectodermal tumors of the peripheral nervous system (also known as neuroepitheliomas). These peripheral primitive neuroectodermal tumors (pPNETs) are not related to central nervous system primitive neuroectodermal tumors (PNETs) but instead share many similarities with Ewing's sarcoma, including immunoreactivity for the MIC2 gene glycoprotein product (p30/32) and a characteristic chromosomal translocation, t11;22 (see Chapter 4). These unique molecular genetic alterations are not found in central nervous system PNETs (173).

Medulloblastoma/Cerebellar PNET

The cerebellar medulloblastoma is by far the most common primitive neuroectodermal tumor and, along with juvenile pilocytic astrocytoma, one of the two most common brain tumors of childhood (Table 1) (70,298). It arises primarily during the first two decades of life but also occurs in smaller numbers in adulthood (44,141,145, 164,236,295). Large series show a male preponderance of approximately 3:2 (70).

A variety of morphologic and differentiation patterns may be exhibited by medulloblastoma. The most common pattern is undifferentiated sheets (Fig. 33A). Neuronal differentiation is more commonly seen than glial differentiation and may be inferred from the presence of certain morphologic patterns such as Homer Wright ("neuroblastic") rosettes (Fig. 33B) or by the presence of apparent maturation into ganglion cells ("cerebellar ganglioneuroblastoma") (95). One recognized variant exhibits streams of rounded nuclei embedded in a fine neurofibrillary mesh resembling neuropil (Fig. 34) and has been referred to as "cerebellar neuroblastoma." Neuronal differentiation may also be reflected by immunopositivity for synaptophysin or a variety of other neuronal markers. Glial differentiation is indicated primarily by immunopositivity for GFAP and less often by morphologic features of astrocytic or, very rarely, ependymal differentiation. Immunoreactivity for GFAP is often only focally present and/or predominantly perivascular in location. Interpretation in such cases is problematic due to the frequent presence of entrapped indigenous reactive astrocytes. Nevertheless, a small percentage of medulloblastomas (about 10%) do exhibit the unimpeachable presence of glial differentiation. Mesenchymal differentiation may appear as either smooth muscle or striated muscle ("medullomyoblastoma") detected either by identification of cross-striated "strap" cells or, more commonly, by immunoreactivity for markers such as desmin, myoglobin, or muscle—specific actin. An additional morphologic variant, termed desmoplastic medulloblastoma, exhibits a vascular, desmoplastic stroma with interspersed reticulin-free "pale islands" (Fig. 35). Tumor cells composing the pale islands may exhibit immunoreactivity for a variety of neuronal and glial markers including synaptophysin and GFAP.

Given the diverse morphologic and differentiation patterns shown by primitive neuroectodermal tumors of the cerebellum, the question arises as to whether the different groups might exhibit differing biologic behavior. Accordingly, several studies have examined the relationship between particular subgroups and clinical outcome, with conflicting results (64,75,127,164,240,277). At present, no definitive association of differentiation with prognosis has been established. However, novel immunohistochemical and molecular genetic markers will

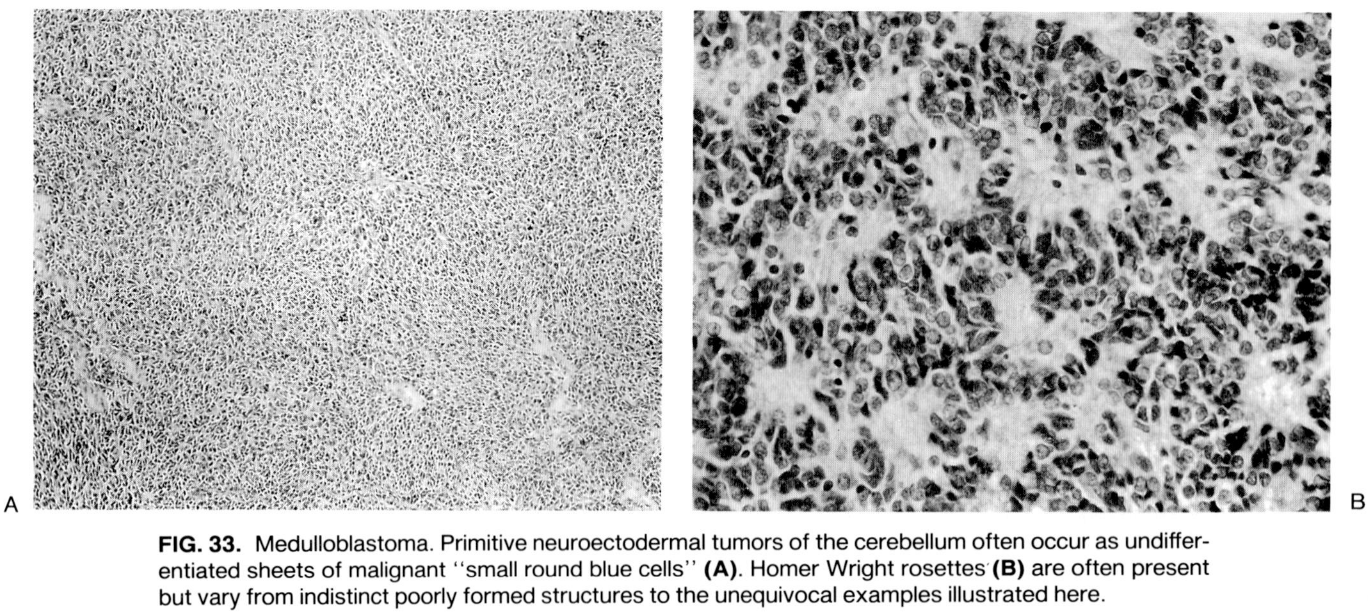

FIG. 33. Medulloblastoma. Primitive neuroectodermal tumors of the cerebellum often occur as undifferentiated sheets of malignant "small round blue cells" **(A)**. Homer Wright rosettes **(B)** are often present but vary from indistinct poorly formed structures to the unequivocal examples illustrated here.

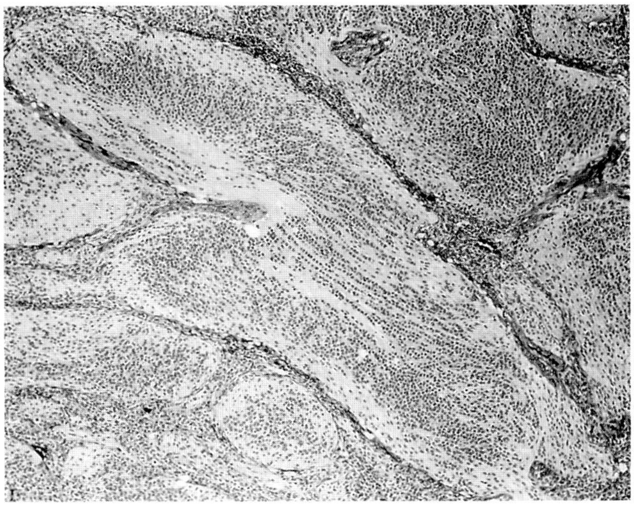

FIG. 34. Medulloblastoma. A nodular growth pattern is seen in many medulloblastomas. There are two principal variants. Illustrated here is the so-called cerebellar neuroblastoma, which displays rounded nuclei streaming in a fine neurofibrillary background. The second pattern is desmoplastic medulloblastoma (Fig. 35).

likely serve as a spur for continued investigation of phenotypic and/or genotypic subsetting for prognostic purposes.

The most common genetic abnormality detected in medulloblastomas is loss of chromosome 17p, yielding isochromosome 17q [i(17q)] by classical cytogenetics. The suspected locus for a putative tumor suppressor gene has been narrowed to the vicinity of or telomeric to 17p13. Because the p53 gene localizes to 17p13, it would be a logical candidate. However, whereas 30–75% of medulloblastomas exhibit i(17q), DNA sequencing studies to date have shown that mutations of exons 5–9 of the p53 gene (which account for at least 95% of reported p53 mutations for all tumor types) are present in only a minority (less than 10%) (3,17,77,267,309,347). Thus, either the p53 gene is altered in a distinctly different fashion compared to other cancers that show a high incidence of p53 mutation or, more likely, a second tumor suppressor gene is colocalized with p53 on the short arm of chromosome 17 (77). The possibility of a novel medulloblastoma tumor suppressor gene in this location is under investigation.

With respect to oncogenes, only about 5% of medulloblastoma biopsies exhibit amplification of known oncogenes (39,112), of which the most common is c-*myc*. Although a large percentage of medulloblastoma cell lines in culture show c-*myc* amplification, the significance of this finding for in vivo tumors is uncertain.

Proliferation indices have also been examined for potential prognostic utility. Data for several marker systems including bromodeoxyuridine (BUdR), PCNA, and Ki-67 confirm high proliferation rates and have permitted characterization of different morphologic populations but have not produced statistically significant patient stratification or correlation with survival time (168,352).

Several model systems are available for study of medulloblastoma and other primitive neuroectodermal tumors, including xenografts of human medulloblastomas and the production of a variety of primitive neuroectodermal tumors in transgenic mice with the simian virus large T antigen. These animal models have been recently reviewed (117,323).

The prognosis for patients with medulloblastoma has improved over the past several decades. Current 5-year progression-free survivals of 50–70% for localized disease can be achieved with irradiation (119,275,318). The recent addition of chemotherapy for patients with subtotal surgical resection or with metastatic disease has yielded exceptional results for these traditionally high-risk groups (275). In contrast, the prognosis for medulloblastoma arising in infants, in whom radiation therapy is generally not acceptable, remains dismal. An additional troubling issue concerns the late effects of treatment. Along with the life-prolonging success of contemporary therapeutic regimens has come risk for a number of deleterious sequelae, including second neoplasms (discussed in Chapter 12). Further study of this problem is needed (275).

Other Primitive Neuroectodermal Tumors

Embryonal neoplasms with morphologic features similar to those of the cerebellar medulloblastoma arise in smaller numbers throughout the neuraxis, occurring in decreasing order of incidence in the pineal gland, cere-

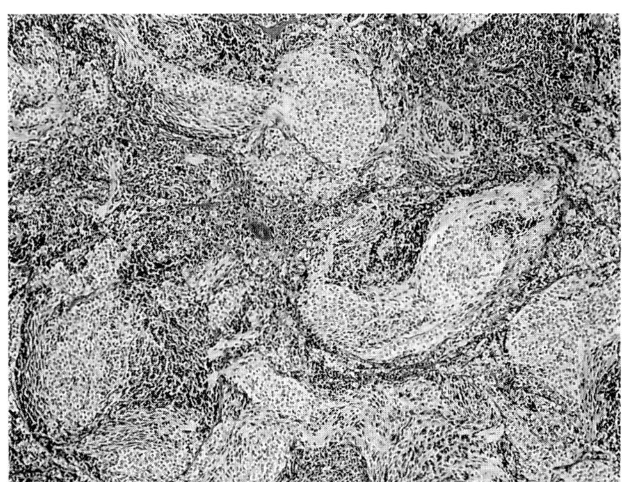

FIG. 35. Desmoplastic medulloblastoma. This nodular variant of medulloblastoma is composed of comparatively hypocellular "pale islands" surrounded by tumor that is densely cellular and reticulin-rich. The pale islands are often positive for neuronal or glial markers such as synaptophysin and GFAP (not shown).

amined so far do not play a role in the genesis of most tumors (47,151,292,365,416). A notable exception in this regard is the finding that approximately one third of GH-producing (somatotropic) adenomas harbor a somatic activating point mutation at one of two hot spots (codons 201 and 227) in the gene encoding the α subunit of guanine nucleotide binding protein (Gs α). This putative oncogene (designated *gsp* for Gs protein) leads to constitutive activation of adenylyl cyclase and marked elevation of intracellular cAMP, thus providing stimulation of tumor cell growth (93,233,366).

Allelic deletions on chromosome 11 have been reported in a minority of adenomas of all hormone classes, suggesting possible involvement of a tumor suppressor gene in a subset of tumors (47). *H-ras* point mutations have been reported in a few pituitary carcinoma metastases and invasive tumors but are otherwise very rare (59,189,292). Thus, while there are a few promising leads, particularly for the subset of somatotropic adenomas harboring a putative *gsp* oncogene, the molecular oncogenic mechanism(s) for the majority of pituitary adenomas remain poorly understood and constitute an area of active investigation.

GERM CELL TUMORS

Intracranial germ cell tumors arise most frequently in childhood and occur principally in midline structures, particularly in the pineal gland, where they constitute the most common neoplasm of that organ, and in the suprasellar region, where they are the second most common tumor after craniopharyngioma. Rare examples of more laterally placed lesions in the basal ganglia and thalamus have also been reported (371,413).

Germinoma

Germinoma is the most common of the intracranial germ cell tumors and is found most commonly in the pineal, followed by the suprasellar region. Some patients present with both pineal and suprasellar tumors, and these are occasionally joined by diffuse spread along the walls of the third ventricle. Approximately 50% of suprasellar tumors are accompanied by pineal lesions, whereas pineal germinomas are more often solitary. There is a male preponderance for pineal tumors, but the M/F ratio is 1:1 for suprasellar germinomas.

The signs and symptoms at clinical presentation are determined by anatomic location of the tumor. Pineal germinomas, like other tumors of this region, tend to compress the midbrain tectum and cerebral aqueduct, producing obstructive hydrocephalus and sometimes paresis of upward gaze (Parinaud's syndrome); they may also produce precocious puberty. Suprasellar tumors, on the other hand, may disrupt normal function of the pituitary and optic pathways, resulting in the classic triad of diabetes insipidus, loss of visual acuity, and hypopituitarism.

Germinomas exhibit a characteristic biphasic cellular composition: large, anaplastic germinoma cells with large nuclei and prominent nucleoli contrast sharply with interspersed collections of small lymphocytes (Fig. 39). An additional feature seen in some specimens is the presence of granulomatous inflammation (207). A majority of germinomas are immunopositive for placental alkaline phosphatase (PLAP) and negative for keratins and epithelial membrane antigen.

Teratoma

Teratoma is the second most common intracranial germ cell tumor; immature, mature, and mixed forms occur in this location. The neuroanatomic distribution of teratomas is broader than that of germinomas: in addition to midline sites such as the pineal, cases arise throughout the neuraxis (e.g., intraventricularly and in the cerebellopontine angle cistern). Immature teratomas are more common than purely mature forms. Cases of both types exhibit characteristic derivatives of the three germ layers as seen in similar tumors arising at other body sites (see Chapter 10).

Teratomas frequently occur as a component of mixed germ cell tumors. The combination of teratoma and embryonal carcinoma has been referred to as "teratocarcinoma." Besides harboring other germ cell components (mixed germ cell tumors), teratomas may also give rise to malignant elements such as adenocarcinoma or sarcoma (teratoma with malignant transformation).

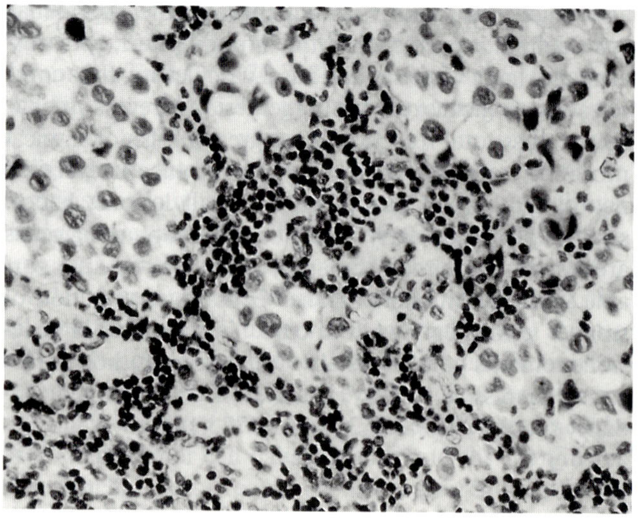

FIG. 39. Germinoma. Germinomas exhibit a characteristic biphasic cellular population composed of large mitotically active tumor cells with prominent nucleoli and zones of small reactive chronic inflammatory cells.

Congenital massive immature teratoma is a well-recognized entity that is diagnosable in utero by ultrasonography (375,405). These enormous tumors may occupy a cerebral hemisphere or entirely fill the intracranial cavity with complete replacement of all brain parenchyma (258,266,268). The majority are lethal, but increased survival has been achieved surgically in rare cases (100,102).

Intracranial Fetus-In-Fetu

A rare occurrence, fetus-in-fetu is considered by many investigators to be a form of incomplete twinning (included monozygous twin). Most examples present as retroperitoneal masses in the first few months of life (183). Exceptional cases of intracranial fetus-in-fetu have been reported (4,165,197,253,382,410).

The distinction between highly organized mature teratoma ("fetiform teratoma") and fetus-in-fetu is somewhat controversial (96,147,273). The reported intracranial examples have satisfied Willis's requirement of axial (vertebral) skeletal development for a diagnosis of fetus-in-fetu (406). Molecular analyses have recently been brought to bear on the issue. Hing et al. (155) used PCR techniques to demonstrate identical heterozygous alleles for multiple loci from four chromosomes in both an infant and its included fetus, and karyotypic and protein polymorphism studies from several other cases have yielded similar findings. These data, however, are compatible with either a monozygotic twin or complex teratoma of premeiosis 1 stem cell origin, so that the issue remains unsettled.

Embryonal Carcinoma, Yolk Sac Carcinoma, and Choriocarcinoma

The remaining germ cell neoplasms (embryonal carcinoma, yolk sac carcinoma, and choriocarcinoma) are much rarer than germinoma and teratoma (41,158,333,349). The morphologic features exhibited by instances of these tumors that arise within the central nervous system are similar to those of corresponding neoplasms that occur in other organs (see Chapter 10).

Embryonal carcinoma is the most poorly differentiated of the germ cell tumors and occurs more commonly as a component of mixed germ cell tumors than in pure form (276). The tumor comprises sheets, nests, and cords of large anaplastic cells with amphophilic cytoplasm, large nuclei, and prominent nucleoli. In contrast to germinoma, to which it may bear some resemblance, embryonal carcinoma is strongly immunopositive for cytokeratins (in contrast to only about 10% of germinomas) and is also positive for the Ki-1 (CD30) antigen (280).

Yolk sac (endodermal sinus) tumors also occur intracranially as components of mixed tumors or, rarely, as pure tumors (22,109). The morphologic features are identical to those of tumors arising in other body locations and include the presence of Schiller–Duval (yolk sac) bodies in some examples. Yolk sac tumors are immunopositive for α-fetoprotein (AFP).

Choriocarcinoma is the least common germ cell tumor occurring intracranially. As at other body sites, the tumor is composed of cytotrophoblasts and syncytiotrophoblasts, with the latter component exhibiting immunoreactivity for β-human chorionic gonadotropin (β-hCG). It should be recalled that other germ cell tumors, including germinoma, embryonal carcinoma, and yolk sac tumor, may contain scattered syncytiotrophoblast cells that react strongly to β-hCG.

HEMANGIOBLASTOMA

Hemangioblastoma occurs both in association with von Hippel–Lindau disease and as a sporadic neoplasm. In both forms it is primarily a tumor of adults in the third through fifth decades, although occasional examples arise during childhood. The Childhood Brain Tumor Consortium reported 6 cases, all of which arose in the posterior fossa, from a total of 3,291 pediatric cases involving brain tumors (70). A cerebellar tumor occurring in childhood is far more likely to be either medulloblastoma or juvenile pilocytic astrocytoma than hemangioblastoma. The morphologic and immunohistochemical features are the same as for hemangioblastomas arising in adults (Fig. 40). Preliminary studies suggest that at least some sporadic hemangioblastomas have mutations of the von Hippel–Lindau tumor suppressor gene on the short arm of chromosome 3 (184).

ATYPICAL TERATOID/RHABDOID TUMOR

Primary central nervous system atypical teratoid/rhabdoid tumors occur primarily in infants and young children but may also be seen in adolescents (5,38,73, 78,136,170,222,239,254,326,344,391,400). These neoplasms arise either in the posterior fossa (cerebellum) or supratentorially where the cerebral hemispheres and lateral ventricles may be involved. Salient phenotypic characteristics include clusters and sheets of epithelioid cells with large pale nuclei, prominent nucleoli, and moderate amounts of eosinophilic cytoplasm (Fig. 41). Immunostaining typically reveals strong diffuse positivity for vimentin and focal positivity for epithelial markers such as cytokeratins and epithelial membrane antigen. Occasional cells may exhibit positivity for various neuroectodermal markers, including GFAP and neurofilament proteins. Ultrastructural examination of tumor cells that exhibit globular cytoplasm shows whorls of intermediate filaments, presumably vimentin.

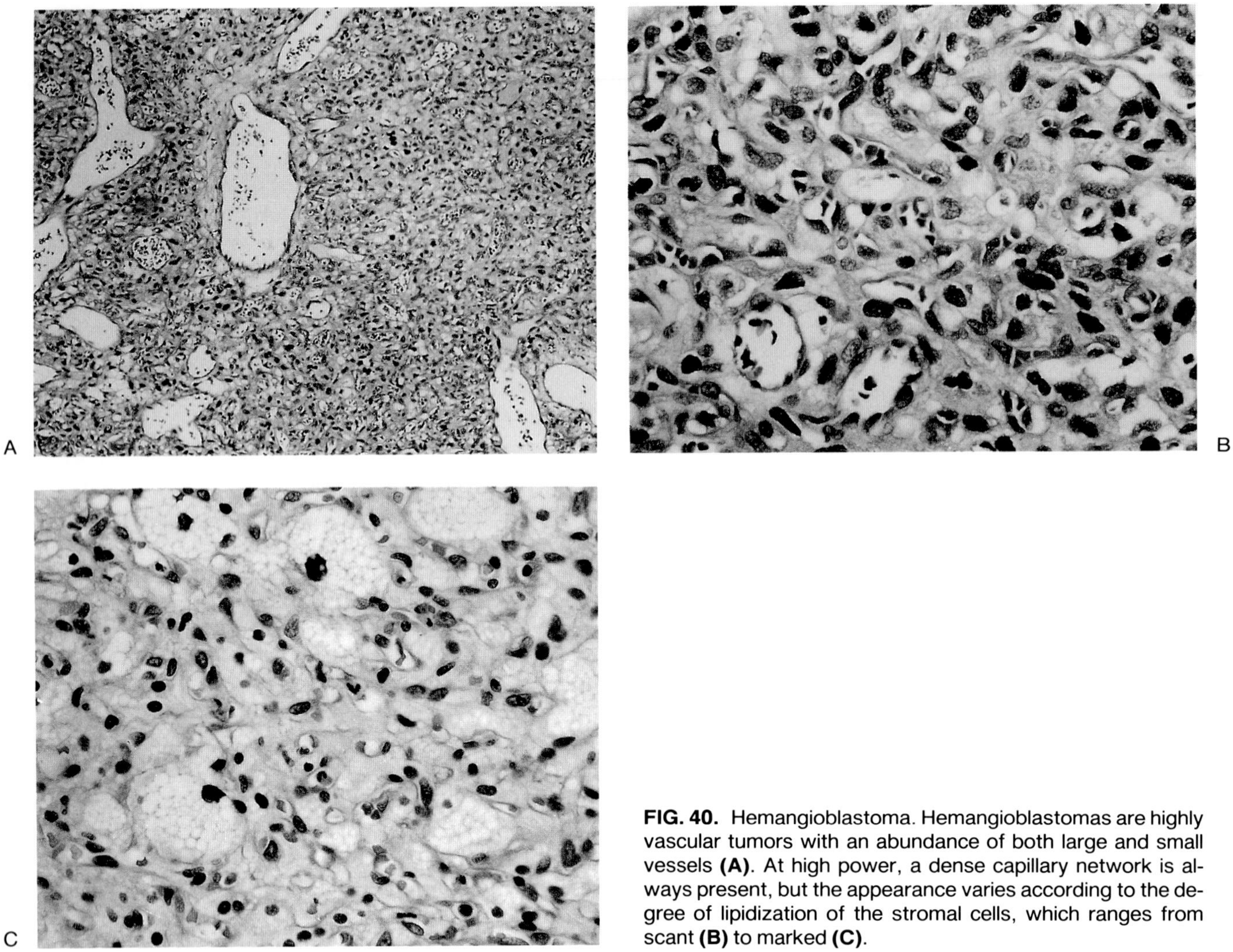

FIG. 40. Hemangioblastoma. Hemangioblastomas are highly vascular tumors with an abundance of both large and small vessels **(A)**. At high power, a dense capillary network is always present, but the appearance varies according to the degree of lipidization of the stromal cells, which ranges from scant **(B)** to marked **(C)**.

The overall histologic impression is that of a malignant neoplasm in which the cells are larger and have more cytoplasm than is seen in a typical PNET but are more epithelioid in appearance than most malignant gliomas. Recognition of rhabdoid tumor requires an awareness of the entity, followed by a high index of suspicion that should be aroused when the observed morphologic features don't quite fit with those of more commonly encountered tumors such as medulloblastoma or glioblastoma.

The histogenesis of these tumors has not been resolved, and the existence of atypical teratoid/rhabdoid tumor as a legitimate nosologic entity sui generis remains controversial. The arguments are similar to those surrounding the diagnosis of soft tissue hemangiopericytoma, with the principal gravamen being that a number of other primary tumors may exhibit rhabdoid-like features. Thus, in a review of 42 neoplasms diagnosed as extrarenal rhabdoid tumors, Parham et al. (283) found evidence for neural or glial differentiation in a majority of the intracranial cases and therefore advocated use of the term "poorly differentiated neoplasm with rhabdoid features" for undifferentiated tumors that exhibit a rhabdoid phenotype but in which immunohistochemical and ultrastructural studies fail to reveal a more specific diagnosis. Based on the presence of neuroglial differentiation, Weeks et al. (400) concluded that intracranial rhabdoid tumors likely represent a distinctive type of neuroectodermal neoplasm but are related more closely to primitive brain tumors than to rhabdoid tumors of the kidney.

As with many other nosologic disputes, molecular genetic analyses are likely to be enlightening and may ultimately serve as final arbiter. The limited cytogenetic and molecular studies performed to date show a high incidence of chromosome 22 deletions in rhabdoid tumors of the central nervous system, implicating possible involvement of a tumor suppressor gene on 22q (35,37,414). Similar chromosome 22 alterations have also been reported for some renal rhabdoid tumors (358) (see Chapter 3).

Atypical teratoid/rhabdoid tumors of the central ner-

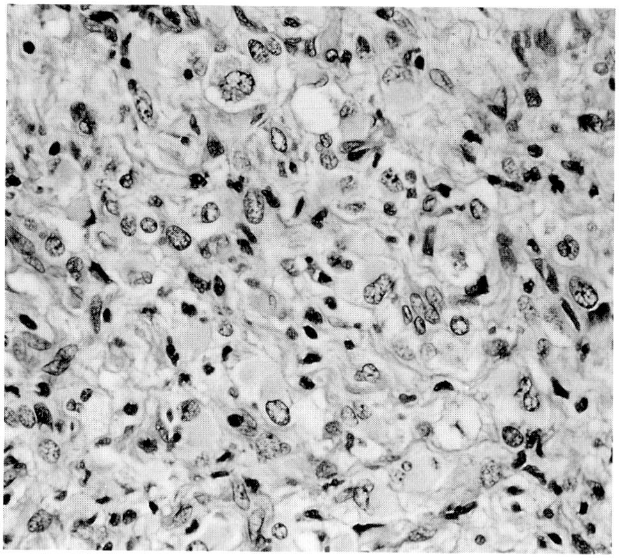

FIG. 41. Atypical teratoid/rhabdoid tumor. Rhabdoid tumors of the central nervous system typically show large cells with more cytoplasm than seen in PNETs and a more pronounced epithelioid appearance than usually seen in glioblastoma.

vous system are aggressive tumors that often disseminate within the nervous system and carry a uniformly dismal prognosis.

MENINGEAL AND PARENCHYMAL MESENCHYMAL NEOPLASMS

The meningeal coverings of the central nervous system are traditionally divided into three layers: the dura mater (pachymeninx), arachnoid, and pia mater. The dura is a thick, heavily collagenized membrane whose principal cellular constituents are fibroblasts. In addition, the dura contains large venous sinuses, meningeal arteries, and peripheral nerve fascicles. Dural venous sinuses receive venous blood via draining parenchymal veins and cerebrospinal fluid via arachnoid villi. The arachnoid consists of a continuous thin sheet of cells (arachnoid barrier cell layer) that is intimately applied to the inner aspect of the dura (dural border cell layer) (134,135). Based on descriptive and experimental ultrastructural investigations of the meninges in animals and humans, it is now generally accepted that the dura and subjacent arachnoid exist in vivo as a physically continuous tissue with sparse but unequivocal intercellular junctions that link the arachnoid barrier cell layer with the dural border cell layer (107,134,135,271). Thus, there is no interposed "subdural space," and it has been recommended that the term "spatium subdurale" be eliminated from the standardized nomenclature of Nomina Anatomica (135). The arachnoid extends delicate trabeculae that fuse with the pia. The arachnoid and pia thus enclose the cerebrospinal fluid-filled subarachnoid space and are often considered together as a single anatomic compartment (the leptomeninges or pia-arachnoid). Melanocytes are also normally present in the pia.

Several types of neoplasms arise from the varied cellular constituents of the meninges during childhood. Meningeal connective tissue elements may give rise to a number of rare primary sarcomas (161,205,256) and leptomeningeal melanocytes are associated with a variety of rare melanocytic lesions (discussed below). As in the adult population, however, the most common tumor of the meninges in children is meningioma. Meningeal hemangiopericytomas also occur in the pediatric population.

Meningioma

Meningiomas arise from the arachnoid and may therefore arise at any site where arachnoid cells are present. Prominent collections of arachnoid cells ("arachnoid cap cells") are found covering the arachnoid villi that project into all dural venous sinuses. This correlates well with the high frequency of meningiomas at these sites, particularly in the parasagittal region adjacent to the superior sagittal sinus (which receives the greatest number of arachnoid villi of all venous sinuses). As mentioned in the discussion of choroid plexus tumors, nests of arachnoid cells are commonly present in the fibrovascular stromal cores of choroid plexus villi and account for the occurrence of intraventricular meningiomas (Fig. 42). Heterotopic nests of meningothelial cells may be displaced during development into the formative cranium and soft tissues of the head and neck region, including the orbit, accounting for meningiomas arising at those sites. Arachnoid also lines the dural sheath of the optic

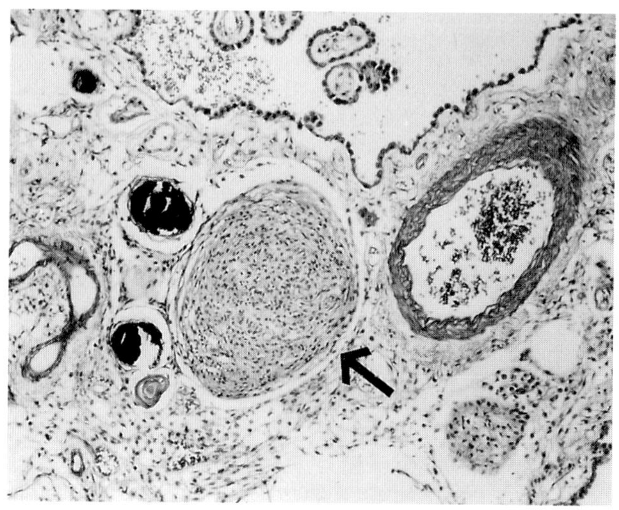

FIG. 42. Arachnoid cell rest in choroid plexus. The presence of meningothelial cell rests in normal choroid plexus *(arrow)* explains the occurrence of intraventricular meningiomas.

nerves and rare pediatric meningiomas have been reported in this location (367).

Pediatric meningiomas exhibit both similarities and differences compared with the much more common tumors of adulthood. Histologically, a similar spectrum of the familiar morphologic subtypes is seen. Most pediatric meningiomas are thus easily recognized as such and exhibit the same immunohistochemical and ultrastructural characteristics as their adult counterparts (Fig. 43; *see figure in color plate section*). In addition, atypical and frankly malignant tumors with invasion of brain parenchyma are also seen in children. Features associated with aggressive behavior include the presence of numerous, readily identifiable mitotic figures and foci of tumor necrosis (Fig. 44A). As for other central nervous system neoplasms, the use of a number of different proliferation markers as potential prognostic aides is under investigation by many laboratories (111) (Fig. 44B).

As in adults, even benign meningiomas may express a strong tendency for invasion of mesenchymal tissues such as the dura and cranial bones. Although this property is not a major therapeutic obstacle in many laterally placed convexity tumors where the calvarial bone and meninges can be excised in toto, it is a significant complicating factor in parasagittal tumors that extensively permeate the superior sagittal venous sinus, and it is the principal cause of morbidity and eventual mortality in skull base meningiomas that defy complete resection.

Despite the many similarities, there are also significant differences between childhood and adult meningiomas, including male/female incidence, various aspects of gross morphology and anatomic distribution, and, most importantly, the relative contribution of specific etiologic factors.

In contrast to meningiomas in adult patients, there is no female predominance in the pediatric population. In fact, a male predominance is reported in some series, particularly for those tumors arising in infancy. This discordance presumably reflects the influence of chronic exposure to steroid hormones in the adult female cohort. Very large, cystic meningiomas are comparatively more common in children than in adult patients, as are intraventricular meningiomas (101,342).

A unique morphologic variant of meningioma that exhibits extensive sclerotic changes has been exclusively described in children (85,161), and a potentially aggressive histologic subtype termed clear cell meningioma has been recently characterized with several examples described in children (417).

With respect to etiology, a significant percentage of pediatric meningiomas is associated with either previous radiation therapy or a genetic disorder, particularly neurofibromatosis type 2. The role of radiation therapy in the induction of meningiomas is well documented (139,321). Because of the typically long latency period, most meningiomas that arise secondary to childhood radiation therapy present decades later in adulthood. However, with exposure to high levels of ionizing radiation, pediatric patients treated early in the first decade of life may present with meningiomas in the second decade (19,121,169).

The largest group of documented radiation-induced meningiomas are those occurring in patients who received low-dose radiation therapy for tinea capitis according to the Keinböck–Adamson irradiation protocol. This regimen was introduced in 1909 (1) and was employed worldwide until efficacious drug therapy (griseofulvin) was introduced in 1960 (139). Keinböck–Adamson treatment produced a

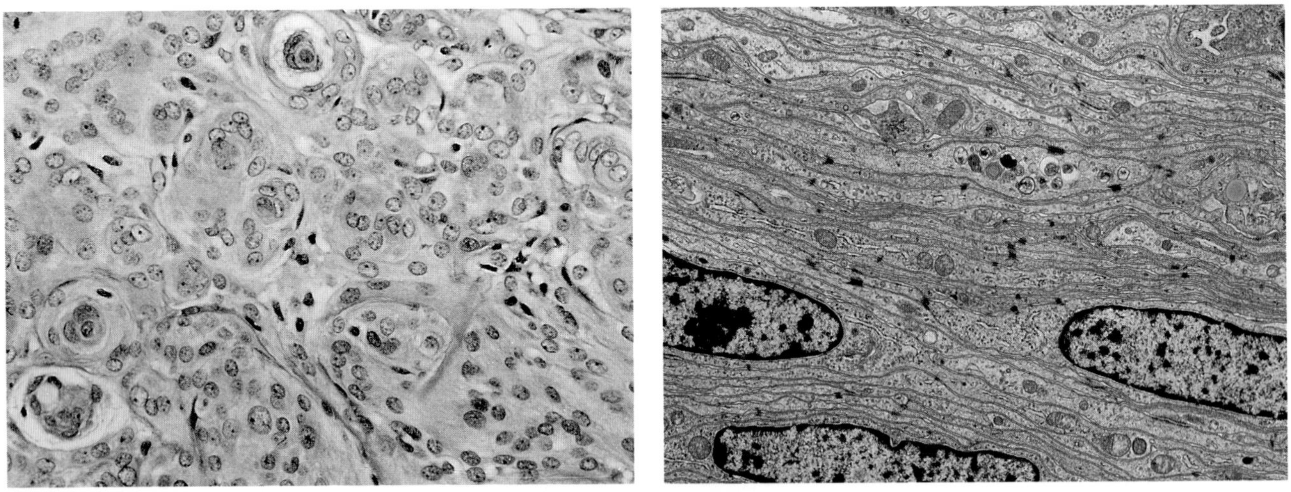

A C

FIG. 43. Meningioma. Meningiomas in children often show classical features such as whorl formation in the transitional variant **(A)**. Although a wide range of meningioma morphologic subtypes occurs, most forms exhibit immunopositivity for epithelial membrane antigen (EMA), as illustrated in the xanthomatous meningioma **(B)** *(see color plate section)* and virtually all tumors examined ultrastructurally exhibit prominent cell processes joined by numerous desmosomes **(C)**.

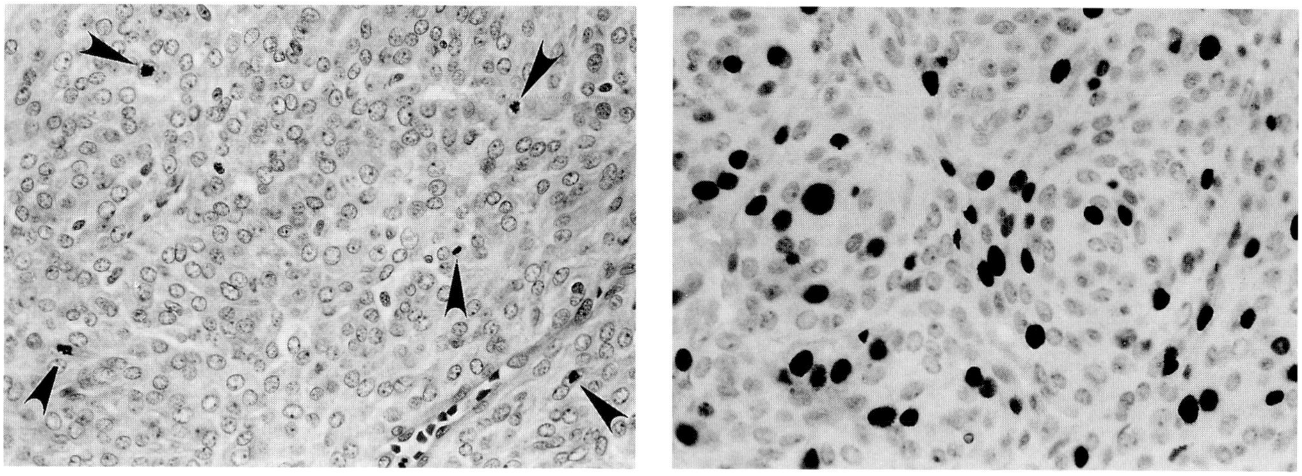

FIG. 44. Atypical meningioma. Numerous mitotic figures are seen (*arrowheads*, **A**). Foci of necrosis are often seen. The presence of brain parenchyma invasion by the tumor warrants a diagnosis of malignant meningioma. Proliferation markers, such as the MIB-1 monoclonal antibody that recognizes the KI-67 antigen in routinely processed formalin-fixed tissue **(B)**, are under study as potential aids in predicting aggressive behavior.

brain surface exposure of approximately 140 rads. The average interval between treatment and meningioma presentation is about 35 years (139). In contrast, the higher doses administered for other conditions, including very high doses given for tumors, result in a significantly shorter latency period (average 20–25 years), and cases with latencies as short as 5–10 years have been documented. It is within this latter group that radiation-associated meningiomas may arise during childhood in children previously treated for other malignancies (19,121,169).

Meningiomas also arise in childhood in association with a number of genetic disorders, most commonly neurofibromatosis type 2 (36,294). An association with basal cell nevus (Gorlin's) syndrome has been reported (6). Rare familial multiple meningioma syndromes have also been described (57,92,246,307).

The primary cytogenetic abnormality identified in adult meningiomas is loss of chromosome 22 (89,90, 338,339). Monosomy 22 occurs in up to 80% of meningiomas. Deletions of portions of chromosome 22, always including the NF2 gene locus, have also been found. Somatic mutations of the NF2 gene have been identified in some sporadic meningiomas (248,282). A number of other chromosome abnormalities have been reported, but none have the prevalence and apparent importance of the NF2 locus on chromosome 22 (302). Investigation of pediatric meningiomas has revealed a similar association with the NF2 locus (36).

Meningeal Hemangiopericytoma

Hemangiopericytomas also frequent the meninges in children, rarely including infants (Fig. 45) (13,154,190, 290,409). These tumors were formerly lumped together with hemangioblastomas and vascular meningiomas (angiomatous meningiomas) under the rubric "angioblastic meningioma," a nonspecific anachronism that should be abandoned. Classification of meningeal hemangiopericytomas has been a subject of considerable debate. The current consensus of opinion is that these tumors warrant separation from meningiomas on both clinical and biologic grounds. Among the factors supporting this distinction are the following: (a) Their light microscopic, ultrastructural, and immunohistochemical features are distinct from those of meningioma and are identical to those of hemangiopericytomas arising at other body locations. (b) Their clinical behavior is uni-

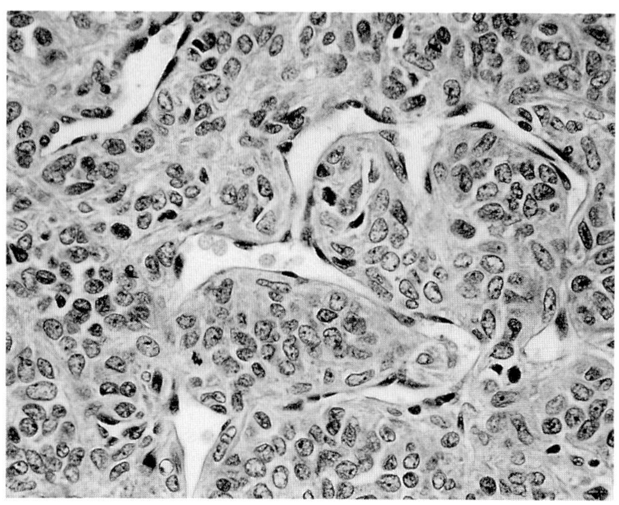

FIG. 45. Hemangiopericytoma. These meningeal tumors are highly vascular and exhibit a characteristic arciform vascular pattern ("staghorn" branching).

formly more aggressive than that of ordinary meningiomas, with higher frequencies of local recurrence and distant metastasis. (c) There is no female predeliction in the adult population as is seen with meningiomas. (d) There is no comparable association with prior radiation therapy as is seen with meningiomas. (e) Perhaps most importantly, the cytogenetic and molecular genetic evidence associating a large percentage of meningiomas with the NF2 tumor suppressor gene locus on chromosome 22 is not found with hemangiopericytomas (149, 150,179,238,293,368).

Hemangiopericytomas of the soft tissues that arise during infancy (infantile hemangiopercytomas) are distinct from those of adulthood in that they exhibit a comparatively benign clinical behavior despite the presence of anaplastic histologic features, including necrosis and a high mitotic rate (see Chapter 8) (97). Whether intracranial hemangiopericytomas that arise during infancy are similar in this regard requires clinical follow-up of additional cases of this rare neoplasm.

Meningioangiomatosis

Brief mention of this lesion is included for completeness because of its focal meningeal origin and predominant occurrence in the pediatric population. Meningioangiomatosis is a childhood hamartomatous lesion of the meninges and vasculature of the superficial cortex that occurs as one of the stigmata of neurofibromatosis type 2 or, rarely, as an isolated sporadic form (45, 137,203,230). As might be predicted from involvement of the cerebral cortex, affected children typically present with a history of seizures. Morphologic findings reveal prominence of cortical blood vessels surrounded by cuffs of spindled cells whose appearance ranges from meningothelial to fibroblastic (Fig. 46). The nature of these perivascular cells has been the subject of debate (55). The association of many cases with NF2 would appear to favor a meningothelial origin (230). Molecular genetic analysis of the NF2 gene in sporadic cases has not yet been reported (due to the rarity of these lesions) and is eagerly awaited.

PRIMARY MELANOCYTIC TUMORS

As mentioned previously, melanocytes are normal constituents of the leptomeninges (114). These cells are true dendritic melanocytes akin to those found in other body locations and are quite distinct from and unrelated to the pigmented neurons of the brainstem, whose pigment ("neuromelanin") is a byproduct of catecholaminergic neurotransmitter synthesis. Leptomeningeal melanocytes are found in greatest numbers in the pia covering the upper cervical cord, medulla, pons, cerebellum, crus cerebri, interpeduncular fossa, medial aspects of the temporal lobes, and gyri recti of the frontal lobes. Focal superficial extension into neural parenchyma along the perivascular Virchow–Robin spaces is common. The distribution of leptomeningeal melanocytes correlates well with that of many of the rare primary melanocytic lesions of the central nervous system, which tend to preferentially involve the leptomeninges and superficial parenchyma (26). There are three major categories: melanosis (most frequently associated with neurocutaneous melanosis), primary malignant melanoma (including diffuse melanomatosis), and melanocytoma. The first and second categories are closely linked in children.

Diffuse leptomeningeal melanosis is a proliferation of

A

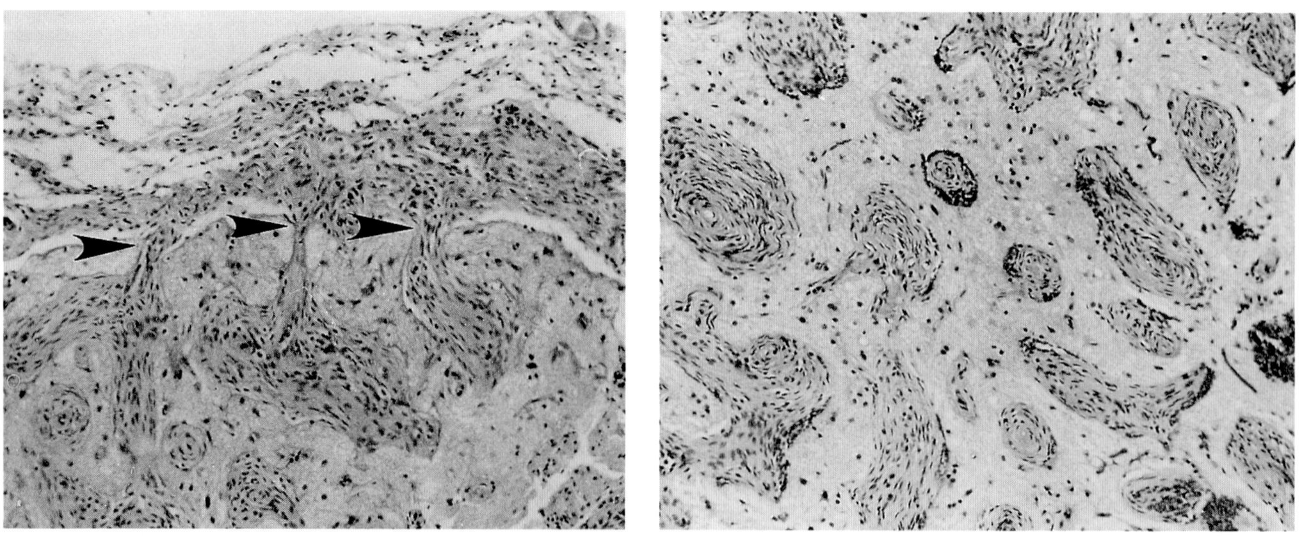

B

FIG. 46. Meningioangiomatosis. This lesion typically shows a cellular proliferation in the leptomeninges **(A)** which is contiguous via perivascular Virchow–Robin spaces (*arrowheads,* **A**) with cuffs surrounding prominent vessels in the underlying cortex **(B)**.

leptomeningeal melanocytes (with marked potential for malignant transformation) most commonly found in children with neurocutaneous melanosis. The association of pigmented skin lesions, commonly giant hairy nevi, with excessive leptomeningeal pigmentation was termed "neurocutaneous melanosis" by Van Bogaert in 1948 (385). Children with this syndrome have a poor prognosis and often present with hydrocephalus secondary to obstruction of cerebrospinal fluid flow in the basal cisterns by melanocytic proliferation (181). An association with congenital cerebellar abnormalities, including Dandy–Walker malformation, has been reported (180,202). The tendency for malignant transformation warrants close surveillance of this patient group (99). Melanomatosis arising in the clinical setting of neurocutaneous melanosis accounts for most cases of primary central nervous system melanoma in childhood. Exceptional cases with peritoneal dissemination of melanoma through a ventriculoperitoneal shunt and with systemic metastases have been reported (99,187). The biologic mechanisms and molecular basis for neurocutaneous melanosis are poorly understood at present.

Melanocytomas (also termed cellular blue nevi of the leptomeninges) are benign, focal proliferations of melanocytes most often located in the leptomeninges of the spinal cord or posterior fossa (217,303,383). Melanocytomas are not associated with neurocutaneous melanosis and the overwhelming majority of cases present in adulthood, although a rare childhood example arising in a 9-year-old boy has been reported (407).

Other Melanotic Tumors

Melanin-containing variants of several different types of primary neoplasms of the nervous system also occur, including medulloblastoma (melanotic medulloblastoma) and schwannoma (melanotic schwannoma). A psammomatous variant of the latter tumor may occur as a component of the Carney complex (65,242,384). Based on ultrastructural and immunohistochemical findings, a majority of the rare examples of so-called melanotic meningiomas appear to be misdiagnosed melanocytomas (224). Very rare examples of melanotic choroid plexus papillomas (218) and ependymomas (245) have also been described. An exceptional melanotic neuroectodermal tumor of infancy (melanotic progonoma) may arise as an intracranial mass (186) (see Chapter 4).

Chordoma

Clival chordomas are rare in childhood but do occur (76) (see Chapter 9). Rare cases may present in infancy (305) and, exceptionally, as an intracranial mass without bony involvement (262).

Intraparenchymal Mesenchymal Tumors

In addition to tumors of the dura and leptomeninges, a wide variety of benign and malignant mesenchymal neoplasms akin to those of the soft tissues infrequently arise in the central nervous system parenchyma (72,176,198,289). Of the very rare sarcomas, rhabdomyosarcoma (Fig. 47; see 47B in color plate section) and undifferentiated sarcomas are among the most commonly reported (34,304,360,372,376). Rhabdomyosarcomas occurring in pure form are generally diagnosed as such; however, it is to be recalled that rhabdomyosarcomatous differentiation may also be encountered in otherwise typical medulloblastoma (medullomyoblastoma).

There is one terminologic caveat concerning central nervous system sarcomas: Readers of the older literature are likely to encounter the terms "arachnoidal cell sarcoma" and "reticulum cell sarcoma." These are obsolete misnomers for desmoplastic medulloblastoma and central nervous system lymphoma, respectively.

INTRATHECAL SCHWANNOMA AND NEUROFIBROMATOSIS TYPE 2

Neurofibromatosis type 2 (NF2, bilateral acoustic neurofibromatosis, central neurofibromatosis) is an autosomal dominant inherited disorder with greater than 95% penetrance that predisposes affected individuals to a variety of nervous system tumors, including intracranial schwannomas, meningiomas, and spinal cord ependymomas (228). The *NF2* gene on chromosome 22 was recently characterized and its protein product (merlin, schwannomin) shown to have sequence homology to a

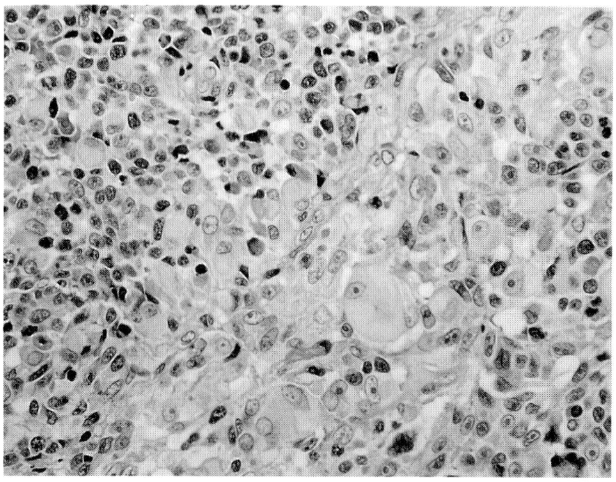

A

FIG. 47. Primary rhabdomyosarcoma of the central nervous system. A wide variety of sarcomas arise rarely as primary tumors within the central nervous system, including rhabdomyosarcoma **(A)** which shows strong, diffuse cytoplasmic immunoreactivity for desmin **(B)** *(see color plate section).*

family of proteins (moesin, ezrin, radixin, talin) that are postulated to mediate interactions between the cytoskeleton and cell membrane (328,380). In addition to patients with NF2, loss of heterozygosity for chromosome 22 loci and mutations in the coding region of the NF2 gene have also been found in a high percentage of sporadically occurring schwannomas and meningiomas. These data suggest that the NF2 gene functions as a tumor suppressor gene and that its inactivation is important in the genesis of a significant percentage (but not all) of both sporadic schwannomas and meningiomas as well as those arising in NF2 patients (89,338,339).

Bilateral vestibular schwannomas (neurilemmoma, acoustic neuroma, neurinoma) are the hallmark of NF2 and develop in the vast majority of patients. Contemporary neuroimaging techniques, particularly gadolinium-enhanced magnetic resonance imaging, permit early detection of these lesions in asymptomatic young children at risk (244,286). Schwannomas may also develop in other cranial nerves, including the trigeminal, glossopharyngeal, vagal, spinal accessory, and hypoglossal nerves (255).

SPORADIC INTRATHECAL SCHWANNOMA

Sporadic schwannomas may rarely arise during childhood in the absence of NF2 from the eighth nerve, other cranial and spinal nerves, and ubiquitous smaller peripheral nerve fascicles distributed throughout the neuraxis (68). Rare examples have been reported in association with the intracranial segments of the oculomotor nerves (oculomotor, trochlear, and abducens) (223). Intraventricular choroid plexus schwannomas likely arise from small nerve fibers of the autonomic nervous system from which the choroid receives its innervation (297). Intraparenchymal schwannomas arising in the cerebral hemispheres, cerebellum, and brainstem have occasionally been reported in the pediatric population (108). A single case of subfrontal schwannoma in an adolescent has been documented (390). Subfrontal and olfactory groove schwannomas are rare tumors of the anterior cranial fossa that may arise from a number of potential sources, including meningeal branches of the trigeminal nerve, the intracranial segment of the anterior ethmoidal nerve, or the terminal nerve (113,138,167). In the spinal cord, schwannomas arise preferentially from the dorsal (sensory) roots. Spinal nerve root neurofibromas also occur in children, usually in association with NF1 but occasionally as sporadic tumors (357).

The histologic features are similar in both sporadic and NF2-associated schwannomas and consist of various combinations of hypercellular Antoni type A tissue and hypocellular Antoni type B tissue (Fig. 48A).

A large number of diverse tumors may arise from the vicinal tissues of the cerebellopontine angle. The most common, however, are vestibular schwannoma and cerebellopontine angle meningioma. These neoplasms may closely resemble one another on hematoxylin and eosin–stained tissue sections. In particular, the issue of distinguishing areas of fibroblastic meningioma from Antoni type A tissue of schwannoma occasionally arises. This diagnostic dilemma can usually be settled by application of immunohistochemistry or electron microscopy. In general, schwannomas show strong diffuse immunoreactivity for S-100 protein, whereas a majority of meningiomas are immunopositive for epithelial membrane anti-

A 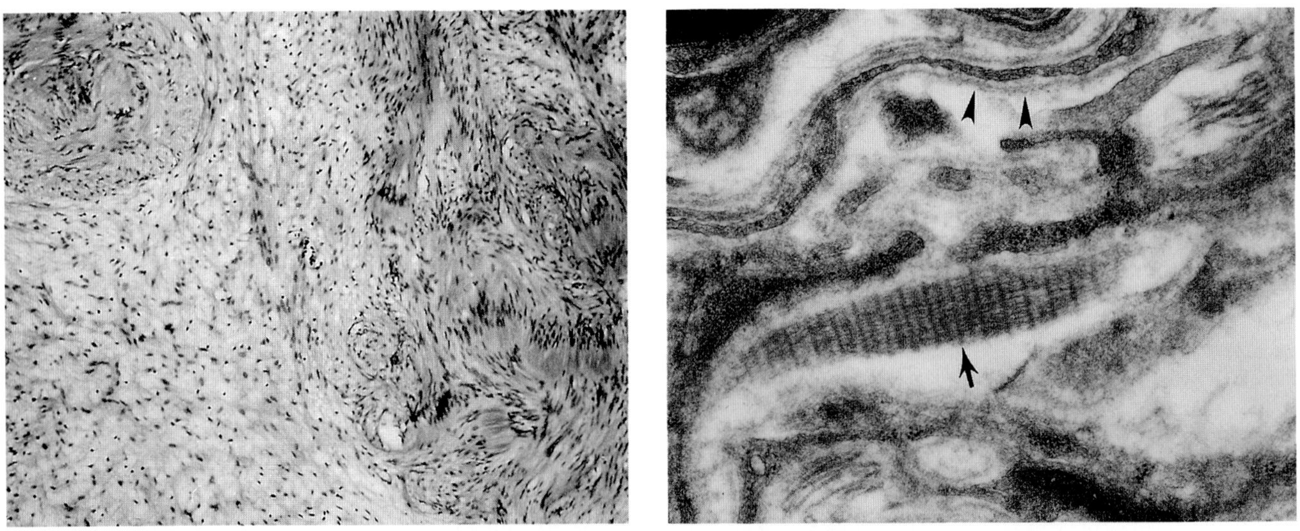 B

FIG. 48. Schwannoma. The typical biphasic architecture consists of densely cellular Antoni type A tissue (often with prominent nuclear palisading) interspersed with hypocellular Antoni type B tissue **(A)**. Ultrastructural examination reveals elongated cell processes covered with basement membrane material (*arrowheads*, **B**) and often long-spacing collagen (Luse bodies) (*arrow*, **B**).

gen. The ultrastructural characteristics of schwannoma are quite distinct compared to those of meningioma, with the principal features being the presence of prominent basal laminae and long-spacing collagen and an absence of the abundant intercellular desmosomal junctions seen in meningiomas (Fig. 48B).

METASTASIS OF SYSTEMIC NEOPLASMS TO THE CENTRAL NERVOUS SYSTEM

Metastatic brain tumors are rare in the pediatric age group compared to the adult population. Metastases from the neoplasms that produce a majority of lesions in adults (lung, breast, kidney, and colon carcinomas, and metastatic melanoma) are exceptionally rare in children (14). Rather, metastases reflect the composition of primary malignancies that are common in childhood. Thus, hematopoietic malignancies constitute the largest group responsible for central nervous system metastatic disease in children. Isolated central nervous system relapse has been reported in as many as 9% of pediatric patients with acute lymphoblastic leukemia (210).

Of the solid tumors, metastatic sarcomas are more common than carcinomas, again reflecting the composition of pediatric tumors. Osteosarcoma (23,40,129,241) and rhabdomyosarcoma (51,129,389) are frequent sources for brain metastases in children (Fig. 49). Instances of metastasis from a wide variety of other sarcoma subtypes have been reported, including leiomyosarcoma (274,289), liposarcoma (201), angiosarcoma (129,216), alveolar soft part sarcoma (234), fibrosarcoma (291), and chondrosarcoma (208). Ewing's sarcoma/peripheral primitive neuroectodermal tumor may also spread to the nervous system by hematogenous dissemination (40,379), and occasional cases of metastatic Wilms' tumor (389), neuroblastoma (291,356,389), melanoma (129,389), germ cell tumor (129), hepatic carcinoma (291,389), ovarian carcinoma (389), and congenital mesoblastic nephroma (146) have been reported.

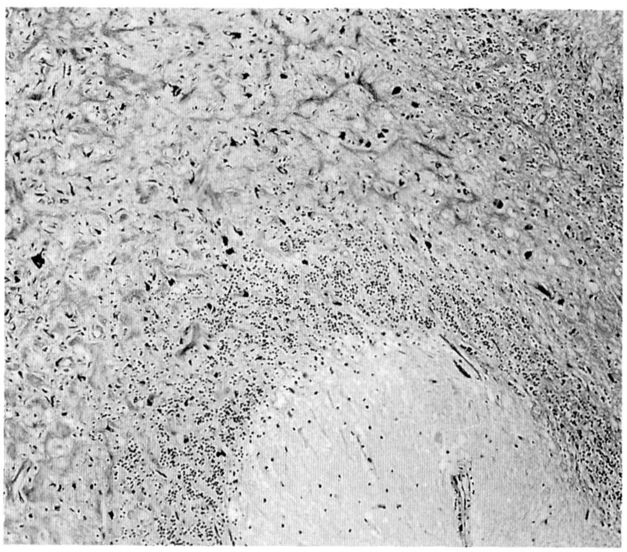

FIG. 49. Metastatic ostesarcoma. In contrast to metastases in adults, sarcomas are more common than carcinomas among pediatric solid tumors that metastasize to the central nervous system. Illustrated is osteosarcoma metastatic to the cerebellum. Note the infiltration of tumor cells through neural parenchyma without formation of a sharp "pushing" interface as is typical of most metastatic tumors.

In a majority of cases, nervous system metastases occur late in the course of the disease and usually in the presence of widespread systemic metastasis, especially to the lungs which may serve as the seeding site for brain metastases. In this regard, the rarity of central nervous system metastases from neuroblastoma compared to the high frequency of this tumor in the pediatric population may in part reflect a preference for liver, bone, lymph nodes, and skin as metastatic sites compared to lung (129).

It has been noted that whereas approximately 50% of metastases in adult patients are multiple, around 75% of metastases in children are solitary (291). Although prognosis is often dependent on the extent of control of extracranial disease, long-term survival has been reported for some pediatric patients following excision of single brain metastases (241,404).

METASTASIS OF PRIMARY BRAIN TUMORS TO SYSTEMIC ORGANS

Medulloblastoma is by far the most common pediatric brain tumor to metastasize outside of the central nervous system, followed distantly by the gliomas, meningeal tumors, and germ cell tumors (62,125,159,363). The majority of metastases of all histologic types occur in patients who have undergone an invasive procedure such as craniotomy, laminectomy, ventricular tap, or intracranial shunt, although spontaneous metastasis may rarely occur (159). Peritoneal metastasis, followed by systemic dissemination, is seen in patients with ventriculoperitoneal shunts, most frequently with medulloblastoma but also with gliomas and other primary brain tumors (159).

The most common sites for medulloblastoma metastases are bone, bone marrow, and lymph nodes (62,159). Metastases have also been reported to liver, lungs, retroperitoneum, pancreas, and adrenal gland (31,200). A single case of tumor-to-tumor metastasis of a medulloblastoma metastasizing to a fibroadenoma in a 17-year-old girl has been described (52).

In contrast to medulloblastoma, glioma metastases preferentially involve lung and lymph nodes rather than bone (62,159). Most glioma metastases arise from ependymomas or high-grade astrocytomas (159,287), although exceptional instances of hematogenous metastasis (227) and ventriculoperitoneal shunt dissemination (301) by low-grade astrocytomas have also been described.

PERSPECTIVE

Pediatric neuro-oncology is a dynamic field in rapid evolution. Advances continue to be made in therapeutic strategies with significant extention of survival for many types of brain tumors. The study of pediatric brain tumor pathology is no less vibrant as illustrated by the spirited debate over primitive neuroectodermal tumors and reflected in the fact that all four of the "new" tumor entities recognized in the revised WHO classification of tumors (desmoplastic infantile ganglioglioma, dysembryoplastic neuroepithelial tumor, pleomorphic xanthoastrocytoma, and central neutrocytoma) arise predominantly in children and young adults (199). Perhaps most exciting is recent progress in dissecting the molecular alterations found in the various hereditary brain tumor syndromes, which in turn contribute to an understanding of the oncogenesis of brain tumors in general (230). Further advances along these lines are ineluctable and eagerly anticipated.

REFERENCES

1. Adamson HG. A simplified method of x ray application for the cure of ringworm of the scalp: Keinböck's method. *Lancet* 1909;1:1378–1380.
2. Adamson TE, Weistler OD, Kleihues P, Yasargil MG. Correlation of clinical and pathological features in surgically treated craniopharyngiomas. *J Neurosurg* 1990;73:12–17.
3. Adesina AM, Nalbantoglu J, Cavenee WK. p53 gene mutation and mdm2 gene amplification are uncommon in medulloblastoma. *Cancer Res* 1994;54:5649–5651.
4. Afshar F, King TT, Berry CL. Intraventricular fetus-in-fetu. Case report. *J Neurosurg* 1982;56:845–849.
5. Agranovich AL, Ang L-C, Griebel RW, Kobrinsky NL, Lowry N, Tchang SP. Malignant rhabdoid tumor of the central nervous system. *Surg Neurol* 1992;37:410–414.
6. Albrecht S, Goodman JC, Rajagopolan S, Levy M, Cech DA, Cooley LD. Malignant meningioma in Gorlin's syndrome: cytogenetic and p53 gene analysis. Case report. *J Neurosurg* 1994;81:466–471.
7. Albrecht S, Rouh E, Becker LE, Bruner J. Transthyretin immunoreactivity in choroid plexus neoplasms and brain metastases. *Mod Pathol* 1991;4:610–614.
8. Albright AL, Packer RJ, Zimmerman R, Rorke LB, Boyett J, Hammond GD. Magnetic resonance scans should replace biopsies for the diagnosis of diffuse brain stem gliomas: a report from the Children's Cancer Group. *Neurosurgery* 1993;33:1026–1029.
9. Albright AL, Wisoff JH, Zeltzer P, et al. Prognostic factors in children with supratentorial (nonpineal) primitive neuroectodermal tumors. A neurosurgical perspective from the Children's Cancer Group. *Pediatr Neurosurg* 1995;22:1–7.
10. Alderson LM, Castleberg RL, Harsh GR 4th, Louis DN, Henson JW. Human gliomas with wild-type p53 express bcl-2. *Cancer Res* 1995;55:999–1001.
11. Allegranza A, Ferraresi S, Bruzzone M, Giombini S. Cerebromeningeal pleomorphic xanthoastrocytoma. Report on four cases: clinical, radiologic and pathological features. (Including a case with malignant evolution). *Neurosurg Rev* 1991;14:43–49.
12. Alvord Jr. EC. Is necrosis helpful in the grading of gliomas? Editorial opinion. *J Neuropathol Exp Neurol* 1992;127–132.
13. Aouad N, Vital C, Rivel J, Ramsoubramanian K, Santosh S, Chowdry O. Giant supratentorial meningeal haemangiopericytoma in a newborn. *Acta Neurochir (Wien)* 1991;112:154–156.
14. Aronson SM, Garcia JH, Aronson BE. Metastatic neoplasms of the brain: Their frequency in relation to age. *Cancer* 1964;17:558–563.
15. Auer RN, Becker LE. Cerebral medulloepithelioma with bone, cartilage, and striated muscle. *J Neuropathol Exp Neurol* 1983;42:256–267.
16. Bader JL, Meadows AT, Zimmerman LE, et al. Bilateral retinoblastoma with ectopic intracranial retinoblastoma: trilateral retinoblastoma. *Cancer Genet Cytogenet* 1982;5:203–213.
17. Badiali M, Iolascon A, Loda M, et al. p53 gene mutation in medulloblastoma. Immunochemistry, gel shift analysis, and sequencing. *Diagn Mol Pathol (United States)* 1993;2:23–28.
18. Bailey P, Cushing HA. *A Classification of the Tumors of the Glioma Group on a Histogenetic Basis with a Correlated Study of Prognosis.* Philadelphia: JB Lippincott; 1926.
19. Balasubramaniam C, Armstrong D, Cheek W, Laurent J. Postradiation meningioma in a child. *Pediatr Neurosci* 1988;14:319–323.
20. Bale PM. Ependymal rests and subcutaneous sacrococcygeal ependymoma. *Pathology (Australia)* 1980;12:237–243.
21. Balko MG, Blisard KS, Samaha FJ. Oligodendroglial gliomatosis cerebri. *Hum Pathol* 1992;23:706–707.
22. Bamberg M, Metz K, Alberti W, Heckemann R, Schulz U. Endodermal sinus tumor of the pineal region. Metastases through a ventriculoperitoneal shunt. *Cancer* 1984;54:903–906.
23. Baram TZ, van Tassel P, Jaffe NA. Brain metastases in osteosarcoma: Incidence, clinical and neuroradiological findings and management options. *J Neuro-oncol* 1988;6:47–52.
24. Barbosa MD, Balsitis M, Jaspan T, Lowe J. Intraventricular neurocytoma: a clinical and pathological study of three cases and review of the literature. *Neurosurgery* 1990;26:1045–1054.
25. Barkovich AJ. *Pediatric Neuroimaging.* 2nd ed. New York: Raven Press; 1995.
26. Barkovich AJ, Frieden IJ, Williams ML. MR of neurocutaneous melanosis. *Am J Neuroradiol* 1994;15:859–867.
27. Becker LE, Hinton D. Primitive neuroectodermal tumors of the central nervous system. *Hum Pathol* 1983;14:538–550.
28. Becker LE. An appraisal of the World Health Organization classification of tumors of the central nervous system. *Cancer* 1985;56:1858–1864.
29. Becker LE. Primitive neuroectodermal tumors: views on a working classification. In: Fields WS, ed. *Primary Brain Tumors: A Review of Histologic Classification.* New York: Springer-Verlag; 1989.
30. Bello MJ, Vaquero J, de Campos JM, et al. Molecular analysis of chromosome 1 abnormalities in human gliomas reveals frequent loss of 1p in oligodendroglial tumors. *Int J Cancer* 1994;57:172–175.
31. Berger MS, Baumeister B, Geyer JR, Milstein J, Kanev PM, Le Roux PD. The risks of metastases from shunting in children with primary central nervous system tumors. *J Neurosurg* 1991;74:872–877.
32. Bergsagel DJ, Finegold MJ, Butel JS, Kupsky WJ, Garcea RL. DNA sequences similar to those of simian virus 40 in ependymomas and choroid plexus tumors of childhood. *N Engl J Med* 1992;326:988–993.
33. Best PV. Posterior fossa medulloepithelioma. Report of a case. *J Neurol Sci* 1974;22:511–518.
34. Bhatia S, Sarker C, Mahapatra A. Primary cerebral rhabdomyosarcoma. *Indian J Pediatr* 1989;56:151–154.
35. Biegel JA, Burk CD, Parmiter AH, Emanuel BS. Molecular analysis of a partial deletion of 22q in a central nervous system rhabdoid tumor. *Genes Chrom Cancer* 1992;5:104–108.
36. Biegel JA, Parmiter AH, Sutton LN, Rorke LB, Emanuel BS. Abnormalities of chromosome 22 in pediatric meningiomas. *Genes Chrom Cancer* 1994;9:81–87.
37. Biegel JA, Rorke LB, Packer RJ, Emanuel BS. Monosomy 22 in rhabdoid or atypical tumors of the brain. *J Neurosurg* 1990;73:710–714.

38. Biggs PJ, Garen PD, Powers JM, Garvin AJ. Malignant rhabdoid tumor of the central nervous system. *Hum Pathol* 1987;18:332–337.
39. Bigner SH, Vogelstein B. Cytogenetics and molecular genetics of malignant gliomas and medulloblastoma. *Brain Pathol* 1990;1:12–18.
40. Bindal RK, Sawaya RE, Leavens ME, Taylor SH, Guinee VF. Sarcoma metastatic to the brain: results of surgical treatment. *Neurosurgery* 1994;35:185–191.
41. Bjornsson J, Scheithauer BW, Okazaki H, Leech RW. Intracranial germ cell tumors: pathobiological and immunohistochemical aspects of 70 cases. *J Neuropathol Exp Neurol* 1985;44:32–46.
42. Blach LE, McCormick B, Abramson DH, Ellsworth RM. Trilateral retinoblastoma—incidence and outcome: A decade of experience. *Int J Radiat Biol Phys* 1994;29:729–733.
43. Bleyer WA. The impact in the United States and the world of central nervous system cancer during childhood. In: Packer RJ, Bleyer WA, Pochedly C, eds. *Pediatric Neuro-oncology: New Trends in Clinical Research.* Chur, Switzerland: Harwood Academic; 1992:1–7.
44. Bloom HJ, Bessell EM. Medulloblastoma in adults: a review of 47 patients treated between 1952 and 1981. *Int J Radiat Oncol Biol Phys* 1990;18:763–772.
45. Blumenthal D, Berho M, Bloomfield S, Schochet SS Jr, Kaufman HH. Childhood meningioma associated with meningioangiomatosis. Case report. *J Neurosurg* 1993;78:287–289.
46. Boesel CP, Paulson GW, Kosnik EJ, Earle KM. Brain hamartomas and tumors associated with tuberous sclerosis. *Neurosurgery* 1979;4:410–417.
47. Boggild MD, Jenkinson S, Pistorello M, et al. Molecular genetic studies of sporadic pituitary tumors. *J Clin Endocrinol Metab* 1994;78:387–392.
48. Bonnin JM, Rubinstein LJ. Astroblastoma: A pathological study of 23 tumors, with a postoperative follow-up in 13 patients. *Neurosurgery* 1989;25:6–13.
49. Borit A, Blackwood W, Mair WG. The separation of pineocytoma from pineoblastoma. *Cancer* 1980;45:1408–1418.
50. Bruner JM, Langford LA, Fuller GN. Neuropathology, cell biology, and newer diagnostic methods. *Curr Opin Oncol* 1993;5:441–449.
51. Bryant BM, Wiltshaw E. Central nervous system involvement in sarcoma. *Eur J Cancer* 1980;16:1503–1507.
52. Brydon HL, Carey MP. Medulloblastoma metastasizing to a breast fibroadenoma: A case report. *Br J Neurosurg* 1991;5:73–75.
53. Burger PC, Fuller GN. Pathology – Trends and pitfalls in histologic diagnosis, immunopathology, and applications of oncogene research. *Neurol Clin* 1991;9:249–272.
54. Burger PC, Scheithauer BW, Vogel FS. *Surgical Pathology of the Nervous System and Its Coverings.* 3rd ed. New York: Churchill Livingstone; 1991.
55. Burger PC, Scheithauer BW. *Atlas of Tumor Pathology. Third Series, Fascicle 10. Tumors of the Central Nervous System.* Washington, DC: Armed Forces Institute of Pathology; 1994.
56. Burger PC, Vogel FS, Green SB, Strike TA. Glioblastoma multiforme and anaplastic astrocytoma. Pathologic criteria and prognostic implications. *Cancer* 1985;56:1106–1111.
57. Butti G, Assietti R, Casalone R, Paoletti P. Multiple meningiomas: A clinical, surgical and cytogenetic analysis. *Surg Neurol* 1989;31:255–260.
58. Caccamo DV, Herman MM, Rubinstein LJ. An immunohistochemical study of the primitive and maturing elements of human cerebral medulloepitheliomas. *Acta Neuropathol (Berl)* 1989;79:248–254.
59. Cai WY, Alexander JM, Hedley-White ET, et al. Ras mutations in human prolactinomas and pituitary carcinomas. *J Clin Endocrinol Metab* 1994;78:89–93.
60. Cairncross G, Macdonald D, Ludwin S, et al. Chemotherapy for anaplastic oligodendroglioma. *J Clin Oncol* 1994;2:2013–2021.
61. Cairncross JG, Macdonald DR, Ramsay DA. Aggressive oligodendroglioma: a chemosensitive tumor. *Neurosurgery* 1992;31:78–82.
62. Campbell AN, Chan HSL, Becker LE, Daneman A, Park TS, Hoffman HJ. Extracranial metastases in childhood primary intracranial tumors. A report of 21 cases and review of the literature. *Cancer* 1984;53:974–981.
63. Canning CR, McCartney AC, Hungerford J. Medulloepithelioma (diktyoma). *Br J Ophthalmol* 1988;72:764–767.
64. Caputy AJ, McCullough DC, Manz HJ, Patterson K, Hammock MK. A review of the factors influencing the prognosis of medulloblastoma. The importance of cell differentiation. *J Neurosurg* 1987;66:80–87.
65. Carney JA. Psammomatous melanotic schwannoma. A distinctive, heritable tumor with special associations, including cardiac myxoma and the Cushing syndrome. *Am J Surg Pathol* 1990;14:206–222.
66. Celli P, Scarpinati M, Nardacci B, Cervoni L, Cantore GP. Gangliogliomas of the cerebral hemispheres. Report of 14 cases with long-term follow-up and review of the literature. *Acta Neurochir (Wien)* 1993;125:52–57.
67. Chamberlain MC, Murovic JA, Levin VA. Absence of contrast enhancement on CT brain scans of patients with supratentorial malignant gliomas. *Neurology* 1988;38:1371–1374.
68. Chen TC, Maceri DR, Giannotta SL, Shih L, McComb JG. Unilateral acoustic neuromas in childhood without evidence of neurofibromatosis: case report and review of the literature. *Am J Otol* 1992;13:318–322.
69. Cheng TM, Coffey RJ, Gelber BR, Scheithauer BW. Simultaneous presentation of symptomatic subependymomas in siblings: case reports and review. *Neurosurgery* 1993;33:145–150.
70. Childhood Brain Tumor Consortium. A study of childhood brain tumors based on surgical biopsies from ten North American institutions: sample description. *J Neuro-oncol* 1988;6:9–23.
71. Chiu JK, Woo SY, Ater J, et al. Intracranial ependymoma in children: analysis of prognostic factors. *J Neuro-oncol* 1992;13:283–290.
72. Cho BK, Chi JG, Wang KC, Chang KH, Choi KS. Intracranial mesenchymal chondrosarcoma: a case report and literature review. *Childs Nerv Syst* 1993;9:295–299.
73. Chou SM, Anderson JS. Primary CNS malignant rhabdoid tumor (MRT): report of two cases and review of literature. *Clin Neuropathol* 1991;10:1–10.
74. Ciraldo AV, Platt MS, Agamanolis DP, Boeckman CR. Sacrococcygeal myxopapillary ependymomas and ependymal rests in infants and children. *J Pediatr Surg* 1986;21:49–52.
75. Coffin CM, Braun JT, Wick MR, Dehner LP. A clinicopathologic and immunohistochemical analysis of 53 cases of medulloblastoma with emphasis on synaptophysin expression. *Mod Pathol* 1990;3:164–170.
76. Coffin CM, Swanson PE, Wick MR, Dehner LP. Chordoma in childhood and adolescence. A clinicopathologic analysis of 12 cases. *Arch Pathol Lab Med* 1993;117:927–933.
77. Cogen PH, Daneshvar L, Metzger AK, Duyk G, Edwards MSB, Sheffield VC. Involvement of multiple chromosome 17p loci in medulloblastoma tumorigenesis. *Am J Hum Genet* 1992;50:584–589.
78. Cossu A, Massarelli G, Manetto V, et al. Rhabdoid tumours of the central nervous system. Report of three cases with immunocytochemical and ultrastructural findings. *Virchows Arch A Histopathol Anat* 1993;422:81–85.
79. Courville CB, Broussalian SL. Plastic ependymomas of the lateral recess. *J Neurosurg* 1961;18:792–799.
80. Crotty TB, Scheithauer BW, Young WF Jr. Papillary craniopharyngioma: a clinicopathological study of 48 cases. *J Neurosurg* 1995;83:206–214.
81. Cruz-Sanchez FF, Haustein J, Rossi ML, Cervos-Navarro J, Hughes JT. Ependymoblastoma: a histological, immunohistochemical and ultrastructural study of five cases. *Histopathology* 1988;12:17–27.
82. Daumas-Duport C. Dysembryoplastic neuroepithelial tumours. *Brain Pathol* 1993;3:283–295.
83. Daumas-Duport C, Scheithauer BW, Chodkiewicz J-P, Laws ER, Vedrenne C. Dysembryoplastic neuroepithelial tumor: a surgically curable tumor of young patients with intracrable partial seizures. *Neurosurgery* 1988;23:545 556.
84. Daumas-Duport C, Scheithauer B, O'Fallon J, et al. Grading of astrocytomas. A simple and reproducible method. *Cancer* 1988;62:2152–2165.

85. Davidson GS, Hope JK. Meningeal tumors in childhood. *Cancer* 1989;63:1205–1210.
86. Davis RL. Grading of gliomas. In: Fields WS, ed. *Primary Brain Tumors. A Review of Histologic Classification.* New York: Raven Press; 1989:150–158.
87. De Potter P, Shields CL, Shields JA. Clinical variations of trilateral retinoblastoma: a report of 13 cases. *J Pediatr Ophthalmol Strabismus* 1994;31:26–31.
88. Deck JH. Cerebral medulloepithelioma with maturation into ependymal cells and ganglion cells. *J Neuropathol Exp Neurol* 1969;28:442–454.
89. Deprez RHL, Bianchi AB, Groen NA, et al. Frequent NF2 gene transcript mutations in sporadic meningiomas and vestibular schwannomas. *Am J Hum Genet* 1994;54:1022–1029.
90. Deprez RHL, Riegman PH, Van Drunen E, et al. Cytogenetic, molecular genetic and pathological analysis in 126 meningiomas. *J Neuropathol Exp Neurol* 1995;54:224–235.
91. Dietlein M, Schroder R, Widemann B, Benz-Bohm G. Dysplastic gangliocytoma of cerebellum in a newborn. Diagnosis by ultrasonography and MRI. *Pediatr Radiol* 1992;22:131–133.
92. Domenicucci M, Santoro A, D'Osvaldo DH, Delfini R, Cantore GP, Guidetti B. Multiple intracranial meningiomas. *J Neurosurg* 1989;70:41–44.
93. Drews DT, Gravel RA, Collu R. Identification of G protein alpha subunit mutations in human growth hormone (GH)- and GH/prolactin-secreting pituitary tumors by single-strand conformation polymorphism (SSCP) analysis. *Mol Cell Endocrinol (Netherlands)* 1992;87:125–129.
94. Duffner PK, Burger PC, Cohen ME, et al. Desmoplastic infantile gangliogliomas: An approach to therapy. *Neurosurgery* 1994;34: 583–589.
95. Durity FA, Dolman CL, Moyers PD. Ganglioneuroblastoma of the cerebellum: Case report. *J Neurosurg* 1968;28:270–273.
96. Eng HL, Chuang JH, Lee TY, Chen WJ. Fetus in fetu: A case report and review of the literature. *J Pediatr Surg* 1989;24:296–299.
97. Enzinger FM, Weiss SW. *Soft Tissue Tumors.* 3rd ed. St Louis: Mosby; 1995:725–726.
98. Epstein FJ, Farmer J-P. Brain-stem glioma growth patterns. *J Neurosurg* 1993;78:408–412.
99. Faillace WJ, Okawara S-H, McDonald JV. Neurocutaneous melanosis with extensive intracerebral and spinal cord involvement. Report of two cases. *J Neurosurg* 1984;61:782–785.
100. Fearson JA, Munro IR, Bruce DA, Whitaker LA. Massive teratomas involving the cranial base: treatment and outcome—A two center report. *Plast Reconstr Surg* 1993;91:223–228.
101. Ferrante L, Acqui M, Artico M, Mastronardi L, Fortuna A. Paediatric intracranial meningiomas. *Br J Neurosurg* 1989;3:189–196.
102. Ferriera J, Eviatar L, Schneider S, Grossman R. Prenatal diagnosis of intracranial teratoma. Prolonged survival after resection of a malignant teratoma diagnosed prenatally by ultrasound: a case report and literature review. *Pediatr Neurosurg* 1993;19:84–88.
103. Figarella-Branger D, Gambarelli D, Perez-Castillo M, Gentet JC, Grisoli F, Pellissier JF. Ectopic intrapelvic medulloepithelioma: case report. *Neuropathol Appl Neurobiol* 1992;18:408–414.
104. Figarella-Branger D, Pellissier JF, Daumas-Duport C, et al. Central neurocytomas: critical evaluation of a small cell neuronal neoplasm. *Am J Surg Pathol* 1992;16:97–109.
105. Forsyth PA, Shaw EG, Scheithauer BW, et al. Supratentorial pilocytic astrocytomas. A clinicopathologic, prognostic, and flow cytometric study of 51 patients. *Cancer* 1993;72:1335–1342.
106. Fraioli B, Ferrante L, Celli P. Pituitary adenomas with onset during puberty. Features and treatment. *J Neurosurg* 1983;59:590–595.
107. Frederickson RG. The subdural space interpreted as a cellular layer of meninges. *Anat Rec* 1991;230:38–51.
108. Frim DM, Ogilvy CS, Vonsattal J-P, Chapman PH. Is intracerebral schwannoma a developomental tumor of children and young adults? Case report and review. *Pediatr Neurosurg* 1992;18:190–194.
109. Fujiwara T, Honjo Y, Nagao S, Honda C, Baba Y, Ohmoto T. Primary cerebellar yolk sac tumor: Case report. *Surg Neurol* 1994;42:121–124.
110. Fulham MJ, Melisi JW, Nishimiya J, Dwyer AJ, Di Chiro G. Neuroimaging of juvenile pilocytic astrocytomas: an enigma. *Radiology* 1993;189:221–225.
111. Fuller GN. Assessment of brain tumor proliferation potential. In: Wilkins RH and Rengachary SS, eds. *Neurosurgery.* 2nd ed. New York: McGraw-Hill; 1996.
112. Fuller GN, Bigner SH. Amplified cellular oncogenes in neoplasms of the human central nervous system. *Mutat Res* 1992;276:299–306.
113. Fuller GN, Burger PC. Nervus terminalis (cranial nerve zero) in the adult human. *Clin Neuropathol* 1990;9:279–283.
114. Fuller GN, Burger PC. Central nervous system. In: Sternberg SS, ed. *Histology for Pathologists.* 2nd ed. New York: Raven Press; 1996.
115. Fuller GN, Burger PC. Gliomas: pathology. In: Wilkins RH, Rengachary SS, eds. *Neurosurgery.* 2nd ed. New York: McGraw-Hill; 1995.
116. Fuller GN, Burger PC. Classification and biology of brain tumors. In: Youmans JR, ed. *Neurological Surgery.* 4th ed. Philadelphia: WB Saunders; 1996.
117. Fung K-M, Trojanowski JQ. Animal models of medulloblastomas and related primitive neuroectodermal tumors. A review. *J Neuropathol Exp Neurol* 1995;54:285–296.
118. Gajjar A, Bhargava R, Jenkins JJ, et al. Low-grade astrocytoma with neuraxis dissemination at diagnosis. *J Neurosurg* 1995;83: 67–71.
119. Garton GR, Schomberg PJ, Scheithauer BW, et al. Medulloblastoma—prognostic factors and outcome of treatment: review of the Mayo Clinic experience. *Mayo Clin Proc* 1990;65:1077–1086.
120. Ghim TT, Davis P, Seo JJ, Crocker I, O'Brien M, Krawiecki N. Response to neoadjuvant chemotherapy in children with pineoblastoma. *Cancer* 1993;72:1795–1800.
121. Ghim TT, Seo JJ, O'Brien M, Meacham L, Crocker I, Krawiecki N. Childhood intracranial meningiomas after high-dose irradiation. *Cancer* 1993;71:4091–4095.
122. Gilles FH, Sobel EL, Leviton A, et al. Histologic feature reliability in childhood neural tumors. *J Neuropathol Exp Neurol* 1994;53: 559–571.
123. Gilles FH. Classification of childhood brain tumors. *Cancer* 1985;56:1850–1857.
124. Glasser RS, Rojiani AM, Mickle JP, Eskin TA. Delayed occurrence of cerebellar pleomorphic xanthoastrocytoma after supratentorial pleomorphic xanthoastrocytoma removal. *J Neurosurg* 1995;82:116–118.
125. Glasuer FE, Yuan RHP. Intracranial tumors with extracranial metastases. Case report and review of the literature. *J Neurosurg* 1968;20:474–493.
126. Globus JH, Strauss I. Spongioblastoma multiforme: a primary malignant form of brain neoplasm. Its clinical and anatomic features. *Arch Neurol Psychiat* 1925;14:139–191.
127. Goldberg-Stern H, Gadoth N, Stern S, Cohen IJ, Zaizov R, Sandbank U. The prognostic significance of glial fibrillary acidic protein staining in medulloblastomas. *Cancer* 1991;68:568–573.
128. Graham PH, Gattamaneni HR, Birch JM. Paediatric craniopharyngiomas: A regional review. *Br J Neurosurg* 1992;6:187–193.
129. Graus F, Walker RW, Allen JC. Brain metastases in children. *J Pediatr* 1983;103:558–561.
130. Gupta RK, Pratap D. Metastasizing congenital subcutaneous sacrococcygeal ependymoma. *Ind J Cancer* 1992;29:76–81.
131. Gururangan S, Heideman RL, Kovner EH, Sanford RA, Kun LE. Peritoneal metastases in two patients with pineoblastoma and ventriculo-peritoneal shunts. *Med Pediatr Oncol* 1994;22:417–420.
132. Haddad SF, Moore SA, Schelper RL, Goecken JA. Vascular smooth muscle hyperplasia underlies the formation of glomeruloid vascular structures of glioblastoma multiforme. *J Neuropathol Exp Neurol* 1992;51:488–492.
133. Haddad SF, Van Gilder JC, Menezes AH. Pediatric pituitary tumors. *Neurosurgery* 1991;29:509–514.
134. Haines DE, Harkey HL, Al-Mefty O. The "subdural" space: A new look at an outdated concept. *Neurosurgery* 1993;32:111–120.

135. Haines DE. On the question of a subdural space. *Anat Rec* 1991;230:3–21.
136. Hanna SL, Langston JW, Parham DM, Douglass EC. Primary malignant rhabdoid tumor of the brain: clinical, imaging, and pathologic findings. *Am J Neuroradiol* 1993;14:107–115.
137. Harada K, Inagawa T, Nagasako R. A case of meningioangiomatosis without von Recklinghausen's disease. Report of a case and review of 13 cases. *Childs Nerv Syst* 1994;10:126–130.
138. Harada T, Kawauchi M, Watanabe M, Kyoshima K, Kobayashi S. Subfrontal schwannoma. Case report. *Neurol Med Chir (Tokyo)* 1992;32:957–960.
139. Harrison MJ, Wolfe DE, Lau T-S, Mitnick RJ, Sachdev VP. Radiation-induced meningiomas: experience at the Mount Sinai Hospital and review of the literature. *J Neurosurg* 1991;75:564–574.
140. Hart MN, Petito CK, Earle KM. Mixed gliomas. *Cancer* 1974;33:134–140.
141. Hartsell WF, Montag AG, Lydon J, Galinsky DL, Sarin P. Treatment of medulloblastoma in adults. *Am J Clin Oncol* 1992;15:207–211.
142. Hassoun J, Gambarelli D, Grisoli F, et al. Central neurocytoma. An electron-microscopic study of two cases. *Acta Neuropathol* 1982;56:151–156.
143. Hassoun J, Soylemezoglu F, Gambarelli D, Figarella-Branger D, von Ammon K, Kleihues P. Central neurocytoma: a synopsis of clinical and histological features. *Brain Pathol* 1993;3:297–306.
144. Hayosteck CJ, Shaw EG, Scheithauer B, et al. Astrocytomas of the cerebellum: a comparative clinicopathologic study of pilocytic and diffuse astrocytomas. *Cancer* 1993;73:856–868.
145. Hazuka MB, De Boise DA, Henderson RH, Kinzie JJ. Survival results in adult patients treated for medulloblastoma. *Cancer* 1992;69:2143–2148.
146. Heidelberger KP, Ritchey ML, Dauser RC, McKeever PE, Beckwith JB. Congenital mesoblastic nephroma metastatic to the brain. *Cancer* 1993;72:2499–2502.
147. Heifetz SA, Alrabeeah A, Brown BS, Lau H. Fetus in fetu: a fetiform teratoma. *Pediatr Pathol* 1988;8:215–226.
148. Helwig EB, Stern JB. Subcutaneous sacrococcygeal myxopapillary ependymoma. A clinicopathologic study of 32 cases. *Am J Clin Pathol* 1984;81:156–161.
149. Henn W, Wullich B, Thonnes M, Steudel WI, Feiden W, Zang KD. Recurrent t(12;19) (q13;q13.3) in intracranial and extracranial hemangiopericytoma. *Cancer Genet Cytogenet* 1993;71:151–154.
150. Herath SE, Stalboerger PG, Dahl RJ, Parisi JE, Jenkins RB. Cytogenetic studies of four hemangiopericytomas. *Cancer Genet Cytogenet* 1994;72:137–140.
151. Herman V, Drazin NZ, Gonsky, Melmed S. Molecular screening of pituitary adenomas for gene mutations and rearrangements. *J Clin Endocrinol Metab* 1993;77:50–55.
152. Herpers MJHM, Budka H. Glial fibrillary acidic protein (GFAP) in oligodendroglial tumors: gliofibrillary oligodendroglioma and transitional oligoastrocytoma as subtypes of oligodendroglioma. *Acta Neuropathol* 1984;64:265–272.
153. Herrick MK, Rubinstein LJ. The cytological differentiating potential of pineal parenchymal neoplasms (true pineolomas): a clinicopathological study of 28 tumours. *Brain* 1979;102:289–320.
154. Herzog CE, Leeds NE, Bruner JM, Baumgartner JE. Intracranial hemangiopericytomas in children. *Pediatr Neurosurg* 1995;22:274–279.
155. Hing A, Cortville J, Foglia RP, Bliss DP Jr, Donis-Keller H, Dowton SB. Fetus in fetu: molecular analysis of a fetiform mass. *Am J Med Genet* 1993;47:333–341.
156. Hirose T, Scheithauer BW, Lopes BS, VandenBerg SR. Dysembryoplastic neuroepithelial tumor (DNT): An immunohistochemical and ultrastructural study. *J Neuropathol Exp Neurol* 1994;53:184–195.
157. Hitotsumatsu T, Iwaki T, Fukui M, Tateishi J. Cytoplasmic inclusions of astrocytic elements of glial tumors: special reference to round granulated body and eosinophilic hyaline droplets. *Acta Neuropathol* 1994;88:501–510.
158. Ho DM, Liu HC. Primary intracranial germ cell tumor. Pathologic study of 51 patients. *Cancer* 1992;70:1577–1584.
159. Hoffman HJ, Duffner PK. Extraneural metastases of central nervous system tumors. *Cancer* 1985;56:1778–1782.
160. Honan WP, Anderson M, Carey MP, Williams B. Familial subependymomas. *Br J Neurosurg* 1987;1:317–321.
161. Hope JK, Armstrong DA, Babyn PS, et al. Primary meningeal tumors in children: correlation of clinical and CT findings with histologic type and prognosis. *Am J Neuroradiol* 1992;13:1353–1364.
162. Hopwood NJ, Kenny FM. Incidence of Nelson's syndrome after adrenalectomy for Cushing's disease in children: results of a nationwide survey. *Am J Dis Child* 1977;131:1353–1356.
163. Horvath E. Ultrastructural markers in the pathologic diagnosis of pituitary adenomas. *Ultrastruct Pathol* 1994;18:171–179.
164. Hubbard JL, Scheithauer BW, Kispert DB, Carpenter SM, Wick MR, Laws ER. Adult cerebellar medulloblastomas: the pathological, radiologic, and clinical disease spectrum. *J Neurosurg* 1989;70:536–544.
165. Hung CF, Lam MS. Intracranial fetus in fetu: report of a case. *J Formos Med Assoc* 1993;92:920–922.
166. Husain AN, Leestma JE. Cerebral astroblastoma: immunohistochemical and ultrastructural features. Case report. *J Neurosurg* 1986;64:657–661.
167. Husain M, Mishra UK, Newton G, Husain N. Isolated olfactory groove neurilemmoma. *Surg Neurol* 1992;37:115–117.
168. Ito S, Hoshino T, Prados MD, Edwards MS. Cell kinetics of medulloblastomas. *Cancer* 1992;70:671–678.
169. Iyer RS, Soman CS, Nair CN, et al. Brain tumors following cure of acute lymphoblastic leukemia. *Leuk Lymphoma* 1994;13:183–186.
170. Jakate SN, Marsden HB, Ingram L. Primary rhabdoid tumor of the brain. *Virchows Arch A Histopathol Anat* 1988;412:393–397.
171. Jansen GH, Troost D, Dingemans KP. Polar spongioblastoma: an immunohistochemical and electron microscopical study. *Acta Neuropathol* 1990;81:228–232.
172. Jay V, Edwards V, Squire J, Rutka J. Astroblastoma: report of a case with ultrastructural, cell kinetic, and cytogenetic analysis. *Pediatr Pathol* 1993;13:323–332.
173. Jay V, Pienkowska M, Becker L, Zielenska M. Primitive neuroectodermal tumors of the cerebrum and cerebellum: absence of t(11;22) translocation by RT-PCR analysis. *Modern Pathol* 1995;8:488–491.
174. Jay V, Squire J, Becker LE, Humphreys R. Malignant transformation in a ganglioglioma with anaplastic neuronal and astrocytic components. Report of a case with flow cytometric and cytogenetic analysis. *Cancer* 1994;73:2862–2868.
175. Jellinger K. Cerebral medulloepithelioma. *Acta Neuropathol (Berl)* 1972;22:95–101.
176. Jellinger K, Paulus W. Mesenchymal, non-meningothelial tumors of the central nervous system. *Brain Pathol* 1991;1:79–87.
177. Jenkin D, Greenberg M, Hoffman H, Hendrick B, Humphreys R, Vatter A. Brain tumors in children: long-term survival after radiation treatment. *Int J Radiat Oncol Biol Phys* 1995;31:445–451.
178. Johannsson JH, Retake HL, Roessmann U. Gangliogliomas: pathological and clinical correlation. *J Neurosurg* 1981;54:58–63.
179. Joseph JT, Lisle DK, Jacoby LB, et al. NF2 gene analysis distinguishes hemangiopericytoma from meningioma. *Am J Pathol* 1995 (in press).
180. Kadonaga JN, Barkovich AJ, Edwards MS, Frieden IJ. Neurocutaneous melanosis in association with the Dandy–Walker complex. *Pediatr Dermatol* 1992;9:37–43.
181. Kadonaga JN, Frieden IJ. Neurocutaneous melanosis: definition and review of the literature. *J Am Acad Dermatol* 1991;24:747–755.
182. Kane LA, Leinung MC, Scheithauer BW, et al. Pituitary adenomas in childhood and adolescence. *J Clin Endocrinol Metab* 1994;79:1135–1140.
183. Kang YK, Suh YL, Kim CW, Chi JG. Fetus in fetu: a case with complete umbilical cord and fetal sac. *Pediatr Pathol* 1994;14:411–419.
184. Kanno H, Kondo K, Ito S, et al. Somatic mutations of the von Hippel–Lindau tumor suppressor gene in sporadic central ner-

vous system hemangioblastomas. *Cancer Res* 1994;54:4845–4847.
185. Kanter SL, Mickle JP, Hunter SB, Rhoton AL. Pituitary adenomas in pediatric patients: Are they more invasive? *Pediatr Neurosci* 1986;12:202–204.
186. Kapadia SB, Frisman DM, Hitchcock CL, Popek EJ. Melanotic neuroectodermal tumors of infancy. Clinicopathological, immunohistochemical, and flow cytometric study. *Am J Surg Pathol* 1993;17:566–573.
187. Kaplan AM, Itabashi HH, Hanelin LG, Lu AT. Neurocutaneous melanosis with malignant leptomeningeal melanoma. A case with metastases outside the nervous system. *Arch Neurol* 1975;32:669–671.
188. Karch SB, Urich H. Medulloepithelioma: definition of an entity. *J Neuropathol Exp Neurol* 1972;31:27–53.
189. Karga HJ, Alexander JM, Hedley-White ET, Klibanski A, Jameson JL. Ras mutations in human pituitary tumors. *J Clin Endocrinol Metab* 1992;74:914–919.
190. Kauffman SL, Stout AP. Hemangiopericytoma in children. *Cancer* 1981;47:906–914.
191. Kepes JJ, Rubinstein LJ, Ansbacher L, Schreiber DJ. Histopathological features of recurrent pleomorphic xanthoastrocytomas: further corroboration of the glial nature of this neoplasm. A study of 3 cases. *Acta Neuropathol* 1989;78:585–593.
192. Kepes JJ, Rubinstein LJ, Eng LF: Pleomorphic xanthoastrocytoma: a distinctive meningocerebral glioma of young subjects with relatively favorable prognosis. A study of 12 cases. *Cancer* 1979;44:1839–1852.
193. Kepes JJ. Pleomorphic xanthoastrocytoma: the birth of a diagnosis and a concept. *Brain Pathol* 1993;3:269–274.
194. Kernohan JW, Maybon RF, Svien HJ, Adson AW. A simplified classification of the gliomas. *Proc Staff Meet Mayo Clin* 1949;24:71–75.
195. Khajavi K, Comair YG, Prayson RA, et al. Childhood gangliogliomas and medically intractable epilepsy. A clinicopathological study of 15 patients and a review of the literature. *Pediatr Neurosurg* 1995;22:181–188.
196. Khatib ZA, Heideman RL, Kovnar EH, et al. Predominance of pilocytic histology in dorsally exophytic brain stem tumors. *Pediatr Neurosurg* 1994;20:2–10.
197. Kimmel DL, Moyer EK, Peale AR, Winborne LW, Gotwals JE. A cerebral tumor containing five human fetuses. *Anat Rec* 1950;106:141–165.
198. Kirk IR, Dominguez R, Castillo M. Congenital primary cerebral angiosarcoma: CT, US, and MR findings. *Pediatr Radiol* 1992;22:134–135.
199. Kleihues P, Burger PC, Scheithauer BW. *Histological Typing of Tumours of the Central Nervous System*. 2nd ed. Berlin: Springer-Verlag; 1993.
200. Kleinman GM, Hochberg FH, Richardson EP Jr. Systemic metastases from medulloblastoma: report of two cases and review of the literature. *Cancer* 1981;48:2296–2309.
201. Knowles CHR, Huggill PH. Liposarcoma: with report of a case in a child. *J Pathol* 1954;68:235–245.
202. Ko SF, Wang HS, Lui TN, Ng SH, Ho YS, Tsai CC. Neurocutaneous melanosis associated with inferior vermian hypoplasia: MR findings. *J Comput Assist Tomogr* 1993;17:691–695.
203. Kollias SS, Crone KR, Ball WS Jr, Prenger EC, Ballard ET. Meningiomatosis of the brain stem. Case report. *J Neurosurg* 1994;80:732–735.
204. Kondziolka D, Lunsford D, Martinez AJ. Unreliability of contemporary neurodiagnostic imaging in evaluating suspected adult supratentorial (low-grade) astrocytoma. *J Neurosurg* 1993;79:533–536.
205. Korinthenberg R, Edel G, Palm DMuller KM, Brandt M, Muller RP. Primary rhabdomyosarcoma of the leptomeninx.Clinical, neuroradiological and pathological aspects. *Clin Neurol Neurosurg* 1984;86:301–305.
206. Kovalic JJ, Flaris N, Grigsby PW, Pirkowski M, Simpson JR, Roth KA. Intracranial ependymoma long term outcome, patterns of failure. *J Neuro-oncol* 1993;15:125–131.
207. Kraichoke S, Cosgrove M, Chandrasoma PT. Granulomatous inflammation in pineal germinoma: A cause of diagnostic failure at stereotaxic brain biopsy. *Am J Surg Pathol* 1988;12:655–660.
208. Kramer ED, Lewis D, Raney B, Womer R, Packer RJ. Neurologic complications in children with soft tissue and osseous sarcoma. *Cancer* 1989;64:2600–2603.
209. Kraus JA, Koopman J, Kaskel P, et al. Shared allelic losses on chromosome 1p and 19q suggest a common origin of oligodendroglioma and oligoastrocytoma. *J Neuropathol Exp Neurol* 1995;54:91–95.
210. Kreuger A, Garwicz S, Hertz H, et al. Central nervous system disease in childhood acute lymphoblastic leukemia: Prognostic factors and results of treatment. *Pediatr Hematol Oncol* 1991;8:291–299.
211. Kros JM, De Jong AAW, Van Der Kwast Th H. Ultrastructural characterization of transitional cells in oligodendrogliomas. *J Neuropathol Exp Neurol* 1992;51:186–193.
212. Kros JM, Van Eden CG, Stefanko SZ, Waayer-Van Batenburg M, Van Der Kwast Th H. Prognostic implications of glial fibrillary acidic protein containing cell types in oligodendrogliomas. *Cancer* 1990;66:1204–1212.
213. Krouwer HG, Davis RL, McDermott MW, Hoshino T, Prados MD. Gangliogliomas: a clinicopathological study of 25 cases and review of the literature. *J Neuro-oncol* 1993;17:139–154.
214. Krouwer HGJ, Davis RL, Silver P, Prados M. Gemistocytic astrocytomas: a reappraisal. *J Neurosurg* 1991;74:399–406.
215. Kun LE, Kovnar EH, Sanford RA. Ependymomas in children. *Pediatr Neurosci* 1988;14:57–63.
216. Kuratsu J, Seto H, Kochi M, Itoyama Y, Uemura S, Ushio Y. Metastatic angiosarcoma of the brain. *Surg Neurol* 1991;35:305–309.
217. Lach B, Russell N, Benoit B, Atack D. Cellular blue nevus ("melanocytoma") of the spinal meninges: electron microscopic and immunohistochemical features. *Neurosurgery* 1988;22:773–780.
218. Lana-Peixoto MA, Lagos J, Silbert SW. Primary pigmented carcinoma of the choroid plexus: a light and electron microscopic study. *J Neurosurg* 1977;47:442–450.
219. Lang FF, Epstein FJ, Ransohoff J, et al. Central nervous system gangliogliomas. 2. Clinical outcome. *J Neurosurg* 1993;79:867–873.
220. Langford LA. The ultrastructure of the ependymoblastoma. *Acta Neuropathol* 1986;71:136–141.
221. Langford LA, Camel MH. Palisading pattern in cerebral neuroblastoma mimicking the primitive polar spongioblastoma. An ultrastructural study. *Acta Neuropathol* 1987;73:153–159.
222. Lefkowitz IB, Rorke LB, Packer RJ, Sutton LN, Siegel KR, Katnick RJ. Atypical teratoid tumor of infancy: definition of an entity. *Ann Neurol* 1987;22:448–449 (Abstract).
223. Leunda G, Vaquero J, Cabezudo J, Garcia-Uria J, Bravo G. Schwannoma of the oculomotor nerves. Report of four cases. *J Neurosurg* 1982;57:563–565.
224. Limas C, Tio FO. Meningeal melanocytoma ("melanotic meningioma"). Its melanocytic origin revealed by electron microscopy. *Cancer* 1972;30:1286–1294.
225. Listernick R, Charrow J, Greenwald M, Mets M. Natural history of optic pathway tumors in children with neurofibromatosis type 1: a longitudinal study. *J Pediatr* 1994;125:63–66.
226. Litofsky NS, Hinton D, Raffel C. The lack of a role for p53 in astrocytomas in pediatric patients. *Neurosurgery* 1994;34:967–972.
227. Longee DC, Friedman HS, Phillips PC, et al. Osteoblastic metastases from astrocytomas: a report of two cases. *Med Pediatr Oncol* 1991;19:318–324.
228. Louis DN, Ramesh V, Gusella JF. Neuropathology and molecular genetics of neurofibromatosis 2 and related tumors. *Brain Pathol* 1995;5:163–172.
229. Louis DN, Rubio M-P, Correa KM, Gusella JF, von Deimling A. Molecular genetics of pediatric brain stem gliomas. Application of PCR techniques to small and archival brain tumor specimens. *J Neuropathol Exp Neurol* 1993;52:507–515.
230. Louis DN, von Deimling A. Hereditary tumor syndromes of the nervous system: overview and rare syndromes. *Brain Pathol* 1995;5:145–151.
231. Louis DN, von Deimling A, Dickersin GR, Dooling EC, Seizinger BR. Desmoplastic cerebral astrocytomas of infancy: a histopathologic, immunohistochemical, ultrastructural, and molecular genetic study. *Hum Pathol* 1992;23:1402–1409.

232. Lund AM, Skovby F. Optic gliomas in children with neurofibromatosis type 1. *Eur J Pediatr* 1991;150:835–838.
233. Lyons J, Landis CA, Harsh G, et al. Two G protein oncogenes in human endocrine tumors. *Science* 1990;249:655–659.
234. Macfarlane A, Macgregor AR, Malignant non-chromaffin paraganglioma of the thigh. *Arch Dis Child* 1958;33:55–57.
235. Maira G, Anile C. Pituitary adenomas in childhood and adolescence. *Can J Neurol Sci* 1990;17:83–87.
236. Maleci A, Cervoni L, Delfini R. Medulloblastoma in children and in adults: a comparative study. *Acta Neurochir (Wein)* 1992;119:62–67.
237. Mamalis N, Font RL, Anderson CW, Monson MC, Williams AT. Concurrent benign teratoid medulloepithelioma and pineoblastoma. *Ophthalmic Surg* 1992;23:403–408.
238. Mandahl N, Orndal C, Heim S, et al. Aberrations of chromosome segment 12q13-15 characterize a subgroup of hemangiopericytomas. *Cancer* 1993;71:3009–3013.
239. Manhoff DT, Rorke LB, Yachnis AT. Primary intracranial atypical teratoid/rhabdoid tumor in a child with Canavan disease. *Pediatr Neurosurg* 1995;22:214–222.
240. Maraziotis T, Perentes E, Karamitopoulou E, et al. Neuron-associated class III beta-tubulin isotype, retinal S-antigen, synaptophysin, and glial fibrillary acidic protein in human medulloblastomas: a clinicopathological analysis of 36 cases. *Acta Neuropathol (Berl)* 1992;84:355–363.
241. Marina NM, Pratt CB, Shema SJ, Brooks T, Rao B, Meyer WH. Brain metastases in osteosarcoma. Report of a long-term survivor and review of the St. Jude Children's Research Hospital Experience. *Cancer* 1993;71:3656–3660.
242. Martin-Reay DG, Shattuck, Guthrie FW Jr. Psammomatous melanotic schwannoma: an additional component of Carney's complex. *Am J Clin Pathol* 1991;95:484–489.
243. Matsui I, Tanimura M, Kobayashi N, Sawada T, Nagahara N, Akatsuka J. Neurofibromatosis type 1 and childhood cancer. *Cancer* 1993;72:2746–2754.
244. Mautner VF, Tatagiba M, Guthoff R,Samii M, Pulst SM. Neurofibromatosis 2 in the pediatric age group. *Neurosurgery* 1993;33:92–96.
245. McClosky JJ, Parker JC Jr, Brooks WH, Blacker HM. Melanin as a component of cerebral gliomas: the melanotic cerebral glioma. *Cancer* 1976;37:2373–2379.
246. McDowell JR. Familial meningioma. *Neurology* 1990;40:312–314.
247. McLendon RE, Burger PC. The primitive neuroectodermal tumor: a cautionary view. *J Pediatr Neurosci* 1987;3:1–8.
248. Mérel P, Hoang-Xuan K, Sanson M, et al. Predominant occurrence of somatic mutations of the NF2 gene in meningiomas and schwannomas. *Genes Chromosom Cancer* 1995;13:211–216.
249. Miller DC, Lang FF, Epstein FJ. Central nervous system gangliogliomas. 1. Pathology. *J Neurosurg* 1993;79:859–866.
250. Mori K, Kurisaka M. Brain tumors in childhood: Statistical analysis of cases from the Brain Tumor Registry of Japan. *Childs Nerv System* 1986;2:233–237.
251. Mørk SJ, Rubinstein LJ. Ependymoblastoma. A reappraisal of a rare embryonal tumor. *Cancer* 1985;55:1536–1542.
252. Mørk SJ, Rubinstein LJ, Kepes JJ. Patterns of epithelial metaplasia in malignant gliomas. I. Papillary formations mimicking medulloepithelioma. *J Neuropathol Exp Neurol* 1988;47:93–100.
253. Mukherjee J, Das S, Das S, Mustafi M, Adhikari SS. Intracranial foetus in fetu. *J Ind Med Assc* 1992;90:130–131.
254. Muller M, Hubbard SL, Provias J, Greenberg M, Becker LE, Rutka JT. Malignant rhabdoid tumour of the pineal region. *Can J Neurol Sci* 1994;21:273–277.
255. Mulvihill JJ, Parry DM, Sherman JL, Pikus A, Kaiser-Kupfer MI, Eldridge R. Neurifibromatosis 1 (Recklinghausen disease) and neurofibromatosis 2 (bilateral acoustic neurofibromatosis). An update. *Ann Intern Med* 1990;113:39–52.
256. Nakamura Y, Becker LE. Meningeal tumors of infancy and childhood. *Pediatr Pathol* 1985;3:341–358.
257. Nakamura Y, Becker LE, Mancer K, Gillespie R. Peripheral medulloepithelioma. *Acta Neuropathol* 1982;57:137–142.
258. Nanda A, Schut L, Sutton LN. Congenital forms of intracranial teratoma. *Childs Nerv Syst* 1991;7:112–114.
259. Nelson JS, Tsukada Y, Schoenfeld D., Fulling K, Lamarche J, Peress N. Necrosis as a prognostic criterion in malignant supratentorial, astrocytic gliomas. *Cancer* 1983;52:550–554.
260. Nevin S. Gliomatosis cerebri. *Brain* 1938;61:170–191.
261. Ng HK, Tang NL, Poon WS. Polar spongioblastoma with cerebrospinal fluid metastases. *Surg Neurol* 1994;41:137–142.
262. Niida H, Tanaka R, Tamura T, Takeuchi S. Clival chordoma in early childhood without bone involvement. *Childs Nerv Syst* 1994;10:533–535.
263. Nijssen PC, Deprez RH, Tijssen CC, et al. Familial anaplastic ependymoma: Evidence of loss of chromosome 22 in tumor cells. *J Neurol Neurosurg Psychiatry* 1994;57:1245–1248.
264. O'Brien JM, Marcus DM, Bernards R, et al. A transgenic mouse model for trilateral retinoblastoma. *Arch Ophthalmol* 1990;108:1145–1151.
265. O'Brien JM, Marcus DM, Niffenegger AS, et al. Trilateral retinoblastoma in transgenic mice. *Trans Am Ophthalmol Soc* 1990;87:301–322.
266. Odell JM, Allen JK, Badura RJ, Weinberger E. Massive congenital intracranial teratoma: a report of two cases. *Pediatr Pathol* 1987;7:333–340.
267. Ohgaki H, Eibl RH, Wiestler OD, Yasargil MG, Newcomb EW, Kleihues P. p53 mutations in nonastrocytic human brain tumors. *Cancer Res* 1991;51:6202–6205.
268. Oi S, Tamaki N, Kondo T, et al. Massive congenital intracranial teratoma diagnosed in utero. *Childs Nerv Syst* 1990;6:459–461.
269. Ojeda VJ, Spagnolo DV, Vaughan RJ. Palisades in primary cerebral neuroblastoma simulating so-called polar spongioblastoma. A light and electron microscopical study of an adult case. *Am J Surg Pathol* 1987;11:316–322.
270. Oppenheim JS, Strauss RC, Mormino J, Sachdev VP, Rothman AS. Ependymomas of the third ventricle. *Neurosurgery* 1994;34:350–353.
271. Orlin JR, Osen KK, Hovig T. Subdural compartment in pig: A morphologic study with blood and horseradish peroxidase infused subdurally. *Anat Rec* 1991;230:22–37.
272. Otsubo H, Hoffman HJ, Humphreys RP, et al. Detection and management of gangliogliomas in children. *Surg Neurol* 1992;38:371–378.
273. Ouimet A, Russo P. Fetus in fetu or not? (letter) *J Pediatr Surg* 1989;24:926–927.
274. Ownby P, Lyon G, Spock A. Primary leiomyosarcoma of the lung in childhood. *Am J Dis Child* 1976;130:1132–1133.
275. Packer RJ, Sutton LN, Elterman R, et al. Outcome for children with medulloblastoma treated with radiation and cisplatin, CCNU, and vincristine chemotherapy. *J Neurosurg* 1994;81:690–698.
276. Packer RJ, Sutton LN, Rorke LB, et al. Intracranial embryonal cell carcinoma. *Cancer* 1984;54:520–524.
277. Packer RJ, Sutton LN, Rorke LB, et al. Prognostic importance of cellular differentiation in medulloblastoma of childhood. *J Neurosurg* 1984;61:296–301.
278. Painter MJ, Pang D, Ahdab-Barmada M, Bergman I. Connatal brain tumors in patients with tuberous sclerosis. *Neurosurgery* 1984;14:570–573.
279. Palaoglu S, Akbay A, Mocan G, et al. Ossified adamantinomatous type craniopharyngiomas. A series of 13 patients. *Acta Neurochir (Wein)* 1994;127:166–169.
280. Pallesen G, Hamilton-Dutoit SJ. Ki-1 (CD30) antigen is regularly expressed by tumor cells of embryonal carcinoma. *Am J Pathol* 1988;133:446–450.
281. Palma L, Celli P, Cantore G. Supratentorial ependymomas of the first two decades of life. Long-term follow-up of 20 cases (including two subependymomas). *Neurosurgery* 1993;32:169–175.
282. Papi L, De Vitis LR, Vitelli F, et al. Somatic mutations in the neurofibromatosis type 2 gene in sporadic meningiomas. *Hum Genet* 1995;95:347–351.
283. Parham DM, Weeks DA, Beckwith JB. The clinicopathologic spectrum of putative extrarenal rhabdoid tumors. An analysis of 42 cases studied with immunohistochemistry or electron microscopy. *Am J Surg Pathol* 1994;18:1010–1029.
284. Parisi JE, Scheithauer BW. Pituitary tumors. In: Nelson JS, Parisi JE, Schochet SS Jr., eds. *Principles and Practice of Neuropathology*. St. Louis: Mosby; 1993:267–295.
285. Partington MD, Davis DH, Laws ER Jr, Scheithauer BW. Pitu-

itary adenomas in childhood and adolescence. Results of transphenoidal surgery. *J Neurosurg* 1994;80:209–216.
286. Pastores GM, Michels VV, Jack CR Jr. Early childhood diagnosis of acoustic neuromas in presymptomatic individuals at risk for neurofibromatosis 2. *Am J Med Genet* 1991;41:325–329.
287. Pasquier B, Pasquier D, N'Golet A, Panh MH, Couderc P. Extraneural metastases of astrocytomas and glioblastomas. Clinicopathological study of two cases and review of the literature. *Cancer* 1980;45:112–125.
288. Paulus W, Scholte W, Perentes E, Jacobi G, Warmuth-Metz M, Roggendorf W. Desmoplastic supratentorial neuroepithelial tumours of infancy. *Histopathology* 1992;21:43–49.
289. Paulus W, Slowik F, Jellinger K. Primary intracranial sarcomas: histopathological features of 19 cases. *Histopathology* 1991;18: 395–402.
290. Peace RJ. A congenital neoplasm of the brain of a newborn infant. *Am J Clin Pathol* 1954;24:1272–1275.
291. Pedersen H, McConnell J, Harwood-Nash DC, Fitz CR, Chuang SH. Computed tomography in intracranial, supratentorial metastases in children. *Neuroradiology* 1989;31:19–23.
292. Pei L, Melmed S, Scheithauer B, Kovacs K, Prager D. H-ras mutations in human pituitary carcinoma metastases. *J Clin Endocrinol Metab* 1994;78:842–846.
293. Perez-Atayde AR, Kozakewich HW, McGill T, Fletcher JA. Hemangiopericytoma of the tongue in a 12-year -old child: ultrastructural and cytogenetic observations. *Hum Pathol* 1994;25: 425-429.
294. Perilongo G, Sutton LN, Goldwein JW, et al. Childhood meningiomas. Experience in the modern imaging era. *Pediatr Neurosurg* 1992;18:16–23.
295. Peterson K, Walker RW. Medulloblastoma/primitive neuroectodermal tumor in 45 adults. *Neurology* 1995;45:440–442.
296. Pierre-Kahn A, Hirsch JF, Vinchon M, et al. Surgical management of brain-stem tumors in children: Results and statistical analysis of 75 cases. *J Neurosurg* 1993;78:845–852.
297. Pimentel J, Tavora L, Cristina ML, Antunes JAFL. Intraventricular schwannoma. *Childs Nerv Syst* 1988;4:373–375.
298. Pollack IF. Brain tumors in children. *N Engl J Med* 1994;331: 1500–1507.
299. Pollack IF, Claassen D, Al-Shboul Q, Janosky JE, Deutsch M. Low-grade gliomas of the cerebral hemispheres in children: an analysis of 71 cases. *J Neurosurg* 1995;82:536–547.
300. Pollack IF, Hoffman HJ, Humphreys RP, Becker LE. The long term outcome after surgical treatment of dorsally exophytic brain-stem gliomas. *J Neurosurg* 1993;78:859–863.
301. Pollack IF, Hurtt M, Pang D, Albright AL. Dissemination of low grade intracranial astrocytomas in children. *Cancer* 1994;73: 2869–2878.
302. Poulsgård L, REDnne M, Schmidek HH. The cytogenetic and molecular genetic analysis of meningiomas. In: Levine AJ, Schmidek HH, eds. *Molecular Genetics of Nervous System Tumors*. New York: Wiley-Liss; 1993:249–254.
303. Prabhu SS, Lynch PG, Keogh AJ, Parekh HC. Intracranial meningeal melanocytoma: a report of two cases and a review of the literature. *Surg Neurol* 1993;40:516–521.
304. Preissig SH, Smith MT, Huntington HW. Rhabdomyosarcoma arising in a pineal teratoma. *Cancer* 1979;44:281–284.
305. Probst EN, Zanella FE, Vortmeyer AO. Congenital clivus chordoma. *Am J Neuroradiol* 1993;14:537–539.
306. Pulitzer DR, Martin PC, Collins PC, Ralph DR. Subcutaneous sacrococcygeal ("myxopapillary") ependymal rests. *Am J Surg Pathol* 1988;12:672–677.
307. Pulst SM, Rouleau GA, Marineau C, Fain P, Sieb JP. Familial meningioma is not allelic to neurofibromatosis 2. *Neurology* 1993;43:2096–2098.
308. Punnett HH, Tomczak EZ, de Chadarevian JP, Kanev PM. Cytogenetic analysis of a choroid plexus papilloma. *Genes Chrom Cancer* 1994;10:282–285.
309. Raffel C, Thomas GA, Tishler DM, Lassoff S, Allen JC. Absence of p53 mutations in childhood central nervous system primitive neuroectodermal tumors. *Neurosurgery* 1993;33:301–306.
310. Rainho CA, Rogatto SR, de Moraes LC, Barbieri-Neto J. Cytogenetic study of a pineocytoma. *Cancer Genet Cytogenet* 1992;64: 127–132.
311. Ransom DT, Ritland SR, Kimmel DW, et al. Cytogenetic and loss of heterozygosity studies in ependymomas, pilocytic astrocytomas, and oligodendrogliomas. *Genes Chrom Cancer* 1992;5: 348–356.
312. Raymond AA, Halpin SFS, Alsanjari N, et al. Dysembryoplastic neuroepithelial tumor. Features in 16 patients. *Brain* 1994;117: 461–475.
313. Rea GL, Akerson RD, Rockswold GL, Smith SA. Subependymoma in a 2 1/2-year old boy. Case report. *J Neurosurg* 1983;59: 1088–1091.
314. Regine WF, Kramer S. Pediatric craniopharyngiomas: long term results of combined treatment with surgery and radiation. *Int J Radiat Oncol Biol Phys* 1992;24:611–617.
315. Reifenberger J, Reifenberger G, Liu L, James CD, Wechsler W, Collins VP. Molecular genetic analysis of oligodendroglial tumors shows preferential allelic deletions on 19q and 1p. *Am J Pathol (United States)* 1994;145:1175–1190.
316. Richmond IL, Wilson CB. Pituitary adenomas in childhood and adolescence. *J Neurosurg* 1978;49:163–168.
317. Ringertz N. Grading of gliomas. *Acta Pathol Microbiol Scand* 1950;27:51–64.
318. Roberts RO, Lynch CF, Jones MP, et al. Medulloblastoma: a population-based study of 532 cases. *J Neuropathol Exp Neurol* 1991;134–144.
319. Robertson PL, Muraszko KM, Brunberg JA, Axtell RA, Dauser RC, Turrisi AT. Pediatric midbrain tumors: a benign subgroup of brainstem gliomas. *Pediatr Neurosurg* 1995;22:65–73.
320. Rogatto SR, Casartelli C, Rainho CA, Barbieri-Neto J. Chromosomes in the genesis and progression of ependymomas. *Cancer Genet Cytogenet* 1993;69:146–152.
321. Ron E, Modan B, Boice JD, et al. Tumors of the brain and nervous system after radiotherapy in childhood. *N Engl J Med* 1988;319:1033–1039.
322. Rorke LB, Gilles FH, Davis RL, Becker LE. Revision of the World Health Organization classification of brain tumors for childhood brain tumors. *Cancer* 1985;56:1869–1886.
323. Rorke LB. Experimental production of primitive neuroectodermal tumors and its relevance to human neuro-oncology. *Am J Pathol* 1994;144:444–448.
324. Rorke LB. Primitive neuroectodermal tumors. In: Nelson JS, Parisi JE, Schochet SS, eds. *Principles and Practice of Neuropathology*. St. Louis: Mosby; 1993:185–202.
325. Rorke LB. The cerebellar medulloblastoma and its relationship to primitive neuroectodermal tumor. *J Neuropathol Exp Neurol* 1983;42:1–15.
326. Rosemberg S, Nenezes Y, Sousa MR, Plese P, Ciquini O. Primary malignant rhabdoid tumor of the spinal dura. *Clin Neuropathol* 1994;13:221–224.
327. Rossitch E Jr, Zeidman SM, Burger PC, et al. Clinical and pathological analysis of spinal cord astrocytomas in children. *Neurosurgery* 1990;27:193–196.
328. Rouleau GA, Merel P, Lutchman M, et al. Alteration in a new gene encoding a putative membrane-organizing protein causes neuro-fibromatosis type 2. *Nature* 1993;363:515–521.
329. Rousseau P, Habrand J-L, Sarrazin D, et al. Treatment of intracranial ependymomas of children: review of a 15-year experience. *Int J Radiat Oncol Biol Phys* 1993;28:381–386.
330. Rubinstein LJ. A commentary on the proposed revision of the World Health Organization Classification of brain tumors for childhood brain tumors. *Cancer* 1985;56:1887–1888.
331. Rubinstein LJ. Embryonal central neuroepithelial tumors and their differentiating potential: a cytogenetic view of a complex neuro-oncological problem. *J Neurosurg* 1985;62:795–805.
332. Rubinstein LJ, Herman MM. The astroblastoma and its possible cytogenetic relationship to the tanycyte. An electron microscopic, immunohistochemical, tissue- and organ-culture study. *Acta Neuropathol* 1989;78:472–483.
333. Rueda-Pedraza ME, Heifetz SA, Sesterhenn IA, Clark GB. Primary intracranial germ cell tumors in the first two decades of life. A clinical, light-microscopic and immunohistochemical analysis of 54 cases. *Perspect Pediatr Pathol* 1987;10:160–207.
334. Rushing EJ, Rorke LB, Sutton L. Problems in the nosology of desmoplastic tumors of childhood. *Pediatr Neurosurg* 1993;19: 57–62.

335. Russell DS, Rubinstein LJ. *Pathology of Tumours of the Nervous System*. 5th ed. Baltimore: Williams & Wilkins; 1989.
336. Rutka JT, Giblin JR, Apodaca G, et al. Inhibition of growth and induction of differentiation in a malignant human glioma cell line by normal leptomeningeal extracellular matrix proteins. *Cancer Res* 1987;47:3515–3522.
337. Rutka JT. Effects of extracellular matrix proteins on the growth and differentiation of an anaplastic glioma cell line. *Can J Neurol Sci* 1986;13:301306.
338. Ruttledge MH, Sarrazin J, Rangaratnam S, et al. Evidence for the complete inactivation of the NF2 gene in the majority of sporadic meningiomas. *Nat Genet* 1994;6:180–184.
339. Ruttledge MH, Xie YG, Han FY, et al. Deletions on chromosome 22 in sporadic meningioma. *Genes Chrom Cancer* 1994;10: 122–130.
340. Ryken TC, Robinson RA, Van Gilder JC. Familial occurrence of subependymoma. Report of two cases. *J Neurosurg* 1994;80: 1108–1111.
341. Sanford RA, Muhlbauer MS. Craniopharyngioma in children. *Neurol Clin* 1991;9:453–465.
342. Sano K, Wakai S, Ochiai C, Takakura K. Characteristics of intracranial meningiomas in childhood. *Childs Brain* 1981;8:98–106.
343. Sara A, Bruner JM, Mackay B. Ultrastructure of ependymomas. *Ultrastruct Pathol* 1994;18:33–42.
344. Satoh H, Goishi J, Sogabe T, Uozumi T, Kiya K, Migita K. Primary malignant rhabdoid tumor of the central nervous system: case report and review of the literature. *Surg Neurol* 1993;40: 429–434.
345. Satoh H, Uozumi T, Arita K, et al. Spontaneous rupture of craniopharyngioma cysts. A report of five cases and review of the literature. *Surg Neurol* 1993;40:414–419.
346. Sawyer JR, Sammartino G, Husain, Boop FA, Chadduck WM. Chromosome aberrations in four ependymomas. *Cancer Genet Cytogenet* 1994;74:132–138.
347. Saylors RL 3d, Sidransky D, Friedman HS, et al. Infrequent p53 gene mutations in medulloblastomas. *Cancer Res* 1991;51:4721–4723.
348. Scheithauer BW, Rubinstein LJ. Cerebral medulloepithelioma. Report of a case with multiple divergent neuroepithelial differentiation. *Childs Brain* 1979;5:62–71.
349. Scheithauer BW. Neuropathology of pineal region tumors. *Clin Neurosurg* 1985;32:351–383.
350. Scheithauer BW. Symptomatic subependymoma. Report of 21 cases with review of the literature. *J Neurosurg* 1978;49:689–696.
351. Scherer HJ. Structural development in gliomas. *Am J Cancer* 1938;34:333–351.
352. Schiffer D, Cavalla P, Chio A, et al. Tumor cell proliferation and apoptosis in medulloblastoma. *Acta Neuropathol (Berl)* 1994;87: 362–370.
353. Schiffer D, Cravioto H, Giordana MT, Migheli A, Pezzulo T, Vigliani MC. Is polar spongioblastoma a tumor entity? *J Neurosurg* 1993;78:587–591.
354. Schild SE, Scheithauer BW, Schomberg PJ, et al. Pineal parenchymal tumors. Clinical, pathologic, and therapeutic aspects. *Cancer* 1993;72:870–880.
355. Schwartz AM, Ghatak NR, Laine FJ. Intrasellar primitive neuroectodermal tumor (PNET) in familial retinoblastoma: a variant of "trilateral retinoblastoma." *Clin Neuropathol* 1990;9:55–59.
356. Sener RN. CT of diffuse leptomeningeal metastasis from primary extracerebral neuroblastoma. *Pediatr Radiol* 1993;23:402–403.
357. Seppälä M, Haltia MJJ, Sanila RJ, Jääskeläinen JE, Heiskanen O. Long-term outcome after removal of spinal neurofibroma. *J Neurosurg* 1995;82:572–577.
358. Shashi V, Lovell MA, von Kap-herr C, Waldron P, Golden WL. Malignant rhabdoid tumor of the kidney: involvement of chromosome 22. *Genes Chromosom Cancer* 1994;10:49–54.
359. Shaw EG, Scheithauer BW, O'Fallon JR, Tazelaar HD, Davis DH. Oligodendrogliomas: the Mayo Clinic experience. *J Neurosurg* 1992;76:428–434.
360. Shin KH, Whitehead VM. Rhabdomyosarcoma of the brain. *Can J Surg* 1980;23:576–578.
361. Shyn PB, Campbell GA, Guinto FC Jr, Crofford MJ. Primary intracranial ependymoblastoma presenting as spinal cord compression due to metastasis. *Childs Nerv Syst* 1986;2:323–325.
362. Sinson G, Sutton LN, Yachnis AT, Duhaime A-C, Schut L. Subependymal giant cell astrocytomas in children. *Pediatr Neurosurg* 1994;20:233–239.
363. Smith DR, Hardman JM, Earle KM. Metastasizing neuroectodermal tumors of the central nervous system. *J Neurosurg* 1969;31:50–58.
364. Smith MT, Ludwig CL, Godfrey AD, Armbrustmacher VW. Grading of the oligodendrogliomas. *Cancer* 1983;52:2107–2114.
365. Spada A, Vallar L, Faglia G. Cellular alterations in pituitary tumors. *Eur J Endocrinol* 1994;130:43–52.
366. Spada A, Vallar L, Faglia G. G-proteins and hormonal signalling in human pituitary tumors: genetic mutations and functional alterations. *Front Neuroendocrinol* 1993;14:214–232.
367. Spittaler PJ, Johnston IH. Multiple extracranial meningiomas in a child. *Childs Nerv Syst* 1992;8:144–146.
368. Sreekantaiah C, Bridge JA, Rao UN, Neff JR, Sandberg AA. Clonal chromosomal abnormalities in hemangiopericytoma. *Cancer Genet Cytogenet* 1991;54:173–181.
369. Sreekantaiah C, Jockin H, Brecher ML, Sandberg AA. Interstitial deletion of chromosome 11q in a pineoblastoma. *Cancer Genet Cytogenet* 1989;39:125–131.
370. Svien JH, Mabon RF, Kernohan JW, Adson AW. Astrocytomas. *Proc Staff Mtg Mayo Clinic* 1949;25:54–64.
371. Tamaki N, Lin T, Shirataki K, et al. Germ cell tumors of the thalamus and the basal ganglia. *Childs Nerv Syst* 1990;6:3–7.
372. Taratuto AL, Molina HA, Diez B, Zuccaro G, Monges J. Primary rhabdomyosarcoma of brain and cerebellum. Report of four cases in infants: an immunohistochemical study. *Acta Neuropathol* 1985;66:98–104.
373. Taratuto AL, Monges J, Lylyk P, Leiguarda R. Superficial cerebral astrocytoma attached to dura. Report of six cases in infants. *Cancer* 1984;54:2505–2512.
374. Taratuto AL, Pomata H, Sevlever G, Gallo G, Monges J. Dysembryoplastic neuroepithelial tumor: morphological, immunocytochemical, and deoxyribonucleic acid analyses in a pediatric series. *Neurosurgery* 1995;36:474–481.
375. ten Broeke ED, Verdonk GW, Roumen FJ. Prenatal ultrasound diagnosis of an intracranial teratoma influencing management: case report and review of the literature. *Eur J Obstet Gynecol Reprod Biol* 1992;45:210–214.
376. Tomei G, Grimoldi N, Cappricci E, et al. Primary intracranial rhabdomyosarcoma: report of two cases. *Childs Nerv Syst* 1989;5:246–249.
377. Tomita T, McLone DG. Radical resections of childhood craniopharyngiomas. *Pediatr Neurosurg* 1993;19:6–14.
378. Treip CS. A congenital medulloepithelioma of the midbrain. *J Pathol Bacteriol* 1957;74:357–363.
379. Trigg ME, Glaubiger D, Nesbit ME Jr. The frequency of isolated CNS involvement by Ewing's sarcoma. *Cancer* 1982;49:2404–2409.
380. Trofatter JA, MacCollin MM, Rutter JL, et al. A novel moesin-, ezrin-, radixin-like gene is a candidate for the neurofibromatosis 2 tumor suppressor. *Cell* 1993;72:791–800.
381. Troost D, Jansen GH, Dingemans KP. Cerebral medulloepithelioma: electron microscopy and immunohistochemistry. *Acta Neuropathol (Berl)* 1990;80:103–107.
382. Tsai CH, Lin JS, Tsai FJ. Intraventricular fetus in fetu: report of one case. *Acta Paediatr Sin* 1993;34:143–150.
383. Uematsu Y, Yukawa S, Yokote H, Itakura T, Hayashi S, Komai N. Meningeal melanocytoma: magnetic resonance imaging characteristics and pathological features. *J Neurosurg* 1992;76:705–709.
384. Utiger CA, Headington JT. Psammomatous melanotic schwannoma. A new cutaneous marker for Carney's complex. *Arch Dermatol* 1993;129:202–204.
385. Van Bogaert LC. La mélanose neurocutanée diffuse hérédofamiliale. *Bull Acad Roy Med Belg* 1948;13:397–427.
386. VandenBerg SR, May EE, Rubinstein LJ, et al. Desmoplastic supratentorial neuroepithelial tumors of infancy with divergent differentiation potential ("desmoplastic infantile gangliogliomas"). Report on 11 cases of a distinctive embryonal tumor with a favorable prognosis. *J Neurosurg* 1987;66:58–71.

387. VandenBerg SR. Desmoplastic infantile ganglioglioma and desmoplastic cerebral astrocytoma of infancy. *Brain Pathol* 1993;3: 275–281.
388. Vandertop WP, Hoffman HJ, Drake JM, et al. Focal midbrain tumors in children. *Neurosurgery* 1992;31:186–194.
389. Vannucci RC, Baten M. Cerebral metastatic disease in childhood. *Neurology* 1974;24:981–985.
390. Vassilouthis J, Richardson AE. Subfrontal schwannoma. Report of a case. *Acta Neurochir* 1980;53:259–266.
391. Velasco ME, Brown JA, Kini J, Ruppert ES. Primary congenital rhabdoid tumor of the brain with neoplastic hydranencephaly. *Childs Nerv Syst* 1993;9:185–190.
392. Vinchon M, Blond S, Lejeune JP, et al. Association of Lhermitte-Duclos and Cowden disease: report of a new case and review of the literature. *J Neurol Neurosurg Psychiatry* 1994;57:699–704.
393. von Deimling A, Janzer R, Kleihues P, Wiestler OD. Patterns of differentiation in central neurocytoma. An immunohistochemical study of eleven biopsies. *Acta Neuropathol* 1990;79:473–479.
394. von Deimling A, Louis DN, Menon AG, et al. Deletions on the long arm of chromosome 17 in pilocytic astrocytoma. *Acta Neuropathol* 1993;86:81–85.
395. von Deimling A, Louis DN, von Ammon K, et al. Association of epidermal growth factor gene amplification with loss of chromosome 10 in human glioblastoma multiforme. *J Neurosurg* 1992;77:295–301.
396. von Deimling A, Louis DN, von Ammon K, Petersen I, Wiestler OD, Seizinger BR. Evidence for a tumor suppressor gene on chromosome 19q associated with human astrocytomas, oligodendrogliomas, and mixed gliomas. *Cancer Res (United States)* 1992;52: 4277–4279.
397. von Deimling A, Nagel J, Bender B, et al. Deletion mapping of chromosome 19 in human gliomas. *Int J Cancer (United States)* 1994;57:676–680.
398. von Deimling A, von Ammon K, Schoenfeld D, Weistler OD, Seizinger BR, Louis DN. Subsets of glioblastoma multiforme defined by molecular genetic analysis. *Brain Pathol* 1993;3:19–26.
399. Wagle VG, Hall A, Voytek T, Silberstein H, Uphoff DF. Aqueductal (pencil) glioma presenting as neurogenic pulmonary edema: a case report. *Surg Neurol* 1990;34:435–438.
400. Weeks DA, Malott RL, Zuppan CW, Liwnics BH, Beckwith JB. Primitive cerebral tumor with rhabdoid features: a case of phenotypic rhabdoid tumor of the central nervous system. *Ultrastruct Pathol* 1994;18:23–28.
401. Wells GB, Lasner TM, Yousem DM, Zager EL. Lhermitte-Duclos disease and Cowden's syndrome in an adolescent patient. Case report. *J Neurosurg* 1994;81:133–136.
402. Wesseling P, Schlingemann RO, Rietveld FJR, Link M, Burger PC, Ruiter DJ. Early and extensive contribution of pericytes/vascular smooth muscle cells to microvascular proliferation in glioblastoma multiforme: An immuno-light and immuno-electron microscopic study. *J Neuropathol Exp Neurol* 1995;54:304–310.
403. Wesseling P, Vandersteenhoven JJ, Downey BT, Ruiter DJ, Burger PC. Cellular components of microvascular proliferation in human glial and metastatic brain neoplasms. A light microscopic and immunohistochemical study of formalin-fixed, routinely processed material. *Acta Neuropathol* 1993;85:508–514.
404. Wexler LH, DeLaney TF, Saris S, Horowitz ME. Long-term survival after central nervous system relapse in a patient with osteosarcoma. *Cancer* 1993;72:1203–1208.
405. Weyerts LK, Catanzarite V, Jones MC, Mendoza A. Prenatal diagnosis of a giant intracranial teratoma associated with pulmonary hypoplasia. *J Med Genet* 1993;30:880–882.
406. Willis RA. The structure of teratomata. *J Pathol Bacteriol* 1953;40:1–36.
407. Winston KR, Sotrel A, Schnitt SJ. Meningeal melanocytoma. Case report and review of the clinical and histological features. *J Neurosurg* 1987;66:50–57.
408. Wolf M, Santiago H, Duby MM. Delayed distant metastasis from a subcutaneous sacrococcygeal ependymoma. Case report, with tissue culture, ultrastructural observations, and review of the literature. *Cancer* 1972;30:1046–1067.
409. Wyler AR, Hered J, Smith JR, Loeser JD. Subarachnoid hemorrhage in infancy due to brain tumor. *Arch Neurol* 1973;29:447–448.
410. Yang ST, Leow SW. Intracranial fetus-in-fetu: CT diagnosis. *Am J Neuroradiol* 1992;13:1326–1329.
411. Yasargil MG, Curcic M, Kis M, Siegenthaler G, Teddy PJ, Roth P. Total removal of craniopharyngiomas. Approaches and long-term results in 144 patients. *J Neurosurg* 1990;73:3–11.
412. Yasargil MG, von Ammon K, von Deimling A, Valavanis A, Wichmann W, Wiestler OD. Central neurocytoma: histopathological variants and therapeutic approaches. *J Neurosurg* 1992; 76:32–37.
413. Yasue M, Tanaka H, Nakajima M, et al. Germ cell tumors of the basal ganglia and thalamus. *Pediatr Neurosurg* 1993;19:121–126.
414. Yu I-T, Burger PC, Griffin CA, et al. Monosomy for chromosome 22 in rhabdoid tumors of the brain by fluorescence in situ hybridization. *Modern Pathol* 1995;8:8P (abstract).
415. Zhang S, Feng X, Koga H, Ichikawa T, Abe S, Kumanishi T. p53 gene mutations in pontine gliomas of juvenile onset. *Biochem Biophys Res Commun* 1993;196:851–857.
416. Zhu J, Leon SP, Beggs AH, Busque L, Gilliland DG, Black PM. Human pituitary adenomas show no loss of heterozygosity at the retinoblastoma gene locus. *J Clin Endocrinol Metab* 1994;78: 922–927.
417. Zorludemir S, Scheithauer BW, Hirose T, Van Houten CV, Meyer FB. Clear cell meningioma. A clinicopathologic study of a potentially aggressive variant of meningioma. *Am J Surg Pathol* 1995;19:493–505.
418. Zulch KJ. *Histological Typing of Tumours of the Central Nervous System.* Geneva: World Health Organization; 1979.

Pediatric Neoplasia: Morphology and Biology, edited by David M. Parham.
Lippincott-Raven Publishers, Philadelphia © 1996.

CHAPTER 8

Soft Tissue Tumors Other Than Rhabdomyosarcoma and Peripheral Neuroepithelioma

Bruce L. Webber and David M. Parham

INTRODUCTION

Tumors of soft tissue compose an extremely heterogeneous group of lesions that vary widely in both morphologic and clinical features. This diversity is associated with the production of extracellular matrix proteins such as collagen, laminin, or chondroitin sulfate; cytoskeletal elements such as vimentin or keratin; and energy-storing and enzymatic proteins such as myoglobin or creatine kinase. The relation between the cytoskeleton and the extracellular matrix defines the shape of the tumor cells: dense collagen compresses them into narrow, elongated structures; a chondroid matrix surrounds them in lacunar fashion; and a watery, myxoid matrix allows them to expand polygonally. This interaction is also affected by the transformation that occurs with the induction of tumorigenesis (20). These cell shapes and their spatial organization define the morphologic composition used for histologic diagnosis.

Complex structures such as blood vessels or epithelial-lined slits may be produced by the tumor or induced from the surrounding mesenchymal tissues. Varying numbers of inflammatory cells are also recruited into the lesion. The tumors forming these diverse patterns likely develop from primitive, resting mesenchymal cells that differentiate along specific lines and not from mature tissues such as striated muscle or fat cells. This would explain why tumors forming synovium rarely arise from an actual synovial membrane, but often near one.

B. L. Webber: MidSouth Pathology Group, Inc., Memphis, Tennessee 38146.

D. M. Parham: Department of Pathology, Arkansas Children's Hospital, Little Rock, Arkansas 72202.

Histologic diagnosis is therefore made based on the pattern produced by the organization of the cellular elements and their interaction with the surrounding nonneoplastic milieu. Distinguishing characteristics may be sufficiently recognizable at the light microscopic level or require enhancement with electron microscopy or immunohistochemistry. Chromosomal abnormalities may also be characteristic of specific soft tissue tumors and thus helpful in diagnosis (63).

The variety of tools available for diagnosis make apportionment increasingly important at the time of the initial biopsy. Aliquots optimally include portions frozen and stored for immunohistochemistry or genetic analysis, fixed for electron microscopy, and maintained in sterile tissue culture medium for cytogenetic study, as well as immersed in formalin or other fixative. Having said this, however, the point at which the primary diagnosis is made remains the hematoxylin and eosin (H&E)—stained section. Many if not most diagnoses of soft tissue lesions can be made by experienced pathologists using light microscopy alone, and, if not, histologic features will suggest which ancillary tests may be most helpful, given the limited tissue often available. Because identification of soft tissue tumors is often difficult, ancillary testing can be extremely helpful for this purpose.

Besides pathologic characteristics, the diagnostician must consider the clinical and radiologic features of the tumor. Important features in the clinical history include age of the patient, location of the lesion, degree and type of discomfort that the tumor induces, and rate of tumor growth. Rapidly growing, painful lesions are often paradoxically benign, whereas malignant tumors usually grow over a period of months. Paresthesias may be produced by neural tumors. Diagnostic imaging may indicate foci of calcification within neoplasms such as synovial sarcoma or calcifying aponeurotic fibroma (179).

Soft tissue tumors present two major problems in diagnosis. The first and more pressing is the distinction between sarcomas and benign mimics. The unfortunate mistake that sometimes occurs at this juncture may bode disastrous consequences for the affected child. The second problem is the identification of specific sarcoma types. Some (69,162) have arguably said that histology is not as clinically important as grade, but in our grading schema for pediatric sarcomas histologic diagnosis is the primary element taken into account (207). Thus, prognostication of pediatric soft tissue tumors requires both histologic definition and assessment of factors such as necrosis and mitotic index (207). Another primary consideration is to separate rhabdomyosarcomas from nonrhabdomyosarcomatous entities, a feat that may require close attention to histologic detail (see Chapter 5).

The biology of pediatric soft tissue neoplasms in many respects recapitulates that of actively developing or regenerating mesenchyme. Growth factors interact with plasmalemmal receptors, which subsequently internalize these signals and transport them to intranuclear transcription centers, to be read by DNA strands as instructions for either cell division or differentiation. Extracellular matrix components actively participate in the process. Messages directing cell motility and cytoskeletal contraction are complemented by signals directing the participation of leukocytes in areas of regeneration and repair. Orchestration of mesenchymal growth, migration, and orientation begins as soon as the mesodermal component of the primitive embryonic disk is formed and continues in a complex and interwoven fashion throughout fetal development. Components of these embryonic signals recur in areas of postnatal tissue injury but normally are squelched when repair is complete, contrasting with the ongoing autonomous growth of neoplastic tissue.

In recent years the existence of recurring nonrandom areas of genetic alteration have been identified in a number of soft tissue neoplasms (91,134,159,184). Many if not most of these cytogenetic aberrations have been found to be specific for various histologic categories of mesenchymal tumors (184). Techniques such as fluorescence in situ hybridization (FISH) thus offer novel approaches to sarcoma diagnosis (144). Other genetic abnormalities that tend to affect sarcomas involve either proto-oncogenes such as c-*sis* (the gene for platelet-derived growth factor) (148) or tumor suppressor genes such as *p53* or the retinoblastoma gene (15,263,301). Cytogenetic alterations seen in sarcomas often involve translocations that transpose sequences encoding signals for soft tissue development. Duplication of specific chromosomes, probably giving rise to amplified growth signals, may also be seen. In this chapter we will relate findings involving the biology of soft tissue neoplasms to their morphology. Fine dissection of the genotype of these tumors continues at a rapid pace.

The clinical behavior of soft tissue tumors falls roughly into three categories: benign, intermediate, and fully malignant. We shall therefore categorize and discuss them in the context of these three broad groups. The benign tumors will not metastasize and usually do not recur locally. The intermediate ones have a propensity to recur locally if inadequately excised but only rarely metastasize. The fully malignant tumors will recur locally if inadequately excised and have a significant propensity for metastasis.

BENIGN LESIONS

Fibrous Lesions

Scar

A lesion as mundane as a scar can create diagnostic problems for clinicians, and a limited biopsy may show marked cellularity that may be mistaken for a sarcoma if taken out of context. We have seen a case of intramuscular scarring that was mistaken for recurrent Hodgkin's disease clinically but was the result of intensive football training. Grossly it resembled a scar within the muscle, but microscopically it was cellular and mitotically active. It is thus critical to take all parameters into account when making a diagnosis; in this instance the gross appearance was the most helpful parameter in coming to a correct diagnosis.

The biologic basis for the formation of scar tissue may serve as a paradigm for the understanding of soft tissue tumor development, particularly the growth and differentiation of fibrous lesions. In fact, neoplasms in general have been referred to as nonhealing scars (66), and nonmesenchymal tumors such as scirrhous carcinoma of the breast are often characterized by the exuberance of their associated fibrous tissue growth. The growth of this carcinoma-associated scar tissue is perpetuated by the paracrine secretion of growth factors by the tumor cells and is analogous to the secretion of leukokines and the recruitment of inflammatory cells by mesenchymal malignancy and repair (267). A number of specific growth factors, receptors, and intracellular transport proteins (also known as "second messengers" or "signal transduction factors") initiate and carry signals for growth or differentiation from the extracellular milieu to the nucleus, where they interact with transcription factors. Transcription factors in turn modulate the production of RNA, which produces proteins associated with cellular division, differentiation, and programmed death (or "apoptosis"). This incredibly complex series of cellular exchanges is controlled by negative and positive feedback loops. In normal scar tissue, the end result is a hypocellular scar formed primarily from mature collagen and tautened by the cytoskeletal framework of participating myofibroblasts. Conversely, in fibrous neoplasms the process fails to draw a histologic conclusion but remains in a cycle of cell renewal, invasion, and necrosis. Exogenous bloodborne growth factors that typify postnatal development also modulate the development of reactive pediatric soft tissue lesions, thus forming a contrast with adult soft tissue tumors.

A number of the growth factors and related proteins involved in connective tissue proliferation have been characterized. A partial listing is found in Table 1. Detailed discussion of these molecules and their effect on cell proliferation is beyond the scope of this text, so that the reader is referred to other books and reviews such as those by Alberts (4) and Darnell (53) for further reading. The first discovery of these factors was that of Peyton Rous, who in 1910 found that cell-free filtrates of sarcomatous tissue in fowls could produce sarcomas when inoculated into other chickens. This Rous sarcoma virus protein, or src, was subsequently discovered to be a perverse form of the normal host cellular machinery by Nobel prize winners Varmus and Bishop in 1976 (259). In this manner the first discoveries of an oncogene (v-*src*), or cancer-causing gene, and a proto-oncogene (c-*src*), or normal host counterpart of an oncogene, were made. V-src (please note that genes are italicized and their corresponding proteins are not) has unique phosphorylating properties, primarily affecting tyrosine-containing membrane-associated proteins and leading to cell transformation, a conformational metamorphosis associated with neoplastic development. Thus, in cell cultures one observes rounding of the cell body, nuclear enlargement, and loss of contact inhibition following transfection or forced expression of oncogenes (59,195,198,276,277).

Besides c-src, growth factors involved in wound healing interact in a complex and intercommunicative manner to modulate the biochemical events of repair. Leukokines such as interleukin 1 (IL-1) and tumor necrosis factor (45) play a critical role by recruitment of inflammatory cells that secrete their own paracrine factors affecting the stromal cell component. Growth factors or their corresponding receptors are also proto-oncogenes; for example, PDGF (platelet-derived growth factor) is also c-*sis*, which causes osteosarcoma in humans when overexpressed (45). Similarly, the gene encoding the EGF (epidermal growth factor) receptor is also *erb*, which causes a number of human neoplasms by overexpression or amplification (45). Active angiogenesis is another critical component of wound healing and gives rise to the erythema that the ancients grossly recognized as "proud flesh." Tumor angiogenesis factors analogous to those of repair are expressed by developing neoplasms and are critical to their propagation (57). These components lead to the development of endothelial sprouts that arise from neighboring blood vessels. Through progressive elongation and lumen formation, capillary buds permeate the injured tissues.

TABLE 1. *Growth factors affecting normal and neoplastic soft tissue proliferation in childhood*

Human growth factor
Insulin-like growth factors I and II
Insulin
Epidermal growth factor
Fibroblastic growth factors
Transforming growth factors
Platelet-derived growth factor
Tumor angiogenesis factors

Simultaneously, fibroblasts migrate, proliferate, and produce collagens, as well as generating a tensile force through microfilament contraction. This force is the basis for wound contracture and generates an action potential that can be measured by electrochemical techniques and induced by pharmacologic agents such as serotonin or epinephrine (243). Thus, inherent in scar formation are not only growth and cell division but motility and cell migration, i.e., factors that affect tumor metastasis.

Nodular Fasciitis

In our experience, nodular fasciitis is the lesion that causes the most difficulty in distinguishing between benign and malignant soft tissue lesions. It is a lesion that occurs over a wide age range, affecting children more commonly in the head and neck area and adults in the extremities. It may even affect newborns, in whom it often presents as a mass involving the skull (cranial fasciitis). Allen (7) has pointed out the great variety of histologic appearances it may assume, as it may mimic malignant fibrous histiocytoma, fibrosarcoma, granulation tissue, or giant cell tumor of tendon sheath. Patients with nodular fasciitis who are misdiagnosed as having sarcoma may be inappropriately treated with radical surgery, radiation therapy, and toxic chemotherapy, so that it behooves the surgical pathologist to be keenly aware of this lesion.

One feature of nodular fasciitis that is particularly helpful in diagnosis is the short clinical history, which is usually measured in weeks rather than months. The lesions tend to grow rapidly over a short period of time, whereas sarcomas generally have a more indolent clinical course measured in months or even years. Another feature is the small size of the tumors, as they are usually in the neighborhood of 2 cm in diameter and rarely over 5.0 cm (Fig. 1).

Histologically, the typical case of nodular fasciitis is composed of active, spindle-shaped cells that are loosely arranged in a tissue culture–like pattern that usually imperceptibly blends into the surrounding tissues (Fig. 2).

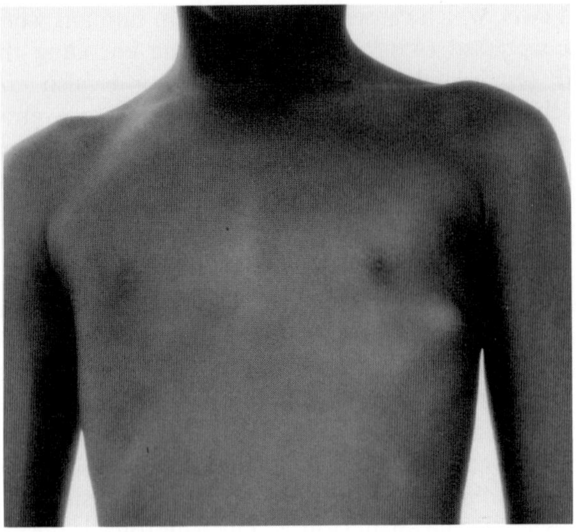

FIG. 1. Nodular fasciitis. A small subcutaneous nodule arises in the left chest wall of this adolescent male.

There may be a few intermingled inflammatory cells, but despite the name this is usually not a conspicuous feature. The tissue culture-like appearance may be subtle in more compact tumors. A most helpful feature stressed in Allen's paper (7) is the presence of shallow S-shaped curves in the bundles of spindle cells. Another helpful feature is the presence of larger polygonal cells with basophilic cytoplasm and prominent nucleoli, these cells somewhat resembling ganglion cells.

As its name implies, nodular fasciitis typically occurs on the deep fascia and usually extends into the overlying subcutaneous fat or underlying muscle. The different patterns seen include a storiform pattern, a giant cell pattern with numerous osteoclastlike giant cells, a granulation tissue-like pattern with prominent vessels, a very myxoid pattern, and a solid cellular pattern in which the cells are closely packed (7). It is this latter pattern that most closely resembles a sarcoma. The histology also depends on the age of the lesion, as older lesions tend to become more fibrous in their appearance and acquire keloidlike collagen bundles.

The cells of nodular fasciitis have the features of myofibroblasts under the electron microscope. Not unexpectedly, positive immunohistochemical staining with some muscle markers may occur, creating further diagnostic confusion. Montgomery and Meis (185) found that CD56 (KP1; a histiocytic marker), smooth muscle actin, muscle-specific actin, and vimentin are positive, whereas desmin, cytokeratin, and S-100 are negative. One should thus recognize that these tumors may stain with both smooth muscle and histiocytic markers to avoid misdiagnosing them as sarcomas with muscle or histiocytic differentiation.

Other lesions strongly resembling nodular fasciitis may be associated with the production of osteoid. These variants have been termed ossifying fasciitis or periosteal fasciitis (Fig. 3). Another lesion that may be quite disturbing is intravascular fasciitis, in which the lesion grows within a vein (211). It may at first resemble organized thrombosis within the vessel, but in fact it is an intravascular lesion that closely resembles typical nodular fasciitis. This lesion is also benign in spite of its location.

Demonstration of mutations of the tumor suppressor gene *p53* as the responsible causative agent for the sarcoma-associated Li–Fraumeni syndrome (149) gave rise to hypotheses concerning use of this phenomenon in differential diagnosis of soft tissue lesions. Immunohistochemistry has been found to be useful in identification of these mutations, for typically the ineffectual p53 protein product is overexpressed in affected tumor cells

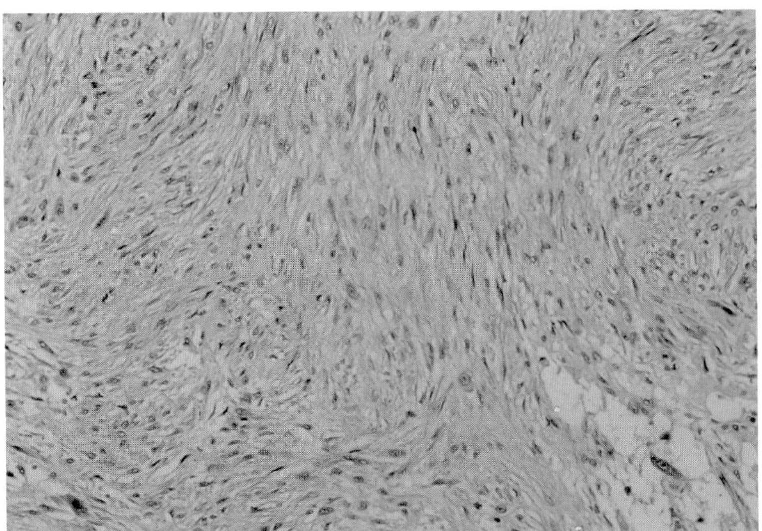

FIG. 2. Nodular fasciitis. The lesion is composed of bland spindle cells arranged in vague S-shaped fascicles.

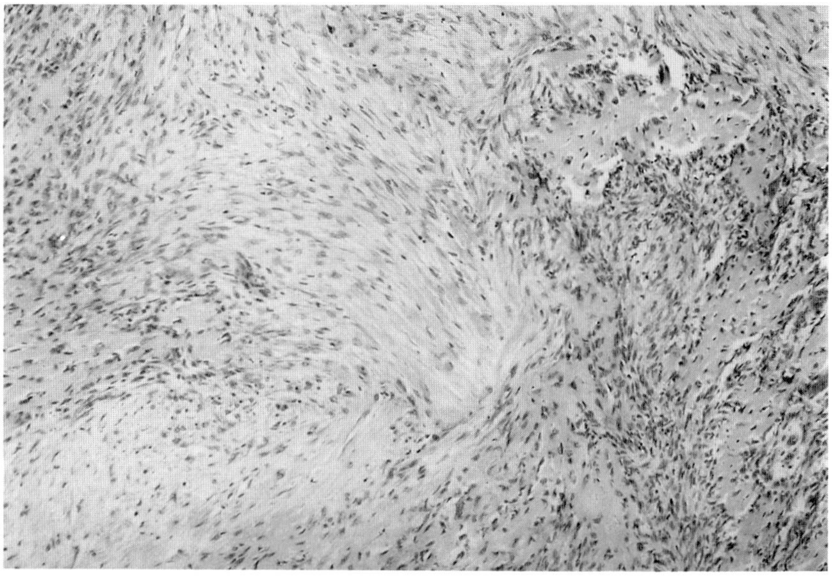

FIG. 3. Ossifying fasciitis. Areas of typical nodular fasciitis **(center)** merge with areas of ossification **(right)**.

(215) and can be identified using antigen retrieval methods and monoclonal antibodies. Hopes for using p53 immunohistochemistry to separate benign proliferative processes such as nodular fasciitis from malignant tumors were dashed with the discovery that positively staining cells could be found in roughly 50% of reactive conditions (56). However, a more recent study indicates that the number of p53-positive cells in benign proliferative lesions such as nodular fasciitis was considerably lower than that found in sarcomas (254). Thus, although not reliable as a sole diagnostic criterion, the presence of more than 1% positively staining cells in a soft tissue suggests malignancy rather than a reactive process.

Investigation of ploidy status and proliferative index has also been performed on nodular fasciitis. All cases examined to date have been diploid (70,200). Determination of proliferative index using Ki-67 nuclear antigen (200) has revealed a DNA content intermediate between that of dermatofibrosarcoma protuberans and malignant fibrous histiocytoma. These findings are consonant with the rapid growth but benign behavior of these lesions.

Proliferative Fasciitis and Myositis

Proliferative fasciitis and myositis was once thought to present exclusively during adulthood (78,172). The youngest patient with proliferative myositis in Enzinger's earlier series (76) was 22 years old and the median age was 50 years. However, Meis and Enzinger (172) recently reported a series of pediatric cases, many of which were initially diagnosed as rhabdomyosarcomas and overtreated as a result (133,209). Similar cases had been previously documented (133,209). It is therefore important to recognize that this entity can present during childhood, although as a very rare occurrence. The childhood lesions are well circumscribed, lobulated, and more cellular than the adult cases, have frequent mitoses, and are often associated with acute inflammation and necrosis. They also have a less myxoid stroma and lack the long, delicate fibroblasts seen in adult cases.

The finding of short spacing and native collagen fibrils within dilated cisternae of rough endoplasmic reticulum led to an electron microscopic diagnosis of one pediatric case of proliferative myositis/fasciitis (99). An immunohistochemical analysis of six examples of proliferative myositis and/or fasciitis revealed α–smooth muscle actin positivity and other features of myofibroblastic differentiation in the spindle cell component (156a). The giant cells were actin-negative and appeared to represent a divergent form of differentiation. These tumors are primarily diploid in cases reported thus far (70,156a), although tetraploidy may be seen in the giant cells (156a).

Myositis Ossificans

Myositis ossificans is a common pseudosarcomatous lesion that primarily affects young boys. Most frequently it occurs on the lower extremity and is preceded by a history of trauma in slightly less than one half of cases. Myositis ossificans begins as a reparative process that is very cellular and contains mitoses (occasionally atypical) and plump myofibroblastlike cells. The important feature of this lesion is its eventual evolution into an osteogenic mass, with new bone being initially formed at the periphery. Thus the most mature bone is found at the circumference and the most cellular and atypical tissue is found at the center of the lesion (Fig. 4A). Diagnostic imaging is often very valuable in these cases, as one can visualize the rim of bone at the edge of the lesion (Fig. 4B).

A 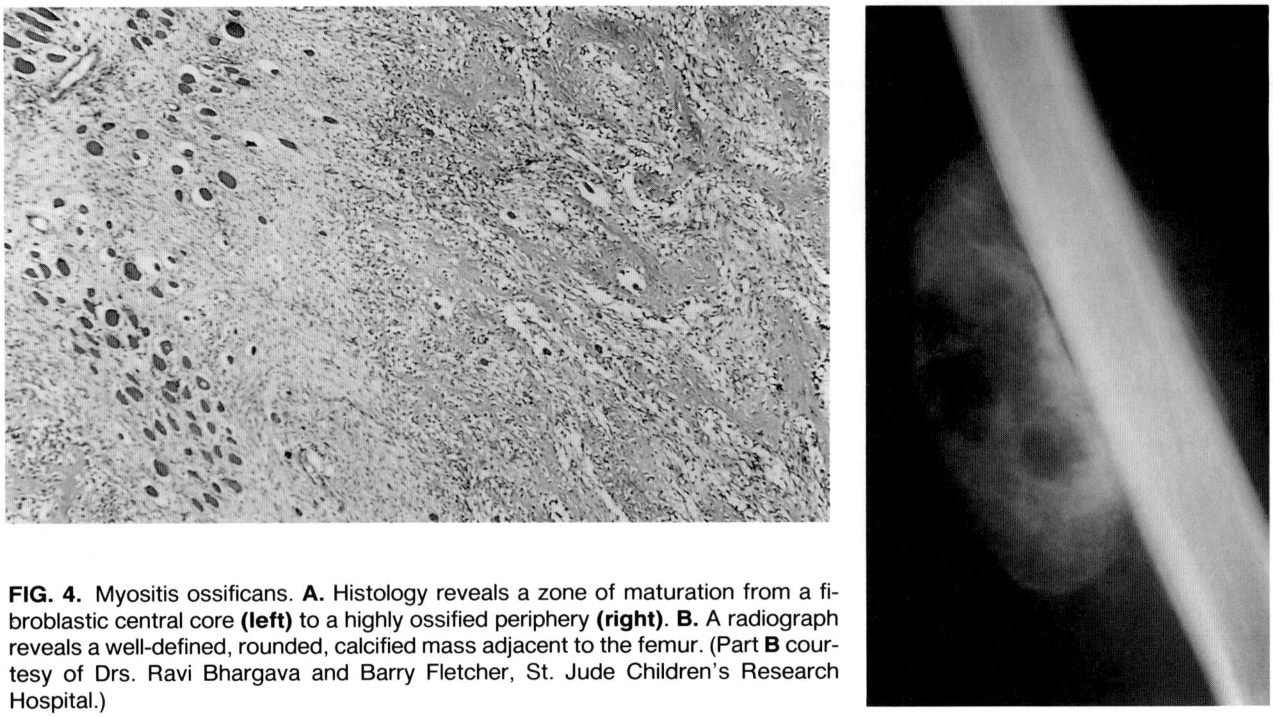 B

FIG. 4. Myositis ossificans. **A.** Histology reveals a zone of maturation from a fibroblastic central core **(left)** to a highly ossified periphery **(right)**. **B.** A radiograph reveals a well-defined, rounded, calcified mass adjacent to the femur. (Part **B** courtesy of Drs. Ravi Bhargava and Barry Fletcher, St. Jude Children's Research Hospital.)

Lesions closely related to myositis ossificans occur in the subcutaneous tissues, particularly in the fingers or toes, and may also be mistaken for bone-forming malignancies. Dupree and Enzinger (65) described 21 such cases. The lesions may appear suddenly or slowly and have growth spurts. Many have pain and mimic an infection clinically. They are well circumscribed and firm with gross evidence of calcification. Microscopically they are multinodular and have ill-defined margins. They consist of a fibroblastic proliferation that may show atypia, together with benign-appearing osteoid and bone produced in a haphazard fashion. The bone does not show the zoning seen with myositis ossificans, and no residual muscle is seen entrapped within the lesions. Spjut and Dorfman (258) felt that this represented a reactive periostitis, but Dupree and Enzinger (65) pointed out that the lesion is centered outside the periosteum and in the subcutaneous tissues, tendons, tendon sheaths, and ligaments.

Fibrodysplasia Ossificans Progressiva

Fibrodysplasia ossificans progressiva is a genetic disease that not infrequently presents as a rapidly growing soft tissue mass. Biopsy yields a somewhat confusing histologic picture, so that it is difficult to make the diagnosis from the histology alone. To this end, clinical and radiologic findings are often helpful.

Affected patients present with a solitary or multiple soft tissue masses, usually in the neck/parotid region, around the scapula, or in the back (Fig. 5A). There may be a history of similar masses that grow and then recede. The lesion grows very rapidly, i.e., too rapidly for this to be a typical malignant tumor! For example, a case that the authors studied started as a small nodule in the parotid region of a 3-year-old and grew to fill the whole side of the neck as well as the upper back within 2 weeks of onset! The biopsy showed nonspecific features: adipose tissue lobules surrounded by proliferating fibroblasts and containing extravasated red blood cells. The correct diagnosis was made by examining the feet and hands of the unfortunate patient, as the vast majority of these children have deformed first metatarsal bones with hallux valgus (Fig. 5B). Examination of the extremities will thus clinch the diagnosis in spite of the nonspecific nature of the histology. In fact, trauma exacerbates the disease, and biopsy may be detrimental.

Fibrodysplasia ossificans progressiva eventually progresses, with exacerbations and remissions, to ossification of large areas, causing severe difficulties that arise from immobilization of various parts of the body (Fig. 5C, D). The thoracic region is a particular site of morbidity, leading to eventual respiratory embarrassment and death.

A genetic basis for this condition is apparent because it is inherited in an autosomal dominant fashion with variable penetrance in some cases, has been reported in monozygotic twins, and appears more frequently with advanced paternal age (40,128). The maldevelopmental features of the disease are similar to those induced in the fruit fly, *Drosophila melanogaster,* by mutation of the decapentaplegic (*dpp*) locus. This gene shares significant

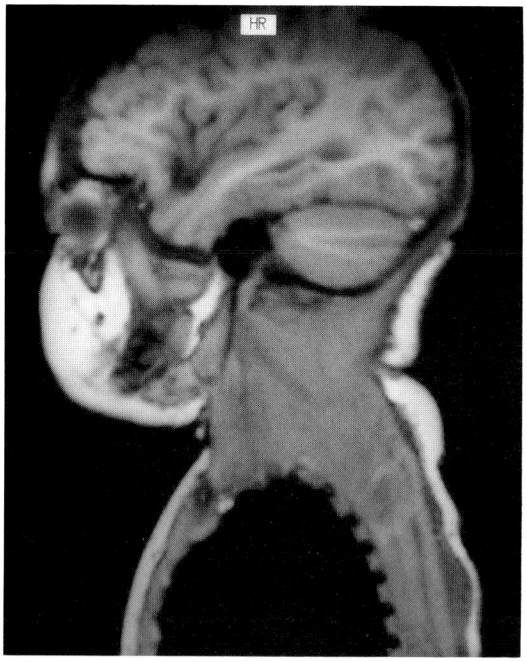

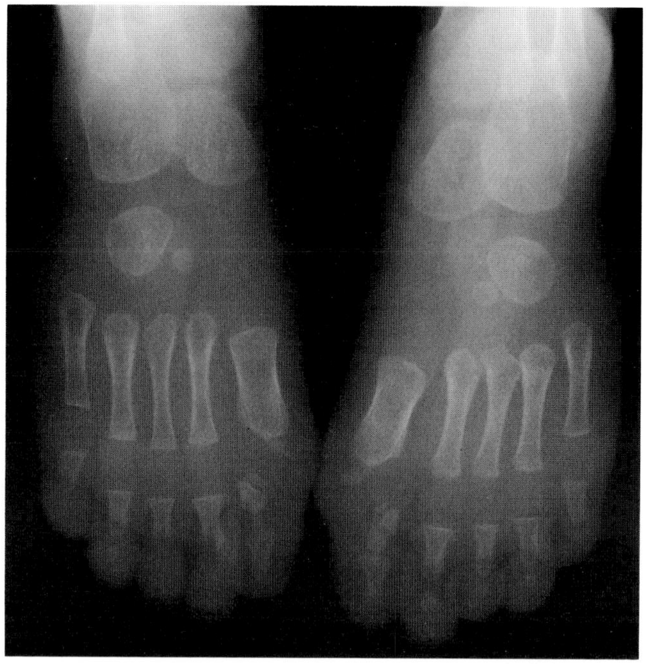

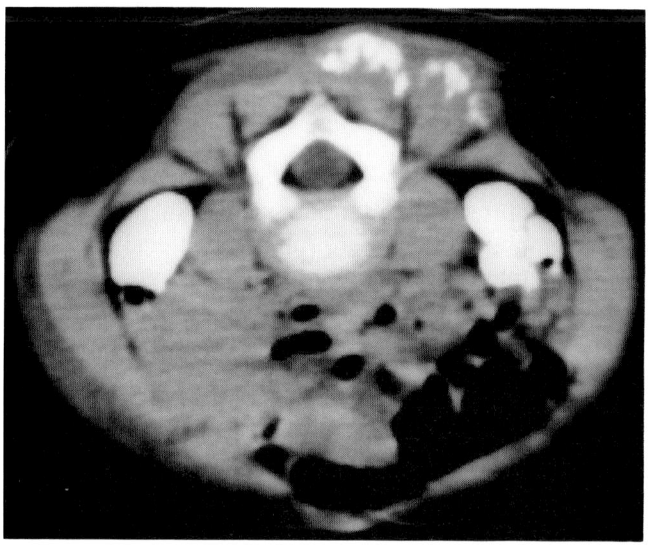

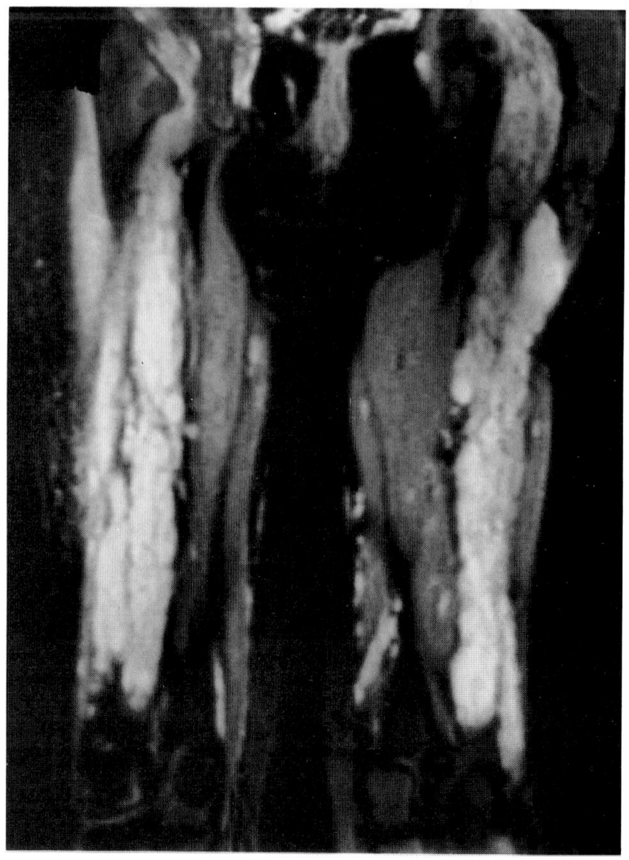

FIG. 5. Fibrodysplasia ossificans progressiva. **A.** An MR scan reveals a large, soft tissue mass that fills and expands the subcutis in the neck. **B.** Bilaterally deformed first metatarsal bones with hallux valgus are apparent on a plain radiograph. **C.** Progressive disease in the paraspinal musculature, apparent on an MR scan as calcified masses. **D.** Progressive disease is also seen bilaterally in the soft tissue of the thighs, which is remarkably calcified on MR scans. (Courtesy of Drs. Ravi Bhargava and Barry Fletcher, St. Jude Children's Research Hospital.)

homology with the human *BMP-2* genes, whose protein products are capable of inducing in vivo ossification (129), suggesting that fibrodysplasia ossificans progressive might be a similar disorder. Some evidence of this hypothesis derives from the characteristic nonrandom order of soft tissue ossification (37,229).

Fibromatosis Colli

Fibromatosis colli is a spindle cell proliferation occurring exclusively in the sternocleidomastoid muscle of very young infants. It is not present at birth, but makes its appearance and gradually enlarges 2–5 weeks afterward. Fibromatosis colli affects the lower portion of the sternocleidomastoid, especially the sternal head, and only rarely the upper half (285). It consists of a very bland fibroblastic proliferation that entraps and destroys myofibers, produces a mass, and eventually goes on to contract. This process may cause the muscle to shorten, resulting in a wry neck. Local excision may be necessary to avert this complication; however, most cases do not develop torticollis and therefore do not require surgical removal.

Juvenile Hyalin Fibromatosis

Juvenile hyalin fibromatosis is an autosomal recessive inherited condition that occurs in siblings but not in subsequent generations (132,168). The lesions usually develop between 2 and 5 years of age as papules evolving into nodules and masses in the skin and subcutaneous tissues of the head, back, and extremities. The tumors may affect the joints and the gums and also develop in the bones as multiple lytic lesions, but they do not affect the viscera—a point of distinction from infantile myofibromatosis (78). Histologically the nodules consist of fascicles of spindle cells separated by varying amounts of periodic acid–Schiff (PAS)–positive, hyaline, lightly eosinophilic material that consists of fibrils and occasional bundles of mature and long-spaced collagen. Electron microscopic examination and phase contrast microscopy also reveal intracytoplasmic collagen secretion granules (132). In view of their demonstration of chondroitin sulfate in older lesions, Mayer-da-Silva et al. (168) postulated that this is a disorder of mesenchymal cells differentiating toward chondroid tissue.

Clinically, the musculoskeletal manifestations of this disease may be quite severe, with the production of crippling and painful joint contractures in addition to the bony abnormalities (197). These joint abnormalities appear to result from the presence of the characteristic tumors in the capsular regions. Excision of the involved tissues may result in exuberant recurrence. The masses produced by juvenile hyalin fibromatosis may be disfiguring, requiring surgical resection for cosmesis, but they tend to remain static for long periods of time.

Soft Tissue Myofibroblastoma

Myofibroblastoma is a solitary benign tumor composed of proliferating myofibroblasts. Sites of involvement include breast, meninges, subcutaneous tissues, tunica vaginalis testis, inguinal lymph nodes, and miscellaneous soft tissues. These are well-circumscribed soft tissue tumors characterized by short, intersecting, or criss-crossing fascicles of spindle cells. There may be necrosis, and mitoses are limited to less than 3 per 10 high-power fields. Myofibroblastomas stain positively for vimentin, actin, and desmin and show myofibroblastic differentiation by electron microscopy. They are clinically benign lesions, thus far described only in males, that do not recur or metastasize after adequate excision. They may recur if incompletely excised and should therefore be removed with wide margins if practical. Herrera et al. (113) described a congenital case.

Calcifying Fibrous Pseudotumor

Calcifying fibrous pseudotumor is a benign fibrous lesion involving subcutaneous and deep soft tissues and containing abundant hyalinized collagen, psammomatous or dystrophic calcifications, and a lymphoplasmacytic infiltrate including occasional germinal centers (Fig. 6). The tumors may become very large, are usually well circumscribed, but may entrap structures such as neurovascular bundles. Multinucleated giant cells rarely may be present adjacent to the calcification. Calcifying fibrous pseudotumors are found in both children and adults, the median age being 18.5 years (86). Sites of involvement include the extremities, trunk, scrotum, groin, neck, and axilla. The lesions rarely may recur after incomplete excision.

Differential diagnosis of calcifying fibrous pseudotumor includes nodular fasciitis, which shows greater cellularity, more mitotic activity, a myxoid matrix with a tissue culture–like appearance, and S-shaped fascicles. The lymphocytes are more diffusely scattered in nodular fasciitis than in calcifying fibrous pseudotumor, where they are more aggregated. Calcification does not occur in typical nodular fasciitis but is seen in some variants. Desmoids may sometimes mineralize but have much less inflammation, more prominent myofibroblasts, more infiltration of surrounding tissues, and much less propensity to calcify. Other lesions to consider include

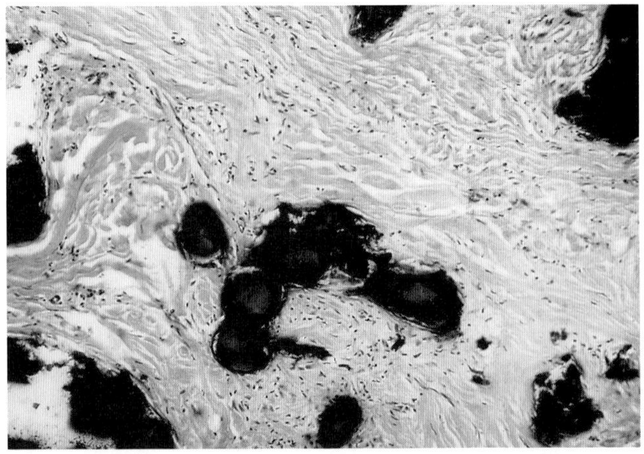

FIG. 6. Calcifying fibrous pseudotumor. Dystrophic calcifications are embedded in a heavily collagenized matrix containing a sprinkling of lymphocytes.

fibro-osseous pseudotumor of the digits (65), ossifying fibromyxoid tumor (176,242), and childhood fibrous tumor with psammoma bodies (234).

Angiofibroma

Angiofibroma is a proliferation of fibrovascular elements arising almost exclusively in the nasal passages or nasopharynx of adolescent males who present with epistaxis or obstruction (298). Often there is invasion of adjacent structures (298). These tumors are composed of bland fibrous tissue intersected by thin-walled, haphazardly organized blood vessels of varying sizes (Fig. 7). The vessels either contain no smooth muscle/pericytic lining or show local padlike thickenings composed of actin-positive muscular tissue (12). The stromal cells are predominantly fibroblasts exhibiting only vimentin positivity, although occasional actin-positive cells may be found. Areas of hyalinization, fibrosis, and myxoid change may also be found. The proliferating vessels have an attenuated lining lacking elastic tissue, resulting in a propensity for severe hemorrhage during surgical procedures (12). Biologically these are benign lesions that may spontaneously regress (293), although sarcomatous transformation has also occurred (25).

Because of the propensity for the lesion to occur during adolescence and almost exclusively in boys, a hormonal influence appears to be operative in their growth. Intracellular estradiol may be demonstrated by immunohistochemistry (136,137), but detection of testosterone is not universal by this method (136). The tumors may respond to estrogen therapy (143) and contain cytosolic androgen receptors, suggesting that the estrogens work as antiandrogens (143). However, androgens do not stimulate tumor growth in nude mice and cell cultures (248), indicating that other factors are operative. Tumor extracts contain a factor that stimulates endothelial cell proliferation; this molecule is immunologically identical to basic fibroblast growth factor (bFGF). As with desmoid tumors, there appears to be an association with the familial adenomatosis polyposis gene, as these lesions are 25 times more frequent in these patients (100).

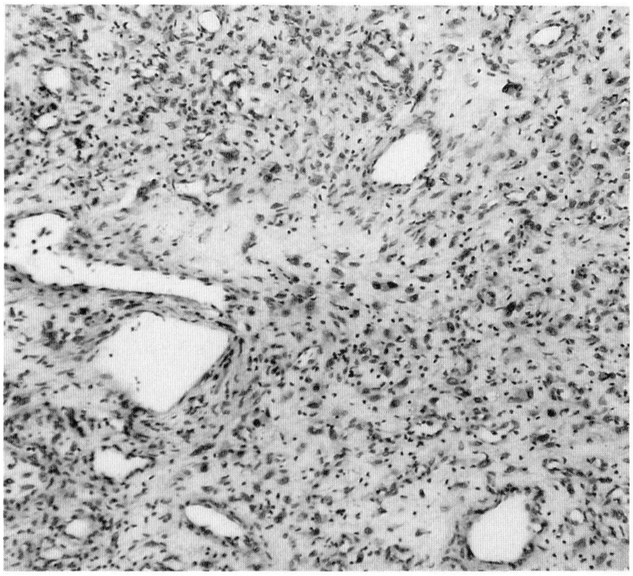

FIG. 7. Nasal angiofibroma. Numerous blood vessels of varying caliber intersect an inflamed fibroblastic stroma.

Inflammatory Myofibroblastic Tumor

Inflammatory myofibroblastic tumors (also known as inflammatory pseudotumors, plasma cell granulomas, inflammatory fibromyxoid tumors, and fibroxanthomas) are benign lesions characterized by a mixed proliferation of fibroblastic/myofibroblastic cells and inflammatory cells, particularly lymphocytes and plasma cells. They are analogous to the plasma cell granuloma of the lung (see Chapter 14) and to nodular fasciitis, but occur in other locations. These locations comprise a wide variety of anatomic sites, including brain, spleen, abdomen, esophagus, liver, stomach, bowel, urinary bladder (Fig. 8A), lymph node, and ear (19,127,246,269,279). Because inflammatory myofibroblastic tumors occur as growing masses composed of spindle cell elements, they may be misdiagnosed as sarcoma, and the potential for this error is further compounded in pleomorphic examples. Patients affected by these tumors may show systemic manifestations such as microcytic anemia, thrombocytosis, hyperglobulinemia, and an elevated erythrocyte sedimentation rate. These symptoms resolve following tumor resection.

Inflammatory myofibroblastic tumors contain a variable mixture of constituent spindle cell and inflammatory cells, resulting in predominately fibrous or markedly inflamed lesions. Similarly to nodular fasciitis, the spindle cells are recognized by their similarity to fibroblasts growing in tissue culture and may form gentle S-shaped curves or a storiform pattern. Although straplike cells are common, the cytoplasm is purplish rather than brick red in H&E-stained sections, offering a distinct difference from rhabdomyosarcoma (Fig. 8B). The nuclei may be immature-appearing with prominent nucleoli and show moderate degrees of pleomorphism. The inflammatory cells are predominately lymphocytes and plasma cells, but macrophages, mast cells, neutrophils, and eosinophils may also be present. There should be a low mitotic rate, not exceeding five per ten high-power fields; indices above this point should raise a suspicion of sarcoma (5).

By immunohistochemistry and electron microscopy, it is apparent that the spindle cells of these lesions are mostly myofibroblasts, as a peripheral web of actin-positive microfilaments is evident (Fig. 8C) (5,279). This

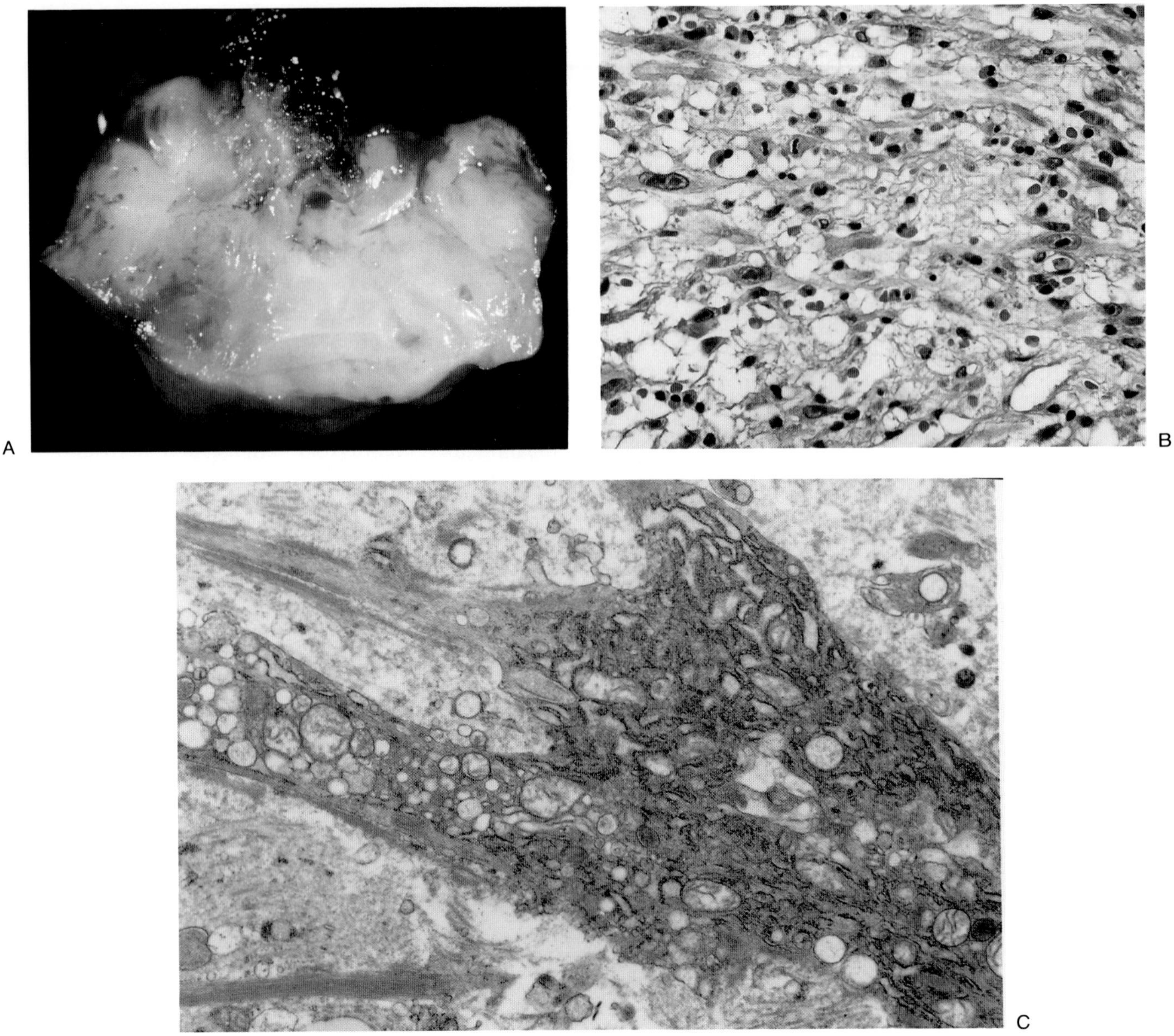

FIG. 8. Inflammatory myofibroblastic tumor. **A.** A transmural fibrous mass expands the urinary bladder in this transverse section of a surgical excision. **B.** Plump fibroblastic cells and inflammatory cells permeate a myxoid stroma. Mitotic activity is apparent. **C.** A myofibroblast with abundant rough endoplasmic reticulum and peripheral microfilaments is seen in this electron micrograph. Bundles of anchoring filaments (fibronexus junctions) run parallel to the plasmalemma in cytoplasmic projections **(left)**. (Parts **A** and **C** courtesy of Dr. Alfredo Pinto, Alberta Children's Hospital, Calgary, Alberta.)

facet of the tumors may lead to a misdiagnosis of leiomyosarcoma, particularly in lesions of the urinary bladder. Thus one should take careful note of the presence of inflammatory cells, particularly plasma cells.

Flow cytometry reveals a diploid population (127), so that the presence of aneuploidy may be an ominous sign. Some of these tumors may progress or transform into sarcomas, as evidenced by the histologically similar diagnostic entity, inflammatory fibrosarcoma (171). Cytogenetic analysis supports this contention, as a chromosomal translocation, t(2;9)(q1.3;p2.2), was noted in an omental case (271).

Fibrohistiocytic Lesions

Benign Fibrous Histiocytoma

Enzinger and Weiss (78) recognize two categories of benign fibrous histiocytoma: cutaneous and deep. Cutaneous fibrous histiocytoma is a common lesion also

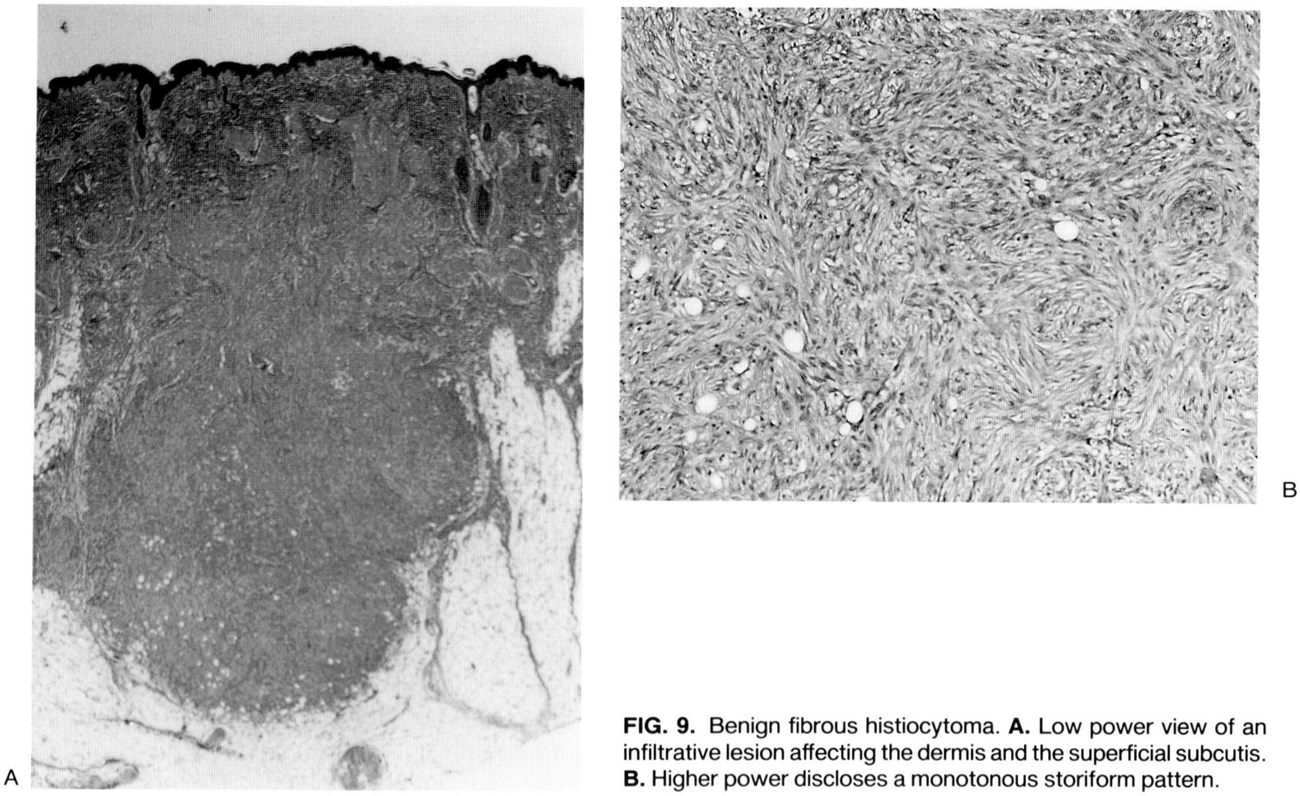

FIG. 9. Benign fibrous histiocytoma. A. Low power view of an infiltrative lesion affecting the dermis and the superficial subcutis. B. Higher power discloses a monotonous storiform pattern.

known as dermatofibroma, nodular subepidermal fibrosis, or sclerosing hemangioma of skin. Deep fibrous histiocytoma is a microscopically similar tumor located in subcutaneous or deeper soft tissue. These tumors are larger, have a prominent storiform pattern, and exhibit a slightly increased potential for local recurrence as compared to the cutaneous fibrous histiocytoma.

Franquemont et al. (96) reported benign fibrous histiocytomas involving the subcutis of eight patients, three of whom were 20 years old or younger. These lesions involved the dermis as well as the subcutaneous tissue (Fig. 9A), were frequently multinodular, and had a diffuse, monotonous, storiform pattern (Fig. 9B). Satellite foci, multinucleated giant cells, foamy macrophages, and hemosiderin deposition were seen. The multinodular growth pattern and the involvement of the subcutaneous tissue helped to distinguish the lesion from cutaneous fibrous histiocytoma (dermatofibroma). Three of six patients with follow-up data suffered recurrences.

Benign fibrous histiocytoma has rarely been inherited (228); in one family the proband died of a malignant fibrous histiocytoma (228). Deep lesions reportedly show no immunohistochemical evidence of true monocyte–macrophage differentiation and thus have an uncertain histogenesis (88).

The differential diagnosis of benign fibrous histiocytoma includes dermatofibrosarcoma protuberans (96), giant cell tumor of tendon sheath, fibroma of tendon sheath, palmar and plantar fibromatoses, silica reaction (291), juvenile xanthogranuloma, plexiform fibrohistiocytic tumor, Hodgkin's disease–associated fibrohistiocytic lesion of bone (46), and xanthoma.

Giant Cell Fibroblastoma

Giant cell fibroblastoma is a benign, pseudosarcomatous lesion that presents as a slowly growing mass, often attached to the overlying skin. It occurs primarily in the first two decades of life; 87% of Shmookler's cases occurred prior to age 12 (251). Giant cell fibroblastoma affects males twice as commonly as females and typically involves the trunk or other sites such as the thigh, axilla, wrist, foot, or ankle. The lesion is prone to recur if incompletely excised, with this event occurring in 42% of Shmookler's cases. However, it does not demonstrate frankly malignant behavior and is cured by reexcision (78).

Giant cell fibroblastomas range in size from 0.8 to 8.0 cm and are rubbery with ill-defined borders. Microscopically they are spindle cell lesions with sinusoidlike spaces lined by either pleomorphic large atypical cells or giant cells with peripheral overlapping nuclei and basophilic central cytoplasm (Fig. 10). The pleomorphic spindle cells may be dispersed elsewhere in the lesion. The tumor infiltrates the surrounding tissue but surrounds adnexal structures without destroying them. Mitoses are rare. Dense fibrovascular cores may project into

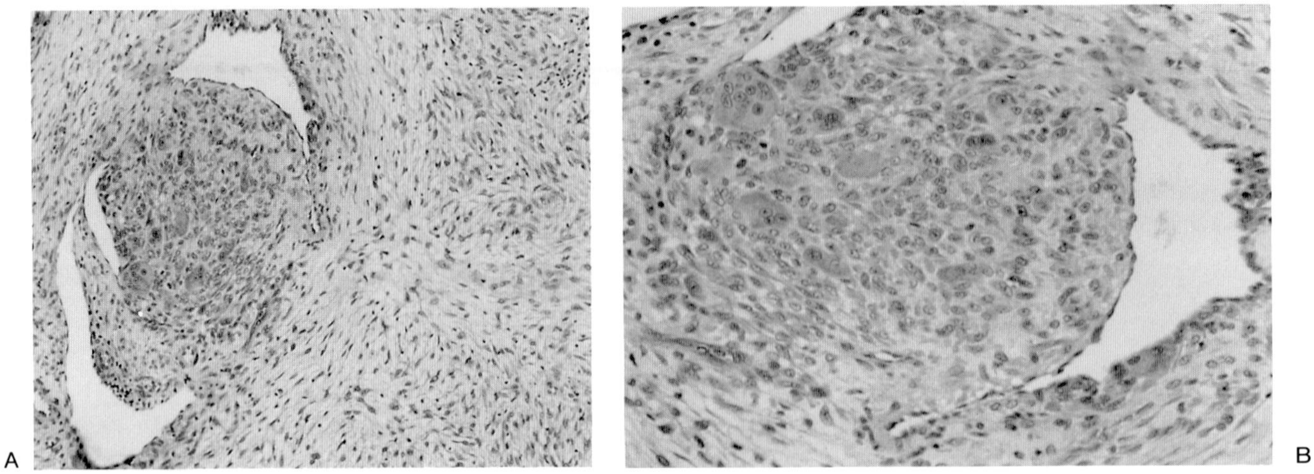

FIG. 10. Giant cell fibroblastoma. Dilated vascular spaces are found in an inflamed fibroblastic tumor with a vague storiform configuration (**A**). There are giant cells and plump histiocytes adjacent to the dilated vessels (**B**).

the sinusoidlike spaces. Areas of the tumor may contain dense, hyaline collagen. Ultrastructurally, the giant cell nuclei have a peculiar segmented appearance, the segments being attached by strands of nuclear membrane material. The cytoplasm contains abundant rough endoplasmic reticulum (251).

Giant cell fibroblastoma was considered by Shmookler and Enzinger (251) to be a juvenile form of dermatofibrosarcoma protuberans (DFSP). The two lesions have many features in common, including disposition as a subcutaneous lesion attached to the epidermis, truncal distribution, tendency to recurrence, and storiform pattern with myxoid areas and sparing of the adnexal structures. Some pediatric giant cell fibroblastomas have evolved into DFSP in adulthood (6) and vice versa (11,47). Thus, while the two lesions are likely closely related, the theory that giant cell fibroblastoma is a childhood variant of DFSP is probably an oversimplification (11).

Plexiform Fibrohistiocytic Tumor

Plexiform fibrohistiocytic tumor is a lesion most commonly affecting the deep dermis and subcutaneous tissue of children, especially females. In Enzinger and Zhang's series (79), the median age was 14.5 years and 67.7% of the affected patients were under 20 years. It usually involves the upper extremities, particularly the elbow region, forearm, wrist, hand, and shoulder. It may also affect the lower extremity, trunk, head, and neck and presents clinically as a small, deep-seated, firm, rubbery, solitary nodule.

Grossly plexiform fibrohistiocytic tumors are irregular, gray–white, and trabeculated, usually measuring between 1 and 3 cm (79). Histologically they show two basic patterns: a fibrohistiocytic pattern composed of polygonal histiocytic cells often surrounded by a rim of collagen, and a fibroblastic pattern composed of spindle cells arranged in a plexiform pattern of intertwining fascicles (Fig. 11). In the series of Enzinger and Zhang (79), 43% of the tumors consisted of fibrohistiocytic nodules, 40% were a mixture of the two patterns, and 17% were predominantly fibroblastic. The fibrohistiocytic nodules frequently contain osteoclastlike giant cells scattered among rounded histiocytic cells. Small hemorrhages, hemosiderin deposition, and chronic inflammation are frequent accompaniments. Osseous metaplasia may be seen in fibrous areas. The lesions do not have a storiform pattern but may contain foam cells. Mitoses are unusual,

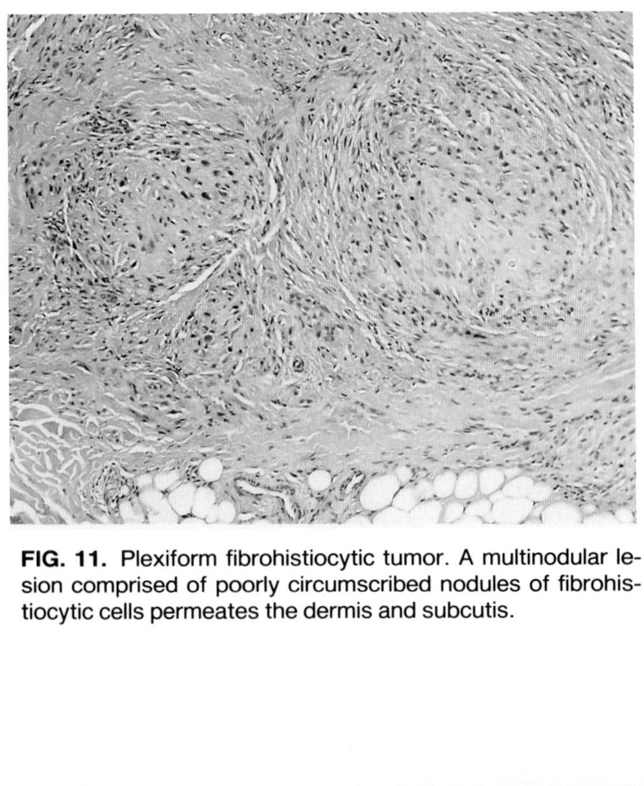

FIG. 11. Plexiform fibrohistiocytic tumor. A multinodular lesion comprised of poorly circumscribed nodules of fibrohistiocytic cells permeates the dermis and subcutis.

but may be found in small numbers; vascular invasion may be seen as well. Necrosis is not a feature of these tumors.

Immunoperoxidase stains of plexiform fibrohistiocytic tumors show positive results for α_1-antitrypsin and α_1-antichymotrypsin but negativity for S-100 protein (79). Immunohistochemical analysis of these lesions has also revealed positivity for smooth muscle actin. This finding in combination with ultrastructural findings indicates that it is a myofibroblastic lesion. On the other hand, evidence that bone marrow–derived histiocytes form a substantial part of these tumors is slim (119).

The lesion was cured by adequate local excision in two thirds of the cases reported by Enzinger and Zhang (79). Further surgery was required in one third of cases for local recurrence. In two patients regional lymph node metastases occurred subsequent to the development of local relapse. One patient was alive and well after 10 months, whereas the second patient was lost to follow-up. No other metastases were noted in this series.

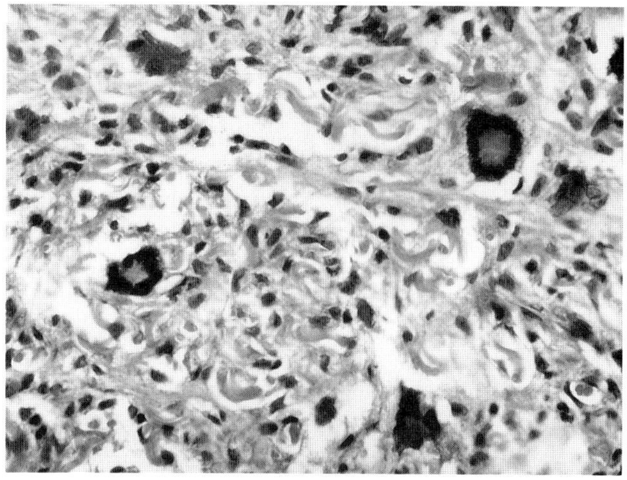

FIG. 12. Juvenile xanthogranuloma. This fibrohistiocytic lesion contains Touton giant cells with multiple nuclei arrayed in peripheral wreaths.

Juvenile Xanthogranuloma

Juvenile xanthogranulomas have been reported under a variety of synonyms, including congenital xanthoma multiplex, nevoxanthoma, and nevoxanthoendothelioma (169,170). They usually present as skin nodules, either solitary or multiple, in young children aged 6 months to 2 years. Fifteen percent occur in adults. Both sexes are affected equally. Solitary lesions are twice as common as multiple ones. Juvenile xanthogranulomas most commonly affect the head and neck (123) or extremities (54). They may also present as deep soft tissue masses within either subcutaneous tissue or skeletal muscle and rarely involve organs such as the lung, eye, epicardium, oral cavity, and testis (123).

Grossly, the deep juvenile xanthogranuloma is a firm, yellow–tan mass with a fairly well-circumscribed border. This macroscopic picture is reflected by the lesion's microscopic composition of sheets of polygonal, mononuclear, histiocytic cells and variable numbers of eosinophils, lymphocytes, and plasma cells, intersected by a delicate capillary network. Many, but not all, juvenile xanthogranulomas contain Touton-type giant cells. Touton giant cells are distinctive large multinucleated cells whose nuclei form a peripheral wreath (Fig. 12). Janney et al. (123) noted that deep-seated tumors differed slightly from dermal cases by showing more circumscription, fewer Touton giant cells, and abundant eosinophils.

By electron microscopy, the Birbeck granules typical of Langerhans cell histiocytosis are not seen in juvenile xanthogranuloma (54). With immunohistochemistry the tumor cells generally stain for HAM-56, muscle-specific actin (HHF-35), and vimentin, but not for S-100 protein, MAC-387, or Factor XIIIa (123). However, single cases reported by De Graaf (54) and O'Laughlin et al. (196) did stain with MAC-387. These findings indicate phenotypic similarity to myofibroblastic cells, monocyte-derived cells, and fixed tissue macrophages such as tingible body macrophages, interdigitating dendritic cells, and Kupffer cells. Conversely, the negative stain for Factor XIIIa indicates a lack of kinship with dermal dendrocytes. Janney et al. (123) thus concluded that juvenile xanthogranuloma may be derived from a migrant population of macrophagic myofibroblasts. De Graaf et al. (54) noted CD1a staining in the tumor cells. This antibody stains Langerhans cells, which contain Birbeck granules (see Chapter 16) and dermal indeterminate cells, which lack them. The latter cells are thought to represent precursors of Langerhans cells. De Graaf thus postulated that the cells of juvenile xanthogranuloma are of indeterminate cell lineage because the tumors also stain with CD1a, do not stain with S-100, and do not have Birbeck granules. O'Laughlin et al. (196) found that the cells in juvenile xanthogranuloma lacked antigens detected by the 25F9 antibody and showed no expression of CD16, CD35, or CD21, in contrast to the histiocytes in most other tested lesions.

These lesions, both in skin and deeper soft tissues, are clinically indolent and do not recur even if incompletely excised. In fact, they often undergo spontaneous regression (54). One of De Graaf's cases (54) had hypercalcemia but no increase in serum parathormone.

Xanthoma

Xanthomas occur as deep soft tissue masses or skin lesions and consist of aggregates of macrophages with foamy cytoplasm and in some instances with extracellular cholesterol. Xanthomas are not true neoplasms (78).

Xanthomas are frequently associated with various types of hyperlipidemia and are divided into eruptive, tuberous, tendinous, plane, and xanthelasmatous types. The eruptive form frequently involves the buttocks, arises acutely as multiple skin papules, and consists histologically of sheets of nonfoamy macrophages with a few foamy macrophages and inflammatory cells. The tuberous and tendinous forms consist of aggregates of foamy macrophages, an inflammatory infiltrate, extracellular cholesterol, and, in older lesions, fibrosis. They involve the subcutaneous and tendinous tissues, respectively. The tendinous form may be associated with the syndrome of cerebrotendinous xanthomatosis in which lipids are deposited in the brain, causing ataxia and other central nervous system (CNS) signs and symptoms. The plane xanthoma and xanthelasma consist of sheets of foamy macrophages, without fibrosis or inflammation. They both arise in either normolipemic or hyperlipemic individuals. Plane xanthoma occurs in the skin creases, particularly the palms.

It is important to biopsy deeper lesions adequately, as other lesions such as giant cell tumor, pigmented villonodular synovitis, and even sarcomas may contain sheets of foam cells. These latter lesions should not be confused with xanthomas, which usually require only conservative treatment (78) and may even slowly respond to dietary measures.

Deposition of lipid in the soft tissues in these conditions proceeds via the bloodstream (208) and is probably facilitated by increased permeability of vessels as occurs at sites of repetitive local trauma (78). All types of xanthomas occur with type III hyperlipidemia, whereas eruptive xanthomas do not occur with type II disease, only eruptive and tendinous xanthomas occur with type IV disease, and only eruptive xanthomas occur with type V disease (78).

Tenosynovial Giant Cell Tumor

Tenosynovial giant cell tumor comprises a controversial group of lesions that are uncommon in children under 10 years (55). They involve both intra- and extra-articular locations and may be further classified as localized or diffuse tenosynovial giant cell tumor or localized or diffuse pigmented villonodular synovitis. Localized tenosynovial giant cell tumors (also known as giant cell tumors of tendon sheath) most commonly involve the fingers, originating in the tendon sheaths of the interphalangeal joints and forming well demarcated, lobulated, soft tissue nodules. They are composed of varying proportions of rounded or polygonal histiocytes, foam cells, siderophages, and osteoclast-type giant cells. Varying degrees of fibrosis may be seen. Localized tenosynovial giant cell tumors are partially encapsulated, unlike the diffuse form, but may recur in 10–15% of cases after local excision (55). When they are highly cellular with prominent mitotic activity, they may be confused with malignant tumors.

Diffuse tenosynovial giant cell tumors are the most aggressive of the group. They invade the extra-articular tissues, sometimes without involving adjacent joints; presumably they arise in a bursa in these situations. Diffuse tenosynovial giant cell tumors may become large and destroy adjacent structures such as bone. Histologically, they are cellular and contain less osteoclast-type giant cells than localized lesions. Cleftlike spaces may be seen, and there may be prominent mitotic activity. Blood vessel invasion has a similar connotation to that occurring in giant cell tumors of bone and does not indicate a propensity for bloodborne metastasis (1). Although they are locally aggressive, only an exceptionally rare case of diffuse tenosynovial giant cell tumor has metastasized (78). However, in one study (1) three of seven cases were aneuploid, a point in favor of the present consensus that these are neoplastic lesions. Fairly radical excision, even amputation, may be required in some cases for tumor control. Diffuse tenosynovial giant cell tumor tends to occur at a younger age than other members of the group. Unlike the localized lesions that predominantly affect the fingers, diffuse tumors involve larger weight-bearing joints such as the knee, sacroiliac joint, or ankle (1).

Pigmented villonodular synovitis, diffuse-type, is a lesion of the synovium of large joints. This term should be confined only to articular lesions (1) to distinguish them from the more aggressive extra-articular diffuse tenosynovial giant cell tumor. Trisomy 7 has been identified in one case (221), supporting the neoplastic nature of these lesions. However, trisomy 7 mosaicism also has been noted in short-term cultures of normal tissues (221). It is of interest that the oncogenes c-*erb* B, which codes for the EGF receptor, and c-*sis,* which codes for PDGF, are both located on chromosome 7 (221).

Pigmented villonodular synovitis, localized type, is a nodular intra-articular lesion with the same cytologic composition as the giant cell tumor of tendon sheath. It is localized and therefore more resectable than the diffuse lesions.

Rarely, frankly malignant tenosynovial giant cell tumors have been described. To make this diagnosis, the malignancy must arise from an associated or previously resected benign tenosynovial giant cell tumor (78).

Benign Cartilaginous Lesions of Soft Tissue

Benign chondromas of soft tissue occur in children, particularly during the second decade (213). The vast majority (96%) occur in the hands and feet (29), and they occasionally are found around the knee (213). They are solitary nodules associated with tendons, tendon sheaths, joint capsules, or synovium. Histologically they may be cellular and atypical, so that care must be taken not to mistake them for chondrosarcoma.

Vascular Lesions

The term "benign vascular tumor" refers to a benign mass-forming lesion in which there is an increase in normal- or abnormal-appearing vessels (78). The contents of its constituent vascular channels generally determines whether the lesion is classified as a hemangioma or a lymphangioma (35). These tumors constitute 25% of all soft tissue masses in childhood, and the vast majority of them are benign. They involve many sites, such as the skin, somatic soft tissues, liver, spleen, and parotid gland (22). There is a wide diversity of lesional types (Table 2).

The question has been raised for decades as to whether hemangiomas represent hamartomatous lesions or true neoplasms. Willis (297) was of the opinion that these are hamartomatous dysmorphogenetic lesions that grow because of their blood flow-related expansile nature. Certainly they are not derived exclusively of one cell type, as pericytes (191), adipose tissue (220,306), and even glomus cells (220) may form integral parts of these lesions. This phenomenon indicates either a field defect affecting multiple cell types or, more unlikely, a lesion in a primitive cell capable of multipotential differentiation. At times vascular overgrowths may occur in association with other tumors, particularly in the central nervous system (68), perhaps as a result of the secretion of tumor-related angiogenesis factors (13).

Regardless of whether they are neoplasms or congenital anomalies, vascular tumors and malformations form a prominent component of a number of inheritable syndromes and are the dominant manifestation of some (210,217,223,238). Table 3 lists some of the genetic conditions associated with these lesions. Some of these conditions, such as von Hippel–Lindau disease, Cowden's syndrome, and Sturge–Weber syndrome, are associated with a propensity to develop tumors affecting other cell types, such as carcinomas or gliomas. Congenital vascular lesions may also appear as a result of an intrauterine accident rather than a genetic mishap, as indicated by their occasional occurrence in only one of monozygotic twins (245). They may result in untoward somatic effects such as limb defects (86a) or pathophysiologic abnormalities such as intravascular coagulation (Kassabach–Merritt syndrome) (306). Although angiomas usually show no histologic progression (220) and may in certain manifestations even progress to sclerosis (223), occasional angiosarcomas can arise in connection with these congenital defects (275).

In contradistinction to certain benign fibrous tumors (see above), steroid hormones do not appear to play a role in the development of hemangiomas (191).

TABLE 2. *Benign vascular lesions of childhood*

Hemangiomas
Capillary
Cavernous
Venous
Arteriovenous
Angiomatosis
Targetoid hemosiderotic hemangioma
Tufted angioma
Epithelioid hemangioma
Lobular hemangioma
Intramuscular hemangioma
Angiomyomatous hamartoma
Synovial hemangioma
Neural hemangioma
Diffuse (systemic) hemangiomatosis
Lymphangiomas
Benign lymphangioendothelioma
Lymphangiomatosis
Glomus tumor

TABLE 3. *Genetic conditions associated with vascular malformations*

von Hippel–Lindau disease
Familial angiomatosis of soft tissues
Aicardi syndrome
Bannayan–Zonona syndrome
Familial nevi flammei
Familial angiomatosis of bones
Blue rubber-bleb-nevus syndrome
Cowden's syndrome
Sturge–Weber syndrome
Ataxia-telangiectasia
Proteus syndrome
Familial cavernous malformations

Hemangiomas

Capillary Hemangiomas

Capillary hemangiomas composed 32% of vascular tumors in one series (35). Most of these are present at birth or early in life, occurring on the skin and mucous membranes of the head and neck (Fig. 13; see figure in color plate section) and in the parotid gland (193). They tend to disappear spontaneously, two thirds having regressed by 7 years (193). As the lesions persist their vascular channels become wider, with thrombi tending to form and organize. It is this process that is thought to explain the spontaneous involution of this form of hemangioma (35).

Immature Hemangioma

Immature hemangiomas form solid cellular masses in which there may be only focal formation of vascular channels, sometimes making the angiomatous nature of the lesion difficult to recognize. Worse yet, they may be mitotically active and therefore mistaken for a malignant tumor (Fig. 14). Focal spindle cell growth added to the solid areas may be mistaken for Kaposi's sarcoma (22). Immature hemangiomas tend to form more vascular channels with time and eventually undergo fibrosis and regression (193). Gonzalez-Crussi and Reyes-Mugica (104) have shown that these lesions contain Factor XIIIa–positive spindle cells, thought to be collagen-associated dendrocytes (192) and located outside the vascular structures. They also contain many mast cells that probably exert angiogenic stimuli (104). By electron microscopy immature hemangiomas do not show Weibel–Palade bodies, but the endothelial cells do contain dense, paracrystalline intracytoplasmic inclusions (104). The vascular channels can be outlined by PAS and reticulin stains, the endothelium is positive for Factor VIII–related antigen and binds *Ulex europaeus*-1 lectin, and the surrounding pericytes stain with actin antibodies (22).

Mature Hemangioma

Mature hemangiomas are easily recognized as vascular tumors by virtue of their content of small, open, blood-filled capillaries. These lesions tend to occur in older infants and young children (35).

Cavernous Hemangioma

Cavernous hemangiomas may occur in childhood, usually during the second decade (35) but also later in life (193). They tend to be larger than capillary hemangiomas and are either localized or more diffuse. The upper part of the body is affected more frequently, and the lesions may occur in the deep soft tissues. Cavernous hemangiomas are the major type of hemangioma affecting the liver, intestine, bone, and skeletal muscle. They do not regress as frequently as do capillary hemangiomas (126).

Histologically, cavernous hemangiomas consist of large, dilated, thin-walled, erythrocyte-laden vessels. The walls occasionally may contain areas of fibrosis and even smooth muscle (193), and the lesions may have an associated capillary component.

Venous Hemangioma

Venous hemangiomas occur predominantly in adults (193), but Weiss (289) recently described a form of this lesion in the feet of two children with Turner's syndrome. The tumors consisted of large, misshapen, thick-walled veins with endothelial webs or miniature vessels replacing the vascular lumina as well as herniation of the endothelium through the muscle coat into the adventitia. The mural thickening may be due to either arteriovenous shunting with increased intraluminal pressure or malformative development.

Arteriovenous Hemangioma (Cirsoid Aneurysm)

Arteriovenous hemangiomas are composed of a conglomerate of medium or large arteries with thick walls and veins. The superficial type, also known as acral arteriovenous tumor, occurs on the head, especially the face, and is not usually associated with shunting (193). The deep type may contain proliferating capillaries in addition to the arteries and veins and conversely often presents signs of shunting of blood. Deep arteriovenous hemangiomas occur in young people and are considered

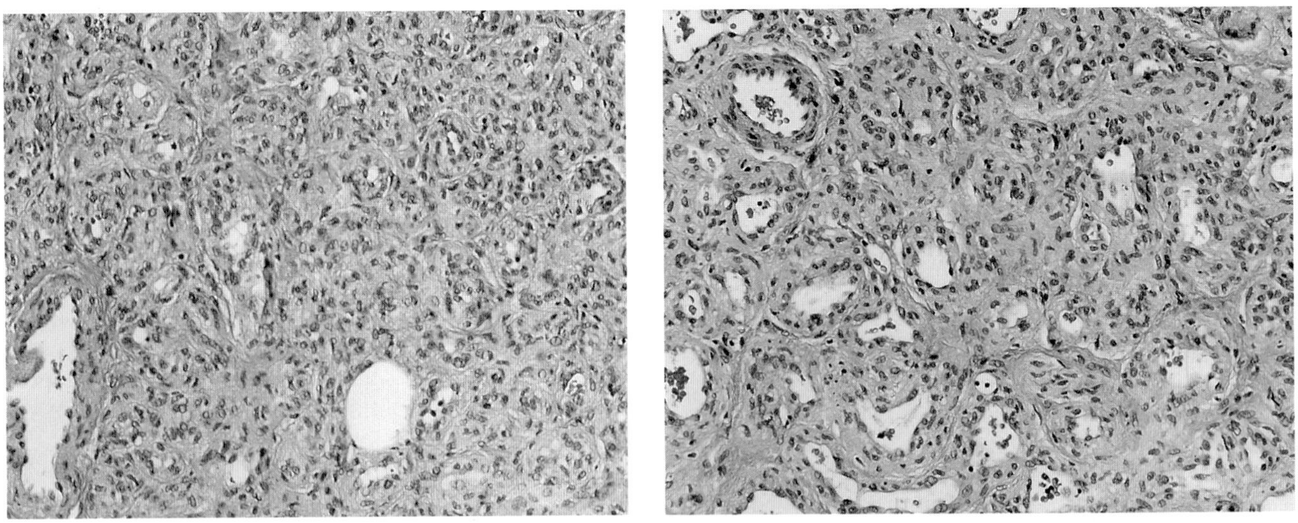

A B

FIG. 14. Immature hemangioma. **A.** Portions of this congenital lesion contain cellular areas with marked endothelial cell proliferation, inapparent lumina, and occasional feeder vessels. **B.** In other areas the vascular nature of the lesion is more apparent.

to be a congenital malformation rather than a true neoplasm. They are located almost exclusively about the face and neck and within the central nervous system. The diagnosis is not easy by pathology alone but usually requires attention to clinical and diagnostic imaging findings that delineate the type of circulation and the extent of the lesion. When there is shunting, the veins are varicose and thick-walled. These lesions may contain spindled microscopic foci resembling Kaposi's sarcoma (165).

Angiomatosis of Soft Tissue

Angiomatosis of soft tissue represented 4% of childhood vascular tumors in Coffin and Dehner's series (35). Approximately equal numbers occur in the first and second decades. Angiomatosis is a histologically benign lesion that extensively involves a body region or several different tissue types in a contiguous fashion (78). Involvement may be of two types: extensive vertical involvement of multiple tissue planes or extensive involvement of tissues of the same type (220). Most cases of angiomatosis have occurred during childhood and probably began in utero or the neonatal period. The most common sites of involvement are the extremities and trunk (Fig. 15).

Two histologic patterns were noted in the series of Rao and Weiss (220). The first is a haphazard proliferation of vessels of varying sizes, particularly veins with large attenuated walls and intimal redundancies. The most distinctive feature in this type is the presence of clusters of capillary vessels residing within or just adjacent to vein walls. Tumors having the second pattern display clusters of capillary-sized vessels that infiltrate the soft tissues and often contain a large central vessel. Both types of the lesion contain large amounts of fat, suggesting that the responsible abnormality is a generalized mesenchymal disturbance rather than a purely vascular lesion. No case progressed to sarcoma in the series of Rao and Weiss (220), but there was a high recurrence rate of nearly 90%. Proper management requires balancing the need to cure against the excessive morbidity of total excision.

Targetoid Hemosiderotic Hemangioma

Targetoid hemosiderotic hemangiomas affect the trunk or extremities of young or middle-aged individuals, predominantly males. They present as small, solitary, circular lesions measuring less than 1 cm (274). The reference to targets is an apt one, as the lesions contain a raised, purple center surrounded by successively clear and ecchymotic haloes that expand centrifugally over time.

Histologically, targetoid hemosiderotic hemangiomas contain irregularly dilated vascular channels lined by epithelioid endothelial cells that focally form papillary projections. There are also narrow, anastomosing, lymphaticlike vascular channels that dissect dermal collagen and concentrate around sweat glands (274). The endothelial cells of the lymphaticlike channels are flat. Extravasated erythrocytes and siderophages are often present. In its late phase the lesion is composed almost exclusively of narrow, empty, thin-walled, anastomosing channels located in the dermis and hypodermis. Collapse of the vascular lumina can create the impression of fibroblastic proliferation.

Tufted Angioma

Tufted angiomas occur in infants and young children of either sex as a slowly growing erythematous macule, plaque, or cluster of papules. They are particularly prone to arise on the neck or upper trunk but may also occur on an extremity. Tufted angiomas do not regress but rather progressively enlarge up to 10 cm or more. They are often painful on palpation (274).

Histologically, tufted angiomas appear to be a variant of the lobular hemangioma described below. They con-

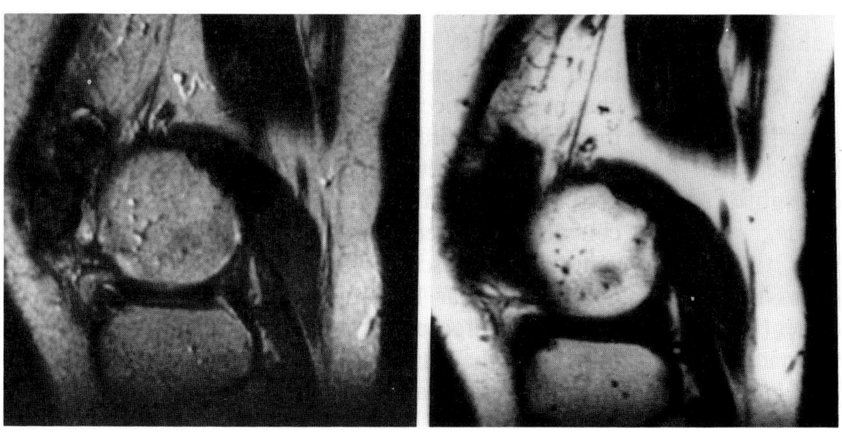

FIG. 15. Angiomatosis of soft tissue. Congeries of abnormal dilated vessels traverse the lower thigh and knee region on these MR images, creating a soft tissue mass medial to the patella. (Courtesy of Drs. Ravi Bhargava and Barry Fletcher, St. Jude Children's Research Hospital.)

volve the affected area, which includes skin, subcutis, and even bone. The vessels are thin-walled and accompanied by large amounts of mature fat. They are not usually associated with local edema but rather shunt large amounts of blood causing complications such as cardiac failure.

Diffuse hemangiomatosis may cause death in neonates because of its space-occupying effects or associated consumption coagulopathy. In older patients the lesions are prone to recur after excision.

Lymphangiomas

Lymphangiomas composed 26% of the pediatric vascular tumors in Coffin and Dehner's series (35). Eighty-six percent occurred in the first decade. Most involve the head and neck, the latter being the site of cystic hygroma, a synonymous lesion. Others may occur within the mesentery (Fig. 18). Most cases in Coffin and Dehner's series (35) were poorly demarcated. They may be very large, up to 15 cm. Histologically they consist of thin-walled vascular channels lined by a single layer of flattened endothelial cells and surrounded by lymphoid aggregates. The vascular channels may take on a slitlike appearance, particularly in recurrent lesions.

Benign Lymphangioendothelioma

Benign lymphangioendothelioma, or progressive lymphangioma, is a rare benign tumor of lymph vessels that histologically mimics low-grade angiosarcoma (274). Often it is been present for many years before the patient seeks clinical advice. Macroscopically the lesion is a pink or reddish brown macule or plaque that tends to enlarge with time. These neoplasms may be large (e.g., 30 cm) but are cured by excision.

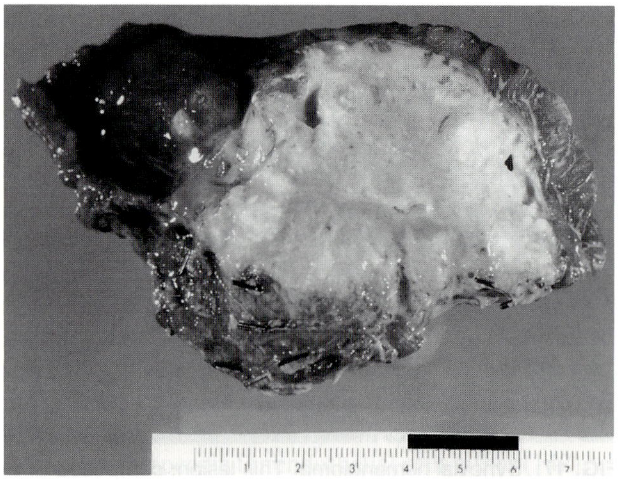

FIG. 18. Mesenteric lymphangioma. This pale yellow, ill-defined lesion abuts the jejunum **(top and right)** and exudes a milky fluid.

Histologically benign lymphangioendothelioma occurs in the upper dermis and may extend into the deeper dermis. The lesion consists of thin-walled spaces lined by endothelium that is horizontally oriented in the superficial field of involvement. In the deeper areas the vessels dissect the collagen similar to an angiosarcoma, but there is no atypia or cellular tuft formation (274). The differential diagnosis also includes Kaposi's sarcoma, but lymphangioendotheliomas are solitary lesions containing no erythrocytes or hemosiderin and few plasma cells.

Lymphangiomatosis

Lymphangiomatosis is a disorder characterized by a multifocal proliferation of lymphatic channels lined by benign endothelial cells and diffusely involving bone and/or soft tissues in children or young adults (218). The patients do well if only bone is involved (except cervical vertebrae), but they have a worse outlook if vital organs are affected, particularly serosal surfaces and viscera. In the series of Ramani and Shah (218) the endothelial cells stained with Factor VIII–related antigen and CD31 were only scantily positive with *Ulex europaeus*-1 and were negative with CD34. The differential diagnosis includes lymphangioleiomyomatosis, persistent interstitial pulmonary emphysema, and pulmonary lymphangiectasia.

Glomus Tumor

Glomus tumors are uncommon in childhood, composing 1% of pediatric vascular tumors in Coffin and Dehner's series (35). They are well known in adults as small, painful tumors that typically occur subungually on the fingers. Glomangiomas consist of masses of uniform, round cells with round nuclei and eosinophilic cytoplasm associated with vascular lumina. These cells may blend into smooth muscle cells within the lesion, and if this is prominent the tumor may be termed a glomangiomyoma. If the vascular spaces are prominent and large, the lesion is termed a glomangioma. The latter lesions tend to be multicentric and to occur at sites other than the typical subungual location.

Intravascular Papillary Hyperplasia

Intravascular papillary hyperplasia, also known as Masson's pseudoangiosarcoma or Masson's vegetant intravascular hemangioendothelioma, occurred particularly on the fingers of boys in the second decade in the series of Coffin and Dehner (35). These lesions represent a form of organizing thrombus in an ectatic vessel. They form a small, purplish, rubbery mass that histologically consists of papillae of endothelial cells confined to the lumen of the involved vessel (Fig. 19). There is no necrosis, invasion, or atypia of the cells. The lesions may be mistaken for an angiosarcoma if their intravascular location is not appreciated, and they may extend beyond the parent vessel into surrounding tissue with rupture of the vessel. Some occur within hematomas.

Smooth Muscle Lesions

Vascular Leiomyoma

Vascular leiomyomas are solitary tumors involving the skin and subcutaneous tissue. They are more common in females and are frequently painful. They form discreet, firm, rubbery nodules that consist of vascular channels surrounded by abundant benign smooth muscle. Geddy et al. (98) recently examined the lesions for mast cells and nerves in an attempt to explain the cause of pain. The painful lesions had fewer mast cells than the nonpainful lesions, but all contained small nerves. They thus hypothesized that mechanisms similar to those seen in the triple response (ie, release of substance P from sensory nerves, close contact between nerves and mast cells, and mast cell degranulation) may explain the pain. The lower number of mast cells in the painful lesions may have been caused by active degranulation due to increased mast cell activity.

Nerve Sheath Lesions

In a series of 139 peripheral neurogenic tumors of soft tissues in 122 children and adolescents, Coffin and Dehner (33) found that 60% were benign and 40% were malignant.

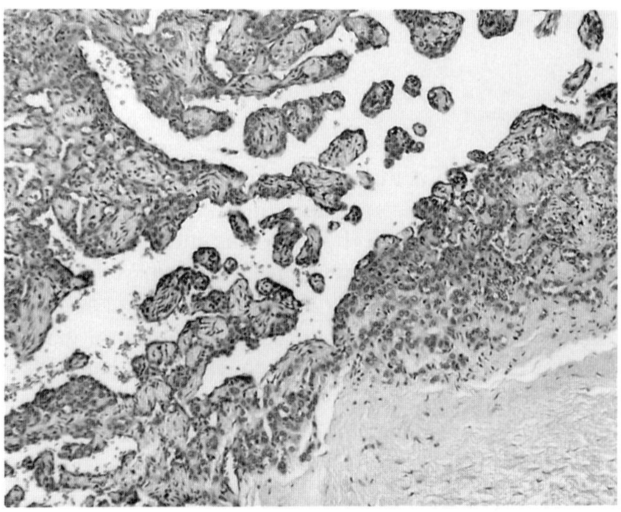

FIG. 19. Intravascular papillary hyperplasia. Papillae lined by bland endothelial cells project into the lumen of this vessel.

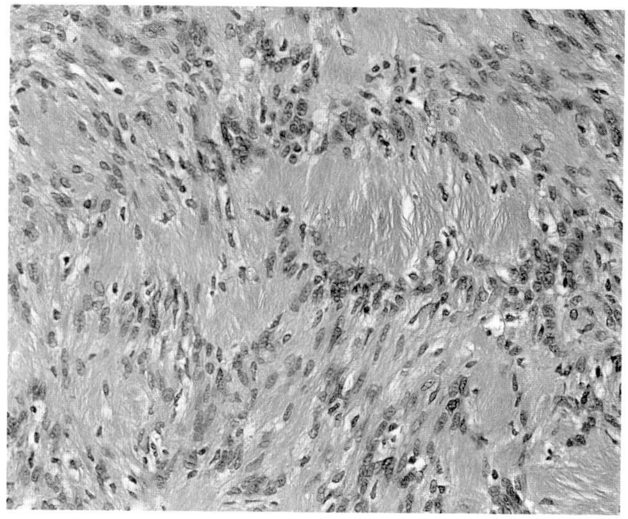

FIG. 20. Schwannoma. Verocay bodies, comprised of rows of palisaded nuclei separated by anuclear zones, are prominent in this lesion.

Schwannoma

Schwannomas, or neurilemmomas, are tumors composed exclusively of cells with the ultrastructure and immunostaining properties of Schwann cells (299). They primarily occur during the middle decades and affect women more often than men. Schwannomas are unusual in children, comprising only 5% of the neurogenic tumors in Coffin and Dehner's series (33). Schwannomas are usually solitary and affect the head and neck and flexor surfaces of the upper and lower extremities, a common site being the acoustic nerve. The latter lesions may occur as part of neurofibromatosis type 2 in which they are bilateral (193).

Grossly schwannoma is a rubbery, well-demarcated mass involving small and medium-sized nerves, although often no nerve is identified (299). Foci of hemorrhage and lipid deposits are often seen (299). They may rarely be plexiform (5%) (78).

Histologically schwannoma is encapsulated and consists of two tissue patterns: a dense, compact growth of spindle cells with areas of nuclear palisading (Antoni type A), and loose, less orderly, myxoid tissue consisting of cells that are widely separated and have multiple, slender processes (Antoni type B). The two patterns occur in varying proportions. Another characteristic feature is the Verocay body, which is made up of at least two rows of palisaded nuclei separated by an anuclear zone (Fig. 20). Nuclear hyperchromatism may be seen as may scattered mitotic figures, but these tumors are almost invariably benign, with only rare cases of malignant transformation having been described (299). It is thus important to separate them from neurofibroma, in which mitoses may portend a more ominous prognosis. The vessels in schwannoma tend to be large and have thick, hyalinized walls. They may contain organizing thrombi. Schwannomas that have been present for a long time (so-called ancient schwannomas) may contain degenerative changes such as nuclear pleomorphism and hyperchromatism that mimic malignancy, but mitoses are absent. Schwannomas stain for S-100 protein more strongly and consistently than neurofibromas (78).

By electron microscopy, the spindle cells of schwannoma have long intertwining processes enveloped by a prominent basal lamina in Antoni A areas and a fragmented basal lamina in Antoni B areas (78,80). The cells form pseudomesaxons that wrap around collagen fibers or other tumor cells, as there are no axons present. Luse bodies may be found in the stroma (157); these consist of long-spaced collagen but are not specific for neurogenic tumors. Skeinoid fibers have also been described in neurogenic tumors and neurogenic gut stromal tumors (181). Skeinoid fibers consist of eosinophilic, stromal masses that are PAS-positive and are composed of tangles of curved 45-nm fibers with indistinct borders and alternating light and dark cross-bands with a 41- to 48-nm periodicity.

Cellular Schwannoma

Like the usual schwannoma, cellular schwannoma primarily is a tumor of middle-aged adults, but it does occur in children (90,294). It presents as either an asymptomatic mass or pain or nerve dysfunction, and it occurs most commonly in the paravertebral region, retroperitoneum, pelvis, or mediastinum (294). Cellular schwannomas grossly resemble typical schwannomas, may be infiltrative or cystic with hemorrhage, but with few exceptions do not have necrosis. A few cases are associated with neurofibromatosis type 1 (294,300). Some cases have associated bony erosion.

Histologically, cellular schwannomas are densely cellular tumors that do not contain the Verocay bodies seen in typical schwannomas. However, nuclear palisading may be seen. The cellularity, occasional presence of nuclear hyperchromatism, and mitotic activity make them difficult to distinguish from sarcoma. The cells are arranged in fascicles and may even have a storiform pattern. Cellular whorls are seen in one fourth of the cases. Cellular schwannomas may resemble smooth muscle tumors, but the nuclei of the former lesion are wavy, thin, and tapered, unlike those of smooth muscle cells (90). Myxoid change is seen, and in a few cases it may be marked. Mitotic activity may be present, but it was never more than 5 per 20 high-power fields in Fletcher's series and never atypical (90). Circumscribed nongeographic areas of necrosis may be seen (294). Nuclear pleomorphism may be focally present, usually associated with degeneration such as hyalinization or cyst formation, but not with mitoses. Cellular schwannoma may be quite vascular, and the hyalinization of the vessels may furnish an important clue to the lesion's benignity (90). The tumor itself may also contain areas of hyalinization. Antoni B areas typical of schwannomas are also helpful in recognition of this difficult lesion. Peripheral aggregates of lymphocytes are often conspicuous, and usually mast cells are scattered throughout the tumor, sometimes with lymphocytes or aggregates of foamy macrophages.

Cellular schwannomas almost invariably stain with S-100 protein antibodies, a very useful feature in differential diagnosis (90). A proportion will also stain with Leu 7, myelin basic protein, and epithelial membrane antigen (294). The differentiation of these lesions from malignancies is critical, as cellular schwannomas may recur if incompletely excised, but never metastasize (294,300). The rounded gross appearance, presence of Antoni B areas, foamy macrophages, and lymphocytes should alert one to the possibility of a benign cellular schwannoma.

Psammomatous Melanotic Schwannoma

Psammomatous melanotic schwannoma is a black, melanin-containing Schwann cell tumor that frequently also contains psammoma bodies. It stains with S-100 protein antibodies and has been reported to stain with antimelanoma antibody, HMB-45. Psammomatous melanotic schwannoma occurs over a wide age range, particularly involves the spinal nerve roots and soft tissues, but also has been reported in the stomach, heart, and acoustic nerve (131). Most such schwannomas are indolent in their behavior, but some recur and a few patients have died with metastatic tumor. Carney (16) reported a familial complex of psammomatous melanotic schwannomas, cardiac and cutaneous myxomas, spotty pigmentation (lentigines and blue nevi), pigmented nodular adrenocortical disease, and large cell calcifying Sertoli cell tumors of the testis. The tumors were multiple in 19% of cases.

Neurofibroma

Neurofibroma is the most common tumor of peripheral nerves and occurs most frequently as a sporadic, solitary, cutaneous lesion. It is also the most common tumor seen in patients with neurofibromatosis 1, or von Recklinghausen's disease (299). Neurofibromatosis 1 is one of the most common autosomal dominant genetic diseases and has an estimated frequency of 1 per 2,500–3,300 births (166). The diagnosis of neurofibromatosis 1 is derived from a constellation of clinical signs (Table 4). The neurofibromas in neurofibromatosis 1 are frequently larger and affect large, deep-seated nerves more frequently than those seen in sporadic cases (299). Neurofibromatosis type 1 is also associated with a higher in-

TABLE 4. *Diagnosis of neurofibromatosis 1*[a]

1. On examination in room light, at least five cafe-au-lait macules over 5 mm in greatest diameter; if prepubertal, six cafe-au-lait macules over 15 mm in greatest diameter
2. Based on clinical or histologic grounds, two or more neurofibromas of any type, or one plexiform neurofibroma
3. Multiple freckles in the axillary or inguinal regions
4. Sphenoid wing dysplasia or congenital bowing or thinning of long-bone cortex, with or without pseudoarthrosis
5. Bilateral optic pathway gliomas
6. Two or more iris Lisch nodules on slit-lamp examination
7. A first-degree relative (parent, sibling, or offspring) with von Recklinghausen's neurofibromatosis, by the above criteria

[a] Two or more findings must be present, provided that no other disease could be the cause of the findings.
(From *Neurofibromatosis Research Newsletter,* Ref. 188.)

cidence of CNS gliomas, optic nerve gliomas, rhabdomyosarcomas, malignant peripheral nerve sheath tumors, and acute myelogenous leukemia. One percent of gliomas, 12% of optic gliomas, and 31% of neurofibrosarcomas in Matsui's series (166) were associated with neurofibromatosis type 1. Neurofibromatosis type 2, which is usually not recognized in childhood, is genotypically characterized by alterations in chromosome 22 and phenotypically distinguished by bilateral acoustic schwannomas, intracranial or spinal cord meningiomas, and spinal cord ependymomas (see Chapter 7) (300).

The neurofibroma is composed of a variety of cell types including perineuriallike cells, cells intermediate between fibroblasts and perineurial cells, and Schwann cells (300). The lesion is typically permeated by axons, in contradistinction to the schwannoma, which pushes them aside. Neurofibromas stain for Factor XIIIa and S-100 protein (300). The tumor cells grow along the nerves causing fusiform rather than globoid swelling (Fig. 21A; see figure in color plate section). When multiple nerves are involved, the lesion is plexiform in appearance. The tumor cells may extend outside small nerves into the surrounding tissues to form nodules in the skin, or diffuse neurofibromas may involve large areas causing localized gigantism. No fat deposits are noted on the cut surface (cf. nerve sheath hamartoma).

Histologically neurofibromas consist of delicate cells with angulated, pointed nuclei. The cells lie between separated bands of collagen and varying amounts of myxoid matrix (Fig. 21B). The tumors may be densely collagenized. Mast cells are frequently present but are not specific.

Neurofibromas, particularly those associated with neurofibromatosis and occurring in large deep-seated nerves, are prone to malignant change.

Neurofibroma cells elaborate an abundant extracellular matrix that produces either a myxoid or a fibrous appearance in histologic sections. Expression of the genes producing extracellular matrix proteins, collagen, fibronectin, and laminin is variable among the three cell types (122). Production of a basal lamina, which is a key ultrastructural feature, is dependent on the cell composition (122), as Schwann cells and perineurial cells are the primary manufacturers of the basement membrane–related proteins, type IV collagen, and laminin. Expression of the c-*kit* gene, which encodes the receptor for the hematopoietic stem cell factor, SCF, is also increased in neurofibroma cells (116). SCF induces the development of mast cells, so that this observation indicates a possible mechanism for the increased numbers of mast cells seen in these tumors.

Neurofibromatosis type 1 (NF1) is characterized by a high spontaneous mutation rate (3) and a susceptibility to various tumors, including nonneural neoplasms such as rhabdomyosarcoma and leukemia (166). Using the technique of positional cloning (101), the gene responsible for NF1, correspondingly called *NF1,* has been isolated and characterized. This gene, located on chromosome 17q11.2, is quite large, spanning approximately 300,000 base pairs (39,163). This great size accounts for the high spontaneous mutation rate, as the likelihood of having miscoding accidents mathematically increases with the breadth of the susceptible nucleotide span. Thus, a variety of genetic alterations have been recorded (278,286). A few recurring mutations have been found (3,81), indicating that some loci are at increased risk. There is also evidence of parental imprinting, as paternal alleles appear to be affected more often than their maternal counterparts (262). However, this observation is controversial, as other data indicate no parental effect but rather a simple haploid insufficiency of the encoded protein (130). Methylation of nucleosides flanking or within the gene appears to effect its mutability (195). The variable expression of the NF1 phenotype among af-

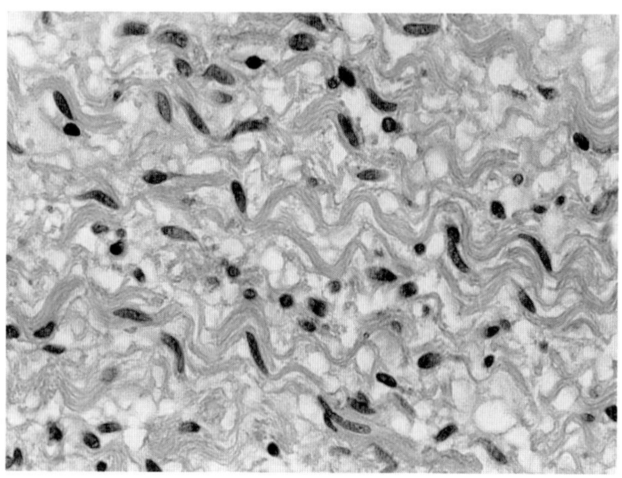

B

FIG. 21. Neurofibroma. **A.** The lesion forms a fusiform, heterogeneous mass (see photo in color plate section). **B (above).** Tumor cells with slender, curved nuclei and wavy cytoplasm are separated by a myxoid matrix.

fected individuals appears to be a result of other as-yet-unidentified "modifying" genes (67).

NF1 encodes a protein known as neurofibromin. This protein appears to be a key link in the second-messenger (or signal transduction) system of molecules that transport receptor-linked signals from the cell membrane to the nucleus. It operates as a guanoside triphosphatase–activating protein, or GAP, by affecting the phosphorylation status of the guanoside triphosphate (GTP) bound to the protein encoded by the *ras* proto-oncogene (101,194). In this manner, the GTP bound to ras is converted to GDP, and ras is inactivated (Fig. 22). The ras protein is a fundamental element in cellular growth and differentiation; thus *ras* acts as an oncogene and *NF1* acts as a tumor suppressor gene (195). Data suggest that neurofibromin may also interact with ras in a GAP-independent manner (125).

Neurofibromin is present in all adult tissues, not just neural tissue, and is highly conserved among species (101,108). In the hamster, it appears to be particularly important for Schwann cell development and differentiation (189). A number of neurofibromatosis patients have mutations in the *NF1* gene resulting in the insertion of a stop codon; as a result the protein is truncated, or shortened, and is thus ineffective (247,278). Other mutations involve insertion or deletion of a base, resulting in a frameshift in the reading of RNA transcripts and formation of a structurally altered neurofibromin molecule (18,39). Neurofibromin appears to be primarily associated with cytoplasmic microtubules (106) and may be altered in malignant peripheral nerve sheath tumors (146,225) as well as unrelated tumors occurring in NF1 patients (150) and in neuroblastomas (268). Recent data suggest that it may even play a critical role as an altered tumor suppressor gene in a variety of sporadic tumors in the general population (244). The complexity of the *NF1* gene creates problems in testing (141), and the potential for confusion is compounded by related sequences (or "pseudogenes") on other chromosomes (147). Nevertheless, gene testing on susceptible individuals may allow detection of affected individuals at a young age prior to the development of the clinically recognized phenotype (117).

Fibrolipomatous Hamartoma of Nerve

Fibrolipomatous hamartoma of nerve, or intraneural lipoma, usually affects the median nerve in the wrist, palm, or finger of patients under 30. There is fusiform enlargement of the nerve by fibrofatty tissue that may be associated with macrodactyly or the carpal tunnel syndrome, but the lesion usually presents as a slowly enlarging mass (299).

Neuromuscular Choristoma

Neuromuscular choristoma (or benign triton tumor) occurs in the brachial plexus of infants and consists of bundles of benign skeletal muscle intermingled with nerve (299).

Perineurioma

Perineurioma is a heretofore rarely documented neoplasm of peripheral nerve. Grossly, it is a well-demarcated, firm mass. Microscopically it consists of spindle cells with markedly elongated, bipolar cell processes separated by abundant collagen or myxoid tissue (273) (Fig. 23). It may be more frequently diagnosed with increasing knowledge that perineurial cells normally stain with epithelial membrane antigen but not with S-100 protein. Perineuriomas recapitulate this staining

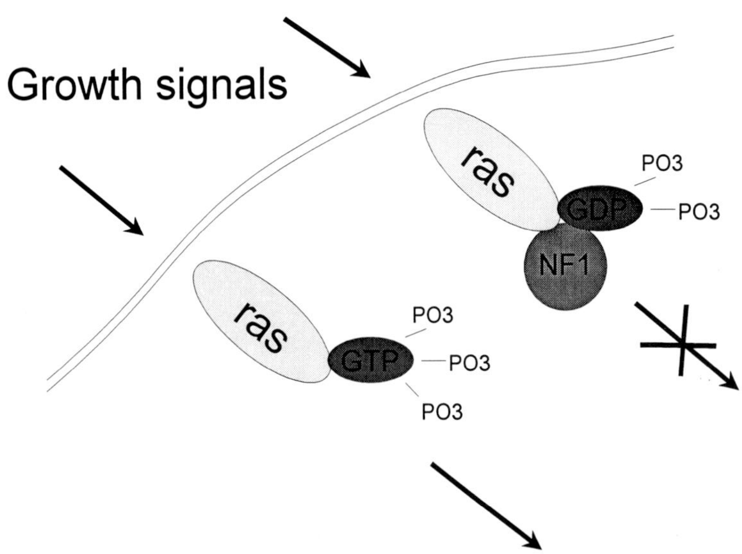

FIG. 22. Schematic diagram of molecular action of NF1 (neurofibromin). The molecule binds to ras, converting the attached GTP to GDP and inactivating the signal transduction pathway.

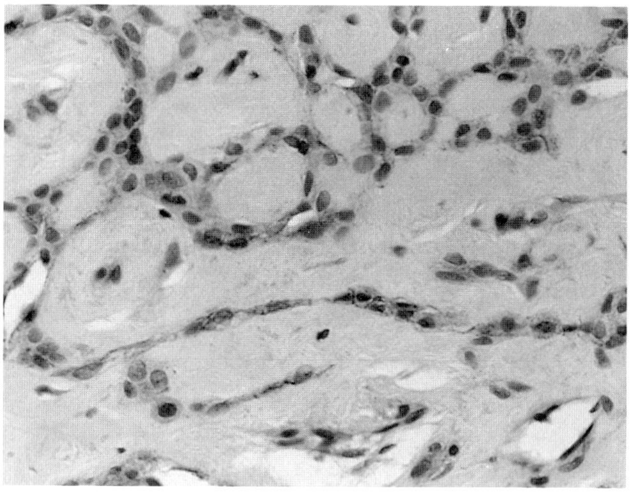

FIG. 23. Perineurioma. Strands of spindle cells circumscribe acellular collagenous areas. The cells were EMA-positive, S-100-negative by immunohistochemistry (not shown).

pattern and also show the typical electron microscopic features of perineurial cells, ie, discontinuous basal lamina, electron-dense cytoplasm, and pinocytotic vesicles (273). Most reported cases have been benign (299), and they have not been associated with neurofibromatosis (273). Rare malignancies have also been reported (115).

Fatty Lesions

Lipoblastoma/Lipoblastomatosis

Lipoblastoma is a tumor of fat that occurs in young children, with 88% being less than 3 years of age (27). The tumor may be either superficial or deep and occurs most commonly on the extremities, as well as in the retroperitoneum, mediastinum, chest wall, and neck (27,174). It may be a well-demarcated lesion, i.e., a lipoblastoma, or a diffuse lesion that permeates adjacent tissue planes or striated muscle, i.e., lipoblastomatosis. The latter lesion is more commonly found in the deep soft tissues. These are benign lesions that may recur if inadequately excised (174). They may show clonal karyotypic changes (236).

The cut surface of these tumors is lobulated and yellow to myxoid in appearance (Fig. 24A). Microscopically lipoblastomas and lipoblastomatosis also have a lobulated appearance, the lobules being separated by fibrous septa and consisting of fat cells in various stages of maturation (Fig. 24B, C). The most mature cells are at the center of the lobules. The tumors are populated by spindle or stellate cells in a myxoid matrix, both uni- and multivacuolated lipoblasts, and mature fat cells. Some cells may be identical to those of the tumor of brown fat, or hibernoma. The septa are often rich in capillaries and venules that may be arranged in a plexiform pattern. The combination of the plexiform vascular pattern, immature fat cells, and myxoid areas may bear a striking resemblance to myxoid liposarcoma; however, liposarcomas are rare in children and have at least occasional hyperchromatic atypical cells. Mitoses are seen in lipoblastomatosis but

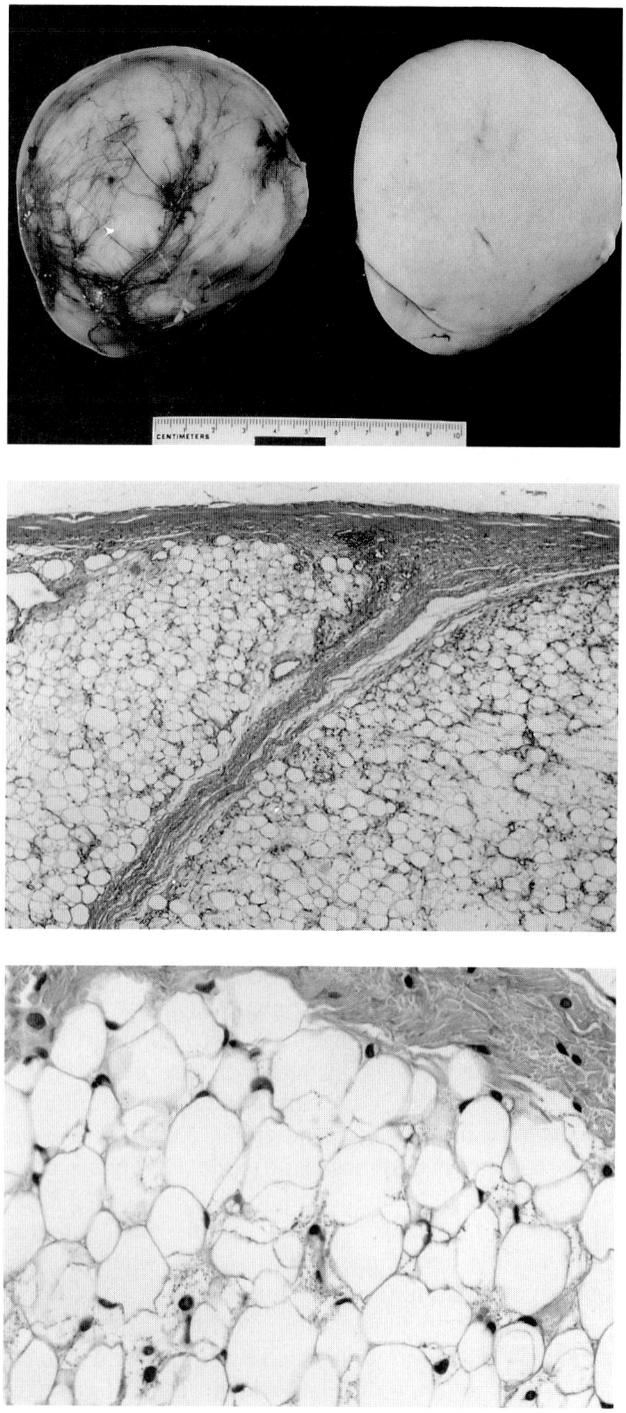

A B C

FIG. 24. Lipoblastoma. **A.** A well-circumscribed globular mass has a homogenous, fatty cut surface **(right)**. **B.** At low magnification, the lobularity of the lesion is apparent. **C.** At higher magnification, the lesion is composed of a mixture of mature adipocytes and immature lipoblasts.

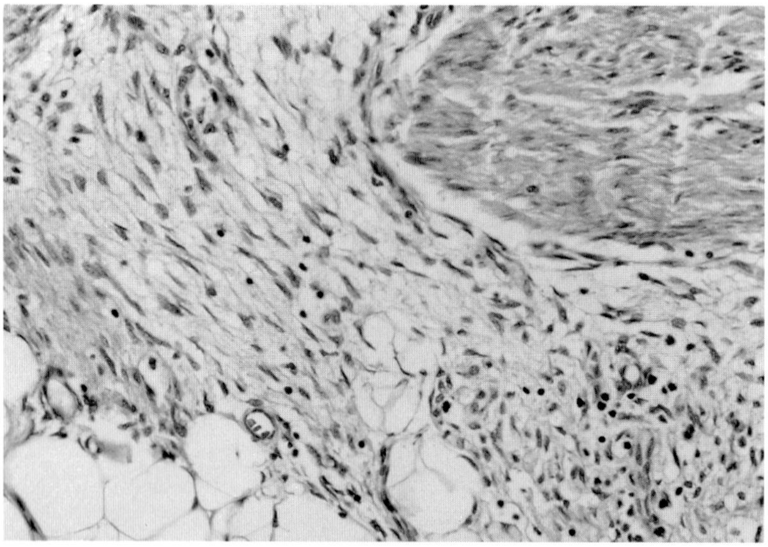

FIG. 25. Fibrous hamartoma of infancy. The tumor contains a mixture of fat **(lower left),** immature mesenchyme **(middle),** and collagenous tissue **(upper right).**

are not atypical (27,174). The tumor will exhibit progressive maturation of the fat cells with time, so that these lesions may thus mature into mature lipomata in later childhood (281).

In diagnosing fatty neoplasms in children, one must remember that mature fat cells are frequently found in pediatric tumors that are not primarily tumors of adipose tissue. Examples include intramuscular hemangioma, infantile musculoaponeurotic fibromatosis, fibrous hamartoma of infancy, neural choristomas, and even Wilms' tumors. It is important that the true nature of the lesion be recognized in spite of the prominent fatty component.

Fibrous Hamartoma of Infancy

Fibrous hamartoma of infancy was first described in 1956 by Reye (224), who termed it "subdermal fibromatous tumor of infancy." Enzinger (73) subsequently described 30 cases and renamed it fibrous hamartoma of infancy. It is a rapidly growing lesion that presents in the first 2 years of life, has a striking male predominance, and is very rare in black patients (73,227). The commonest site of occurrence is the axilla. Other sites of involvement include the subcutaneous tissues of the upper arm, shoulder, thigh, inguinal region, back, forearm, perianal area, and scrotum (78,107,227), where it is frequently attached to the overlying skin.

Grossly fibrous hamartoma consists of a mixture of firm, gray, poorly circumscribed tissue and fat. Histologically it is composed of varying proportions of three tissue types: bands of collagenous fibrous tissue; primitive mesenchymal cells in a vascular, mucoid matrix; and mature adipose tissue (Fig. 25). The dense fibrous tissue may form a dense mass at the center of the lesion (107). Immunohistochemically the cells in the fibrous bands and the primitive mesenchyme show features of myofibroblasts (107).

In spite of its rapid growth fibrous hamartoma is benign. It may recur if inadequately excised but will not metastasize and should be treated conservatively.

LESIONS OF INTERMEDIATE CLINICAL BEHAVIOR

Fibromatoses

An abbreviated classification of childhood fibromatoses is listed in Table 5. Because of their generally benign behavior, some of these lesions have already been discussed in the preceding chapter. Others, such as musculoaponeurotic fibromatosis, are aggressive lesions that may lead to the demise of an unfortunate patient by virtue of their tendency for local recurrence and insinuation. Of particular interest in recent years has been the association of some lesions with well-defined genetic syndromes and tumor suppressor genes.

TABLE 5. *Fibromatoses of childhood*

Digital fibromatosis
Myofibromatosis
Solitary
Multicentric
Fibromatosis, desmoid type
Immature
Mature
Calcifying aponeurotic fibroma
Fibromatosis colli
Juvenile hyaline fibromatosis
Fibrous hamartoma of infancy

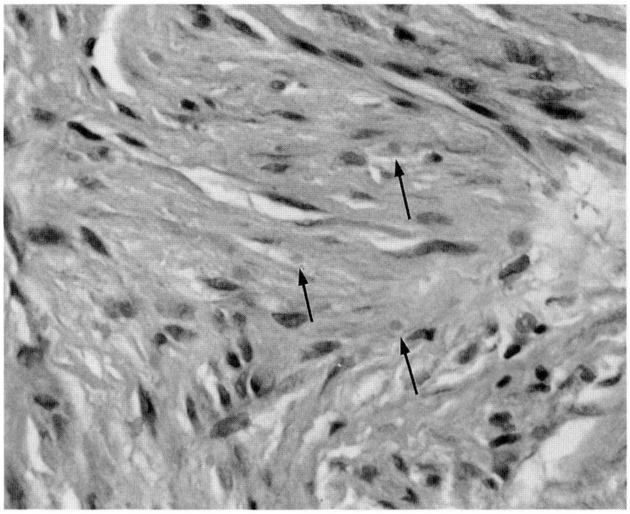

FIG. 26. Infantile digital fibromatosis. Proliferating fibroblasts contain small globular cytoplasmic inclusions *(arrows)*.

Infantile Digital Fibromatosis

Infantile digital fibromatosis, or simply digital fibromatosis, is a fibrous proliferation that presents as a solitary or multiple nodules located on the fingers or toes of infants. It also rarely occurs in older individuals. The major clinical importance lies in the fact that the nodules are prone to recur after attempts at resection.

Histologically, infantile digital fibromatoses are composed of bland, fibroblastic tissues containing myofibroblasts that have a characteristic morphologic marker—rounded, eosinophilic, cytoplasmic inclusions visible by light microscopy (Fig. 26). By electron microscopy the inclusion consists of an amorphous electron-dense mass without a limiting membrane but continuous with bundles of actin filaments. Following pretreatment with potassium hydroxide or formic acid followed by trypsin, Mukai et al. (186) demonstrated immunostaining of the inclusions for actin.

Infantile (Desmoid-type) Fibromatosis

Infantile (desmoid-type) fibromatosis occurs in immature and mature forms. The immature type occurs in the first 2 years of life and consists of a diffuse proliferation of plump fibroblasts and adipose tissue that infiltrate skeletal muscle. There is no significant cytologic atypia, and mitoses are absent or infrequent. The mature type generally occurs in children over 2 years of age and consists of a diffuse growth of interlacing bundles of fibroblasts and varying amounts of collagen (Fig. 27). Some are identical to the typical musculoaponeurotic fibromatosis, or desmoid tumor, seen in adults, in terms of both behavior and morphology.

Desmoid-type fibromatosis lesions are prone to recur locally if incompletely excised but will not metastasize (219). They therefore require wide excision if feasible. Recently, Yokohama et al. (302) and Schmidt et al. (239) found that behavior of desmoid-type fibromatoses can be predicted based on the number of blood vessels and undifferentiated mesenchymal cells. Yokohama noted that 92% of cases with a high vascularity recurred, compared to 24% of those with a low vascularity. Immunohistochemistry assisted in the identification of the undifferentiated mesenchymal cells, which stained only for vimentin and not for muscle-specific actin or desmin.

Cytogenetic analyses of desmoid tumors have indicated that clonal abnormalities are not unusual (14). Deletions of 5q and mutations of the *apc* gene, the region affected in familial polyposis of the colon, occur in these tumors (14,183,199,303), indicating that they share genetic abnormalities as might be predicted by their mu-

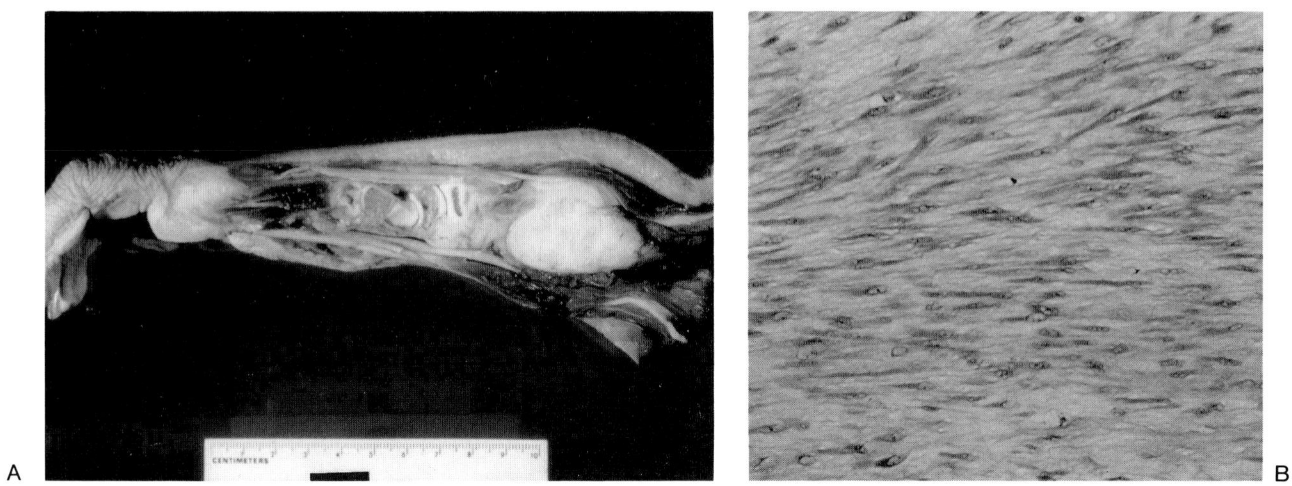

FIG. 27. Extra-abdominal fibromatosis, desmoid type. **A.** A poorly circumscribed, pale gray, fibrous lesion diffusely infiltrates the soft tissues of the proximal forearm in this amputation specimen. **B.** The tumor is composed of homogeneous bundles of bland fibroblasts.

tual occurrence in Gardner's syndrome (see Chapter 12). Abnormalities of the Y chromosome and telomeric fusion may also occur (14). The observation that some desmoids exhibit trisomy 8 has implied a relationship with other fibromatoses, such as Dupuytren's contracture and Peyronie's disease, that show similar findings (51). This finding may be demonstrable with FISH but not with standard techniques, possibly due to tumor heterogeneity (51).

Control of desmoids by sex hormones has been documented in several studies (111), with estrogen receptors being found in the tumor cytosol. This phenomenon may explain the more aggressive growth of these tumors in fertile women (110) and has been successfully used for antiestrogen therapy (295).

Infantile Myofibromatosis

Infantile myofibromatosis is a well-demarcated lesion that may be solitary or multicentric, most frequently affects the skin, and may involve the subcutaneous and deeper tissues including bone and viscera. It affects infants predominantly: 54% are congenital and 89% occur during the first 2 years of life (30); but the lesions have been seen in a variety of ages (10).

Infantile myofibromatosis arises as a rounded nodule consisting of a cellular center with features resembling hemangiopericytoma surrounded by spindle cells with features of myofibroblasts (30) or smooth muscle cells (89) (Fig. 28). It is this combination of the two components that is diagnostic. The pericytomatous and leiomyomatous cells occur in variable proportions and may be associated with necrosis, mitoses, myxoid change, or calcification (30). The presence of a familial occurrence in some instances suggests an autosomal recessive or autosomal dominant mode of inheritance, the latter with reduced penetrance (284).

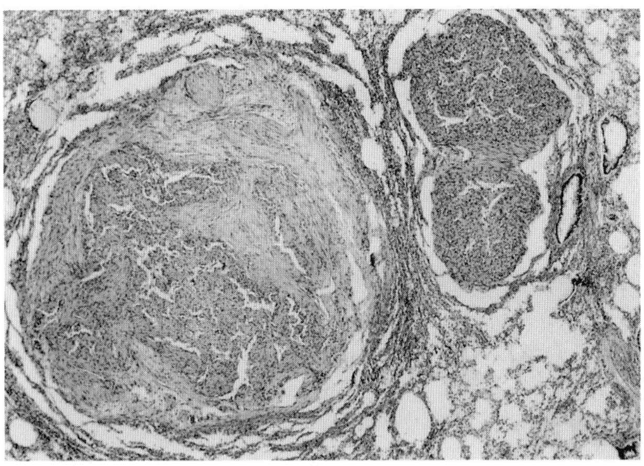

FIG. 28. Infantile myofibromatosis. These intrapulmonary nodules are composed of a vascular, hemangiopericytomalike core and a myofibroblastic shell.

Multicentric lesions composed 26% of the AFIP cases (30). These lesions occur in the neonatal period and involve the underlying soft tissues, bone, and/or viscera as well as the skin. The prognosis depends on the extent of involvement. Multicentric infantile myofibromatoses may therefore be divided into multiple or generalized types, the latter having visceral involvement. Those patients whose deep viscera are involved have the worst prognosis and are likely to die of their disease. If the patients survive their disease the lesions may undergo spontaneous regression, but new nodules occasionally develop during follow-up (30).

Cell culture studies of fibroblasts removed from myofibromatosis nodules reveal that there are no abnormalities in the ability to synthesize collagen or contract a gel. Rather the striking abnormality is a decreased synthesis of collagen and increased cell division following an initial lag phase (21).

Calcifying Aponeurotic Fibroma

Calcifying aponeurotic fibroma occurs predominantly in children but may affect adults. It arises in either the hand (palm or fingers) or foot (sole or ankle) (78). Calcifying aponeurotic fibroma presents as an ill-defined mass that often shows calcification, frequently visible on radiographs (Fig. 29A). Grossly it is intimately associated with the adjacent fascia, tendon sheaths, and other complex fibrous tissues. Because it is not well circumscribed, attempts at excision may be difficult and followed by local recurrence. The lesion frequently cuts with a gritty sensation due to the calcification.

Histologically calcifying aponeurotic fibroma is ill defined with tongues of cells extending into adjacent fat and fibrous tissue. The component cells are either spindle-shaped or rounded and are often arranged in long parallel rows. They palisade around hypocellular areas that undergo calcification. The lesion is quite cellular but mitoses are rare. There is frequently a cartilaginous component with a sulfated mucopolysaccharide matrix that becomes more prominent in older lesions. Giant cells may be found near areas of calcification.

In younger children calcifying aponeurotic fibroma must be differentiated from infantile myofibromatosis and in older children from soft tissue chondroma. Although these lesions are prone to recur, they do not metastasize, so that excision should be conservative and repeated if necessary (78).

Vascular Lesions of Intermediate Behavior

Epithelioid Hemangioendothelioma

Epithelioid hemangioendothelioma is a distinctive, low-grade malignancy of endothelium intermediate be-

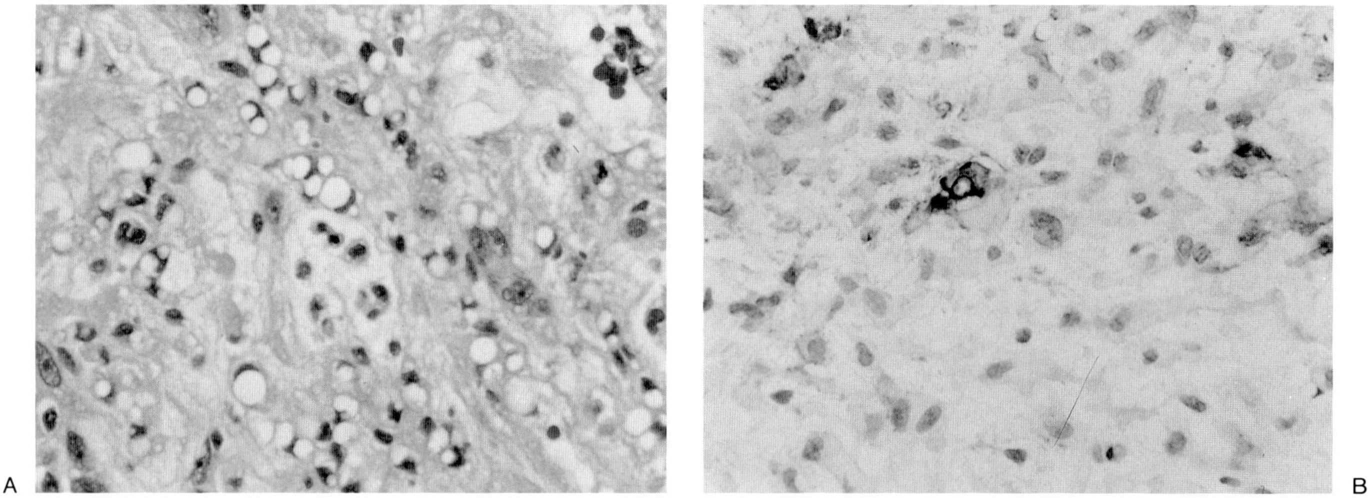

FIG. 29. Epithelioid hemangioendothelioma. A. This hepatic lesion is composed of cells with prominent cytoplasmic vacuoles. B. Scattered tumor cells display strong Factor VIII–related antigen positivity.

tween hemangioma and angiosarcoma in its behavior. It consists of a solitary, slightly painful mass in either the superficial or deep soft tissues. Half of the lesions clearly arise from a vessel and may resemble an organizing thrombus (292).

Histologically epithelioid hemangioendothelioma consists of strands or nests of uniform, epithelioid cells, many of which have round vacuoles in their cytoplasm. These vacuoles are intracytoplasmic lumina by electron microscopy and occasionally contain erythrocytes identifiable by light microscopy (Fig. 29A). The strands of tumor cells lie in an abundant matrix consisting either of acid mucopolysaccharides or hyaline material. The tumors fill the lumen of involved vessels and extend through their walls into surrounding tissues (292). The cells appear bland, with little in the way of mitotic activity in most cases, but in about 25% of cases foci of atypia with mitotic activity, spindle cells, and necrosis are present. It is these latter cases that tend to pursue a more aggressive course (292).

Immunohistochemically the tumor cells stain for Factor VIII–related antigen (Fig. 29B), particularly around the edge of the intracytoplasmic lumina, and show binding of *Ulex europaeus*-1 lectin. They are variably negative with cytokeratin immunostains and consistently negative with mucicarmine stains. They may contain Weibel–Palade bodies by electron microscopy. The differential diagnosis includes metastatic carcinoma, melanoma, and epithelioid sarcoma.

This neoplasm is relatively indolent in its behavior. In the series of Weiss et al. (292), 13% of the tumors recurred locally and 31% metastasized to regional lymph nodes, lung, liver, and bone, although less than half of their cases with metastases died of their disease. They accounted for this by the fact that many of the metastases were in regional lymph nodes that were resected with the primary tumor. It is of interest that important primary sites for the tumor besides soft tissue include lung, liver, and bone. The common involvement of regional lymph nodes should be considered in the surgical management of these cases.

Spindle and histiocytoid (epithelioid) hemangioendothelioma was described by Silva et al. in 1986 (252). Chan et al. (22) consider this lesion to be a variant of epithelioid hemangioendothelioma with a significant number of spindle cells.

Spindle Cell Hemangioendothelioma

Spindle cell hemangioendothelioma was initially considered to be a low-grade angiosarcoma by Weiss (290). However, this is controversial in that other authors question the malignant nature of the lesion, considering it to be a nonneoplastic or benign lesion (61,95). Spindle cell hemangioendothelioma principally affects the skin or the superficial subcutis of the distal extremities and may involve the chest and abdominal walls. The peak incidence is in the second and third decades. Single lesions do not tend to recur, but patients with multiple lesions tend to develop additional lesions (274). The lesions may slowly progress over many years to involve large areas of the body if not controlled (290). They may be associated with other syndromes such as Milroy's disease, Maffucci's syndrome, angiosarcoma, and epithelioid hemangioendothelioma (290).

Grossly, spindle cell hemangioendotheliomas consist of single or multiple, well-circumscribed, red or blue nodules that are sometimes tender. Histologically they consist of thin-walled dilated vascular spaces resembling cavernous hemangioma combined with solid spindle cell areas (Fig. 30). They may be within vessels, resembling

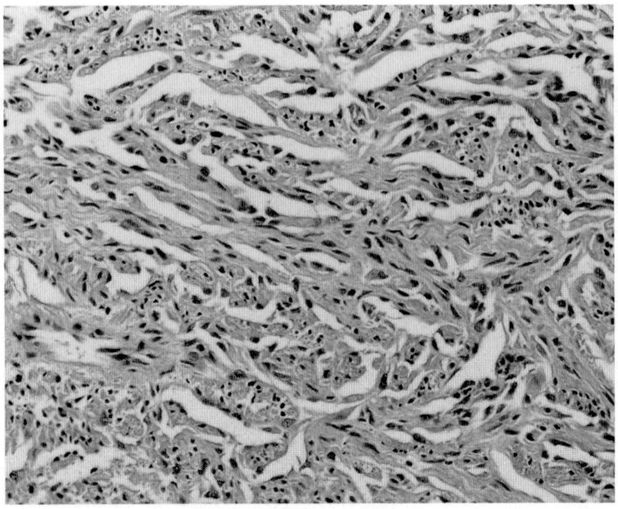

FIG. 30. Spindle cell hemangioendothelioma. A proliferation of spindle cells subtends slitted lumina.

a combination of cavernous hemangioma and Kaposi's sarcoma. The vessels are lined by a single layer of flat endothelial cells and often contain organizing thrombi (274). They are partially surrounded by a reactive myxoid zone containing lymphocytes. Mitoses are absent or scanty. The endothelial cells are sometimes plump and rounded in the spindle cell areas, giving the lesion a biphasic appearance (290). They are sometimes vacuolated. Weibel–Palade bodies and Factor VIII–related antigen staining are seen in the cells lining the cavernous spaces. The latter marker was noted in the plump cells, but neither was seen in the spindle cells (290).

Recurrent nodules generally occur in the vicinity of the original tumor but may be located some distance away. Only one of Weiss and Enzinger's cases (290) metastasized to regional lymph nodes and recurred as a conventional angiosarcoma after radiotherapy. This "metastasis" may have actually been a second malignancy. The lesions have many features similar to those of Kaposi's sarcoma but differ in that they have cavernous vessels and plump, sometimes vacuolated, Factor VIII–associated protein-positive endothelial cells (290). The young age of the patients and lack of known risk factors also set it apart from Kaposi's sarcoma. Treatment would be wide excision of solitary or localized lesions. The efficacy of radiotherapy, chemotherapy, or hormonal therapy is not established.

Giant Cell Angioblastoma

Giant cell angioblastoma is a rare congenital lesion with an extensive, infiltrative growth pattern. It is composed of nodules of concentrically oriented bland, plump cells and multinucleated giant cells. Factor VIII–related antigen-positive flattened endothelium is present at the center of the nodules. The blood vessels are lined by plump cells with eosinophilic cytoplasm and occasional cytoplasmic vacuoles. The lesions may resemble plexiform fibrohistiocytic tumor, but the nodules are smaller, whorled, and consistently have a central blood vessel (274).

Kaposi's Sarcoma

Kaposi's sarcoma is rare in childhood in the United States. Coffin and Dehner (35) found 1 case among 222 patients with vascular tumors in childhood. It does affect young boys in Africa. Tumors in the latter patients are not associated with immunosuppression and are aggressive forms of Kaposi's sarcoma affecting lymph nodes and internal organs such as the bowel and spleen.

Kaposiform Hemangioendothelioma of Infancy and Childhood

Kaposiform hemangioendothelioma of infancy and childhood is a rare pediatric tumor with a histologic appearance intermediate between Kaposi's sarcoma and capillary hemangioma (272,306). Most cases occur in the first decade and present as a soft tissue mass. In Zukerberg's series (306) the lesions involved the upper extremity, retroperitoneum, chest wall, mediastinum, and scalp (306). Three of their nine cases had lymphangiomatosis, and four developed the Kasabach–Merritt syndrome. The two patients who died did so from disease-associated syndromes, either lymphangioma compromising the upper airway or intracerebral hemorrhage related to the Kasabach–Merritt syndrome, and not from tumor burden. The tumors grow as nodular masses in the deep soft tissues and occasionally the skin. They may be locally aggressive and metastasize locally, but no distant metastases were noted in Zukerberg's series (306).

Kaposiform hemangioendotheliomas grow in a nodular fashion and do not contain the plasmacellular infiltrate seen with Kaposi's sarcoma. They consist of areas of spindle cell proliferation with crescentic vascular spaces resembling Kaposi's sarcoma together with areas resembling capillary hemangioma (272,306). The vascular spaces are lined by thin, spindle cells with darkly staining nuclei similar to normal endothelial cells. They form plump, rounded, glomeruloid nests of cells with hemosiderin and hyaline globules in their cytoplasm, particularly in the skin. Weibel–Palade bodies have not been identified by electron microscopy in these tumors (306). Like Kaposi's sarcoma these tumors express CD34 and either lack or weakly express Factor VIII–related antigen (272,306). However, they are surrounded by a population of Factor XIIIA–positive cells and in the skin by dense hyaline fibrosis (306). The deeper lesions extensively involve adjacent structures such as bone, intestine, biliary system, pancreas, intestine, and perinodal soft tissues. Atypia is minimal and mitoses are relatively infrequent (<3 per 10 high power fields).

Malignant Endovascular Papillary Angioendothelioma (Dabska Tumor)

Dabska tumor is an exceedingly rare lesion described by Maria Dabska in 1969 (49). It composed 2% of childhood vascular tumors in Coffin and Dehner's series (35). Grossly it forms a diffuse subcutaneous tumor or localized intradermal mass in children and adults. On low-power microscopic examination the lesion resembles a cavernous lymphangioma. At higher power one observes papillary tufts projecting into vascular lumens. The cells lining the papillae range from lymphocytelike to cuboidal to columnar in shape and typically contain nuclei polarized away from the basement membrane. The papillae surround a central hyaline core formed from basement membrane material. The cells mark as endothelial cells immunohistochemically (Factor VIII–related antigen and *Ulex europaeus*-1 lectin–positive, HLA-DR–negative (78). Numerous lymphocytes may be found in the lumen of the vessels.

Such tumors may deeply invade underlying structures, such as the cranial cavity. They have metastasized to regional lymph nodes in a few patients, but the overall prognosis appears to be excellent following wide excision. They do not respond to radiation therapy (49).

Angiomatoid Malignant Fibrous Histiocytoma

Angiomatoid malignant fibrous histiocytoma is an unusual tumor that is often misdiagnosed (44). It was first described by Enzinger in 1979 (75) and is morphologically and clinically distinct from other forms of malignant fibrous histiocytoma. One primary distinction is its usual occurrence in young people with a mean age of 17 years (44). It involves the extremities in 65% of cases, the trunk in 28%, and the head and neck in 7%. The lesions are superficial and slow growing. A minority of the cases are associated with constitutional symptoms including anemia, weight loss, fever, and polyclonal gammopathy. Clinically it is often felt to be a benign cyst (44).

Grossly angiomatoid malignant fibrous histiocytomas are cystic in 82% of cases (44). The cysts are well-demarcated and filled with blood or blood-stained fluid. Histologically the lesions consist of sheets of spindled or rounded cells that have a somewhat bland cytologic appearance. They were myxoid in 13% of cases in Costa's series (44). There is frequent and abundant hemosiderin deposition within the tumor, along with other features of organizing hemorrhage such as a foam and spindle cell proliferation. The nodule is surrounded in virtually all cases by a mantle of chronic inflammation composed of lymphocytes, plasma cells, and a pseudocapsule (Fig. 31). Germinal centers are often present. The inflammation is a distinctive feature and may invite confusion of this lesion with a lymph node metastasis. Angiomatoid malignant fibrous histiocytomas are usually easily cured by wide excision. In the series of Costa and Weiss (44), 11% had a local recurrence, 4% had local metastases, and only 1% had presumed distant metastases. There was only one death from tumor after 19 years. Three features correlate with more aggressive behavior: an irregular histologic border, deep location, and involvement of the head and neck. Mitotic activity and nuclear pleomorphism are not useful predictors of survival or recurrence.

There is controversy as to the nature of the cells making up angiomatoid malignant fibrous histiocytoma. They originally were thought to be fibrohistiocytic by Enzinger (75), but the immunohistochemical studies of Fletcher (92) suggest muscle differentiation. Fletcher thus prefers to name the lesion an angiomatoid myosarcoma and notes an immunohistochemical similarity to alveolar soft part sarcoma.

Fibrosarcoma of Infancy

As the name implies, infantile fibrosarcoma arises during the first 4 years of life, usually during the first year and in some cases congenitally (28). It presents as a painless mass, often attaining a large size over a relatively short time. Infantile fibrosarcoma differs from the typical adult fibrosarcoma in that it tends to affect the more distal portions of the extremities rather than the proximal extremities or the trunk and has a much better prognosis than its adult counterpart (28).

Infantile fibrosarcomas are poorly demarcated, fleshy tumors with areas of hemorrhage and necrosis on gross examination (Fig. 32A, B). Histologically they consist of

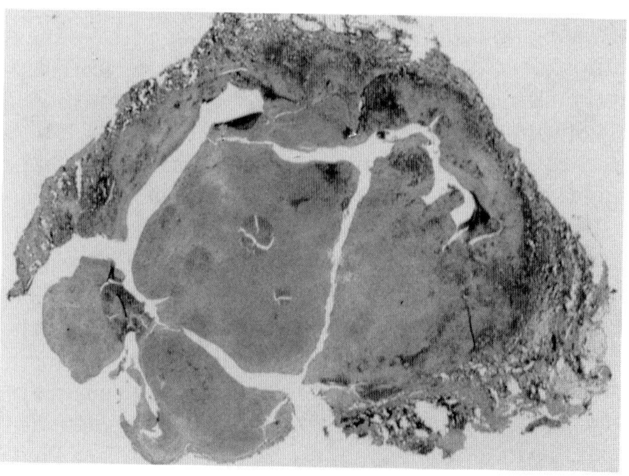

FIG. 31. Angiomatoid malignant fibrous histiocytoma. Low magnification of a subcutaneous nodule reveals irregular spaces and an inflamed periphery, yielding resemblance to a lymph nodal metastasis.

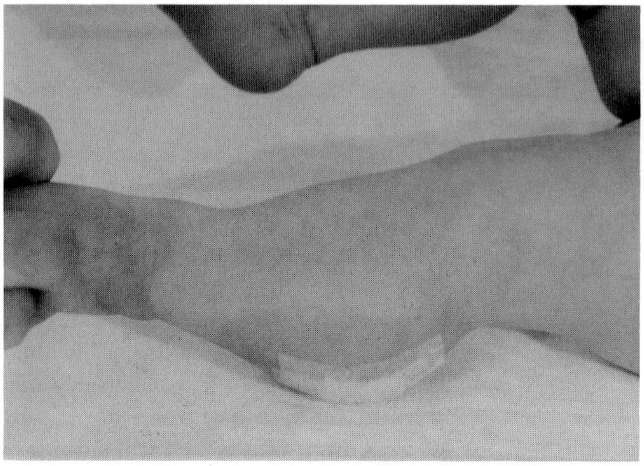
A
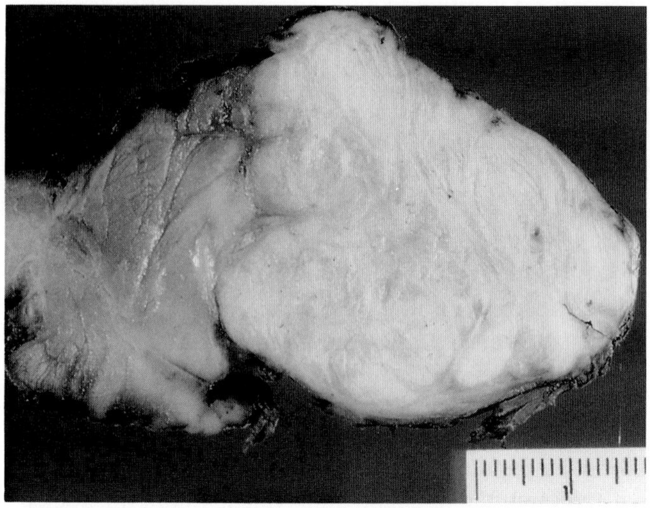
B
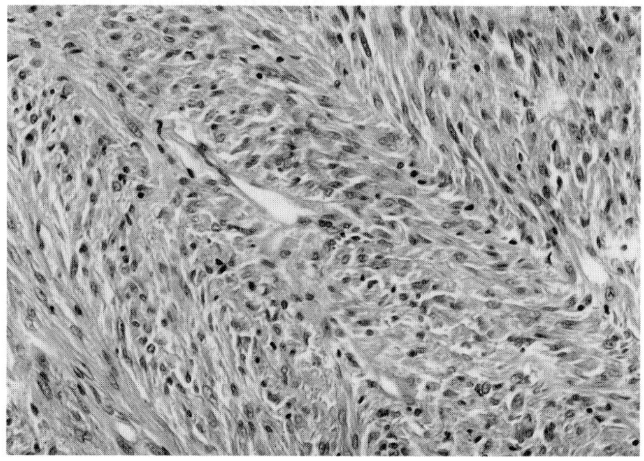
C

FIG. 32. Infantile fibrosarcoma. **A.** A rapidly growing mass distends the leg of this infant. **B.** A section through the lesion discloses a whorled, fibrous tumor with infiltrating borders. **C.** The tumor is composed of a cellular fibroblastic proliferation arranged in herringbonelike fascicles.

spindle cells arranged in densely packed fascicles (Fig. 32C). If there is relatively little collagen production, the tumor cells tend to be more rounded and closely packed, whereas with increased collagen they are more spindled. They are arranged in a typical herringbone pattern of interlacing fascicles. They are very cellular with frequent mitoses but do not generally have much nuclear pleomorphism, and giant cells are rare. They do not show a significant amount of glycogen on special stains. There may be scattered inflammatory cells, and areas may be quite vascular.

In Chung and Enzinger's series (28) only 4 of 48 patients with infantile fibrosarcoma died of metastatic tumor; overall there was a 5-year survival rate of 84%. This is much better than the outlook for adult fibrosarcomas, whose 5-year survival is approximately 50%. The treatment is wide excision, but in view of the small chance of metastasis, it is justifiable to be relatively conservative in resecting these lesions and thus avoid the sacrifice of major structures. Some cases will require amputation by virtue of their size.

Chromosomal analyses of infantile fibrosarcomas have revealed recurring trisomies of chromosomes 8, 11, 17, and 20 (50). This genotypic feature may be demonstrated in interphase cells by use of fluorescence in situ hybridization (FISH) using centromeric probes and may also be seen in cellular fibromatosis (241).

Dermatofibrosarcoma Protuberans; Bednar Tumor (Storiform Neurofibroma)

Dermatofibrosarcoma protuberans and Bednar tumor are closely related if not variants of the same neoplasm. They are unusual in children. It has been postulated that they represent the adult end-product of childhood giant cell fibroblastomas (6,8,251). Recent observations on their immunopositivity for CD34 appear to link them more closely to neural tumors than to fibrohistiocytic ones (36), and it has been the authors' experience that subcutaneous pediatric lesions with a marked storiform pattern are often actually neurofibromas or low-grade malignant peripheral nerve sheath tumors.

MALIGNANT LESIONS

Sarcomas other than rhabdomyosarcoma are uncommon tumors in childhood (216), so that it has been difficult to prospectively examine a sufficient number of cases to obtain meaningful data with regard to their natural history and optimal treatment. A randomized study was thus undertaken under the auspices of the Pediatric Oncology Group (POG) in order to better understand these neoplasms. One of the parameters studied was tumor grade (124). The grading system used was derived from that of Enzinger and Weiss (78) and Costa et al. (43). Features used to grade these tumors included histologic category, age, necrosis, mitotic index, pleomorphism, and differentiation (Table 6). Using these criteria in the evaluation of 75 prospectively randomized cases, grades 1 and 2 patients had a 91.7% disease-free survival at 3 years, whereas grade 3 patients had a disease-free survival of only 75.1% ($p = 0.018$). Thus a grading scheme including histologic type of sarcoma was of great value in predicting outcome in these cases (207).

An estimate of the relative incidence of tumors of this type can also be gleaned from the POG study, as listed in Table 7. These figures are similar to those obtained from a similar study in Germany (139).

Synovial Sarcoma

Excluding rhabdomyosarcoma and peripheral neuroepithelioma, synovial sarcoma is the commonest sarcoma in patients under 20 years of age (240). It composed 31% of the cases in a POG study of nonrhabdomyosarcomatous sarcomas of soft tissue (124). Synovial sarcoma involves the lower extremity most frequently, followed by the upper extremity, and much less commonly the head, neck, and abdominal wall (78,240). Recent cases have also been reported in the thorax. In the lower extremity the tissue around the knee and the lower thigh is the most frequent tumor site, followed by the foot and ankle. Tissue around the elbow is often involved as well. Synovial sarcoma presents as a mass, painful in about half of the cases. In children it is most frequent in the teenage years (78). The mass may have been present for a long time in some patients. Particularly in longstanding cases, the tumors appear well encapsulated but are actually delimited by a pseudocapsule (102). This is often confusing to the surgeon, who may consider the lesion a benign cyst or other innocuous lesion.

TABLE 6. *The POG nonrhabdomyosarcoma soft tissue sarcoma grading schema*

Grade 1
Myxoid and well-differentiated liposarcoma
Deep-seated dermatofibrosarcoma protuberans
Well-differentiated or infantile (age ≤4 years) fibrosarcoma
Well-differentiated or infantile (age ≤4 years) hemangiopericytoma
Well-differentiated malignant peripheral nerve sheath tumor
Extraskeletal myxoid chondrosarcoma
Angiomatoid malignant fibrous histiocytoma

Grade 2
Sarcomas not specifically included in grades 1 or 3 and in which <15% of the surface area shows necrosis or the mitotic count is ≤5 per 10 high-power fields using a 40× objective

Grade 3
Pleomorphic or round cell liposarcoma
Mesenchymal chondrosarcoma
Extraskeletal osteosarcoma
Malignant triton tumor
Alveolar soft part sarcoma
Sarcomas not included in grade 1 and in which >15% of the surface area shows necrosis or the mitotic count is >5/10 high-power fields using a 40× objective
Marked atypia or cellularity are less predictive but may be used in borderline cases to place them into either grade 2 or 3

TABLE 7. *Relative incidence of nonrhabdomyosarcoma, nonperipheral neuroepithelioma soft tissue sarcomas treated on the POG study, 1986–1991*[a]

Tumor type	Percent
Synovial sarcoma, biphasic	20
Synovial sarcoma, monophasic	11
Malignant peripheral nerve sheath tumor	13
Malignant fibrous histiocytoma	12
Leiomyosarcoma	8
Fibrosarcoma	5
Sarcoma, not otherwise specified	8
Miscellaneous[b]	23

[a] Total number of cases = 75.
[b] Miscellaneous sarcomas included alveolar soft part sarcoma, chondrosarcoma, clear cell sarcoma, ectomesenchymoma, epithelioid sarcoma, infantile fibrosarcoma, liposarcoma, malignant mesenchymoma, and extrarenal rhabdoid tumor.

Diagnostic imaging may be useful in diagnosis in that about 30% of cases contain calcification (78,282) (Fig. 33). In rare cases the calcification may be very extensive, a feature found to be associated with a much improved prognosis (282). Although the lesions often occur in adjacent tissues, they almost never arise within the synovium of a joint. Most authorities thus believe that the tumors arise from primitive mesenchymal cells with the capability of variably differentiating into both epithelial and spindle cells. There is controversy as to whether the spindle cells blend via intermediate cells into the epithelial cells or whether they are two completely separate lines of differentiation. More recent articles suggest that the latter is the case (52), a point in favor of calling these neoplasms soft tissue carcinosarcomas (52,178). The epithelial cells do not share the usual immunohistochemical or electron microscopic features of synovial cells, which are cytokeratin-negative (178).

Grossly synovial sarcoma is often well demarcated with a pseudocapsule and a variable cut surface that may be cystic. It is often densely adherent to tendon sheaths and other adjacent structures (Fig. 34). Histologically four variants are recognized: biphasic with glandular ep-

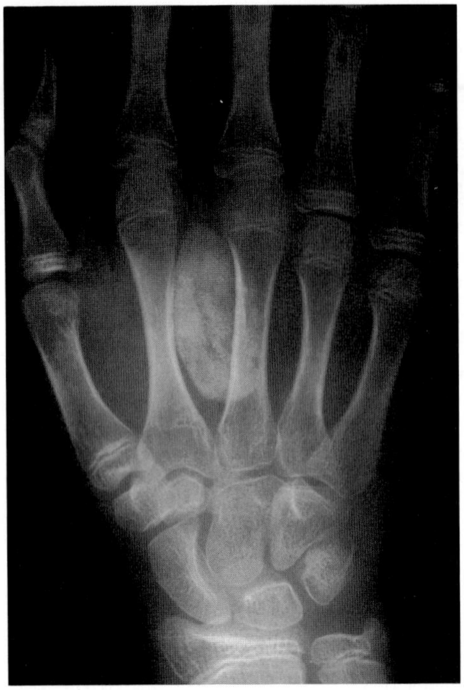

FIG. 33. Synovial sarcoma. An intermetacarpal lesion reveals extensive calcification on a plain radiograph.

ithelium or solid epithelial islands, monophasic spindle cell, monophasic epithelial cell, and anaplastic (Fig. 35). The biphasic tumors are generally the commonest (approximately 60%), followed by the monophasic spindle cell (approximately 30%) (240). The biphasic tumors consist of both epithelial and spindle cell elements. The epithelial elements may form glands with lumina, solid islands, or both and may form cysts. They vary from low cuboidal to tall columnar in appearance. Mucin may be demonstrated in their lumina with PAS, colloidal iron, and alcian blue stains.

With immunohistochemistry, synovial sarcomas usually stain positively for cytokeratin (Fig. 36) and epithelial membrane antigen, and bind *Ulex europaeus-1* and peanut agglutinin lectins (178,240). Miettinen found that keratins 7 and 19 and desmoplakin are highly associated with morphologically observable epithelial differentiation and are restricted to synovial sarcoma among spindle cell sarcomas (175). A basement membrane can be outlined with immunostaining for type IV collagen (240). The tumor cells may also be positive for Leu 7, Ki M7, S-100 protein, neuron-specific enolase, and carcinoembryonic antigen (201,240).

The epithelial elements may be very subtle, requiring a careful search for clusters of cells with slightly more rounded contours and more cohesion than the surrounding spindle cells. They may be very sparse and only found after searching many slides. However, visualization of the epithelial components may be enhanced by immunohistochemical or reticulin stains. Squamous metaplasia may be noted occasionally (240,288). The spindle cell elements are plump, closely packed with ill-defined cytoplasm and arranged either as compact bundles or as loose, myxoid areas. A very helpful feature is the presence of hemangiopericytomalike areas with gaping, staghorn-type vessels separating densely cellular tissue. Calcification is frequently present and can also be diagnostically useful (Fig. 35A). There may even be metaplastic bone formation, inviting confusion with osteogenic sarcoma (179). Mast cells are often present in large numbers.

In the biphasic tumors the epithelial elements stain with epithelial markers but not carcinoembryonic antigen or vimentin, and the spindle cell elements stain with vimentin but not epithelial markers (52). By electron microscopy, the epithelial cells enclose glandular lumina with juxtaluminal tight junctions and desmosomes (201). A basal lamina is recognizable between the epithelial cells and the spindle cells (78). The spindle cells contain prominent rough endoplasmic reticulum, and there are more intercellular junctions and less extracellular collagen than in fibrosarcomas of similar appearance (52,178). Unlike mesothelioma, the epithelial cells do not have a significant amount of glycogen in their cytoplasm.

A specific cytogenetic abnormality has been identified in the majority of synovial sarcoma, namely t(X:18)(p11.2;q11.2) (Fig. 37). In a series of 32 cases reported by Linman, there were abnormalities in Xp11 or 18q11

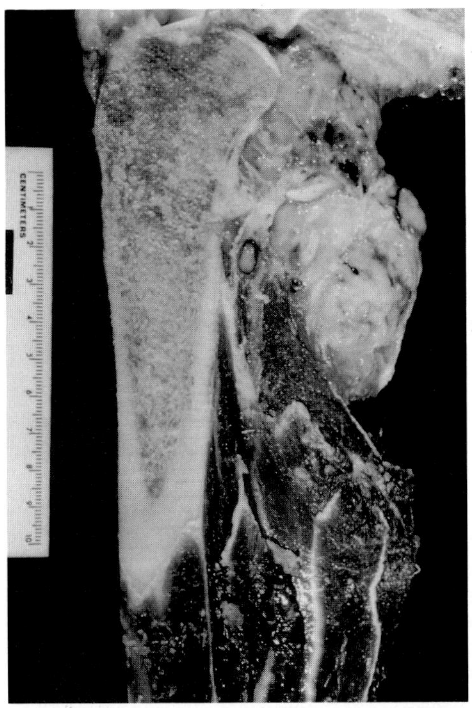

FIG. 34. Synovial sarcoma. There is extensive invasion of the popliteal soft tissues by this fleshy tumor. Vascular invasion is grossly apparent in the center of the photograph.

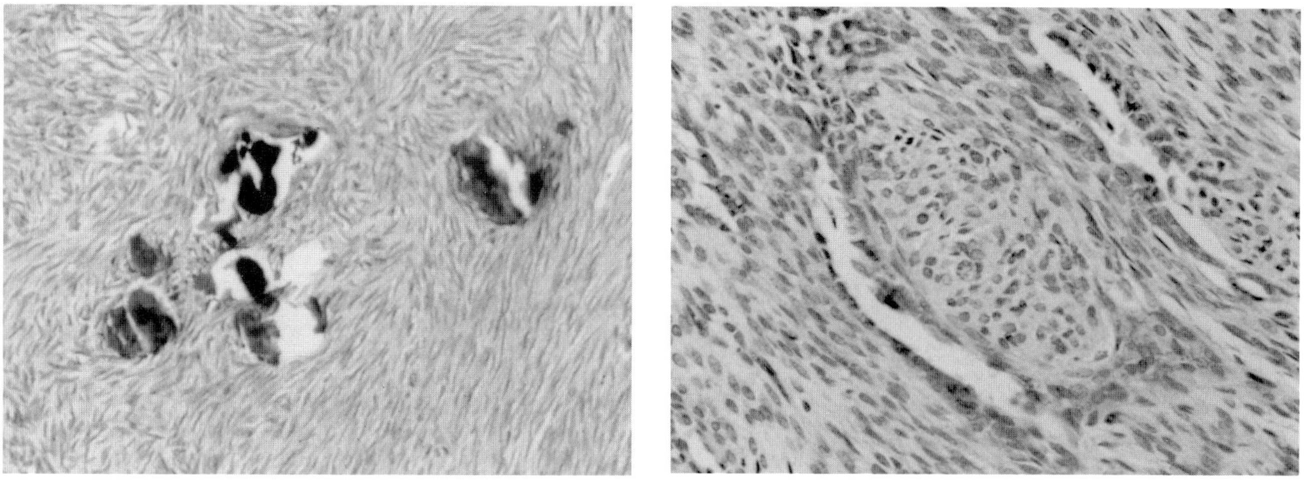

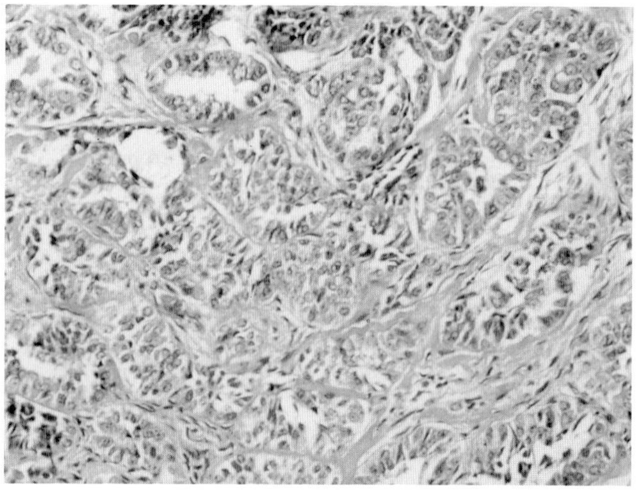

FIG. 35. Synovial sarcoma. The tumor can exist in a variety of histologic forms, including monophasic spindle cell **(A),** biphasic **(B),** and monophasic epithelial cell **(C).** Microcalcifications, an important clue to the diagnosis, are apparent in panel A. In panel B, elongated glandular spaces coexist with spindle cell fascicles.

in all but two cases, and the karyotype did not differ between monophasic or biphasic tumors (154). Shipley mapped the t(X;18) breakpoint, locating at least two separate loci on chromosome X (249). Recently, a gene termed *SYT* on chromosome 18 and one termed *SSX* on chromoxome X were identified in a hybrid transcript (32). FISH has been used to delineate the abnormality in tissue sections (135). Recurrent tumors contain additional genetic aberrations consistent with tumor progression (154). A tendency to transformation from biphasic to monophasic tumors with progression has also been noted (154).

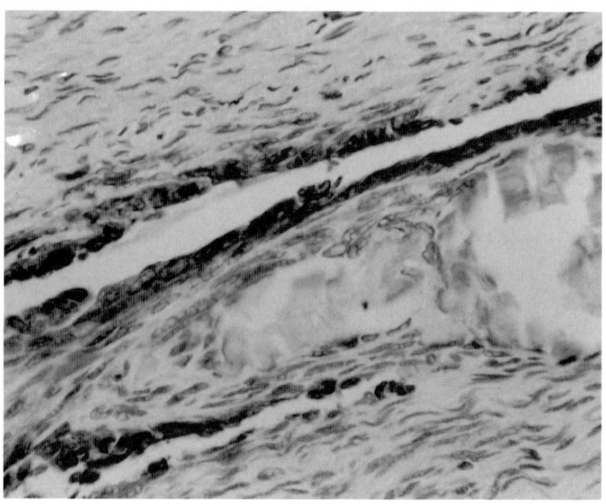

FIG. 36. Synovial sarcoma. Epithelial cells displayed marked cytokeratin positivity.

Features of prognostic importance include the patient's age, tumor size, aneuploidy, mitotic activity, necrosis, extensive calcification, and anaplastic histology. Children appear to have a better survival in general than adults (71,204). Synovial sarcomas metastasize primarily to the lung via the bloodstream but may spread to regional lymph nodes or bones (78). Metastases may occur very late, so that prolonged follow-up is necessary. It is also worthwhile to resect amenable pulmonary metastases.

Hemangiopericytoma

Hemangiopericytoma is a rare tumor in childhood (77). Most are benign in their clinical behavior, but the criteria differentiating benign from malignant are not

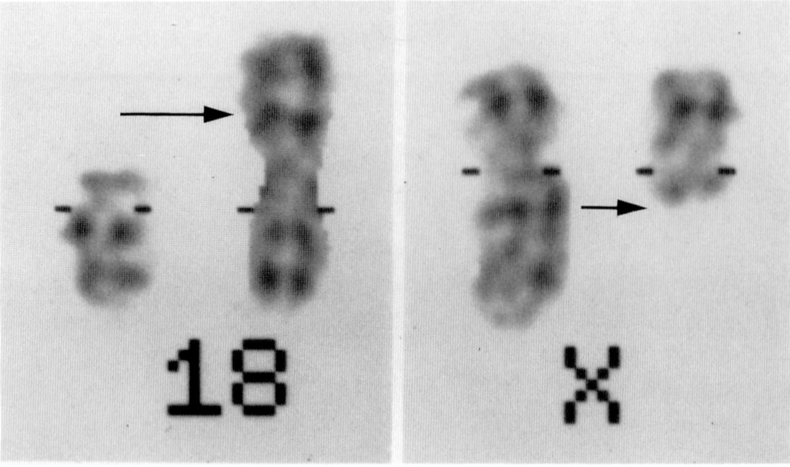

FIG. 37. Synovial sarcoma. There is a reciprocal translocation between the long arm of chromosome X and the short arm of chromosome 18 [the t(X;18)(p11.2;q11.2)] (*arrows*). (Courtesy of Marc Valentine, St. Jude Children's Research Hospital.)

clearly defined. As with fibrosarcomas in infancy, a tumor with the histologic features of a hemangiopericytoma occurs in infancy but in spite of aggressive features behaves in a benign fashion. Enzinger and Smith (77) discuss eight cases occurring in patients from newborn to 7 months of age. Unlike typical adult hemangiopericytomas, these tumors occurred exclusively in the subcutaneous tissue, often had intra- or perivascular growth outside the main tumor, had more collagen than usual, and showed endothelial proliferation into vascular spaces. They had disturbing histologic features, namely, mitoses and foci of necrosis, but they all behaved in a benign manner. Yu et al. (304) had one patient who was still alive at 2 years in spite of a high proliferative index, which is usually a poor prognostic feature in adult lesions.

The more typical hemangiopericytoma is a cellular tumor with oval- to spindle-shaped cells packed between uniformly distributed vessels (Fig. 38A). The vessels are typically branching with a characteristic staghorn pattern (77). The cells are surrounded by reticulin fibers and separated from the endothelium of the vessels by a basement membrane (Fig. 38B). The spindle cells are never arranged in long fascicles or bundles as seen in fibrosarcomas or synovial sarcomas.

Many other lesions mimic hemangiopericytoma, such as synovial sarcoma, mesenchymal chondrosarcoma, vascular smooth muscle tumors, glomus tumors, malignant fibrous histiocytomas, malignant peripheral nerve sheath tumors, and the periphery of many large mesenchymal tumors of various types, but the pattern is not uniform throughout these lesions (77,190). It is important to make the distinction among these tumor types, as hemangiopericytoma is rare and tends to be overdiagnosed.

Until recently there were no known specific markers for hemangiopericytoma, and the diagnosis was based on the architectural pattern of the tumor. Nemes's cases (190) stained for Factor XIIIa and variably stained with HLA-DR, markers that did not stain synovial sarcomas,

A 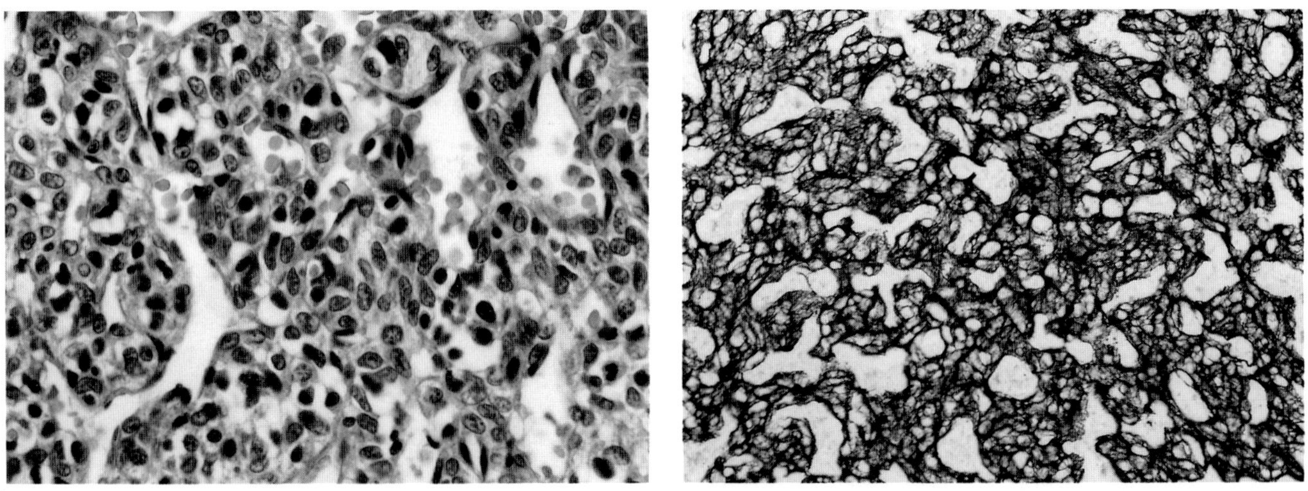 B

FIG. 38. Hemangiopericytoma. **A.** Tumor cells are separated by uniformly distributed small vessels. **B.** There is a characteristic investment of individual tumor cells by reticulin fibers, as seen in this Gordon–Sweet reticulin stain. The vascular framework is prominent.

liposarcomas, leiomyosarcomas, malignant peripheral nerve sheath tumors, or meningiomas. However, malignant fibrous histiocytomas did express these antigens. Porter et al. (214) found that hemangiopericytomas do not stain for muscle-specific actin, unlike the normal pericyte. Cytogenetic analyses have indicated that abnormalities of chromosome segment 12q13-15 are seen in some hemangiopericytomas (161), contrasting with the t(X;18) of synovial sarcoma.

Hemangiopericytomas in older children are well-demarcated lesions that behave in a benign manner if they are not very cellular and do not contain necrosis or mitoses (77). Tumors larger than 6.5 cm or having a high cellularity, more than 3 mitoses per 10 high-power fields, or necrosis behave in a more malignant manner. Recurrence or metastasis sometimes occurs after a long interval. Fifteen percent metastasize, typically to lung or bone.

Malignant Peripheral Nerve Sheath Tumors

Malignant peripheral nerve sheath tumors compose any malignant tumor arising from a component of the nerve sheath. One half of patients with a malignant nerve sheath tumor have neurofibromatosis type 1 (Fig. 39), and 2% of patients with neurofibromatosis type 1 will develop one during their lifetime (256,299). Two thirds of patients develop their neurofibrosarcoma from a neurofibroma (299), and most of the remainder arise from a grossly identifiable peripheral nerve, usually a large nerve such as the sciatic nerve, brachial plexus, or spinal or sacral nerve root (78,299). These tumors are thus most common in the proximal upper and lower extremities and trunk. They may rarely develop in a ganglioneuroma or ganglioneuroblastoma, usually after radiotherapy (226). In the pediatric series of the AFIP (173), 38% of malignant nerve sheath tumors were associated with a nerve trunk, neurofibroma, or neurofibromatosis type 1.

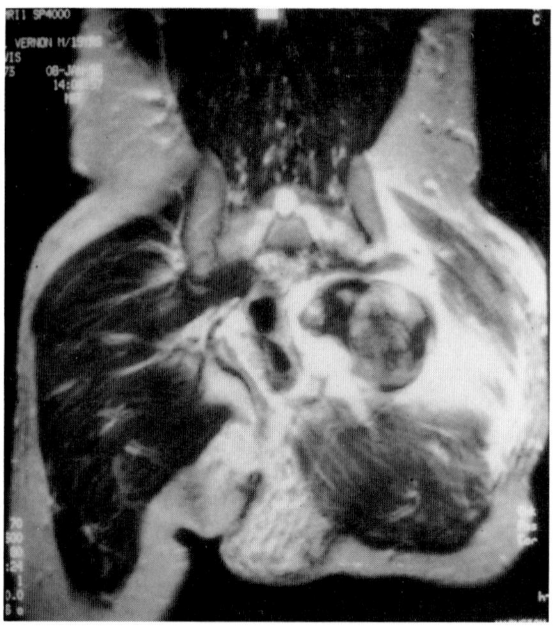

FIG. 39. Malignant peripheral nerve sheath tumor. An MR scan demonstrates an expansile mass that arises from the right pelvic soft tissues in this NF1 patient. Note the marked distortion of the gluteal soft tissues and the multiple, small, plexiform neurofibromas in the paraspinal tissues and subcutis. (Courtesy of Dr. Barry Fletcher, St. Jude Children's Research Hospital.)

Grossly malignant peripheral nerve sheath tumors form large, deep-seated, fusiform or globoid masses, often arising from a large peripheral nerve. They often appear well circumscribed with a thick pseudocapsule and on cut surface are firm with areas of necrosis (299) (Fig. 40). They may extend long distances along the parent nerve beyond the actual mass (78).

Malignant peripheral nerve sheath tumors are strikingly variable by light microscopy. Some have a low-grade, bland appearance, resembling a neurofibroma but with mitotic activity and cellular areas, whereas others are highly anaplastic, obviously malignant tumors with little differentiation (Fig. 41A). Meis et al. (173) noted that the pediatric examples have a more primitive microscopic appearance than those of adults and not infrequently overlap with primitive neuroepithelial tumors. Typically they are spindle cell neoplasms, with the nuclei often having a curved, buckled, comma shape and a wavy growth pattern. The cells are usually arranged in fascicles but may show a storiform pattern or aggregate into foci resembling abortive tactile corpuscles (78,173) (Fig. 41B). A minority (10%) contain palisaded nuclei. Hyalinized cords or nodules of collagen may be present, and the cells may be arranged in whorls or a plexiform pattern. They may show a peculiar subendothelial growth with herniation into vascular lumina. The presence of alternating cellular and myxoid areas is a helpful diagnostic feature.

It can be difficult to tell whether a tumor is malignant or not if it is low grade. Mitoses are critical. The presence of more than three or four mitoses in a slide indicates that the lesion has malignant potential (78). We have seen a case in which a tumor resembled a neurofibroma but had scattered mitoses. One year later it recurred as a high-grade neurofibrosarcoma, fully malignant. The presence of cellular areas should engender a search for mitotic activity. Coffin and Dehner (34) report nine cases designated cellular neurofibromas in a series of 139 peripheral nerve sheath tumors. Two of these cellular tumors recurred and one of them eventually metastasized to the lung. Four of the affected patients had associated neurofibromatosis 1, including the case with lung metastases. They stress that although it is important not to overdiagnose malignancy in neurogenic tumors, the presence of increased cellularity and mitotic activity are

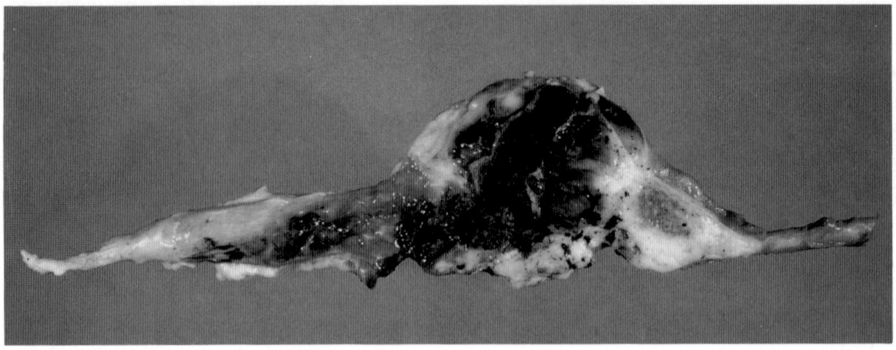

FIG. 40. Malignant peripheral nerve sheath tumor. A longitudinal section highlights an irregular, hemorrhagic, fusiform mass that arises from a large peripheral nerve.

warning signs of possible aggressive behavior. Geographic necrosis is also an important feature of malignant nerve sheath tumors (121) but is often not present in childhood cases (173). Nuclear pleomorphism per se does not indicate malignancy in a nerve sheath tumor unless accompanied by mitotic activity (2), as atypia may be due to degenerative change. Malignant peripheral nerve sheath tumors commonly show evidence of tumor progression histologically and contain both low- and high-grade foci. Tumor progression is accompanied by mutations in the *p53* gene (145).

Divergent differentiation may be seen in approximately 14–28% of malignant peripheral nerve sheath tumors (64,173,233,299). This may include the presence of intestinal-type glandular elements, even with neuroendocrine differentiation. Chondroid tissue, bone, and striated muscle may be seen, the latter element being present in neoplasms termed "malignant triton tumor" (Fig. 41C). The glandular elements tend to be more mature and discreet than those in synovial sarcoma. Angiosarcomas may also arise from a plexiform neurofibroma (24). Even brain tumor–like elements, such as glia or medulloepithelial canals (Fig. 41D), may be seen rarely. The latter tumors have been referred to as "peripheral medulloepitheliomas."

Epithelioid malignant peripheral nerve sheath tumor is a malignant nerve sheath tumor that mostly consists of cells resembling primitive epithelium or melanoma (140). The cells are often arranged in nests or cords. They do not stain with HMB45 but are vimentin– and S-100 protein–positive (140). Ten percent of Meis's childhood cases (173) were of this type. Type IV collagen is a useful marker to distinguish between epithelioid malignant peripheral nerve sheath tumors and malignant melanomas (140). Epithelioid tumors have a lower association with neurofibromatosis type 1 than other malignant peripheral nerve sheath tumors. Those lesions located superficially are smaller at presentation and have a much better prognosis due to their small size and ease of complete resection. It appears that they do not metastasize to lymph nodes as frequently as do melanomas (140).

Electron microscopy may be useful in the diagnosis of malignant peripheral nerve sheath tumor. The cells may show discontinuous portions of surrounding basal lamina and form long, slender, intertwining processes (Fig. 42A) (80). They may show attempts at mesaxon formation ("pseudomesaxons") and long-spaced collagen (Luse bodies; Fig. 42B). Primitive cell junctions are noted. The pseudomesaxons may envelop collagen bundles in lieu of the normally enwrapped axons. Fibroblastic cells with dilated cisternae of rough endoplasmic reticulum are often prominent (Fig. 42C).

Immunohistochemistry may be helpful as a majority of tumors show focal positivity for S-100 protein, myelin basic protein, Leu 7, glial fibrillary acidic protein, or epithelial membrane antigen. Positivity for the latter marker is suggestive of perineurial differentiation. Staining for either Leu 7 or S-100 was positive in 76% of cases in the series of Meis et al. (173) and 40% of their cases were positive for muscle-specific actin. They may also be positive for elements of the basal lamina such as laminin and type IV collagen. One must be aware that Leu 7 or S-100 positivity may occur in rhabdomyosarcomas, so that the findings must be placed in the proper morphologic context. The differential diagnosis also includes fibrosarcoma, synovial sarcoma, and leiomyosarcoma.

Meis et al. (173) found that patient age ≥7 years, male sex, presence of neurofibromatosis type 1, central tumor location, larger tumor size (≥6 cm), or tumor necrosis (≥25%) had a negative impact on survival. Forty-seven percent were dead of disease at 4–86 months, 14% were alive with disease at 4–72 months, and 30% showed no evidence of disease at 7–230 months. Generally, this is a tumor with a poor prognosis in children, although the reported survival including all ages is somewhat worse.

Epithelioid Sarcoma

Epithelioid sarcoma, first described by Enzinger in 1970 (74), is an uncommon but not rare tumor in childhood. Its diagnosis may elicit confusion, both clinically and pathologically. Cases under 20 years of age consti-

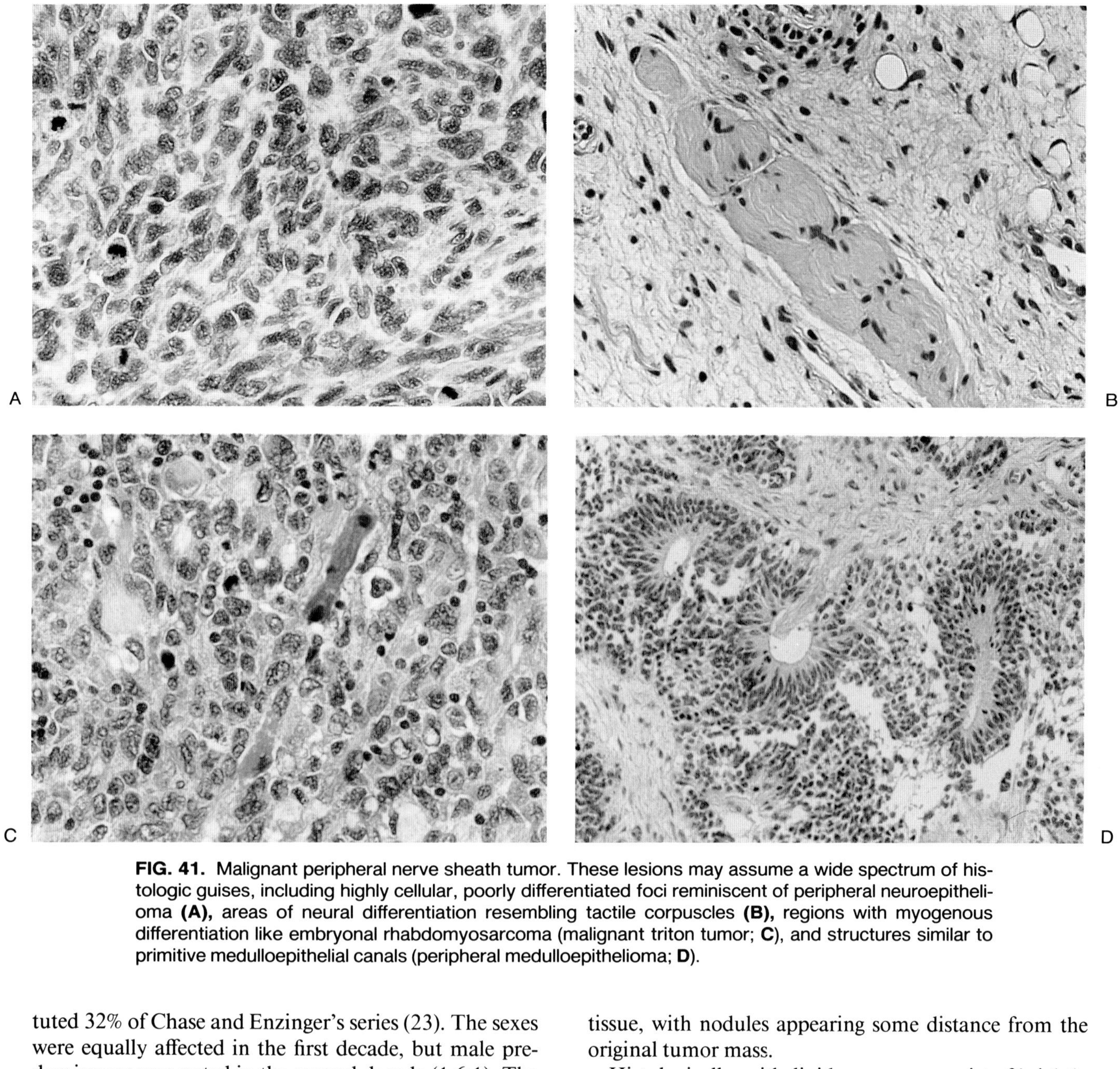

FIG. 41. Malignant peripheral nerve sheath tumor. These lesions may assume a wide spectrum of histologic guises, including highly cellular, poorly differentiated foci reminiscent of peripheral neuroepithelioma **(A),** areas of neural differentiation resembling tactile corpuscles **(B),** regions with myogenous differentiation like embryonal rhabdomyosarcoma (malignant triton tumor; **C**), and structures similar to primitive medulloepithelial canals (peripheral medulloepithelioma; **D**).

tuted 32% of Chase and Enzinger's series (23). The sexes were equally affected in the first decade, but male predominance was noted in the second decade (1.6:1). The commonest site was the distal upper extremity (58%), followed by the distal lower extremity (15%) and then the proximal extremities. It presents as a mass in the skin, subcutaneous tissue, or deep soft tissues such as tendons, fascia, or aponeuroses. The skin lesions may be ulcerated. There is often a long interval between diagnosis and the first appearance of the lesion, as it frequently has a very indolent but relentless course over many years (23).

Grossly epithelioid sarcoma has a nodular growth pattern, the nodules having central areas of necrosis or hyalinization and becoming confluent into multinodular masses. The tumors involve the skin in 24% of cases and may ulcerate or present as chronic draining sinuses. They tend to spread widely and insidiously through the tissue, with nodules appearing some distance from the original tumor mass.

Histologically epithelioid sarcomas consist of brightly eosinophilic, polygonal, epithelioid cells that merge gradually into more fusiform bodies. These do not form long fascicles. The nodules of tumor often have central necrosis or hyalinization and so may mimic granulomata (Fig. 43). The tumors may have a storiform pattern in areas. Giant cells may be seen but are sparse and never highly pleomorphic like those of malignant fibrous histiocytoma. The tumor cell cytoplasm may contain vacuoles giving some resemblance to lipoblasts or primitive endothelial cells, and it often contains glycogen. Intracytoplasmic mucin is not seen (180), but areas of alcian blue–positive myxoid degeneration may be noted in the center of the nodules (23). Hemosiderin pigment may be noted.

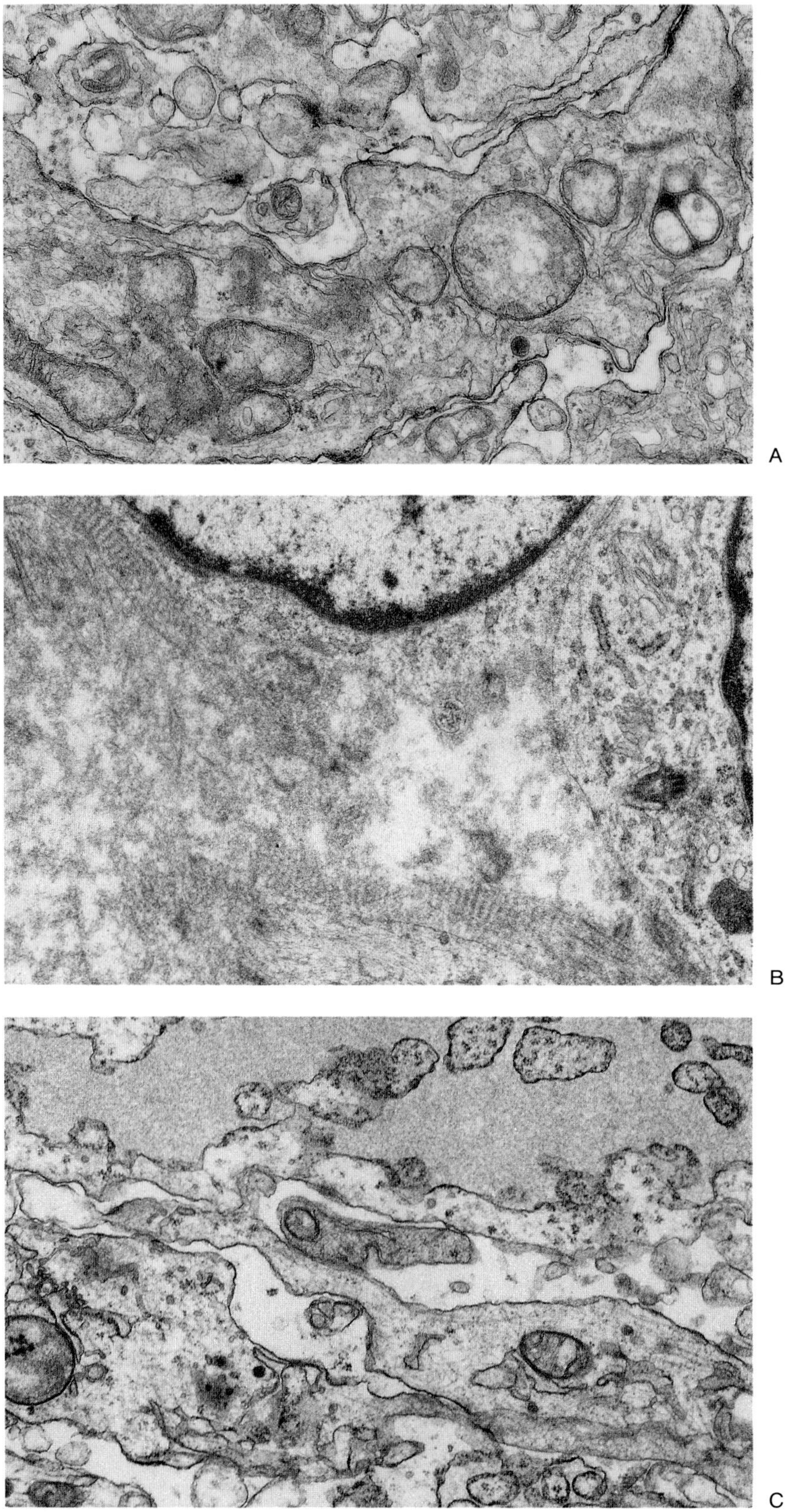

FIG. 42. Malignant peripheral nerve sheath tumor. Tumor cells form attenuated intertwining processes reminiscent of mesaxon formation **(A).** Long-spaced collagen **(B)** and fibroblastic cells with dilated rough endoplasmic reticulum **(C)** may be prominent.

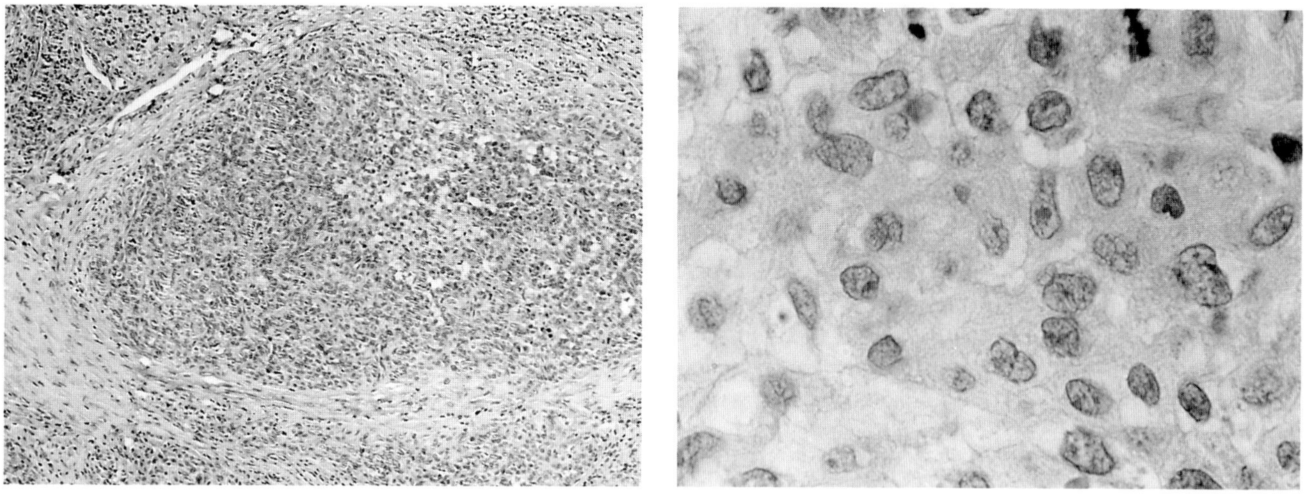

A B

FIG. 43. Epithelioid sarcoma. **A.** At low magnification there is a multinodularity with a resemblance to granulomatous inflammation. **B.** The lesion is composed of polygonal, epithelioid cells with abundant cytoplasm and well-defined plasma membranes.

Immunostaining is very useful in the diagnosis of these tumors, as most stain positively with antibodies to low molecular weight keratin and vimentin (23,180). Some also stain for carcinoembryonic antigen, and the vast majority are negative for S-100 protein. The differential diagnosis of epithelioid sarcoma includes necrobiotic granuloma, giant cell tumor of tendon sheath, malignant fibrous histiocytoma, invasive squamous cell carcinoma, malignant melanoma, clear cell sarcoma, synovial sarcoma, and epithelioid hemangioendothelioma. Recently Mirra et al. (182) described a fibroma variant of epithelioid sarcoma which lacked the typical necrobiotic nodular epithelioid pattern but had a deceptively bland, fibroma-like or dermatofibroma-like appearance. This variant involved bone more frequently than the usual epithelioid sarcoma, and the features useful in diagnosis were the presence of myoid cells and positive cytokeratin staining.

In the study of Chase and Enzinger (23), 7% of epithelioid sarcomas recurred and 45% metastasized. In the cases with metastases, 48% went to lymph nodes, 25% initially to lung, 10% to the scalp, and 6% to nonscalp skin. The high recurrence rate is due to the wide and insidious spread of the tumor. It is important to follow these patients for prolonged periods, as 5% of the cases died as long as 18–19 years after diagnosis. The tumor is best treated with early, aggressive surgery with very wide margins including amputation if necessary (23). Features tending to predict a good prognosis are location in a distal part of an extremity; female sex; young age (<10 years); small size (<1 cm); superficial location; low mitotic index (<2 mitoses per 10 high-power fields); absence of necrosis, hemorrhage, or vascular invasion; and presence of a lymphoid response (23).

Cytogenetic studies of epithelioid sarcoma have revealed deletion of chromosome 1 (260), a t(8;22)(q22;q11) (42), and no abnormalities (255). The t(8;22)(q22;q11) raises interesting speculation regarding its relationship to Ewing's sarcoma, which may share the chromosome 22 breakpoint.

Malignant Fibrous Histiocytoma

Twelve percent of cases accessioned on POG Study 8653 were classified as malignant fibrous histiocytoma (124). This is a somewhat higher incidence than in other series in which the incidence varies from 2% to 6% (38). Malignant fibrous histiocytoma comprises a controversial group of tumors that originally were thought to show divergent differentiation into both fibroblasts and histiocytes (202). Popular theories at the present time are that it represents the end result of dedifferentiation of various other types of sarcoma or a convenient diagnosis for pathologists when a pleomorphic sarcoma cannot be placed in a more specific category (93).

Malignant fibrous histiocytoma has been divided into five different histologic types: storiform pleomorphic, inflammatory, myxoid, giant cell, and angiomatoid. All of these except the angiomatoid variant are tumors predominantly of adult life, but the angiomatoid variety typically occurs in children and young adults (see above). Cole et al. (38), however, found that malignant fibrous histiocytoma was similar in childhood and adulthood in the overall incidence of subtypes and behavior. Two occurred in the orbit of patients previously treated for retinoblastoma with radiotherapy. Zuppan et al. (307) also reported a series of pediatric malignant fibrous histiocytomas that were pathologically similar to those in adults occurred in children.

Malignant Fibrous Lesions

Fibrosarcoma, Adult Type

In a review of 110 cases of fibrosarcoma in infants and children, Soule and Pritchard (257) found two age peaks, one under 5 years (fibrosarcoma of infancy) and one over 10 years (adult-type fibrosarcoma). The importance of separating these two groups lies in the fact that the infantile fibrosarcoma has a much better overall prognosis than that occurring in the older age group. In their series, the survival rate in the older group was 50% and therefore approximated that of adult fibrosarcomas, as opposed to the infantile fibrosarcomas in which the chance of dying from the disease was only 7.3%.

Histologically these tumors are spindle cell lesions typically with a herringbone pattern and no evidence of differentiation other than varying amounts of collagen production. They are more cellular than fibromatoses, show significant mitotic activity and nuclear atypia, and may be partially difficult to differentiate from malignant nerve sheath tumors and synovial sarcomas. Immunohistochemistry and electron microscopy may be very helpful in making these distinctions. The histologic grade is important in deciding the likely behavior of these tumors and therefore the intensity of therapy necessary for cure, as these tumors vary widely from low- to high-grade lesions.

Inflammatory Fibrosarcoma

Meis and Enzinger (171) recently published a series of cases termed inflammatory fibrosarcoma of the mesentery and retroperitoneum, a tumor closely simulating inflammatory pseudotumor. Seventy-nine percent of their 38 patients were under 21 years of age. They presented with abdominal pain, anemia, fever, a mass, or intestinal obstruction and had tumors involving the bowel, mesentery, retroperitoneum, mediastinum, or liver. The neoplasms often formed multiple lesions and invaded through the bowel wall into the mucosa, forming occasionally ulcerated polypoid masses. Histologically the lesions resembled inflammatory myofibroblastic tumors, as they contained a proliferation of fibroblasts, myofibroblasts, and histiocytoid cells arranged in loose, sweeping fascicles (Fig. 44). The tumor cells had vesicular nuclei with prominent nucleoli, and numerous inflammatory cells, mostly plasma cells and some lymphocytes, were present. However, neutrophils and eosinophils were not a feature. Meis and Enzinger speculated that a number of lesions published under other names, such as the omental myxoid hamartoma of Gonzalez-Crussi (103), are actually variants of this tumor.

Myofibrosarcoma

Myofibroblasts are found in many reactive and neoplastic conditions (62). Tumors that do not show specific diagnostic features of other sarcomas and consist for the most part of myofibroblasts may be designated as myofibrosarcoma (83). Immunohistochemistry may be helpful in identifying this cell type in that it is α-smooth

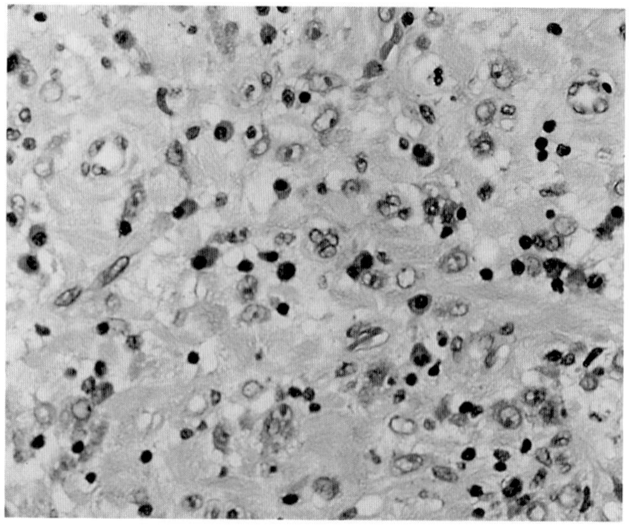

FIG. 44. Inflammatory fibrosarcoma. This lesion, which arose in the abdominal cavity of an infant, is composed of a mixture of plump, histiocytoid cells, fibroblasts, plasma cells, and lymphocytes.

muscle actin–positive, vimentin-positive, and usually desmin-negative, but the diagnosis is usually made by electron microscopy (83). Relatively few cases have been described thus far. Most have occurred in adults between 65 and 85 years of age (83), although children with this tumor have been described (156,283). Most of the initially reported tumors occurred in the superficial soft tissue and tended to be low grade sarcomas (83). More recently, Smith et al. (253) described six myofibrosarcomas occurring in the head and neck of adolescents. These tended to be deeper invasive lesions that killed the patients by repeated recurrences and local extension; only two patients have survived. These head and neck lesions were remarkable for the wide diversity of histologic patterns they exhibited, as they resembled malignant fibrous histiocytoma, fibrosarcoma, rhabdoid tumor, spindle cell rhabdomyosarcoma, and leiomyosarcoma.

Electron microscopic features of the myofibroblasts making up the majority of myofibrosarcoma include spindled contours, abundant rough endoplasmic reticulum, prominent Golgi apparatus, tracts of fine myofilaments with focal densities, fibronexus junctions (anchoring filaments), collagen secretion granules, and micropinocytotic vesicles (83). The fibronexus is an interesting structure thought to be responsible for the attachment of these contractile cells to the connective tissue matrix and possibly to neighboring cells (82). It consists of a plasmalemmal plaque continuous with focally condensed microfilaments on the cytoplasmic side and dense fibrils with extension into interstitial matrix on the extracellular side (Fig. 8C). The fibers outside the cell have been shown to be at least partially composed of fibronectin (85). The fibronexus is postulated as being essential for the diagnosis of a myofibroblast (82). Collagen secretion granules are another ultrastructural feature of myofibrosarcomas and consist of membrane-bound vacuoles containing longitudinally oriented fibrillar material that comprises collagen precursors being packaged for extracellular export (83).

The presence of varying degrees of myofibroblastic differentiation is relatively common in fibrosarcomatous lesions (87,264). Many myofibrosarcomas have thus likely been designated as fibrosarcomas in the past. The differential diagnosis also includes leiomyosarcoma, monophasic synovial sarcoma, neurofibrosarcoma, and malignant fibrous histiocytoma. The main distinction from fibrosarcoma is that the majority of the tumor is made up of myofibroblasts. Leiomyosarcoma differs from this tumor in that its constituent cells contain a greater abundance of myofilaments with focal densities, a better defined basal lamina, and few if any fibronexus junctions with the stroma (84). In addition, smooth muscle cells have relatively inconspicuous rough endoplasmic reticulum and Golgi apparatus as compared with myofibroblasts. Some malignant fibrous histiocytomas are probably forms of myofibrosarcoma (93).

Alveolar Soft Part Sarcoma

Alveolar soft part sarcoma is a rare sarcoma constituting about 1% of all soft tissue sarcomas (78). It was first described in 1952 by Christopherson et al. (26). In children it tends to occur in the head and neck, particularly the tongue and the orbit, whereas in adults it is more common in the lower extremity. The peak age range is between 15 and 35 years (78). The tumor presents as a rather indolent, painless mass that grossly is ill-defined, soft, and friable, often with areas of hemorrhage and necrosis. It may bleed excessively at the time of surgery.

Microscopically, alveolar soft part sarcoma consists of nests of large, rounded, or polygonal cells with abundant eosinophilic cytoplasm, round nuclei, and single, prominent nucleoli (Fig. 45A). The cells are better preserved at the periphery of the nests and tend to degenerate at their center. Each nest is surrounded by thin-walled capillaries, and the tumor as a whole is divided into lobules by fibrous septa. There are prominent vessels in the tissue surrounding the tumor. The tumor cells contain variable amounts of glycogen, but the diagnostic feature is the presence of cytoplasmic PAS-positive, diastase-resistant crystals, found in 80% of cases (Fig. 45B) (78).

By electron microscopy the crystals have a characteristic appearance. They are membrane-bound and rhomboid or rod-shaped with a fine lattice pattern of 60 angstroms periodicity (Fig. 45C). The tumor cells may also contain granular PAS-positive, diastase-resistant material, even in the absence of the crystals; these are seen as electron-dense, membrane-bound granules by electron microscopy (78). A basal lamina is present between the tumor cells and the surrounding capillaries, and desmosomes or hemidesmosomes are seen.

The histogenesis of this tumor is somewhat controversial. Four major theories have been proposed: a granular cell tumor origin, a paraganglioma origin, a muscle origin, and an angioreninoma origin (151,231). Immunoperoxidase staining shows actin, desmin, MyoD, and Z-protein positivity in some tumors (114,177,187,231), cited as support of the myogenic tumor theory. Other lesions (48) do not express muscle markers and appear to be neural in origin. De Schryver-Kecskemeti et al. (58) felt that the crystalloids resembled renin by electron microscopy and obtained renin immunoreactivity in tumor cells. Crystalloids similar to those in alveolar soft part sarcoma have been noted in the muscle spindle, so that this is another possible origin of the neoplasm (17,231). However, similar crystals have been found in a paraganglioma (120) and in a gastric schwannoma (164). Alveolar soft part sarcomas do bear some resemblance to paragangliomas, and Heller et al. (112) reported a case with features of both alveolar soft part sarcoma and paraganglioma. However, S-100 stains the chief cells of alveolar soft part sarcoma but only the sustentacular cells of paragangliomas, and alveolar soft part sarcomas do not stain with argyrophil stains such as Grimelius (151). It is generally accepted that this is not a malignant granular cell tumor (151).

Lieberman et al. (151) in studying the Memorial Sloan-Kettering Hospital experience with this tumor found a number of features to be of prognostic significance; these included patient age and tumor size. Local recurrence was not a major problem provided that the tumor could be excised with a wide margin. Alveolar soft part sarcoma metastasizes to the lung, bone, and brain. Metastases can occur as late as 33 years after diagnosis (152), with 38% occurring 10 years after the diagnosis (151).

Clear Cell Sarcoma of Tendons and Aponeuroses

Clear cell sarcoma of tendons and aponeuroses, also known as malignant melanoma of soft parts, was first described by Enzinger in 1965 (72). It affects the foot, ankle, and the region around the knee (78,237). It may also affect the hand, but the head, neck, and trunk are only rarely involved. The age range is very wide, but most cases occur in young adults (median age 27 years). The neoplasm commonly presents as a slow-growing mass, sometimes having been present for as long as 20 years. It is deep-seated and frequently attached to tendons or aponeuroses (78). It does not arise in the skin but may extend to the dermis (237).

Microscopically, the tumor consists of plump spindle cells or epithelioid cells arranged in nests separated by fine and coarse collagen bundles. Mitoses are infrequent but tumor giant cells are not. The cells contain prominent nucleoli and clear, glycogenated cytoplasm (Fig. 46A). Using the Fontana–Masson stain (Fig. 46B), intracytoplasmic melanin is noted in more than 50% of cases

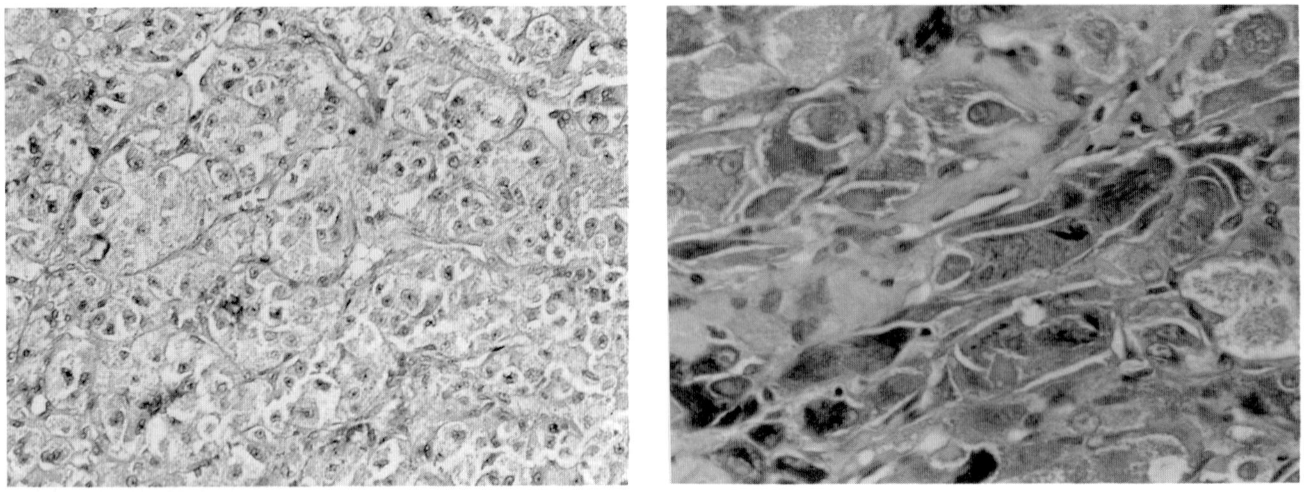

A B

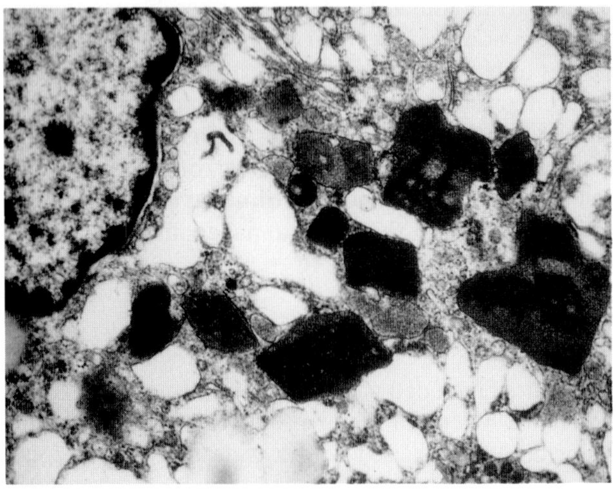

C

FIG. 45. Alveolar soft part sarcoma. **A.** The lesion has an easily recognizable low power pattern comprised of small nests of cells with regular nuclei and abundant cytoplasm. **B.** Periodic acid–Schiff stains reveal the presence of needle-shaped cytoplasmic crystals. **C.** Electron microscopy discloses the typical rhomboidal crystals in the tumor cell cytoplasm. (Part **C** courtesy of Dr. J. O. Palmer, St. John Medical Center, Tulsa, OK.)

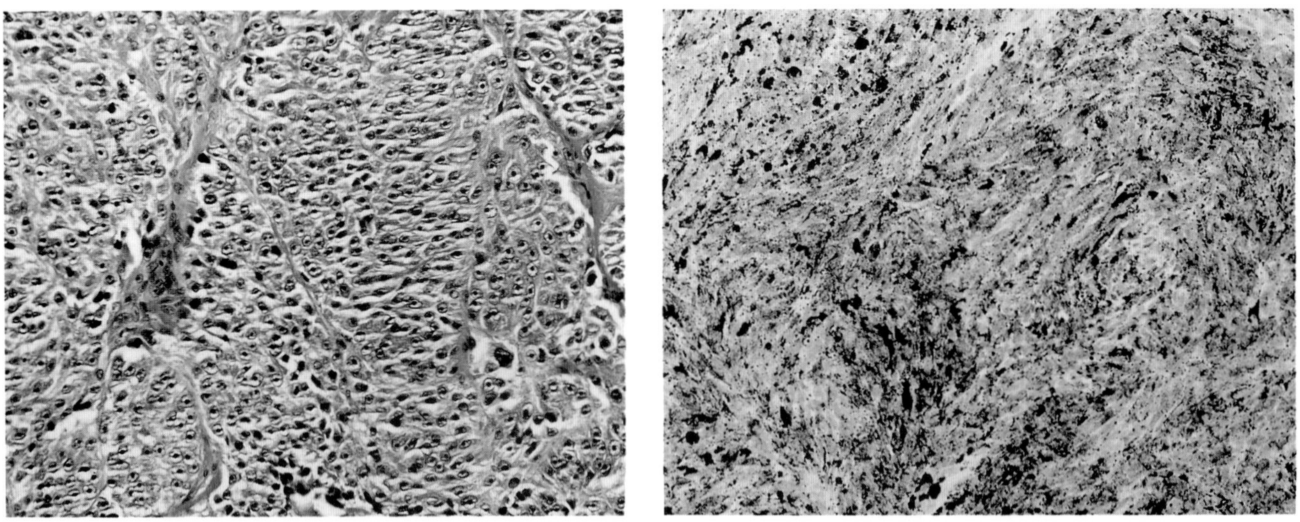

A B

FIG. 46. Clear cell sarcoma of soft tissue. **A.** The tumor is composed of nests of cells with large oval nuclei, prominent nucleoli, and clear to amphophilic cytoplasm. **B.** A Fontana stain reveals abundant intracytoplasmic melanin, visible as darkly staining granules.

(78). Most cases have cells containing premelanosomes on electron microscopy or staining with S-100 protein and HMB-45 (Fig. 46B) (78,155,203).

Clear cell sarcoma is a highly malignant tumor (155,237). It metastasizes to regional lymph nodes, lung, and bone. Metastases may occur as late as 29 years after surgery (31). Sara et al. (237) noted a relationship between an epithelioid phenotype and the presence of lymph node metastases. Tumor size, necrosis, and regional lymph node metastases are also major prognostic factors (155,237).

Two recurring genetic aberrations, t(12;22)(q13;q13) and trisomy 8, are found in clear cell sarcomas (153,222,230,261,270). These abnormalities are distinct from those seen in malignant melanoma (see Chapter 12) and confirm that these are histologically similar but unrelated tumors. The breakpoint involved in the t(12;22) fuses the *EWS* gene on chromosome 22 with the *ATF-1* gene on chromosome 12 (305), thus indicating a genetic relatedness to Ewing's sarcoma.

Angiosarcoma

Angiosarcoma composes 1% of childhood vascular tumors and usually occurs in older teenagers (35). Pediatric angiosarcomas have been reported with neurofibromatosis type 1, angiomatosis, congenital hypertrophy of the extremities, and postradiotherapy (24,35). They have the same histologic appearance as those in adults, namely, anastomosing vascular channels lined by atypical endothelium with mitotic activity and a tendency to protrude into the lumen (Fig. 47). The vascular channels can be followed continuously for long distances across the slide (SW Weiss, personal communication). There may be a deceptively solid appearance in areas, making differentiation from carcinoma or melanoma difficult.

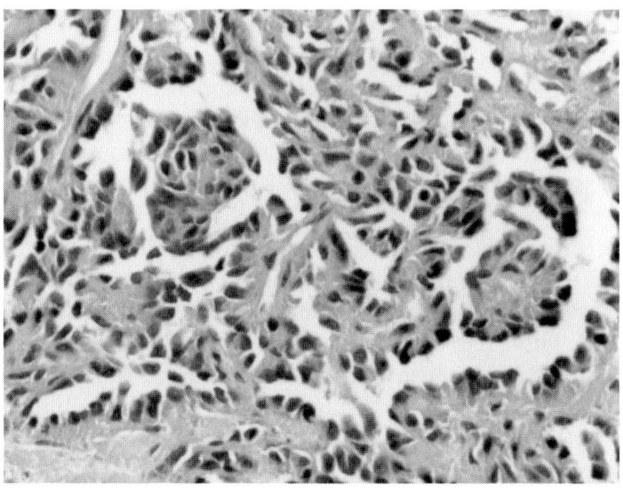

FIG. 47. Angiosarcoma. Anastomosing vascular channels are lined by cuboidal neoplastic endothelial cells that protrude into the lumen.

Invasion of the surrounding dermis occurs by insinuation of tumor cells between the collagen fibers forming clefts, and in these areas it may be difficult to identify the tumor as a malignancy.

It has been said that angiosarcomas in childhood have a better prognosis than in adults. Fukunaga et al. (97) had four cases of pediatric angiosarcoma among their 20 cases; two of these children died of their disease. DNA ploidy analysis was not very useful as a predictor of outcome, and size was not as reliable in predicting behavior as had been previously found (118).

Liposarcoma

Liposarcoma is common in adults but is a rare tumor in childhood. However, it may occur in patients between 10 and 15 years of age (250). Shmookler and Enzinger (250) found 17 cases in children under 15 years of age among a total of 2,500 liposarcomas accessioned at the AFIP. Almost all fatty tumors occurring in children under 10 years are lipoblastomas (78). Lipoblastomas show distinct lobular compartmentalization (see above) whereas liposarcomas do not, and lipoblastomas do not show the microcystic change commonly present in liposarcoma (250). As in adults, the thigh is a very common site for childhood liposarcoma, but the retroperitoneum is a very uncommon site. Children have a higher proportion of low-grade lesions than adults and have a better outlook overall (138,250). Myxoid liposarcomas are relatively more common and well-differentiated liposarcomas relatively less common than in adults (250). La Quaglia et al. (138) confirmed that patients with completely excised tumors had an excellent prognosis. However, all four patients with gross residual disease died from tumor progression. Other features affecting survival include site (lesions on the extremities doing better) and size (with tumors 5 cm in diameter or more having a significantly worse prognosis).

Leiomyosarcoma

Leiomyosarcomas are rare in children. In the authors' experience (9) they have been most common in the gastrointestinal tract and have not occurred in the uterus. Immunohistochemical stains show overlap with rhabdomyosarcoma, as desmin, vimentin, and muscle-specific actin are positive. Myoglobin stains will separate better differentiated examples of rhabdomyosarcoma from leiomyosarcoma; the authors' experience with MyoD in the latter tumor is limited (266) but suggests that it may be useful in less differentiated sarcomas. The issue is complicated by the fact that both rhabdomyosarcoma and developing skeletal muscle may express a smooth muscle phenotype, including expression of α-smooth muscle actin and a newer marker, cortactin (206), and peripheral condensates of microfilaments punctuated by dense bodies (205). Nevertheless, we treat childhood leiomyosarcoma on nonrhabdomyosarcoma soft tissue sarcoma protocols and find that it behaves in a fashion similar to that of other tumors of this group (167). Another emerging issue has been its separation from myofibroblastic tumors, which may bear a close resemblance to smooth muscle neoplasms (see above).

Another highly pertinent observation has been the recent emergence of pediatric leiomyosarcomas as a complication of human immunodeficiency virus–1 infection (280).

Extraskeletal Mesenchymal Chondrosarcoma

Extraskeletal mesenchymal chondrosarcoma may occur within skeletal muscle and affects young adults predominantly from 15 to 35 years of age (78). It presents as a circumscribed, lobulated mass that may have spiculated calcification on radiographs. Histologically it consists of sheets of small cells with inconspicuous cytoplasm, separated by prominent vascular channels frequently arrayed in a hemangiopericytomalike pattern (Fig. 48). A varying amount of chondroid differentiation is observed, from rare spicules of fairly well-differentiated cartilage to fairly frequent islands of cartilage. The chondroid areas stain for S-100 protein and Leu 7 antigen (265).

It is important to distinguish this tumor from hemangiopericytoma and synovial sarcoma. The former does not show cartilaginous differentiation and the latter shows a biphasic pattern or cytokeratin staining at least focally. These tumors are highly malignant and metastasize to the lungs. A Ewing's sarcoma–type cytogenetic abnormality, the t(11;22)(q24;q12), has been reported (235).

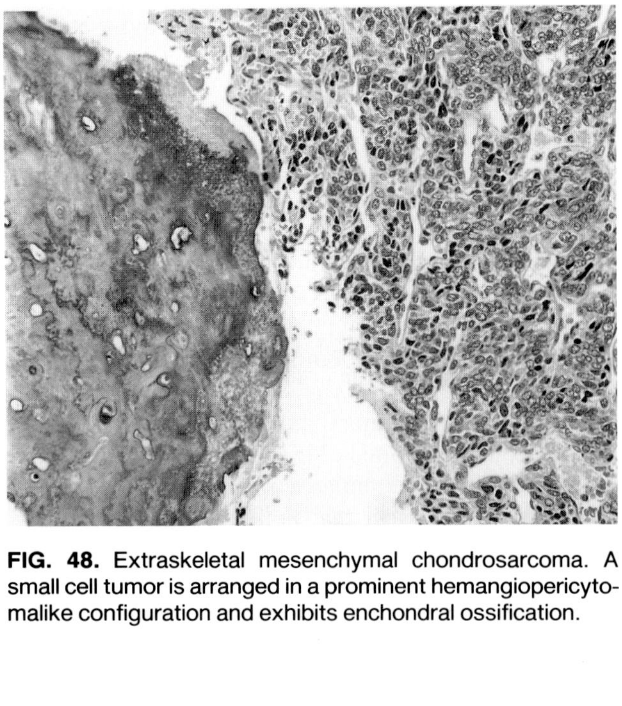

FIG. 48. Extraskeletal mesenchymal chondrosarcoma. A small cell tumor is arranged in a prominent hemangiopericytomalike configuration and exhibits enchondral ossification.

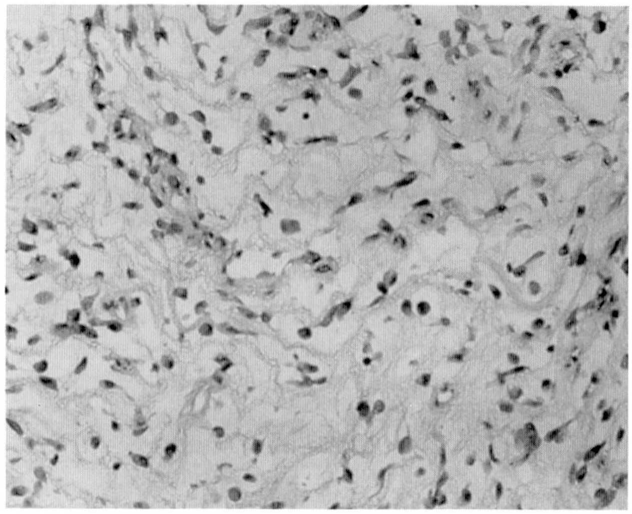

FIG. 49. Extraskeletal myxoid chondrosarcoma. Loose cords and trabeculae of chondrocytic cells lie in an abundant myxoid matrix.

Extraskeletal Myxoid Chondrosarcoma

Extraskeletal myxoid chondrosarcoma is a very rare soft tissue sarcoma in childhood. In a literature review, Hachitanda et al. (109) found five cases in children and added two of their own. The neoplasm presents as a mass most commonly in the lower extremity or buttock. Other cases involve the chest wall, the upper arm, and the scalp. We have observed a case involving the epiglottis (296). Histologically the tumors have a lobulated configuration, the lobules being separated by fibrous septa. The lobules contain abundant myxoid matrix between small rounded tumor cells that lie in cords or form sheets (Fig. 49). The matrix stains with alcian blue dye at pH 2.5 in a hyaluronidase-resistant manner. The tumor cells are uniform with relatively little cytoplasm. They may have eosinophilic cytoplasmic inclusions that push the nucleus to one side. The cytoplasm contains glycogen. The cells stain positively for S-100 protein and vimentin but are negative for cytokeratin, EMA, carcinoembryonic antigen, neuron-specific enolase, desmin, and Leu 7 (109). By electron microscopy some cells contain dilated cisternae of rough endoplasmic reticulum, sometimes filled with characteristic arrays of microtubules (109). The t(9;22) has been found to characterize this tumor cytogenetically (160). Differential diagnosis includes rhabdomyosarcoma, malignant extrarenal rhabdoid tumors, neurothekioma, chordoma, myxoid liposarcoma, and myxoid malignant fibrous histiocytoma.

In adults these tumors have been considered to be relatively innocuous in their behavior. However, they have been very aggressive in some pediatric cases; five of seven reported children died of their disease within months of diagnosis (109).

ACKNOWLEDGMENT

Supported in part by Cancer Center Support CORE grant P30 CA21765 and American Lebanese Syrian Associated Charities (ALSAC).

REFERENCES

1. Abdul-Karim FW, El-Naggar AK, Joyce MJ, Makley JT, Carter JR. Diffuse and localized tenosynovial giant cell tumor and pigmented villonodular synovitis: a clinicopathologic and flow cytometric DNA analysis. *Hum Pathol* 1992;23:729–735.
2. Ackerman LV, Taylor FH. Neurogenous tumors within the thorax. A clinicopathological evaluation of forty-eight cases. *Cancer* 1951;4:669–691.
3. Ainsworth PJ, Rodenhiser DI, Costa MT. Identification and characterization of sporadic and inherited mutations in exon 31 of the neurofibromatosis (NF1) gene. *Hum Genet* 1993;91:151–156.
4. Alberts B, Bray D, Lewis J, Raff M, Roberts K, Watson JD. *Molecular Biology of the Cell.* 2nd ed. New York: Garland; 1989.
5. Albores-Saavedra J, Manivel JC, Essenfeld H, Dehner LP, Drut R, Gould E, Rosai J. Pseudosarcomatous myofibroblastic proliferations in the urinary bladder of children. *Cancer* 1990;66: 1234–1241.
6. Alguacil-Garcia A. Giant cell fibroblastoma recurring as dermatofibrosarcoma protuberans. *Am J Surg Pathol* 1991;15:798–801.
7. Allen PW. Nodular fasciitis. *Pathology* 1972;4:9–26.
8. Allen PW, Zwi J. Giant cell fibroblastoma transforming into dermatofibrosarcoma protuberans. *Am J Surg Pathol* 1992;16: 1127–1128.
9. Angel CA, Gant LL, Parham DM, Rao BN, Douglass EC, Lobe T, Philippe PG. Leiomyosarcomas in children: clinical and pathologic characteristics. *Pediatr Surg Int* 1992;7:116–120.
10. Beham A, Badve S, Suster S, Fletcher CDM. Solitary myofibroma in adults: clinicopathological analysis of a series. *Histopathology* 1993;22:335–341.
11. Beham A, Fletcher CDM. Dermatofibrosarcoma protuberans with areas resembling giant cell fibroblastoma: report of two cases. *Histopathology* 1990;17:165–167.
12. Beham A, Fletcher CDM, Kainz J, Schmid C, Humer U. Nasopharyngeal angiofibroma: an immunohistochemical study of 32 cases. *Virchows Arch A Histopathol Anat* 1993;423:281–285.
13. Brem S, Tsanaclis AMC, Gately S, Gross JL, Herblin WF. Immunolocalization of basic fibroblast growth factor to the microvasculature of human brain tumors. *Cancer* 1993;70:2673–2680.
14. Bridge JA, Sreekantaiah C, Mouron B, Neff JR, Sandberg AA, Wolman SR. Clonal chromosomal abnormalities in desmoid tumors. Implications for histopathogenesis. *Cancer* 1992;69:430–436.
15. Cance WG, Brennan MF, Dudas ME, Huang C-M, Cordon-Cardo C. Altered expression of the retinoblastoma gene product in human sarcomas. *N Engl J Med* 1990;323:1457–1462.
16. Carney JA. Psammomatous melanotic schwannoma. A distinctive, heritable tumor with special associations, including cardiac myxoma and the Cushing syndrome. *Am J Surg Pathol* 1990;14: 206–222.
17. Carstens PHB. Membrane-bound cytoplasmic crystals, similar to those in alveolar soft part sarcoma, in a human muscle spindle. *Ultrastruct Pathol* 1990;14:423–428.
18. Cawthon RM, Weiss R, Xu GF, et al. A major segment of the neurofibromatosis type 1 gene: cDNA sequence, genomic structure, and point mutations. *Cell* 1990;62:193–201.
19. Celasun B, Seçkin B, Harmankaya Ç, Pabusçu Y, Finci R. A pseudotumour of the bladder. *Scand J Urol Nephrol* 1993;27: 127–128.
20. Chambers AF, Tuck AB. Oncogene transformation and the metastatic phenotype. *Anticancer Res* 1988;8:861–871.
21. Chamson A, Frey J, Frappaz D, Damon G, Freycon F, Lauras B. Collagen biosynthesis in a case of infantile myofibromatosis. *Clin Physiol Biochem* 1988;6:57–63.
22. Chan JK, Frizzera G, Fletcher CD, Rosai J. Primary vascular tumors of lymph nodes other than Kaposi's sarcoma. Analysis of 39 cases and delineation of two new entities. *Am J Surg Pathol* 1992;16:335–350.
23. Chase DR, Enzinger FM. Epithelioid sarcoma. Diagnosis, prognostic indicators, and treatment. *Am J Surg Pathol* 1985;9:241–263.
24. Chaudhuri B, Ronan SG, Manaligod JR. Angiosarcoma arising in a plexiform neurofibroma: a case report. *Cancer* 1980;46:605–610.
25. Chen KTK, Bauer FW. Sarcomatous transformation of nasopharyngeal angiofibroma. *Cancer* 1982;49:369–371.
26. Christopherson WM, Foote FW, Stewart FW. Alveolar soft part sarcomas. Structurally characteristic tumors of uncertain histogenesis. *Cancer* 1952;5:100–111.
27. Chung EB, Enzinger FM. Benign lipoblastomatosis. An analysis of 35 cases. *Cancer* 1973;32:482–492.
28. Chung EB, Enzinger FM. Infantile fibrosarcoma. *Cancer* 1976;38:729–739.
29. Chung EB, Enzinger FM. Chondroma of soft parts. *Cancer* 1978;41:1414–1424.
30. Chung EB, Enzinger FM. Infantile myofibromatosis. *Cancer* 1981;48:1807–1818.
31. Chung EB, Enzinger FM. Malignant melanoma of soft parts. A reassessment of clear cell sarcoma. *Am J Surg Pathol* 1983;7:405–413.
32. Clark J, Rocques PJ, Crew AJ, et al. Identification of novel genes, SYT and SSX, involved in the t(X; 18)(p11.2;q11.2) translocation found in human synovial sarcoma. *Nat Genet* 1994;7:502–508.
33. Coffin CM, Dehner LP. Peripheral neurogenic tumors of the soft tissues in children and adolescents: a clinicopathologic study of 139 cases. *Pediatr Pathol* 1989;9:387–407.
34. Coffin CM, Dehner LP. Cellular peripheral neural tumors (neurofibromas) in children and adolescents: a clinicopathological and immunohistochemical study. *Pediatr Pathol* 1990;10:351–361.
35. Coffin CM, Dehner LP. Vascular tumors in children and adolescents: a clinicopathologic study of 228 tumors in 222 patients. *Pathol Annu* 1993;28 Pt 1:97–120.
36. Cohen PR, Rapini RP, Farhood AI. Expression of the human hematopoietic progenitor cell antigen CD34 in dermatofibrosarcoma protuberans, other spindle cell tumors, and vascular lesions. *J Am Acad Dermatol* 1994;30:147–148.
37. Cohen RB, Hahn GV, Tabas JA, et al. The natural history of heterotopic ossification in patients who have fibrodysplasia ossificans progressiva. A study of forty-four patients. *J Bone Joint Surg Am* 1993;75:215–219.
38. Cole CH, Magee JF, Gianoulis M, Rogers PCJ. Malignant fibrous histiocytoma in childhood. *Cancer* 1993;71:4077–4083.
39. Colman SD, Collins FS, Wallace MR. Characterization of a single base-pair deletion in neurofibromatosis type 1. *Hum Mol Genet* 1993;2:1709–1711.
40. Connor JM, Skirton H, Lunt PW. A three generation family with fibrodysplasia ossificans progressiva. *J Med Genet* 1993;30:687–689.
41. Cooper PH, McAllister HA, Helwig EB. Intravenous pyogenic granuloma. A study of 18 cases. *Am J Surg Pathol* 1979;3:221–228.
42. Cordoba JC, Parham DM, Meyer WH, Douglass EC. A new cytogenetic finding in an epithelioid sarcoma, t(8;22)(q22;q11). *Cancer Genet Cytogenet* 1994;72:151–154.
43. Costa J, Wesley RA, Glatstein E, Rosenberg SA. The grading of soft tissue sarcomas. Results of a clinicohistopathologic correlation in a series of 163 cases. *Cancer* 1984;53:530–541.
44. Costa MJ, Weiss SW. Angiomatoid malignant fibrous histiocytoma: A follow-up study of 108 cases with evaluation of possible

histologic predictors of outcome. *Am J Surg Pathol* 1990;14: 1126–1132.

45. Cotran RS, Kumar V, Robbins SL. *Robbins Pathologic Basis of Disease.* 5th ed. Philadelphia: WB Saunders; 1994.
46. Cox JV, Balaban EP, Demian SE, Sheehan RG. An eosinophilic fibrohistiocytic lesion of bone marrow in a patient with Hodgkin's disease: A potential for morphologic confusion. *Cancer* 1991;68: 1824–1827.
47. Coyne J, Kaftan SM, Craig RDP. Dermatofibrosarcoma protuberans recurring as a giant cell fibroblastoma. *Histopathology* 1992;21:184–187.
48. Cullinane C, Thorner PS, Greenberg ML, Ng YK, Kumar M, Squire J. Molecular genetic, cytogenetic, and immunohistochemical characterization of alveolar soft-part sarcoma: implications for cell of origin. *Cancer* 1992;70:2444–2450.
49. Dabska M. Malignant endovascular papillary angioendothelioma of the skin in childhood. Clinicopathologic study of 6 cases. *Cancer* 1969;24:503–510.
50. Dal Cin P, Brock P, Casteels-Van Daele M, De Wever I, Van Damme B, Van Den Berghe H. Cytogenetic characterization of congenital or infantile fibrosarcoma. *Eur J Pediatr* 1991;150: 579–581.
51. Dal Cin P, Sciot R, Aly MS, et al. Some desmoid tumors are characterized by trisomy 8. *Genes Chrom Cancer* 1994;10:131–135.
52. Dardick I, Ramjohn S, Thomas MJ, Jeans D, Hammar SP. Synovial sarcoma. Inter-relationship of the biphasic and monophasic subtypes. *Pathol Res Pract* 1991;187:871–885.
53. Darnell J, Lodish H, Baltimore D. *Molecular Cell Biology.* New York: Scientific American Books; 1986.
54. De Graaf JH, Timens W, Tamminga RYJ, Molenaar WM. Deep juvenile xanthogranuloma: a lesion related to dermal indeterminate cells. *Hum Pathol* 1992;23:905–910.
55. Dehner LP. *Pediatric Surgical Pathology.* 2nd ed. Baltimore: Williams and Wilkins; 1987.
56. Dei Tos AP, Doglioni C, Laurino L, Barbareschi M, Fletcher CDM. p53 protein expression in non-neoplastic lesions and benign and malignant neoplasms of soft tissue. *Histopathology* 1993;22:45–50.
57. Denekamp J. Review article: angiogenesis, neovascular proliferation and vascular pathophysiology as targets for cancer therapy. *Br J Radiol* 1993;66:181–196.
58. DeSchryver-Kecskemeti K, Kraus FT, Engleman W, Lacy PE. Alveolar soft-part sarcoma—a malignant angioreninoma: Histochemical, immunocytochemical, and electron-microscopic study of four cases. *Am J Surg Pathol* 1982;6:5–18.
59. Deuel TF. Polypeptide growth factors: roles in normal and abnormal cell growth. *Annu Rev Cell Biol* 1987;3:443–492.
60. Devaney K, Vinh TN, Sweet DE. Synovial hemangioma: a report of 20 cases with differential diagnostic considerations. *Hum Pathol* 1993;24:737–745.
61. Ding J, Hashimoto H, Imayama S, Tsuneyoshi M, Enjoji M. Spindle cell haemangioendothelioma: probably a benign vascular lesion not a low-grade angiosarcoma. A clinicopathological, ultrastructural and immunohistochemical study. *Virchows Arch A Histopathol Anat* 1992;420:77–85.
62. Dominguez-Malagon H. Proliferative disorders of myofibroblasts. *Ultrastruct Pathol* 1993;17:211–220.
63. Donner LR. Cytogenetics and molecular biology of small round-cell tumors and related neoplasms. Current status. *Cancer Genet Cytogenet* 1991;54:1–10.
64. Ducatman BS, Scheithauer BW. Malignant peripheral nerve sheath tumors with divergent differentiation. *Cancer* 1984;54: 1049–1057.
65. Dupree WB, Enzinger FM. Fibro-osseous pseudotumor of the digits. *Cancer* 1986;58:2103–2109.
66. Dvorak HF. Tumors: wounds that do not heal. Similarities between tumor stroma generation and wound healing. *N Engl J Med* 1986;315:1650–1659.
67. Easton DF, Ponder MA, Huson SM, Ponder BA. An analysis of variation in expression of neurofibromatosis (NF) type 1 (NF1): evidence for modifying genes. *Am J Hum Genet* 1993;53:305–313.
68. Ecklund J, Schut L, Rorke L. Associated vascular malformations and neoplasms in children. *Pediatr Neurosurg* 1993;19:196–201.
69. El-Jabbour JN, Akhtar SS, Kerr GR, McLaren KM, Smyth JF, Rodger A, Leonard RCF. Prognostic factors for survival in soft tissue sarcoma. *Br J Cancer* 1990;62:857–861.
70. El-Jabbour JN, Wilson GD, Bennett MH, Burke MM, Davey AT, Eames K. Flow cytometric study of nodular fasciitis, proliferative fasciitis, and proliferative myositis. *Hum Pathol* 1991;22:1146–1149.
71. El-Naggar AK, Ayala AG, Abdul-Karim FW, et al. Synovial sarcoma: A DNA flow cytometric study. *Cancer* 1990;65:2295–2300.
72. Enzinger FM. Clear cell sarcoma of tendons and aponeuroses: an analysis of 21 cases. *Cancer* 1965;18:1163–1174.
73. Enzinger FM. Fibrous hamartoma of infancy. Cancer 1965;18: 241–248.
74. Enzinger FM. Epithelioid sarcoma. A sarcoma simulating a granuloma or a carcinoma. *Cancer* 1970;26:1029–1041.
75. Enzinger FM. Angiomatoid malignant fibrous histiocytoma: a distinct fibrohistiocytic tumor of children and young adults simulating a vascular neoplasm. *Cancer* 1979;44:2147–2157.
76. Enzinger FM, Dulcey F. Proliferative myositis. Report of thirty-three cases. *Cancer* 1967;20:2213–2223.
77. Enzinger FM, Smith BH. Hemangiopericytoma. An analysis of 106 cases. *Hum Pathol* 1976;7:61–82.
78. Enzinger FM, Weiss SW. *Soft Tissue Tumors.* 2nd ed. St. Louis: Mosby; 1988.
79. Enzinger FM, Zhang RY. Plexiform fibrohistiocytic tumor presenting in children and young adults. An analysis of 65 cases. *Am J Surg Pathol* 1988;12:818–826.
80. Erlandson RA. *Diagnostic Transmission Electron Microscopy of Tumors with Clinicopathological, Immunohistochemical, and Cytogenetic Correlations.* New York: Raven Press; 1994.
81. Estivill X, Lazaro C, Casals T, Ravella A. Recurrence of a nonsense mutation in the NF1 gene causing classical neurofibromatosis type 1. *Hum Genet* 1991;88:185–188.
82. Eyden BP. Brief review of the fibronexus and its significance for myofibroblastic differentiation and tumor diagnosis. *Ultrastruct Pathol* 1993;17:611–622.
83. Eyden BP, Banerjee SS, Harris M, Mene A. A study of spindle cell sarcomas showing myofibroblastic differentiation. *Ultrastruct Pathol* 1991;15:367–378.
84. Eyden BP, Christensen L. Leiomyosarcoma versus myofibrosarcoma: observations and terminology. Ultrastruct *Pathol 1993;*17: 231–239.
85. Eyden BP, Christensen L, Tagore V, Harris M. Myofibrosarcoma of subcutaneous soft tissue of the cheek. *J Submicrosc Cytol Pathol* 1992;24:307–313.
86. Fetsch JF, Montgomery EA, Meis JM. Calcifying fibrous pseudotumor. *Am J Surg Pathol* 1993;17:502–508.

86a. Filling-Katz MR, Levin SW, Patronas NJ, Katz NN. Terminal transverse limb defects associated with familial cavernous angiomatosis. *Am J Med Genet* 1992;42:346–351.

87. Fisher C. The value of electronmicroscopy and immunohistochemistry in the diagnosis of soft tissue sarcomas: A study of 200 cases. *Histopathology* 1990;16:441–454.
88. Fletcher CD. Benign fibrous histiocytoma of subcutaneous and deep soft tissue: a clinicopathologic analysis of 21 cases. *Am J Surg Pathol* 1990;14:801–809.
89. Fletcher CD, Achu P, van Noorden S, McKee PH. Infantile myofibromatosis: a light microscopic, histochemical and immunohistochemical study suggesting true smooth muscle differentiation. *Histopathology* 1987;11:245–258.
90. Fletcher CD, Davies SE, McKee PH. Cellular schwannoma: a distinct pseudosarcomatous entity. *Histopathology* 1987;11:21–35.
91. Fletcher CDM. Recent advances in the pathology of soft tissue tumours. *Diagn Oncol* 1991;1:5–11.
92. Fletcher CDM. Angiomatoid "malignant fibrous histiocytoma": an immunohistochemical study indicative of myoid differentiation. *Hum Pathol* 1991;22:563–568.
93. Fletcher CDM. Pleomorphic malignant fibrous histiocytoma: fact or fiction? A critical reappraisal based on 159 tumors diagnosed as pleomorphic sarcoma. *Am J Surg Pathol* 1992;16:213–228.
94. Fletcher CDM, Beham A, Bekir S, Clarke AMT, Marley NJE. Epithelioid angiosarcoma of deep soft tissue: a distinctive tumor

readily mistaken for an epithelial neoplasm. *Am J Surg Pathol* 1991;15:915–924.

95. Fletcher CDM, Beham A, Schmid C. Spindle cell haemangioendothelioma: a clinicopathological and immunohistochemical study indicative of a non-neoplastic lesion. *Histopathology* 1991;18:291–301.
96. Franquemont DW, Cooper PH, Shmookler BM, Wick MR. Benign fibrous histiocytoma of the skin with potential for local recurrence: a tumor to be distinguished from dermatofibroma. *Mod Pathol* 1990;3:158–163.
97. Fukunaga M, Shimoda T, Nikaido T, Ushigome S, Ishikawa E. Soft tissue vascular tumors. A flow cytometric DNA analysis. *Cancer* 1993;71:2233–2241.
98. Geddy PM, Gray S, Reid WA. Mast cell density and PGP 9.5-immunostained nerves in angioleiomyoma: their relationship to painful symptoms. *Histopathology* 1993;22:387–390.
99. Ghadially FN, Thomas MJ, Jabi M, Rippstein P. Intracisternal collagen fibrils in proliferative fasciitis and myositis of childhood. *Ultrastruct Pathol* 1993;17:161–168.
100. Giardiello FM, Hamilton SR, Krush AJ, Offerhaus JA, Booker SV, Petersen GM. Nasopharyngeal angiofibroma in patients with familial adenomatous polyposis. *Gastroenterology* 1993;105: 1550–1552.
101. Goldberg NS, Collins FS. The hunt for the neurofibromatosis gene. *Arch Dermatol* 1991;127:1705–1707.
102. Golouh R, Vuzevski V, Bracko M, van der Heul RO, Cervek J. Synovial sarcoma: a clinicopathological study of 36 cases. *J Surg Oncol* 1990;45:20–28.
103. Gonzalez-Crussi F, deMello DE, Sotelo-Avila C. Omental-mesenteric myxoid hamartomas. Infantile lesions simulating malignant tumors. *Am J Surg Pathol* 1983;7:567–578.
104. Gonzalez-Crussi F, Reyes-Mugica M. Cellular hemangiomas ("hemangioendotheliomas") in infants. Light microscopic, immunohistochemical, and ultrastructural observations. *Am J Surg Pathol* 1991;15:769–778.
105. Gray MH, Rosenberg AE, Dickersin GR, Bhan AK. Cytokeratin expression in epithelioid vascular neoplasms. *Hum Pathol* 1990;21:212–217.
106. Gregory PE, Gutmann DH, Mitchell A, et al. Neurofibromatosis type 1 gene product (neurofibromin) associates with microtubules. *Somat Cell Mol Genet* 1993;19:265–274.
107. Groisman G, Lichtig C. Fibrous hamartoma of infancy: an immunohistochemical and ultrastructural study. *Hum Pathol* 1991;22:914–918.
108. Gutmann DH, Wood DL, Collins FS. Identification of the neurofibromatosis type 1 gene product. *Proc Natl Acad Sci USA* 1991;88:9658–9662.
109. Hachitanda Y, Tsuneyoshi M, Daimaru Y, Enjoji M, Nakagawara A, Ikeda K, Sueishi K. Extraskeletal myxoid chondrosarcoma in young children. *Cancer* 1988;61:2521–2526.
110. Hayry P, Reitamo JJ, Totterman S, Hopfner-Hallikainen D, Sivula A. The desmoid tumor. II. Analysis of factors possibly contributing to the etiology and growth behavior. *Am J Clin Pathol* 1982;77:674–680.
111. Hayry P, Reitamo JJ, Vihko R, et al. The desmoid tumor. III. A biochemical and genetic analysis. *Am J Clin Pathol* 1982;77:681–685.
112. Heller DS, Frydman CP, Gordon RE, Jagirdar J, Schwartz IS. An unusual organoid tumor: alveolar soft part sarcoma or paraganglioma. *Cancer* 1991;67:1894–1899.
113. Herrera GA, Johnson WW, Lockard VG, Walker BL. Soft tissue myofibroblastomas. *Mod Pathol* 1991;4:571–577.
114. Hirose T, Kudo E, Hasegawa T, Abe J-I, Hizawa K. Cytoskeletal properties of alveolar soft part sarcoma. *Hum Pathol* 1990;21: 204–211.
115. Hirose T, Sumitomo M, Kudo E, et al. Malignant peripheral nerve sheath tumor (MPNST) showing perineurial cell differentiation. *Am J Surg Pathol* 1989;13:613–620.
116. Hirota S, Nomura S, Asada H, Ito A, Morii E, Kitamura Y. Possible involvement of c-kit receptor and its ligand in increase of mast cells in neurofibroma tissues. *Arch Pathol Lab Med* 1993;117:996–999.
117. Hofman KJ, Boehm CD. Familial neurofibromatosis type 1: clinical experience with DNA testing. *J Pediatr* 1992;120:394–398.
118. Holden CA, Spittle MF, Jones EW. Angiosarcoma of the face and scalp, prognosis and treatment. *Cancer* 1987;59:1046–1057.
119. Hollowood K, Holley MP, Fletcher CDM. Plexiform fibrohistiocytic tumour: clinicopathological, immunohistochemical and ultrastructural analysis in favour of a myofibroblastic lesion. *Histopathology* 1991;19:503–513.
120. Horvath KK, Ormos J, Ribari O. Crystals in a jugulotympanic paraganglioma. *Ultrastruct Pathol* 1986;10:257–264.
121. Hruban RH, Shiu MH, Senie RT, Woodruff JM. Malignant peripheral nerve sheath tumors of the buttock and lower extremity. A study of 43 cases. *Cancer* 1990;66:1253–1265.
122. Jaakkola S, Peltonen J, Riccardi V, Chu ML, Uitto J. Type 1 neurofibromatosis: selective expression of extracellular matrix genes by Schwann cells, perineurial cells, and fibroblasts in mixed cultures. *J Clin Invest* 1989;84:253–261.
123. Janney CG, Hurt MA, Santa Cruz DJ. Deep juvenile xanthogranuloma. Subcutaneous and intramuscular forms. *Am J Surg Pathol* 1991;15:150–159.
124. Jenkins JJ, Parham DM, Webber BL, Pratt CB, Salzberg A, Cantor A, Maurer HM. Prognostic value of grading in pediatric non-rhabdomyosarcomatous soft tissue sarcomas (PNRSTS). *Mod Pathol* 1993;6:126A (Abstract).
125. Johnson MR, DeClue JE, Felzmann S, Vass WC, Xu G, White R, Lowy DR. Neurofibromin can inhibit Ras-dependent growth by a mechanism independent of its GTPase-accelerating function. *Mol Cell Biol* 1994;14:641–645.
126. Johnson WC. Pathology of cutaneous vascular tumors. *Int J Dermatol* 1976;15:239–270.
127. Jones EC, Clement PB, Young RH. Inflammatory pseudotumor of the urinary bladder: a clinicopathological, immunohistochemical, ultrastructural, and flow cytometric study of 13 cases. *Am J Surg Pathol* 1993;17:264–274.
128. Kaplan FS, McCluskey W, Hahn G, Tabas JA, Muenke M, Zasloff MA. Genetic transmission of fibrodysplasia ossificans progressiva. Report of a family. *J Bone Joint Surg Am* 1993;75:1214–1220.
129. Kaplan FS, Tabas JA, Zasloff MA. Fibrodysplasia ossificans progressiva: a clue from the fly? *Calcif Tissue Int* 1990;47:117–125.
130. Kayes LM, Burke W, Riccardi VM, Bennett R, Ehrlich P, Rubenstein A, Stephens K. Deletions spanning the neurofibromatosis 1 gene: identification and phenotype of five patients. *Am J Hum Genet* 1994;54:424–436.
131. Killeen RM, Davy CL, Bauserman SC. Melanocytic schwannoma. *Cancer* 1988;62:174–183.
132. Kitano Y, Horiki M, Aoki T, Sagami S. Two cases of juvenile hyalin fibromatosis. Some histological, electron microscopic, and tissue culture observations. *Arch Dermatol* 1972;106:877–883.
133. Kleinman GM, Zelem JD, Sanders FJ. Proliferative myositis in a two-year-old child. *Pediatr Pathol* 1987;7:71–75.
134. Knight JC. The molecular genetics of soft tissue sarcomas. *Eur J Cancer* 1990;26:511–513.
135. Knight JC, Reeves BR, Kearney L, Monaco AP, Lehrach H, Cooper CS. Localization of the synovial sarcoma t(X;18)(p11.2;q11.2) breakpoint by fluorescence in situ hybridization. *Hum Mol Genet* 1992;1:633–637.
136. Kumagami H. Testosterone and estradiol in juvenile nasopharyngeal angiofibroma tissue. *Acta Otolaryngol (Stockh)* 1991;111: 569–573.
137. Kumagami H. Sex hormones in juvenile nasopharyngeal angiofibroma tissue. *Auris Nasus Larynx* 1993;20:131–135.
138. La Quaglia MP, Spiro SA, Ghavimi F, Hajdu SI, Meyers P, Exelby PR. Liposarcoma in patients younger than or equal to 22 years of age. *Cancer* 1993;72:3114–3119.
139. Ladenstein R, Treuner J, Koscielniak E, et al. Synovial sarcoma of childhood and adolescence: report of the German CWS-81 study. *Cancer* 1993;71:3647–3655.
140. Laskin WB, Weiss SW, Bratthauer GL. Epithelioid variant of malignant peripheral nerve sheath tumor (malignant epithelioid schwannoma). *Am J Surg Pathol* 1991;15:1136–1145.
141. Lazaro C, Gaona A, Ravella A, Volpini V, Casals T, Fuentes JJ, Estivill X. Novel alleles, hemizygosity and deletions at an Alu-repeat within the neurofibromatosis type 1 (NF1) gene. *Hum Mol Genet* 1993;2:725–730.
142. Leader M, Collins M, Patel J, Henry K. Staining for factor VIII

related antigen and *Ulex europaeus* agglutinin I (UEA-I) in 230 tumours. An assessment of their specificity for angiosarcoma and Kaposi's sarcoma. *Histopathology* 1986;10:1153–1162.
143. Lee DA, Rao BR, Meyer JS, Prioleau PG, Bauer WC. Hormonal receptor determination in juvenile nasopharyngeal angiofibromas. *Cancer* 1980;46:547–551.
144. Lee W, Han K, Harris CP, Shim S, Kim S, Meisner LF. Use of FISH to detect chromosomal translocations and deletions: analysis of chromosome rearrangement in synovial sarcoma cells from paraffin-embedded specimens. *Am J Pathol* 1993;143:15–19.
145. Legius E, Dierick H, Wu R, Hall BK, Marynen P, Cassiman JJ, Glover TW. TP53 mutations are frequent in malignant NF1 tumors. *Genes Chrom Cancer* 1994;10:250–255.
146. Legius E, Marchuk DA, Collins FS, Glover TW. Somatic deletion of the neurofibromatosis type 1 gene in a neurofibrosarcoma supports a tumour suppressor gene hypothesis. *Nat Genet* 1993;3: 122–126.
147. Legius E, Marchuk DA, Hall BK, Andersen LB, Wallace MR, Collins FS, Glover TW. NF1-related locus on chromosome 15. *Genomics* 1992;13:1316–1318.
148. Leveen P, Claesson-Welsh L, Heldin CH, Westermark B, Betsholtz C. Expression of messenger RNAs for platelet-derived growth factor and its receptors in human sarcoma cell lines. *Int J Cancer* 1990;46:1066–1070.
149. Levine AJ, Momand J, Finlay CA. The p53 tumour suppressor gene. *Nature* 1991;351:453–456.
150. Li Y, Bollag G, Clark R, et al. Somatic mutations in the neurofibromatosis 1 gene in human tumors. *Cell* 1992;69:275–281.
151. Lieberman PH, Brennan MF, Kimmel M, Erlandson RA, Garin-Chesa P, Flehinger BY. Alveolar soft-part sarcoma: a clinicopathologic study of half a century. *Cancer* 1989;63:1–13.
152. Lillehei KO, Kleinschmidt-DeMasters B, Mitchell DH, Spector E, Kruse CA. Alveolar soft part sarcoma: an unusually long interval between presentation and brain metastasis. *Hum Pathol* 1993;24:1030–1034.
153. Limon J, Debiec-Rychter M, Nedoszytko B, Liberski PP, Babinska M, Szadowska A. Aberrations of chromosome 22 and polysomy of chromosome 8 as non-random changes in clear cell sarcoma. *Cancer Genet Cytogenet* 1994;72:141–145.
154. Limon J, Mrozek K, Mandahl N, et al. Cytogenetics of synovial sarcoma: presentation of ten new cases and review of the literature. *Genes Chrom Cancer* 1991;3:338–345.
155. Lucas DR, Nascimento AG, Sim FH. Clear cell sarcoma of soft tissues: Mayo Clinic experience with 35 cases. *Am J Surg Pathol* 1992;16:1197–1204.
156. Lundgren L, Angervall L, Stenman G, Kindblom L-G. Infantile rhabdomyofibrosarcoma: a high-grade sarcoma distinguishable from infantile fibrosarcoma and rhabdomyosarcoma. *Hum Pathol* 1993;24:785–795.
156a. Lundgren L, Kindblom LG, Willems J, Falkmer U, Angervall L. Proliferative myositis and fasciitis. A light and electron microscopic, cytologic, DNA-cytometric and immunohistochemical study. *APMIS* 1992;100:437–448.
157. Luse SA. Electron microscopic studies of brain tumors. *Neurology* 1960;10:881–905.
158. Luthringer DJ, Virmani R, Weiss SW, Rosai J. A distinctive cardiovascular lesion resembling histiocytoid (epithelioid) hemangioma. Evidence suggesting mesothelial participation. *Am J Surg Pathol* 1990;14:993–1000.
159. Malone M. Soft tissue tumours in childhood. *Histopathology* 1993;23:203–216.
160. Mandahl N. Genetic changes in bone and soft tissue tumors (Meeting abstract). Fifth International Workshop on Chromosomes in Solid Tumors, January 1993.
161. Mandahl N, O˙rndal C, Heim S, Wille´n H, Rydholm A, Bauer HCF, Mitelman F. Aberrations of chromosome segment 12q13-15 characterize a subgroup of hemangiopericytomas. *Cancer* 1993;71:3009–3013.
162. Mandard AM, Petiot JF, Marnay J, et al. Prognostic factors in soft tissue sarcomas: A multivariate analysis of 109 cases. *Cancer* 1989;63:1437–1451.
163. Marchuk DA, Saulino AM, Tavakkol R, et al. cDNA cloning of the type 1 neurofibromatosis gene: complete sequence of the NF1 gene product. *Genomics* 1991;11:931–940.
164. Marcus PB, Couch WD, Martin JH. Crystals in a gastric schwannoma. *Ultrastruct Pathol* 1981;2:139–144.
165. Marshall ME, Hatfield ST, Hatfield DR. Arteriovenous malformation simulating Kaposi's sarcoma (pseudo-Kaposi's sarcoma). *Arch Dermatol* 1985;121:99–101.
166. Matsui I, Tanimura M, Kobayashi N, Sawada T, Nagahara N, Akatsuka J. Neurofibromatosis type 1 and childhood cancer. *Cancer* 1993;72:2746–2754.
167. Maurer HM, Cantor A, Salzberg A, Pratt C, Thomas P, Parham D, Webber B, et al. Adjuvant chemotherapy vs observation for localized non-rhabdomyosarcoma soft tissue sarcoma (NRSTS) in childhood. *Proc Am Soc Clin Oncol* 1992;11:363 (Abstract).
168. Mayer-da-Silva A, Poiares-Baptista A, Rodrigo FG, Teresa-Lopes M. Juvenile hyaline fibromatosis: a histologic and histochemical study. *Arch Pathol Lab Med* 1988;112:928–931.
169. McDonagh JER. Spontaneous disappearance of an endothelioma (nevoxanthoma). *Br J Dermatol* 1909;21:254–256.
170. McDonagh JER. A contribution to our knowledge of the naevoxantho-endotheliomata. *Br J Dermatol* 1912;24:85–99.
171. Meis JM, Enzinger FM. Inflammatory fibrosarcoma of the mesentery and retroperitoneum: a tumor closely simulating inflammatory pseudotumor. *Am J Surg Pathol* 1991;15:1146–1156.
172. Meis JM, Enzinger FM. Proliferative fasciitis and myositis of childhood. *Am J Surg Pathol* 1992;16:364–372.
173. Meis JM, Enzinger FM, Martz KL, Neal JA. Malignant peripheral nerve sheath tumors (malignant schwannomas) in children. *Am J Surg Pathol* 1992;16:694–707.
174. Mentzel T, Calonje E, Fletcher CDM. Lipoblastoma and lipoblastomatosis: a clinicopathological study of 14 cases. *Histopathology* 1993;23:527–533.
175. Miettinen M. Keratin subsets in spindle cell sarcomas: keratins are widespread but synovial sarcoma contains a distinctive keratin polypeptide pattern and desmoplakins. *Am J Pathol* 1991;138:505–513.
176. Miettinen M. Ossifying fibromyxoid tumor of soft parts. Additional observations of a distinctive soft tissue tumor. *Am J Clin Pathol* 1991;95:142–149.
177. Miettinen M, Ekfors T. Alveolar soft part sarcoma: immunohistochemical evidence for muscle cell differentiation. *Am J Clin Pathol* 1990;93:32–38.
178. Miettinen M, Lehto VP, Virtanen I. Monophasic synovial sarcoma of spindle-cell type. Epithelial differentiation as revealed by ultrastructural features, content of prekeratin and binding of peanut agglutinin. *Virchows Arch B Cell Pathol* 1983;44:187–199.
179. Milchgrub S, Ghandur-Mnaymneh L, Dorfman HD, Albores-Saavedra J. Synovial sarcoma with extensive osteoid and bone formation. *Am J Surg Pathol* 1993;17:357–363.
180. Mills SE, Fechner RE, Bruns DE, Bruns ME, O'Hara MF. Intermediate filaments in eosinophilic cells of epithelioid sarcoma: a light-microscopic, ultrastructural, and electrophoretic study. *Am J Surg Pathol* 1981;5:195–202.
181. Min K-W. Skeinoid fibers: an ultrastructural marker of neurogenic spindle cell tumors. *Ultrastruct Pathol* 1991;15:603–611.
182. Mirra JM, Kessler S, Bhuta S, Eckardt J. The fibroma-like variant of epithelioid sarcoma: A fibrohistiocytic/myoid cell lesion often confused with benign and malignant spindle cell tumors. *Cancer* 1992;69:1382–1395.
183. Miyaki M, Konishi M, Kikuchi-Yanoshita R, et al. Coexistence of somatic and germ-line mutations of APC gene in desmoid tumors from patients with familial adenomatous polyposis. *Cancer Res* 1993;53:5079–5082.
184. Molenaar WM, DeJong B, Buist J, Idenburg VJS, Seruca R, Vos AM, Hoekstra HJ. Chromosomal analysis and the classification of soft tissue sarcomas. *Lab Invest* 1989;60:266–274.
185. Montgomery EA, Meis JM. Nodular fasciitis: Its morphologic spectrum and immunohistochemical profile. *Am J Surg Pathol* 1991;15:942–948.
186. Mukai M, Torikata C, Iri H, Hata J, Naito M, Shimoda T. Immunohistochemical identification of aggregated actin filaments in formalin-fixed, paraffin-embedded sections: I. A study of infantile digital fibromatosis by a new pretreatment. *Am J Surg Pathol* 1992;16:110–115.
187. Mukai M, Torikata C, Iri H, Mikata A, Hanaoka H, Kato K,

Kageyama K. Histogenesis of alveolar soft part sarcoma: an immunohistochemical and biochemical study. *Am J Surg Pathol* 1986;10:212–218.
188. Mulvihill JJ. Tentative definitions of neurofibromatosis. *Neurofibromatosis Res Newslett* 1986;2:1
189. Nakamura T, Nemoto T, Arai M, et al. Specific expression of the neurofibromatosis type 1 gene (NF1) in the hamster Schwann cell. *Am J Pathol* 1994;144:549–555.
190. Nemes Z. Differentiation markers in hemangiopericytoma. *Cancer* 1992;69:133–140.
191. Nichols GE, Gaffey MJ, Mills SE, Weiss LM. Lobular capillary hemangioma: an immunohistochemical study including steroid hormone receptor status. *Am J Clin Pathol* 1992;97:770–775.
192. Nickoloff BJ, Griffiths CE. Factor XIIIa-expressing dermal dendrocytes in AIDS-associated cutaneous Kaposi's sarcomas. *Science* 1989;243:1736–1737.
193. Ninfo V, Chung EB, Cavazzana AO. *Tumors and Tumorlike Lesions of Soft Tissue.* New York: Churchill Livingstone; 1991.
194. Nishi T, Lee PS, Oka K, Levin VA, Tanase S, Morino Y, Saya H. Differential expression of two types of the neurofibromatosis type 1 (NF1) gene transcripts related to neuronal differentiation. *Oncogene* 1991;6:1555–1559.
195. Nur-E-Kamal MS, Varga M, Maruta H. The GTPase-activating NF1 fragment of 91 amino acids reverses v-Ha-Ras-induced malignant phenotype. *J Biol Chem* 1993;268:22331–22337.
196. O'Laughlin S, Braverman M, Smith-Jefferies M, Buckley P. Macrophages (histiocytes) in various reactive and inflammatory conditions express different antigenic phenotypes. *Hum Pathol* 1992;23:1410–1418.
197. O'Neill DB, Kasser JR. Juvenile hyaline fibromatosis. A case report and review of musculoskeletal manifestations. *J Bone Joint Surg* [Am] 1989;71:941–944.
198. Obom KM, Pogo BG. Tumorigenic conversion of NIH 3T3 cells by transfection with Shope fibroma virus DNA. *Virus Genes* 1989;3:5–10.
199. Okamoto M, Sato C, Kohno Y, et al. Molecular nature of chromosome 5q loss in colorectal tumors and desmoids from patients with familial adenomatous polyposis. *Hum Genet* 1990;85:595–599.
200. Ooe M, Ishiguro N, Kawashima M. Nuclear DNA content and distribution of Ki-67 positive cells in nodular fasciitis. *J Dermatol* 1993;20:214–218.
201. Ordo´n˜ez NG, Mahfouz SM, Mackay B. Synovial sarcoma: an immunohistochemical and ultrastructural study. *Hum Pathol* 1990;21:733–749.
202. Ozello L, Stout AP, Murray MR. Cultural characteristics of malignant histiocytomas and fibrous xanthomas. *Cancer* 1963;16:331–344.
203. Papas-Corden P, Gown AM, Zarbo RJ, Crissman JD. Immunohistochemical characterization of synovial, epithelioid, and clear cell sarcomas. *Surg Pathol* 1989;2:43–58.
204. Pappo AS, Fontanesi J, Luo X, et al. Synovial sarcoma in children and adolescents: the St. Jude Children's Research Hospital experience. *J Clin Oncol* 1994;12:2360–2366.
205. Parham DM, Kelly DR, Donnelly WH, Douglass EC. Immunohistochemical and ultrastructural spectrum of hepatic sarcomas of childhood: evidence for a common histogenesis. *Mod Pathol* 1991;4:648–653.
206. Parham DM, Reynolds AB, Webber BL. Use of monoclonal antibody 1H1, anti-cortactin, to distinguish normal and neoplastic smooth muscle cells: comparison with anti-alpha-smooth muscle actin and anti-muscle specific actin. *Hum Pathol* 1995;26:776–783.
207. Parham DM, Webber BL, Jenkins JJ, Cantor AB, Maurer HM. Nonrhabdomyosarcomatous soft tissue sarcomas of childhood: formulation of a simplified system for grading. *Mod Pathol* 1995;8:705–710.
208. Parker F, Odland GF. Experimental xanthoma. A correlative biochemical, histologic, histochemical, and electron microscopic study. *Am J Pathol* 1968;53:537–565.
209. Pasquel P, Salazar M, Marvan E. Proliferative myositis in an infant: report of a case with electron microscopic observations. *Pediatr Pathol* 1988;8:545–551.
210. Pasyk KA, Wlodarczyk SR, Jakobczak MM, Kurek M, Aughton DJ. Familial medial telangiectatic nevus: variant of nevus flammeus—port-wine stain. *Plast Reconstr Surg* 1993;91:1032–1041.
211. Patchefsky AS, Enzinger FM. Intravascular fasciitis: a report of 17 cases. *Am J Surg Pathol* 1981;5:29–36.
212. Pearl GS, Mathews WH. Congenital retroperitoneal hemangioendothelioma with Kasabach–Merritt syndrome. *South Med J* 1979;72:239–240.
213. Pettrone FA, Stay EJ. Chondroma. An unusual presentation of an extraarticular soft tissue mass about the knee. *Am J Sports Med* 1990;18:536–538.
214. Porter PL, Bigler SA, McNutt M, Gown AM. The immunophenotype of hemangiopericytomas and glomus tumors, with special reference to muscle protein expression: an immunohistochemical study and review of the literature. *Mod Pathol* 1991;4:46–52.
215. Porter PL, Gown AM, Kramp SG, Coltrera MD. Widespread p53 overexpression in human malignant tumors: an immunohistochemical study using methacarn-fixed, embedded tissue. *Am J Pathol* 1992;140:145–153.
216. Pratt CB, Kun LE. Soft tissue sarcomas of children. In: Pinedo HM, Verweij J, Suit H, eds. *Soft Tissue Sarcomas: New Developments in the Multidisciplinary Approach to Treatment.* Boston: Kluwer Academic; 1991:149–165.
217. Radke M, Waldschmidt J, Stolpe HJ, Mix M, Richter I. Blue rubber-bleb-nevus syndrome with predominant urinary bladder hemangiomatosis. *Eur J Pediatr* Surg 1993;3:313–316.
218. Ramani P, Shah A. Lymphangiomatosis: Histologic and immunohistochemical analysis of four cases. *Am J Surg Pathol* 1993;17:329–335.
219. Rao BN, Horowitz ME, Parham DM, et al. Challenges in the treatment of childhood fibromatosis. *Arch Surg* 1987;122:1296–1298.
220. Rao VK, Weiss SW. Angiomatosis of soft tissue: an analysis of the histologic features and clinical outcome in 51 cases. *Am J Surg Pathol* 1992;16:764–771.
221. Ray RA, Morton CC, Lipinski KK, Corson JM, Fletcher JA. Cytogenetic evidence of clonality in a case of pigmented villonodular synovitis. *Cancer* 1991;67:121–125.
222. Reeves BR, Fletcher CDM, Gusterson BA. Translocation t(12;22)(q13;q13) is a nonrandom rearrangement in clear cell sarcoma. *Cancer Genet Cytogenet* 1992;64:101–103.
223. Reid AB, Reid IL, Johnson G, Hamonic M, Major P. Familial diffuse cystic angiomatosis of bone. *Clin Orthop* 1989;211–218.
224. Reye RDK. A consideration of certain subdermal "fibromatous tumors" of infancy. *J Pathol Bacteriol* 1956;72:149–156.
225. Reynolds JE, Fletcher JA, Lytle CH, Nie L, Morton CC, Diehl SR. Molecular characterization of a 17q11.2 translocation in a malignant schwannoma cell line. *Hum Genet* 1992;90:450–456.
226. Ricci A, Parham DM, Woodruff JM, Callihan T, Green A, Erlandson RA. Malignant peripheral nerve sheath tumors arising from ganglioneuromas. *Am J Surg Pathol* 1984;8:19–29.
227. Ritchie EL, Gonzalez-Crussi F, Zaontz MR. Fibrous hamartoma of infancy masquerading as a rhabdomyosarcoma of the spermatic cord. *J Urol* 1988;140:800–801.
228. Roberts JT, Byrne EH, Rosenthal D. Familial variant of dermatofibroma with malignancy in the proband. *Arch Dermatol* 1981;117:12–15.
229. Rocke DM, Zasloff M, Peeper J, Cohen RB, Kaplan FS. Age- and joint-specific risk of initial heterotopic ossification in patients who have fibrodysplasia ossificans progressiva. *Clin Orthop* 1994;243–248.
230. Rodriguez E, Sreekantaiah C, Reuter VE, Motzer RJ, Chaganti RSK. t(12;22)(q13;q13) And trisomy 8 are nonrandom aberrations in clear-cell sarcoma. *Cancer Genet Cytogenet* 1992;64:107–110.
231. Rosai J, Dias P, Parham DM, Shapiro DN, Houghton P. MyoD1 protein expression in alveolar soft part sarcoma as confirmatory evidence of its skeletal muscle nature. *Am J Surg Pathol* 1991;15:974–981.
232. Rosai J, Gold J, Landy R. The histiocytoid hemangiomas. A unifying concept embracing several previously described entities of skin, soft tissue, large vessels, bone, and heart. *Hum Pathol* 1979;10:707–730.
233. Rose DSC, Wilkins MJ, Birch R, Evans DJ. Malignant peripheral nerve sheath tumour with rhabdomyoblastic and glandular

differentiation: immunohistochemical features. *Histopathology* 1992;21:287–290.
234. Rosenthal NS, Abdul-Karim FW. Childhood fibrous tumor with psammoma bodies. Clinicopathologic features in two cases. *Arch Pathol Lab Med* 1988;112:798–800.
235. Sainati L, Scapinello A, Montaldi A, Bolcato S, Ninfo V, Carli M, Basso G. A mesenchymal chondrosarcoma of a child with the reciprocal translocation (11;22)(q24;q12). *Cancer Genet Cytogenet* 1993;71:144–147.
236. Sandberg AA, Gibas Z, Saren E, Li FP, Limon J, Tebbi CK. Chromosome abnormalities in two benign adipose tumors. *Cancer Genet Cytogenet* 1986;22:55–61.
237. Sara AS, Evans HL, Benjamin RS. Malignant melanoma of soft parts (clear cell sarcoma): a study of 17 cases, with emphasis on prognostic factors. *Cancer* 1990;65:367–374.
238. Schmid M, Boltshauser E. Familial multiple naevi flammei. *Helv Paediatr Acta* 1989;43:491–492.
239. Schmidt D, Klinge P, Leuschner I, Harms D. Infantile desmoid-type fibromatosis. Morphological features correlate with biological behaviour. *J Pathol* 1991;164:315–319.
240. Schmidt D, Thum P, Harms D, Treuner J. Synovial sarcoma in children and adolescents: a report from the Kiel Pediatric Tumor Registry. *Cancer* 1991;67:1667–1672.
241. Schofield DE, Fletcher JA, Grier HE, Yunis EJ. Fibrosarcoma in infants and children: application of new techniques. *Am J Surg Pathol* 1994;18:14–24.
242. Schofield JB, Krausz T, Stamp GWH, Fletcher CDM, Fisher C, Azzopardi JG. Ossifying fibromyxoid tumour of soft parts: immunohistochemical and ultrastructural analysis. *Histopathology* 1993;22:101–112.
243. Schürch W, Seemayer TA, Gabbiani G. Myofibroblast. In: Sternberg SS, ed. *Histology for Pathologists.* New York: Raven Press; 1992:109–144.
244. Seizinger BR. NF1: a prevalent cause of tumorigenesis in human cancers? *Nat Genet* 1993;3:97–99.
245. Shamir R, Kohn G, Metzker A. Nevus flammeus. Discordance in monozygotic twins. *Am J Dis Child* 1991;145:85–86.
246. Shek TWH, Ng IOL, Chan KW. Inflammatory pseudotumor of the liver: report of four cases and review of the literature. *Am J Surg Pathol* 1993;17:231–238.
247. Shen MH, Upadhyaya M. A de novo nonsense mutation in exon 28 of the neurofibromatosis type 1 (NF1) gene. *Hum Genet* 1993; 92:410–412.
248. Shikani AH, Richtsmeier WJ. Juvenile nasopharyngeal angiofibroma tumor models. Failure of androgens to stimulate growth in nude mice and in vitro. *Arch Otolaryngol Head Neck Surg* 1992;118:256–259.
249. Shipley JM, Clark J, Crew AJ, et al. The t(X;18)(p11.2;q11.2) translocation found in human synovial sarcomas involves two distinct loci on the X chromosome. *Oncogene* 1994;9:1447–1453.
250. Shmookler BM, Enzinger FM. Liposarcoma occurring in children. An analysis of 17 cases and review of the literature. *Cancer* 1983;52:567–574.
251. Shmookler BM, Enzinger FM, Weiss SW. Giant cell fibroblastoma: a juvenile form of dermatofibrosarcoma protuberans. *Cancer* 1989;64:2154–2161.
252. Silva EG, Phillips MJ, Langer B, Ordonez NG. Spindle and histiocytoid (epithelioid) hemangioendothelioma. Primary in lymph node. *Am J Clin Pathol* 1986;85:731–735.
253. Smith DM, Mahmoud HH, Jenkins JJ, Rao B, Hopkins KP, Parham DM. Myofibrosarcoma of the head and neck in children. *Pediatr Pathol Lab Med* 1995;112:275–281.
254. Soini Y, Vähäkangas K, Nuorva K, Kamel D, Lane DP, Pääkkö P. p53 Immunohistochemistry in malignant fibrous histiocytomas and other mesenchymal tumours. *J Pathol* 1992;168:29–33.
255. Sonobe H, Furihata M, Iwata J, Oka T, Ohtsuki Y, Hamasato S, Fujimoto S. Morphological characterization of a new human epithelioid sarcoma cell line, ES020488, in vitro and in vivo. *Virchows Arch B Cell Pathol* 1993;63:219–225.
256. Sorensen SA, Mulvihill JJ, Nielsen A, Srensen SA. Long-term follow-up of von Recklinghausen neurofibromatosis. Survival and malignant neoplasms. *N Engl J Med* 1986;314:1010–1015.
257. Soule EH, Pritchard DJ. Fibrosarcoma in infants and children: a review of 110 cases. *Cancer* 1977;40:1711–1721.
258. Spjut HJ, Dorfman HD. Florid reactive periostitis of the tubular bones of the hands and feet. A benign lesion which may simulate osteosarcoma. *Am J Surg Pathol* 1981;5:423–433.
259. Stehelin D, Varmus HE, Bishop JM, Vogt PK. DNA related to the transforming gene(s) of avian sarcoma viruses is present in normal avian DNA. *Nature* 1976;260:170–173.
260. Stenman G, Kindblom L-G, Willems J, Angervall L. A cell culture, chromosomal and quantitative DNA analysis of a metastatic epithelioid sarcoma: deletion 1p, a possible primary chromosomal abnormality in epithelioid sarcoma. *Cancer* 1990;65: 2006–2013.
261. Stenman G, Kindblom LG, Angervall L. Reciprocal translocation t(12;22)(q13;q13) in clear-cell sarcoma of tendons and aponeuroses. *Genes Chrom Cancer* 1992;4:122–127.
262. Stephens K, Kayes L, Riccardi VM, Rising M, Sybert VP, Pagon RA. Preferential mutation of the neurofibromatosis type 1 gene in paternally derived chromosomes. *Hum Genet* 1992;88:279–282.
263. Stratton MR, Moss S, Warren W, et al. Mutation of the p53 gene in human soft tissue sarcomas: association with abnormalities of the RB1 gene. *Oncogene* 1990;5:1297–1301.
264. Suh C-H, Ordonez NG, Mackay B. Fibrosarcoma: observations on the ultrastructure. *Ultrastruct Pathol* 1993;17:221–229.
265. Swanson PE, Lillemoe TJ, Manivel JC, Wick MR. Mesenchymal chondrosarcoma: an immunohistochemical study. *Arch Pathol Lab Med* 1990;114:943–948.
266. Tallini G, Parham DM, Dias P, Cordon-Cardo C, Houghton PJ, Rosai J. Myogenic regulatory protein expression in adult soft tissue sarcomas: a sensitive and specific marker of skeletal muscle differentiation. *Am J Pathol* 1994;144:693–701.
267. Taylor HG, Terebelo HR, Gamez A. Lymphocytosis in a patient with malignant fibrous histiocytoma. *Cancer* 1982;50:1563–1567.
268. The I, Murthy AE, Hannigan GE, Jacoby LB, Menon AG, Gusella JF, Bernards A. Neurofibromatosis type 1 gene mutations in neuroblastoma. *Nat Genet* 1993;3:62–66.
269. Thomas RM, Jaffe ES, Zarate-Osorno A, Medeiros LJ. Inflammatory pseudotumor of the spleen: a clinicopathologic and immunophenotypic study of eight cases. *Arch Pathol Lab Med* 1993;117:921–926.
270. Travis JA, Bridge JA. Significance of both numerical and structural chromosomal abnormalities in clear cell sarcoma. *Cancer Genet Cytogenet* 1992;64:104–106.
271. Treissman SP, Gillis DA, Lee CL, Giacomantonio M, Resch L. Omental-mesenteric inflammatory pseudotumor. Cytogenetic demonstration of genetic changes and monoclonality in one tumor. *Cancer* 1994;73:1433–1437.
272. Tsang WYW, Chan JKC. Kaposi-like infantile hemangioendothelioma: a distinctive vascular neoplasm of the retroperitoneum. *Am J Surg Pathol* 1991;15:982–989.
273. Tsang WYW, Chan JKC, Chow LTC, Tse CCH. Perineurioma: An uncommon soft tissue neoplasm distinct from localized hypertrophic neuropathy and neurofibroma. *Am J Surg Pathol* 1992;16:756–763.
274. Tsang WYW, Chan JKC, Fletcher CDM. Recently characterized vascular tumours of skin and soft tissues. *Histopathology* 1991;19:489–501.
275. Tsao CY, Sommer A, Hamoudi AB. Aicardi syndrome, metastatic angiosarcoma of the leg, and scalp lipoma. *Am J Med Genet* 1993;45:594–596.
276. Uehara Y, Hori M, Takeuchi T, Umezawa H. Phenotypic change from transformed to normal induced by benzoquinonoid ansamycins accompanies inactivation of p60src in rat kidney cells infected with Rous sarcoma virus. *Mol Cell Biol* 1986;6:2198–2206.
277. Umezawa K, Tanaka K, Hori T, Abe S, Sekizawa R, Imoto M. Induction of morphological change by tyrosine kinase inhibitors in Rous sarcoma virus-transformed rat kidney cells. *FEBS Lett* 1991;279:132–136.
278. Upadhyaya M, Shen M, Cherryson A, Farnham J, Maynard J, Huson SM, Harper PS. Analysis of mutations at the neurofibromatosis 1 (NF1) locus. *Hum Mol Genet* 1992;1:735–740.

279. Uzoaru I, Chou P, Reyes-Mugica M, Shen-Schwarz S, Gonzalez-Crussi F. Inflammatory myofibroblastic tumor of the pancreas. *Surg Pathol* 1993;5:181–188.
280. Van Hoeven KH, Factor SM, Kress Y, Woodruff JM. Visceral myogenic tumors: a manifestation of HIV infection in children. *Am J Surg Pathol* 1993;17:1176–1181.
281. Van Meurs DP. The transformation of an embryonic lipoma to a common lipoma. *Br J Surg* 1947;34:282–284.
282. Varela-Duran J, Enzinger FM. Calcifying synovial sarcoma. *Cancer* 1982;50:345–352.
283. Vasudev KS, Harris M. A sarcoma of myofibroblasts: an ultrastructural study. *Arch Pathol Lab Med* 1978;102:185–188.
284. Venencie PY, Bigel P, Desgruelles C, Lortat-Jacob S, Dufier JL, Saurat JH. Infantile myofibromatosis. Report of two cases in one family. *Br J Dermatol* 1987;117:255–259.
285. Wakely PE, Jr., Price WG, Frable WJ. Sternomastoid tumor of infancy (fibromatosis colli): diagnosis by aspiration cytology. *Mod Pathol* 1989;2:378–381.
286. Wallace MR, Andersen LB, Saulino AM, Gregory PE, Glover TW, Collins FS. A de novo Alu insertion results in neurofibromatosis type 1. *Nature* 1991;353:864–866.
287. Warner J, Jones EW. Pyogenic granuloma recurring with multiple satellites. A report of 11 cases. *Br J Dermatol* 1968;80: 218–227.
288. Webber BL. Synovial sarcoma of the head and neck. *S Afr Med J* 1975;49:1059
289. Weiss SW. Pedal hemangioma (venous malformation) occurring in Turner's syndrome: an additional manifestation of the syndrome. *Hum Pathol* 1988;19:1015–1018.
290. Weiss SW, Enzinger FM. Spindle cell hemangioendothelioma. A low-grade angiosarcoma resembling a cavernous hemangioma and Kaposi's sarcoma. *Am J Surg Pathol* 1986;10:521–530.
291. Weiss SW, Enzinger FM, Johnson FB. Silica reaction simulating fibrous histiocytoma. *Cancer* 1978;42:2738–2743.
292. Weiss SW, Ishak KG, Dail DH, Sweet DE, Enzinger FM. Epithelioid hemangioendothelioma and related lesions. *Semin Diagn Pathol* 1986;3:259–287.
293. Weprin LS, Siemers PT. Spontaneous regression of juvenile nasopharyngeal angiofibroma. *Arch Otolaryngol Head Neck Surg* 1991;117:796–799.
294. White W, Shiu MH, Rosenblum MK, Erlandson RA, Woodruff JM. Cellular schwannoma. A clinicopathologic study of 57 patients and 58 tumors. *Cancer* 1990;66:1266–1275.
295. Wilcken N, Tattersall MH. Endocrine therapy for desmoid tumors. *Cancer* 1991;68:1384–1388.
296. Wilkinson AH, Beckford NS, Babin RW, Parham DM. Extraskeletal myxoid chondrosarcoma of the epiglottis: case report and review of the literature. *Otolaryngol Head Neck Surg* 1991;104:257–260.
297. Willis RA. *The Borderland of Embryology and Pathology*. 2nd ed. London: Butterworths; 1962.
298. Witt TR, Shah JP, Sternberg SS. Juvenile nasopharyngeal angiofibroma. A 30 year clinical review. *Am J Surg* 1983;146:521–525.
299. Woodruff JM. The pathology and treatment of peripheral nerve tumors and tumor-like conditions. *CA Cancer J Clin* 1993;43: 290–308.
300. Woodruff JM, Godwin TA, Erlandson RA, Susin M, Martini N. Cellular schwannoma: a variety of schwannoma sometimes mistaken for a malignant tumor. *Am J Surg Pathol* 1981;5:733–744.
301. Wunder JS, Czitrom AA, Kandel R, Andrulis IL. Analysis of alterations in the retinoblastoma gene and tumor grade in bone and soft-tissue sarcomas. *JNCI* 1991;83:194–200.
302. Yokoyama R, Shinohara N, Tsuneyoshi M, Masuda S, Enjoji M. Extra-abdominal desmoid tumors: correlation between histologic features and biologic behavior. *Surg Pathol* 1989;2:29–42.
303. Yoshida MA, Ikeuchi T, Iwama T, et al. Chromosome changes in desmoid tumors developed in patients with familial adenomatous polyposis. *Jpn J Cancer Res* 1991;82:916–921.
304. Yu CC-W, Hall PA, Fletcher CDM, Camplejohn RS, Waseem NH, Lane DP, Levison DA. Haemangiopericytomas: the prognostic value of immunohistochemical staining with a monoclonal antibody to proliferating cell nuclear antigen (PCNA). *Histopathology* 1991;19:29–33.
305. Zucman J, Delattre O, Desmaze C, et al. EWS and ATF-1 gene fusion induced by t(12;22) translocation in malignant melanoma of soft parts. *Nat Genet* 1993;4:341–345.
306. Zukerberg LR, Nickoloff BJ, Weiss SW. Kaposiform hemangioendothelioma of infancy and childhood: an aggressive neoplasm associated with Kasabach—Merritt syndrome and lymphangiomatosis. *Am J Surg Pathol* 1993;17:321–328.
307. Zuppan CW, Mierau GW, Wilson HL. Malignant fibrous histiocytoma in childhood: a report of two cases and review of the literature. *Pediatr Pathol* 1987;7:303–318.

Pediatric Neoplasia: Morphology and Biology, edited by David M. Parham.
Lippincott-Raven Publishers, Philadelphia © 1996.

CHAPTER 9

Bone Tumors Other Than Ewing's Sarcoma

Bruce L. Webber and David M. Parham

INTRODUCTION

Tumors of bone in childhood provide some of the most challenging problems in both diagnosis and management. Here more than in any other area of pathology is it essential to carefully correlate the clinical and diagnostic imaging findings before making a diagnosis. Before reviewing the histologic appearance of a bone tumor it is essential to know three things: the site of the lesion within the bone (epiphyseal/metaphyseal/diaphyseal), the radiologic appearance, and the age of the patient. These will narrow down the diagnostic possibilities considerably. Knowledge of the radiologic findings is essential, as they give critical information regarding the gross outline of the lesion and its effect on the host bone. A good working relationship with a radiologist interested in bone lesions is thus advisable. Pathologists should also be familiar with the rudiments of bone radiology so that they can recognize the gross pattern of the lesion. Benign bone tumors generally are well demarcated and often have a sclerotic border. They may cause deformity of the native bone as they slowly distort its growth; this deformity indicates that the lesion has been present for a considerable time. More aggressive tumors have a more destructive growth pattern with irregular margins. Destruction of cortical bone is much more easily seen than destruction of trabecular bone, which must be extensive before it can be recognized on radiographs.

Benign lesions may expand the cortex and elevate the periosteum. Malignant tumors destroy the cortex, elevate the periosteum, and eventually invade through it into the adjacent soft tissues. The periosteum in children is much more loosely attached to the bone than in adults and its reactions tend to be more dramatic. When the periosteum is elevated it deposits bone in layers that are parallel or at an angle to the cortex, producing the so-called sun ray spicules. Highly malignant tumors also permeate the bone diffusely, producing a finely mottled pattern of destruction.

Benign lesions such as aneurysmal bone cysts and eosinophilic granuloma of bone may mimic a malignancy radiologically. Conversely, malignant lesions may occasionally be well demarcated and appear benign, but the radiologic appearance usually gives a good indication of their nature. In bone pathology it is also very important to become familiar with patterns of reaction such as with fracture callus. These reactions may be very cellular and atypical in appearance and can easily be misdiagnosed as malignant, with disastrous consequences.

CARTILAGINOUS LESIONS

Osteochondroma

Osteochondroma is a malformation resulting from a portion of the epiphyseal plate herniating through the periosteum and growing away from the bone by endochondral ossification (174). This results in a mass that has a broad or narrow base, a cartilaginous cap (at least in its initial stages), and a bony stalk whose cortex and medullary space are continuous with those of the parent bone. These latter features are critical in differentiating this lesion from similar lesions such as parosteal osteosarcoma or juxtacortical chondroma.

Osteochondromas are the most common benign tumors of bone (96). They may be either solitary or multiple, with the solitary lesions being very common

B. L. Webber: MidSouth Pathology Group, Inc., Memphis, Tennessee 38146.
D. M. Parham: Department of Pathology, Arkansas Children's Hospital, Little Rock, Arkansas 72202.

and the multiple lesions being inherited as an autosomal dominant with incomplete penetrance in females (83). The solitary lesions occur in males and females equally, whereas the multiple ones have a male predominance (127). As the patient grows, the lesion moves away from the epiphysis and angles toward the shaft of the bone. These lesions appear to originate from abnormal epiphyseal cartilage that separates from the main growth plate and proliferates autonomously (174).

Solitary Osteochondroma

Solitary osteochondromas are very common lesions. Their sex incidence is controversial, with some reports claiming a male predominance of 2:1 and others finding no sex difference (83). These tumors may affect any bone other than the facial bones and arise in long and flat bones roughly equally (90). Osteochondromas develop in about 12% of patients receiving radiation therapy and may be multiple (83), but there is only one report of malignant change in this setting (198). Osteochondromas may produce a mass, pain, or interference with tendon function. The pain may be due to compression of an adjacent nerve (83), development of an overlying bursa (78), fracture of the stalk (60), or infarction (259). Tumors close to a large vessel may cause complications such as thrombosis or erosion of the vessel wall with hemorrhage or the development of a pseudoaneurysm (153).

Osteochondromas are completely covered by periosteum that is continuous with that of the parent bone. They are covered by a cartilage cap that invests a variable amount of the surface of the lesion (Fig. 1); the cap is usually less than 0.5 cm in thickness but may be up to 3.0 cm thick in growing children (83). The cortex and medulla are also continuous with those of the parent bone, a very important point in the diagnosis of this lesion. This observation can be made both radiologically and in the gross specimen, and it may require careful sectioning of the lesion for demonstration. The cartilage cap is not seen on plain radiographs but is visible and can be accurately measured with magnetic resonance imaging (MRI) (50). However, computed tomography (CT) scanning has been shown to be inaccurate in assessing the thickness of the cartilage cap (96). MRI is also helpful in identifying the continuity of the host bone marrow with that of the osteochondroma and thus distinguishing it from a parosteal osteosarcoma (96). Islands of cartilage with associated bone and calcified debris may be present in the stalk of the lesion and persist as the lesion grows (83).

The incidence of malignancy in solitary osteochondromas is not known. It has been estimated as being

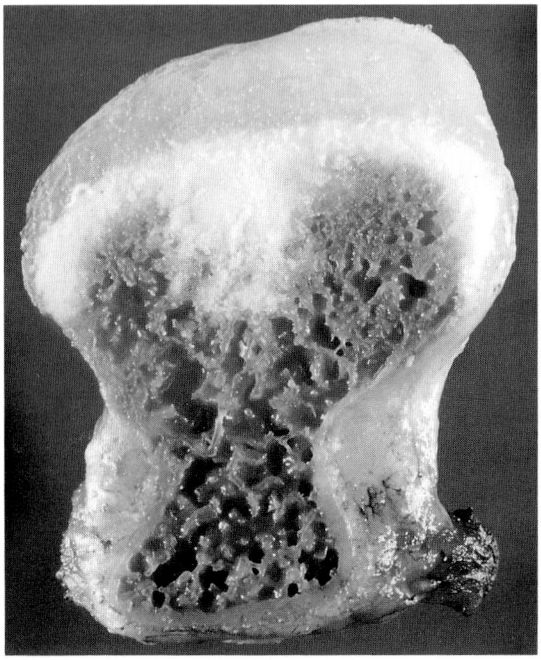
A

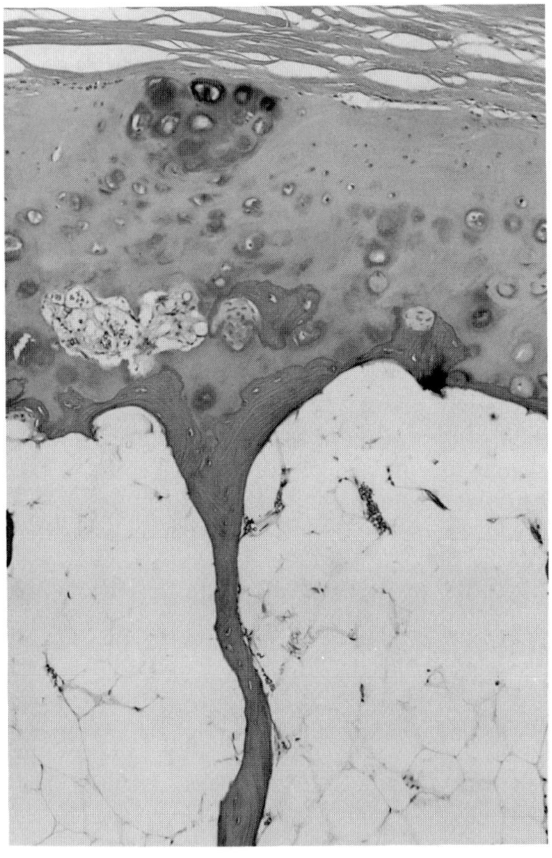
B

FIG. 1. Osteochondroma. **A.** Gross cross-section of tumor composed of medullary bone capped by hyaline cartilage and invested by periosteum. **B.** Microscopically, bland hyaline cartilage is contiguous with trabecular bone and fatty bone marrow.

around 1%, but this figure does not account for the high number of asymptomatic patients (83). The cartilage cap may contain cellular areas with large chondrocytes, but as long as it is less than 3.0 cm in thickness, cellularity or pleomorphism does not indicate malignancy (83). However, a cartilage cap thicker than 3.0 cm is very likely malignant. Other features indicating malignancy include invasion beyond the periosteum into surrounding soft tissue, destructive invasion of the underlying stalk or bone, infiltration of Haversian systems (83,175), exuberant peripheral fibroplasia at the soft tissue interface (175), fibrous bands separating lobules of cartilage (175), and cartilage with high cellularity, many binucleate cells in lacunae, and obvious signs of malignancy. Most malignancies are low grade.

One must be aware of bizarre osteochondromatous growths that may mimic chondrosarcoma. These proliferations, known as "Nora's lesions" (169,185), occur primarily on the distal extremities and exhibit histologically disturbing features such as proliferative activity, irregular cartilage–bone interfaces, and pleomorphic chondrocytes. A distinctive feature is a peculiar blue staining of the constituent bone (169). In spite of their alarming appearance, Nora's lesions have a benign behavior, but recurrences are common (169).

Another osteocartilaginous lesion that may present a disturbing appearance is the chest wall hamartoma, which typically is a congenital lesion affecting the ribs and causing thoracic distortion (66). Histologically these lesions are complex masses of solid and aneurysmal tissues with cartilaginous and osteoblastic differentiation.

Multiple Osteochondromas

Multiple osteochondromas arise from dominantly inherited epiphyseal defects resulting in the formation of multifocal lesions and accompanied by other malformations such as unequal growth and/or widening of radius and ulna or tibia and fibula and abnormalities in the wrists, ankles, and small bones of the hands and feet (83,94). Boys are more commonly affected than girls (7: 3) (127). Any bone other than the facial bones may be affected. Vertebral involvement may result in spinal cord compression. The lesions cease to appear when the patient reaches adulthood.

Malignancy may develop in these cases. Unlike the case of solitary osteochondroma, these chondrosarcomas affect the flat bones more commonly than long bones (83). When kindreds are followed the incidence is around 1% or even less (200,268). In the past, these tumors were considered to have a very high incidence of malignancy (e.g., 25%), but these figures were derived from consultation practices with a strong selection bias toward complicated cases (83). The grade of malignancy tends to be higher than with solitary osteochondromas (90). Ten of 11 high-grade chondrosarcomas arising in osteochondromas in one series were in patients with osteochondromatosis (90). Rarely the malignancy may be an osteosarcoma or a malignant fibrous histiocytoma (163).

Enchondroma

Enchondromas are the second most common benign neoplasm of cartilaginous origin, following osteochondromas (96). They are thought to arise from portions of cartilage arising from the cartilaginous growth plate and remaining within the growing bone (174). They are associated with abnormalities of the growth plate in multiple osteochondromatosis and Maffucci's syndrome (83). Enchondromas arise in bones formed by endochondral ossification (96) and occur in children over 5 years, but mostly in patients between 15 and 40 years of age.

Enchondromas present as incidental asymptomatic radiographic lesions, as hot spots on a bone scan, or as masses (83). They may present with pain if there is cortical thinning with fracture, particularly in the small bones of the hands. The phalanges are affected more commonly in this location than the metacarpals, and the proximal phalanges are affected most commonly. The phalanges of the hand are much more commonly affected than those of the foot. The second most common site is the knee (96).

Radiologically, enchondromas usually present as central masses of variably calcified material in the medullary cavity. They may cause thinning of the cortex, especially in the small bones of the hands and feet, but do not penetrate it and lift the periosteum. They retain a peripheral shell of cortex (83). In the long bones there may be some endosteal scalloping (96). Because cartilage grows in a lobular fashion, often with ossification around the cartilage lobules, the plain radiograph often has the calcium arranged as small circlets; this is a useful radiologic marker of cartilaginous differentiation. Enchondromas may occasionally be eccentric within the bone.

Microscopically, enchondromas usually consist of lobules of hyaline cartilage, often surrounded by a bony rim. In the long bones, the cartilage is very similar to normal hyaline cartilage with relatively low cellularity, few foci with more than one cell in a lacuna, no atypia or hyperchromatism, and no myxoid areas (Fig. 2A). Necrosis may be present (83). In the small bones of the hands and feet, one can allow for a larger degree of cellularity, binucleate cells, and even some nuclear atypia. These features are often seen in this location in tumors that are perfectly benign. The site of the tumor is therefore critical in histologic assessment and diagnosis.

Great difficulty is experienced in the differential diagnosis between enchondroma and low-grade chondrosarcoma. The site, size, radiographic appearance, and a his-

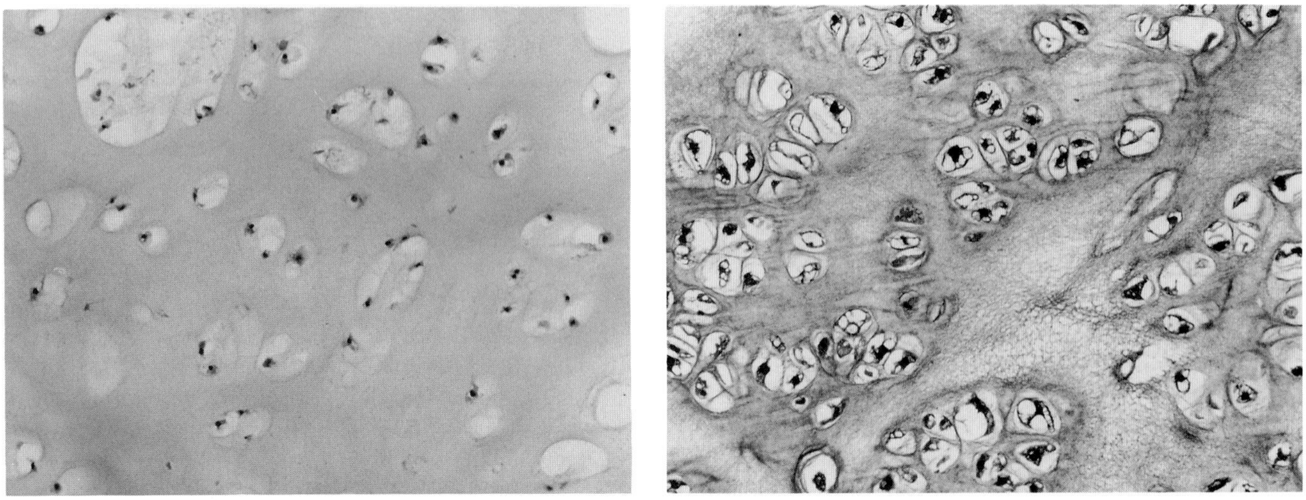

A B

FIG. 2. Cartilagious neoplasms. **A.** Enchondroma comprises innocuous-appearing chondrocytes with small, bland nuclei. With few exceptions, single cells lie within lacunae. **B.** Chondrosarcoma is composed of abundant, atypical chondrocytes with enlarged, pleomorphic nuclei. Widened lacunae containing multiple cells are frequent.

tory of pain in the absence of a fracture (in long-bone lesions) are useful clues that the tumor may be malignant. If the lesion has broken through the cortex and elevates the periosteum, it is very likely malignant, especially in the long bones. A tumor in the pelvis or upper end of the femur is much more likely to be malignant than one in the small bones of the hands and feet or even the lower end of the femur. Myxoid change may be seen in enchondromas but should raise the possibility of malignancy. Higher grade tumors with high cellularity and nuclear pleomorphism are easier to recognize as malignant and usually present no problem (Fig. 2B). MRI may

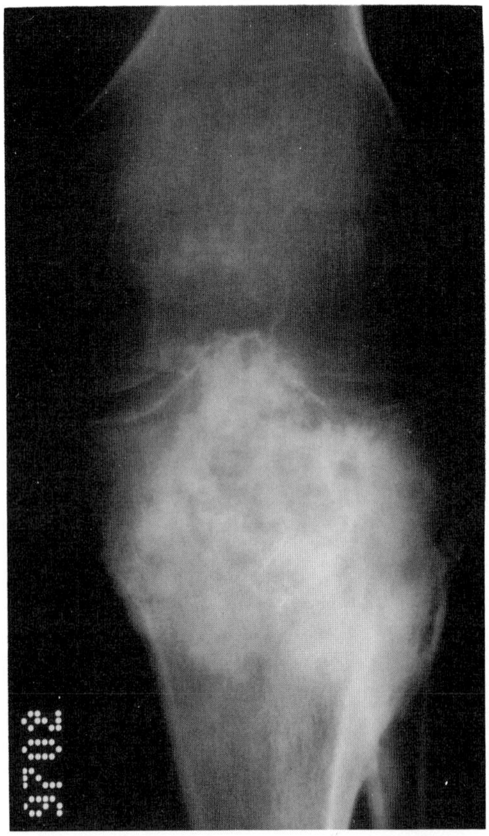

A

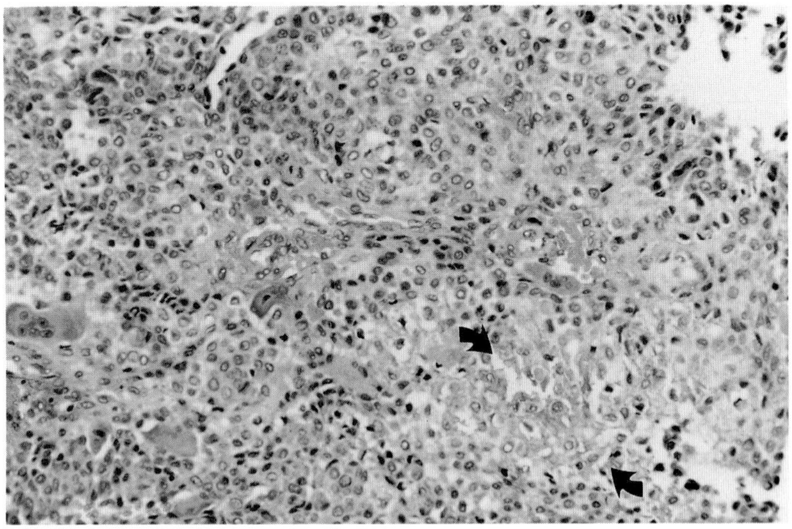

B

FIG. 3. Chondroblastoma. **A.** Plain radiograph shows a lytic lesion with marginal sclerosis in the proximal tibial epiphysis. **B.** The lesion is composed of mononuclear cells and osteoclasts containing a subtle focus of "chicken-wire" calcification *(arrows).* (Part **A** courtesy of Dr. Barry Fletcher, St. Jude Children's Research Hospital [SJCRH].)

be useful in that enchondromas are usually homogeneous in appearance, whereas chondrosarcomas are inhomogeneous due to the presence of fibrous bands coursing between lobules of tumor (96). Bone scans are useful for the detection of multiple lesions (96).

Multiple enchondromatosis (Ollier's disease) is a nonhereditary disease in which multiple chondromas develop. These vary in number and are often confined to one extremity (83). Histologically they are more cellular and exhibit more atypia than solitary enchondromas (83). Affected patients are prone to develop malignancy in one or more lesions (43,83).

Maffucci's syndrome is a disorder in which there are multiple enchondromas associated with hemangiomatosis, usually cavernous in type. These patients are also prone to develop malignancies such as chondrosarcomas (151). Unlike solitary enchondroma, which has an equal sex distribution, both Ollier's disease and Maffucci's syndrome have a male predominance. Besides the propensity for cartilaginous lesions, patients with Maffucci's syndrome and Ollier's disease suffer an apparent tendency for endocrine and brain neoplasms, suggesting a genetic abnormality with pleiotropic effects (10,173).

Chondroblastoma

Chondroblastoma is typically a benign tumor affecting the epiphysis (48%) or epiphysis and metaphysis (52%), predominantly in patients in their second and third decades (256). It constitutes about 1% of all bone tumors (76). Males are more commonly affected than females, 1.5–1 (76,145,147). Chondroblastomas present with pain in the joint, joint stiffness, joint effusion (243), a soft tissue mass, muscle atrophy, or, in the case of the temporal bone, hearing loss. Radiologically there is a rounded, lytic lesion that variably contains speckled calcifications (220). The epicenter is in the epiphysis of long bones (66%) or in the flat bones (30%), including the temporal bone, pelvis, and ribs (Fig. 3A). The margin of the lesion is well defined in 74% of cases, fairly well defined in 20%, and ill defined in 3%. Marginal sclerosis is common (256), and a periosteal reaction is seen in 20.4–50% of cases (76,274). Intramedullary and peritumoral edema make the neoplasm appear aggressive on MRI scan (274). The most common bones involved are the proximal tibia, proximal humerus, and femur (both proximal and distal) (243,256). In view of the usual site of origin, this tumor appears to arise in relation to epiphyseal cartilage (76,256). It may invade the adjacent joint, usually along either a cruciate ligament or the ligamentum teres (243).

Histologically chondroblastoma consists of sheets of round, but occasionally spindled, mononuclear cells, often with grooved nuclei (59). Intranuclear cytoplasmic inclusions are also seen (9). These cells show focal cartilage matrix production (256), which most typically takes the form of pericellular, chicken wire calcification, although the latter is present in only one third of cases (145). More frequently, there is an amorphous, eosinophilic, chondroid or fibrochondroid matrix with a somewhat granular appearance (76,145), and typical hyaline cartilage may also be seen (147). Numerous osteoclast-type giant cells are a prominent feature (Fig. 3B). In fact, chondroblastoma was originally classified with giant cell tumors of bone until Jaffe and Lichtenstein defined it as a distinct entity (128). The tumor cells often appear atypical, but this does not indicate malignancy (145,256). The tumor may also be mitotically active (145). Secondary aneurysmal bone cyst changes and necrosis may be present (256). There may be a focal hemangiopericytomatous pattern (76), particularly in tumors involving the small bones of the hands and feet (145).

Immunohistochemical staining shows the tumor cells to be positive for vimentin and S-100 protein (76,179). Both cytoplasmic and nuclear S-100 staining must be present to consider the lesion positive (179). The chondroid matrix is positive for type II and type VI collagen. Anticytokeratin stains are positive in a small number of tumor cells in just under half of the cases, and epithelial membrane antigen may also be positive (76,228). Osteoclast-type giant cells stain positively with CD68 (KP1) and CD45 (76). MAC 387 is negative, however.

Chondroblastomas gradually expand if not treated, destroying the surrounding bone. An 18% local recurrence rate has been noted (256). There is a higher recurrence rate in flat bone lesions (particularly temporal bone) than in long bone disease (256). Patients with this tumor have rarely developed pulmonary metastases (147). Two of Turcotte et al.'s cases (256) developed pulmonary metastases, possibly due to dedifferentiation of the tumor following radiation therapy. Kahn et al. (135) reported malignant behavior in two cases. The lung and liver metastases in one of their cases resembled benign chondroblastoma histologically. The second case had extensive local joint and soft tissue invasion with lymphatic vessel invasion and tumor nodules in the soft tissue away from the surgical scar, necessitating amputation. It is possible that vigorous curettage of the primary tumor may result in lung deposits through embolization of tumor cells (147). Metastatic tumor may result in the demise of the patient, but pulmonary metastases have remained quiescent for many years or have been successfully removed surgically (147).

The differential diagnosis includes eosinophilic granuloma, clear cell chondrosarcoma (96), other types of chondrosarcoma, bone-forming lesions including osteosarcoma and osteoblastoma, chondromyxoid fibroma, giant cell tumor, aneurysmal bone cyst, osteitis fibrosa cystica, and chondroma (59) [particularly with fine needle aspirations (179)], inflammatory diseases such as Brodie's abscess, and subchondral or degenerative cysts (96).

Chondromyxoid Fibroma

Chondromyxoid fibromas are uncommon, benign chondroid tumors that present as chronic pain or a mass in young people in their second and third decades. They arise in long bones, particularly the proximal tibia, but also the proximal fibula, distal femur, distal tibia, and small bones of the feet. Flat bones such as the pelvis may also be involved (96). They rarely involve the upper humerus, unlike many other tumors affecting the bones around the knee (175). When they affect the ribs, chondromyxoid fibromas tend to occur posteriorly in the equivalent of the metaphysis (291). There is a male predominance of about 2:1 in some series (83). In one series 71% occurred in the lower extremity (96). The tumor is metaphyseal and eccentric in location, expanding the bone and having a sclerotic rim and lobulated contour (Fig. 4A). In the small bones of the hands and feet, the tumor is central, expanding the bone symmetrically (83,221). Matrix mineralization is infrequent (96). CT scans show cortical integrity around the lesions, which exhibit increased radionuclide activity on bone scan (96). The radiologic differential diagnosis includes simple bone cyst, giant cell tumor, enchondroma, fibroxanthoma, fibrous dysplasia, eosinophilic granuloma, hemangioma, and nonossifying fibroma (96,175). Lesions of the vertebral body may extend beyond the periosteum and thus have a more malignant appearance than the usual chondromyxoid fibroma (291).

Histologically chondromyxoid fibroma consists of lobules of myxoid tissue surrounded by bands of more cellular spindle and/or round cell components (Fig. 4B). Variable numbers of osteoclast-type giant cells and fibrous trabeculae separate lobules of tumor, but these fibrous bands are not as conspicuous as the name would imply (83). The tumor cells may show significant nuclear pleomorphism that may lead to a mistaken diagnosis of malignancy, particularly in the small bones of the hands and feet (129,221), but mitoses are rare. Necrosis may be

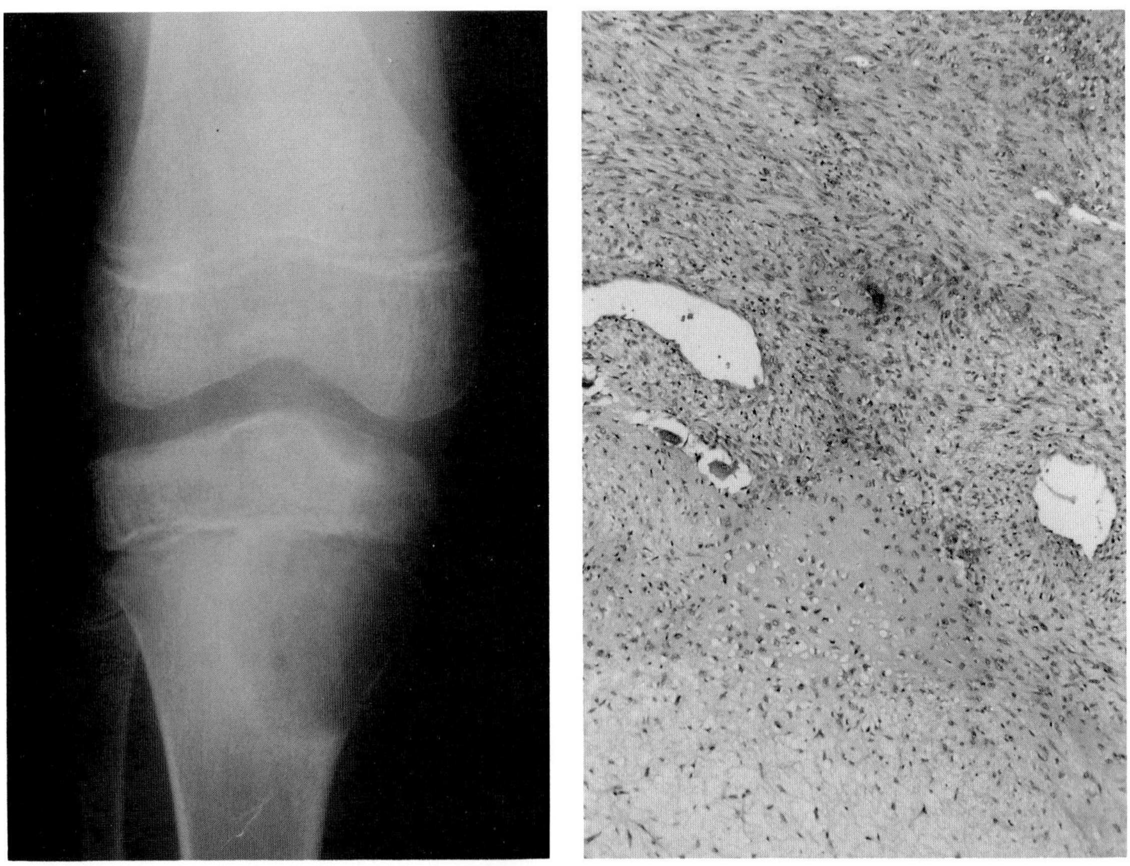
A B

FIG. 4. Chondromyxoid fibroma. **A.** Plain radiograph discloses a sharply defined, eccentric, lytic lesion of the proximal tibial metaphysis. **B.** The lesion is composed of bundles of fibroblastic tissue **(top)**, ill-defined chondroid matrix **(middle)**, and myxoid stroma **(bottom).** (Part **A** courtesy of Dr. Barry Fletcher, SJCRH.)

present but is unusual (83). Osteoid may be produced in the tissue surrounding the lobules (83). Like osteoid osteoma and osteoblastoma, this lesion does not permeate the adjacent bone (175). The major microscopic differential diagnosis is chondrosarcoma, including dedifferentiated and mesenchymal types (129). Production of typical hyaline cartilage by the tumor (129) and the presence of more than a rare mitosis should alert the observer that the lesion is something other than a chondromyxoid fibroma (129,175). Secondary aneurysmal bone cyst formation may occur (291). These tumors stain positively with antibodies to S-100 protein (19,278).

Chondromyxoid fibroma is treated by curettage and bone chips and is usually cured by this procedure, with a recurrence rate of 10–15%, particularly in patients under 15 years (83,129). It is rare for these tumors to undergo malignant change, although it has been reported (96,129). Pulmonary metastases have also occurred, but usually only after previous surgery (96). Chondromyxoid fibroma may be implanted in the soft tissues at the time of surgery (146).

Periosteal Chondroma

Periosteal chondromas occur mostly in patients in the second and third decades (83) and show a male preponderance (2.3:1) (175). They involve the extremities in the majority of cases, especially the metaphyses of long bones (2/3) and the diaphyses (1/3), and they also involve the phalanges (83,175). They present as an incidental finding in many instances, but there may be pain, particularly if the lesion has eroded the cortex with the formation of stress fractures in the weakened cortex (175), and they may present as a swelling.

Radiologically, periosteal chondromas are seen as a lucency in the cortex with a sclerotic rim on the bony side and a buttress of new bone overlying the edges where periosteal new bone has been formed (175). One third of cases show intralesional calcification with the popcorn configuration of cartilaginous lesions (Fig. 5) (68). The lesion is characteristically elongated in the long axis of the bone, indicating its concurrent development with skeletal growth (83).

Histologically periosteal chondromas are usually typical hyaline cartilage. They have a pushing margin with the adjacent tissues and do not infiltrate them, often being flanked by a layer of lamellar bone (83,175). Some may be cellular with a significant number of binucleate cells, some nuclear enlargement, but no mitotic activity (83). Some show varying degrees of myxoid change (83), which may lead to a mistaken diagnosis of chondrosarcoma. One must therefore allow for a significant degree of atypia before making the diagnosis of malignancy. The radiographic appearance with its sclerotic rim is very helpful in most instances.

Periosteal chondroma is usually curable by marginal excision and has a low recurrence rate. If possible, en bloc excision is preferable and will cure it completely. The main differential diagnosis is periosteal chondrosar-

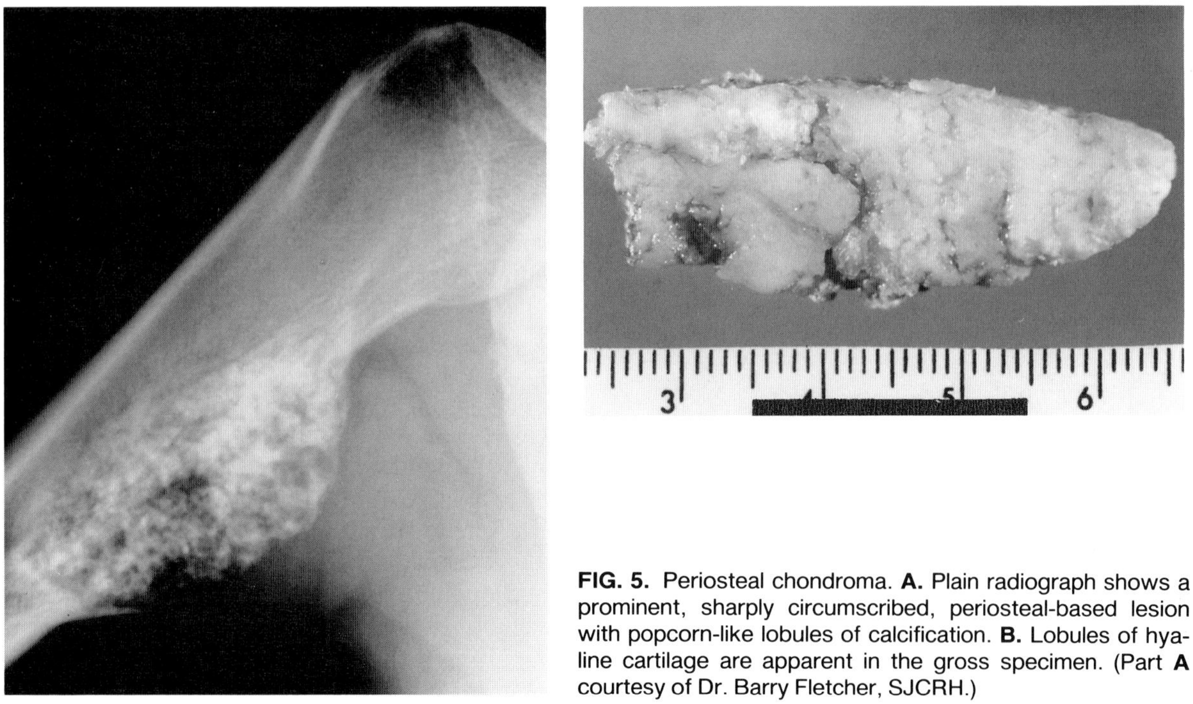

A B

FIG. 5. Periosteal chondroma. **A.** Plain radiograph shows a prominent, sharply circumscribed, periosteal-based lesion with popcorn-like lobules of calcification. **B.** Lobules of hyaline cartilage are apparent in the gross specimen. (Part **A** courtesy of Dr. Barry Fletcher, SJCRH.)

coma. The degree of atypia must be substantial for one to make this diagnosis, and ancillary data must be taken into account.

Chondrosarcoma

Chondrosarcoma is rare in childhood; most malignant pediatric tumors with a cartilaginous component are chondroblastic osteosarcomas. The former tend to occur at a younger age when there is an underlying predisposition such as Ollier's disease, Maffucci's syndrome, or multiple osteochondromatosis (96). Most are detected after 10 years of age (66). Primary chondrosarcomas also may arise de novo and occur at a younger age. They may be intramedullary or surface in their distribution and often arise in unusual sites such as the skull (48,57). Most adult chondrosarcomas are thought to arise from a preexisting benign lesion (96). The histologic grading of these tumors is of great prognostic importance, but it is difficult to obtain good concordance among pathologists in this regard (96).

Chondrosarcomas consist of hyaline cartilage with or without myxoid areas and show increased cellularity, nuclear atypia, permeation of bony trabeculae, and fibrous bands separating lobules of tumor (Fig. 2B). The tumors present with either local pain or swelling. The site of the tumor is of great importance in distinguishing benign from malignant cartilaginous tumors. Those in the hands or feet are almost invariably benign (see above), whereas those arising in the proximal femora and humeri, pelvis, scapuli, ribs, sternum, and spine are more likely to be malignant, possibly because they are able to attain a larger size before detection. It is said that all sternal cartilage tumors are malignant, and in fact any cartilaginous tumor in the above sites has a much greater chance of being malignant than more distal lesions of the same histologic degree of atypia (96). Surface chondral tumors tend to occur on the midhumerus, midfemur, or more distally. They probably arise from osteochondromas. When the cartilaginous cap of an osteochondroma is thicker than 2–3 cm, it is more likely to be malignant, although there is considerable overlap (96).

Mesenchymal Chondrosarcoma

Mesenchymal chondrosarcoma is an uncommon tumor that typically occurs in the spine or nonpelvic flat bones. It is often a large neoplasm and has a propensity to metastasize to lungs, lymph nodes, or other bones. Radiologically these tumors are predominantly lytic, but 75% have some matrix mineralization (96).

Histologically mesenchymal chondrosarcomas consist of sheets of small undifferentiated cells, often with a hemangiopericytomatous pattern of vasculature associated with scattered, often well-differentiated islands of cartilage. It is these islands of cartilage that are diagnostic. The undifferentiated areas correspond to the most primitive condensations of cells in cartilage-forming areas in the developing embryo (266). The average patient age is 25 years (96). These tumors frequently occur in an extraosseous location and are also discussed in Chapter 8.

Clear Cell Chondrosarcoma

Clear cell chondrosarcoma is rare. It was first described by Unni and colleagues in 1976 and constitutes about 2% of all chondrosarcomas (18,261). It is particularly prone to occur in the proximal epiphyses of the femur and humerus. About half of cases are lytic, and many have a sclerotic rim on radiographs that can mimic a chondroblastoma. One third of cases are mineralized. They have a mortality rate of about 15% (96).

Histologically clear cell chondrosarcoma consists of sheets of clear cells in a background of islands of conventional chondrosarcomatous tissue, prominent multinucleated giant cells, a very vascular stroma, and very conspicuous trabecular osteoid and bone formation. The tumor cells contain abundant glycogen and are S-100 protein–positive. The bony trabeculae are reactive in nature and not part of the neoplasm (277).

The importance of this neoplasm lies in the fact that it must be considered in the differential diagnosis of chondroblastoma and even giant cell tumor. Biopsies of these latter tumors must therefore be performed in such a manner as to not compromise a subsequent resection, should the lesion turn out to be clear cell chondrosarcoma (277).

Molecular Biology of Cartilaginous Tumors

Cartilaginous tumors present a confusing array of genetic abnormalities that are present in benign as well as malignant lesions (Table 1). Aneuploidy may be present in low-grade and benign lesions, but the presence of a high proliferative index or S-phase fraction is generally indicative of malignancy (2,3). Clonal cytologic aberrations have been described for chondromyxoid fibroma (25,31,252), chondroblastoma (25,160), enchondroma (25,28), osteochondroma (25), and periosteal chondroma (156,158). In situ hybridization of these lesions may reveal anomalies such as trisomy that are not apparent with standard cytogenetic techniques and indicate the presence of tumor cell heterogeneity (142).

A variety of chromosomal abnormalities, generally nonreciprocal translocations and deletions, are present in chondrosarcomas (69,156,192). Clonal karyotypic evolution may be associated with tumor cell heterogeneity (191). A unique reciprocal translocation, the t(9;22)(q22;q12), has been primarily described with extraskeletal myxoid chondrosarcoma (116,189,255) and

TABLE 1. *Chromosomal arrangements in cartilaginous tumors*[a]

Chromosome	Abnormality	Ref.
1	1p rearr.; −; 1 rearr.; 1q21 rearr.; 1 rearr.	156, 191, 192, 245, 289
2	−; t(2;13)(p14;q33),t(2;13(q21;p12); abn.	25, 31, 245
3	−; abn.	25, 245
4	−; 4 rearr.	156, 245
5	abn.; +; ins(5;2)(q13)(p21p25); 5q13 rearr.; deletion, rearr.	25, 31, 156, 191, 252
6	t(6;12)(q25;q13); −; −, rearr.	117, 156, 191
7	abn; +; +,7p11 rearr.	25, 117, 191
8	−; abn.; +; complex trans., deletion	25, 117, 156, 245
9	−; t(9;22;15)(q31;q12.2;q25); t(9;22)(q22;q11); t(922)(q34;q11–12); t(9;22)(q22;q12); 9p13–22 abn.; rearr.	116, 130, 156, 189, 245, 253, 255
10	−; 10q21.1 rearr., deletion of 10q21–q23; −; −	156, 191, 231, 245
11	−; +; −	117, 156, 245
12	abn.; t(6;12)(q25;q13),t(12;19)(q13;q13); complex trans., rearr.	25, 117, 156
13	−; t(2;13)(p14;q33),t(2;13)(q32;p12); −; complex trans., −	31, 156, 191, 245
14	−	245
15	−; +; rearr.	69, 156, 245
16	−; der(21)t(16;21)(q11;p11)	69, 245
17	−; −	117, 245
18	−; −	156, 245
19	+; 19p abn.; +,t(12;19)(q13;q13)	69, 117, 149
20	+,20q11 rearr.; rearr.	156, 191
21	der(21)t(16;21)(q11;p11)	69
22	−; 22q breakpt.; +; −; t(9;22)(q34;q11); −,t(9;22)(q34;q11–12)	116, 117, 156, 160, 231, 253
X	−; complex trans.	156, 245
Y	−	191

Abbreviations: Abn., abnormality; der, derivative chromosome; trans., translocation; breakpt., breakpoint; rearr., rearrangement; −, monosomy; +, trisomy.
[a] Abnormalities are separated by brackets corresponding to references in adjacent column.

has been used for the confirmation of this diagnosis in a fine needle aspiration sample (189). However, it has also been observed in a dedifferentiated chondrosarcoma without myxoid foci (253), and alterations of chromosome 9 may not be observed in myxoid tumors (231). Abnormalities of chromosome 9, however, are frequent in chondrosarcoma (130), and microcell transfer of a normal chromosome 9 may induce senescence in an affected chondrosarcoma cell line (131). The common involvement of 9p13-22 may affect the familial atypical mole–melanoma locus, *MLM* (130), and in fact an association between melanoma and chondrosarcoma has been noted in some families (107).

Although they appear to be genetic diseases, Maffucci's syndrome and Ollier's disease to date have shown a surprising lack of constitutional cytogenetic abnormalities (79). Neural abnormalities with resultant growth factor release have been postulated as being responsible for the proliferation of the hemangiomas and enchondromas associated with the former syndrome (212). On the other hand, multiple osteochondromatosis has been well characterized molecularly. Three loci, termed *EXT1, EXT2,* and *EXT3,* have been described on chromosomes 8, 11, and 19, respectively. Loss of heterozygosity for these genetic regions may be demonstrated in chondrosarcomas arising from affected patients as well as in sporadic tumors (109,149,207). Overexpression and mutation of *p53* may also be demonstrated by immunohistochemistry in sporadic high-grade lesions (70).

OSSEOUS LESIONS

Bone Island

A bone island, or enostosis, is an island of dense cortical-like bone occurring in the medullary portion of a bone. It is diagnosed radiologically as an intramedullary radiodense lesion having radiating bony spicules and blending with the surrounding bone (20). It is usually cold on bone scan (20,99), but some lesions appear "hot" (99,100). Histologically it is an island of dense intramedullary cortical bone with no other distinguishing features. It may be multiple and should be distinguished from osteoblastic metastases or osteopoikilosis (20).

Osteoid Osteoma

Osteoid osteoma is a fairly common benign lesion of bone (10% of benign tumors) and can be very frustrating both in diagnosis and in treatment. It affects young people, especially late teenage years, and has a male/female ratio of 2:1 (20). Osteoid osteoma arises in long bones, especially the femur and tibia, as well as the posterior elements of the vertebrae, humerus, hand, and the foot, particularly the talus. When located in the cortex, osteoid osteoma is associated with a prominent sclerotic reaction in the surrounding bone and periosteum. In this situation it usually occurs in the diaphysis of the long bones. When it occurs in the medullary portion of the bone or when the lesion is adjacent to or within a joint, it may not exhibit circumferential sclerosis. In the latter situation it may be associated with a chronic inflammatory reaction and thus mimic arthritis. It may also occur subperiosteally with no sclerosis. When in the spinal column it may be associated with scoliosis with the concavity toward the lesion. There may also be limb length discrepancy (20).

Osteoid osteoma should be less than 2.0 cm in maximum diameter and may be purely lytic, focally ossified, or totally ossified. It is very vascular and has been shown to contain many nerve fibers that are thought to account for its usual presentation with pain (175). This pain may be severe, is worse at night, and is dramatically relieved by salicylates. The lesion is best demonstrated by CT scans, technetium bone scans, or gadolinium-enhanced MRI scans (Fig. 6A) (20). The associated edema may be confusing. The tumor must be differentiated from a Brodie abscess, stress fracture, arthritis, bone island, and osteoblastoma (20).

At the time of surgery osteoid osteoma may be very difficult to identify and totally remove. Administration of tetracycline before surgery, use of ultraviolet light during surgery, and performance of an intraoperative technetium scan may help. Specimen radiographs are useful in documenting that the lesion is included with the excision.

Histologically osteoid osteoma consists of a well-demarcated nidus of relatively small osteoid trabeculae surrounded by osteoblasts and separated by a somewhat loose fibrous stroma with a prominent vasculature (Fig. 6B). The osteoid shows varying degrees of ossification. The lesion is sharply delimited from the adjacent sclerotic cortical bone and does not permeate it for any distance—an important point of distinction from the more infiltrative osteosarcoma. Another histologic mimic is the osteoblastoma, which is less common in the long bones, more common in the vertebral column and flat bones, and larger than an osteoid osteoma, being more than 2 cm in size. Osteoblastoma is not associated with surrounding sclerosis.

Osteoblastoma

Osteoblastoma is a tumor of young teenagers with a median age of 16 years. It occurs most commonly in the posterior elements of the spinal column but also involves the long bones, particularly the proximal femur, and the hands and feet, particularly the talus. It is a lytic lesion, usually well demarcated, without the dense sclerosis seen with osteoid osteoma. When located in the vertebral column it often produces neurologic symptoms. When it occurs in long bones, it frequently involves the diaphysis and is usually eccentric and intramedullary, but it may primarily involve the cortex or be central. It often involves the proximal femur (Fig. 7A, B) (20). Histologically osteoblastoma bears a striking resemblance to osteoid osteoma. Some feel that the trabeculae are longer and broader than osteoid osteoma spicules, but this may be

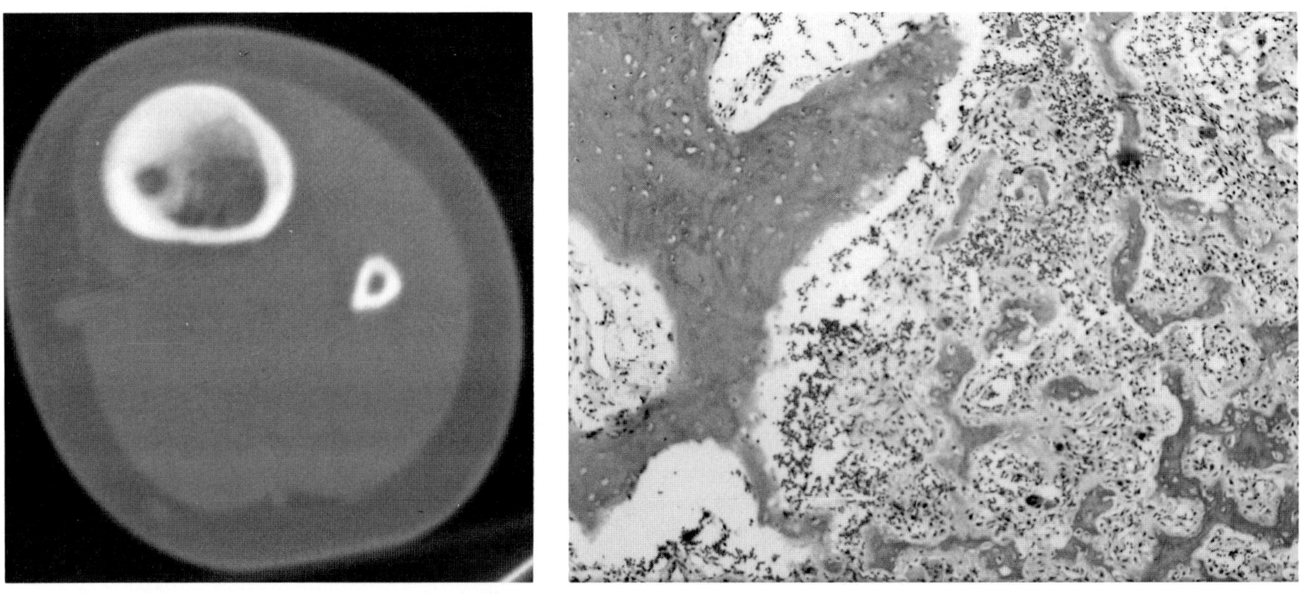

A B

FIG. 6. Osteoid osteoma. **A.** CT reveals a circular, punched-out nidus with circumferential sclerosis in the cortex of the tibia. **B.** A bone-forming nidus sharply abuts densely sclerotic cortical bone. (Part **A** courtesy of Dr. Barry Fletcher, SJCRH.)

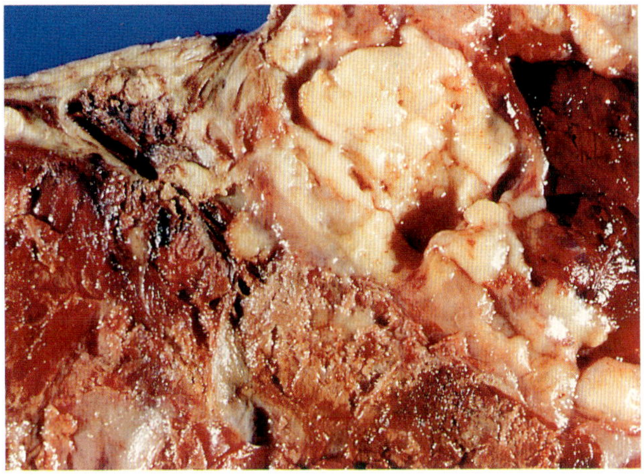

FIG. 2–1. Gross specimen of juvenile cancer containing viable *(upper right)* and necrotic *(lower left)* tissues.

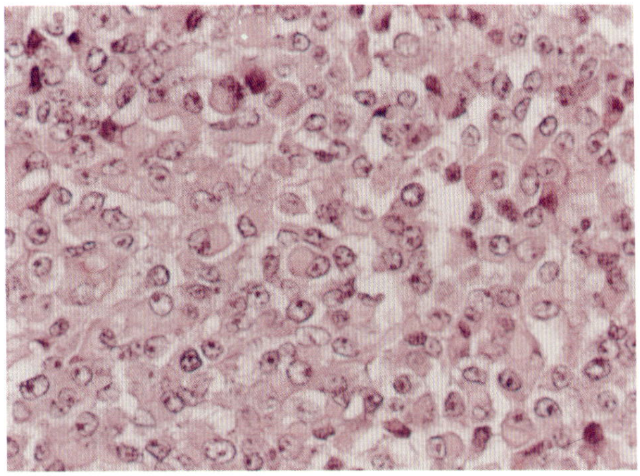

FIG. 3–28. Malignant rhabdoid tumor composed of cells with eccentric nuclei, prominent nucleoli, and hyaline cytoplasmic inclusions.

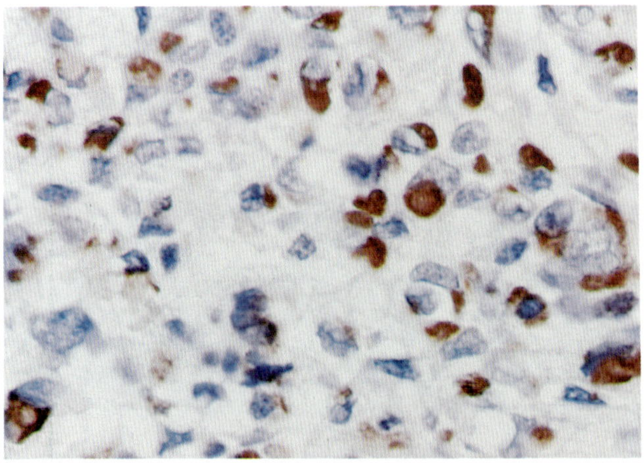

FIG. 3–30. Immunostain of malignant rhabdoid tumor containing prominent cytokeratin-positive inclusions. (Avidin–biotin complex [ABC] technique with hematoxylin counterstain.) (Courtesy of Dr. Bruce Webber, Memphis, TN.)

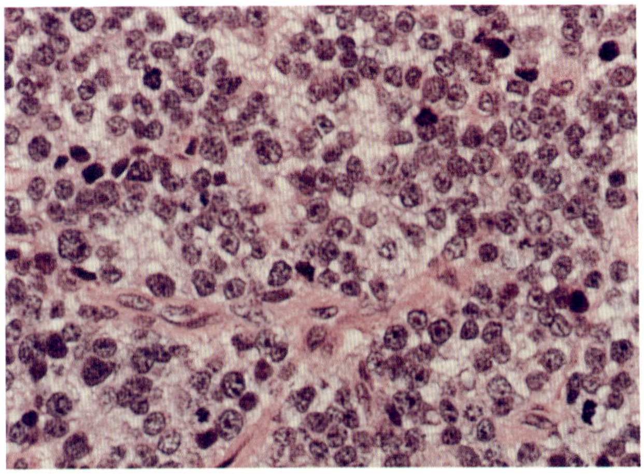

FIG. 4–3. Histologic appearance of "typical" Ewing's sarcoma. There is a diffuse infiltrate of primitive cells with uniform, round nuclei, small to inconspicuous nucleoli, and bubbly, clear cytoplasm. Cell margins are indistinct. Scattered "dark" cells with pyknotic nuclei are apparent.

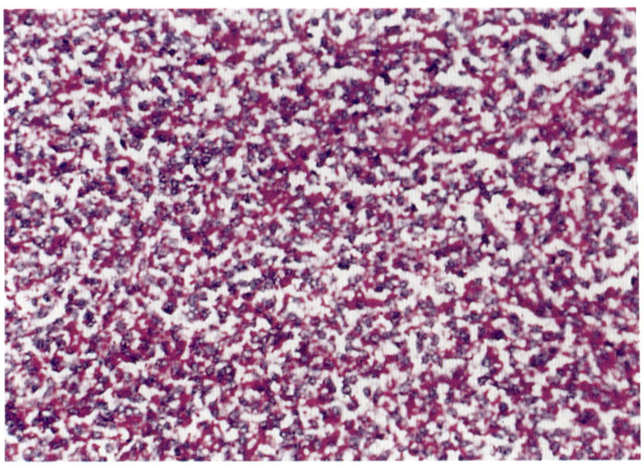

FIG. 4–8A. Histochemical stain for Ewing's sarcoma, illustrating strong periodic acid–Schiff positivity.

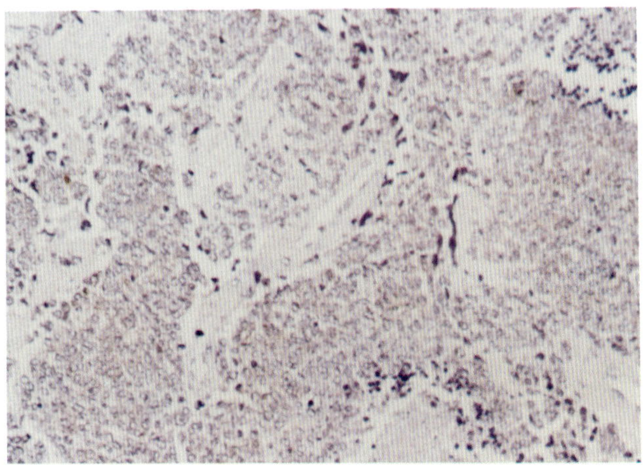

FIG. 4–11. Cytokeratin stain of Ewing's sarcoma of bone. There is weak, diffuse, cytoplasmic positivity. (ABC technique.)

A 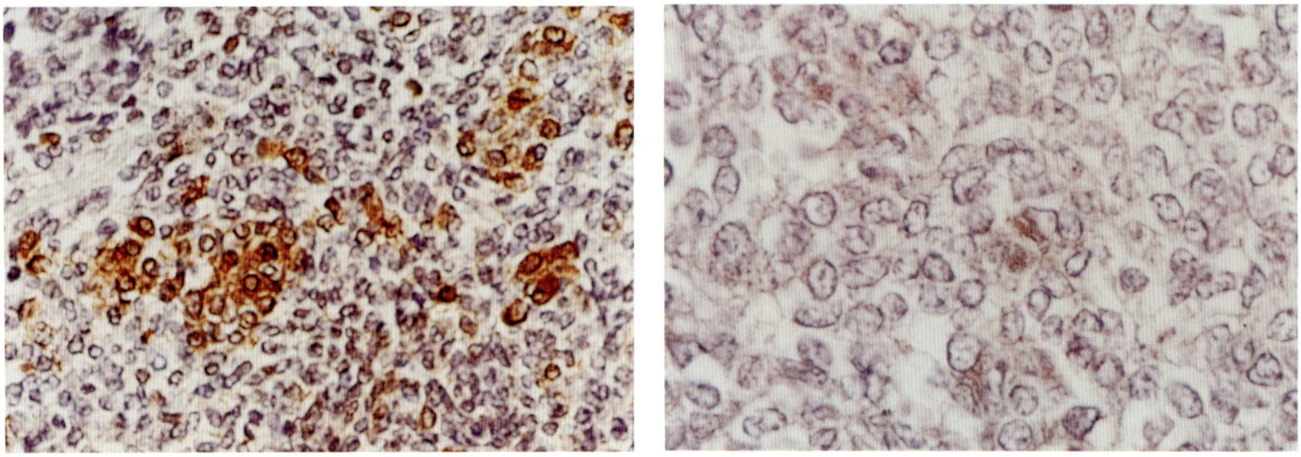 B

FIG. 4–12. Neural marker positivity in Ewing's sarcoma. Both neuron-specific enolase **(A)** and synaptophysin **(B)** show positivity in discrete cell clusters. (ABC technique.)

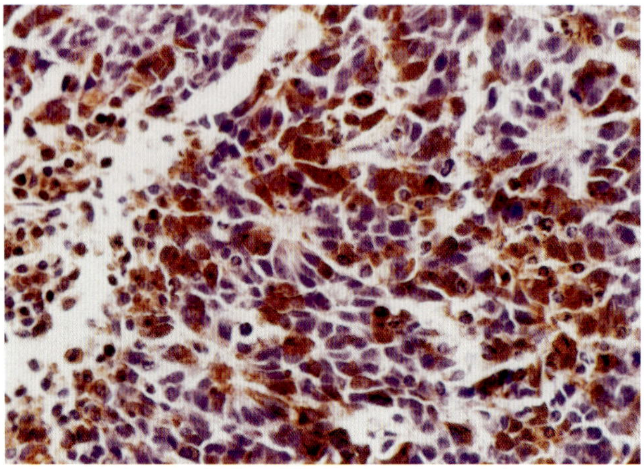

FIG. 4–13. Glial fibrillary acidic protein positivity in metastatic small cell tumor of bone. (From Parham DM et al. *Am J Clin Pathol* 1991;95:166–171, courtesy of American Society of Clinical Pathologists.)

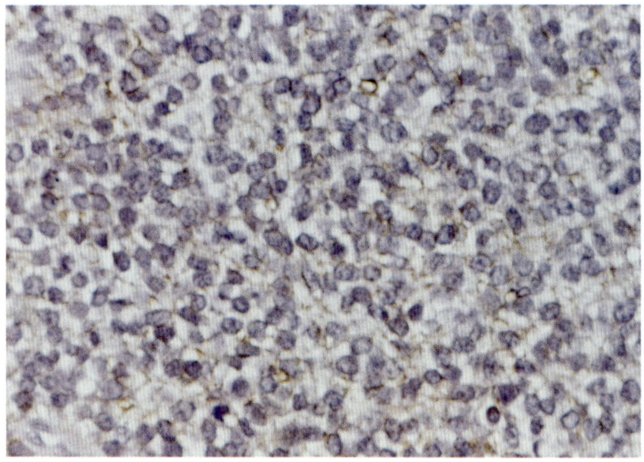

FIG. 4–14. MIC2 positivity in Ewing's sarcoma, as revealed by immunohistochemistry with the HBA71 monoclonal antibody. There is diffuse membranous staining.

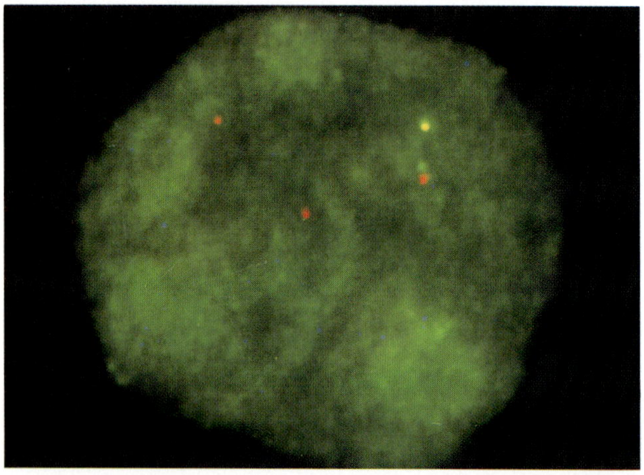

FIG. 4–18. Interphase FISH study of tumor cell nucleus containing a translocation. Two probes that map to the genes affected by the translocation are tested with two color signals: red and green. With normal, untranslocated alleles, there is separation of the two probes *(lower right and middle of cell)*, but the two signals are juxtaposed in translocated chromosomes *(lower left).* This cell contains more than two copies of the affected genes. (Courtesy of Marc Valentine and Drs. Stephen Morris and Prasad Matthew, St. Jude Children's Research Hospital.)

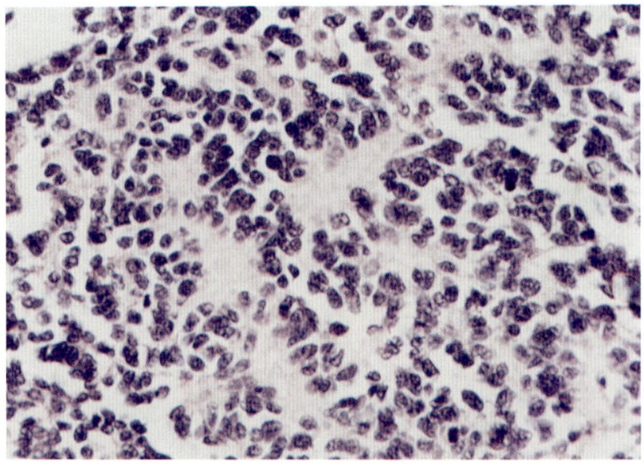

FIG. 4–21. Routine light micrograph of peripheral neuroepithelioma, which contains prominent Homer Wright rosettes with central neurofibrillary cores.

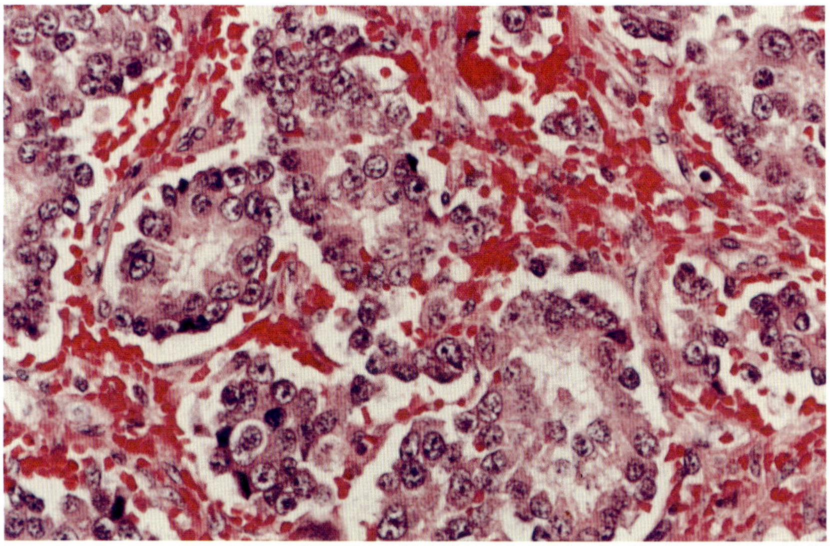

FIG. 4–22. Peripheral neuroepithelioma containing rosettes with central lumens.

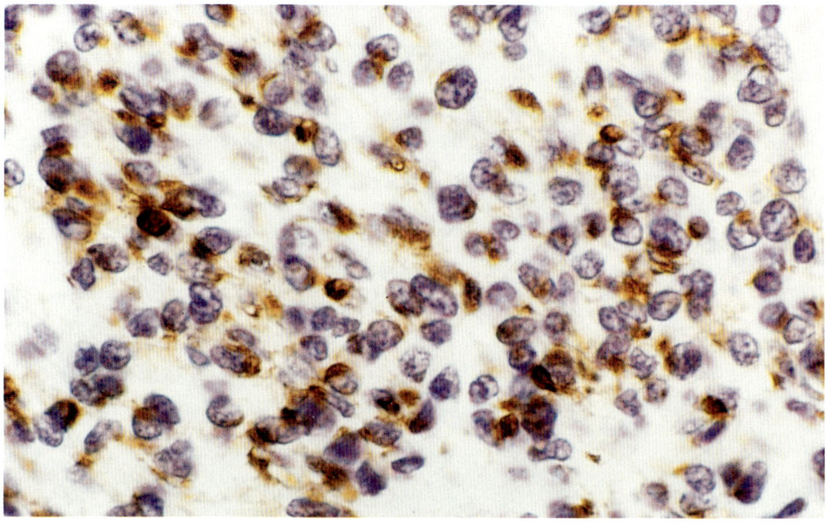

FIG. 4–27. Desmin positivity in peripheral neuroepithelioma. (ABC technique.)

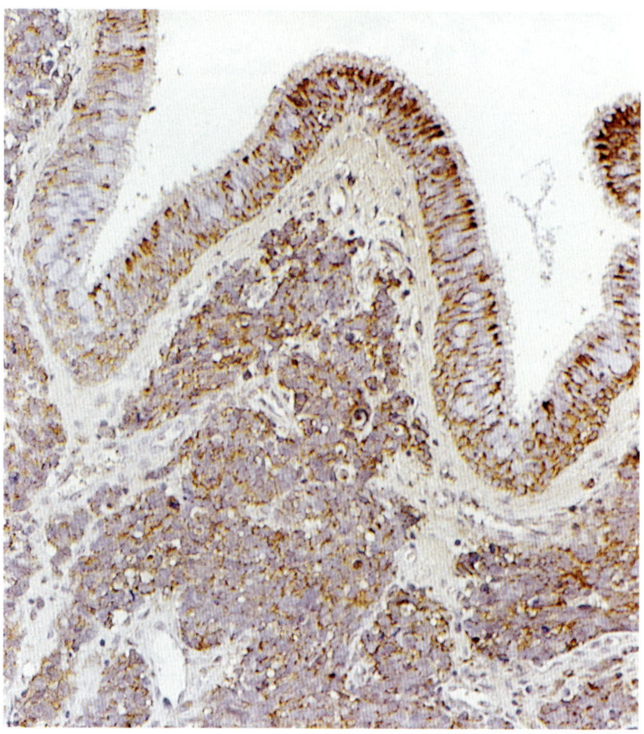

FIG. 4–32. Synaptophysin stain of esthesioneuroblastoma. There is diffuse positivity of the tumor as well as the neuroepithelium in the adjacent mucosa.

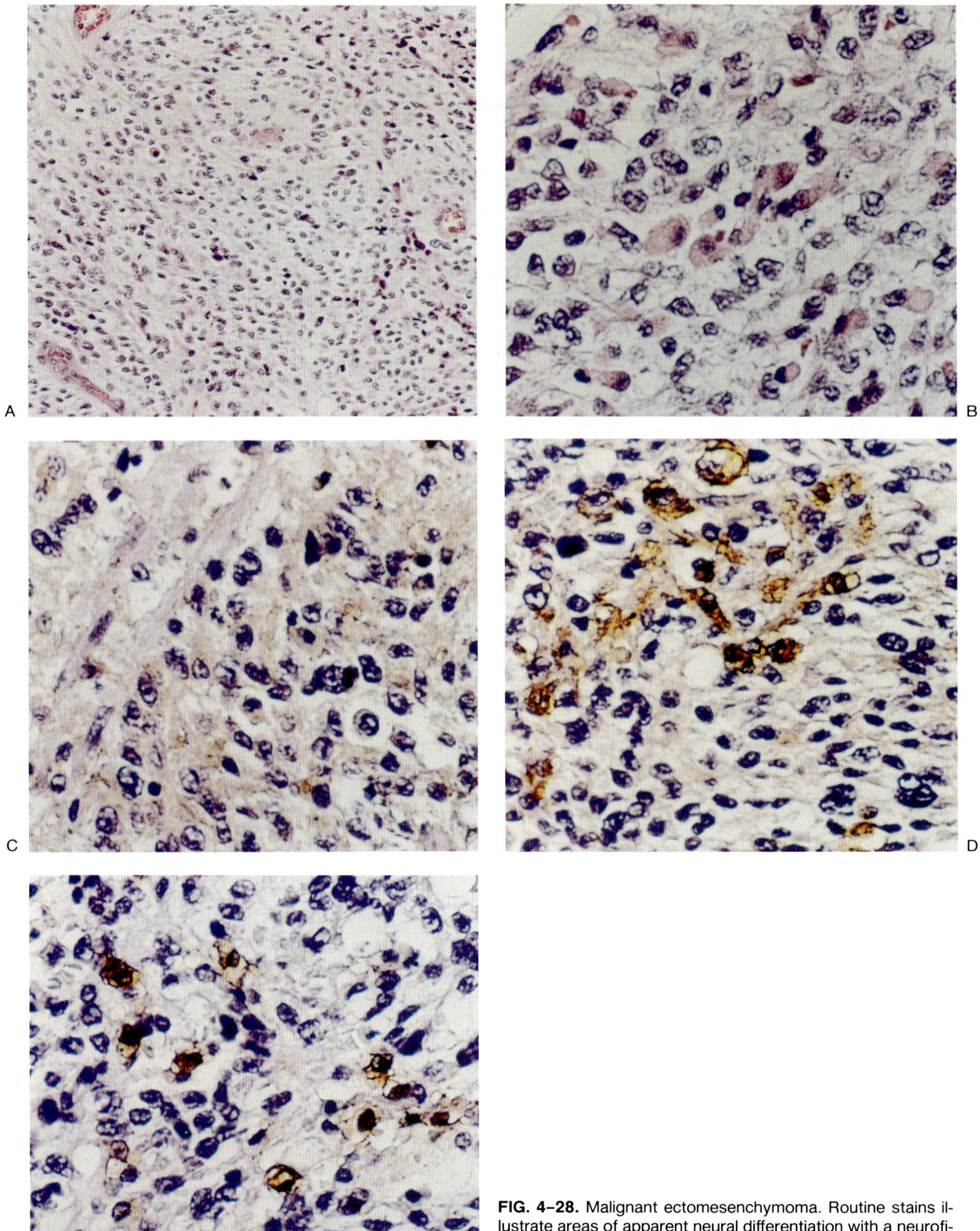

FIG. 4–28. Malignant ectomesenchymoma. Routine stains illustrate areas of apparent neural differentiation with a neurofibrillary matrix **(A)** and myogenic differentiation with rhabdomyoblasts **(B).** Immunostains for neuron-specific enolase **(C)**, desmin **(D)**, and S-100 **(E)** are positive (ABC technique).

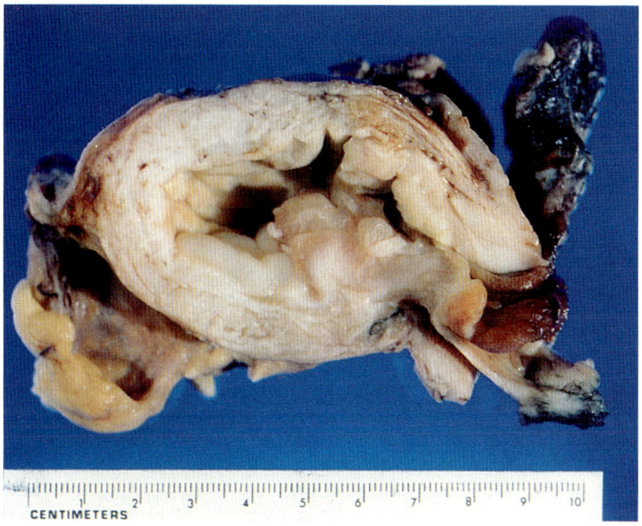

FIG. 5–5A. Botryoid rhabdomyosarcoma of the urinary bladder, presenting as multiple, rounded polypoid lesions on gross examination.

FIG. 5–6. Developing skeletal muscle in midterm fetus, illustrating condensation of myotubes in loose primitive mesenchyme **(A).** Embryonal rhabdomyosarcoma shows similar areas of condensation and myogenesis in loose mesenchymal tissues **(B).**

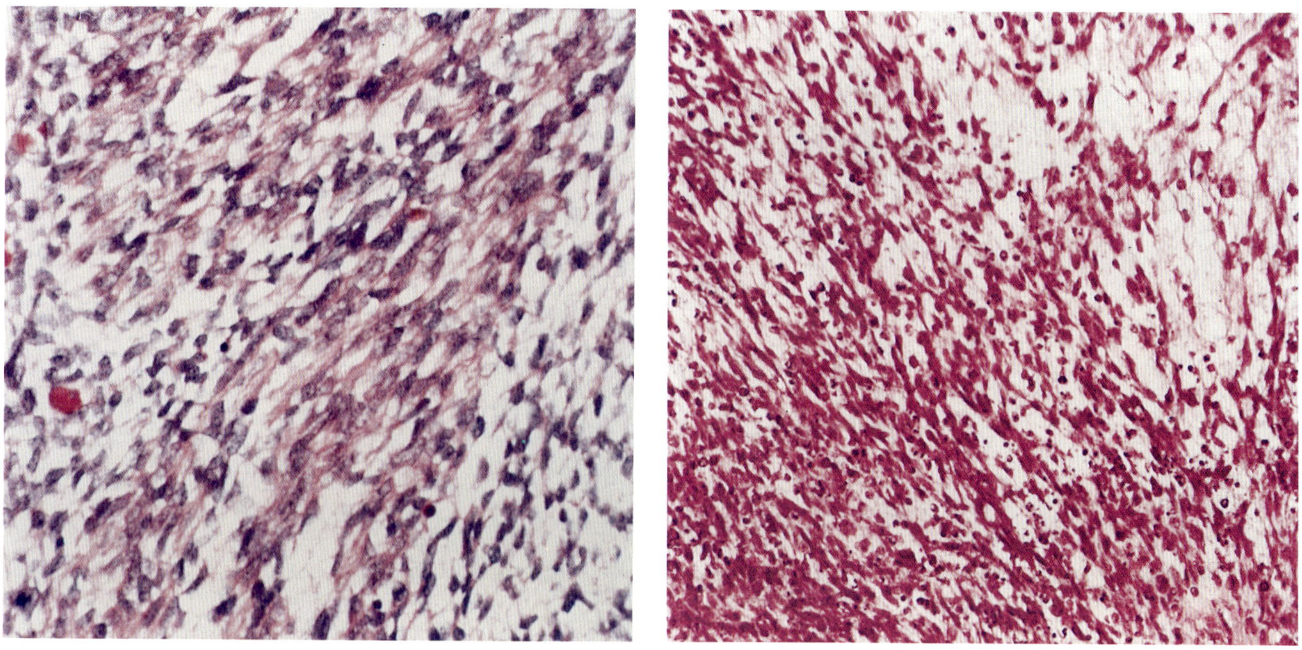

A B

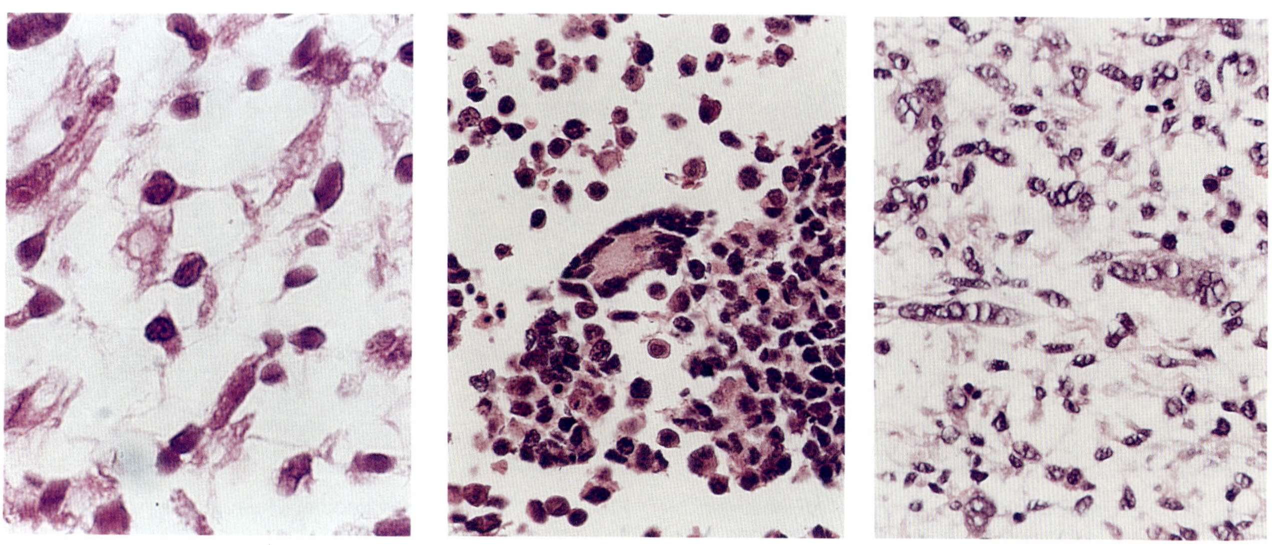

A,B C

FIG. 5–7. Analogy of stages of myogenesis to cell types found in rhabdomyosarcoma. The flow diagram at the figure top on page 90 illustrates the normal stages of embryonic myogenesis. The photomicrographs shown here illustrate compatible features in rhabdomyosarcoma, namely early myoblast formation **(A)**, giant cells resulting from myocyte fusion **(B)**, and tandem cells similar to myofibers **(C)**.

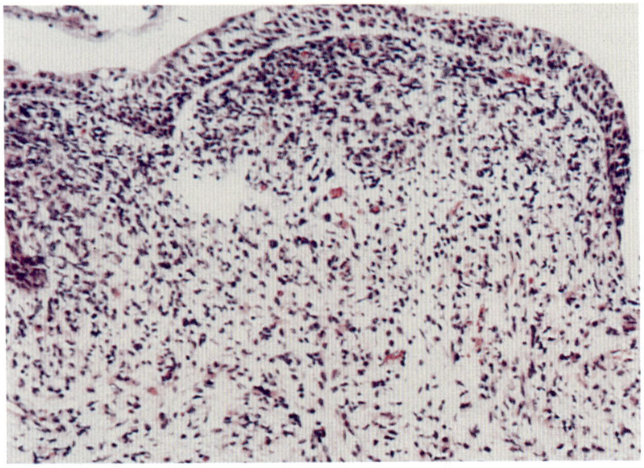

FIG. 5–8. Botryoid rhabdomyosarcoma of urinary bladder. A zone of condensed tumor cells (the cambium layer) is immediately beneath the urothelium.

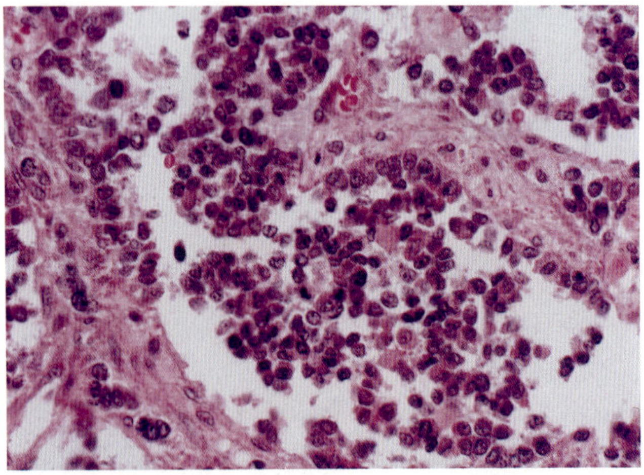

FIG. 5–9. Alveolar rhabdomyosarcoma.Tumor cells form "floating" clusters separated by a prominent framework of stromal cells and collagen. Rows of tumor cells align the fibrous septa in a picket fence fashion.

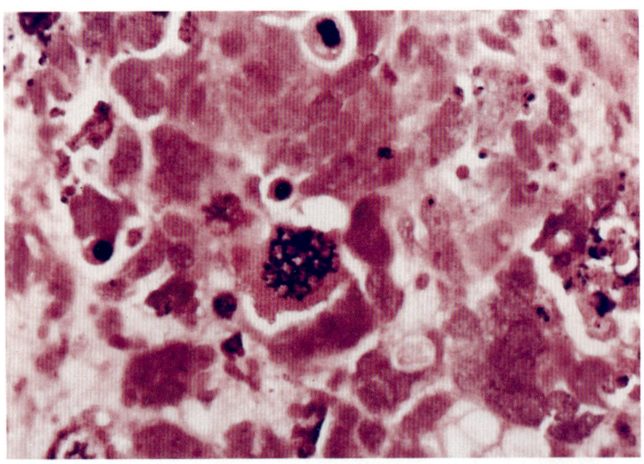

FIG. 5–11. Anaplastic rhabdomyosarcoma. An enlarged bizarre mitosis with a multipolar spindle apparatus is apparent in the center of the figure. (Courtesy of Dr. Bruce Webber, Memphis, TN.)

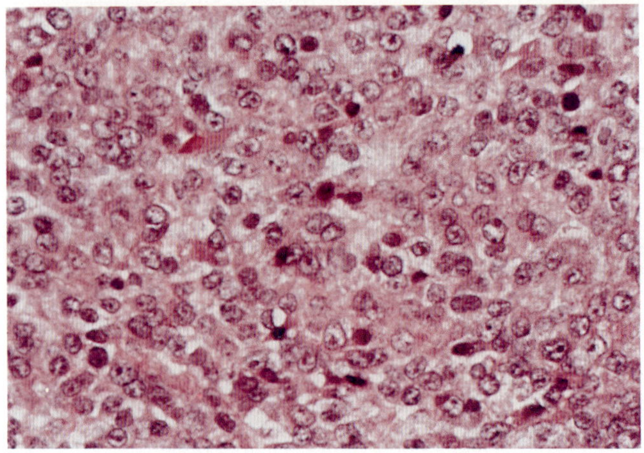

FIG. 5–12. Monomorphous round cell rhabdomyosarcoma. The tumor is composed of diffuse sheets of primitive round cells with central nucleoli. The cytology in this example is also compatible with a diagnosis of solid alveolar rhabdomyosarcoma. (Courtesy of Dr. Bruce Webber, Memphis, TN.)

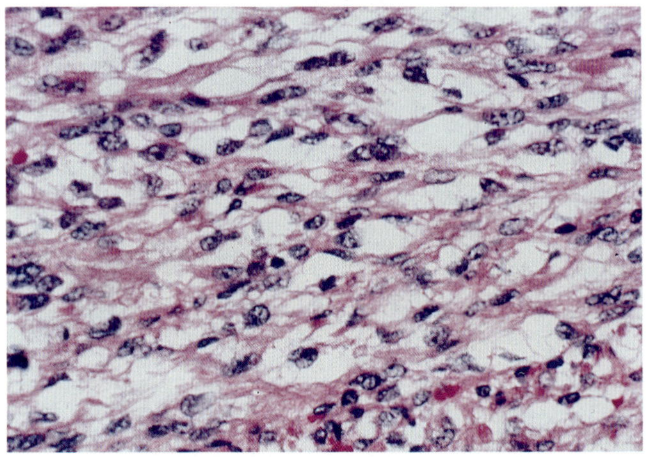

FIG. 5–13. Spindle cell or "type A" rhabdomyosarcoma. This lesion has histologic features reminiscent of leiomyosarcoma. (Courtesy of Dr. Bruce Webber, Memphis, TN.)

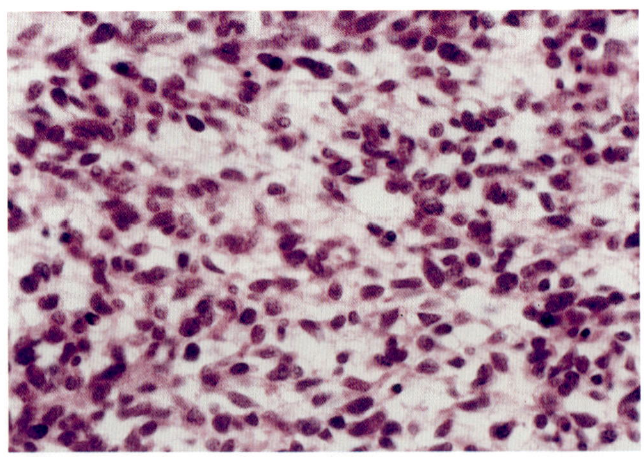

FIG. 5–14. Embryonal sarcoma. The tumor cells appear primitive and show no obvious cytologic evidence of myogenesis. (Courtesy of Dr. Bruce Webber, Memphis, TN.)

A
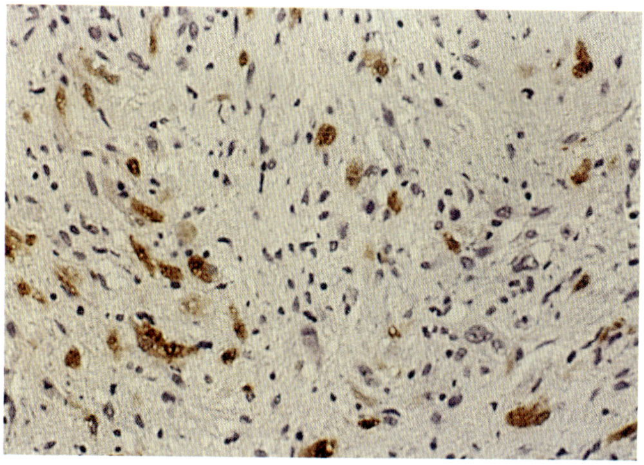

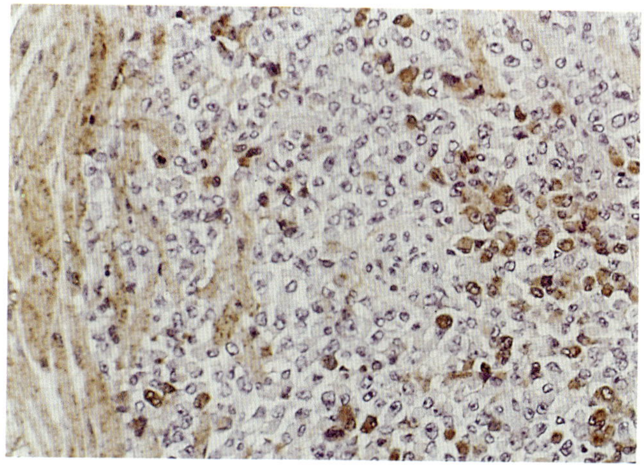
B

C
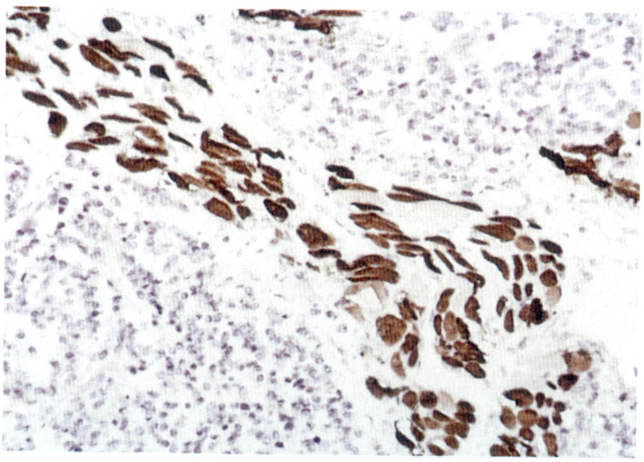

FIG. 5–18. Myoglobin stains showing positivity in **(A)** differentiating rhabdomyosarcoma cells, **(B)** nonrhabdomyosarcoma cells adjacent to skeletal muscle, and **(C)** skeletal muscle fibers entrapped within non-staining tumor. (ABC technique.)

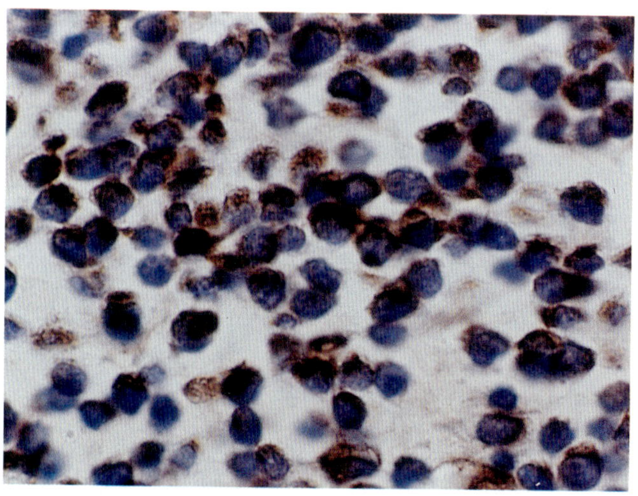

FIG. 5–19. Rhabdomyosarcoma containing round cells that are intensely desmin-positive. (ABC technique.)

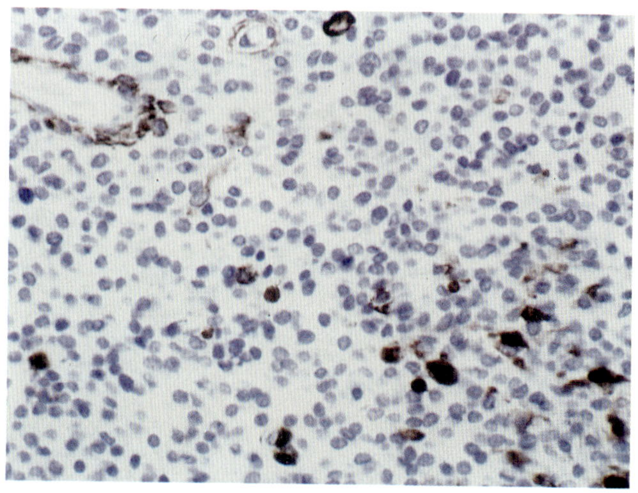

FIG. 5–20. Muscle-specific actin-positive rhabdomyosarcoma cells and pericytes. (ABC technique.)

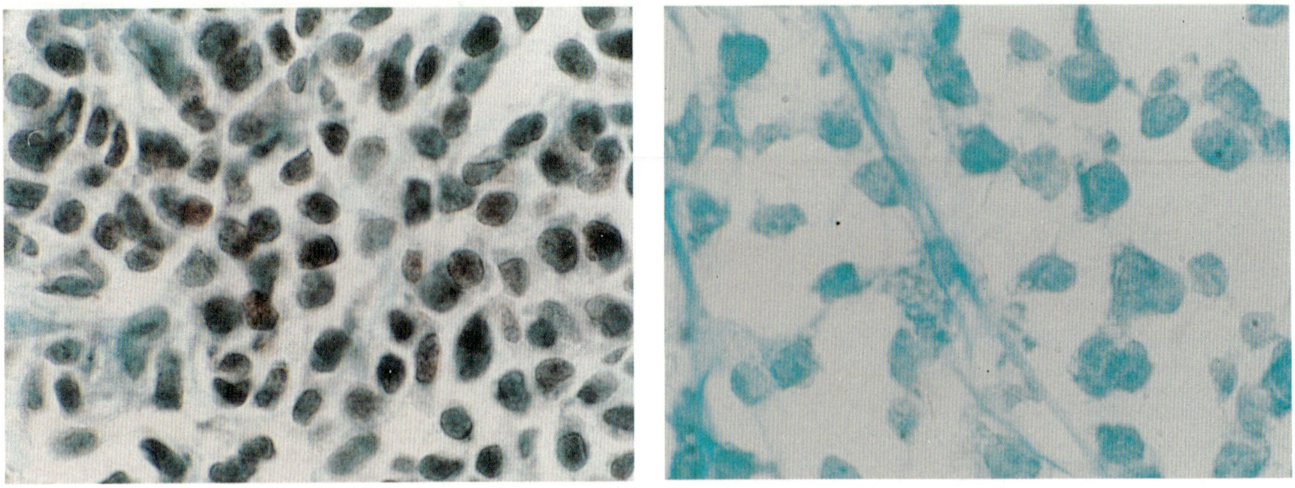

A B

FIG. 5–21. Positive MyoD staining in a rhabdomyosarcoma **(A)**, compared with negative staining in a Ewing's sarcoma **(B).** There is granular dark brown positivity in the rhabdomyosarcoma cell nuclei.

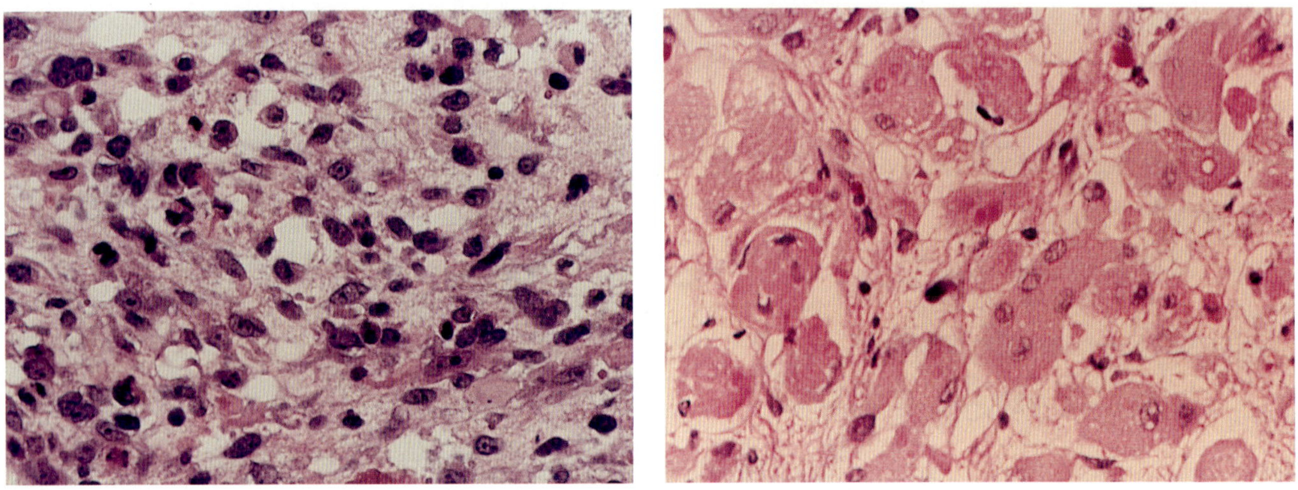

A B

FIG. 5–26. Embryonal rhabdomyosarcoma before **(A)** and after **(B)** therapy. There is marked posttherapy maturation of the tumor cells **(B)**, which contain voluminous amounts of cytoplasm and marginated nuclei. (Courtesy of Dr. Peter Houghton, St. Jude Children's Research Hospital.)

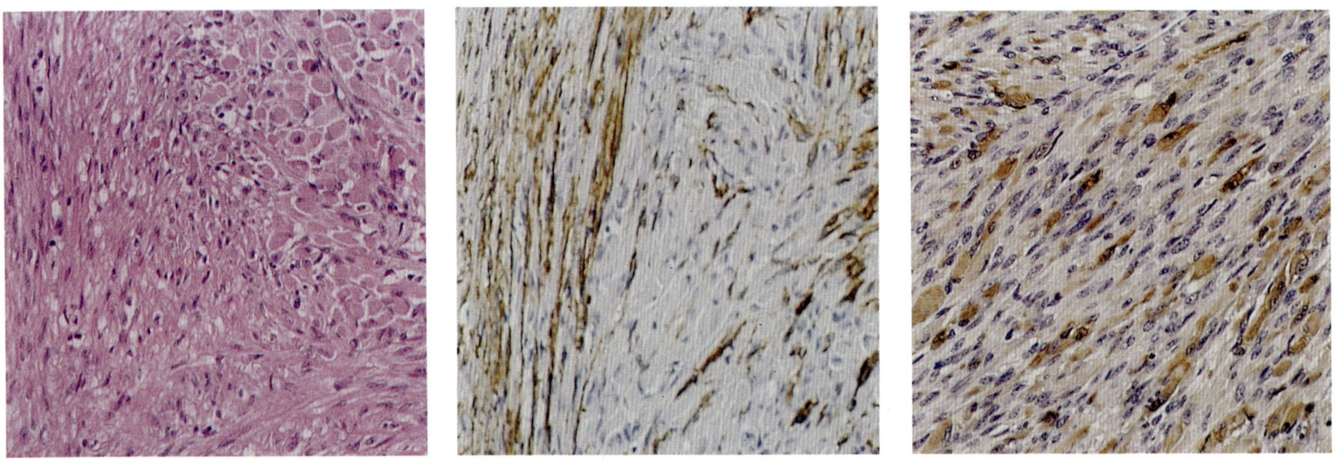

A,B C

FIG. 5–27. Intermediate rhabdomyoma. There is a mixture of smooth muscle-like spindle cells and rhabdomyoblastic round cells **(A).** The cells are respectively positive for α-smooth muscle actin **(B)** and myoglobin **(C).** (A: Hematoxylin and eosin; B,C: ABC technique.)

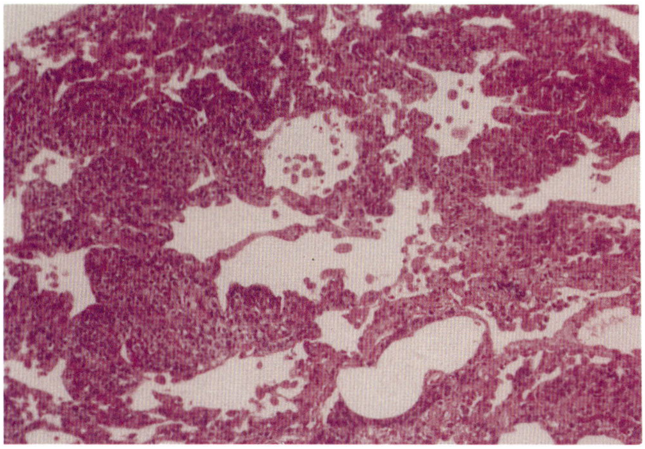

FIG. 6–7. Nodules of metastatic neuroblastoma in the lung of a 3-year-old boy who developed progressive disease after autologous bone marrow transplantation.

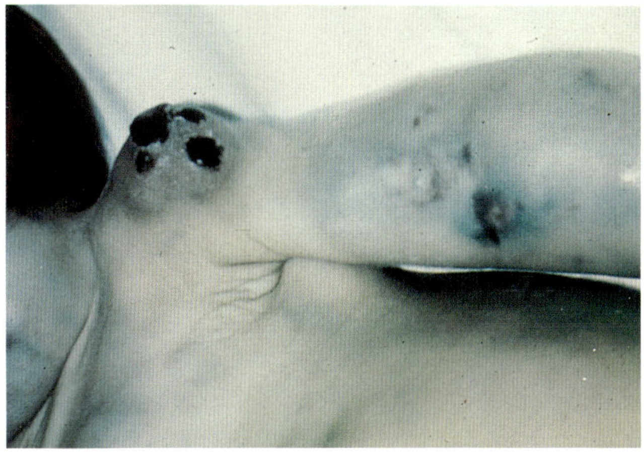

FIG. 6–8. Blueberry muffin baby. (Courtesy of Drs. Laura Bowman and Ann Hayes, St. Jude Children's Research Hospital, Memphis, TN.)

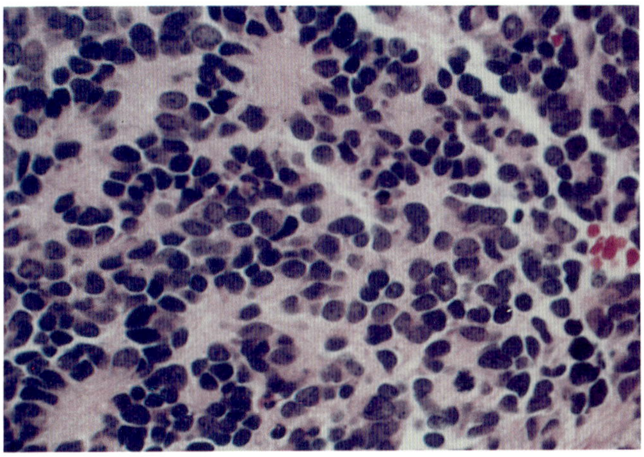

FIG. 6–17. Neuroblastoma with prominent Homer Wright rosettes.

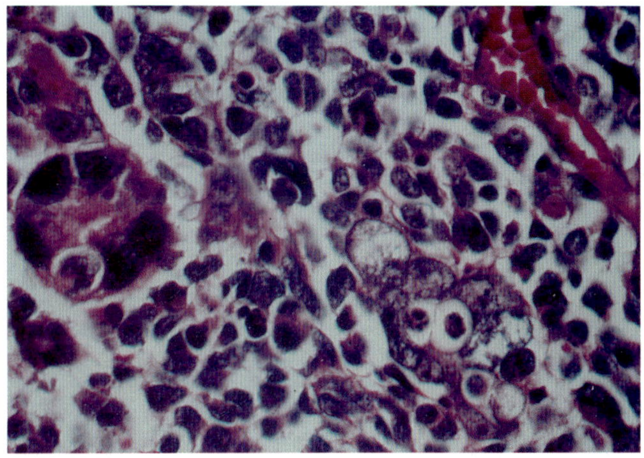

FIG. 6–28. Anaplastic undifferentiated neuroblastoma from the adrenal gland. (Courtesy of Drs. Muoi Arnold and Bruce Beckwith, Loma Linda University, Loma Linda, CA.)

A,B

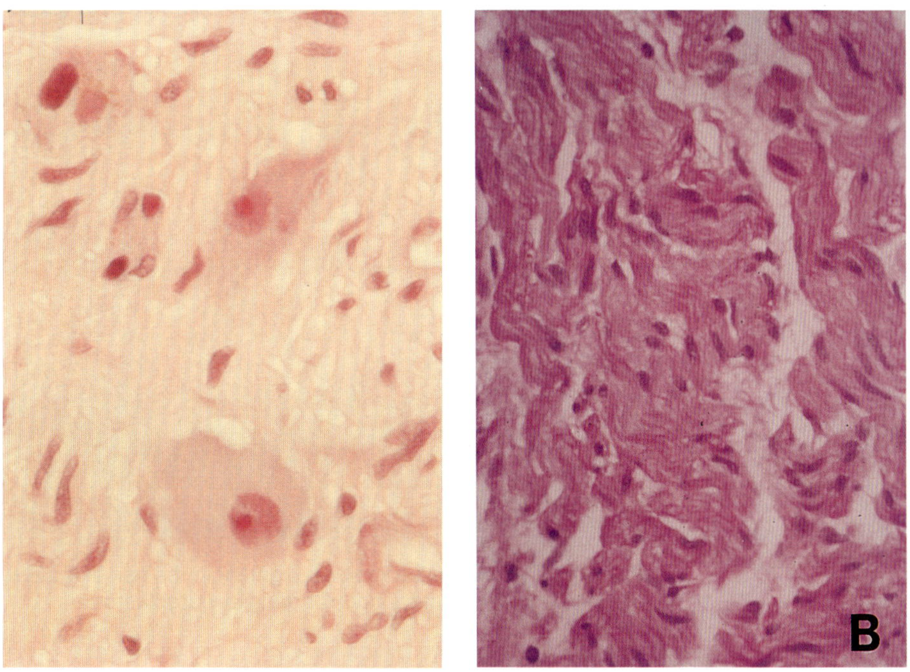

FIG. 6–18. (A,B) Prominent fascicles of neuritic processes, spindle cell (Schwannian) stroma, and occasional ganglion cells in ganglioneuroma.

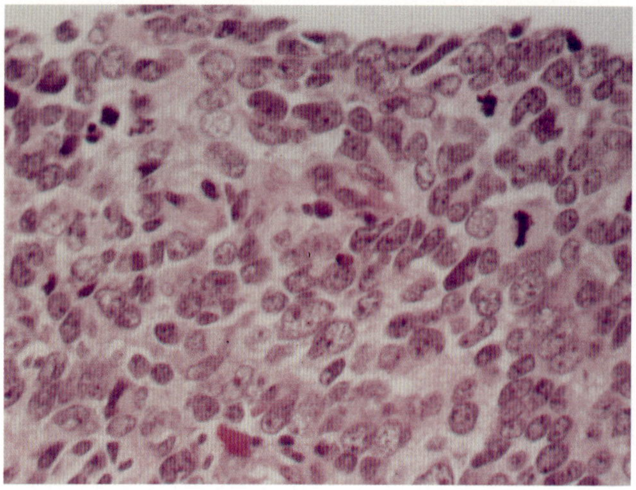

FIG. 6–29. Undifferentiated neuroblastoma from the pelvic region.

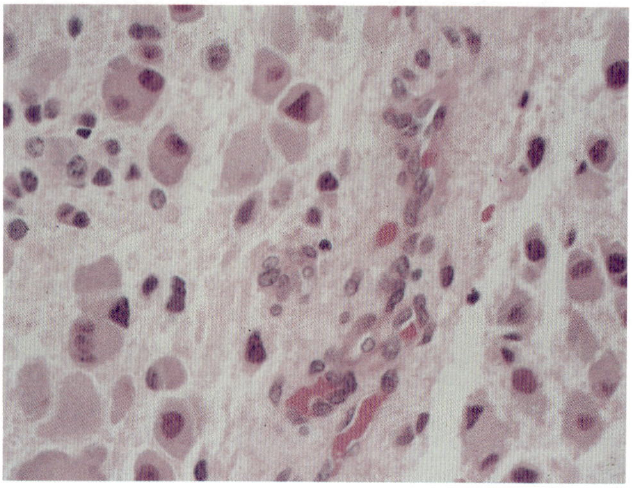

FIG. 6–30. Differentiating neuroblastoma from the thoracic region.

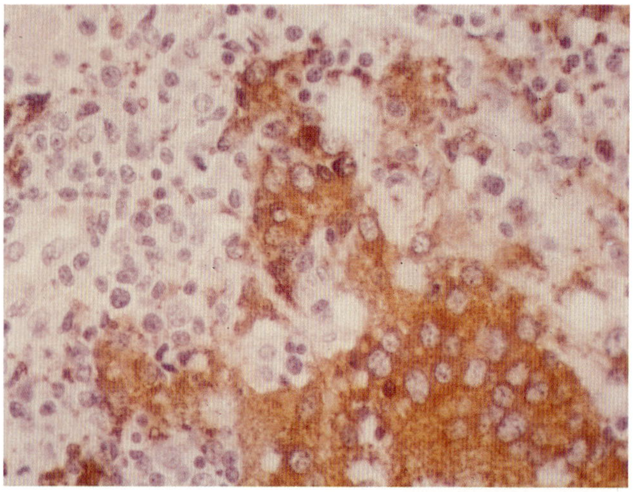

FIG. 6–38. Metastatic neuroblastoma with intense immunoreactivity for neuron-specific enolase in B5-fixed decalcified section (peroxidase-antiperoxidase stain).

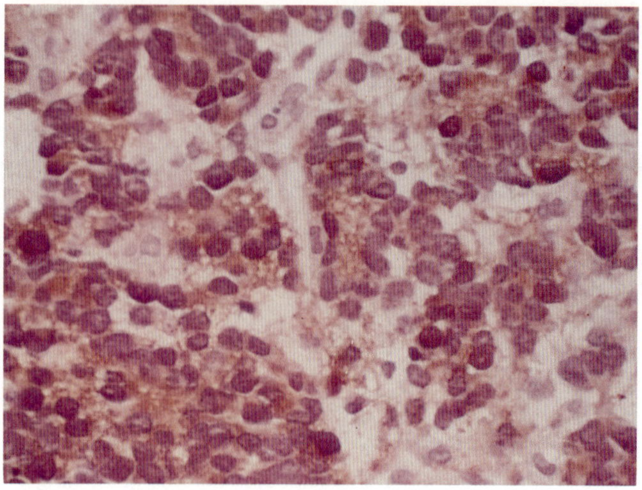

FIG. 6–39. Diffuse immunoreactivity with NSE in a poorly differentiated pelvic neuroblastoma (peroxidase-antiperoxidase stain).

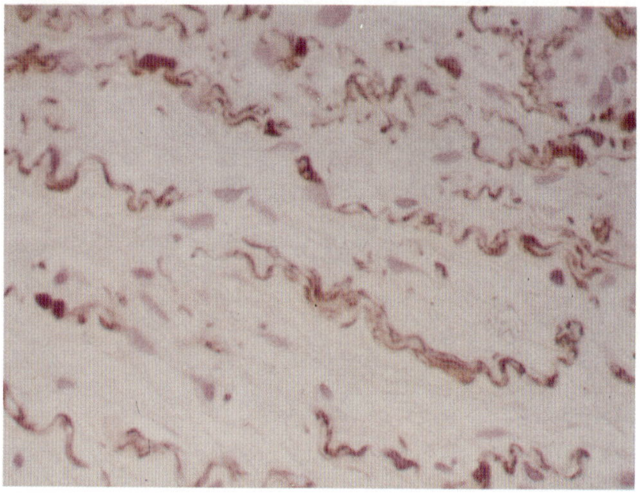

FIG. 6–40. S-100 protein immunoreactivity of the Schwannian stroma in ganglioneuroblastoma (peroxidase-antiperoxidase stain).

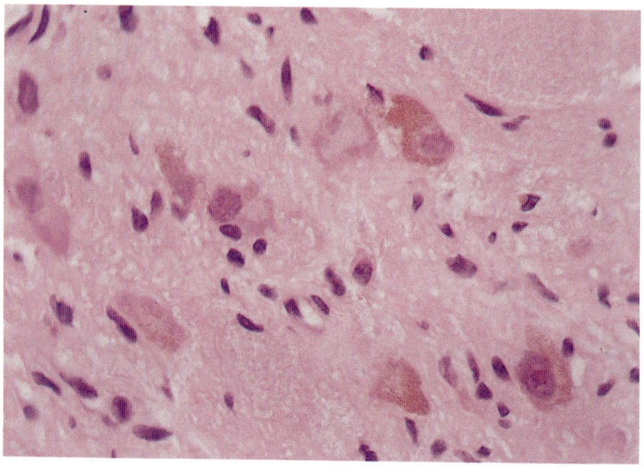

FIG. 6–45. Brown neuromelanin pigment in the ganglion cells of a posterior mediastinal nodular ganglioneuroblastoma.

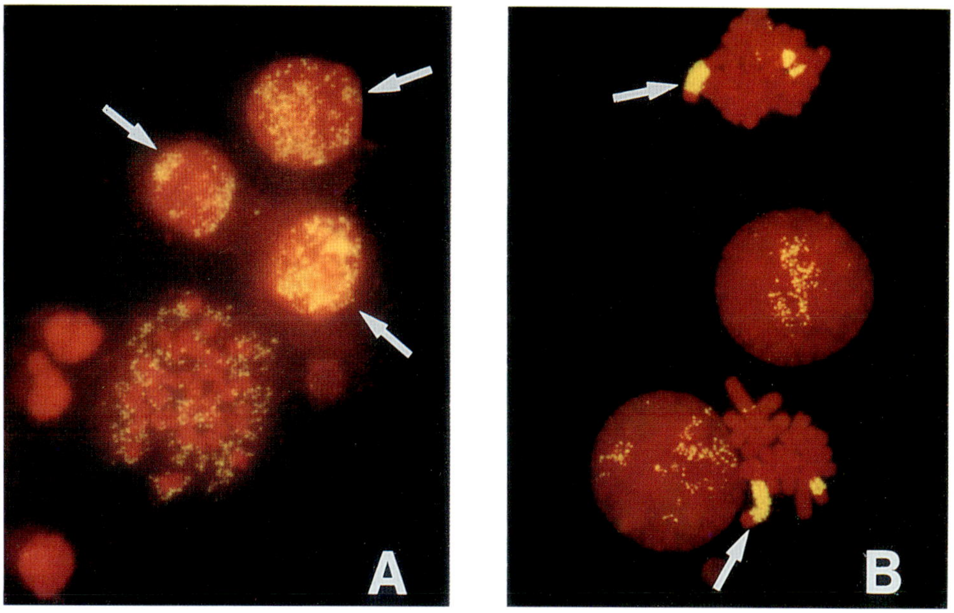

FIG. 6–48. N-*myc* amplification in neuroblastoma cells represented as **(A)** extrachromosomal double-minute chromatin bodies *(arrows)* and **(B)** homogeneously staining regions *(arrows)*. (FISH, courtesy of Dr. David Shapiro and Susan Ragsdale, St. Jude Children's Research Hospital, Memphis, TN.)

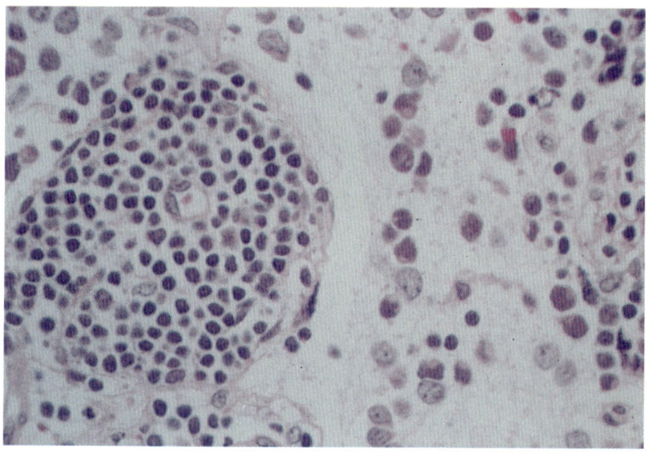

FIG. 6–49. Lymphocytic aggregate in a differentiating neuroblastoma from a second look specimen in a previously treated adrenal tumor.

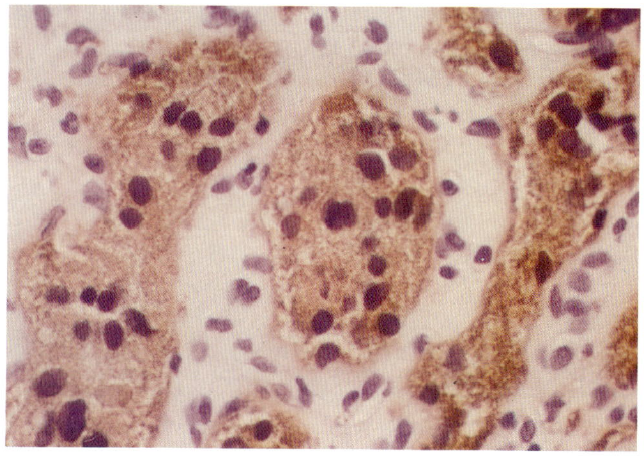

FIG. 6–60. Cordlike trabeculae of tumor cells in metastatic paraganglioma showing diffuse granular cytoplasmic immunoreactivity for synaptophysin (peroxidase-antiperoxidase stain).

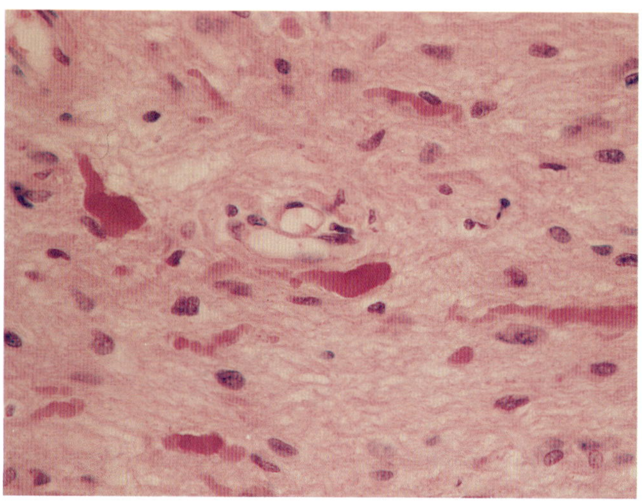

FIG. 7–2A. Juvenile pilocytic astrocytoma. Rosenthal fibers are a prominent feature of most JPAs.

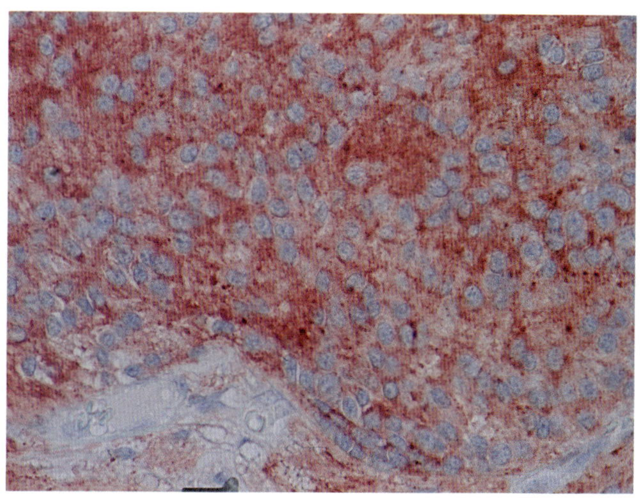

FIG. 7–28B. Central neurocytomas with strong immunopositivity for the neuronal marker synaptophysin.

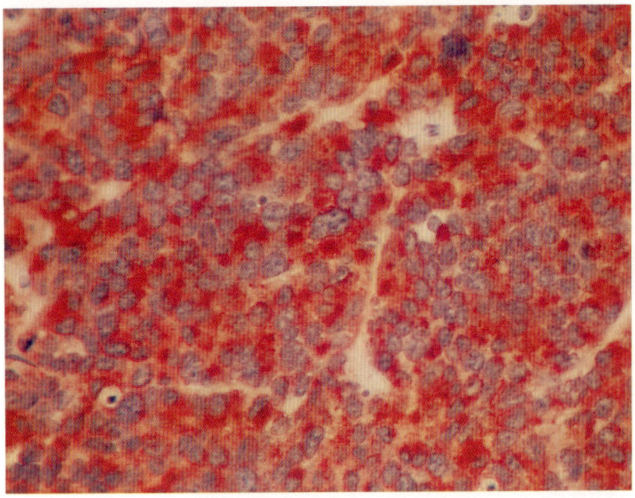

FIG. 7-36B. Pineoblastoma with strong immunopositivity for synaptophysin.

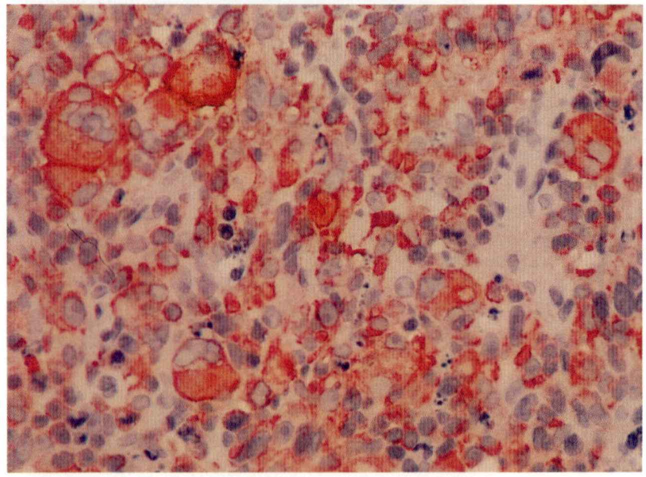

FIG. 7-47B. Primary rhabdomyosarcoma of the central nervous system showing strong, diffuse cytoplasmic immunoreactivity for desmin.

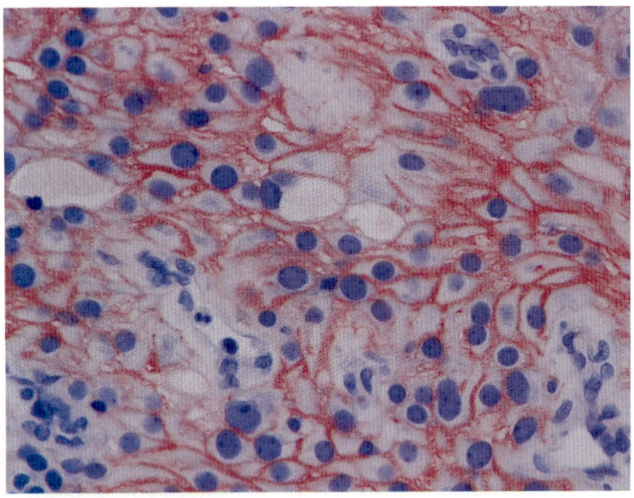

FIG. 7-43B. Meningioma with immunopositivity for epithelial membrane antigen (EMA).

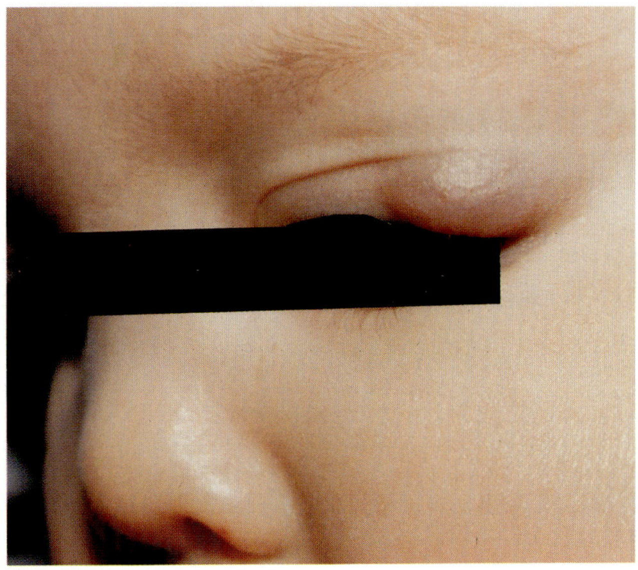

FIG. 8-13. Congenital hemangioma. An erythematous nodule arises from the upper lid of an infant. This particular example had cavernous features histologically.

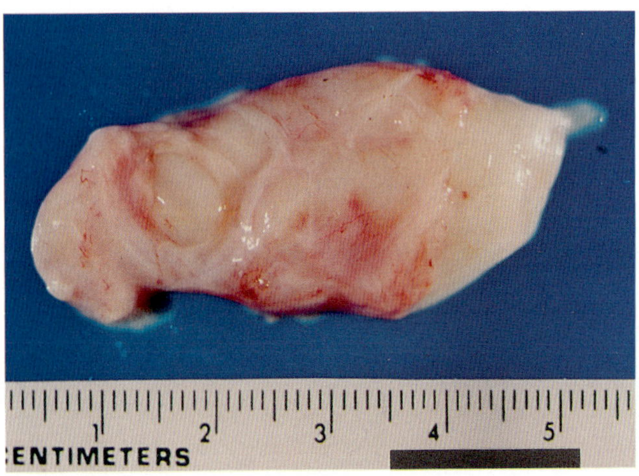

FIG. 8-21A. Neurofibroma. The lesion forms a fusiform, heterogeneous mass.

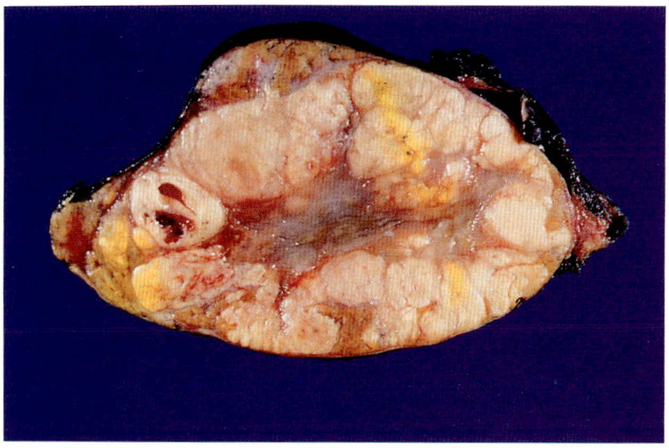

FIG. 12-3. Adrenal cortical carcinoma removed from a child. Note the lobulation, necrosis, and bright yellow foci.

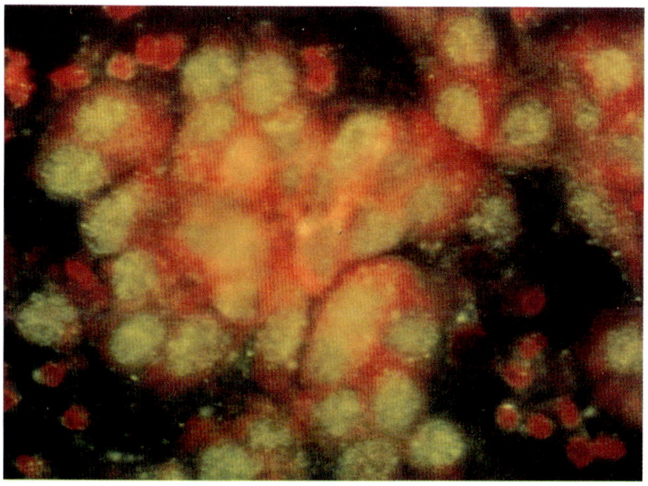

FIG. 12-12C. Undifferentiated nasopharyngeal carcinoma, metastatic to a cervical lymph node. Immunofluorescence of an imprint reveals the presence of EBNA. (Indirect immunofluorescence with anti-EBNA, courtesy of Dr. John Sixbey, St. Jude Children's Research Hospital.)

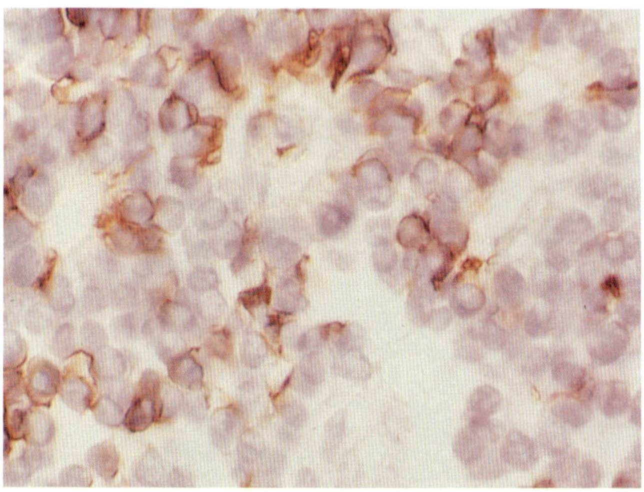

FIG. 13-7. Indirect immunoperoxidase stain of normal human retina showing S-antigen immunoreactivity completely surrounding the photoreceptor cell. (With permission, from *Invest Ophthalmol Vis Sci* 1985;26:561-567.)

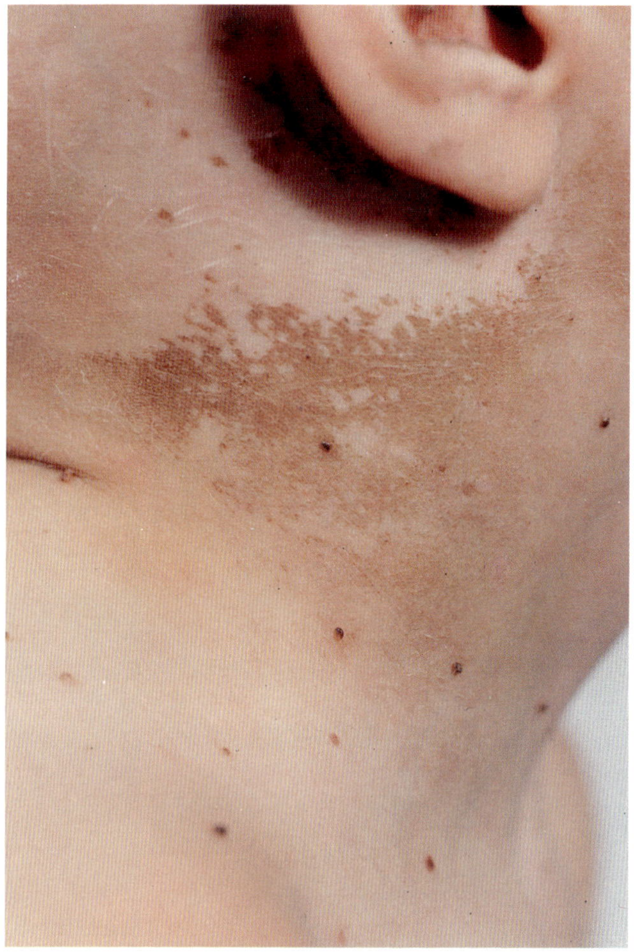

FIG. 12-23. Patient with basal cell nevus syndrome. There are multiple lesions arising in the site of previous radiation. (Courtesy of Dr. Andrew Walter, St. Jude Children's Research Hospital.)

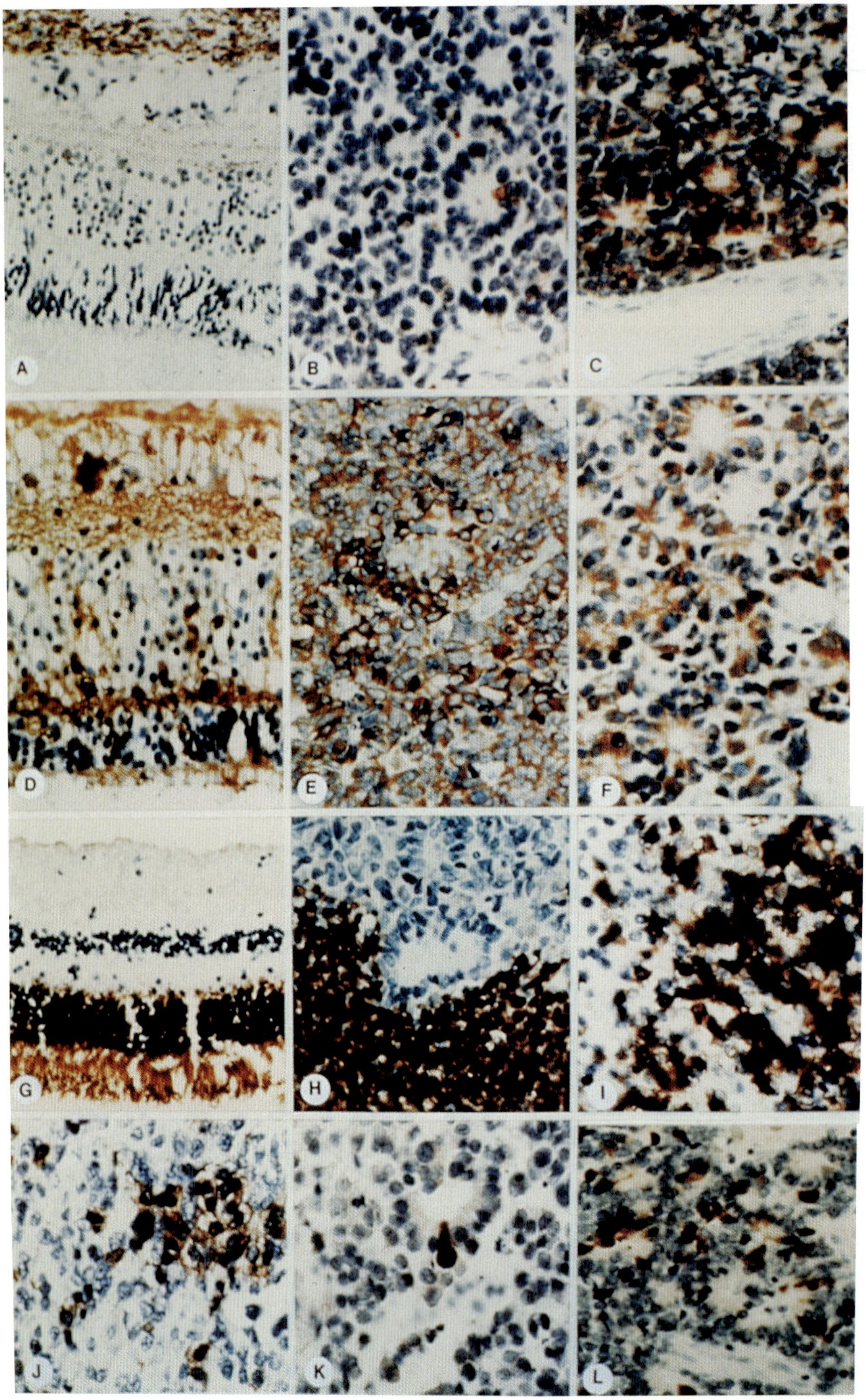

FIG. 13–6. Neural-associated antigens in retinoblastoma. **A–C**: Neurotriplet protein (200-kd subunit). **D–F**: Neuron-specific enolase. **G–L**: S antigen. **A**: Neurofilament (200-kd subunit) in ganglion cell layer of retina. **B, C**: Flexner–Wintersteiner rosettes staining positive for neurofilament protein. **D**: Neuron-specific enolase staining all layers of the normal retina. **E, F**: Neuron-specific enolase staining an undifferentiated **(E)** and differentiated **(F)** retinoblastoma. **G–L**: S-antigen immunoreactivity in a retinoblastoma. (With permission from the *American Journal of Ophthalmology.* © The Ophthalmic Publishing Company. *Am J Ophthalmol* 1987;103:647–658.)

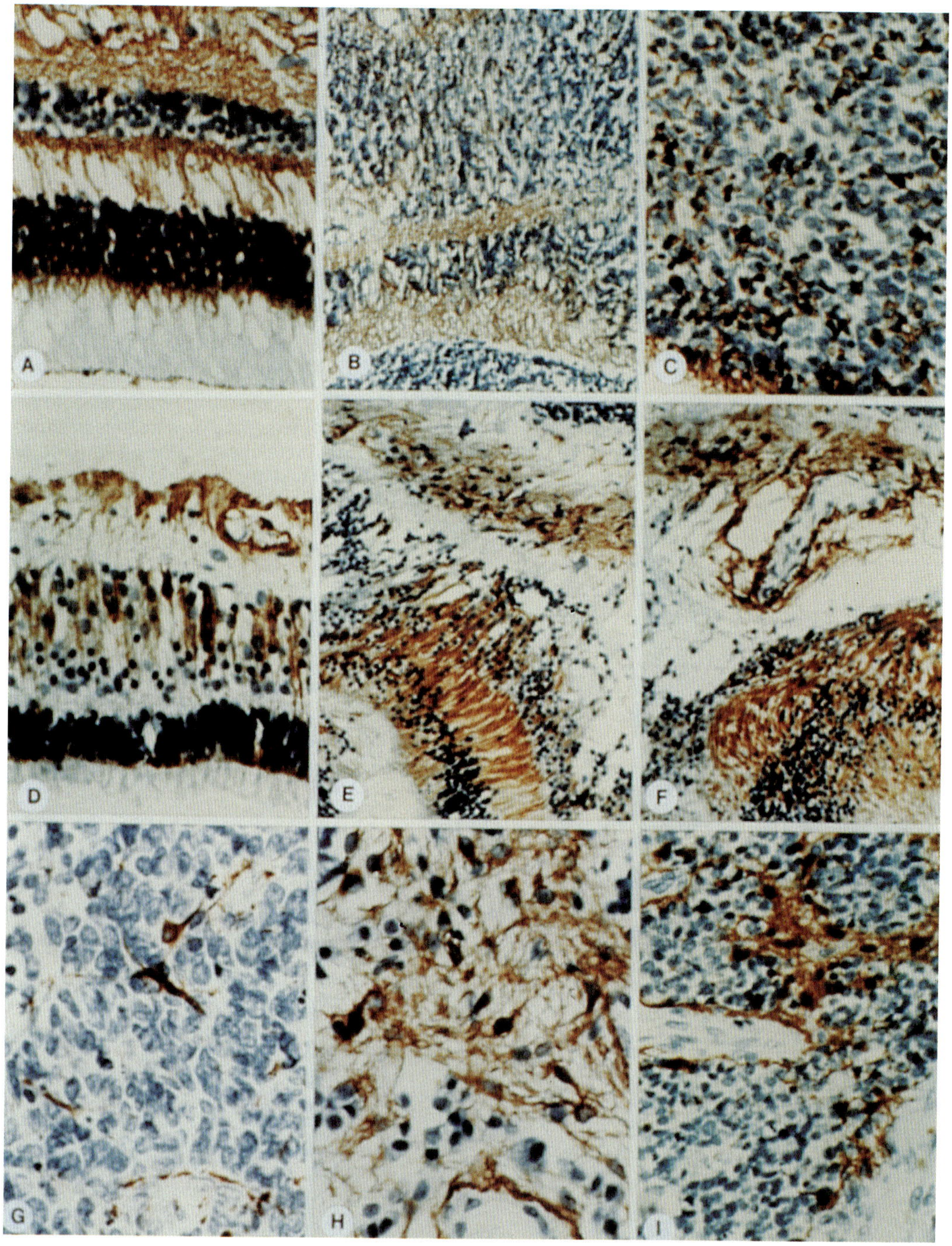

FIG. 13–10. Glial-associated antigens in retinoblastoma. Leu 7 **(A,B,C)**; GFAP **(D–H)**; and S-100 **(I)**. **A**: Staining of all retinal layers by Leu 7 monoclonal antibody. **B, C**: In retinoblastoma all neoplastic cells are Leu 7–negative whereas normal retinal elements are immunopositive. **D**: GFAP staining of normal retina with prominent staining of Muller fibers. **E, F**: Normal retina entrapped within retinoblastoma stain positive for GFAP, as well as reactive astrocytes **(G)** and perivascular glial elements **(H)**. **I**: Perivascular elements in retinoblastoma with positive staining for S-100 protein whereas tumor cells are negative. (With permission from the *American Journal of Ophthalmology*. © The Ophthalmic Publishing Company. *Am J Ophthalmol* 1987; 103:647–658.)

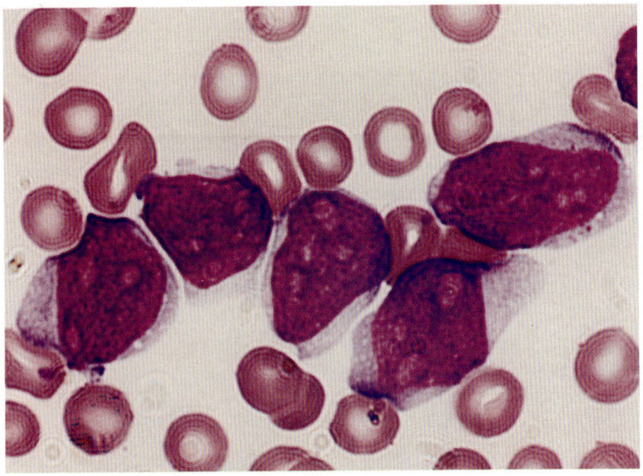

FIG. 15–1. Type I myeloblasts. Acute myeloblastic leukemia, FAB-M1, with partial myeloid differentiation. The blasts have low nucleocytoplasmic ratios and multiple, distinct nuclei. (Wright's stain.)

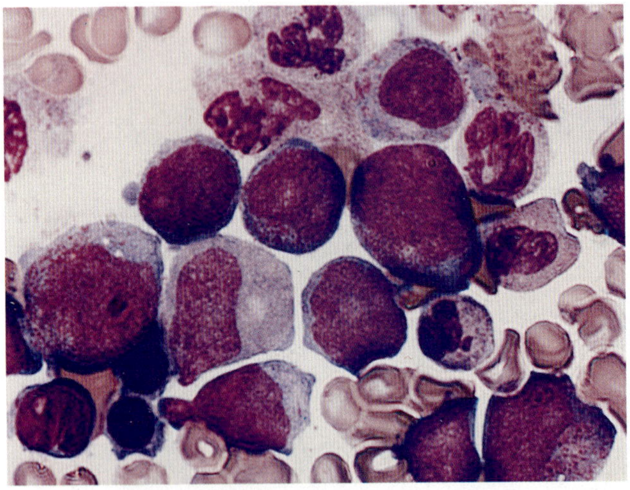

FIG. 15–2. Type II myeloblasts. Acute myelocytic leukemia, FAB-M2, with differentiation. The leukemic population consists of type I and II blasts and promyelocytic and myelocytic forms. (Wright's stain.)

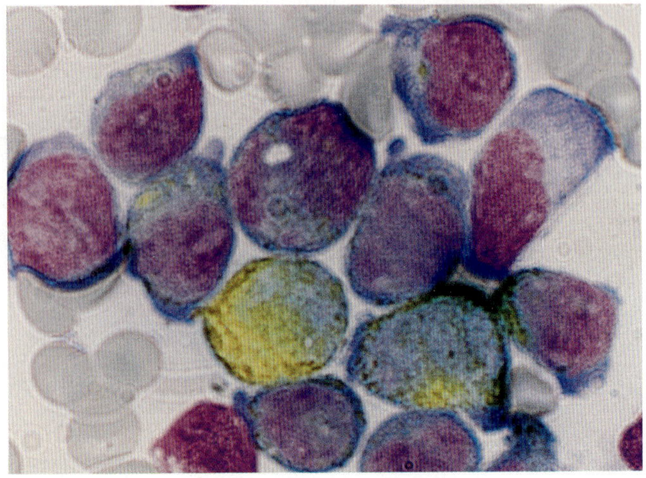

FIG. 15–4. Acute myeloblastic leukemia. Myeloperoxidase enzyme in the cytoplasm of myeloblasts produces a yellow reaction product. [Myeloperoxidase stain (*O*-toluidine/H_2O_2 reaction) with Giemsa counterstain.]

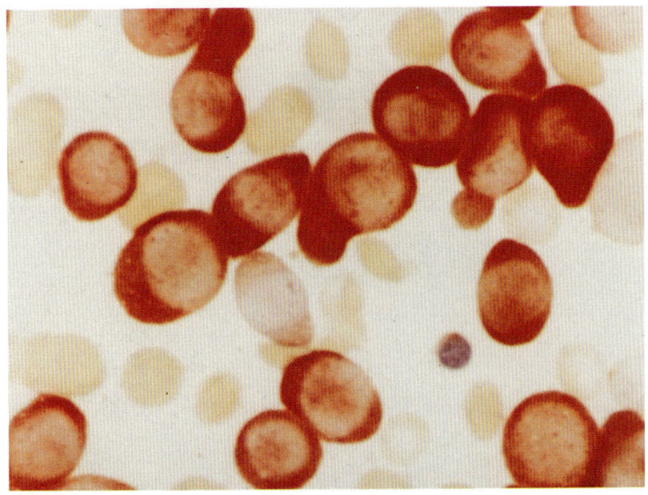

FIG. 15–5. Acute monoblastic leukemia, FAB-M5a. α-Naphthylbutyrate (ANB) esterase enzyme in monoblasts produces an intense, diffuse, red–brown reaction product. (ANB esterase stain.)

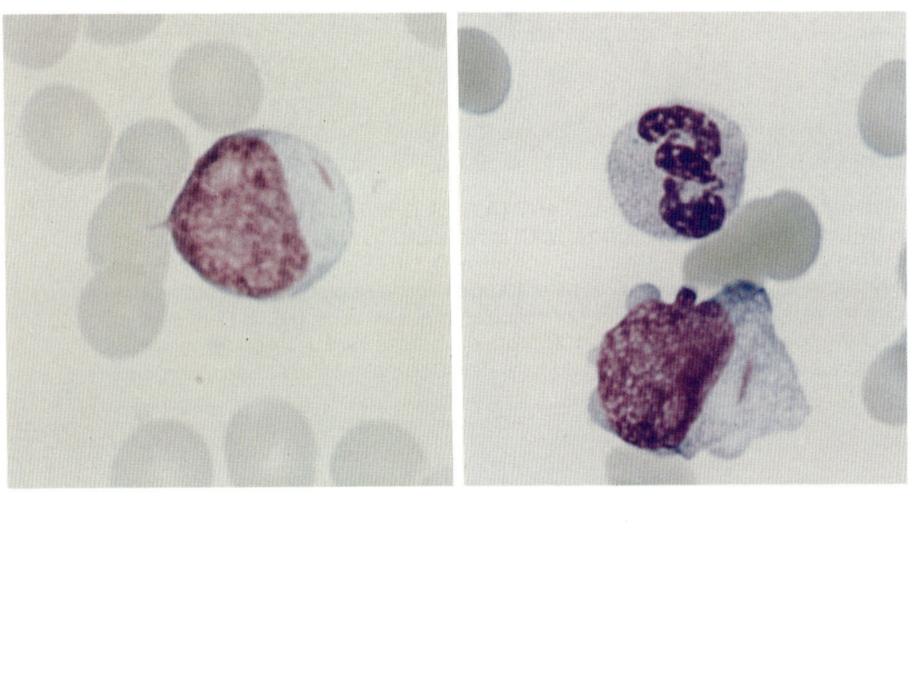

FIG. 15–3. Auer rods. Two blasts from two cases of acute myeloblastic leukemia, containing crystalline rods. (Wright's stain.)

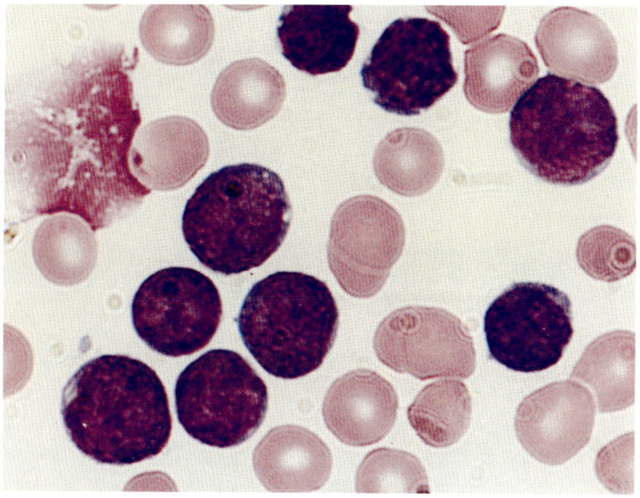

FIG. 15–14. Acute lymphoblastic leukemia, ALL-L1 type. Blasts are small and have high nucleocytoplasmic ratios. (Wright's stain.)

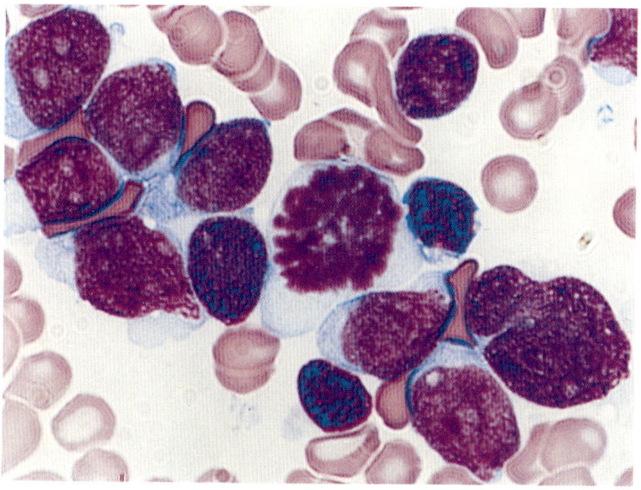

FIG. 15–15. Acute lymphoblastic leukemia, ALL-L2 type. Blasts are large, show low nucleocytoplasmic ratios, and contain several distinct nucleoli. (Wright's stain X100.)

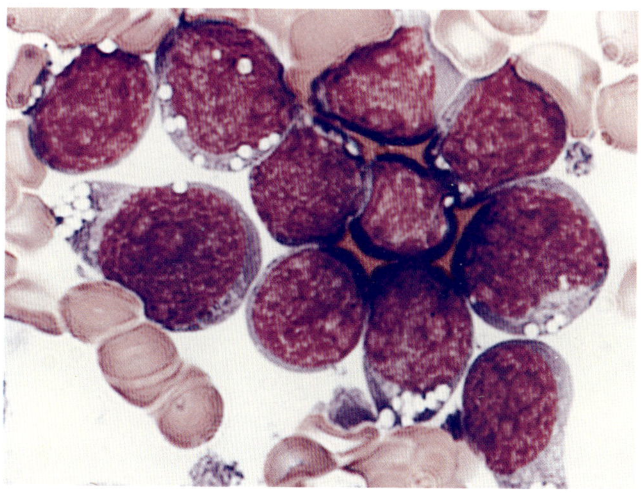

FIG. 15–16. Acute lymphoblastic leukemia, ALL-L3 type. Blasts are large and contain moderate amounts of basophilic cytoplasm, show one to three distinct nucleoli, and frequently display clear cytoplasmic vacuoles. (Wright's stain.)

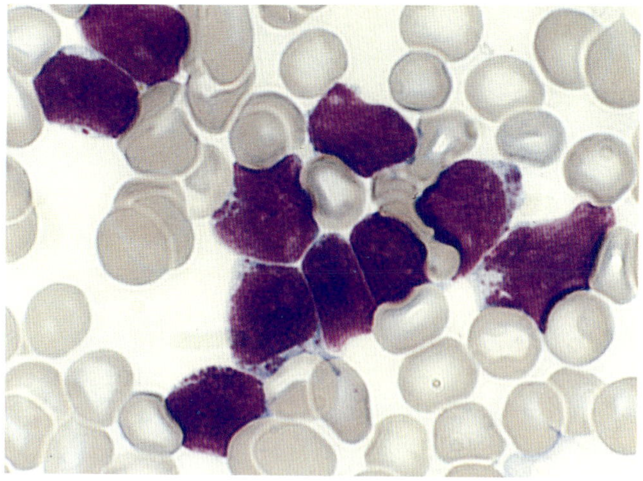

FIG. 15–21. Acute lymphoblastic leukemia, granular variant. Azurophilic cytoplasmic granules are present in many lymphoblasts. (Wright's stain.)

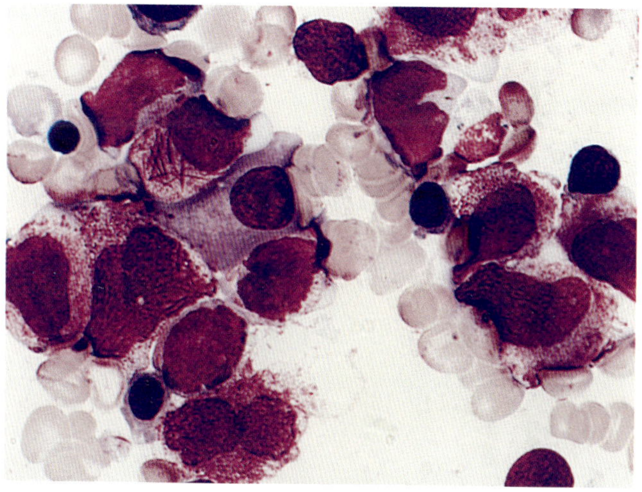

FIG. 15–24. Leukemic cells of acute promyelocytic leukemia, FAB-M3. Large leukemic cells have folded or indented nuclei and heavy azurophilic granulation. One promyelocytic form contains multiple Auer rods and represents a faggot cell. (Wright's stain.)

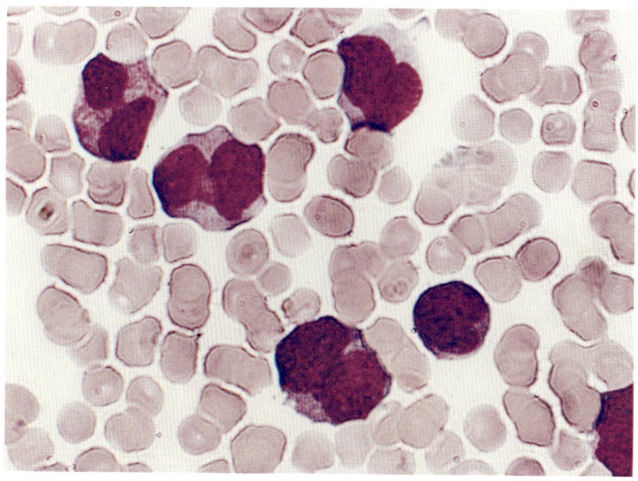

FIG. 15–25. Acute promyelocytic leukemia (FAB-M3), microgranular variant. Leukemic promyelocytes contain only a few fine azurophilic granules. The "monocytoidlike" nuclei are typical of AML-M3. (Wright's stain.)

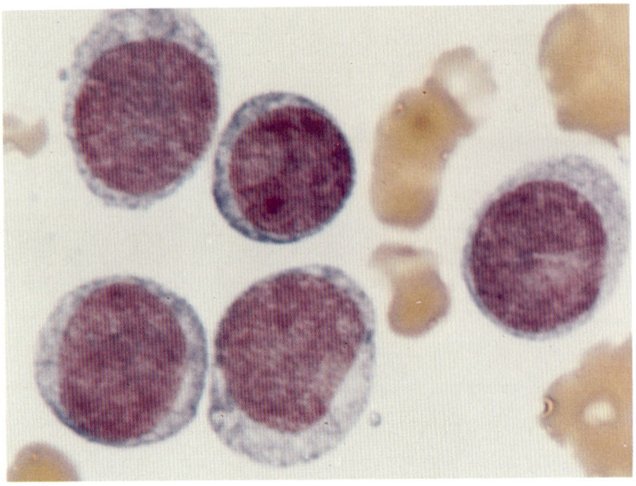

FIG. 15–28. Acute monoblastic leukemia, undifferentiated (FAB-M5a). The large blasts of this leukemia usually have round to reniform nuclei with distinct nucleoli. Fine azurophilic granules may be present. (Wright's stain.)

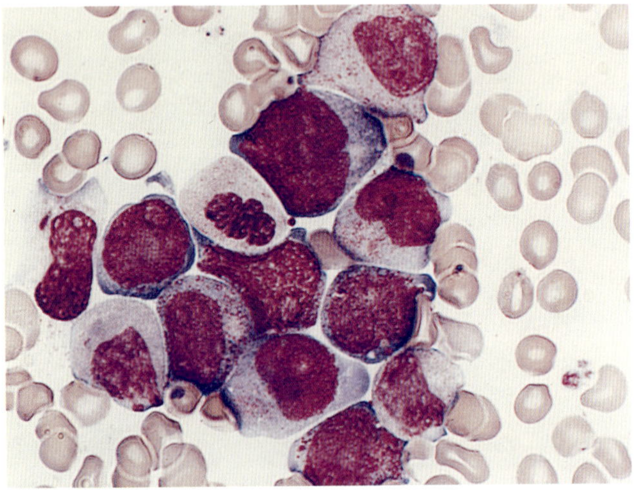

FIG. 15–29. Acute myelomonocytic leukemia, FAB-M4. The leukemic population consists of myeloid and monocytic precursor forms. Monocytic cells have folded or indented nuclei and contain azurophilic granules. (Wright's stain.)

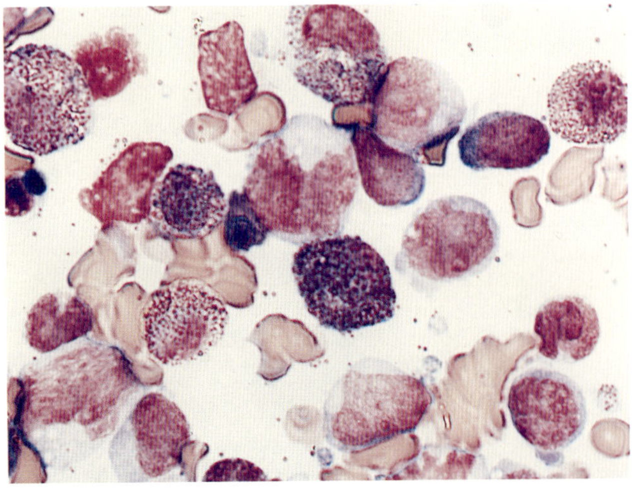

FIG. 15–30. Acute myelomonocytic leukemia with eosinophilia, FAB-M4Eo. The bone marrow contains many eosinophilic precursors in addition to monocytic and myelocytic elements. (Wright's stain.)

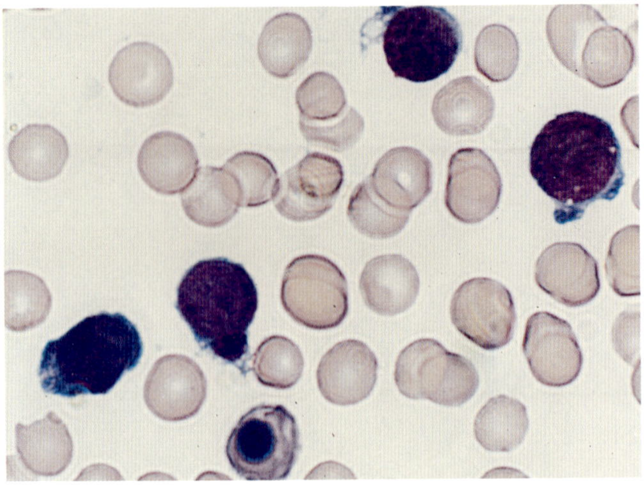

FIG. 15–32. Acute erythroblastic leukemia, blastic variant of FAB-M6. Five leukemic blasts and an orthochromatic normoblast are shown. Leukemic erythroblasts are small and have high nucleocytoplasmic ratios. Nucleoli are not evident. (Wright's stain.)

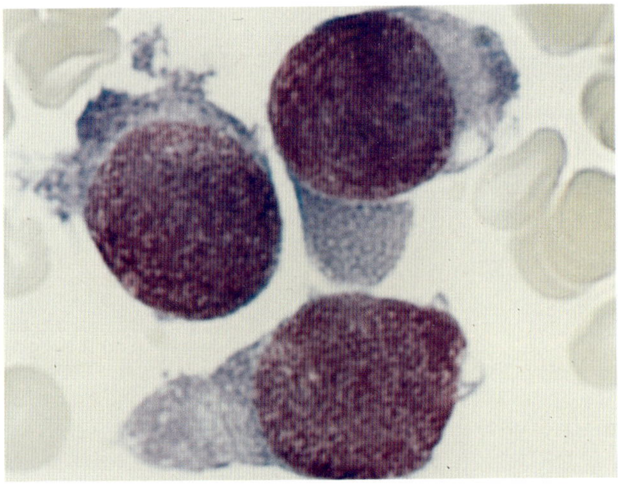

FIG. 15–33. Acute megakaryoblastic leukemia, FAB-M7. Blasts frequently display cytoplasmic blebs and pseudopodia. Their nuclei have a finely reticular chromatin pattern without discernible nuclei. (Wright's stain.)

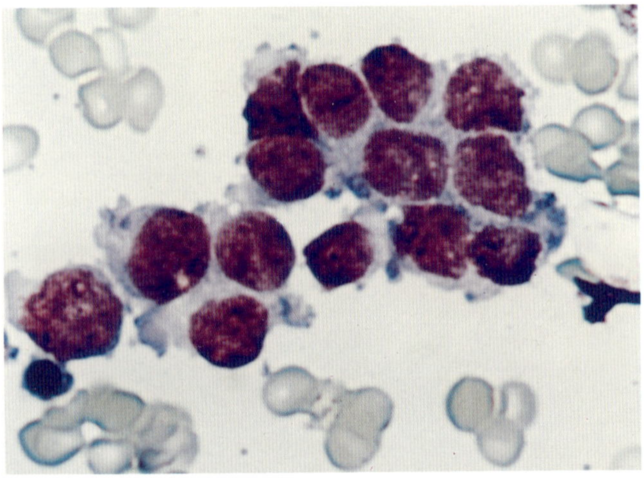

FIG. 15–34. Acute megakaryocytic leukemia, FAB-M7. Leukemic blasts form a tight cohesive cluster resembling metastatic small cell tumor. (Wright's stain.)

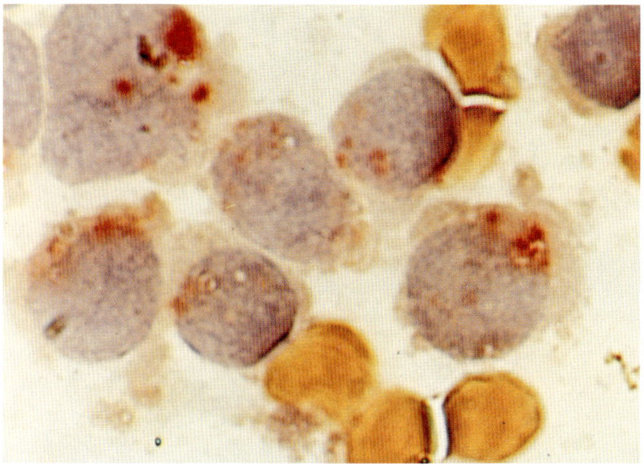

FIG. 15-35. Acute megakaryocytic leukemia, FAB-M7. Leukemic blasts show a characteristic, diffuse, granular α-naphthylacetate (ANA) esterase positivity. (ANA esterase stain with hematoxylin counterstain.)

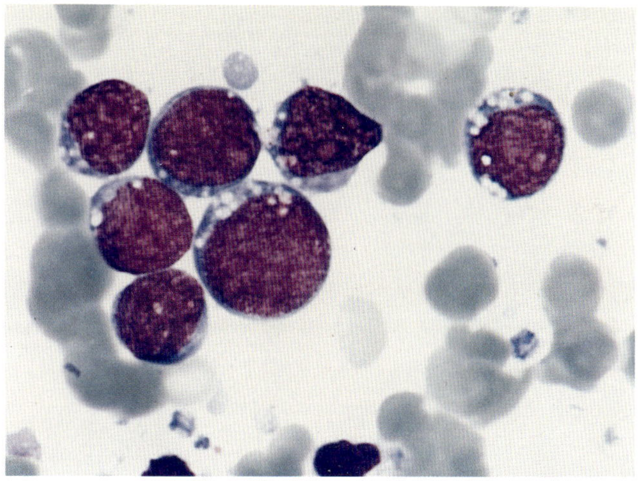

FIG. 16-5. Wright-Giemsa-stained cytologic preparations of Burkitt's lymphoma cells characteristically show medium size blastic cells with moderate chromatin condensation and distinctly basophilic vacuolated cytoplasm.

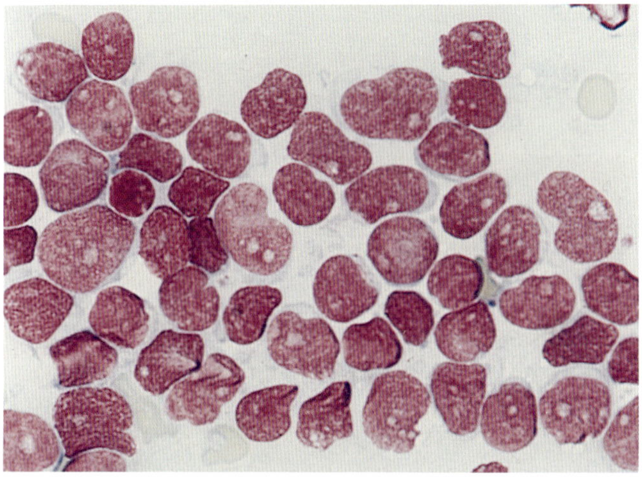

FIG. 16-3. On Wright-Giemsa-stained cytologic preparations, lymphoblasts in lymphoblastic leukemia resemble those of acute lymphoblastic leukemia.

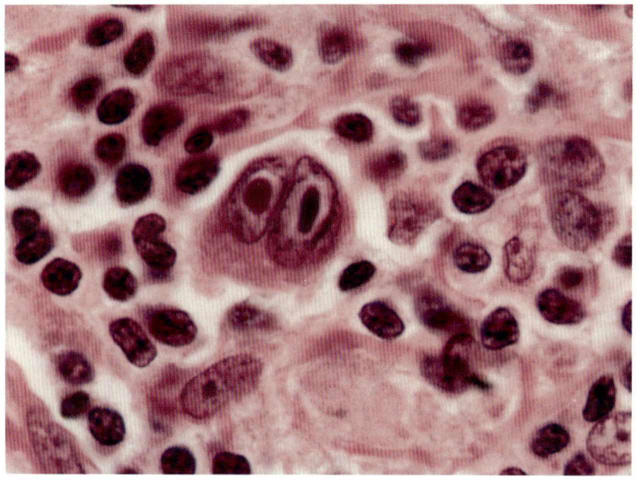

FIG. 16-10. The diagnostic Reed-Sternberg cell of Hodgkin's disease shows a typically bilobed or multilobated nucleus with inclusionlike eosinophilic nucleoli.

A 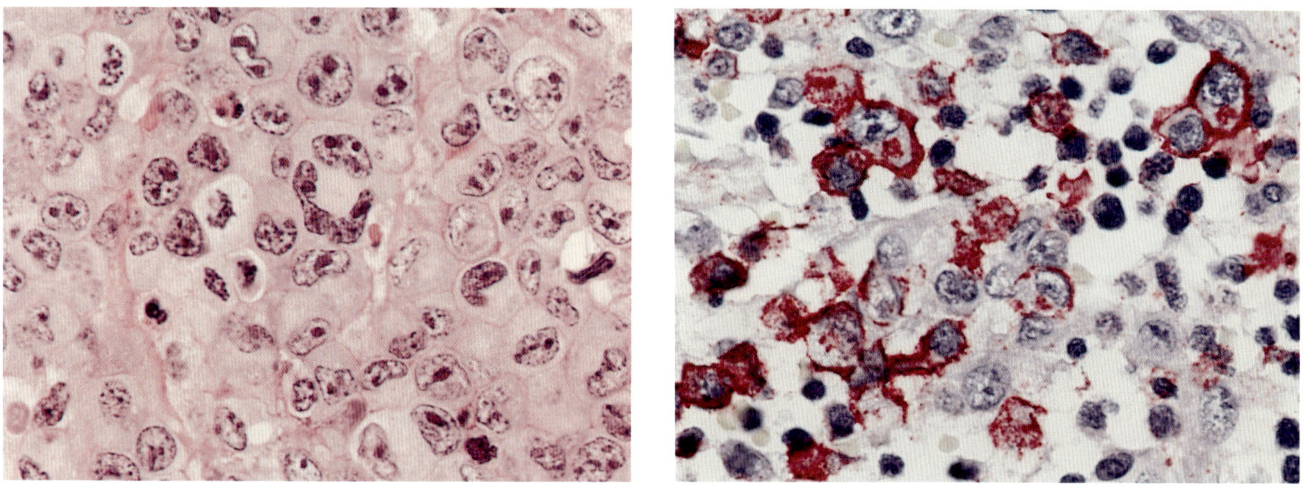 B

FIG. 16-9. (A) Anaplastic large cell lymphoma (ALCL) shows large cells with abundant cytoplasm that often appear in sheets in the paracortex, sinuses, and around follicles. Nuclei are round or indented, often horseshoe-shaped, and sometimes multiple. **(B)** CD30 antigen, detected in paraffin sections with Ber-H2, is localized primarily to the Golgi and cytoplasmic membrane of neoplastic large cells in ALCL.

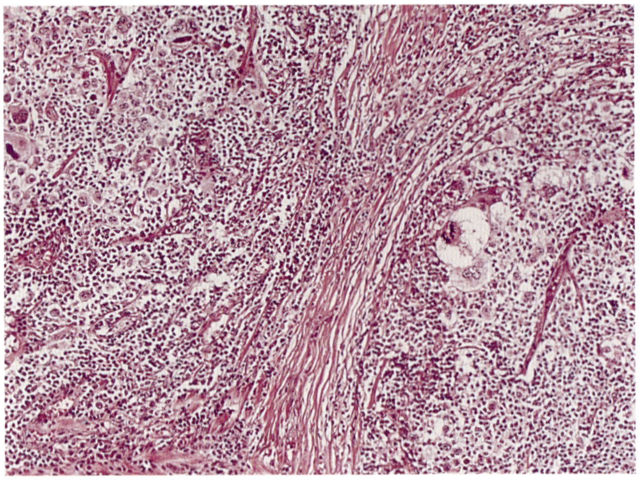

FIG. 16-12. Nodular sclerosis HD shows tumor nodules containing RS cells and lacunar cells surrounded by dense collagen bands.

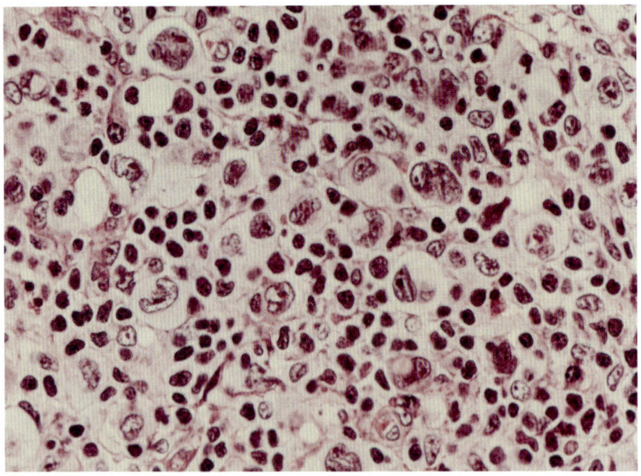

FIG. 16-14. Lymphocyte-depleted Hodgkin's disease contains large numbers of neoplastic cells and relatively few reactive cells.

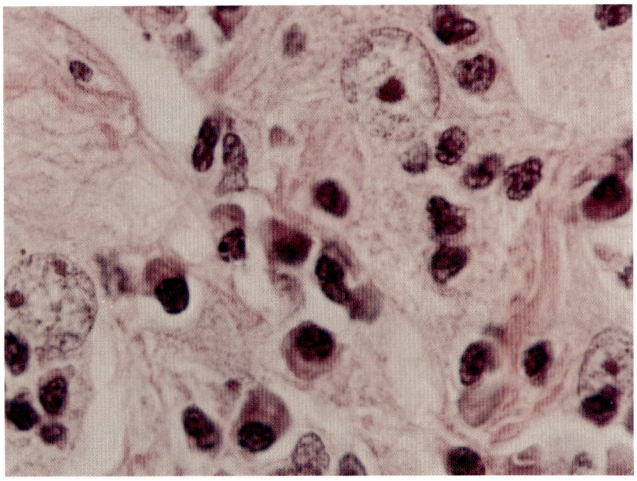

FIG. 16-20. In Rosai-Dorfman disease, benign-appearing macrophages often contain viable leukocytes.

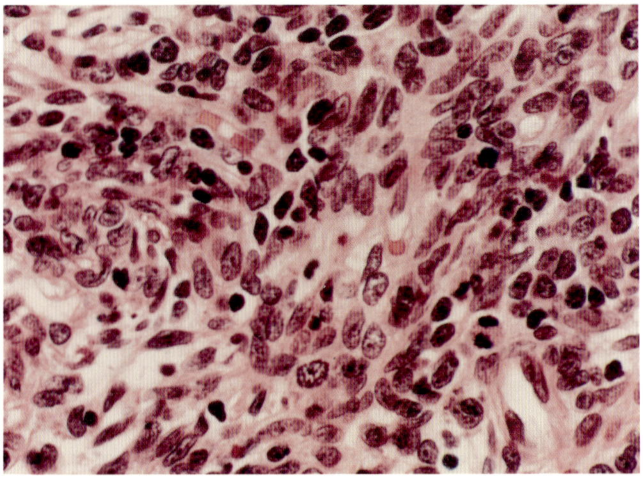

FIG. 16-22. Thymoma showing a mixture of spindled epithelial cells and thymic lymphocytes. Each component predominated in different areas of the tumor. (Photograph courtesy of Dr. Henry Friedman, Syracuse, NY.)

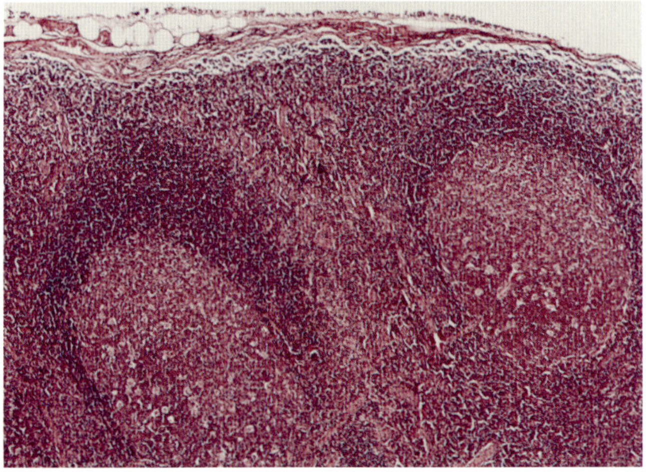

FIG. 16-24. Follicular hyperplasia shows enlargement of intact germinal centers with preservation of mantle zones and other nodal structures.

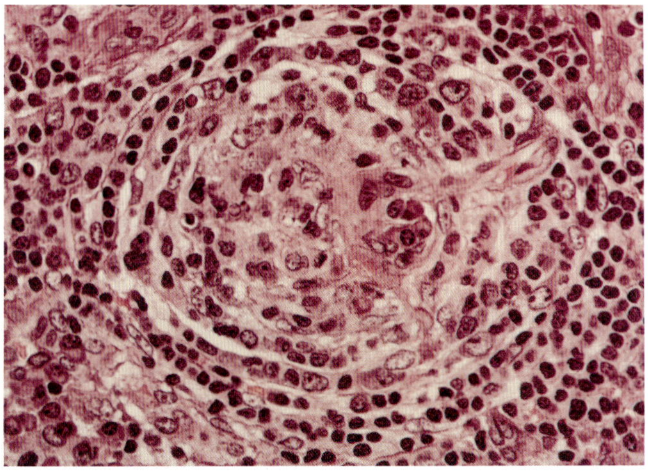

FIG. 16-29. The hyaline-vascular type of Castleman's disease shows altered germinal centers with concentric rings of mantle lymphocytes that impart an "onion skin" appearance. Frequently, a prominent venule is seen penetrating the germinal center. Plasma cells are present in variable numbers.

A 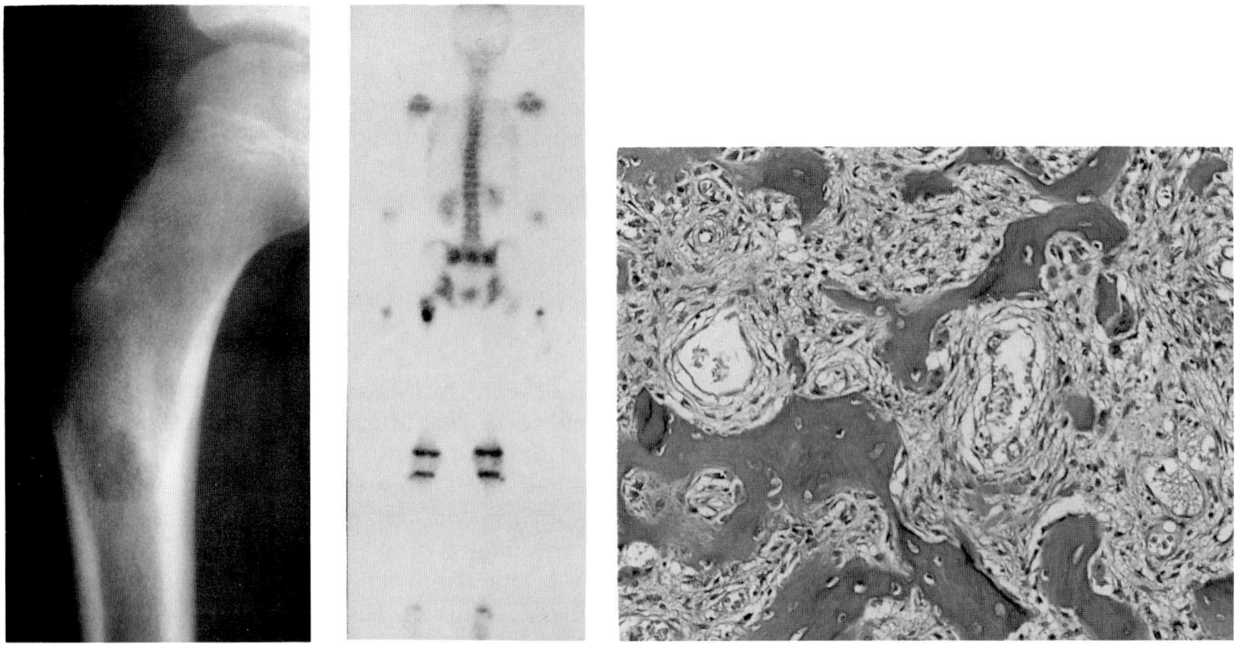 B,C

FIG. 7. Osteoblastoma. A well-defined area of lysis is present in the proximal femur on a plain radiograph **(A)** and shows discrete uptake of radionuclide on bone scan **(B)**. Histologically, the lesion is composed of bony trabeculae embedded in a fibroblastic stroma and invested by osteoblasts **(C)**. (Parts **A** and **B** courtesy of Dr. Barry Fletcher, SJCRH.)

very difficult to apply for diagnosis (20). The trabeculae are covered by a rim of osteoblasts (Fig. 7C). Unlike osteosarcoma, the tumor has a line of sharp demarcation from the surrounding bone, and it almost never contains cartilage unless there is an associated pathologic fracture (83,175).

A lesion termed aggressive osteoblastoma was described by Dorfman in 1973 (73). Schajowicz used the term "malignant osteoblastoma" for the same lesion (222). These tumors often recur but do not metastasize (73,222). Radiologically they are usually well circumscribed with variable marginal sclerosis. Histologically they resemble osteoblastoma, but the cells are larger and more epithelioid, may form small sheets, and show larger, slightly atypical nuclei and scattered mitoses (73). They form osteoid in the form of blue bony spicules (222). Their trabeculae are wider than the usual osteoblastoma, and they may have more osteoclastic giant cells (73,222). They tend to occur at an older age than regular osteoblastoma but do occur in the pediatric age group (73). The distinction between these lesions and osteosarcoma may be problematic in some cases. Helpful points include the following (83): osteoblastomas do not contain cartilage unless there has been an associated fracture; osteoblastomas do not permeate the adjacent normal bone but stop abruptly at their junction with normal bone; and osteoblastomas show osteoblastic rimming of bony spicules and osteoid whereas this is rare in osteosarcomas.

Another variant, termed "benign pseudosarcomatous (pseudomalignant) osteoblastoma," has been described and shows nuclear pleomorphism without mitoses. However, it behaves like an osteoblastoma and must be differentiated from an osteosarcoma (178).

Ossifying Fibroma

Ossifying fibroma is a tumor of the jaws that is prone to recur and consists of bony trabeculae surrounded by osteoblasts and set in a benign fibrous stroma (Fig. 8).

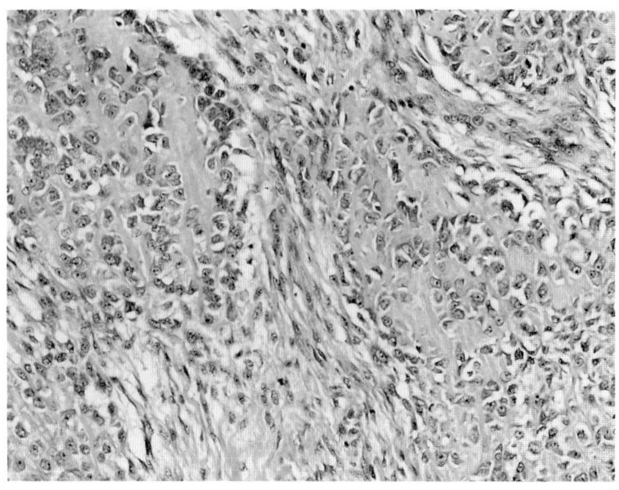

FIG. 8. Ossifying fibroma. An exuberant proliferation of benign-appearing osteoblasts produces spicules of osteoid.

Ossifying fibroma of long bones is synonymous with osteofibrous dysplasia. In Dehner's (et al.) series (65), 4 of 46 histologically benign pediatric jaw lesions were ossifying fibromas. All of these patients had an excellent postoperative course.

Fibrous Dysplasia

Fibrous dysplasia is more a hamartoma of bone than a true neoplasm. It may represent a failure of maturation with focal inability to form lamellar bone. It may occur as a single monostotic lesion but is multicentric (polyostotic) in 20% of patients, causing severe deformity (83). The lesion involves the facial bones, skull, ribs, and long bones, particularly the tibia and the intertrochanteric region of the proximal femur. Fibrous dysplasia begins as an intramedullary lesion that frequently expands the bone, does not invade the adjacent soft tissues, but may break through the cortex (Fig. 9A). In the skull the lesion expands the outer cortex, leaving the inner table intact (175). Pathologic fractures may occur. The polyostotic form of the disease may be associated with flat, irregularly marginated, pigmentary lesions of the skin; precocious puberty; and fibromyxomas of soft tissue (the McCune–Albright syndrome).

Radiologically fibrous dysplasia consists of a homogeneous, ground-glass–appearing lesion that expands the bony cortex. It may be cystic (83). On cut surface it has a dense, fibrous, and gritty appearance.

Histologically fibrous dysplasia consists of a fairly cellular but bland fibroblastic or myxoid stroma containing spicules of bone that appear to arise directly from the stroma and not from osteoblasts, which are absent. The spicules consist of woven bone and have a somewhat unusual curvilinear arrangement, resembling Chinese letters (Fig. 9B). Occasionally cementicles may also be present and constitute a feature quite specific for fibrous dysplasia in bones other than the jaw (175). The cellularity and amount of collagen are variable, but there is usually an abundance of the latter. The stroma may be quite cellular and usually has no mitoses, although a few may be present. Some lesions may have a prominent cartilaginous component (83), which is at times massive and

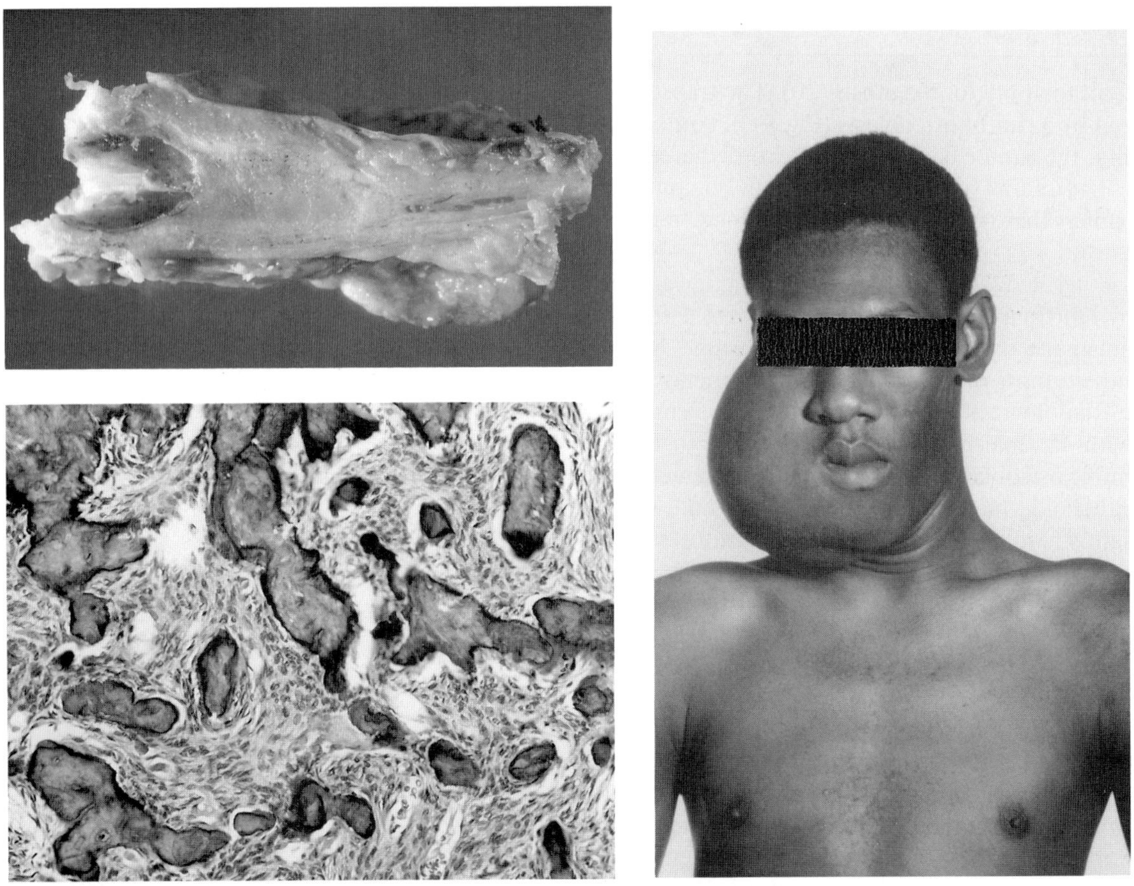

A B C

FIG. 9. Fibrous dysplasia. **A.** Gross view of rib lesion that expands the medullary cavity and has a granular cut surface with cystic change. **B.** The lesion is composed of irregular, curvilinear spicules of osteoid embedded in a fibrous stroma and lacking osteoblastic activity (compare with Fig. 9). **C.** Patient with facial deformity due to expansile lesion of jaw. (Part **C** courtesy of Dr. Charles Pratt, SJCRH.)

may be confused with an enchondroma or chondrosarcoma (125). The lesion may percolate between normal bone spicules and thus entrap lamellar bone. This phenomenon may sometimes create a problem in distinction from a low-grade osteogenic sarcoma. Osteofibrous dysplasia differs from fibrous dysplasia in that its bony spicules are rimmed by osteoblasts and it is almost totally confined to the tibia and fibula.

Fibrous dysplasia is a benign lesion but may cause considerable deformity, particularly about the face (Fig. 9C), and it can be difficult to eradicate because of the extent and site of involvement. It tends to stabilize after puberty but may be reactivated during pregnancy (83). Rarely it may undergo malignant change (0.4%), most commonly in the form of osteosarcoma (83,284). Fibrosarcoma and chondrosarcoma may also develop (175).

Osteofibrous Dysplasia

Osteofibrous dysplasia is an unusual lesion involving almost exclusively the tibia and fibula and occurring in the majority of cases in children under 10 years old (38,39). In the large series reported by Park et al. (196) the median age was 10 years for boys and 13.5 years for girls, with no apparent sexual predilection. Unlike fibrous dysplasia, osteofibrous dysplasia arises intracortically.

Radiologically osteofibrous dysplasia shows lytic foci that tend to be confluent and associated with sclerosis. The lesions involve predominantly the anterior cortex. The cortex is expanded and the tibia shows anterior bowing. Periosteal reaction is rare (196).

Histologically osteofibrous dysplasia consists predominantly of bony lamellae in a fibrous but somewhat myxoid background with a storiform pattern (196,250). The bony lamellae show prominent osteoblastic rimming (Fig. 8), a feature of distinction from fibrous dysplasia. The fibrous tissue is also somewhat looser than that seen in fibrous dysplasia (250). A zoning phenomenon has been noted in these lesions, with a central fibroblastic zone surrounded by concentric zones of fibrous tissue, purely woven bone trabeculae, and lamellar bone that merges with the surrounding reactive bone (175,196).

Osteofibrous dysplasia resembles an adamantinoma radiologically and has a similar stroma; however, the sheets of epithelial cells seen in an adamantinoma are not seen, and an adamantinoma occurs in a somewhat older age group; but there is overlap (250). The presence of a periosteal reaction in the absence of a fracture, extension into the medullary cavity without an endosteal sclerotic bony rim, or the presence of a soft tissue mass should raise the possibility of adamantinoma (250). Immunostaining may show individual cytokeratin-positive cells scattered within the lesion, but this does not constitute evidence that this is an adamantinoma (250). This finding was present in 93% of Sweet et al.'s cases (250) and is a useful feature to distinguish these lesions from fibrous dysplasia. There may be some relationship between osteofibrous dysplasia and adamantinoma, but Sweet et al. (250) were unable to identify a case of progression to adamantinoma when they had adequate biopsy material. Mirra (175) illustrates such a case in his textbook, however. Park et al. (196) also describe two cases with evolution from osteofibrous dysplasia to typical fibrous dysplasia.

Osteofibrous dysplasia may progress before epiphyseal closure or regress spontaneously, but progression ceases after epiphyseal closure (38,39). If an attempt is made to resect the lesion before this age, it will very likely recur. Therefore these lesions should not be resected before age 15 years if possible (39). According to Sweet (250), the radiologic differential diagnosis includes fibroxanthoma (nonossifying fibroma), cortical chondroma, chronic osteomyelitis, and intracortical angioma. The histopathologic differential diagnosis also includes fibroxanthoma, craniofacial ossifying fibroma, and fracture with repair (250).

Osteosarcoma

Osteosarcoma, or osteogenic sarcoma, is a malignant mesenchymal tumor in which bone is formed directly from the sarcomatous elements. Following multiple myeloma, it is the second most common malignant tumor of bone. There is a bimodal age distribution, with one peak during the second decade (median age, 17 years) and a second in older adults (around 70 years) (20,72). Males are affected more commonly than females, 1.25: 1 (20,60). Younger patients have a higher incidence of extremity lesions (72), the most common sites being in the bones around the knee (the lower femoral metaphysis and upper tibial metaphysis), followed by the upper humeral metaphysis (20). Osteosarcoma may also occur in other bones such as the pelvis (20), vertebrae, and craniofacial bones (72). Unlike many of the benign tumors of the spine that tend to involve the posterior elements (e.g., osteoblastoma or aneurysmal bone cyst), osteosarcoma involves the body of the vertebra (175).

Osteosarcoma may be classified into three major categories: intramedullary, juxtacortical, and soft tissue. The last category seldom occurs in childhood. Intramedullary tumors may have several histologic patterns (Table 2). Osteosarcoma may also be categorized as primary or secondary, depending on whether or not there is a demonstrable preexisting lesion. A number of conditions may predispose a patient to the development of osteosarcoma (Table 3).

Osteosarcoma was the most common second malignant neoplasm among more than 300 children studied by the Late Effects Study Group (182). It may arise in

TABLE 2. *Histologic patterns of osteosarcoma*

Type	Incidence (%)	Ref.
Osteoblastic (NOS)	78.3	72
Chondroblastic[a]	4.2	20, 72
Fibroblastic	3.9	72
MFH-like	NA	NA
Giant cell–rich	0.1	NA
Telangiectatic	NA	72
Low-grade intraosseous	0.1	NA
Small cell	NA	72
Juxtacortical		
Parosteal	NA	NA
Periosteal	NA	NA
High-grade surface	NA	NA

Abbreviations: NA, not available; NOS, not otherwise specified; MFH, malignant fibrous histiocytoma.

[a] More than 90% of the tumor must be cartilage.

irradiated or unirradiated bone. Among irradiated tumors 25% were in patients with retinoblastoma (see Chapters 12 and 13).

Clinically osteosarcomas present with bone pain or pain around the knee, and occasional patients will have their knee explored with the clinical diagnosis of a torn meniscus. The tumor is usually large by the time it becomes clinically apparent and often grows at a remarkably rapid pace if left untreated.

TABLE 3. *Conditions predisposing to osteosarcoma*

Hereditary retinoblastoma
Paget's disease (confined to patients over 50 years of age)
Site of previous radiation
Osteomyelitis
Fibrous dysplasia
Osteoblastoma
Bone infarct
Osteogenesis imperfecta
Chondrosarcoma (dedifferentiation)
Enchondroma
Osteochondroma
Giant cell tumor

(From ref. 72, p. 260.)

Osteosarcoma typically arises in the metaphysis of a long bone, although the telangiectatic variety usually arises in the diaphysis. Depending on the amount of tumor bone formed, the lesion may be sclerotic (25%), lytic (25%), or mixed lytic and sclerotic (50%) on plain radiographs (20). Tumor bone has a cumulus cloud appearance and chondroblastic areas have curvilinear or popcorn densities. The tumor has a permeative or geographic appearance on radiographs and almost invariably erodes the cortex by the time it presents, often elevating the periosteum to produce the classical Codman's triangle with sun ray spiculing or a multilamellar appearance (Fig. 10A). It may produce a soft tissue mass

A
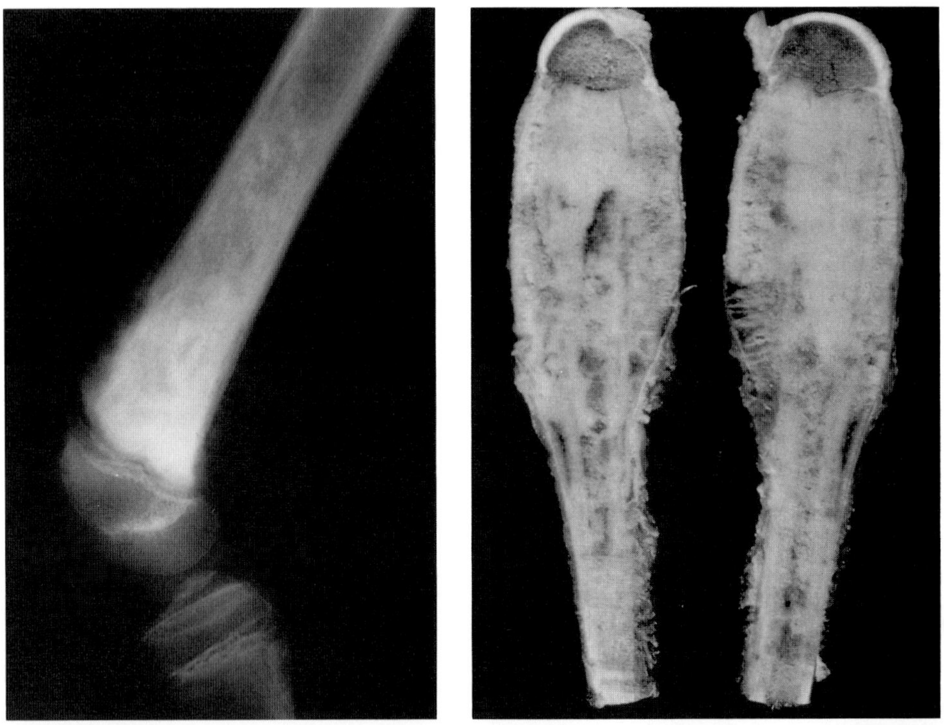
B

FIG. 10. Osteoblastic osteosarcoma. **A.** Lateral view of distal femur discloses a sclerotic metaphyseal lesion with periosteal elevation and irregular, poorly circumscribed margins. **B.** Sagittal sectioning of the femur reveals a densely sclerotic metaphyseal tumor with periosteal elevation. Note that the epiphysis appears spared in both the plain radiograph **(A)** and gross specimen **(B).** (Part **A** courtesy of Dr. Barry Fletcher, SJCRH.)

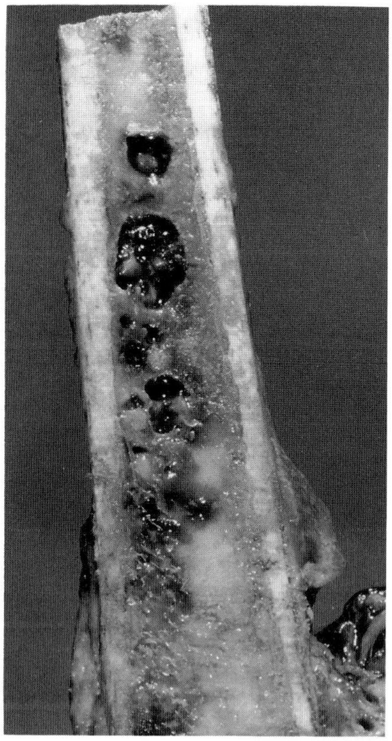

FIG. 11. Telangiectatic osteosarcoma. The medullary cavity of the femur is permeated by cystic, hemorrhagic foci that invade the bone extensively.

and invade the soft tissues beyond the periosteum. In spite of its usual gross appearance, it quite frequently invades through the epiphyseal cartilage into the epiphysis. The articular cartilage forms a more consistent barrier to tumor invasion. It may invade the adjacent joint via the joint capsule or along the cruciate ligaments (20). The telangiectatic variety may appear deceptively bland with a smooth border, thus resembling an aneurysmal bone cyst or even a unicameral bone cyst, and is a purely lytic lesion. A skip lesion may be demonstrated with a completely separate focus from the main tumor within the bone. The incidence of this phenomenon is controversial and ranges from <2% (175) to 20% (81). MRI is useful for the delineation of the extent of the tumor but is not as useful as plain radiographs for the actual diagnosis.

Grossly, the cut surface of osteosarcoma varies considerably with the histologic type. The sclerotic varieties are hard and yellow in appearance (Fig. 10B); the chondroblastic tumor shows abundant, translucent, bluish cartilage matrix; and the telangiectatic lesions contain a mass of hemorrhage within the bone and resemble an aneurysmal bone cyst (Fig. 11). The central intramedullary portion of the tumor is often necrotic, whereas the periphery is a more fleshy, gray color. Arcas of hemorrhage are common. The fibroblastic variety has a white, fibrous, cut surface. The tumor tends to extend further up the medullary portion of the bone than along the periosteum (Fig. 11). The gross extent of the tumor correlates well with the microscopic extent, so that gross evaluation of the medullary resection margin in an amputation specimen is reasonably reliable.

Histologically, the diagnosis of osteosarcoma is based on the finding of tumor osteoid and/or bone that is formed directly from the sarcomatous element without an intervening cartilaginous step (Fig. 12A). The typical intramedullary osteosarcoma shows a sarcomatous stroma with cells varying from spindled to rounded (epithelioid) in appearance. They usually have a relatively large amount of eosinophilic or amphophilic cytoplasm. In addition to osteoid they may produce abundant collagen, cartilage, or bone. The intramedullary portion of the tumor shows extension of the tumor cells between nor-

A

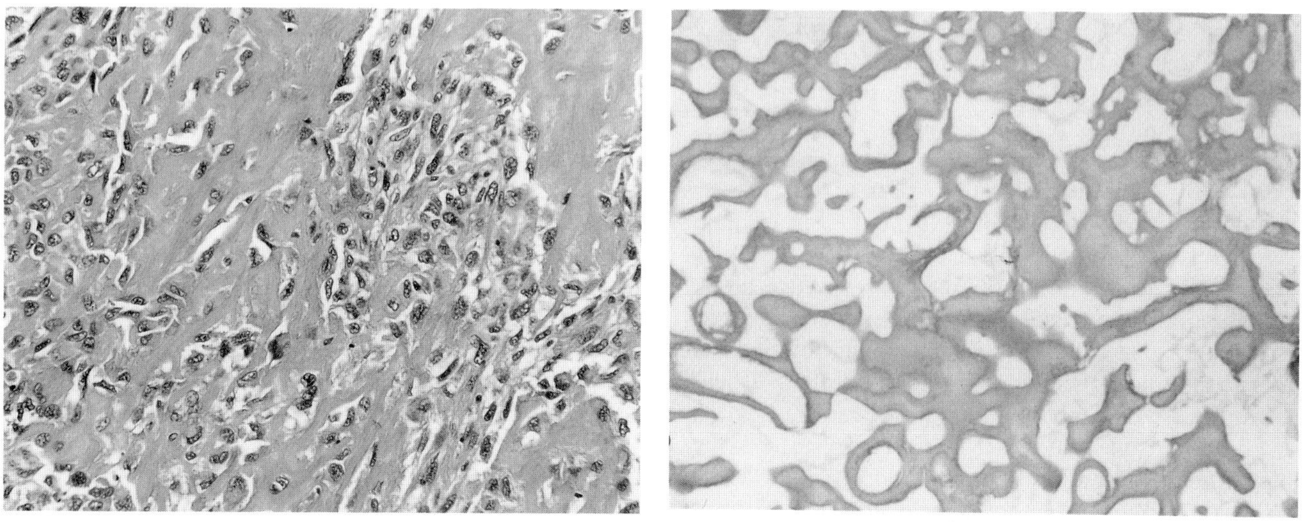

B

FIG. 12. Osteosarcoma. **A.** The tumor is composed of pleomorphic spindle cells that produce irregular clusters of osteoid. **B.** Following combination chemotherapy, there is massive necrosis with obliteration of the cellular compartment and preservation of an acellular osteoid matrix.

mal bony spicules and deposition of tumor osteoid upon the preexisting bony spicules—a characteristic feature of osteosarcoma. Osteoid osteoma and osteoblastoma by contrast do not permeate the adjacent bone for any distance. One variant of osteosarcoma with abundant collagen deposition may have a storiform pattern and pleomorphism like a malignant fibrous histiocytoma, but it is distinguished by the production of tumor bone; conversely, hyalinized collagen in malignant fibrous histiocytoma may closely resemble osteoid. The best way to distinguish the two neoplasms is by finding calcium deposition within the hyaline material, thus confirming its bony nature.

Antibodies to osteonectin may be useful in the differential diagnosis of bone tumors. Serra et al. (229) found that antiosteonectin stained all osteogenic tumors but also stained giant cell tumor and chondroblastoma weakly. Antiosteonectin did not stain any of the other nonosteogenic tumors. It appeared to be most useful in the differential diagnosis of small cell osteosarcoma from other small round cell tumors of bone.

The older portions of osteosarcoma often undergo infarction as a result of vascular compression from growth within the rigid confines of the bone, and the more viable tumor is found at the advancing margin. The latter may not show much osteoid, however, so that selection of a suitable biopsy site requires some thought. The necrotic older tumor will leave footprints in the form of tumor osteoid deposited on preexisting bony trabeculae; this can still be easily recognized even after the actual tumor cells are long gone (Fig. 12B). As the tumor invades through the cortex it elevates the periosteum, producing various periosteal reaction patterns. These result from a combination of reactive bone laid down by the periosteum and bone laid down by the tumor. The Codman triangle consists for the most part of bone formed by the elevated periosteum. Some tumors, particularly chondroblastic ones, may show vascular invasion. We have seen one case in which the tumor extended the length of the femoral vein to the resection margin of an above-knee amputation.

Diagnosis of osteosarcoma must be established by biopsy before definitive treatment is instituted. There is some controversy as to the best way to do this. In major research study protocols, tissue is needed for both diagnosis and research purposes, and thus a wedge biopsy providing adequate tissue is usually requested. This form of biopsy provides the most adequate tissue for diagnosis from a pathologist's standpoint; however, there are disadvantages. The hematoma that forms can track extensively in the soft tissues; we have seen an open biopsy hematoma from a distal femoral lesion track up to the resection margin of the above-knee amputation specimen, so that it has the potential to carry tumor cells to this margin. Less traumatic methods produce less of a chance of hematoma formation but generate less material. A good needle core biopsy may be diagnostic if unequivocal sarcoma with tumor bone formation is seen. A fine needle aspiration generates even less material, although the procedure may sample the lesion more widely. It too may be diagnostic if the cell block contains malignant cells generating tumor osteoid. If successful, these procedures save time and avoid the necessity for general anesthesia and the formation of a large hematoma. It has been suggested that an open procedure may increase the chance of tumor spread via the blood stream or lymphatics. If the diagnosis is based on the more limited procedures, it must be absolutely unequivocal before allowing definitive treatment to proceed. If there is any lingering doubt biopsy should be repeated, and if it persists, a larger one should be taken. MRI may be very helpful in identifying cellular areas, compact bone, or liquefaction within the lesion and thus help to select a more specific site for biopsy. The differential diagnosis includes osteoblastoma, aneurysmal bone cyst, fibrous dysplasia, fracture callus, and myositis ossificans (20).

A popular method of treatment at this time is to establish the diagnosis of osteosarcoma, and if it is a high-grade tumor to then give a course of chemotherapy, after which time a definitive excision is performed. The pathologist then plays a crucial role in evaluating the effect of that chemotherapy by assessing the extent of necrosis within the tumor (Fig. 13). Osteosarcomas not treated with chemotherapy may undergo extensive necrosis (244), so that the tumor death needs to be massive before the treatment can be deemed effective. The response is graded as follows (97): grade I, <50% necrosis; grade II, 50–90% necrosis; grade III, 91–99% necrosis; grade IV, 100% necrosis. Grade III and IV necrosis indicate chemosensitivity and are predictive of good subsequent patient outcome (97,172). The assessment of this parameter requires that a slab of the tumor be taken to include a full cross-section of the tumor in one plane, all the sections assessed semiquantitatively, and the percentage determined (Fig. 13) (161,216). Studies are in progress to determine whether modern diagnostic imaging techniques can be used to predict chemotherapy response (103).

Osteosarcomas typically metastasize to the lung and are found in 20% at the time of diagnosis and are in 80% overall in patients treated by resection only (20,83). Metastases may occur at other bones and, more rarely, at other sites. Until the advent of chemotherapy, the overall survival was around 15–20%. In a recent study using Surveillance, Epidemiology, and End Results (SEER) data, Dorfman (72) found an overall 5-year survival of 41% and, interestingly, noted that in their cohort there was no tendency to improve over the 1973–1987 period of observation. Survival in females was better than in males. Another interesting finding was that survival for craniofacial osteosarcoma was similar to that of long bone tumors, whereas previously the former had been

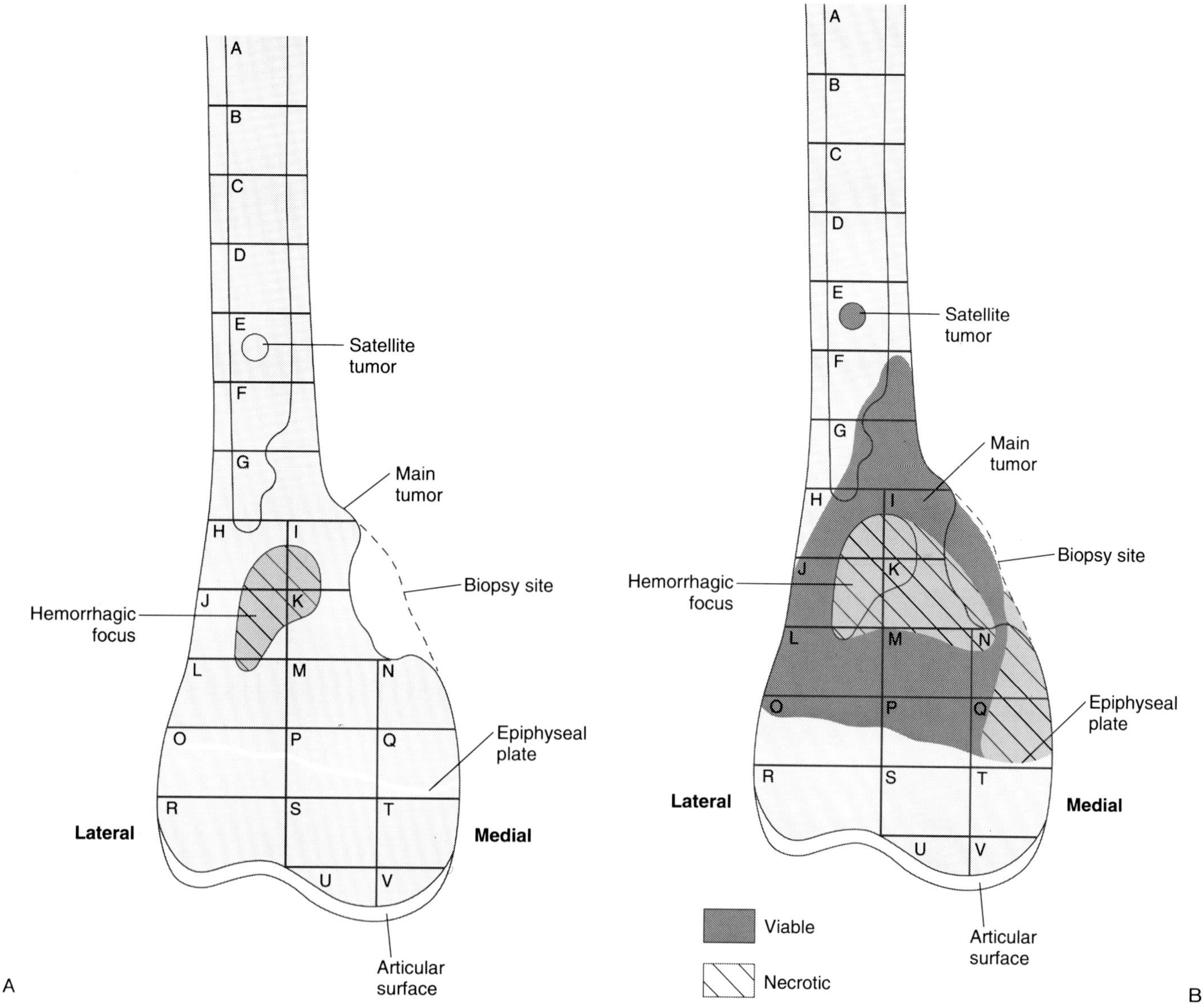

FIG. 13. Osteosarcoma. **A.** A slide map is prepared from a coronal section of tumorous bone. **B.** Following histologic evaluation, the diagram documents the extent and distribution of viable and necrotic tumor. This map shows a grade 1 chemotherapy effect (<50% necrosis) and can be used for radiographic correlation.

considered by most authorities to have a much better prognosis. Pelvic osteosarcoma had a much worse prognosis, with a <20% 5-year survival (72). An overall survival of 70% at 5 years has been noted in some studies (97). Resection of lung metastases has proven worthwhile in that it prolongs the disease-free survival (159), but the long-term survival of these patients is not good (20). With increased survival lengths, metastases are being noted in more unusual sites such as the liver, kidney, small bowel, and peritoneum (20).

Telangiectatic Osteosarcoma

Telangiectatic osteosarcoma occurs in a similar age range and sex ratio as usual osteosarcomas. It does, however, tend to involve the midshaft of long bones, especially the femur, more frequently. The proximal humerus is also commonly involved (20). Radiologically it is by definition a purely lytic lesion that may be either markedly destructive and obviously malignant in its appearance or may mimic a benign lesion such as aneurysmal bone cyst or unicameral bone cyst (20,83). These lesions tend to progress more rapidly and have a pathologic fracture much more frequently than usual osteosarcomas (20,264). Grossly they are typically very hemorrhagic (Fig. 11) with few fleshy or sclerotic areas. Microscopically the resemblance to an aneurysmal bone cyst may be striking, with large blood-filled spaces separated by narrow septa with a cellular stroma and giant cells. It is important to inspect this stroma carefully because the clue to the diagnosis is the finding of unequivocal malignant cells in the septa or more solid parts of the neoplasm and tumor osteoid production. Mitoses are important to identify, as aneurysmal bone cysts may show nuclear atypia as a degenerative phenomenon. Aneurysmal bone cysts may also have a malignant-appearing radiograph, which may add to the confusion. The osteoid in telangiectatic osteosarcoma is more delicate and lacelike than the denser osteoid in aneurysmal bone cysts (83). Telangiectatic osteosarcomas are very aggressive even when compared to usual osteosarcoma, but they appear to be chemoresponsive (20), probably because of the excellent blood supply to individual tumor cells via blood lakes.

Small Cell Osteosarcoma

Small cell osteosarcoma is also a very aggressive tumor that does not respond well to conventional therapy for osteosarcoma. It presents in a similar fashion and is usually a lytic lesion. Histologically it consists of sheets of small cells with a high nucleocytoplasmic ratio, resembling Ewing's sarcoma. In fact, many of the reported cases in earlier series were found among cases classified as Ewing's sarcoma. The difference between the two tumors is the presence of tumor osteoid in osteosarcoma, abundant reticulin in the former tumor, and their sparsity in the latter (83). One study (184) demonstrated a t(11;22)(q24;q12) in a small cell osteosarcoma, suggesting that it may be related more closely to Ewing's sarcoma than was previously realized. The authors have made a similar observation using polymerase chain reaction technology (unpublished data).

The differential diagnosis also includes mesenchymal chondrosarcoma, malignant lymphoma of bone, and primitive neuroectodermal tumor (PNET) (83). The cartilage in mesenchymal chondrosarcoma is better differentiated than that of osteosarcoma, and immunohistochemical markers will help distinguish between small cell osteosarcoma, lymphoma, and PNET. These tumors may respond to Ewing-type chemotherapy, but they have a very poor prognosis at the present time. Their responsiveness to radiotherapy is controversial (83).

Low-Grade Intraosseous Osteosarcoma

Low-grade intraosseous osteosarcoma is a slow-growing tumor of bone with an indolent course and an older age occurrence (median age, 30 years) (20,144). Males and females are affected equally (144). The tumors involve the long bones predominantly (81%) with 15% occurring in flat bones and 4% in the small bones of the hands and feet (144). Eighty-six percent of Kurt et al.'s series (144) were intramedullary, but 14% were intracortical in origin. They more frequently have a pathologic fracture than usual osteosarcoma. On plain radiographs they may be either lytic or sclerotic, and 50% may have a relatively benign appearance with a geographic type of bone destruction (20). MRI may be helpful in identifying cortical destruction, which may be difficult to see on a plain radiograph. Fifty-five percent have soft tissue invasion (144).

Histologically low-grade intraosseous osteosarcomas may have a number of different patterns (144). They basically consist of a rather bland, spindle cell proliferation with abundant collagen, relatively few mitoses, and variable production of tumor osteoid/bone. In 40% of cases they resemble a parosteal osteosarcoma. Fourteen percent resemble fibrous dysplasia, in some instances to a remarkable degree, so that this is the most difficult differential diagnosis. The radiograph may show malignant characteristics, and histologic foci of atypia beyond that of fibrous dysplasia may provide the clue to the diagnosis. Another helpful feature is the presence of an infiltrative growth pattern in osteosarcoma, as opposed to the well-demarcated pattern of fibrous dysplasia in the long bones. One third are very similar to desmoplastic fibroma, with occasional foci of osteoid/bone production making the distinction. The tumors may also have a fibrochondromyxoid pattern. Another differential diagnostic consideration is a solid aneurysmal bone cyst. The latter are more cellular and have more mitotic activity than low-grade osteosarcomas, but they lack atypia in most instances (144).

Low-grade intraosseous osteosarcomas will recur if incompletely excised; thus they require radical surgery for cure. The metastatic rate is much lower than that for regular osteosarcoma. They may, however, undergo dedifferentiation to a higher grade lesion if left alone. This phenomenon occurred in 15% of the cases in Kurt et al.'s series (144), and these cases subsequently behaved like high-grade osteosarcomas.

Juxtacortical (Surface) Osteosarcomas

Juxtacortical, or surface, osteosarcomas compose 4.6 of all osteosarcomas (72). There are three varieties: parosteal, periosteal, and high-grade surface.

Parosteal Osteosarcoma

Parosteal osteosarcoma frequently presents as a slowly growing mass behind the distal femur metaphysis of a female who is somewhat older than the usual osteosarcoma patient. It may also occur around the proximal humeral or proximal tibial metaphysis and occurs almost exclusively in long bones (20). It arises on the surface of the bone and elevates the periosteum to produce a densely sclerotic mass adherent to the underlying cortex. The cortex is not continuous with the mass as in an osteochondroma, nor is there extension of the underlying marrow space into the lesion. It will often wrap itself around the bone, leaving a narrow space between the tumor and the host bone cortex, and be attached to the cortex by only a short stalk. The tumor is usually osteosclerotic and histologically consists of a fairly cellular fibroblastic stroma with abundant collagen and long parallel spicules of bone without osteoblastic rimming. There is very little or no nuclear atypia, and mitoses are sparse (Fig. 14). A small amount of cartilage may be present and may even form a cap over the tumor.

Parosteal osteosarcomas have a slowly progressive course with enlargement over years. They will recur if incompletely removed and thus require radical surgery for cure. They rarely metastasize but may undergo dedifferentiation into a high-grade sarcoma, at which time the prognosis becomes decidedly worse. This may be signaled by the development of a lytic area in a formerly osteosclerotic portion of the tumor.

Periosteal Osteosarcoma

Periosteal osteosarcoma, unlike most other osteosarcomas, occurs more frequently in the midshaft of long bones, particularly the tibia. It affects the same age range as usual osteosarcoma and is a somewhat more aggressive tumor than parosteal osteosarcoma, but less so than usual osteosarcoma (20). It arises as a mass on the surface of the bone and on plain radiographs shows an area in which the cortex appears faintly scooped out. It elevates the periosteum and forms a mass lipped by periosteal new bone at either end (Fig. 15). Varying amounts of curvilinear or popcornlike calcification, indicative of a high content of malignant cartilage, are present. Histologically it is a clearly malignant, bone-forming tumor but with a very prominent malignant cartilaginous component (20). It has a metastatic potential between that of parosteal and regular osteosarcoma and must be completely excised to prevent local recurrence. It may be possible to obtain a margin of normal bone around the tumor and thus salvage the limb.

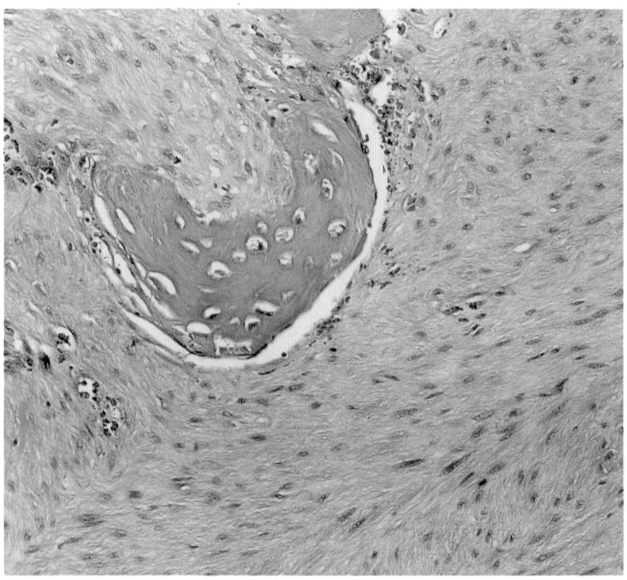

FIG. 14. Parosteal osteosarcoma. This periosteal lesion is composed of a relatively bland proliferation of spindle cells associated with bony trabeculae. There is minimal atypia in this field.

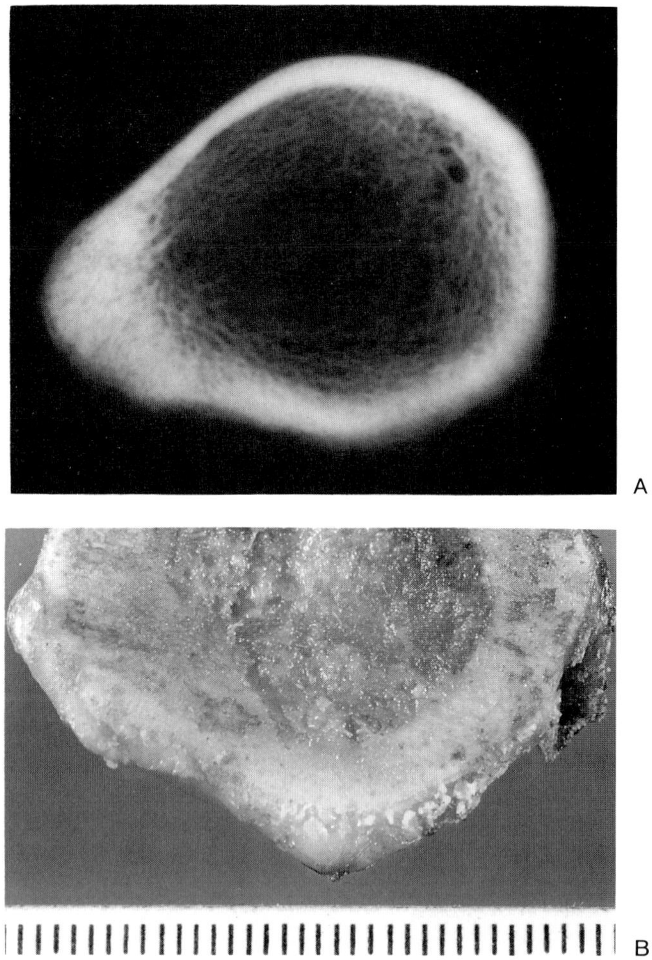

FIG. 15. Periosteal osteosarcoma. **A.** CT scan of the proximal tibia shows ill-defined feathering and loss of the bony contour in the lower half of the photograph. **B.** The gross specimen contains a periosteal lesion that elevates the surface of the bone. (Part **A** courtesy of Dr. Barry Fletcher, SJCRH.)

High-Grade Surface Osteosarcoma

High-grade surface osteosarcomas occur in a slightly older age range than the usual osteosarcoma (third decade), but show histologically similar high grade features and are situated on the surface of the cortex rather than in the medulla. They behave in a similar fashion to the usual osteogenic sarcoma and require similar radical treatment, including chemotherapy.

Multifocal Osteosarcoma

Multifocal osteosarcomas compose a controversial and interesting group of cases. The tumors are multicentric and may be synchronous, occurring within 6 months of each other (175), or asynchronous, occurring at a younger age than the usual osteosarcoma. They are often densely sclerotic. The multiple tumors should all be of approximately the same size without a dominant tumor (Fig. 16) (195). Earlier definitions required that these patients not have accompanying pulmonary metastases, but this is no longer required for the definition (20). These patients have a dismal prognosis, especially when they have synchronous tumors.

Molecular Biology of Osseous Tumors

Although a plethora of data exists on the biology of osteosarcoma, there is little information on benign bone-forming neoplasms. A three-way unbalanced translocation involving chromosomes 15, 17, and 20, with loss of 17p sequences, has been described in an osteoblastoma (162). Osteomas of the jaw are typically found in Gardner's syndrome, a form of polyposis coli (193,240). As discussed in Chapter 12, this syndrome is associated with mutations of the *apc* gene, which is located on chromosome 5q (188). Of interest is that osteomas may be found in the unaffected siblings and children of Gardner's syndrome patients (34) and that the incidence of mandibular osteomas is increased in patients with sporadic colorectal carcinoma (239). Because they arise relatively early in life, the presence of osteomas may be used as a diagnostic marker of familial polyposis coli in children who have not developed colonic lesions (45,75).

Although fibrous dysplasia has historically been considered a hamartomatous lesion, the presence of clonal cytogenetic abnormalities suggests that it is neoplastic in nature and develops as a result of somatic mutations (170). One patient with polyostotic fibrous dysplasia and an osteosarcoma had a constitutional 4q-/7p- translocation in his blood lymphocytes (32). Tumors with either multiple aberrations, t(6;11)(q11;p15), or a derivative chromosome 2 have also been reported (170,232).

Extensive biologic studies have been performed in patients with the McCune–Albright syndrome, revealing mutations in the gene encoding the α subunit of Gs, an adenylate cyclase-stimulating protein (232,276). The action of Gs-α on adenyl cyclase results in the production of cyclic AMP and acts in signal transduction. Gs-α mutations are present in a mosaic pattern that results in a mixed population of affected cells and nonaffected cells in both target and nontarget organs (276). It is thus postulated that the mutation would be lethal and lead to intrauterine death if it were present in pure form. This observation would explain the scattered asymmetric distribution of the bone lesions (105). High levels of expression of the proto-oncogene c-*fos* are observed in both sporadic and genetic fibrous dysplasia and are an apparent consequence of increased adenylate cyclase activity. This finding proceeded from the observation of fibrous dysplasialike lesions in the long bones of transgenic mice overexpressing c-*fos*, which leads to marrow fibrosis and increased bone turnover (42).

Osteosarcomas may grow readily in vitro, allowing establishment of cell lines. These cells have furnished the fuel for numerous studies into osteoblast differentiation and function (4,241). Similar to chondrosarcoma, cytogenetic studies have generally revealed complex chromosomal aberrations (17,157,192). Hyperdiploidy is frequent and is indicative of malignancy in bone-forming tumors (14,114). Parosteal osteosarcomas are characterized by a supernumerary ring chromosome (190). As noted above, the t(11;22)(q24;q12) that is characteristic of Ewing's sarcoma has been described in small cell osteosarcoma (184), but it is not universally present (95).

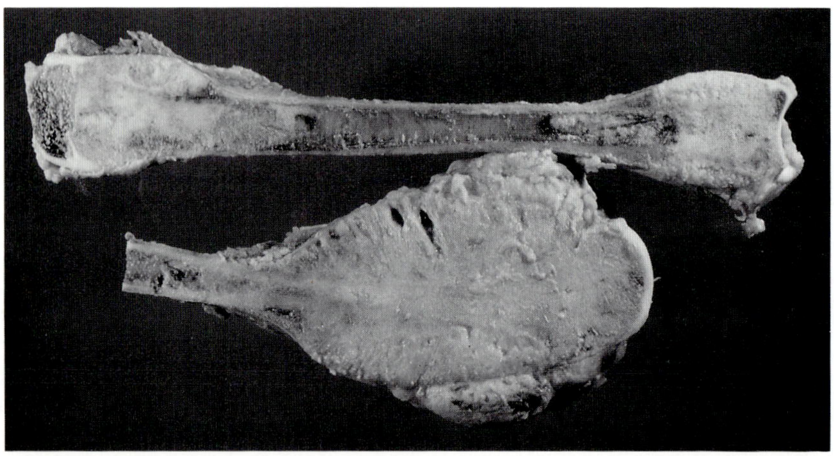

FIG. 16. Multifocal osteosarcoma. The proximal tibia, distal tibia, and distal femur contain large, invasive, densely sclerotic tumors.

Mutations of two genes, *p53* and *RB1*, have particularly been associated with osteosarcoma (104,282). Both of these genes are tumor suppressor genes whose loss or mutation is associated with increased susceptibility to cancer, and alterations in both are characteristically inherited in an autosomal dominant fashion. *p53* is located on chromosome 17p and is mutated in a large proportion of sporadic osteosarcomas, as well as those arising in connection with the Li–Fraumeni cancer susceptibility syndrome (6,152,254,269). Missense mutations of *p53* result in a cytoplasmic accumulation of the effete protein, which may be detected by immunohistochemistry; however, mutations leading to truncated or abnormally spliced RNA lead to absence of staining (6,269). The frequent occurrence of osteosarcoma as a secondary neoplasm in patients with hereditary retinoblastoma (89) led to recognition of the role of the associated *RB1* gene on chromosome 13q in bone sarcoma development. Loss of heterozygosity within the *RB1* locus is a common event in sporadic osteosarcomas and is frequently associated with a similar abnormality on chromosomes 3, 11, 17, and 22 (223). The association of mutations at chromosomes 13 and 17 suggest that alterations of both *RB1* and *p53* are obligate events in osteosarcoma development (104). Genetic dysfunction at both of these loci may be induced by radiation and lead to osteosarcoma as a second malignancy (23).

Cell cycle disturbance related to the abnormal expression of growth factors may also occur in osteosarcoma. These alterations include amplification of *SAS* (238), *CDK4, GLI,* and *MDM2* (138), overexpression of c-*fos* (283), and elaboration of insulin growth factor–I receptors (204), basic fibroblastlike growth factors (286), and the met proto-oncogene kinase receptor and its ligand (214).

FIBROHISTIOCYTIC NEOPLASMS

Giant Cell Tumor

Giant cell tumor is a fairly common neoplasm, composing 5% of primary bone tumors. It presents after the epiphyses have closed, so that it occurs in patients in late teen years (98) and early adulthood (83,155). In one large series of cases, only 1.7% of giant cell tumors occurred in skeletally immature individuals (203). Giant cell tumors have a slight female preponderance (1.3:1) (83,155) and involve the epiphysis and adjacent metaphysis of long bones, particularly the distal femur, upper tibia, and distal radius (155). They may also involve other bones, such as the vertebral bodies, ulna, fibula, sacrum, pelvis, and small bones of the hands and feet (155). The body of the vertebra rather than the posterior elements is affected (98). Early giant cell tumors arise in the metaphysis, and cases have been described involving the epiphysis alone (155).

Radiologically giant cell tumors are eccentric and lytic with well-demarcated nonsclerotic edges and a soap bubble appearance. They may expand the bone and erode through the cortex or into the joint (Fig. 17A) (155).

Histologically giant cell tumors consist of sheets of mononuclear cells containing uniformly dispersed osteoclast-type giant cells (Fig. 17B). The tumors are very cellular with relatively little collagen deposition. The mononuclear cells are polygonal in shape, may show mitotic activity, but are cytologically benign. A small amount of osteoid may be formed. In an immunohistochemical and histochemical study of nine giant cell tumors, Medeiros et al. (164) demonstrated that the mononuclear cells show histiocytic differentiation, whereas the giant cells have features in common with both histiocytes and normal osteoclasts. These two cell types may be different subsets or different stages of differentiation of otherwise similar cells (164). Brecher et al. (24) also suggested that the giant cells are derived from stromal cells of mononuclear phagocyte lineage.

Giant cell tumor is prone to recur if treated conservatively, as by curettage with or without bone grafting (155). Thus, if the tumor occurs in an expendable bone, and particularly if it can be recognized with a high degree of certainty from imaging studies, it is best to do an immediate en bloc resection of the lesion. If this cannot be done without serious morbidity, the rate of recurrence can be reduced by the use of cryotherapy (83). Giant cell tumors often may extend into adjacent soft tissues and invade blood vessels (83,155). The latter feature does not indicate malignant behavior, as in one series only 11 of 218 patients with blood vessel invasion developed pulmonary metastases (98). They may, however, metastasize to the lungs in rare cases (4–5%), with the lung nodules often showing a rim of either fibrosis or actual bone formation (155). After resection of the lung metastases, the patient may have a normal life span.

Present et al. (206) have proposed a staging system that appears to be predictive of the behavior of these tumors (Table 4). Aside from metastasizing giant cell tumor of the usual morphology, malignant change may be associated with these tumors. Those tumors that recur early tend to maintain their benign morphology. Rare cases may have a sarcomatous pattern together with typical giant cell tumor at diagnosis. More common is the development of a frank sarcoma in the site of the original tumor at varying intervals following radiation therapy, and sarcoma may develop years later in the absence of radiation therapy (the so-called evolutionary giant cell tumor) (155). The evolutionary giant cell tumor usually has the pattern of a malignant fibrous histiocytoma. Sarcomas arising in giant cell tumors following radiation therapy include fibrosarcoma, osteosarcoma, and malignant fibrous histiocytoma (155).

The biology of giant cell tumor is made more complex because of the intermingling of the two main elements,

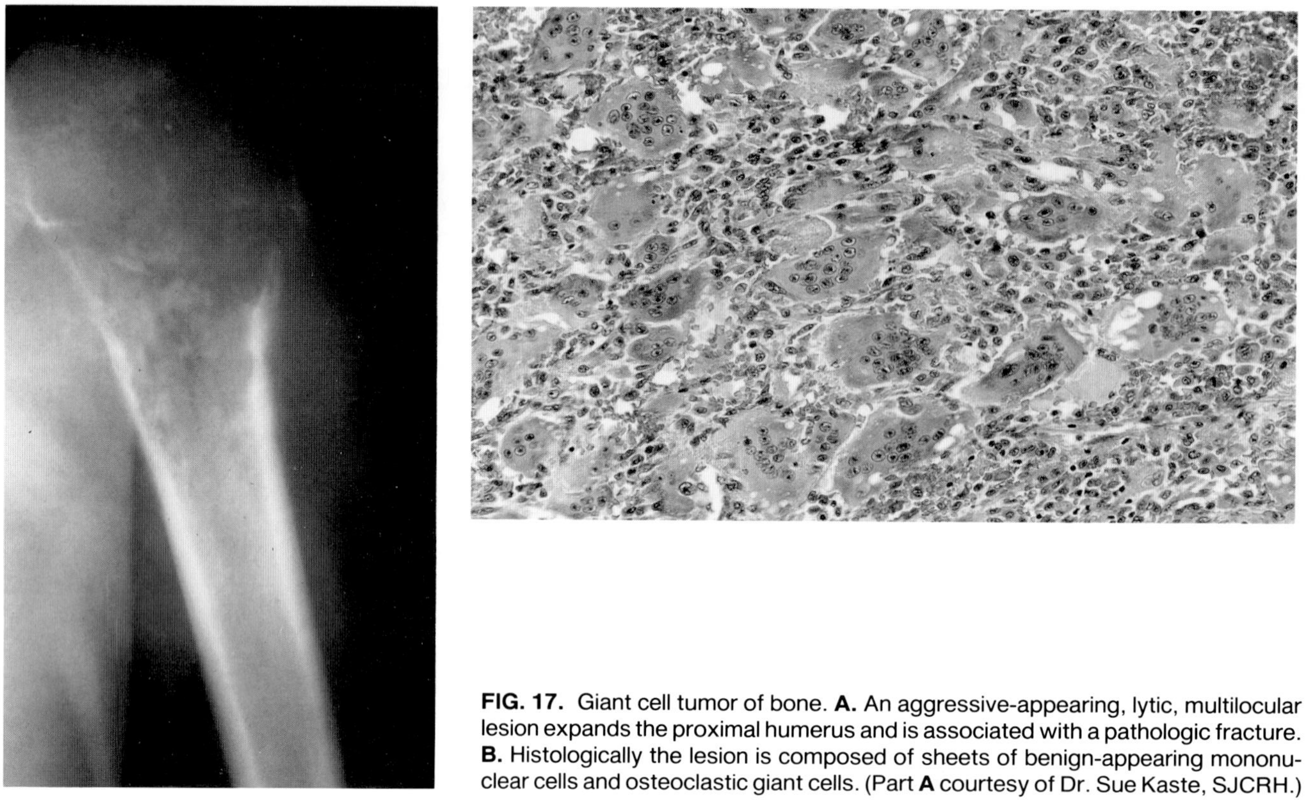

A

B

FIG. 17. Giant cell tumor of bone. **A.** An aggressive-appearing, lytic, multilocular lesion expands the proximal humerus and is associated with a pathologic fracture. **B.** Histologically the lesion is composed of sheets of benign-appearing mononuclear cells and osteoclastic giant cells. (Part **A** courtesy of Dr. Sue Kaste, SJCRH.)

i.e., mononuclear spindle cells and multinuclear giant cells. It is generally accepted that the spindle cells compose the neoplastic component and that the giant cells are osteoclastic in type and reactive in nature (213). The migration and accumulation of giant cells into giant cell tumors results from the elaboration of cytokines, primarily transforming growth factor (TGF), by the spindle cells (211,290). Several cell lines have been established (121,140).

Cytogenetic abnormalities are common in giant cell tumors and are occasionally clonal. Clonal abnormalities include translocations involving 11p15, fus (14p;21p), fus(15p;21p), dic(19;20)(p13;q31), dic(19;22)(q13;q13), and the t(12;19)(q13;q13) (27,183,248). A particularly striking and common feature of giant cell tumors is their tendency for telomeric fusion, or union of the ends of the chromosomes. This phenomenon most frequently involves chromosomes 11p, 13p, 15p, 19q, 20q, and 21p (27,225,226). The telomeric fusion of 19q may be related to the tumor's overexpression of TGF, as the gene for this growth factor is located at the terminus of the long arm of chromosome 19 (225). However, no alterations of this genetic locus were detected in ten tested tumors, although telomeric associations were frequent (36). The activity of telomerase, the enzyme that maintains telomere integrity, is increased in giant cell tumors and may be related to maintenance of the transformed phenotype (227).

The presence of marker chromosomes appears to portend a more aggressive clinical behavior for giant cell tumors (58,248). However, ploidy studies have no apparent value in prognosticating the behavior of this

TABLE 4. *Giant cell tumor staging (205)*

	Stage I	Stage II	Stage III
Symptoms	Absent	Absent	Present
Radiologic findings	Quiescent appearing	Active appearing, i.e., with expansion of bone but no extension beyond cortex	Aggressive appearing, with permeative bony destruction, extension beyond cortex, and formation of a soft tissue mass, extension to the subchondral cortex, or invasion of a joint
Histologic findings	Benign	Benign	Benign
Metaphases	Absent	Absent	Present
Periosteal reaction	Absent	Absent	Present
Distant metastases	Absent	Absent	Present

enigmatic neoplasm, as aneuploidy may be observed in nonaggressive tumors and diploidy in metastasizing ones (88,112,148).

Benign Fibrous Histiocytoma

Benign fibrous histiocytoma is a rare tumor of bone that is histologically identical to nonossifying fibroma but occurs at an older age or in sites unusual for nonossifying fibroma. These include the ilium, ribs, and fibula, the majority being in the ilium (83). Affected patients as young as 5 years have been described (154). In the long bones they tend to occur near the ends in the epiphyses and metaphyses, to be eccentric, and to have a sclerotic rim with expansion of the cortex (122). Unlike nonossifying fibroma, these lesions are painful and may recur (83). Like nonossifying fibroma, they are spindle cell lesions containing a storiform pattern, osteoclast-type giant cells, cholesterol clefts, hemosiderin deposition, and foamy macrophages (122).

Nonossifying Fibroma/Fibrous Cortical Defect

Nonossifying fibromas and fibrous cortical defects are extremely common lesions affecting up to 30–40% of children, particularly boys (122). They occur at a relatively young age (4–8 years) and can be diagnosed with confidence radiologically and thus be managed without surgery in the majority of cases (122). The lesions occur in the metaphyses of long bones, particularly the distal femoral metaphysis and distal and proximal tibia at the sites of tendinous insertions (83). They are eccentric, lytic lesions eroding the cortex, with a sclerotic rim (Fig. 18A)(122).

Histologically fibrous cortical defects are spindle cell lesions, often with a storiform pattern and osteoclast-type giant cells. Foam cells, cholesterol clefts, and hemosiderin deposition are frequently seen (Fig. 18B). Mitoses are usually absent.

Nonossifying fibroma is a less common, larger lesion occurring between 2 and 20 years of age and involving the medullary portion of the bone. Conversely, the subperiosteal fibrous cortical defect is, as its name implies, subperiosteal and within the cortex. Both lesions have identical histology as described above. If the lesion involves more than half the diameter of the bone or is more than 33 mm in length, surgery is indicated to avoid pathologic fracture (7).

Nonossifying fibromas have been described as the cause of hypophosphatemic rickets (11) and may be familial and multiple (82). Fibrous cortical defects may be multiple in 8% of cases. This phenomenon may be associated with neurofibromatosis type 1 in 5% of cases with multiple lesions (180) or with cafe au lait spots and other anomalies outside the skeleton (Jaffe–Campanacci syndrome) (177).

Malignant Fibrous Histiocytoma

Malignant fibrous histiocytoma is an uncommon malignant bone tumor. It affects mostly adults but is seen in

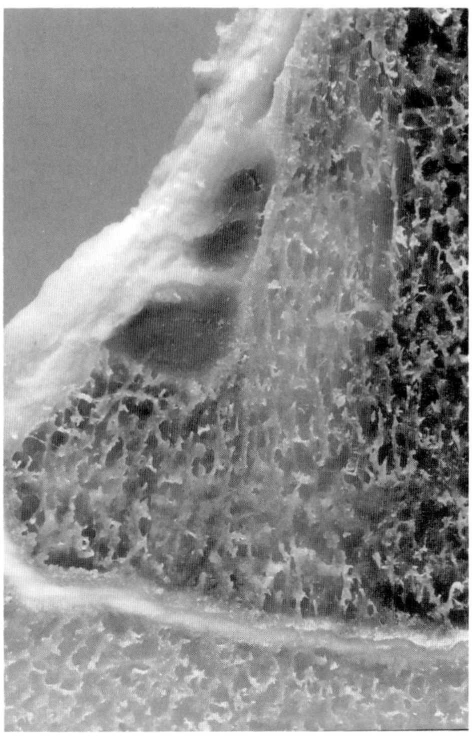

A

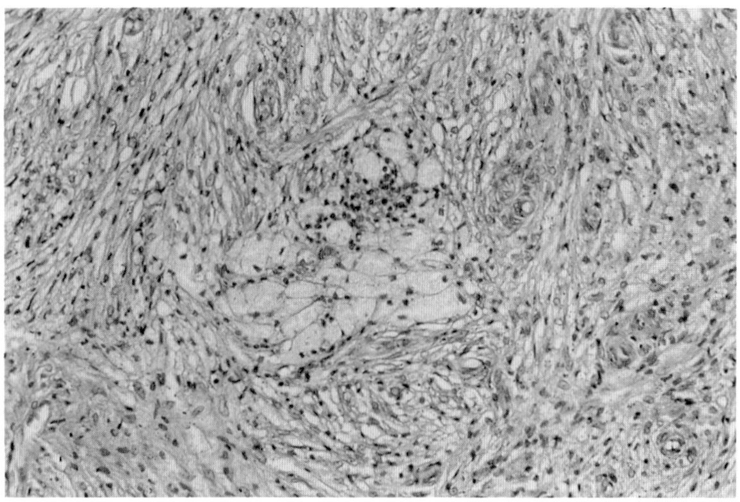

B

FIG. 18. Nonossifying fibroma. **A.** An eccentric, lytic, well-circumscribed lesion erodes the cortex of the distal femoral metaphysis. **B.** The lesion is composed of swirling fascicles of bland spindle cells and foam cells.

older children with a male-to-female ratio of 1.5:1.0. It affects the distal femur predominantly, but also arises in the proximal tibia, humerus, and pelvis. A relatively large proportion of these tumors arise on the basis of a preexisting condition, such as an infarct, Paget's disease, site of orthopedic device placement, previously irradiated bone, giant cell tumor, enchondroma, or osteomyelitis (44,53,56,91,101,122,176).

Radiologically malignant fibrous histiocytoma is a lytic lesion with geographic, moth-eaten, or permeative patterns of bone destruction (122). It invades through the cortex, elevates the periosteum, and eventually breaks through into the soft tissues forming a soft tissue mass (122).

Grossly malignant fibrous histiocytoma varies from a firm, fibrous mass to a softer, fleshy tumor, depending on the amount of stromal collagen. Microscopically it is a spindle cell tumor with a storiform pattern and marked nuclear pleomorphism. There are often giant cells present, sometimes with a Touton appearance. Foam cells may also be seen. Areas of necrosis and hemorrhage are frequent. There may be abundant collagen, which may be indistinguishable from osteoid in the absence of calcification. This latter feature makes the distinction from osteogenic sarcoma very difficult, especially as there is a variant of osteogenic sarcoma that has the same overall growth pattern as malignant fibrous histiocytoma (288). They may occasionally have a predominantly histiocytic appearance in that the cells have a plump, polygonal shape and are closely packed in sheets.

The biologic differences between osteosarcoma and malignant fibrous histiocytoma may be more perceived than real, as both share unique tendencies to show amplification of *SAS,* mutation of *p53,* and increased expression of transin, c-fos, and c-jun (6,119,167,269). Familial cases of malignant fibrous histiocytoma of bone have been reported (84).

Central Giant Cell Granuloma

Central giant cell granuloma, also known as reparative giant cell granuloma, is a fibrohistiocytic lesion that primarily affects the maxilla and mandible (118,235), and, less frequently, other bones of the skull and extremities (1,194). It is particularly prone to occur in children, in whom it is one of the most common benign jaw tumors (65,118). The mandible, particularly its anteriormost portion, is most frequently affected (118) (Fig. 19A).

Central giant cell granuloma is a destructive lesion that acquires a multiloculated "soap bubble" roentgenographic appearance as it progresses (Fig. 19A). Typically these tumors are painless, so that the presence of a large mass may call their attention to the patient. Extragnathic spread and "floating teeth" are not unusual. However, their course is benign, and they are usually adequately treated by curettage (118).

Histologically, central giant cell granuloma is composed of a mixture of spindle cells and giant cells (Fig. 19B). The spindle cells are proliferating myofibroblasts that are embedded in a myxoid to cellular stroma with reparative features. Similarly to the "brown tumors" of hyperparathyroidism (see below), microhemorrhages and hemosiderosis are frequent. Bone and osteoid production may be present, particularly at the boundaries of the lesion. The giant cells are osteoclastic in nature (22,85) and contain multiple, benign-appearing nuclei. These lesions may appear very similar to giant cell tu-

A

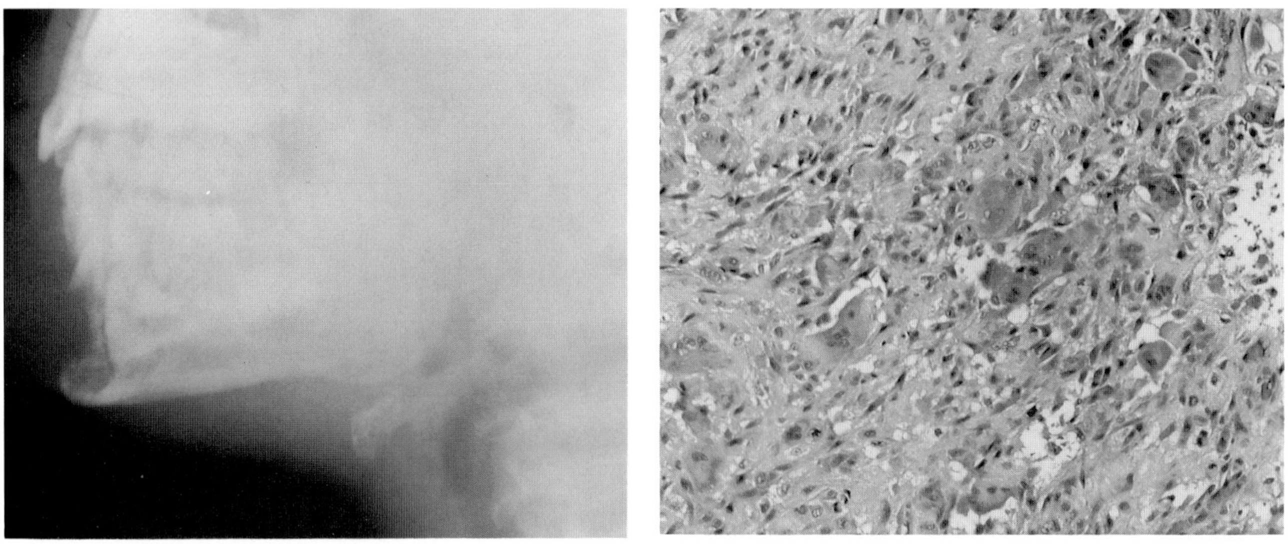

B

FIG. 19. Central giant cell granuloma. **A.** A destructive, lytic lesion erodes the anterior mandible. **B.** The lesion is composed of a mixture of bland spindle cells and multinucleated giant cells, embedded in a loose stroma. (Part **A** courtesy of Dr. Barry Fletcher, SJCRH.)

mors, which also may affect the skull (15,236). The latter tumors lack the fibrogenic collagenous stroma and hemorrhage of giant cell granulomas and possess a more diffuse proliferation of giant cells. However, in jaw lesions, the distinction may be impossible (15).

The biologic nature of central giant cell granuloma has fueled heated debate (246). As the name implies, a nonneoplastic reactive process has been historically considered as its etiology (1,41). Others consider it to be a neoplasm (118). Tender for the former contention has recently come from biologic studies showing that identical lesions are seen with elevated serum levels of parathyroid hormone–related peptide (63) and with vitamin D–resistant rickets (46). These findings could imply that central giant cell granulomas and the histologically identical brown tumor are related phenomena. Other authors using ultrastructural data have come to a similar conclusion (67). Another related observation is that administration of calcitonin may induce regression of the lesions (106). In spite of their predilection for females, central giant cell granulomas do not appear to possess estrogen or progesterone receptors (280).

Regardless of the biologic nature of central giant cell granuloma, a tendency to develop these lesions may be inherited (62,275). These tumors may also occur in association with cherubism (136,197,275), ossifying fibroma (197), prior irradiation (86), neurofibromatosis (262), and a Noonan-like syndrome characterized by multiple phenotypic anomalies (16,51). Multifocal lesions should suggest the possibility of hyperparathyroidism (141,208,237,262) but may be evidence of an underlying biologic abnormality (62,63,237,262).

FIBROUS TUMORS

Desmoplastic Fibroma

Desmoplastic fibroma is the intraosseous equivalent to the desmoid tumor of soft tissue. It behaves in a similar manner to that tumor in that it is locally aggressive but does not metastasize. It is rare, comprising <0.1% of bone tumors overall (124). Forty-six percent of cases occur in the second decade, and there is a slight male predominance (249).

Radiologically, desmoplastic fibroma will usually show a destructive, malignant appearance and is typically quite large at the time of diagnosis. The gross appearance is that of a firm, white mass invading and destroying the bone. The histologic appearance often comes as a surprise after the malignant-appearing radiograph, in that the tumor contains abundant collagen production with a somewhat hypocellular appearance and widely separated, bland-appearing fibroblasts and myofibroblasts with few or no mitoses. It is the combination of this desmoidlike histology with a usually aggressive radiographic appearance that is diagnostic of this entity.

The differential diagnosis includes low-grade fibrosarcoma and low-grade intraosseous osteosarcoma. The former is a more cellular tumor with more prominent mitotic activity, at least some nuclear pleomorphism, and a herringbone growth pattern. We have had difficulty in distinguishing low-grade intraosseous osteosarcoma from this tumor, the difference being the production of tumor osteoid or bone by the tumor in osteosarcoma. It may be difficult to distinguish between entrapped preexisting bone/reactive bone and true tumor bone in this setting.

These tumors are locally aggressive with progressive destructive growth within the bone as well as extension outside the bone. It is therefore important to resect them with a wide margin of normal tissue if possible. They do not metastasize. Their response to radiation therapy is not well documented, although desmoid tumors of soft tissue have been shown to respond to radiotherapy. The role of chemotherapy is unknown.

Cytogenetic analysis of a desmoplastic fibroma arising in an adolescent revealed trisomies of chromosomes 3 and 5 (30).

Fibrosarcoma

Fibrosarcomas of bone are rare in the first decade but are more common in the second (83). They present as purely lytic lesions in the distal femoral metaphysis, proximal tibial metaphysis, and proximal humeral metaphysis and have a permeative or geographic destructive pattern on plain radiographs (83). Approximately 25% of fibrosarcomas of bone arise on the basis of a preexisting lesion such as giant cell tumor, Paget's disease, enchondroma, osteochondroma, chronic osteomyelitis, fibrous dysplasia, or bone infarct (40,83).

Grossly, fibrosarcomas vary from firm, fibrous masses in well-differentiated tumors to softer, fleshy masses with necrosis in the higher grade tumors. Histologically they are malignant spindle cell lesions that vary in the degree of cellular atypia and the amount of collagen production, depending on the grade. By definition there should be no bone or cartilage production by the tumor. They frequently have a herringbone pattern of growth and may have myxoid areas, particularly the higher grade lesions (83).

The behavior of fibrosarcomas correlates with the grade of the tumor. They metastasize to the lungs and spread to extrapulmonary sites in a higher proportion of cases than osteosarcomas (83,132).

It is important to distinguish between intramedullary lesions and eccentric lesions centered on the cortex or periosteum, as the latter may represent invasion of the bone by a soft tissue fibrosarcoma. These eccentric lesions are noted to have a better prognosis than the medullary lesions (83,123,251).

HEMATOLOGIC LESIONS

Eosinophilic Granuloma

Eosinophilic granuloma is an important lesion of bone in childhood and represents a localized form of Langerhans cell histiocytosis, which is discussed in Chapter 16. Eosinophilic granuloma is a relatively common osseous neoplasm of children, representing 6% of all bone tumors in one pediatric series (218). It can appear quite aggressive on radiologic study and may closely mimic Ewing's sarcoma (108) (Fig. 20). Lesions in the cranium may present as scalp nodules (287).

Diagnosis of eosinophilic granuloma is possible with fine needle aspiration (80,230), which may be combined with therapy by intralesional instillation of corticosteroids (77,80,230). Ancillary techniques such as anti-S-100 and peanut agglutinin staining and electron microscopy can be confirmatory (80,139,210). One caveat is to not confuse the lesion with chronic osteomyelitis, which may have a similar cytologic composition but should not include abundant Langerhans cells (230). Other diagnostic considerations include xanthoma, sinus histiocytosis with massive lymphadenopathy (Rosai–Dorfman disease) (5,271), and an eosinophilic lesion associated with Hodgkin's disease (54).

Lymphoma

Malignant lymphoma of bone is an important tumor that is included in the differential diagnosis of small round cell tumors of bone. It may be easily confused with entities such as Ewing's sarcoma by those unaccustomed to seeing these lesions on a frequent basis. However, it is uncommon in childhood; the majority of cases of primary bone lymphoma occur in adults (83).

Lymphomas of bone show lytic, sclerotic, or mixed

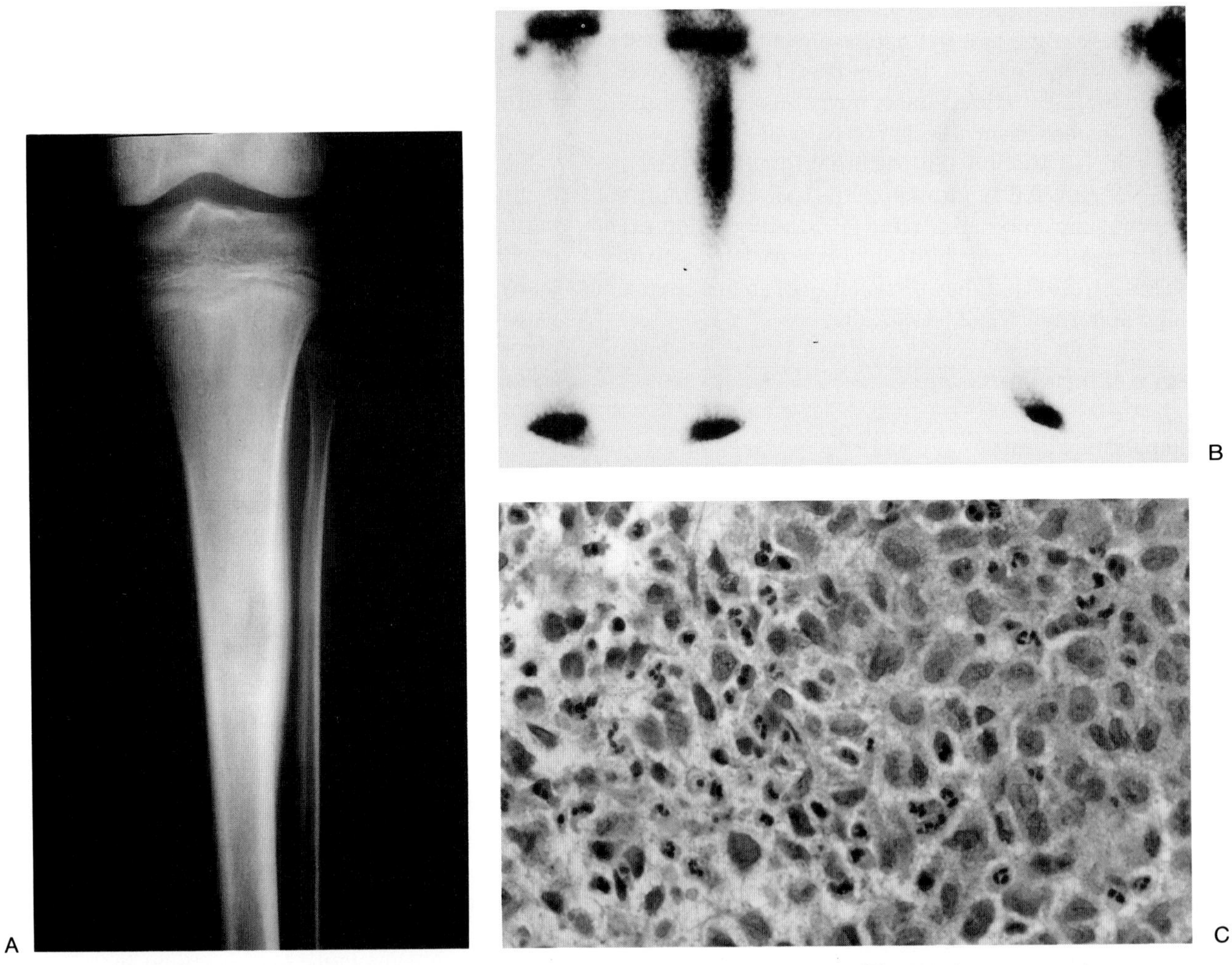

FIG. 20. Eosinophilic granuloma. A plain radiograph **(A)** and bone scan **(B)** reveal an aggressive-appearing, extensive lesion involving the tibial diaphysis. Histologically **(C)**, the lesion is composed of infiltrates of Langerhans cells and eosinophils. The Langerhans cells are mononuclear cells with oblong, grooved nuclei. (Parts **A** and **B** courtesy of Dr. Barry Fletcher, SJCRH.)

appearances on radiographic studies and have a permeative, malignant pattern, often involving the bone extensively to a degree which the radiographs underestimate (83). With extraosseous extension, they may generate a periosteal reaction and a soft tissue mass. The soft tissue mass may be quite large with a paradoxical minimum of cortical bone destruction. This latter effect is postulated to be due to tumor cytokine production causing stimulation of osteoclasts and formation of cortical channels of tumor egress (113). Grossly these tumors resemble lymphomas of lymph nodes and have a fleshy appearance.

Histologically, the majority of non-Hodgkin's lymphomas are diffuse large cell lymphomas, usually of the B-cell type (83,201,281). Lymphoblastic lymphomas are frequent in children (52). In large cell lymphomas, smaller lymphoid cells are present between the more atypical, large cells. Their nuclei show prominent folding, lobulation, and irregularity of outline. The cytoplasm is usually free of stainable glycogen, and the majority of cases have fairly plentiful reticulin between the cells. These features are in contrast to Ewing's sarcoma in which the cells appear more closely packed and have more uniform, round nuclei with a finer, more even chromatin distribution, plentiful cytoplasmic glycogen, and very little intercellular reticulin. In addition, immunostaining is very helpful, in that most large cell lymphomas will stain with leukocyte common antigen, while Ewing's sarcoma stains with antibodies against MIC2. However, one must beware lymphoblastic lymphomas of bone, which often display MIC2 positivity (209).

Other pediatric tumors that must be differentiated from non-Hodgkin's lymphomas of bone include chloroma, osteomyelitis, sarcomas, sinus histiocytosis with massive lymphadenopathy, and eosinophilic granuloma. Hodgkin's disease may also come to clinical attention because of bony involvement (92). Radiation therapy and chemotherapy are the preferred methods of treatment for these lesions.

CYSTIC LESIONS

Solitary Bone Cyst

Solitary, or unicameral, bone cyst is an interesting and not uncommon pediatric lesion that mimics a bone tumor on plain radiographs and represents about 3.0% of biopsied bone lesions (83). There is some evidence that it may develop on the basis of previous bone infarction or in relation to previous injury (83). There is a male predominance (3:1) (83). The most frequent site is the upper humeral metaphysis, followed by the upper femoral metaphysis. Eighty-five percent occur in the childhood years, mostly during the teens (83,186). Radiographs demonstrate a central bone lesion that is purely lytic with thinning of the adjacent cortex. With the development of a pathologic fracture, a flake of bone may break free and, because the cyst is unilocular, float to the inferior end of the lesion, producing the fallen leaf sign on plain radiographs (247). As the child grows older and the limb expands, the lesion becomes situated further and further away from the epiphysis.

Grossly solitary bone cysts consist of unilocular cysts lined by a thin fibrous membrane and situated in the central portion of the bone. In the event of a previous pathologic fracture, they may be filled with bloody or brown fluid; otherwise they are filled with clear fluid. Histologically, the amount of biopsy material is usually small and somewhat anticlimactic in that it consists of fibrous tissue often admixed with homogeneous, basophilic material and some reactive new bone. If there has been a pathologic fracture, the reaction to this will be evident and include hemosiderin-laden macrophages, osteoclast-type giant cells, and granulation tissue. Injection of steroids into the cyst will often result in filling by loose fibrous tissue and eventual ossification without the necessity of surgical intervention. If this endeavor fails it may be necessary to operate on the patient, remove the lining, and pack the cyst with bone chips to effect a cure.

Simple bone cysts have been considered to arise from blockage of venous blood and lymphatic flow (47, 143,273), resulting in relative ischemia and accumulation of bone-resorbing free radicals (143). They have been associated with aneuysmal bone cyst (115) and osteoblastomas (8), perhaps because of the venous obstruction related to these space-occupying lesions.

Simple bone cysts may lead to pathologic fracture (186), so that one should be aware that the histologic features of callus formation may accompany those of bone cysts. Familiarity with the radiologic features of each individual lesion is key to making this distinction.

Aneurysmal Bone Cyst

Aneurysmal bone cyst is an important and not uncommon lesion in childhood. It presents as a sometimes quite rapidly expanding mass that may involve the posterior elements of the vertebrae, where it may involve contiguous vertebral spines, or the long bones, particularly the distal femur and proximal tibia, usually in the peripheral metaphysis (83). On radiographs it has a smooth outline within the bone, giving it a predominantly benign appearance. Occasional cases may destroy the cortex in a manner that can mimic malignancy, particularly in the early or incipient phase (83). As aneurysmal bone cysts expand the cortex, they elevate the periosteum, resulting in a thin shell of new bone bulging out from the original cortex.

Grossly aneurysmal bone cysts are hemorrhagic lesions traversed by multiple fibrous septa (Fig. 21A). At surgery the blood within them is not clotted but actively flowing. This blood may be under significant pressure and result in substantial hemorrhage.

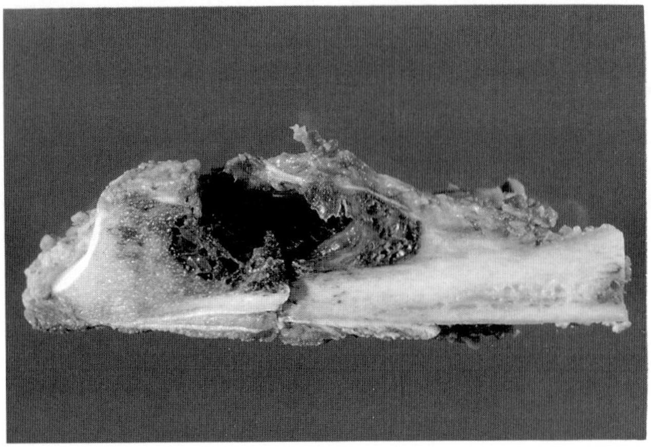

A

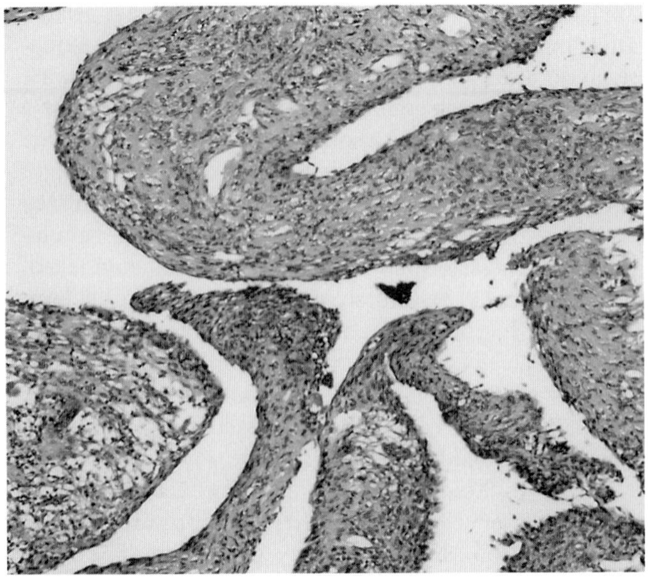

B

FIG. 21. Aneurysmal bone cyst. **A.** A hemorrhagic, cystic, sharply marginated tumor expands a rib. **B.** Microscopically the lesion is composed of bland, osteoid-forming, fibrohistiocytic tissues that comprise variably sized septa.

Histologically aneurysmal bone cysts consist of large lakes filled with blood surrounded by membranes with numerous mononuclear histiocytic cells and osteoclast-type giant cells but without an endothelial lining (Fig. 21B). Hemosiderin may be plentiful, and a variable amount of collagen deposition is noted. They may contain an osteoid or chondroid matrix (83). In rare examples some nuclear pleomorphism may occur in the absence of mitoses, adding to the potential confusion with malignancy.

A significant proportion of these lesions arise on the basis of an underlying lesion such as a chondroblastoma, giant cell tumor, or osteoblastoma, so that these should be sought in any case in which the diagnosis of aneurysmal bone cyst is contemplated. Aneurysmal bone cysts are thought to arise on the basis of an arteriovenous malformation that may be acquired as a result of the underlying lesion or for some other reason such as a previous fracture (83).

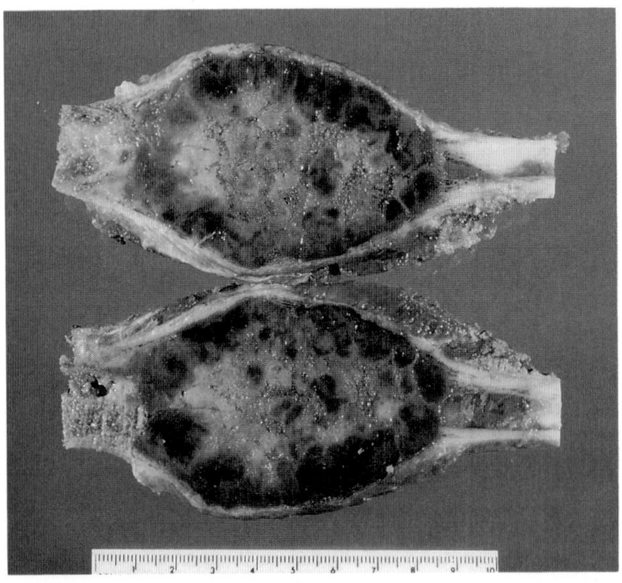

FIG. 22. Solid aneurysmal bone cyst. A hemorrhagic, solid, well-circumscribed lesion expands the midportion of the tibia. No cystic areas are apparent in this lesion, which otherwise contained cells similar to "typical" aneurysmal bone cyst.

An aneurysmal bone cyst must be differentiated from a telangiectatic osteogenic sarcoma, which may also have similar blood lakes, but a careful search of the latter lesion will usually show malignant cells, atypical mitoses, and tumor osteoid production. A solid variant of aneurysmal bone cyst has been described in which the blood lakes are absent or a minor component (Fig. 22), but the cell types present are otherwise similar and comprise mononuclear histiocytic cells, osteoclast-type giant cells, fibroblasts, osteoid, and calcifying fibromyxoid tissue (219). It resembles central giant cell granuloma (83). Aneurysmal bone cysts must also be differentiated from giant cell tumor of bone, with which they may be associated. They occur at a younger age than most giant cell tumors and do not have as many nuclei in the giant cells as the typical giant cell tumor (83).

Aneurysmal bone cysts are benign but are prone to recur after curettage and packing with bone chips. The initial treatment should be conservative but thorough to prevent this recurrence.

Aneurysmal bone cysts are karyotypically normal (202). Familial inheritance has been described (265).

EPITHELIAL TUMORS

Adamantinoma

Adamantinoma is a rare and curious low-grade malignant tumor that involves the tibia in the vast majority of cases, with or without involvement of the adjacent fibula. In children it is commonest in the second decade and is rare prior to this age (83). It is typically a midshaft lesion but may involve the upper metaphysis. Radiographs show a destructive, eccentric, lytic lesion that appears well demarcated but often with extensive surrounding sclerosis (Fig. 23A). It has a lobulated appearance on radiographs and in the gross specimen. In a minority of cases it penetrates the cortex and has a soft tissue component (83).

Histologically adamantinoma of bone shows epithelial differentiation with a pattern very reminiscent of the adamantinoma of the jaw (Fig. 23B). This is composed of lobules of cells that peripherally palisade, have a high nucleocytoplasmic ratio, and surround a central, more stellate area. Sometimes the epithelial component consists of strands of small polygonal cells arrayed in single files within the surrounding fibrous tissue. In other areas or cases there is frank squamous epithelial differentiation. The tumor may also form glandlike spaces, and the epithelium may be spindle-shaped and difficult to recognize without epithelial markers (83). The second important component is the stroma, which is fibroblastic with abundant collagen, resembling in many instances that of fibrous dysplasia. There may be new bone formation, but unlike fibrous dysplasia, the bone is rimmed by active osteoblasts. The mesenchymal component is thus identical to osteofibrous dysplasia, which is thought by some to be a forme fruste or end result of regressed adamantinoma (55).

Adamantinomas are locally aggressive, very slowly progressive, and not infrequently metastasizing, sometimes very late in the course of the disease (83). They metastasize to regional lymph nodes, lungs, and bones (83,137) and thus require radical surgery.

Cytogenetic analysis of adamantinoma in one patient revealed a complex karyotype primarily with multiple aberrations of chromosomes 7 and 13. A t(7;13)(q32;q14) was found in the peripheral blood lymphocytes of the patient and his unaffected father, as well as in the patient's tumor (242). The related lesion, osteofibrous dysplasia, has been reported to contain trisomy 12 in one case and trisomy 7, 8, and 22 in another; trisomy 7 and 12 have also been reported in adamantinoma (26).

Cases of adamantinoma that bear a close resemblance to Ewing's sarcoma have been reported (126,165,263). Because Ewing's sarcomas and peripheral neuroepitheliomas have a capacity for epithelial differentiation (102,233), this is an intriguing observation. However, no cases with alterations of chromosome 22q12, the site of the *EWS* gene, have been reported to date.

Chordoma

Chordoma is an uncommon tumor occurring mostly in adults and sometimes in children (49,187). It accounts

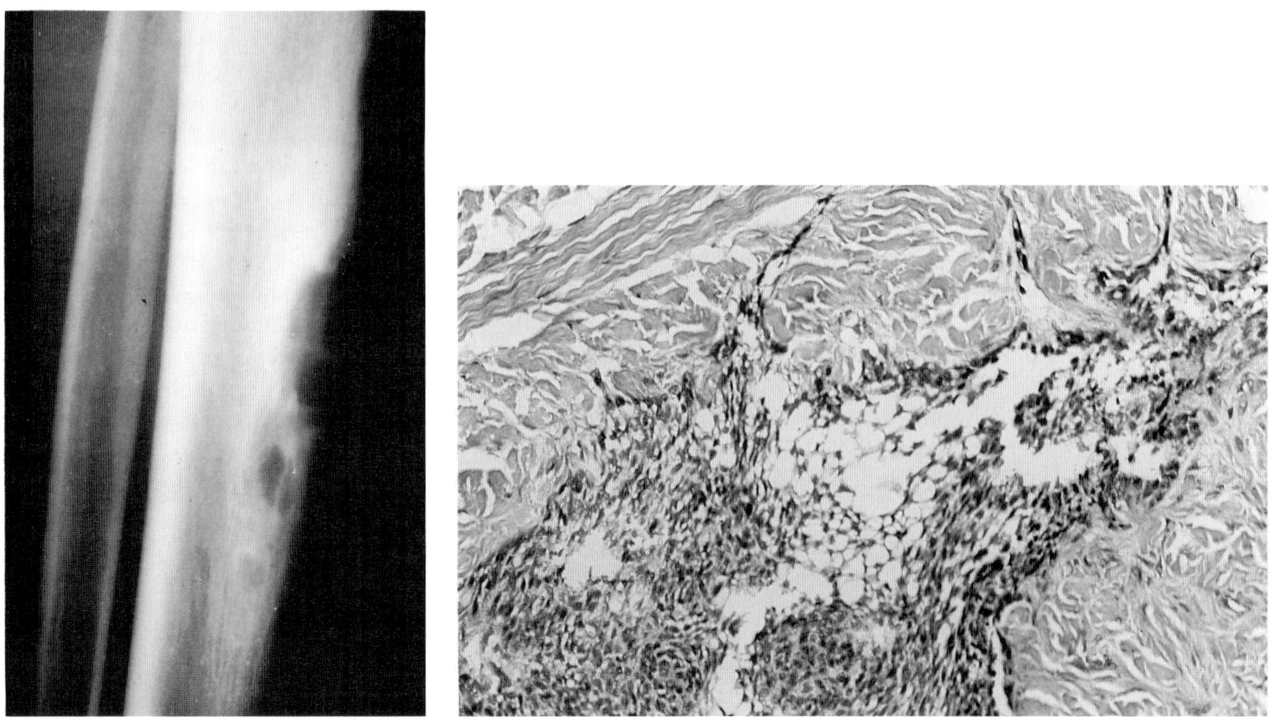

A B

FIG. 23. Adamantinoma of bone. **A.** A destructive, lytic lesion permeates the tibial diaphysis. **B.** Histologically the lesion is composed of nests of epithelial cells embedded in a fibrous stroma. Stellate reticulin, similar to that seen in ameloblastoma and craniopharyngioma, is apparent in the midportion of this epithelial nest. (Part **A** courtesy of Dr. Barry Fletcher, SJCRH.)

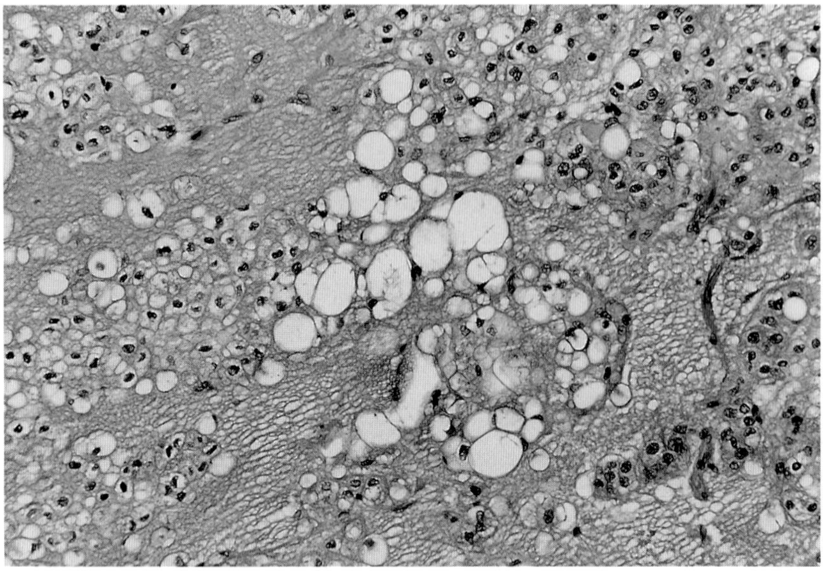

FIG. 24. Chordoma. Cells with clear cytoplasm, focally with a bubblelike configuration, are embedded in a gelatinous matrix.

for 1–4% of all primary bone neoplasms (110,133). The origin of this lesion from notochord remnants is suggested by their common location in the axial skeleton and immunohistochemical and histologic similarities (35,258). Chordomas involve the clival region of the skull, the sacrum, and occasionally the cervical or thoracic vertebrae. Heffelfinger et al. (110) described a neoplasm occurring at the base of the skull that had both chordomatous and chondromatous features and felt that these chondroid chordomas were a separate clinicopathologic entity in that they occurred at a younger age and had a better prognosis. Others have subsequently disputed this hypothesis (33). Nevertheless, intracisternal microtubular aggregates, an ultrastructural feature of myxoid chondrosarcoma, has been described in chordoma and underscores the possible relatedness of these lesions (134,257).

Grossly, chordoma presents as a gelatinous, lobulated mass. Histologically it consists of cords of cohesive epithelioid cells lying in a mucoid matrix and having abundant cytoplasm. Many show marked vacuolation and are called physaliferous cells (Fig. 24). These cells contain glycogen and are positive for epithelial markers such as low molecular weight keratin and epithelial membrane antigen, as well as for S-100 protein, but are negative for vimentin (33). The literature contains conflicting reports of staining patterns of chondroid chordoma, with some claiming that they are all negative for epithelial markers and are therefore low-grade chondrosarcomas (33,272), whereas others demonstrate epithelial positivity in many or all or their cases and claim them to be related to chordomas (133).

In a review of a substantial number of pediatric chordomas, Coffin et al. (49) noted that atypical, high-grade histologic features were sometimes present. They based the diagnosis of these cases primarily on tumor immunophenotype. However, the true identity of these lesions has been questioned (61).

Chordomas are low-grade malignant neoplasms that by virtue of their location are frequently lethal after many years. They may occasionally metastasize or dedifferentiate into a high-grade spindle cell sarcoma (120).

A variety of chromosomal abnormalities have been reported in chordoma. In one study numeric and structural aberrations were present in two cases; both shared rearrangements of chromosome 21q22 (93). Another study of two additional tumors failed to confirm these findings but instead revealed no abnormalities in one case and two separate abnormal clones in another (199). Other cases in older men have revealed complex abnormalities with marker chromosomes (29,64). A series of seven chordomas revealed no abnormalities in three tumors, a t(1;6)(q44;q11) in one, del(2)(p21), del(9)(p13), -10, rearrangements of 12q13, and add(19)(p13) in one, and numerous numeric and structural aberrations in the other two (171). Although there appear to be no common cytogenetic threads as yet, the presence of abnormal ploidy appears to be predictive of behavior (224) or the presence of malignant spindle cells (120).

VASCULAR LESIONS

Hemangioma

Hemangiomas of bone are frequently asymptomatic but may create problems in differential diagnosis. If operated on unawares, they may result in catastrophic hemorrhage.

The typical hemangioma of bone is seen in a vertebral

body in which the radiograph shows coarse vertical striation. On a CT scan this has a coarse, punctate appearance. In other locations such as the facial bones or the skull, the lesion may extend through the cortex and elevate the periosteum to produce a sun ray spiculated appearance very like that seen in osteosarcoma. Hemangiomas may be multiple. Histologically they usually consist of cavernous vascular channels, replacing the normal marrow and lined by a single layer of flattened endothelial cells. It is often difficult to differentiate telangiectasis from a true hemangioma on histologic grounds alone.

Angiomatous change in bone may be associated with marked resorption of bone and replacement by angiomas and fibrosis. This condition is known as "massive osteolysis," "disappearing bone disease," or Gorham's disease (217). In children this condition may have a variety of clinical consequences, including respiratory distress (166), and affects a wide range of bones (111). Most patients show involvement of either the femur or ribs alone or with vertebral disease (234). The disease is generally progressive but may be self-limited (74). Because of the severe bone destruction and frequent multifocality of the process, malignancy may be a prime diagnostic consideration (168). However, the lesion consists of a nonneoplastic-appearing proliferation of stromal and vascular tissues (87).

Epithelioid Hemangioendothelioma/Histiocytoid Hemangioma

A curious fact about some cases termed hemangioendothelioma in the past was that in spite of their being multicentric they had a better prognosis than other vasoformative lesions that were solitary. Subsequently, vasoformative tumors with plump endothelial cells that had a tendency to recur and behave in an aggressive but low-grade manner were included under the blanket term of histiocytoid hemangioma by Rosai (215) and as hemangioendotheliomas by other workers (279). Others have used the term hemangioendothelioma as synonymous with angiosarcoma. There is, however, a group of vascular neoplasms with behavior intermediate between hemangioma and angiosarcoma that are best designated as hemangioendothelioma. They are frequently multicentric and consist of arborizing vascular structures lined by plump epithelioid or histiocytoid endothelial cells. These vessels are usually accompanied by an infiltrate of inflammatory cells including many eosinophils as well as lymphocytes. The inflammatory cells may obscure the true nature of the lesion resulting in its confusion with an inflammatory lesion such as chronic osteomyelitis. These tumors tend to recur if incompletely excised and are often multicentric. The prognosis in these patients is generally excellent.

Angiosarcoma of Bone

Angiosarcoma of bone is a rare malignant tumor. A smattering of pediatric cases have been described (21,267,285). Some cases appear to have arisen from chronic osteomyelitis (12). The radiographic appearance is that of multiple coalescing lytic defects with a permeative, destructive pattern. Histologically they show the features of fully malignant angiosarcoma of soft tissue, with variably developed, arborizing vascular channels and solid sheets of epithelioid cells. In the channels they are often multilayered and have a cobblestone appearance. They show nuclear atypia and mitoses are usually readily recognizable. They may stain for endothelial markers such as CD31, Factor VIII–related antigen, and CD34 and are to be distinguished from metastatic carcinoma. Treatment needs to be radical surgical resection, if feasible, and/or radiation therapy. Chemotherapy may also be useful. There is, however, insufficient information available for one to know the effectiveness of either radiation therapy or chemotherapy (83).

REACTIVE BONE CONDITIONS THAT SIMULATE NEOPLASMS

A variety of reactive bone lesions, such as osteomyelitis or fracture callus, may simulate neoplasia and in fact are far more common. Typically, clinical or historical information such as recent trauma or fever calls attention to the true nature of these lesions. Nevertheless, on occasion there may be unrealized trauma or infection, so that the surgical pathologists must be ever astute as to the histologic features of these lesions. In these instances, there is an unfortunate opportunity for the treatment to be far worse than the disease, and a number of malpractice suits have been based on this fact.

The prototypic reactive condition is the fracture callus. This reparative lesion proceeds from acute trauma that disrupts the cortex and leads to both scarring and osteogenesis. As the wound heals, there is osteoid formation that begins with the remnants of periosteum and may be accompanied by chondroid metaplasia of the reparative tissues. One cardinal feature is the presence of hemorrhage from the traumatic episode, and this sign persists for a prolonged period as hemosiderosis. The osteoid formation can be exuberant and lead to disturbing radiographic features (108) and an even more unsettling proliferation of reactive osteoblasts and young bone (Fig. 25). These features can trap an unwary pathologist into a diagnosis of osteosarcoma, which can be avoided if one pays careful attention to the reactive, nonneoplastic cytologic features of the osteoblasts and the presence of adjacent fibrosis and hemosiderosis.

A related lesion is periostitis ossificans, which is a similar traumatic lesion produced by periosteal injury. The

A

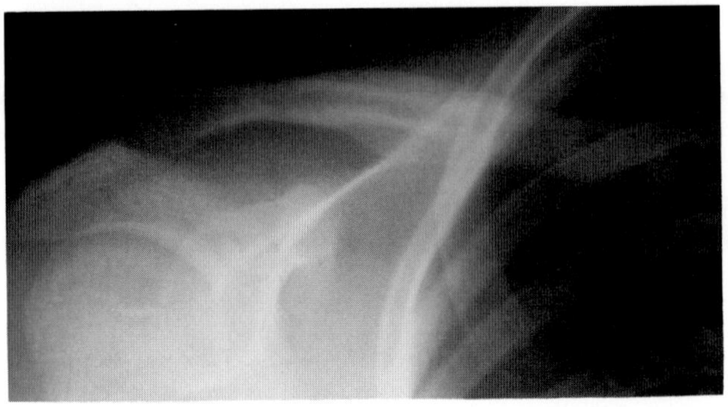

B

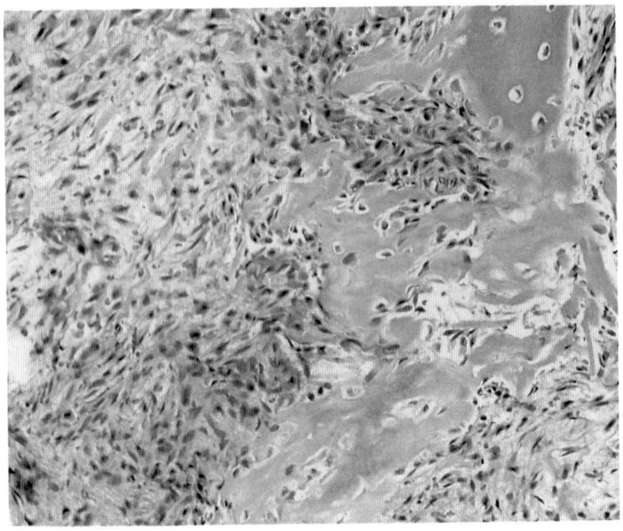

FIG. 25. Fracture callus simulating malignancy. **A.** A lesion causes marked periosteal elevation in the midclavicle. **B.** Osteoid formation is associated with reactive-appearing granulation tissue. Further questioning of this adolescent female revealed that she was a saxophone player in a marching band and carried her instrument strapped across this shoulder. (Part **A** courtesy of Dr. Barry Fletcher, SJCRH.)

disrupted periosteum again reacts by bone formation, and the resultant spiculation may yield a disturbing radiographic picture (71). Again, the presence of reactive changes in the biopsied tissues and the lack of malignant cytologic atypia are histologic clues to the true nature of this lesion.

Osteomyelitis, particularly chronic osteomyelitis, may also produce a fibrotic, reactive lesion with periosteal elevation, irregular spiculation, and poorly defined sclerosis and lysis (37,181). The nidus of these infections may come from a variety of clinically unrecognized sources, and a host of organisms may be causative (270). Staphylococci are frequent initiators of childhood osteomyelitis, and salmonella infections may be seen with hemoglobinopathies. Multifocal involvement may be recognized on bone scans and resemble metastatic disease. On the other hand, neoplasms such as Ewing's sarcoma may mimic osteomyelitis and lead to delayed diagnosis, so that early biopsy is advisable in questionable cases. Histologically, one encounters the classic features of osteomyelitis: sequestrum, or necrotic bone, and involucrum, or the surrounding reactive bone. Thus, there is a mixture of bony trabeculae with fragmentation and empty lacunae (necrosis), widened trabeculae with osteoblastic rimming (reactive new bone), and chronic inflammatory cells (lymphocytes and plasma cells) and fibrosis. Attempts to isolate a microbial culprit may be negative (270).

Another reactive, tumorlike condition is osteitis fibrosa cystica, or the brown tumor. This often unifocal lesion is a consequence of primary or secondary hyperparathyroidism and results from focal bony resorption (13). Microfractures in the weakened bone lead to hemorrhage, and the resultant hemosiderosis gives the lesion its name, "brown tumor" (150). The synonym, osteitis fibrosa cystica, graphically describes the histologic features of these lesions, which contain a mixed inflammatory cell and fibroblastic infiltrate and are often cystic. Multinucleated osteoclasts are prominent features and create a close simulation of central giant cell granuloma or giant cell tumor. Thus, one must always check the patient's serum calcium, phosphorus, and parathormone to avoid unnecessary surgery on these lesions (141,262).

ACKNOWLEDGMENT

Supported in part by Cancer Center Support CORE grant P30 CA21765 and by American Lebanese Syrian Associated Charities (ALSAC).

REFERENCES

1. Alappat JP, Pillai AM, Prasanna D, Sambasivan M. Giant cell reparative granuloma of the craniofacial complex: case report and review of the literature. *Br J Neurosurg* 1992;6:71–74.
2. Alho A, Skjeldal S, Melvik JE, Pettersen EO, Larsen TE. The clinical importance of DNA synthesis and aneuploidy in bone and soft tissue tumours. *Anticancer Res* 1993;13:2383–2387.
3. Alho A, Skjeldal S, Pettersen EO, Melvik JE, Larsen TE. Aneuploidy in benign tumors and nonneoplastic lesions of musculoskeletal tissues. *Cancer* 1994;73:1200–1205.
4. Ali NN, Harrison MA, Rowe J, Teich NM. Spectrum of osteoblastic differentiation in new cell lines derived from spontaneous murine osteosarcomas. *Bone* 1993;14:847–858.
5. Allegranza A, Barbareschi M, Solero CL, Fornari M, Lasio G. Primary lymphohistiocytic tumour of bone: a primary osseous localization of Rosai–Dorfman disease. *Histopathology* 1991;18: 83–86.
6. Andreassen A, Oyjord T, Hovig E, et al. p53 Abnormalities in different subtypes of human sarcomas. *Cancer Res* 1993;53: 468–471.
7. Arata MA, Peterson HA, Dahlin DC. Pathological fractures through non-ossifying fibromas. Review of the Mayo Clinic experience. *J Bone Joint Surg* 1981;63:980–988.
8. Asada Y, Suzuki I, Suzuki M, Fukushima M. Atypical multiple benign osteoblastomas accompanied by simple bone cysts. A case report. *J Craniomaxillofac Surg* 1991;19:166–171.
9. Ascoli V, Facciolo F, Muda AO, Martelli M, Nardi F. Chondroblastoma of the rib presenting as an intrathoracic mass Report of a case with fine needle aspiration biopsy, immunocyto-

chemistry and electron microscopy. *Acta Cytol* 1992;36: 423–429.

10. Asirvatham R, Rooney RJ, Watts HG. Ollier's disease with secondary chondrosarcoma associated with ovarian tumour. A case report. *Int Orthop* 1991;15:393–395.
11. Asnes RS, Berdon WE, Bassett CA. Hypophosphatemic rickets in an adolescent cured by excision of a nonossifying fibroma. *Clin Pediatr (Phila)* 1981;20:646–648.
12. Bacchini P, Calderoni P, Gherlinzoni F, Gualtieri G. Angiosarcoma in chronic osteomyelitis. *Ital J Orthop Traumatol* 1984;10: 393–398.
13. Bassler T, Wong ET, Brynes RK. Osteitis fibrosa cystica simulating metastatic tumor: an almost-forgotten relationship. *Am J Clin Pathol* 1993;100:697–700.
14. Bauer HCF, Kreicbergs A, Silfverswärd C, Tribukait B. DNA analysis in the differential diagnosis of osteosarcoma. *Cancer* 1988;61:2532–2540.
15. Bertoni F, Unni KK, Beabout JW, Ebersold MJ. Giant cell tumor of the skull. *Cancer* 1992;70:1124–1132.
16. Betts NJ, Stewart JC, Fonseca RJ, Scott RF. Multiple central giant cell lesions with a Noonan-like phenotype. *Oral Surg Oral Med Oral Pathol* 1993;76:601–607.
17. Biegel JA, Womer RB, Emanuel BS. Complex karyotypes in a series of pediatric osteosarcomas. *Cancer Genet Cytogenet* 1989;38:89–100.
18. Bjornsson J, Unni KK, Dahlin DC, Beabout JW, Sim FH. Clear cell chondrosarcoma of bone. Observations in 47 cases. *Am J Surg Pathol* 1984;8:223–230.
19. Bleiweiss IJ, Klein MJ. Chondromyxoid fibroma: report of six cases with immunohistochemical studies. *Mod Pathol* 1990;3: 664–666.
20. Bloem JL, Kroon HM. Osseous lesions. *Radiol Clin North Am* 1993;31:261–278.
21. Bollobas B, Hauk I. Nebenhohlen-Angiosarkom in der Pubertat. *HNO* 1966;14:343–346.
22. Bonetti F, Pelosi G, Martignoni G, et al. Peripheral giant cell granuloma: evidence for osteoclastic differentiation. *Oral Surg Oral Med Oral Pathol* 1990;70:471–475.
23. Brachman DG, Hallahan DE, Beckett MA, Yandell DW, Weichselbaum RR. p53 gene mutations and abnormal retinoblastoma protein in radiation-induced human sarcomas. *Cancer Res* 1991;51:6393–6396.
24. Brecher ME, Franklin WA, Simon MA. Immunohistochemical study of mononuclear phagocyte antigens in giant cell tumor of bone. *Am J Pathol* 1986;125:252–257.
25. Bridge JA, Bhatia PS, Anderson JR, Neff JR. Biologic and clinical significance of cytogenetic and molecular cytogenetic abnormalities in benign and malignant cartilaginous lesions. *Cancer Genet Cytogenet* 1993;69:79–90.
26. Bridge JA, Dembinski A, DeBoer J, Travis J, Neff JR. Clonal chromosomal abnormalities in osteofibrous dysplasia. Implications for histopathogenesis and its relationship with adamantinoma. *Cancer* 1994;73:1746–1752.
27. Bridge JA, Neff JR, Mouron BJ. Giant cell tumor of bone. Chromosomal analysis of 48 specimens and review of the literature. *Cancer Genet Cytogenet* 1992;58:2–13.
28. Bridge JA, Persons DL, Neff JR, Bhatia P. Clonal karyotypic aberrations in enchondromas. *Cancer Detect Prev* 1992;16: 215–219.
29. Bridge JA, Pickering D, Neff JR. Cytogenetic and molecular cytogenetic analysis of sacral chordoma. *Cancer Genet Cytogenet* 1994;75:23–25.
30. Bridge JA, Rosenthal H, Sanger WG, Neff JR. Desmoplastic fibroma arising in fibrous dysplasia. Chromosomal analysis and review of the literature. *Clin Orthop* 1989;272–278.
31. Bridge JA, Sanger WG, Neff JR. Translocations involving chromosomes 2 and 13 in benign and malignant cartilaginous neoplasms. *Cancer Genet Cytogenet* 1989;38:83–88.
32. Brodeur GM, Caces J, Williams DL, Look AT, Pratt CB. Osteosarcoma, fibrous dysplasia, and a chromosomal abnormality in a 3- year-old child. *Cancer* 1980;46:1197–1201.
33. Brooks JJ, LiVolsi VA, Trojanowski JQ. Does chondroid chordoma exist? *Acta Neuropathol (Berl)* 1987;72:229–235.
34. Bulow S, Holm NV, Sondergaard JO, Witt IN, Tetens G, Sndergaard JO. Mandibular osteomas in unaffected sibs and children of patients with familial polyposis coli. *Scand J Gastroenterol* 1986;21:744–748.
35. Burger PC, Makek M, Kleihues P. Tissue polypeptide antigen staining of the chordoma and notochordal remnants. *Acta Neuropathol (Berl)* 1986;70:269–272.
36. Butler MG, Dahir GA, Schwartz HS. Molecular analysis of transforming growth factor beta in giant cell tumor of bone. *Cancer Genet Cytogenet* 1993;66:108–112.
37. Cabanela ME, Sim FH, Beabout JW, Dahlin DC. Osteomyelitis appearing as neoplasms. A diagnostic problem. *Arch Surg* 1974;109:68–72.
38. Campanacci M. Osteofibrous dysplasia of long bones a new clinical entity. *Ital J Orthop Traumatol* 1976;2:221–237.
39. Campanacci M, Laus M. Osteofibrous dysplasia of the tibia and fibula. *J Bone Joint Surg [Am]* 1981;63:367–375.
40. Campanacci M, Olmi R. Fibrosarcoma of bone. A study of 114 cases. *Ital J Orthop Traumatol* 1977;3:199–206.
41. Campannaci M. *Bone and Soft Tissue Tumors.* Wien: Springer-Verlag, 1990.
42. Candeliere GA, Glorieux FH, Prud'homme J, St-Arnaud R. Increased expression of the c-fos proto-oncogene in bone from patients with fibrous dysplasia. *N Engl J Med* 1995;332:1546–1551.
43. Cannon SR, Sweetnam DR. Multiple chondrosarcomas in dyschondroplasia (Ollier's disease). *Cancer* 1985;55:836–840.
44. Capanna R, Bertoni F, Bacchini P, Bacci G, Guerra A, Campanacci M. Malignant fibrous histiocytoma of bone. The experience at the Rizzoli Institute: report of 90 cases. *Cancer* 1984;54: 177–187.
45. Carl W, Herrera L. Dental and bone abnormalities in patients with familial polyposis coli. *Semin Surg Oncol* 1987;3:77–83.
46. Chadwick BL, Aldred MJ. An unusual giant cell lesion in a child with vitamin D-resistant rickets. *Int J Paediatr Dent* 1992;2: 41–45.
47. Chigira M, Maehara S, Arita S, Udagawa E. The aetiology and treatment of simple bone cysts. *J Bone Joint Surg [Br]* 1983;65: 633–637.
48. Chou P, Mehta S, Gonzalez-Crussi F. Chondrosarcoma of the head in children. *Pediatr Pathol* 1990;10:945–958.
49. Coffin CM, Swanson PE, Wick MR, Dehner LP. Chordoma in childhood and adolescence: a clinicopathologic analysis of 12 cases. *Arch Pathol Lab Med* 1993;117:927–933.
50. Cohen EK, Kressel HY, Frank TS, Fallon M, Burk DL, Jr., Dalinka MK, Schiebler ML. Hyaline cartilage-origin bone and soft-tissue neoplasms: MR appearance and histologic correlation. *Radiology* 1988;167:477–481.
51. Cohen MM, Jr., Gorlin RJ. Noonan-like/multiple giant cell lesion syndrome. *Am J Med Genet* 1991;40:159–166.
52. Coppes MJ, Patte C, Couanet D, et al. Childhood malignant lymphoma of bone. *Med Pediatr Oncol* 1991;19:22–27.
53. Cossetto D, Nade S, Blackwell J. Malignant fibrous histiocytoma in Paget's disease of bone. A report of seven cases. *Aust N Z J Surg* 1992;62:52–55.
54. Cox JV, Balaban EP, Demian SE, Sheehan RG. An eosinophilic fibrohistiocytic lesion of bone marrow in a patient with Hodgkin's disease: a potential for morphologic confusion. *Cancer* 1991;68: 1824–1827.
55. Czerniak B, Rojas-Corona RR, Dorfman HD. Morphologic diversity of long bone adamantinoma. The concept of differentiated (regressing) adamantinoma and its relationship to osteofibrous dysplasia. *Cancer* 1989;64:2319–2334.
56. Czerwinski E, Skolarczyk A, Frasik W. Malignant fibrous histiocytoma in the course of chronic osteomyelitis. *Arch Orthop Trauma Surg* 1991;111:58–60.
57. Çolak A, Berker M, Saglam S, Önol B. Chondrosarcoma of the temporal bone in an infant: Case report and review of the literature. *Neurosurgery* 1992;31:956–957.
58. Dahir GA, Vnencak-Jones CL, Schwartz HS, Butler MG. Dosage and allelic restriction fragment studies and PCR analysis of the H-ras locus in giant cell tumor of bone. *Cancer Genet Cytogenet* 1994;74:95–98.
59. Dahlin DC, Ivins JC. Benign chondroblastoma. A study of 125 cases. *Cancer* 1972;30:401–413.

60. Dahlin DC, Unni KK. *Bone Tumors: General Aspects and Data on 8,542 Cases.* 4th ed. Springfield, IL: Charles C Thomas; 1986.
61. Dahlin DC, Unni KK. Chordoma (letter). *Arch Pathol Lab Med* 1994;118:596–597.
62. Davis GB, Tideman H. Multiple recurrent central giant cell granulomas of the jaws. Case report. *J Maxillofac Surg* 1977;5:127–129.
63. Davis JP, Archer DJ, Fisher C, Wimalawansa SJ, Baldwin D. Multiple recurrent giant cell lesions associated with high circulating levels of parathyroid hormone-related peptide in a young adult. *Br J Oral Maxillofac Surg* 1991;29:102–105.
64. DeBoer JM, Neff JR, Bridge JA. Cytogenetics of sacral chordoma. *Cancer Genet Cytogenet* 1992;64:95–96.
65. Dehner LP. Tumors of the mandible and maxilla in children. I. Clinicopathologic study of 46 histologically benign lesions. *Cancer* 1973;31:364–384.
66. Dehner LP. *Pediatric Surgical Pathology.* 2nd ed. Baltimore: Williams and Wilkins; 1987.
67. Desai P, Steiner GC. Ultrastructure of brown tumor of hyperparathyroidism. *Ultrastruct Pathol* 1990;14:505–511.
68. deSantos LA, Spjut HJ. Periosteal chondroma: a radiographic spectrum. *Skeletal Radiol* 1981;6:15–20.
69. Dijkhuizen T, Van den Berg E, Molenaar WM, et al. Cytogenetics as a tool in the histologic subclassification of chondrosarcomas. *Cancer Genet Cytogenet* 1994;76:100–105.
70. Dobashi Y, Sugimura H, Sato A, et al. Possible association of p53 overexpression and mutation with high-grade chondrosarcoma. *Diagn Mol Pathol* 1993;2:257–263.
71. Donoghue V, Daneman A, Mancer K, Krajbich I. CT features of reactive periostitis in the humerus: a lesion resembling myositis ossificans. *J Comput Assist Tomogr* 1985;9:401–403.
72. Dorfman HD, Czerniak B. Bone cancers. *Cancer* 1995;75:203–210.
73. Dorfman HD, Weiss SW. Borderline osteoblastic tumors: problems in the differential diagnosis of aggressive osteoblastoma and low-grade osteosarcoma. *Semin Diagn Pathol* 1984;1:215–234.
74. Dunbar SF, Rosenberg A, Mankin H, Rosenthal D, Suit HD. Gorham's massive osteolysis: the role of radiation therapy and a review of the literature. *Int J Radiat Oncol Biol Phys* 1993;26:491–497.
75. Duncan BR, Dohner VA, Priest JH. The Gardner syndrome: need for early diagnosis. *J Pediatr* 1968;72:497–505.
76. Edel G, Ueda Y, Nakanishi J, et al. Chondroblastoma of bone. A clinical, radiological, light and immunohistochemical study. *Virchows Arch A Histopathol Anat* 1992;421:355–366.
77. Egeler RM, Thompson RC, Jr., Voute PA, Nesbit ME, Jr. Intralesional infiltration of corticosteroids in localized Langerhans' cell histiocytosis. *J Pediatr Orthop* 1992;12:811–814.
78. El-Khoury GY, Bassett GS. Symptomatic bursa formation with osteochondromas. *AJR* 1979;133:895–898.
79. Elmore SM, Cantrell WC. Maffucci's syndrome. Case report with a normal karyotype. *J Bone Joint Surg [Am]* 1966;48:1607–1613.
80. Elsheikh T, Silverman JF, Wakely PE, Jr., Holbrook CT, Joshi VV. Fine-needle aspiration cytology of Langerhans' cell histiocytosis (eosinophilic granuloma) of bone in children. *Diagn Cytopathol* 1991;7:261–266.
81. Enneking WF, Kagan A. "Skip" metastases in osteosarcoma. *Cancer* 1975;36:2192–2205.
82. Evans GA, Park WM. Familial multiple non-osteogenic fibromata. *J Bone Joint Surg [Br]* 1978;60-B:416–419.
83. Fechner RE, Mills SE. *Tumors of the Bones and Joints.* Fascicle 8. Washington, DC: Armed Forces Institute of Pathology; 1993.
84. Finci R, Günhan Ö, Uçmakli E, Sarlak Ö. Multiple and familial malignant fibrous histiocytoma of bone. *J Bone Joint Surg [Br]* 1990;72A:295–298.
85. Flanagan AM, Nui B, Tinkler SMB, Horton MA, Williams DM, Chambers TJ. The multinucleate cells in giant cell granulomas of the jaw are osteoclasts. *Cancer* 1988;62:1139–1145.
86. Forte V, Shimotakahara S, Crysdale WS, Thorner P. Recurring giant-cell granuloma at the site of previous radiation therapy. *J Otolaryngol* 1990;19:285–287.
87. Frederiksen NL, Wesley RK, Sciubba JJ, Helfrick J. Massive osteolysis of the maxillofacial skeleton: a clinical, radiographic, histologic, and ultrastructural study. *Oral Surg Oral Med Oral Pathol* 1983;55:470–480.
88. Fukunaga M, Nikaido T, Shimoda T, Ushigome S, Nakamori K. A flow cytometric DNA analysis of giant cell tumors of bone including two cases with malignant transformation. *Cancer* 1992;70:1886–1894.
89. Gallie BL, Dunn JM, Chan HS, Hamel PA, Phillips RA. The genetics of retinoblastoma. Relevance to the patient. *Pediatr Clin North Am* 1991;38:299–315.
90. Garrison RC, Unni KK, McLeod RA, Pritchard DJ, Dahlin DC. Chondrosarcoma arising in osteochondroma. *Cancer* 1982;49:1890–1897.
91. Gaucher AA, Regent DM, Gillet PM, Pere PG, Aymard BM, Clement V. Case report 656: Malignant fibrous histiocytoma in a previous bone infarct. *Skeletal Radiol* 1991;20:137–140.
92. Gaudin P, Juvin R, Rozand Y, et al. Skeletal involvement as the initial disease manifestation in Hodgkin's disease: a review of 6 cases. *J Rheumatol* 1992;19:146–152.
93. Gibas Z, Miettinen M, Sandberg AA. Chromosomal abnormalities in two chordomas. *Cancer Genet Cytogenet* 1992;58:169–173.
94. Giedion A, Kesztler R, Muggiasca F. The widened spectrum of multiple cartilaginous exostosis (MCE). *Pediatr Radiol* 1975;3:93–100.
95. Giovannini M, Selleri L, Biegel JA, Scotlandi K, Emanuel BS, Evans GA. Interphase cytogenetics for the detection of the t(11;22)(q24; q12) in small round cell tumors. *J Clin Invest* 1992;90:1911–1918.
96. Giudici MA, Moser RP, Jr., Kransdorf MJ. Cartilaginous bone tumors. *Radiol Clin North Am* 1993;31:237–259.
97. Glasser DB, Lane JM, Huvos AG, Marcove RC, Rosen G. Survival, prognosis, and therapeutic response in osteogenic sarcoma: The Memorial Hospital experience. *Cancer* 1992;69:698–708.
98. Goldenberg RR, Campbell CJ, Bonfiglio M. Giant-cell tumor of bone. An analysis of two hundred and eighteen cases. *J Bone Joint Surg [Am]* 1970;52:619–664.
99. Greenspan A. Bone island (enostosis): current concept—a review. *Skeletal Radiol* 1995;24:111–115.
100. Greenspan A, Steiner G, Knutzon R. Bone island (enostosis): clinical significance and radiologic and pathologic correlations. *Skeletal Radiol* 1991;20:85–90.
101. Haag M, Adler CP. Malignant fibrous histiocytoma in association with hip replacement. *J Bone Joint Surg [Br]* 1989;71:701
102. Hachitanda Y, Tsuneyoshi M, Enjoji M, Nakagawara A, Ikeda K. Congenital primitive neuroectodermal tumor with epithelial and glial differentiation: An ultrastructural and immunohistochemical study. *Arch Pathol Lab Med* 1990;114:101–105.
103. Hanna SL, Parham DM, Fairclough DL, Meyer WH, Le AH, Fletcher BD. Assessment of osteosarcoma response to preoperative chemotherapy using dynamic FLASH gadolinium-DTPA-enhanced magnetic resonance mapping. *Invest Radiol* 1992;27:367–373.
104. Hansen MF. Molecular genetic considerations in osteosarcoma. *Clin Orthop* 1991;237–246.
105. Happle R. The McCune–Albright syndrome: a lethal gene surviving by mosaicism. *Clin Genet* 1986;29:321–324.
106. Harris M. Central giant cell granulomas of the jaws regress with calcitonin therapy. *Br J Oral Maxillofac Surg* 1993;31:89–94.
107. Hartley AL, Birch JM, Marsden HB, Harris M. Malignant melanoma in families of children with osteosarcoma, chondrosarcoma, and adrenal cortical carcinoma. *J Med Genet* 1987;24:664–668.
108. Hayes CW, Conway WF, Sundaram M. Misleading aggressive MR imaging appearance of some benign musculoskeletal lesions. *Radiographics* 1992;12:1119–1134.
109. Hecht JT, Hogue D, Strong LC, Hansen MF, Blanton SH, Wagner M. Hereditary multiple exostosis and chondrosarcoma: linkage to chromosome 11 and loss of heterozygosity for EXT-linked markers on chromosomes 11 and 8. *Am J Hum Genet* 1995;56:1125–1131.
110. Heffelfinger MJ, Dahlin DC, MacCarty CS, Beabout JW. Chordomas and cartilaginous tumors at the skull base. *Cancer* 1973;32:410–420.
111. Heffez L, Doku HC, Carter BL, Feeney JE. Perspectives on mas-

sive osteolysis. Report of a case and review of the literature. *Oral Surg Oral Med Oral Pathol* 1983;55:331–343.

112. Helio H, Karaharju E, Bohling T, Nordling S. Giant cell tumours of bone. A DNA-flow cytometric study. *Eur J Surg Oncol* 1994;20:200–206.
113. Hicks DG, Gokan T, O'Keefe RJ, et al. Primary lymphoma of bone: correlation of magnetic resonance imaging features with cytokine production by tumor cells. *Cancer* 1995;75:973–980.
114. Hiddemann W, Roessner A, Wormann B, et al. Tumor heterogeneity in osteosarcoma as identified by flow cytometry. *Cancer* 1987;59:324–328.
115. Hillerup S, Hjorting-Hansen E. Aneurysmal bone cyst—simple bone cyst, two aspects of the same pathologic entity? *Int J Oral Surg* 1978;7:16–22.
116. Hinrichs SH, Jaramillo MA, Gumerlock PH, Gardner MB, Lewis JP, Freeman AE. Myxoid chondrosarcoma with a translocation involving chromosomes 9 and 22. *Cancer Genet Cytogenet* 1985;14:219–226.
117. Hirabayashi Y, Yoshida MA, Ikeuchi T, et al. Chromosome rearrangements at 12q13 in two cases of chondrosarcomas. *Cancer Genet Cytogenet* 1992;60:35–40.
118. Hoffman S, Jacoway JR, Krolls SO. *Atlas of Tumor Pathology. Second Series, Fascicle 24. Intraosseous and Parosteal Tumors of the Jaws.* Washington, DC: Armed Forces Institute of Pathology; 1987.
119. Honoki K, Tsutsumi M, Tsujiuchi T, et al. Expression of the transin, c-fos, and c-jun genes in rat transplantable osteosarcomas and malignant fibrous histiocytomas. *Mol Carcinog* 1992;6:122–128.
120. Hruban RH, Traganos F, Reuter VE, Huvos AG. Chordomas with malignant spindle cell components. A DNA flow cytometric and immunohistochemical study with histogenetic implications. *Am J Pathol* 1990;137:435–447.
121. Huang TS, Green AD, Beattie CW, Das Gupta TK. Monocyte-macrophage lineage of giant cell tumor of bone. Establishment of a multinucleated cell line. *Cancer* 1993;71:1751–1760.
122. Hudson TM, Stiles RG, Monson DK. Fibrous lesions of bone. *Radiol Clin North Am* 1993;31:279–297.
123. Huvos AG, Higinbotham NL. Primary fibrosarcoma of bone. A clinicopathologic study of 130 patients. *Cancer* 1975;35:837–847.
124. Inwards CY, Unni KK, Beabout JW, Sim FH. Desmoplastic fibroma of bone. *Cancer* 1991;68:1978–1983.
125. Ishida T, Dorfman HD. Massive chondroid differentiation in fibrous dysplasia of bone (fibrocartilaginous dysplasia). *Am J Surg Pathol* 1993;17:924–930.
126. Ishida T, Kikuchi F, Oka T, et al. Case report 727. Juxtacortical adamantinoma of humerus (simulating Ewing tumor). *Skeletal Radiol* 1992;21:205–209.
127. Jaffe HL. *Tumors and Tumorous Conditions of the Bones and Joints.* Philadelphia: Lea and Febiger; 1958.
128. Jaffe HL, Lichtenstein L. Benign chondroblastoma of bone: a reinterpretation of the so-called calcifying or chondromatous giant cell tumor. *Am J Pathol* 1942;18:969–991.
129. Jaffe HL, Lichtenstein L. Chondromyxoid fibroma of bone: a distinctive benign tumor likely to be mistaken especially for chondrosarcoma. *Arch Pathol* 1948;45:541–551.
130. Jagasia A, Block J, Diaz M, Olopade O, Nobori T, Gitelis S, Iyer A. Cytogenetic and molecular characterization of human chondrosarcomas (Meeting abstract). *Proc Annu Meet Am Soc Clin Oncol* 1993;12:A297.
131. Jagasia A, Block J, Porterfield B, Diaz M, Olopade O, Gitelis S, Iyer A. Induction of senescence in a chondrosarcoma cell line by microcell transfer of human chromosome 9 (Meeting abstract). *Proc Annu Meet Am Assoc Cancer Res* 1993;34:A630.
132. Jeffree GM, Price CH. Metastatic spread of fibrosarcoma of bone; A report on forty-nine cases, and a comparison with osteosarcoma. *J Bone Joint Surg [Br]* 1976;58-B:418–425.
133. Jeffrey PB, Biava CG, Davis RL. Chondroid chordoma. A hyalinized chordoma without cartilaginous differentiation. *Am J Clin Pathol* 1995;103:271–279.
134. Jeffrey PB, Davis RL, Biava C, Rosenblum M. Microtubule aggregates in a clival chordoma. *Arch Pathol Lab Med* 1993;117:1055–1057.
135. Kahn LB, Wood FM, Ackerman LV. Malignant chondroblastoma. Report of two cases and review of the literature. *Arch Pathol* 1969;88:371–376.
136. Kaugars GE, Niamtu J, 3d, Svirsky JA, Niamtu J. Cherubism: diagnosis, treatment, and comparison with central giant cell granulomas and giant cell tumors. *Oral Surg Oral Med Oral Pathol* 1992;73:369–374.
137. Keeney GL, Unni KK, Beabout JW, Pritchard DJ. Adamantinoma of long bones: a clinicopathologic study of 85 cases. *Cancer* 1989;64:730–737.
138. Khatib ZA, Matsushime H, Valentine M, Shapiro DN, Sherr CJ, Look AT. Coamplification of the CDK4 gene with MDM2 and GLI in human sarcomas. *Cancer Res* 1993;53:5535–5541.
139. Kitano M, Landini G, Semba I, Urago A, Sugihara K, Mukai H, Yamashita S. Eosinophilic granuloma showing rapid regression. Report of a mandibular case with application of a modified PNA staining method for demonstration of Langerhans-type histiocytes. *Acta Pathol Jpn* 1990;40:588–595.
140. Kito M, Moriya H, Mikata A, et al. Establishment of a cell line from a human giant cell tumor of bone. *Clin Orthop* 1993;353–360.
141. Knezevic G, Uglesic V, Kobler P, Svajhler T, Bagatin M. Primary hyperparathyroidism: evaluation of different treatments of jaw lesions based on case reports. *Br J Oral Maxillofac Surg* 1991;29:185–188.
142. Knuutila S, Larramendy M, Ruutu T, Paetau A, Heinonen K, Mahlamaki E. Analysis of phenotype and genotype of individual cells in neoplasms. *Cancer Genet Cytogenet* 1993;68:104–113.
143. Komiya S, Tsuzuki K, Mangham DC, Sugiyama M, Inoue A. Oxygen scavengers in simple bone cysts. *Clin Orthop* 1994;199–206.
144. Kurt AM, Unni KK, McLeod RA, Pritchard DJ. Low-grade intraosseous osteosarcoma. *Cancer* 1990;65:1418–1428.
145. Kurt AM, Unni KK, Sim FH, McLeod RA. Chondroblastoma of bone. *Hum Pathol* 1989;20:965–976.
146. Kyriakos M. Soft tissue implantation of chondromyxoid fibroma. *Am J Surg Pathol* 1979;3:363–372.
147. Kyriakos M, Land VJ, Penning HL, Parker SG. Metastatic chondroblastoma. Report of a fatal case with a review of the literature on atypical, aggressive, and malignant chondroblastoma. *Cancer* 1985;55:1770–1789.
148. Ladanyi M, Traganos F, Huvos AG. Benign metastasizing giant cell tumors of bone. A DNA flow cytometric study. *Cancer* 1989;64:1521–1526.
149. Le Merrer M, Legeai-Mallet L, Jeannin PM, et al. A gene for hereditary multiple exostoses maps to chromosome 19p. *Hum Mol Genet* 1994;3:717–722.
150. Levine MR, Chu A, Abdul-Karim FW. Brown tumor and secondary hyperparathyroidism. *Arch Ophthalmol* 1991;109:847–849.
151. Lewis RJ, Ketcham AS. Maffucci's syndrome: functional and neoplastic significance. Case report and review of the literature. *J Bone Joint Surg [Am]* 1973;55:1465–1479.
152. Li FP, Fraumeni JF, Jr., Mulvihill JJ, Blattner WA, Dreyfus MG, Tucker MA, Miller RW. A cancer family syndrome in twenty-four kindreds. *Cancer Res* 1988;48:5358–5362.
153. Lizama VA, Zerbini MA, Gagliardi RA, Howell L. Popliteal vein thrombosis and popliteal artery pseudoaneurysm complicating osteochondroma of the femur. *AJR* 1987;148:783–784.
154. Magliato HJ, Nastasi A. Non-osteogenic fibroma occurring in the ilium. Report of a case. *J Bone Joint Surg [Am]* 1967;49:384–386.
155. Manaster BJ, Doyle AJ. Giant cell tumors of bone. *Radiol Clin North Am* 1993;31:299–323.
156. Mandahl N, Heim S, Arheden K, Rydholm A, Willen H, Mitelman F. Chromosomal rearrangements in chondromatous tumors. *Cancer* 1990;65:242–248.
157. Mandahl N, Heim S, Brosjö O, Bauer HCF, Tribukait B, Rydholm A, Mitelman F. Cytogenetic and quantitative DNA analysis of primary and xenografted human osteosarcomas. *Cancer Genet Cytogenet* 1989;42:27–34.
158. Mandahl N, Willen H, Rydholm A, Heim S, Mitelman F. Rearrangement of band q13 on both chromosomes 12 in a periosteal chondroma. *Genes Chrom Cancer* 1993;6:121–123.

159. Marina NM, Pratt CB, Rao BN, Shema SJ, Meyer WH. Improved prognosis of children with osteosarcoma metastatic to the lung(s) at the time of diagnosis. *Cancer* 1992;70:2722–2727.
160. Mark J, Wedell B, Dahlenfors R, Grepp C, Burian P. Human benign chondroblastoma with a pseudodiploid stemline characterized by a complex and balanced translocation. *Cancer Genet Cytogenet* 1992;58:14–17.
161. Marroum MC, Huvos AG, Rosen G. Pathologic aspects of chemotherapy response in the treatment of osteogenic sarcoma. An analysis of two cases. *Oncology* 1977;34:273–280.
162. Mascarello JT, Krous HF, Carpenter PM. Unbalanced translocation resulting in the loss of the chromosome 17 short arm in an osteoblastoma. *Cancer Genet Cytogenet* 1993;69:65–67.
163. Matsuno T, Ichioka Y, Yagi T, Ishii S. Spindle-cell sarcoma in patients who have osteochondromatosis. A report of two cases. *J Bone Joint Surg [Am]* 1988;70:137–141.
164. Medeiros LJ, Beckstead JH, Rosenberg AE, Warnke RA, Wood GS. Giant cells and mononuclear cells of giant cell tumor of bone resemble histiocytes. *Appl Immunohistochem* 1993;1:115–122.
165. Meister P, Konrad E, Hubner G. Malignant tumor of humerus with features of "adamantinoma" and Ewing's sarcoma. *Pathol Res Pract* 1979;166:112–122.
166. Meller JL, Curet-Scott M, Dawson P, Besser AS, Shermeta DW. Massive osteolysis of the chest in children: an unusual cause of respiratory distress. *J Pediatr Surg* 1993;28:1539–1542.
167. Meltzer PS, Jankowski S, Guan XY, et al. Molecular cytogenetic analysis of an amplification unit on chromosome 12q (Meeting abstract). Fifth International Workshop on Chromosomes in Solid Tumors, January 1993.
168. Mendez AA, Keret D, Robertson W, MacEwen GD. Massive osteolysis of the femur (Gorham's disease): a case report and review of the literature. *J Pediatr Orthop* 1989;9:604–608.
169. Meneses MF, Unni KK, Swee RG. Bizarre parosteal osteochondromatous proliferation of bone (Nora's lesion). *Am J Surg Pathol* 1993;17:691–697.
170. Mertens F, Albert A, Heim S, Lindholm J, Brosjo O, Mitelman F, Mandahl N. Clonal structural chromosome aberrations in fibrous dysplasia. *Genes Chrom Cancer* 1994;11:271–272.
171. Mertens F, Kreicbergs A, Rydholm A, Willen H, Carlen B, Mitelman F, Mandahl N. Clonal chromosome aberrations in three sacral chordomas. *Cancer Genet Cytogenet* 1994;73:147–151.
172. Meyers PA, Heller G, Healey J, et al. Chemotherapy for nonmetastatic osteogenic sarcoma: the Memorial Sloan-Kettering experience. *J Clin Oncol* 1992;10:5–15.
173. Miki K, Kawamoto K, Kawamura Y, Matsumura H, Asada Y, Hamada A. A rare case of Maffucci's syndrome combined with tuberculum sellae enchondroma, pituitary adenoma and thyroid adenoma. *Acta Neurochir (Wien)* 1987;87:79–85.
174. Milgram JW. The origins of osteochondromas and enchondromas. A histopathologic study. *Clin Orthop* 1983;264–284.
175. Mirra JM. *Bone Tumors: Clinical, Radiologic, and Pathologic Correlations.* Philadelphia: Lea and Febiger; 1989.
176. Mirra JM, Bullough PG, Marcove RC, Jacobs B, Huvos AG. Malignant fibrous histiocytoma and osteosarcoma in association with bone infarcts; report of four cases, two in caisson workers. *J Bone Joint Surg [Am]* 1974;56:932–940.
177. Mirra JM, Gold RH, Rand F. Disseminated nonossifying fibromas in association with cafe-au-lait spots (Jaffe–Campanacci syndrome). *Clin Orthop* 1982;192–205.
178. Mirra JM, Kendrick RA, Kendrick RE. Pseudomalignant osteoblastoma versus arrested osteosarcoma: a case report. *Cancer* 1976;37:2005–2014.
179. Monda L, Wick MR. S-100 protein immunostaining in the differential diagnosis of chondroblastoma. *Hum Pathol* 1985;16:287–293.
180. Moser RP, Jr., Sweet DE, Haseman DB, Madewell JE. Multiple skeletal fibroxanthomas: radiologic-pathologic correlation of 72 cases. *Skeletal Radiol* 1987;16:353–359.
181. Musil HE. Diagnostische und differentialdiagnosttische Erwagungen bei der Osteomyelitis. *Wien Klin Wochenschr* 1976;88:588–590.
182. Newton WA, Jr., Meadows AT, Shimada H, Bunin GR, Vawter GF. Bone sarcomas as second malignant neoplasms following childhood cancer. *Cancer* 1991;67:193–201.
183. Noguera R, Llombart-Bosch A, Lopez-Gines C, Carda C, Fernandez C. Giant-cell tumor of bone, stage II, displaying translocation t(12;19)(q13;q13). *Virchows Arch A Histopathol Anat* 1989;415:377–382.
184. Noguera R, Navarro S, Triche TJ. Translocation (11;22) in small cell osteosarcoma. *Cancer Genet Cytogenet* 1990;45:121–124.
185. Nora FE, Dahlin DC, Beabout JW. Bizarre parosteal osteochondromatous proliferations of the hands and feet. *Am J Surg Pathol* 1983;7:245–250.
186. Norman A, Schiffman M. Simple bone cysts: factors of age dependency. *Radiology* 1977;124:779–782.
187. Oexle K, Dammann O, Bechmann B, Vortmeyer AO, Probst EN. Intracranial chordoma in a neonate. *Eur J Pediatr* 1992;151:336–338.
188. Okamoto M, Sato C, Kohno Y, et al. Molecular nature of chromosome 5q loss in colorectal tumors and desmoids from patients with familial adenomatous polyposis. *Hum Genet* 1990;85:595–599.
189. Orndal C, Carlen B, Akerman M, et al. Chromosomal abnormality t(9;22)(q22;q12) in an extraskeletal myxoid chondrosarcoma characterized by fine needle aspiration cytology, electron microscopy, immunohistochemistry and DNA flow cytometry. *Cytopathology* 1991;2:261–270.
190. Orndal C, Mandahl N, Rydholm A, Willen H, Brosjo O, Heim S, Mitelman F. Supernumerary ring chromosomes in five bone and soft tissue tumors of low or borderline malignancy. *Cancer Genet Cytogenet* 1992;60:170–175.
191. Orndal C, Mandahl N, Rydholm A, Willen H, Brosjo O, Mitelman F. Chromosome aberrations and cytogenetic intratumor heterogeneity in chondrosarcomas. *J Cancer Res Clin Oncol* 1993;120:51–56.
192. Ozisik YY, Meloni AM, Peier A, et al. Cytogenetic findings in 19 malignant bone tumors. *Cancer* 1994;74:2268–2275.
193. Palmer TH, Jr. Gardner's syndrome: six generations. *Am J Surg* 1982;143:405–408.
194. Panico L, Passeretti U, De Rosa N, D'Antonio A, De Rosa G. Giant cell reparative granuloma of the distal skeletal bones. A report of five cases with immunohistochemical findings. *Virchows Arch A* 1994;425:315–320.
195. Parham DM, Pratt CB, Parvey LS, Webber BL, Champion J. Childhood multifocal osteosarcoma. Clinicopathologic and radiologic correlates. *Cancer* 1985;55:2653–2658.
196. Park YK, Unni KK, McLeod RA, Pritchard DJ. Osteofibrous dysplasia: clinicopathologic study of 80 cases. *Hum Pathol* 1993;24:1339–1347.
197. Penfold CN, McCullagh P, Eveson JW, Ramsay A. Giant cell lesions complicating fibro-osseous conditions of the jaws. *Int J Oral Maxillofac Surg* 1993;22:158–162.
198. Perez CA, Vietti T, Ackerman LV, Eagleton MD, Powers WE. Tumors of the sympathetic nervous system in children. An appraisal of treatment and results. *Radiology* 1967;88:750–760.
199. Persons DL, Bridge JA, Neff JR. Cytogenetic analysis of two sacral chordomas. *Cancer Genet Cytogenet* 1991;56:197–201.
200. Peterson HA. Multiple hereditary osteochondromata. *Clin Orthop* 1989;222–230.
201. Pettit CK, Zukerberg LR, Gray MH, Ferry JA, Rosenberg AE, Harmon DC, Harris NL. Primary lymphoma of bone. A B-cell neoplasm with a high frequency of multilobated cells. *Am J Surg Pathol* 1990;14:329–334.
202. Pfeifer FM, Bridge JA, Neff JR, Mouron BJ. Cytogenetic findings in aneurysmal bone cysts. *Genes Chrom Cancer* 1991;3:416–419.
203. Picci P, Manfrini M, Zucchi V, Gherlinzoni F, Rock M, Bertoni F, Neff JR. Giant-cell tumor of bone in skeletally immature patients. *J Bone Joint Surg [Am]* 1983;65:486–490.
204. Pollak MN, Polychronakos C, Richard M. Insulinlike growth factor I: A potent mitogen for human osteogenic sarcoma. *JNCI* 1990;82:301–305.
205. Present D, Bertoni F, Hudson T, Enneking WF. The correlation between the radiologic staging studies and histopathologic findings in aggressive stage 3 giant cell tumor of bone. *Cancer* 1986;57:237–244.
206. Present D, Bertoni F, Hudson T, Enneking WF. The correlation between the radiologic staging studies and histopathologic find-

ings in aggressive stage 3 giant cell tumor of bone. *Cancer* 1986;57:237–244.

207. Raskind WH, Conrad EU, Chansky H, Matsushita M. Loss of heterozygosity in chondrosarcomas for markers linked to hereditary multiple exostoses loci on chromosomes 8 and 11. *Am J Hum Genet* 1995;56:1132–1139.
208. Ratner V, Dorfman HD. Giant-cell reparative granuloma of the hand and foot bones. *Clin Orthop* 1990;251–258.
209. Riopel M, Dickman PS, Link MP, Perlman EJ. MIC2 analysis in pediatric lymphomas and leukemias. *Hum Pathol* 1994;25: 396–399.
210. Robb IA, Jimenez CL, Carpenter BF. Birbeck granules or Birbeck junctions? Intercellular "zipperlike" lattice junctions in eosinophilic granuloma of bone. *Ultrastruct Pathol* 1992;16:423–428.
211. Robinson D, Einhorn TA. Giant cell tumor of bone: a unique paradigm of stromal-hematopoietic cellular interactions. *J Cell Biochem* 1994;55:300–303.
212. Robinson D, Tieder M, Halperin N, Burshtein D, Nevo Z. Maffucci's syndrome—the result of neural abnormalities? Evidence of mitogenic neurotransmitters present in enchondromas and soft tissue hemangiomas. *Cancer* 1994;74:949–957.
213. Roessner A, Vassallo J, Vollmer E, Zwadlo G, Sorg C, Grundmann E. Biological characterization of human bon tumors. X. The proliferation behavior of macrophages as compared to fibroblastic cells in malignant fibrous histiocytoma and giant cell tumor of bone. *J Cancer Res Clin Oncol* 1987;113:559–562.
214. Rong S, Jeffers M, Resau JH, Tsarfaty I, Oskarsson M, Vande Woude GF. Met expression and sarcoma tumorigenicity. *Cancer Res* 1993;53:5355–5360.
215. Rosai J, Gold J, Landy R. The histiocytoid hemangiomas. A unifying concept embracing several previously described entities of skin, soft tissue, large vessels, bone, and heart. *Hum Pathol* 1979;10:707–730.
216. Rosen G, Marcove RC, Caparros B, Nirenberg A, Kosloff C, Huvos AG. Primary osteogenic sarcoma: the rationale for preoperative chemotherapy and delayed surgery. *Cancer* 1979;43: 2163–2177.
217. Ross JL, Schinella R, Shenkman L. Massive osteolysis. An unusual cause of bone destruction. *Am J Med* 1978;65:367–372.
218. Salter DM, Reid R. Bone tumors in a pediatric population: the Scottish Bone Tumour Registry experience (Meeting abstract). *J Pathol* 1993;170:413A.
219. Sanerkin NG, Mott MG, Roylance J. An unusual intraosseous lesion with fibroblastic, osteoclastic, osteoblastic, aneurysmal and fibromyxoid elements. "Solid" variant of aneurysmal bone cyst. *Cancer* 1983;51:2278–2286.
220. Schajowicz F, Gallardo H. Epiphysial chondroblastoma of bone. A clinico-pathological study of sixty-nine cases. *J Bone Joint Surg [Br]* 1970;52:205–226.
221. Schajowicz F, Gallardo H. Chondromyxoid fibroma (fibromyxoid chondroma) of bone. A clinico-pathological study of thirty-two cases. *J Bone Joint Surg [Br]* 1971;53:198–216.
222. Schajowicz F, Lemos C. Malignant osteoblastoma. *J Bone Joint Surg [Br]* 1976;58:202–211.
223. Scheffer H, Kruize YCM, Osinga J, et al. Complete association of loss of heterozygosity of chromosomes 13 and 17 in osteosarcoma. *Cancer Genet Cytogenet* 1991;53:45–55.
224. Schoedel KE, Martinez AJ, Mahoney TM, Contis L, Becich MJ. Chordomas: pathological features; ploidy and silver nucleolar organizing region analysis. A study of 36 cases. *Acta Neuropathol (Berl)* 1995;89:139–143.
225. Schwartz HS, Butler MG, Jenkins RB, Miller DA, Moses HL. Telomeric associations and consistent growth factor overexpression detected in giant cell tumor of bone. *Cancer Genet Cytogenet* 1991;56:263–276.
226. Schwartz HS, Jenkins RB, Dahl RJ, Dewald GW. Cytogenetic analyses on giant-cell tumors of bone. *Clin Orthop* 1989; 250–260.
227. Schwartz HS, Juliao SF, Sciadini MF, Miller LK, Butler MG. Telomerase activity and oncogenesis in giant cell tumor of bone. *Cancer* 1995;75:1094–1099.
228. Semmelink HJF, Pruszczynski M, Wiersma-V.Tilburg A, Smedts F, Ramaekers FCS. Cytokeratin expression in chondroblastomas. *Histopathology* 1990;16:257–263.
229. Serra M, Morini MC, Scotlandi K, et al. Evaluation of osteonectin as a diagnostic marker of osteogenic bone tumors. *Hum Pathol* 1992;23:1326–1331.
230. Shabb N, Fanning CV, Carrasco CH, et al. Diagnosis of eosinophilic granuloma of bone by fine-needle aspiration with concurrent institution of therapy: a cytologic, histologic, clinical, and radiologic study of 27 cases. *Diagn Cytopathol* 1993;9:3–12.
231. Shen WP, Young RF, Walter BN, Choi BH, Smith M, Katz J. Molecular analysis of a myxoid chondrosarcoma with rearrangements of chromosomes 10 and 22. *Cancer Genet Cytogenet* 1990;45:207–215.
232. Shenker A, Weinstein LS, Sweet DE, Spiegel AM. An activating Gs alpha mutation is present in fibrous dysplasia of bone in the McCune–Albright syndrome. *J Clin Endocrinol Metab* 1994;79: 750–755.
233. Shinoda M, Tsutsumi Y, Hata J-I, Yokoyama S. Peripheral neuroepithelioma in childhood: immunohistochemical demonstration of epithelial differentiation. *Arch Pathol Lab Med* 1988;112: 1155–1158.
234. Shives TC, Beabout JW, Unni KK. Massive osteolysis. *Clin Orthop* 1993;267–276.
235. Sidhu MS, Parkash H, Sidhu SS. Central giant cell granuloma of jaws—review of 19 cases. *Br J Oral Maxillofac Surg* 1995;33:43–46.
236. Sidoni A, Monico S, D'Errico P, Simoncelli C. Giant cell reparative granuloma of the maxillary bone: case report and review of diagnostic criteria. *Pathologica* 1994;86:552–556.
237. Smith PG, Marrogi AJ, Delfino JJ. Multifocal central giant cell lesions of the maxillofacial skeleton: a case report. *J Oral Maxillofac Surg* 1990;48:300–305.
238. Smith SH, Weiss SW, Jankowski SA, Coccia MA, Meltzer PS. SAS amplification in soft tissue sarcomas. *Cancer Res* 1992;52: 3746–3749.
239. Sondergaard JO, Svendsen LB, Witt IN, Bulow S, Lauritsen KB, Tetens G, Sndergaard JO. Mandibular osteomas in colorectal cancer. *Scand J Gastroenterol* 1985;20:759–761.
240. Sondergaard JO, Svendsen LB, Witt IN, Bulow S, Lauritsen KB, Tetens G, Sndergaard JO. Mandibular osteomas in the cancer family syndrome. *Br J Cancer* 1985;52:941–943.
241. Sonobe H, Mizobuchi H, Manabe Y, et al. Morphological characterization of a newly established human osteosarcoma cell line, HS-Os-1, revealing its distinct osteoblastic nature. *Virchows Arch B Cell Pathol* 1991;60:181–187.
242. Sozzi G, Miozzo M, Di Palma S, et al. Involvement of the region 13q14 in a patient with adamantinoma of the long bones. *Hum Genet* 1990;85:513–515.
243. Springfield DS, Capanna R, Gherlinzoni F, Picci P, Campanacci M. Chondroblastoma. A review of seventy cases. *J Bone Joint Surg [Am]* 1985;67:748–755.
244. Springfield DS, Schakel ME, Jr., Spanier SS. Spontaneous necrosis in osteosarcoma. *Clin Orthop* 1991;233–237.
245. Sreekantaiah C, Leong SPL, Davis JR, Sandberg AA. Cytogenetic and flow cytometric analysis of a clear cell chondrosarcoma. *Cancer Genet Cytogenet* 1991;52:193–199.
246. Stolovitzky JP, Waldron CA, McConnel FM. Giant cell lesions of the maxilla and paranasal sinuses. *Head Neck* 1994;16:143–148.
247. Struhl S, Edelson C, Pritzker H, Seimon LP, Dorfman HD. Solitary (unicameral) bone cyst. The fallen fragment sign revisited. *Skeletal Radiol* 1989;18:261–265.
248. Su CC, Tzeng CC, Chow NH, Lin CJ. Tissue culture, DNA flow cytometric and cytogenetic studies of a giant cell tumor of bone. *Chung Hua I Hsueh Tsa Chih (Taipei)* 1991;48:419–426.
249. Sugiura I. Desmoplastic fibroma. Case report and review of the literature. *J Bone Joint Surg [Am]* 1976;58:126–130.
250. Sweet DE, Vinh TN, Devaney K. Cortical osteofibrous dysplasia of long bone and its relationship to adamantinoma. A clinicopathologic study of 30 cases. *Am J Surg Pathol* 1992;16:282–290.
251. Taconis WK, Mulder JD. Fibrosarcoma and malignant fibrous histiocytoma of long bones: radiographic features and grading. *Skeletal Radiol* 1984;11:237–245.
252. Tarkkanen M, Bohling T, Helio H, et al. A recurrent chondromyxoid fibroma with chromosome aberrations ins(5;2) (q13;p21p25) and 2p deletion: a case report. *Cancer Genet Cytogenet* 1993;65:141–146.

253. Tarkkanen M, Wiklund T, Virolainen M, Elomaa I, Knuutila S. Dedifferentiated chondrosarcoma with t(9;22)(q34;q11-12). *Genes Chrom Cancer* 1994;9:136–140.
254. Toguchida J, Yamaguchi T, Dayton SH, et al. Prevalence and spectrum of germline mutations of the p53 gene among patients with sarcoma. *N Engl J Med* 1992;326:1301–1308.
255. Turc-Carel C, Dal Cin P, Rao U, Karakousis C, Sandberg AA. Recurrent breakpoints at 9q31 and 22q12.2 in extraskeletal myxoid chondrosarcoma. *Cancer Genet Cytogenet* 1988;30:145–150.
256. Turcotte RE, Kurt A-M, Sim FH, Krishnan Unni K, McLeod RA. Chondroblastoma. *Hum Pathol* 1993;24:944–949.
257. Ueda Y, Nakanishi I, Tsuchiya H, Tomita K. Microtubular aggregates in the rough endoplasmic reticulum of sacrococcygeal chordoma. *Ultrastruct Pathol* 1991;15:77–82.
258. Ueda Y, Oda Y, Kawashima A, Tsuchiya H, Tomita K, Nakanishi I. Collagenous and basement membrane proteins of chordoma: Immunohistochemical analysis. *Histopathology* 1992;21: 345–352.
259. Unger EC, Gilula LA, Kyriakos M. Case report 430: Ischemic necrosis of osteochondroma of tibia. *Skeletal Radiol* 1987;16: 416–421.
260. Unni KK, Dahlin DC. Premalignant tumors and conditions of bone. *Am J Surg Pathol* 1979;3:47–60.
261. Unni KK, Dahlin DC, Beabout JW, Sim FH. Chondrosarcoma: clear-cell variant. A report of sixteen cases. *J Bone Joint Surg* [*Am*] 1976;58:676–683.
262. van Damme PA, Mooren RE. Differentiation of multiple giant cell lesions, Noonan-like syndrome, and (occult) hyperparathyroidism. Case report and review of the literature. *Int J Oral Maxillofac Surg* 1994;23:32–36.
263. van Haelst UJ, de Haas van Dorsser AH. A perplexing malignant bone tumor. Highly malignant so-called adamantinoma or nontypical Ewing's sarcoma. *Virchows Arch A Histopathol Anat* 1975;365:63–74.
264. Vanel D, Tcheng S, Contesso G, Zafrani B, Kalifa C, Dubousset J, Kron P. The radiological appearances of telangiectatic osteosarcoma. A study of 14 cases. *Skeletal Radiol* 1987;16:196–200.
265. Vicenzi G. Familial incidence in two cases of aneurysmal bone cyst. *Ital J Orthop Traumatol* 1981;7:251–253.
266. Vilanova JR, Simon-Marin R, Burgos-Bretones J, Ramirez MM, Rivera-Pomar JM. Non-conventional chondrosarcomas and chondrogenesis. *Histopathology* 1985;9:719–728.
267. Volpe R, Mazabraud A. Hemangioendothelioma (angiosarcoma) of bone: a distinct pathologic entity with an unpredictable course? *Cancer* 1982;49:727–736.
268. Voutsinas S, Wynne-Davies R. The infrequency of malignant disease in diaphyseal aclasis and neurofibromatosis. *J Med Genet* 1983;20:345–349.
269. Wadayama B, Toguchida J, Yamaguchi T, Sasaki MS, Kotoura Y, Yamamuro T. p53 expression and its relationship to DNA alterations in bone and soft tissue sarcomas. *Br J Cancer* 1993;68: 1134–1139.
270. Waldvogel FA, Vasey H. Osteomyelitis: the past decade. *N Engl J Med* 1980;303:360–370.
271. Walker PD, Rosai J, Dorfman RF. The osseous manifestations of sinus histiocytosis with massive lymphadenopathy. *Am J Clin Pathol* 1981;75:131–139.
272. Walker WP, Landas SK, Bromley CM, Sturm MT. Immunohistochemical distinction of classic and chondroid chordomas. *Mod Pathol* 1991;4:661–666.
273. Watanabe H, Arita S, Chigira M. Aetiology of a simple bone cyst. A case report. *Int Orthop* 1994;18:16–19.
274. Weatherall PT, Maale GE, Mendelsohn DB, Sherry CS, Erdman WE, Pascoe HR. Chondroblastoma: classic and confusing appearance at MR imaging. *Radiology* 1994;190:467–474.
275. Wechsler J, Grellet M. Cas familial associant cherubisme, granulomes centro-osseaux a cellules geantes et tumeurs geantes des maxillaires. *Rev Stomatol Chir Maxillofac* 1984;85:337–340.
276. Weinstein LS, Shenker A, Gejman PV, Merino MJ, Friedman E, Spiegel AM. Activating mutations of the stimulatory G protein in the McCune–Albright syndrome. *N Engl J Med* 1991;325:1688–1695.
277. Weiss A-PC, Dorfman HD. Clear-cell chondrosarcoma: a report of ten cases and review of the literature. *Surg Pathol* 1988;1:123–129.
278. Weiss AP, Dorfman HD. S-100 protein in human cartilage lesions. *J Bone Joint Surg* [*Am*] 1986;68:521–526.
279. Weiss SW, Ishak KG, Dail DH, Sweet DE, Enzinger FM. Epithelioid hemangioendothelioma and related lesions. *Semin Diagn Pathol* 1986;3:259–287.
280. Whitaker SB, Bouquot JE. Estrogen and progesterone receptor status of central giant cell lesions of the jaws. *Oral Surg Oral Med Oral Pathol* 1994;77:641–644.
281. Wollner N, Lane JM, Marcove RC, et al. Primary skeletal non-Hodgkin's lymphoma in the pediatric age group. *Med Pediatr Oncol* 1992;20:506–513.
282. Womer RB. The cellular biology of bone tumors. *Clin Orthop* 1991;12–21.
283. Wu J-X, Carpenter PM, Gresens C, Keh R, Niman H, Morris JWS, Mercola D. The proto-oncogene c-fos is over-expressed in the majority of human osteosarcomas. *Oncogene* 1990;5:989–1000.
284. Yabut SM, Jr., Kenan S, Sissons HA, Lewis MM. Malignant transformation of fibrous dysplasia. A case report and review of the literature. *Clin Orthop* 1988;281–289.
285. Yalcm RC, Gavuzoglu K, Koseli I. Hemangio-endothelial sarcoma of the rib in a fourteen year old girl. *Turk J Pediatr* 1966;8: 150–156.
286. Yamada K, Yoshitake Y, Norimatsu H, Nishikawa K. Roles of various growth factors in growth of human osteosarcoma cells which can grow in protein-free medium. *Cell Struct Funct* 1992;17:9–17.
287. Yiannias JA, Brodland DG. Transcranial eosinophilic granuloma manifested by a subcutaneous scalp mass. Differential diagnosis in children. *J Dermatol Surg Oncol* 1993;19:631–634.
288. Yoshida H, Yumoto T, Minamizaki T. Osteosarcoma with features mimicking malignant fibrous histiocytoma. *Virchows Arch A Histopathol Anat* 1992;421:229–238.
289. Zalupski MM, Ensley JF, Ryan J, Selvaggi S, Baker LH, Wolman SR. A common cytogenetic abnormality and DNA content alterations in dedifferentiated chondrosarcoma. *Cancer* 1990;66: 1176–1182.
290. Zheng MH, Fan Y, Wysocki SJ, et al. Gene expression of transforming growth factor-beta 1 and its type II receptor in giant cell tumors of bone. Possible involvement in osteoclast-like cell migration. *Am J Pathol* 1994;145:1095–1104.
291. Zillmer DA, Dorfman HD. Chondromyxoid fibroma of bone: thirty-six cases with clinicopathologic correlation. *Hum Pathol* 1989;20:952–964.

Pediatric Neoplasia: Morphology and Biology, edited by David M. Parham. Lippincott-Raven Publishers, Philadelphia © 1996.

CHAPTER 10

Germ Cell Tumors

Edith P. Hawkins and Elizabeth J. Perlman

INTRODUCTION

Germ cell tumors in children are a disparate group of tumors comprising mature and immature teratomas, germinomas (seminomas, dysgerminomas), embryonal carcinomas, yolk sac tumors (endodermal sinus tumors, orchidoblastomas), and choriocarcinomas (27,58,92, 95,96,158,249). Gonadoblastomas arising in the dysgenetic gonad may also be included (95,212). The general consensus is that these tumors arise from primitive germ cells that have undergone neoplastic transformation; alternatively, some may arise from totipotent embryonal cells. There is increasing evidence that the germ cell tumors occurring in early childhood are different from those occurring in adults. Cytogenetic abnormalities, histopathologic patterns, sites of origin, and tumor behavior are different in infantile and adult tumors (Table 1). It has been suggested that, at least in the testis, adult tumors represent a field defect whereas those in young children are the result of malignant transformation of one or at most a few individual cells (151).

Controversy remains concerning the pathway from the primitive germ cell to the different types of tumor. Most hypothetical pathways are centered around data and observations derived from postpubertal testicular germ cell tumors, as this group has been the most intensively studied. One proposed pathway is illustrated in Fig. 1. This schema is consistent with observed tumors in early childhood (48,165) and can be applied to all sites of tumor origin. A variant of this schema suggests that seminomas branch off separately but that all other nonseminomatous germ cell tumors (NSGCTs) are derived from embryonal carcinoma (15,28,51,128,237). Still others have suggested that the seminoma is an intermediate tumor through which all other NSGCTs must go (30,51,53,149,184). Supportive evidence for this latter hypothesis is based on pathologic observations as well as ploidy, cytogenetic, and immunohistochemical analyses (54,68,146,149,166,245). In particular, mathematical analyses of ploidy data from testicular germ cell tumors show near-tetraploid DNA content in seminomas, with nonrandom chromosomal loss accompanied by decreased DNA content in the triploid to hypotetraploid range for nonseminomatous germ cell tumors (54,68). The near-universal presence of a characteristic cytogenetic abnormality, the isochromosome 12p, in all histologic subtypes of postpubertal testicular germ cell tumors also supports a common lineage (11,24,36,60,81,82, 209). Recent studies utilizing interphase cytogenetics in adult tumors suggest that the atypical germ cells in intratubular germ cell neoplasia (ITGCN) (Fig. 2) show increased numbers of chromosomes as well as the presence of the i(12p) and overexpression of the alkaline phosphatase genes prior to becoming invasive. The degree of numeric increase depends on whether ITGCN is adjacent to seminoma or to embryonal carcinoma. Thus, under the appropriate circumstances, the atypical germ cell may be the precursor for either seminoma or embryonal carcinoma (53,146,246). Similar studies performed in childhood tumors show DNA content to be more commonly euploid (diploid or tetraploid) with no evidence of an i(12p), supporting a different pathogenesis (194). In addition, histopathologic ITGCN is not seen in association with infantile yolk sac tumors. The germ cells in neighboring seminiferous tubules may be enlarged with clear cytoplasm (Fig. 3), but there is no nuclear atypia or placental alkaline phosphatase (PLAP) positivity (94,150,223). A recent case report has purported to show

E. P. Hawkins: Department of Pathology, Baylor College of Medicine and Texas Children's Hospital, Houston, Texas 77030.

E. J. Perlman: Department of Pathology, Johns Hopkins Hospital, Baltimore, Maryland 21287.

TABLE 1. *Differences between infantile and adult germ cell tumors*

Infantile	Adult
Usually pure yolk sac tumor or teratoma	Generally mixed or pure seminoma/germinoma
No malignant non-neural epithelial components	May have malignant epithelial components
Mature teratomas do not metastasize	Mature teratomas may metastasize (testis)
No isochromosome 12p	Many have ischromosome 12p
Often euploid or tetraploid	Usually aneuploid
No testicular ITN: enlarged cells with clear cytoplasm but no nuclear atypia and PIAP negative	Testicular ITN: enlarged cells with nuclear atypia and PLAP positivity
No testicular seminomas	Testicular seminomas common
Extragonadal tumors common	Extragonadal tumors uncommon

(Data from Refs. 15,25,30,31,57,59,62,84,85,92,94,96,109,129,131,132,150,151,168,175, 184,195,215,220,221,223,237,246.)

Abbreviations: ITN, intratubular neoplasia; PLAP, placental alkaline phosphatase.

ITGCN adjacent to a mature teratoma in an infant testis (203). The cells in this report are histopathologically identical to the enlarged clear cells that have been described by others (94,150,223) and are similarly PLAP-negative. However, because immunohistochemical studies showed the cells to be proliferating cell nuclear antigen (PCNA) and p53-positive, it was concluded that they are neoplastic. In the authors' opinion, this conclusion is probably not warranted at the present time, as PCNA is present in all proliferating cells, whether neoplastic or nonneoplastic, and the *p53* gene has been associated with normal spermatogenesis in the experimental animal (4). The p53 protein has also been demonstrated in a discrete tetraploid cell population consistent with midpachytene spermatocytes (211). In addition, two studies have failed to demonstrate mutations in the *p53* gene in testicular germ cell tumors (78,193), although p53 protein has been demonstrated immunohistochemically in both tumors and ITGCN in adults (236). Thus, it seems more likely that the demonstration of PCNA and p53 in these tubular cells is a consequence of cell stimulation by some as yet unidentified tumor growth factor or cytokine akin to the well-recognized angiogenic tumor factor. Therefore the hypothesis that all NSGCTs go through an embryonal carcinoma stage seems less likely for childhood tumors, as pure yolk sac tumors are the most common type of malignant germ cell tumor in early childhood, and embryonal carcinomas are quite unusual.

A recent study of proto-oncogenes in adult testicular tumors has found significant levels of N-*myc* expression in seminomas and embryonal carcinomas, but no expression of N-*myc* in immature teratomas. On the other hand, immature teratomas expressed high levels of *c-erbB-1* and one tumor expressed *c-erbB-2,* whereas neither proto-oncogene was expressed in the majority of the malignant tumors (216). Similarly, significant differences between seminomatous and nonseminomatous germ cell tumors in the expression of the *hist-1, c-kit,*

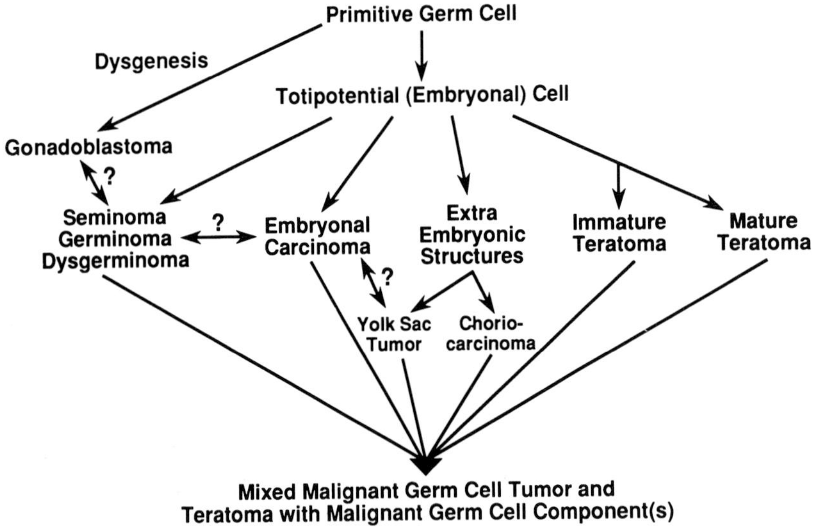

FIG. 1. Proposed pathway from primitive germ cell to various germ cell tumors is consistent with observed tumors of childhood.

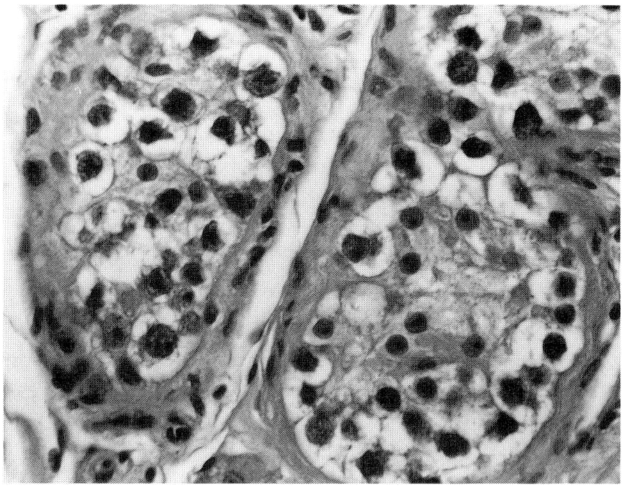

FIG. 2. Intratubular germ cell neoplasia adjacent to a germ cell tumor in an 18-year-old male patient is characterized by the proliferation of large germ cells that have abundant clear cytoplasm and large, occasionally bizarre nuclei with prominent nucleoli.

and *int-2* oncogenes have been reported (226). Whether a similar pattern of expression is present in infantile tumors is not known.

The potential for aggressive behavior of malignant germ cell tumors in children is quite varied and is age- and site-dependent. Germinomas are the least aggressive, and teratomas with malignant neural elements [neuroblastoma, primitive neuroepithelioma, medulloepithelioma (23,58,92,95,96,127,130,225,249)] are the most aggressive. Germinomas generally respond to radiation therapy alone (95,156,237). Tumors with only malignant germ cell elements (yolk sac tumor, embryonal carcinoma, choriocarcinoma) tend to respond to a platinum-containing combination chemotherapeutic regimen (67,75,95,96,153,156,199,200,225,237), whereas those with malignant neural or mesenchymal elements have the same poor prognosis as their somatic counterparts (127,225) (personal observations).

Germ cell tumors, both the benign and malignant forms, are most often gonadal in origin. However, they may be found anywhere in the body, usually along the midline. The percentage of extragonadal tumors is higher in children than in adults (25,57,58,92,95,96). In children, the most common extragonadal sites are sacrococcygeum, mediastinum, and intracranium (6,56,92, 95,112,137), and the most common locations for congenital tumors are sacrococcygeum and intracranium (87,95,173,174,181,207,210). However, tumors have been observed in a host of unusual sites such as face (57,215), neck (113,247), naso- and oropharynx (5,32, 133,202,240), mouth (22,204), sinuses (225), thyroid (22,148), heart (9,46,49,148), stomach (47,133,148, 213), urinary bladder (22), mesentery (112), and liver (43,112,244). Vaginal, other female genital tract, and retroperitoneal yolk sac tumors have also been reported (44,96,112,159,215,249). The majority of ovarian germ cell tumors are thought to arise from germ cells after the first phase of meiosis but before the second phase (117,227), whereas extragonadal tumors appear to arise from mitotic division (100,117,189).

The mitotic rather than meiotic origin of the stem line of extragonadal germ cell tumors has led to questions concerning their germ cell origin. The prevailing hypothesis has been that extragonadal germ cell tumors arise from germ cells that have incompletely or aberrantly migrated. However, extragonadal ectopic germ cells have been only rarely reported to exist in human embryos, and these disappear completely by 8 weeks gestation (111). In addition, ectopic germ cells in humans have never been described outside the abdomen (72), whereas extragonadal germ cell tumors are often located in the mediastinum and central nervous system. In mice, ec-

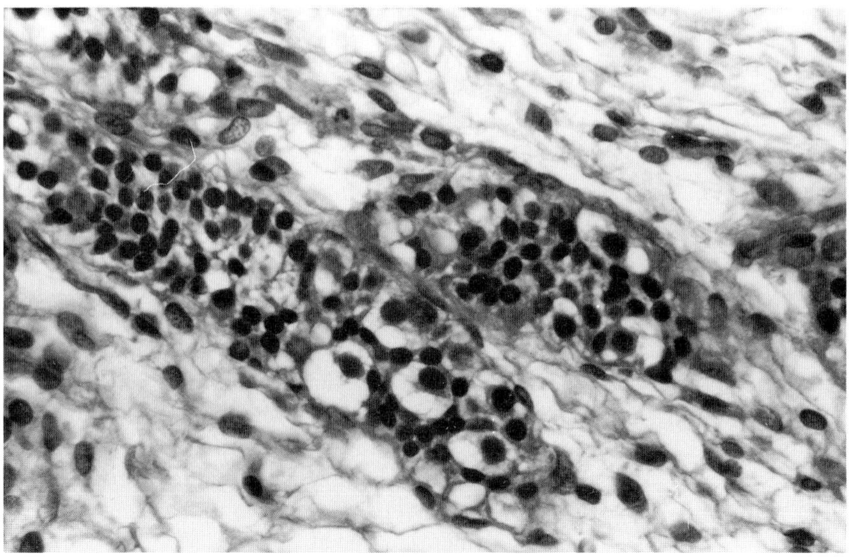

FIG. 3. Germ cells in the seminiferous tubules adjacent to an infantile yolk sac tumor have abundant clear cytoplasm and are increased in number, but the nuclei are not bizarre or enlarged over normal. The seminiferous tubules in an infant are much smaller than those of the postpubertal male (compare with Fig. 2).

topic germ cells are more common; however, these enter meiosis early in gestation, in phase with normal oocytes, regardless of the sex of the animal, and disappear after 3 postnatal weeks (147,239). Therefore, germ cell tumors arising from these ectopic germ cells would be expected to be postmeiotic rather than mitotic in origin. Therefore, other than the histologic similarities to gonadal germ cell tumors, there is little evidence to support a germ cell origin for extragonadal germ cell tumors. An alternative hypothesis suggests that extragonadal germ cell tumors arise from undifferentiated embryonal cells of the primitive streak that have escaped the influence of embryonic organizers (86).

There are a variety of classifications of germ cell tumors (28,58), but none is completely satisfactory when applied to childhood tumors. The most confusion exists concerning the designation of teratomas. When are they benign and when are they malignant? A sensible approach would be to designate a teratoma as one of three types: "mature teratoma," a teratoma with only mature elements; "immature teratoma," a teratoma with immature elements; and "teratoma with malignant elements" (yolk sac tumor, embryonal carcinoma, germinoma, choriocarcinoma, or malignant neural elements such as neuroblastoma). The teratomatous elements in this latter designation may be either mature or immature. The use of this nomenclature would avoid the confusion between immature teratomas and teratomas with true malignant elements and would help to prevent unnecessarily aggressive therapy for children with immature teratomas.

Children with dysgenetic gonads have an increased incidence of germ cell tumors (89,102,107,153,168, 169,201), and infants may have ITGCN in the dysgenetic gonad (107). Gonadoblastomas, a mixture of germ cells and gonadal sex cord cells, may represent totipotential cell derivatives and are the most common tumor seen in dysgenetic gonads (93,95,212,228). These benign tumors may be associated with a malignant germ cell tumor in the same or opposite gonad. Congenital malformations, particularly urogenital anomalies (e.g., cryptorchid testes, anorectal anomalies, sacral agenesis), have a higher than expected association with germ cell tumors (16,87,102,113,153,188,222). The tumors associated with cryptorchid testes tend to be malignant (89), whereas those associated with sacrococcygeal anomalies are usually benign and may be familial (198,222). Germ cell tumors are also associated with certain syndromes such as Klinefelter's syndrome (47,XXY), testicular feminization, trisomy 21, and cutaneous ichthyosis (28,56,218). In children with Klinefelter's syndrome, the tumors may be benign or malignant, but are most often extragonadal, usually occurring in the mediastinum and the central nervous system (8,56,161).

Mediastinal germ cell tumors are associated with the development of hematopoietic malignancies, either simultaneously or within less than 2 years of diagnosis of the germ cell neoplasm. Leukemias, myelodysplastic syndromes, refractory thrombocytopenia, autoimmune hemolytic anemia, mastocytosis, and malignant histiocytosis have all been reported (38,39,65,138,141, 153,176,187,218). Although it has been suggested that hematopoietic growth factors secreted by germ cell tumors result in these hematopoietic malignancies, cytogenetic and immunohistochemical studies indicate that the malignant hematopoietic cells originate from pluripotent germ cells within the germ cell tumor rather than from the host's marrow cells (38,61,138,187). Orazi and coauthors believe that these hematopoietic malignancies only arise from a yolk sac tumor component and that reports of such malignancies arising in germ cell tumors other than yolk sac tumors indicate insufficient sampling of the tumor (187). Support for this concept may be found in normal embryogenesis, during which time the embryonal yolk sac serves as the source of hematopoietic elements that disseminate into the subsequent blood-forming sites of the body (187). The demonstration in yolk sac tumors of hemoglobins F and A offers further confirmation of this hypothesis. However, blood group–related antigens such as the type 1 precursor antigen and blood group antigen H have been found in embryonal carcinomas as well as yolk sac tumors (3,166). There are also rare reports of hematologic malignancies associated with gonadal germ cell tumors (118,153), tumors occurring in a testis and paraovarian tissues in phenotypic females whose constitutional chromosomes were, respectively, 46,XX/46,XY and 46,XY. It has also been suggested that the mast cell malignancies are related either to a cytokine produced by the germ cell tumors or that a stem cell growth factor that is required to grow germ cells in culture can lead to mast cell proliferation (39). However, cytogenetic analysis of the mast cell proliferation shows the presence of the i(12p), supporting their germ cell origin (personal observations).

The estimated incidence of malignant germ cell tumors in children in the United States is 2–3 per 1 million children. The incidence of all germ cell tumors, both benign and malignant, is not as well defined because most estimates are derived from tumor registries that tend to be biased in favor of malignancy. However, one study based on the experience in a primary care hospital suggests that the total incidence is around 4.5 per 1 million children (95). Extragonadal germ cell tumors are 2–3 times more common in girls (25,210), but malignant tumors in the mediastinum are most often present in boys (56,86,135,137,232).

A germ cell tumor may have many different types of tissue, both benign and malignant. The most malignant cell type in the teratoma or mixed malignant germ cell tumor determines the behavior. Thus, the tumor should be sampled extensively. The conventional method has been to recommend taking at least one section per centimeter of greatest diameter. Joshi has recommended a modification that takes the volume of the tumor into consideration and is probably slightly better. He suggests taking sections according to the following formula: 1.5 multiplied by the mean of the three diameters (114). Whatever the method used, the pathologist should not be limited by rigid adherence to a formula. One should carefully examine the complete tumor and then take sections from every site that appears different.

BENIGN GERM CELL TUMORS

Mature Teratoma

Teratomas by definition are neoplasms composed of one or more representatives of all three embryonic germ cell layers: endoderm, mesoderm, and ectoderm (Fig. 4). In mature teratomas all components are mature, and in children these teratomas generally exhibit benign behavior. In those instances in which a "mature" teratoma recurs as a malignancy, a careful review of the original tumor will usually reveal an occult focus of cancer (Fig. 5) (97). On the other hand, in adults, mature teratomas in the testis may metastasize as mature teratomas or as other malignant germ cell elements (237). Mature teratomas in children occur most often in the ovary and the sacrococcygeal area (92,95,96). The mediastinum is the third most common location in this age group (56). In the sacrococcygeal area, the majority of the mature teratomas occur during the neonatal period, whereas the peak incidence for such tumors in the ovary and the mediastinum is in the second decade of life (95,96).

Gonadal mature teratomas are encapsulated, multicystic tumors (Fig. 6) that may have foci of bone and calcification. Ovarian teratomas frequently have teeth and hair as well. The cysts are of varying sizes, and the contents vary depending on the type of epithelial lining. Thus, the contents may be clear, viscous, or mucoid fluid or semisolid, yellow keratinous material. In the ovarian teratomas, this latter material is often associated with hairs. Gray–tan, solid areas suggestive of brain and yellow soft areas of adipose tissue are often interspersed between cysts. Extragonadal mature teratomas have a similar gross appearance on the cut surfaces, but these neoplasms are not encapsulated and tend to blend with the surrounding tissues.

Although all three germ cell layers are present in the majority of tumors, the distribution of tissue types varies somewhat depending on the location of the tumor. Ovarian teratomas have large amounts of skin, skin appendages, adipose tissue, hair, and central nervous system tissue; testicular teratomas tend to be composed primarily of epithelial-lined cysts with little or no neural tissue; mediastinal teratomas often have pancreas (56,66,95); and pancreas may also be seen in occasional sacrococcygeal teratomas (Fig. 7), but has not been reported in gonadal teratomas (115).

The pancreatic tissue may occasionally produce amylase that can be detected in the cystic fluid and/or lead to pericarditis or tissue necrosis secondary to enzymatic activity (56,115). Insulin and growth hormone production have also been reported in association with teratomatous pancreatic tissue (86). Rarely, teratomas have been reported to have other types of endocrine secretions, such as a mediastinal teratoma causing precocious

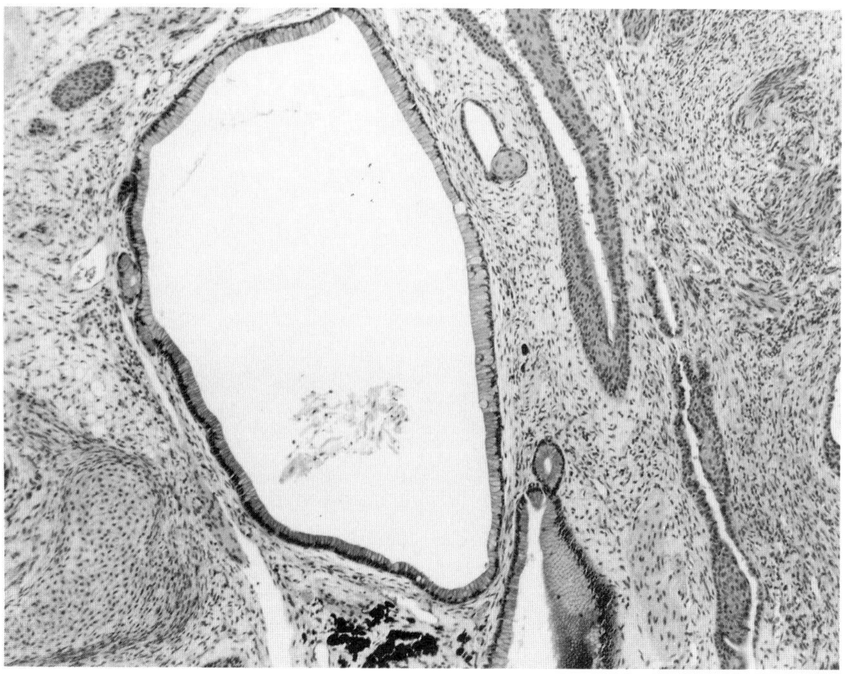

FIG. 4. Mature teratoma has cystic spaces lined by mucus-producing cells (endoderm), mature cartilage (mesoderm), and pigmented retinal epithelium (neuroectoderm).

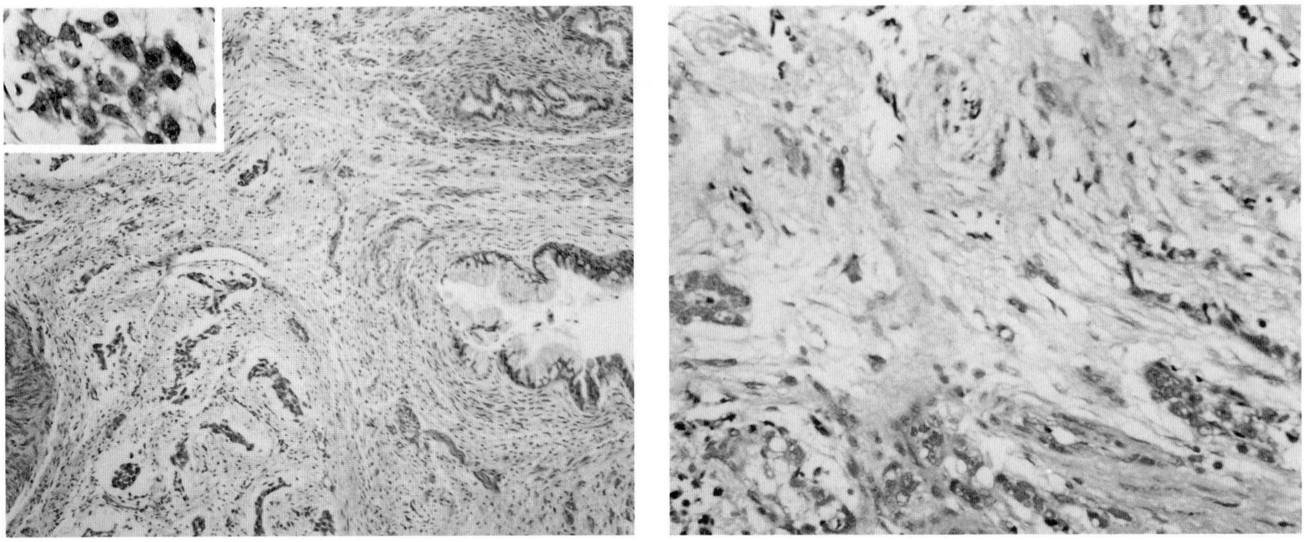

A

B

FIG. 5. A. Collapsed reticular structures in a loose, slightly myxoid background represent a focus of yolk sac tumor in an otherwise mature teratoma. **Inset:** One of the reticular structures is shown at higher magnification. Hematoxylin and eosin. Original magnification 160×. **B**. Similar reticular structures are identified in portions of the recurrent tumor from the patient in part A.

puberty from increased concentrations of testosterone (121), an ovarian teratoma with a prolactin-secreting pituitary gland (74), or a sacrococcygeal teratoma containing pituitary cells and hormones in a hydropic infant (173). In this latter case, the authors postulated that increased concentrations of vasopressin from the tumor may have led to the hydropic state. Bone with fibrotic marrow may be found in teratomas at all sites, but bone with hematopoietic marrow has only been reported in the mediastinum (Fig. 8). However, we recently saw hematopoietic marrow in an ovarian teratoma. Mature representations of virtually all tissues in the body may be found. These include lung, liver, salivary gland, prostate, and intestine (29). Frequently, these are quite well organized (Fig. 9). A recent study has shown that the proliferative index of these mature elements is similar to that of the related normal organs (40). At times the organization of tissues in a mature teratoma is such that the possibility of a fetus-in-fetu is raised. However, most observers will accept this diagnosis only if there is a well-organized axial spine in the specimen (69,116). Immunohistochemical stains on mature teratomas follow the pattern of staining found in normal tissues and are generally not required for diagnosis.

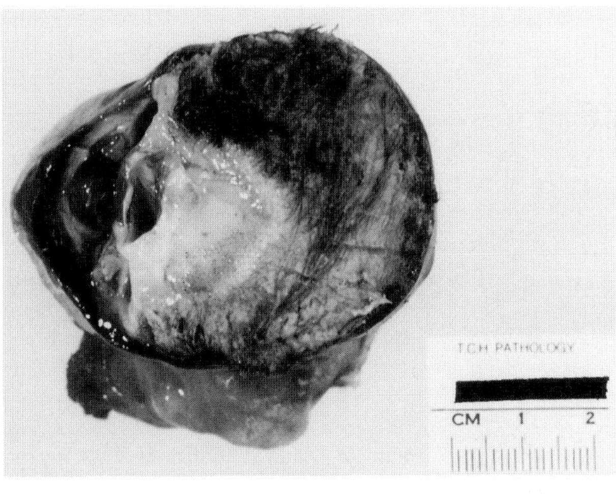

FIG. 6. The cut surface of this encapsulated mature ovarian teratoma has multiple cysts and large amounts of grossly visible hair and adipose tissue.

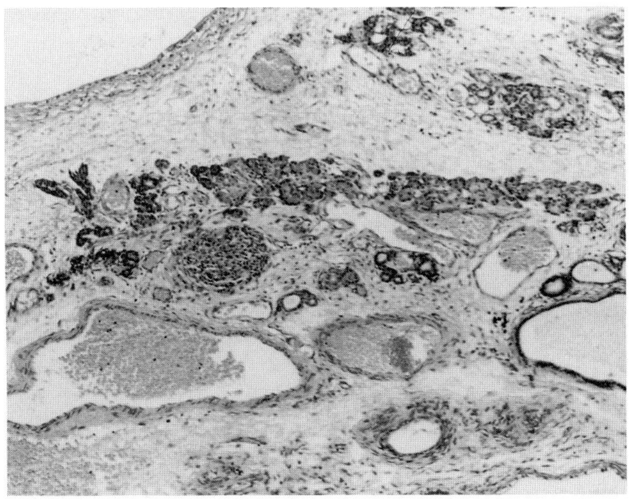

FIG. 7. Pancreatic acini and an islet are present in this mature teratoma from the sacrococcygeum.

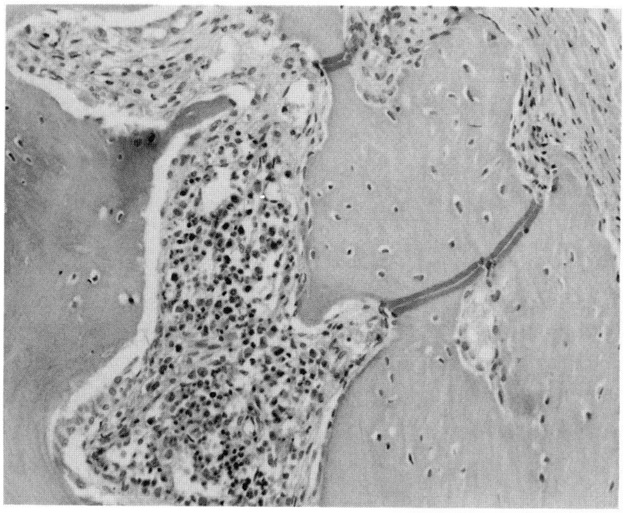

FIG. 8. Hematopoietic bone marrow is identified in a mature teratoma from the mediastinum.

Mature cartilage, osteoid and bone, squamous or mucinous epithelium, striated muscle, and other such mature tissues may occur singly or together in some pediatric neoplasms such as Wilms' tumor and hepatoblastoma. However, the presence of these differentiated tissues does not identify these neoplasms as teratomas, as the cell of origin is the multipotential blastemal cell of the kidney or liver and not a migratory germ cell or uncommitted stem cell (19,248).

Despite the histologic similarities of all mature teratomas, biologic and clinical studies suggest that these tumors show distinct differences depending on the age of the patient and site of tumor involvement. Ovarian mature teratomas have been the most thoroughly studied due to their ample numbers; these studies form a solid database for comparison with teratomas from other sites. Cytogenetic analyses of over 325 cases have shown 95% of ovarian mature teratomas to be karyotypically normal and 5% to have nonrecurrent numeric chromosomal abnormalities (45,143,192,227); genetic studies indicate that the stem cells of the vast majority of these tumors have entered, but have not completed, meiosis (227). This suggests that ovarian mature teratomas are parthenogenic tumors that arise in germ cells due to errors in meiosis.

Testicular teratomas are biphasic, with a peak in early childhood and a second peak in adolescence and young adulthood. Due to their rarity, little is known about teratomas arising in the testes of young children. These tumors behave in a benign fashion regardless of degree of maturity (144); and analogous to their ovarian counterparts, the few that have been analyzed are diploid with a normal 46,XY karyotype (100,120). Conversely, teratomas of the adult/adolescent testis, both mature and immature, are potentially malignant tumors that share genetic features with malignant testicular germ cell tumors, including aneuploid DNA content and the presence of a particular cytogenetic abnormality, the i(12p) (35,186, 205). Adult and childhood testicular teratomas both show genetic evidence for a premeiotic (mitotic) origin (100). Thus, the pathogenesis of testicular teratomas is quite different from mature ovarian teratomas.

Extragonadal mature teratomas are poorly understood. Cytogenetic and genetic studies support a premeiotic (mitotic) stem cell (100,117,154,189). The majority of cytogenetic studies show the tumors to share the constitutional karyotype of their host (79,117,154).

Gonadoblastoma

A second benign germ cell tumor is the gonadoblastoma (93,95,212,228), which is a mixture of immature germ cells and gonadal sex cord cells, usually of the granulosa or Sertoli cell type (Fig. 10) The source of the sex cord cells is unclear. Leydig cells and luteinizing cells may also be seen. Focal calcification is common. Gonadoblastomas are virtually always located in a dysgenetic or streak gonad. Although the majority of patients with gonadoblastomas are phenotypically female, they typically have a Y chromosome, usually with a karyotype consisting of 46,XY or 45,X/46,XY, and exhibit virilization. The benign gonadoblastoma is associated with a germinoma in approximately 50% of patients, and it is sometimes associated with embryonal and extraembryonic malignant germ cell tumors. These malignancies may be found in the same or the contralateral gonad and should always be searched for by careful gross and microscopic examination. The germ cells of the gonadoblastoma have diffuse staining for PLAP in cell mem-

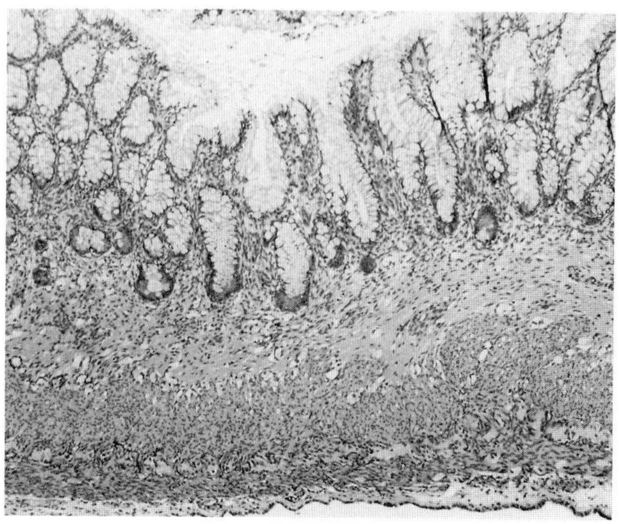

FIG. 9. Well-organized intestine is seen in an immature teratoma of the ovary.

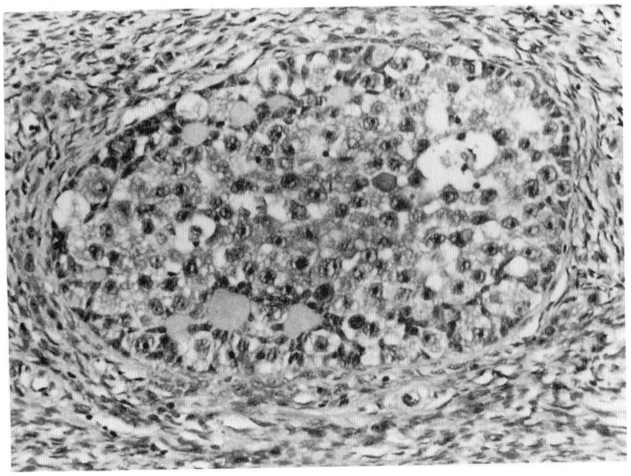

FIG. 10. In this dysgenetic gonad a well-encapsulated nest of primitive germ cells (gonadoblastoma) is surrounded by ovarianlike stroma. A few hyaline bodies are scattered among the germ cells.

branes and focal staining in the cytoplasm, supporting the neoplastic, albeit benign, nature of these tumors (personal observation) (21).

Due to their rarity, little is known about the biology of gonadoblastomas. Ploidy and cytogenetic analysis of a single gonadoblastoma showed a diploid DNA content and a normal 46,XY karyotype (personal observations). The fact that gonadoblastomas have been documented almost exclusively in a subpopulation of patients with 46,XY gonadal dysgenesis has led to the suggestion that the genetic requirements for development of a gonadoblastoma include the presence of a dysgenetic gonad as well as the presence of a portion of the Y chromosome. It may be that a gene residing on the long arm of the Y chromosome codes for an oncogene that, acting in the environment of a dysgenetic gonad, results in this tumor (190). The development of a malignant germ cell tumor within a gonadoblastoma is also poorly understood. However, the resulting malignant germ cell tumors appear to show biologic differences from those arising in normal gonads. The DNA content of the malignant tumors arising in the setting of a dysgenetic gonad are diploid rather than aneuploid (90) (personal observations). Whereas one tumor showed evidence of an i(12p) by routine cytogenetic analysis, two failed to show evidence for an i(12p) by fluorescence in situ hybridization (90) (personal observations).

GERM CELL TUMORS OF INDETERMINATE BEHAVIOR

Immature Teratoma

Like mature teratomas, immature teratomas are also composed of representatives of all three germ cell layers, but some portion of these tissues is immature. The gross appearance of these tumors is similar to that of mature teratomas, and the mature components are similar microscopically. The predominant immature component is usually of neuroepithelial origin (Fig. 11), but all germ cell layers may participate in the immaturity. Immature mesenchyme is frequently prominent (Fig. 12) and renal blastema is not uncommon (Fig. 13) (58,86,95).

Ovarian teratomas are graded by a system proposed by Thurlbeck and Scully (231) and modified by Dehner (58). By this system, a teratoma with no immature tissue

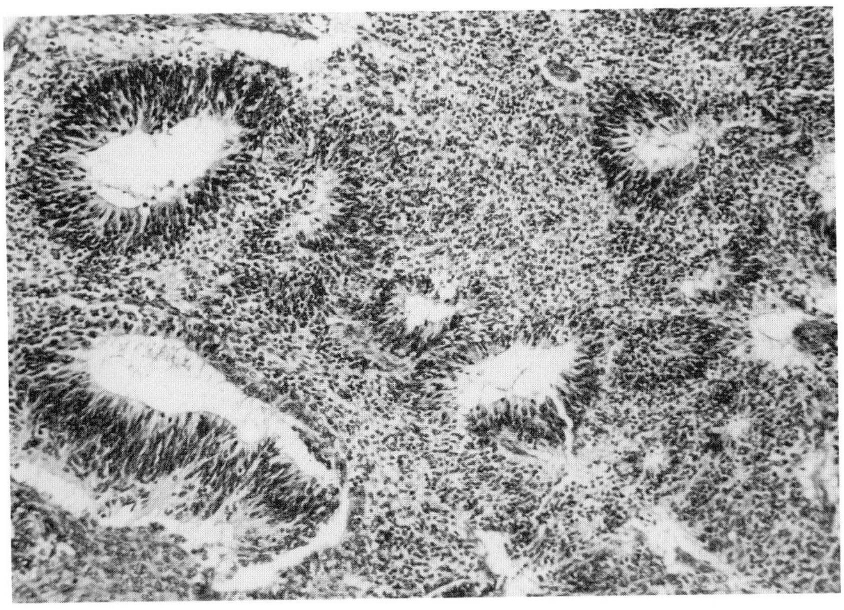

FIG. 11. Immature neural tissue identified this teratoma as immature.

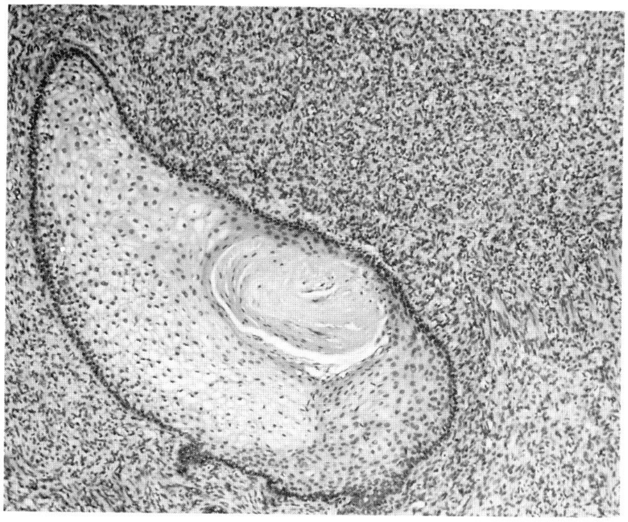

FIG. 12. A mature squamous island is present within a background of immature mesenchyme in this immature teratoma.

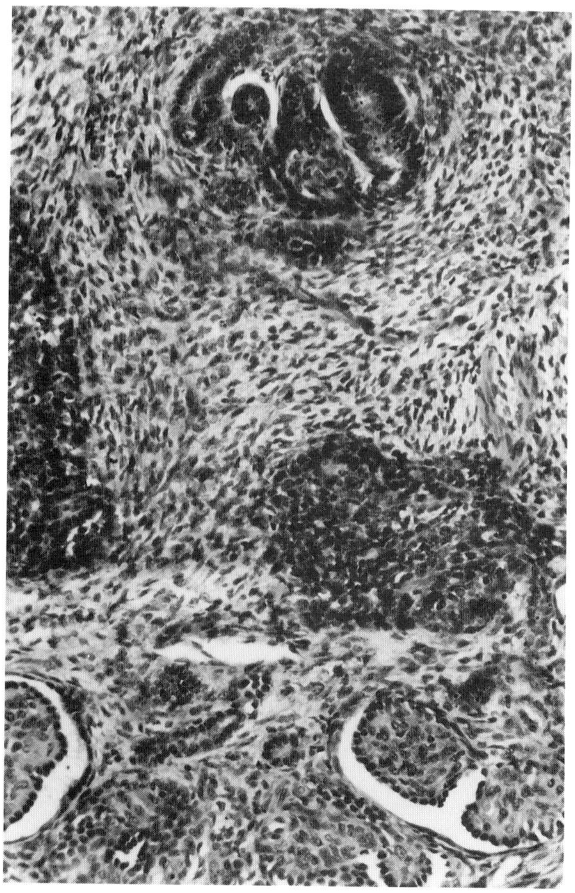

FIG. 13. Small areas of renal blastema are not uncommon in a grade 3 immature teratoma.

is grade 0; a teratoma with the equivalent of no more than one low power field of immature tissue is grade 1; a teratoma with more than one but less than four low-power fields of immature neuroepithelial foci with or without other immature somatic elements is grade 2; and a teratoma with consecutive microscopic fields of immature tissues either neuroepithelial or somatic is grade 3. In the past, using this system, ovarian teratomas of grades 1–3 have been considered malignant. However, virtually all grade 1 and 2 ovarian teratomas occurring in children behave in a benign fashion (95,133,134), and the grade 3 teratomas in children that exhibit malignant behavior tend to have occult foci of yolk sac tumor (Fig. 14) (97,133) or frankly malignant neuroepithelial components (Fig. 15) (87,127) (personal observation). These latter components may be difficult to identify and may not declare themselves until they metastasize. Fortunately, they are extremely rare.

Immature teratomas occurring in extraovarian sites are relatively rare, so that only a small number have been evaluated in a similar fashion (133). In one study, the presence of immature tissues in central nervous system teratomas appeared to be correlated with the age of the patient rather than with malignant potential, being more common in congenital and infantile tumors (207). One review of immature teratomas in children did not find any without some foci of immature neural tissue (133), but in our experience infantile testicular and sacrococcygeal teratomas may have markedly immature mesenchymal components in the absence of immature neural elements.

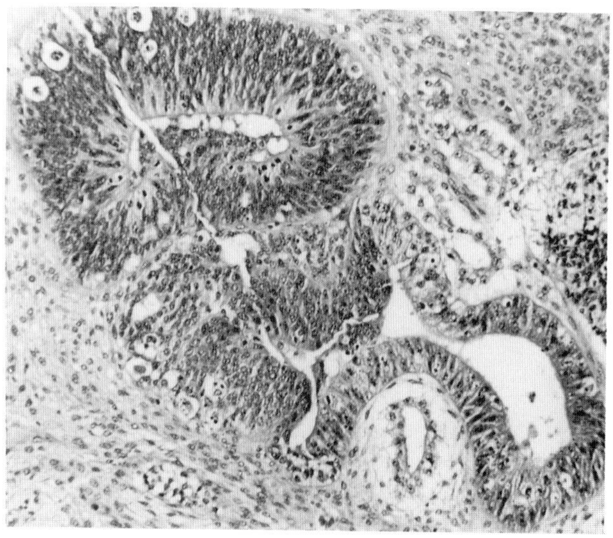

FIG. 14. Small reticular foci of yolk sac tumor are in intimate association with the area of immature neural tissue. The cystic structure emerging from the neural tissue has larger, more vesicular nuclei and represents the enteric pattern of yolk sac tumor.

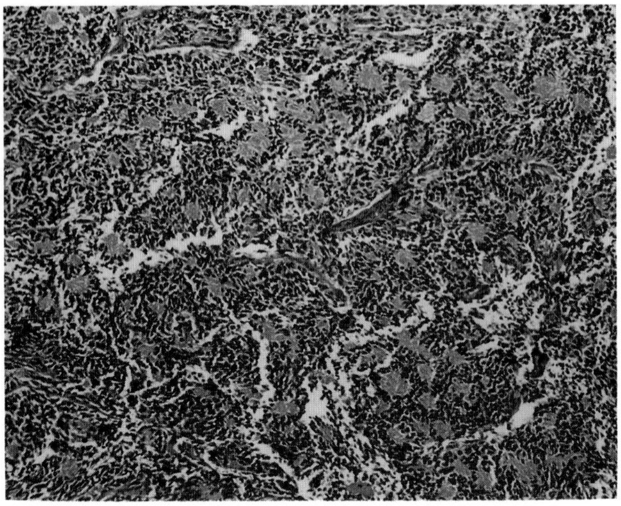

FIG. 15. An area of neuroblastoma is identified in this immature teratoma. The child later developed metastatic neuroblastoma.

It has been stated in the older literature (14,71) that the immature neural tissue in immature teratomas is the probable source of the elevations in serum α-fetoprotein (AFP) concentrations (see below), but more recent studies indicate that small foci of yolk sac tumor can almost invariably be found in those immature teratomas that are associated with elevated serum AFP (97,196). These foci may stain positively for AFP, but usually they do not. Rarely, elevations of serum AFP are associated with small foci of tissue resembling fetal liver (Fig. 16) and staining strongly positive for AFP (237). In the majority of such teratomas, unequivocal yolk sac tumor (Fig. 16) may also be identified, suggesting that at least some of these foci actually represent the hepatoid pattern of yolk sac tumor. However, in occasional teratomas, particularly congenital ones occurring in premature infants, only hepatoid foci can be found. It is presently unclear as to whether these latter foci represent malignant or immature tissue. Recently, there has been a report of teratomas containing immature enteric tissue and having elevated serum AFP, but many of the photographs of the AFP-positive structures in these teratomas appear to represent less well-recognized yolk sac patterns such as the endometrioid (41) and pure intestinal patterns (Fig. 17) (42). The association of yolk sac tumor with hepatoid and enteric structures appears to recapitulate early embryonic development, when the yolk sac is in direct continuity with the primitive gut. This latter structure is sometimes called the secondary yolk sac vesicle and is the source of the hepatobiliary anlage (201).

It seems reasonable to assume that virtually all teratomas associated with elevated serum AFP have yolk sac elements somewhere in the tumor. Whether these elements lead to recurrent or metastatic disease probably depends on the site of the tumor and the stage at the time of diagnosis (27,96). If the tumor is a stage I ovarian teratoma with these small foci, it will likely require no further treatment after complete excision, whereas if it is an extragonadal tumor with no definitive capsule or boundaries, it should probably be treated with chemotherapy. After either therapeutic approach, it would be prudent to monitor serum markers such as AFP concentrations to detect their appearance or recurrence. Even small foci of cells producing AFP or human chorionic gonadotropin (hCG) may have a malignant potential that cannot be predicted at the time of initial diagnosis.

Ovarian teratomas are sometimes associated with

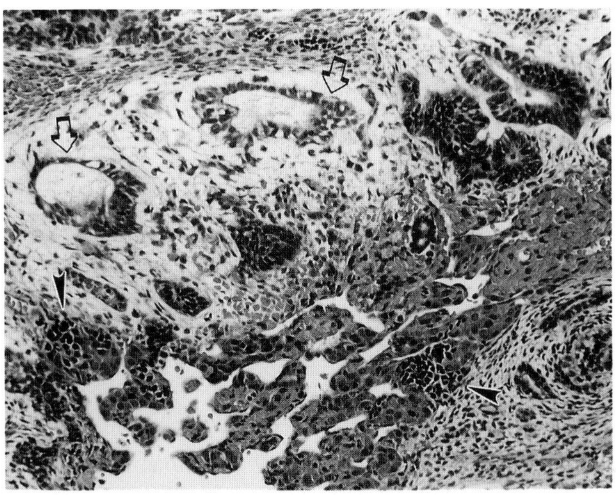

FIG. 16. Fetal liver with extramedullary hematopoiesis *(arrowheads)* is in intimate association with foci of yolk sac tumor *(arrows)* in an immature teratoma from the sacrococcygeum of a premature infant.

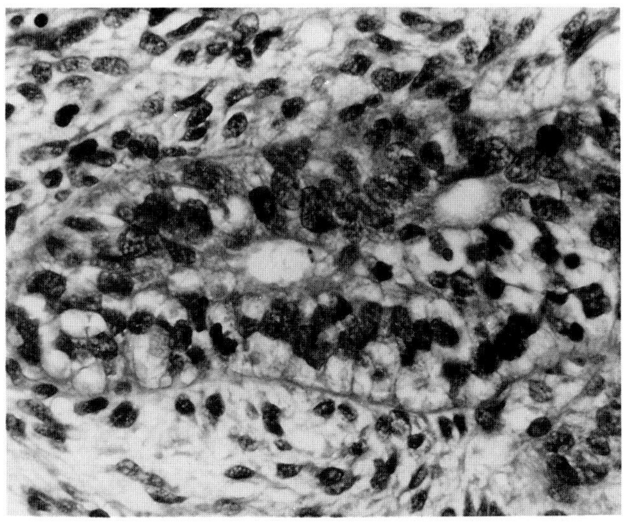

FIG. 17. This primitive tubular structure in a teratoma resembles the "endometrioid" pattern of a yolk sac tumor or a somewhat disorganized early stage of fetal intestinal development.

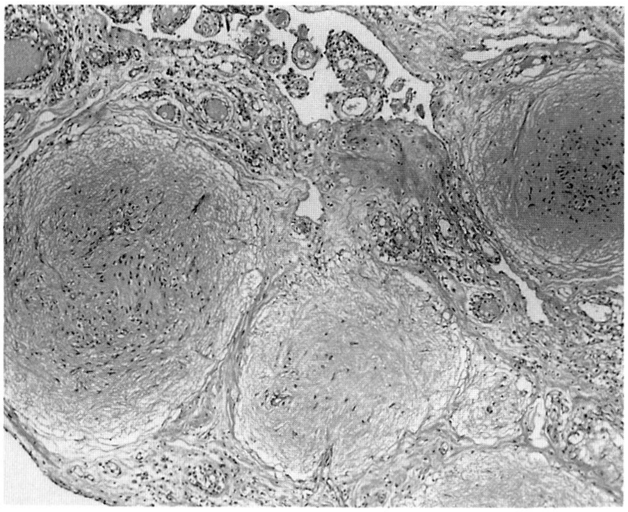

FIG. 18. Gliomatosis peritonei is characterized by intra-abdominal mature glial implants as seen in this biopsy of the mesentery.

peritoneal implants that on microscopic examination contain only mature glial elements (Fig. 18). The presence of these implants, designated gliomatosis peritonei, does not alter the prognosis for the child if they contain no immature or malignant elements (91,95,133,177, 233). However, these implants may recur one or more times, requiring additional surgery. Mature glial nodules have also been reported in rare instances in lymph nodes (197,214) (Fig. 19) and in other abdominal viscera (47), and likewise seem to behave in a benign fashion. Similar nodules have been found in cervical lymph nodes in association with head and neck teratomas; these are also not associated with recurrent tumor (57,247).

Biologic studies of immature teratomas are complex, reflecting their indeterminant clinical behavior as well as their site- and age-related differences. Whereas mature ovarian teratomas show genetic evidence of a postmeiotic origin, similar studies of immature ovarian teratomas show a more mixed picture; euploid tumors appear to arise secondary to meiotic errors, similar to mature teratomas, while some aneuploid cases are premeiotic (i.e., mitotic) in origin (182). Cytogenetic studies show a greater frequency of chromosomal abnormalities in immature teratomas (60%) when compared to mature ovarian teratomas (5%) (83,126,182,252). In addition, there appears to be a relationship between the histologic grade of immaturity and the increased presence of aneuploidy and frequency of structural rearrangements. Ploidy analysis of ovarian teratomas shows the majority of grade 1 and grade 2 immature teratomas to be diploid, with grade 3 immature teratomas being aneuploid in the hyperdiploid range (217). Another study by King and colleagues suggests that euploid grade 3 teratomas do well, whereas aneuploid tumors may not (126). Additional evaluation of the usefulness of such DNA ploidy determinants needs to be performed. Cytogenetic studies have shown no evidence of the i(12p) in these tumors, and there have been no consistent numeric or structural abnormalities identified. The common association between immature teratomas and malignant endodermal sinus tumors in the ovary, as well as in extragonadal sites of young children, suggests a close biologic relationship between these two histologic types. The biologic changes associated with this histologic transformation have not been studied. However, the association of an immature ovarian teratoma, DNA index 1.39, with an endodermal sinus tumor, DNA index 1.70, suggests that this histologic transformation is accompanied by genetic changes (217).

In contrast to ovarian teratomas, all infantile sacrococcygeal, testicular, and central nervous system teratomas, regardless of degree of immaturity, have been reported to be diploid (100,217), in keeping with the clinical observation that the grade of immaturity in these lesions does not seem to correlate with behavior. Similar to ovarian reports, sacrococcygeal teratomas recurring as endodermal sinus tumors are associated with the development of aneuploidy (217). However, central nervous system teratomas in adolescents have been consistently shown to have numeric sex chromosomal abnormalities (34,253). Of six unselected cases, all showed an increased copy of the X chromosome, and two also showed a increased copy of the Y chromosome (253). These studies are of particular interest when considering the high proportion of extragonadal germ cell tumors that arise in patients with Klinefelter's syndrome as well as the increased incidence of extragonadal teratomas in (46,XXY) females (79,136,154).

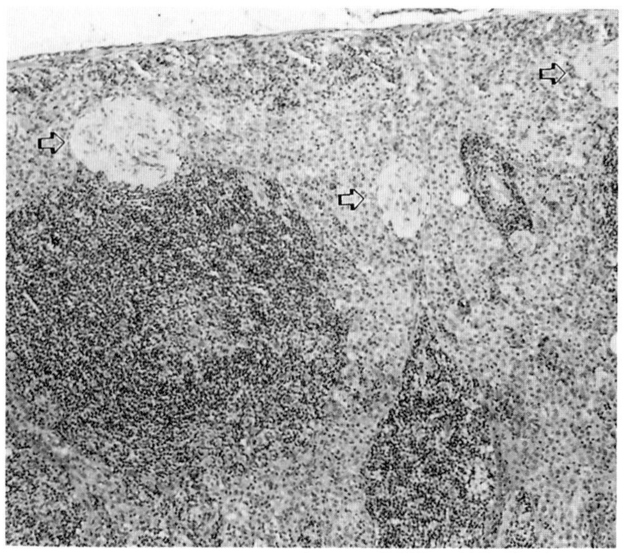

FIG. 19. Small nodules of mature glial tissue *(arrows)* are present in the interfollicular spaces of a para-aortic lymph node from a child with a mature ovarian teratoma.

MALIGNANT GERM CELL TUMORS

Malignant germ cell tumors in children differ from those in adults in both composition and distribution and differ from each other according to site (56,58,65, 92,95,113,133,150,151,170,223). Extragonadal tumors are more common in children than in adults, and sacrococcygeal tumors occur only in very young children. Forty to fifty-five percent of the malignant germ cell tumors of childhood occur in extragonadal sites (95). Testicular tumors in prepubertal males are usually malignant (yolk sac tumors), whereas ovarian tumors in the same age group are usually benign. The overwhelming majority of malignant germ cell tumors in prepubertal children are yolk sac tumors, either pure or mixed with other teratomatous or malignant components. Embryonal carcinomas are rare, and seminomas are not reported to occur in young children. Pure germinomas occur almost exclusively in the ovary (as dysgerminomas) or central nervous system. Children do not have malignant epithelial components (carcinomas) other than neuroepithelial. Sarcomatous components such as rhabdomyosarcomas and angiosarcomas (Fig. 20) are rare in childhood germ cell tumors, but when they occur, they are found most often in mediastinal tumors (152).

Biologic studies of malignant germ cell tumors have in the past largely focused on postpubertal testicular germ cell tumors, due to their large numbers and relative clinical homogeneity. Ploidy analyses show these tumors to fall in the triploid to hypotetraploid range, with seminomas being hypotetraploid and nonseminomatous germ cell tumors showing a lower DNA content (13,68,184). These observations, coupled with mathematical analyses, suggest that all postpubertal testicular germ cell tumors arise in a tetraploid (seminoma) precursor stem line, with subsequent nonrandom chromosomal loss and concomitant nonseminoma histology (54,68). Cytogenetic analyses of testicular germ cell tumors have long shown a characteristic abnormality to be present in the majority of postpubertal germ cell lesions regardless of histology, the isochromosome 12p, or i(12p) (10,11, 24,36,60,81,82,209). The i(12p) is composed of two copies of the short arm of chromosome 12, rather than the usual single short arm and single long arm (Fig. 21). Molecular data demonstrate the i(12p) of testicular tumors to be of uniparental origin (219); other studies show retention of 12q heterozygosity (241). Together these studies provide evidence that aneuploidization or polyploidization precedes i(12p) formation in testicular germ cell tumor. It has been suggested that those tumors lacking cytogenetic evidence of the i(12p) show chromosome 12 abnormalities by molecular analysis (37). The pathogenetically significant material on 12p that is amplified, or on 12q that is deleted, is not known. Fluorescence in situ hybridization (FISH) can be utilized to detect the i(12p) in interphase cells due to the different quantity of repetitive centromeric DNA in the i(12p) (167,205). Fluorescence in situ hybridization has documented the presence of the i(12p) in the tubules adjacent to malignant germ

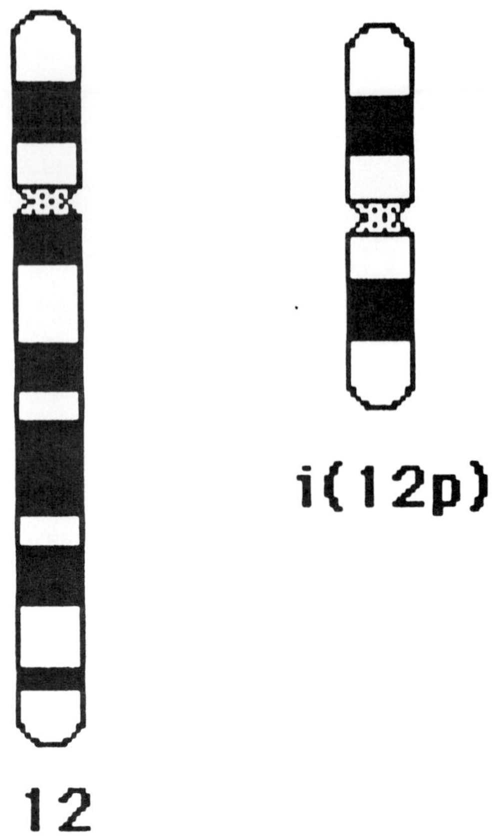

FIG. 21. This schematic diagram shows a normal chromosome 12 (left) and the isochromosome 12p (right), composed of two copies of the short arm of chromosome 12.

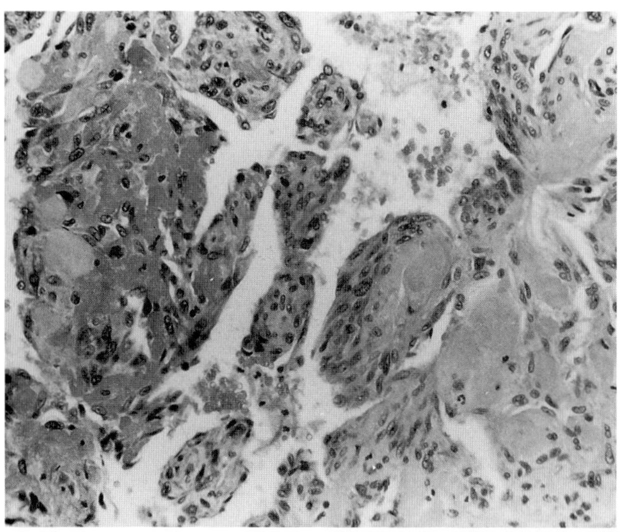

FIG. 20. The focus of angiosarcoma is from a mixed malignant germ cell tumor of the mediastinum in an adolescent boy.

cell tumors showing in situ neoplasia, providing further evidence that this is not a secondary event (145). Furthermore, many germ cell tumors have more than one copy of the i(12p), and increased copy number has been associated with worse prognosis (24). The incidence and frequency of the i(12p) in malignant germ cell tumors at other sites is not known. However, it would appear that some mediastinal malignant germ cell tumors (50), some but not all malignant ovarian germ cell tumors (12,100,110,224), and at least some pineal germinomas (52) have the i(12p). Immature ovarian teratomas have not been shown to carry the i(12p). However, in the germ cell tumors of two patients, the yolk sac tumor component arising in the setting of immature teratomas contained an i(12p) in a minority of cells, suggesting that the genetic alterations accompanying the transition from immature teratoma to yolk sac tumor may include the development of i(12p) (101,224). Other ovarian yolk sac tumors, however, have not shown an i(12p) but have a DNA content ranging from 1.62 to 1.78 and cytogenetic evidence of 6q deletion and chromosome 3 duplication (101,125).

Malignant germ cell tumors arising in the prepubertal testis and in extragonadal sites of young children show significant differences when compared to their postpubertal counterparts. First, they are restricted to the yolk sac (endodermal sinus) tumor histology. Second, ploidy analyses have shown these childhood yolk sac tumors to be most commonly euploid (diploid or tetraploid) and only rarely aneuploid (194,217). Polyploidization is not a pathogenetic requirement in these lesions. Finally, yolk sac tumors of young children do not show the i(12p) but instead show recurrent, non-random chromosomal anomalies, including 1p deletion, 3p duplication, and 6q deletion (185,194). Whether these abnormalities are primary or secondary and whether they are clinically useful or not is yet to be determined.

Germinoma

Germinomas are the least aggressive of the malignant germ cell tumors of childhood and respond well to radiation therapy or chemotherapy. They are relatively uncommon in children and are usually found in the ovary, where they are called dysgerminomas, and in the pineal region of the central nervous system (58,73,92,153, 180). Rarely, they may constitute the malignant component of a teratoma. Germinomas, or seminomas as they are designated when arising in the testis, are not found in the testes of young children, nor are they common in testicular tumors of adolescents (92,102). This is likely due to their slower growth, and hence later detection.

Germinomas are encapsulated, solid, gray–pink tumors that have a rubbery consistency and may have small foci of hemorrhage and necrosis. Microscopically, the tumor cells are arranged in nests or ribbons separated by bands of fibrous tissue in which variable numbers of lymphocytes are identified. The cells are large and round, oval, or polygonal with clear cytoplasm, distinct cell membranes, and large round nuclei with one or two prominent nucleoli. Some of the nucleoli appear elongated and cigar-shaped (Fig. 22). Foreign body and Langerhans giant cells and/or granulomas are frequently scattered throughout the tumor (Fig. 23). The giant cells must be distinguished from syncytiotrophoblasts that

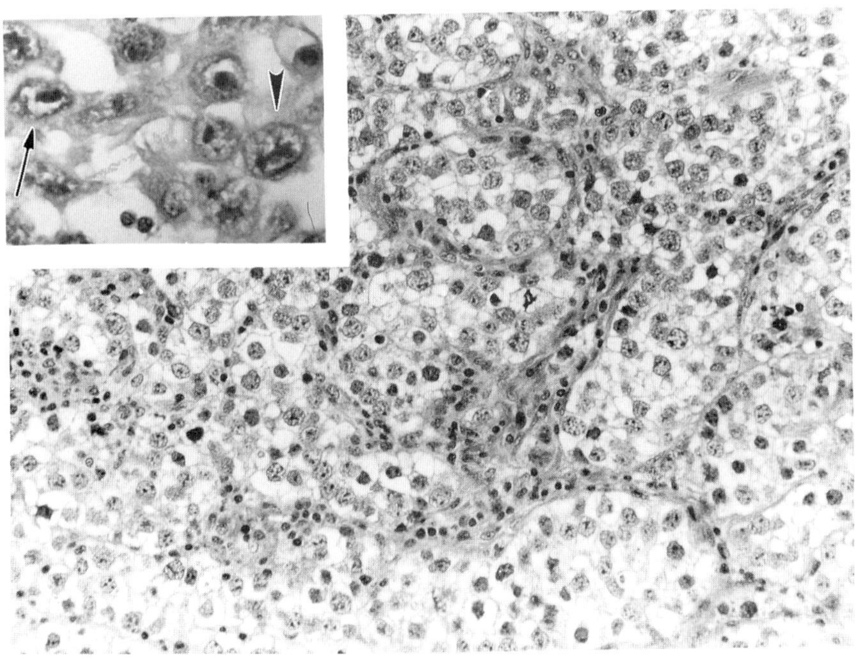

FIG. 22. Germinomas are composed of nests of monomorphic cells with vesicular nuclei and large, prominent nucleoli. The nests are separated by bands of connective tissue infiltrated by variable numbers of lymphocytes. **Inset:** Nucleoli sometimes appear cigar-shaped *(arrow)* or bilobed *(arrowhead)*.

may also be found in germinomas and other nonchoriocarcinomas. These latter cells tend to be scattered individually (unlike the syncytial arrangement in choriocarcinomas), and many have ill-defined, vacuolated cytoplasm. If syncytiotrophoblasts are present, the serum gonadotrophin β-hCG concentration may be mildly elevated, but syncytiotrophoblasts alone do not alter the prognosis of the tumor (229,237). Immunohistochemically, germinomas have diffuse membrane and cytoplasmic staining for PLAP (30,73,99,104), and the syncytiotrophoblasts exhibit positive hCG staining (30,95). Some intracranial germinomas also express epithelial membrane antigen (EMA), cytokeratin, and vimentin, but gonadal germinomas typically do not (170). By electron microscopy, the nuclei are large and round with ribbonlike nucleoli, and there is scant cytoplasm containing abundant glycogen, moderate numbers of organelles, and annulate lamellae (Fig. 24) (70,98,104,163). Germinomas are sometimes difficult to identify due to problems in fixation (Fig. 25). They may at times have large amounts of hyalinized fibrous tissue between nests of cells, and occasionally the cells will form into single "Indian file" rows (Fig. 26). This latter pattern is usually associated with more classical germinoma in other areas and should not often pose a problem in diagnosis. Seminomas in the testes of adolescents have an appearance similar to that of the germinomas seen elsewhere. The anaplastic and spermatocytic variants are not seen in children of any age.

Yolk Sac Tumor (Endodermal Sinus Tumor)

Yolk sac tumor has been called endodermal sinus tumor because of its resemblance to the endodermal sinus of the rat yolk sac (230). It is the most common malignant germ cell tumor in prepubertal children and is the only malignant germ cell component in sacrococcygeal and infantile testicular malignancies (95). The site of origin determines how often it will cause significant morbidity and mortality. Testicular tumors can be diagnosed early, and prepubertal boys with testicular yolk sac tumors have a greater than 90% disease-free survival (96,102,153). On the other hand, the long-term survival of children with extragonadal yolk sac tumors is still reported to be between 40% and 70% (73,96,153). The reduced survival of children with sacrococcygeal tumors may largely be due to inadequate resections. However, intrinsic biologic differences have not been excluded. In adults, there is a suggestion that germ cell malignancies with a yolk sac component have a worse prognosis than those lacking the yolk sac component (237). Because yolk sac tumor is most often the only malignant component in germ cell tumors of childhood, such a comparison cannot be made. However, malignant neural and sarcomatous components appear to be more aggressive than yolk sac components in the tumors of children (127,130,225) (personal observation).

Yolk sac tumor is virtually always associated with elevated concentrations of serum AFP and is probably the only malignant germ cell element that is so characterized. Thus, serum AFP concentration is a useful marker of the presence, recurrence, and/or metastasis of yolk sac tumor (88,102,215,251). However, there are a few instances in which elevations may be misleading. Newborn infants normally may have very high concentrations of AFP in the serum, and these levels may remain above the normal adult range until 8–9 months of age. The elevations are even higher in premature infants, making differentiation between normal and tumor-related con-

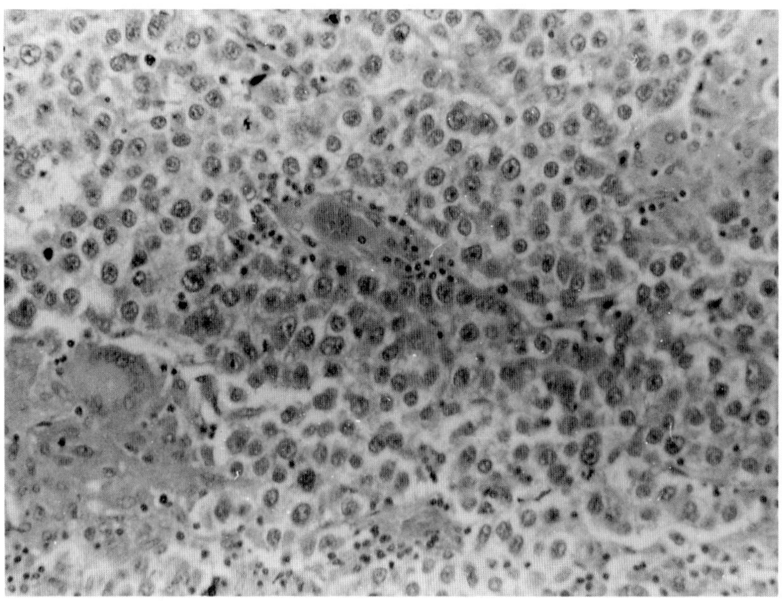

FIG. 23. A histiocytic aggregate and a poorly formed granuloma with a foreign body giant cell are seen in this section from a germinoma.

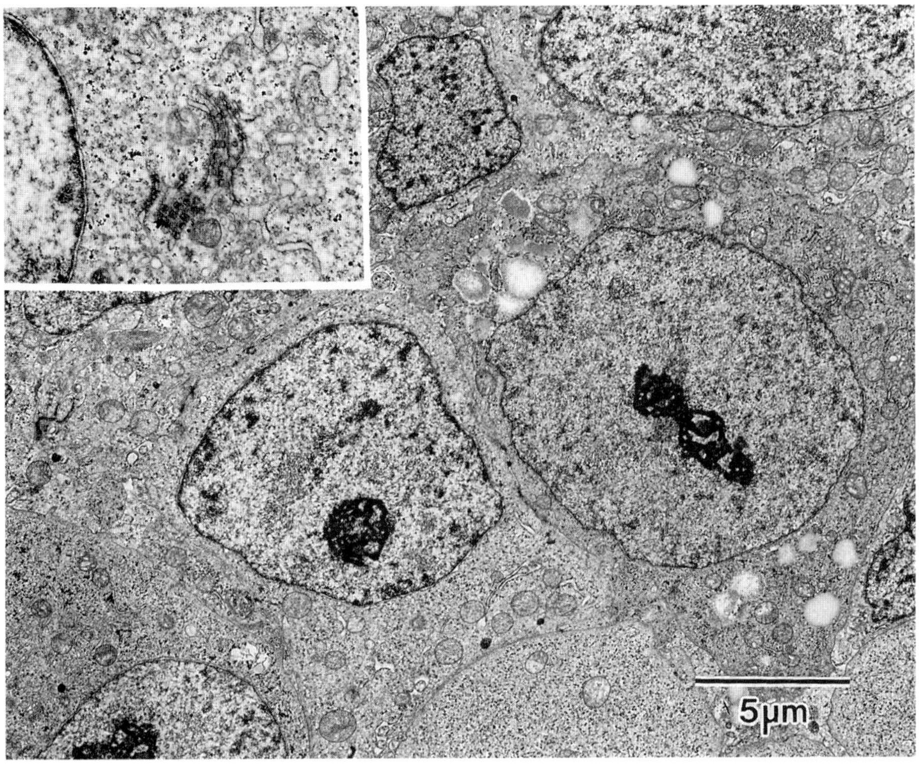

FIG. 24. The germinoma cells have round nuclei with ribbonlike nucleoli ultrastructurally. The cytoplasm has moderate numbers of organelles and glycogen particles scattered throughout. **Inset:** Annulate lamellae, seen here in longitudinal and cross-section, are often present in the cytoplasm.

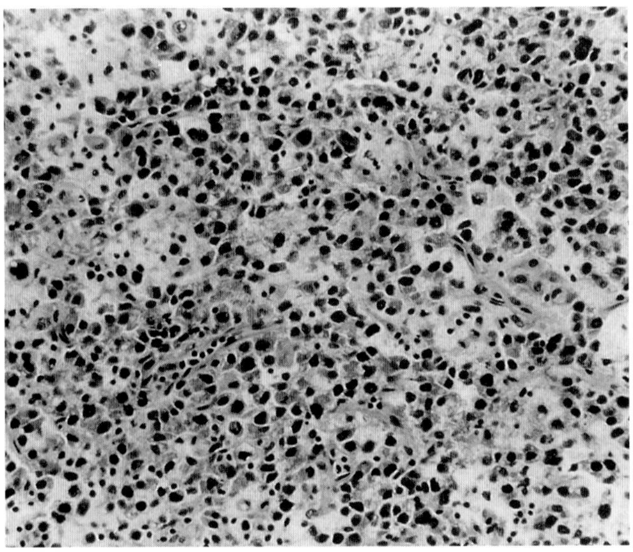

FIG. 25. This poorly fixed, necrotic germinoma has lost all nuclear detail, making a definitive diagnosis difficult. Fortunately, small areas retained sufficient detail to confirm the diagnosis. PLAP staining can be very helpful in diagnosing poorly fixed or necrotic tumor.

centrations difficult (26,97,140,250). Also, because hepatic injury and hepatic tumors may be associated with elevations in serum AFP concentrations, it is not always easy to differentiate between hepatic injury and yolk sac tumor metastatic to the liver (80). In recent years, the separation of fractions of serum AFP by their binding affinity to concanavalin A (Con A) has shown differences between the AFP produced by hepatocellular carcinomas and that produced by yolk sac tumors; that produced by hepatic tumors has a high affinity (75–90%) for Con A, whereas that produced by yolk sac tumors only binds 45–50% (88,140,157,183). Unfortunately, the only study that has investigated the binding characteristics of serum AFP in infancy has found that by the age of 6 months the majority of the normally produced AFP does not bind to Con A (140). Thus, the separation by binding characteristics may not help in differentiating between yolk sac tumor and hepatic injury in the infant. One study has used immunohistochemical methods to demonstrate the Con A binding differences in tissue. This study found that yolk sac tumors stained for AFP but did not stain for Con A, whereas hepatocellular carcinomas

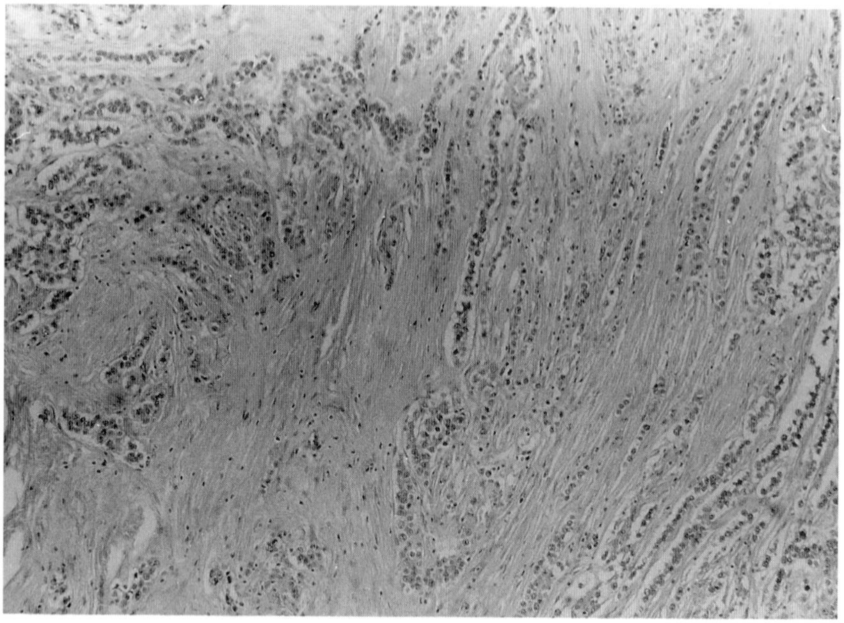

FIG. 26. Broad bands of hyalinized stroma extend between nests and single rows "Indian file" of germinoma cells. Hematoxylin and eosin. Original magnification 63×.

and fetal hepatoblasts stained for both (183). Perhaps this technique could be applied to the foci of fetal liver/hepatoid pattern of yolk sac tumor in immature teratomas to better characterize the malignant potential of these foci. A study from Japan found that serum AFP reacted with *Ricinus communis* agglutinin–I (RCA-I) when produced by a malignancy (either hepatic or germ cell in origin) but did not react with RCA-I when produced by benign hepatic diseases or fetal hepatocytes (105). This technique might also prove useful in the diagnosis of tumors occurring in infancy, but it needs to be tested further.

There are reports of elevated serum AFP concentrations associated with different types of germ cell tumors (99,123), but other studies suggest that in the majority of these cases, foci of yolk sac tumor have been either misinterpreted or overlooked (97,237). There are also rare cases of elevated serum AFP associated with so-called immature enteric glands (103,196). Earlier reports suggested that the immature neural components in immature teratomas were the source of the elevated AFP (14,71), but this suggestion has not been supported by more recent studies (196) (personal observations).

Yolk sac tumors are generally encapsulated or well circumscribed. They are composed of friable, pale gray, mucoid tissue in which variable amounts of hemorrhage and necrosis are identified (Fig. 27). Microscopically they are quite varied. The individual cells may be small and pale with scanty cytoplasm, round to oval nuclei, and inapparent nucleoli (Fig. 28), or they may be medium-sized to large with clear vesicular nuclei and prominent nucleoli, resembling embryonal carcinoma or germinoma (Fig. 29). In some tumors, the cells have abundant cytoplasm that is generally clear. Mitoses range from few to many (95).

Four general patterns with many individual variations have been recognized. These patterns are pseudopapillary or festoon, microcystic or reticular, solid, and polyvesicular vitelline (58,95,234,237). More recently, it was recognized that yolk sac tumors may have a number of additional patterns. These include endometrioid, intestinal, hepatoid, and mesenchymelike (41,42,162,171,201,234). The pseudopapillary pattern is one of the two

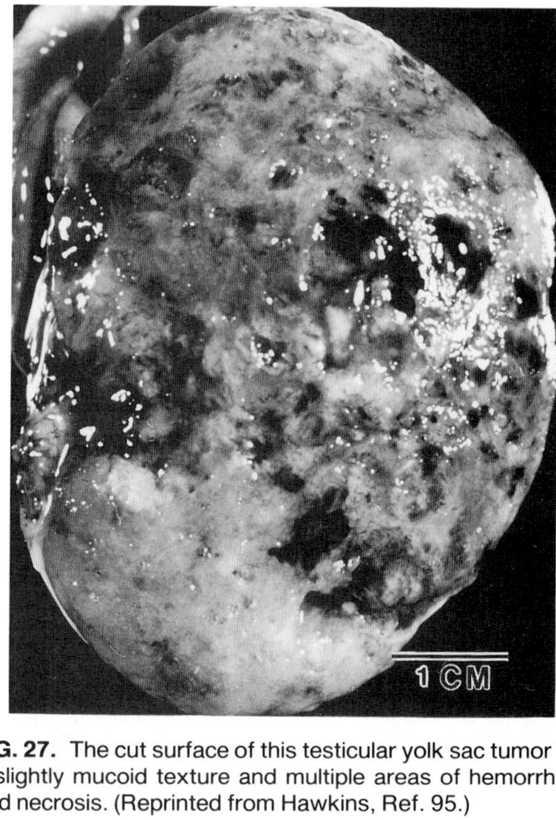

FIG. 27. The cut surface of this testicular yolk sac tumor has a slightly mucoid texture and multiple areas of hemorrhage and necrosis. (Reprinted from Hawkins, Ref. 95.)

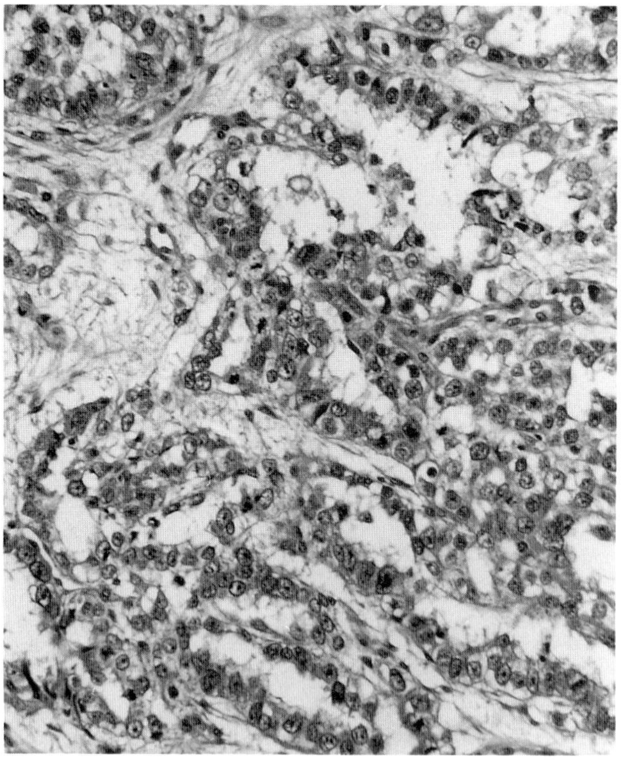

FIG. 28. The cells in this yolk sac tumor are uniformly small with small, round nuclei and modest nucleoli.

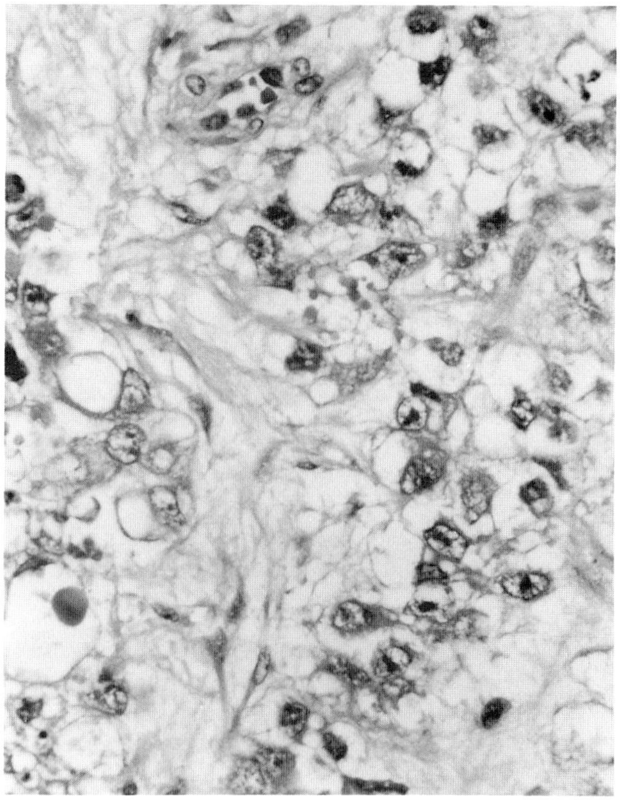

FIG. 29. The cells in this yolk sac tumor have large vesicular nuclei and prominent nucleoli.

most common and most widely recognized (Fig. 30) (92,95,234). It is one of the two patterns with which the classic Schiller–Duval body is usually associated (the microcystic pattern is the other). This structure was originally described as glomerularlike, or resembling an outpouching of the yolk sac endoderm around allantoic blood vessels (230). A classic Schiller–Duval body (Fig. 31) has a central blood vessel covered by an inner rim of tumor cells and separated from an outer rim of tumor cells by a space. Partial or pseudo-Schiller–Duval bodies that lack the outer rim of tumor cells (Fig. 32) are much more common and are the structures frequently identified as Schiller–Duval bodies. It must be emphasized, however, that neither classic nor pseudo-Schiller–Duval bodies are necessary for the diagnosis of yolk sac tumor. They are rarely, if ever, seen in association with any patterns other than pseudopapillary and microcystic. The pseudopapillary pattern has a wide variety of appearances, and the cells may vary from medium-sized to quite large. Occasionally, the intervening stroma is widened by dense, hyalinized material. It has been reported that the pseudopapillary pattern is one of the patterns that seems to persist in tumors in which chemotherapy is ineffective (235,237).

The microcystic or reticular pattern (Fig. 33) is characterized by a delicate reticular arrangement of cells forming small cysts. At times the cysts may be somewhat larger, and this pattern is occasionally associated with cells that have large, bizarre, hyperchromatic nuclei (Fig. 34). Schiller–Duval bodies also may be seen with this pattern. Eosinophilic, hyaline, intracytoplasmic, and extracytoplasmic globules and strands are most often found in the portions of the tumor exhibiting this pat-

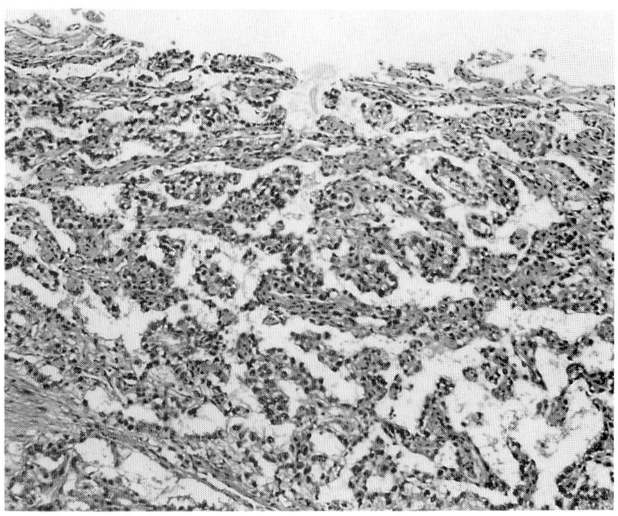

FIG. 30. The pseudopapillary (festoon) pattern of yolk sac tumor is characterized by tumor cells lining a central hyaline core. Small vascular spaces are present in some of the cores. Hematoxylin and eosin.

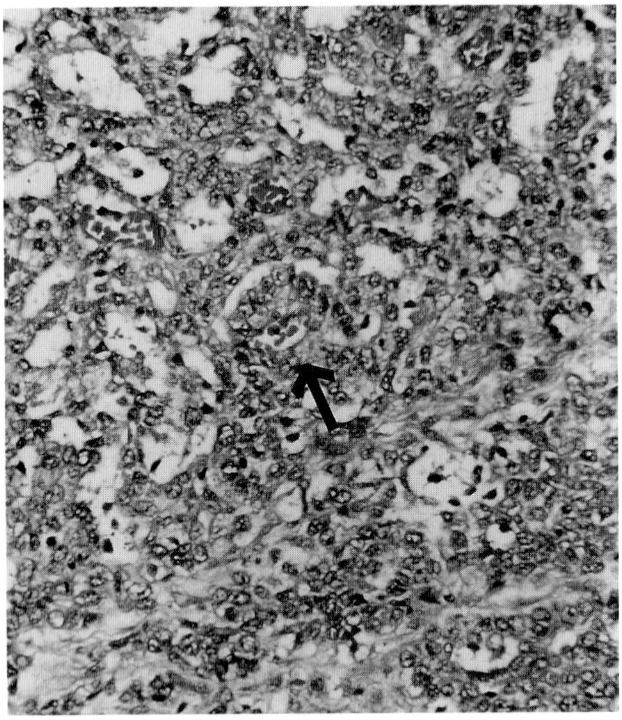

FIG. 31. The Schiller–Duval body *(arrow)* has a central vascular core lined by tumor cells, a space, and then an outer rim of tumor cells resembling a glomerulus with Bowman's capsule.

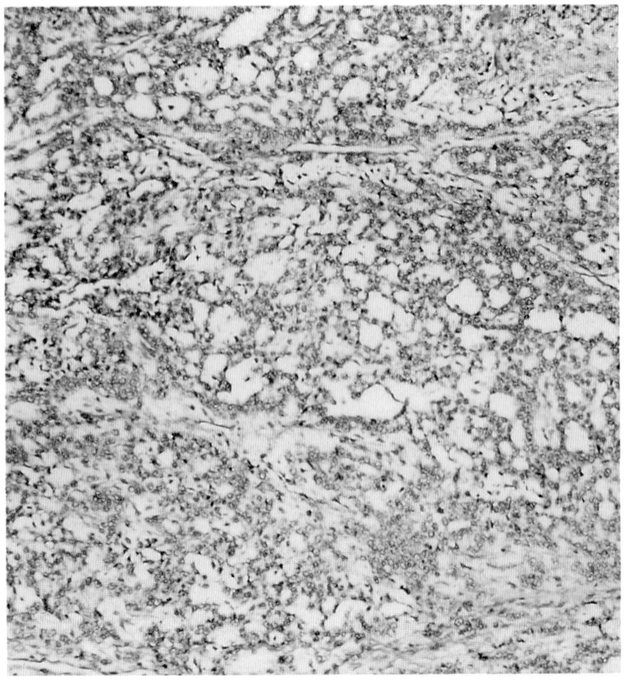

FIG. 33. This microcystic pattern of yolk sac tumor has small uniform cells forming microscopic cysts.

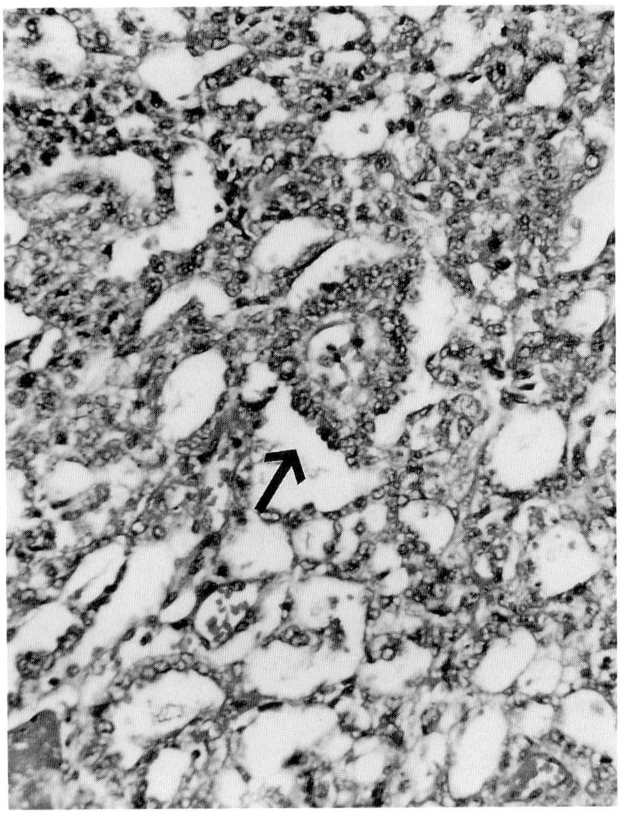

FIG. 32. The pseudo–Schiller–Duval body *(arrow)* has a central vascular core lined by tumor cells, but no second, outer rim of tumor cells.

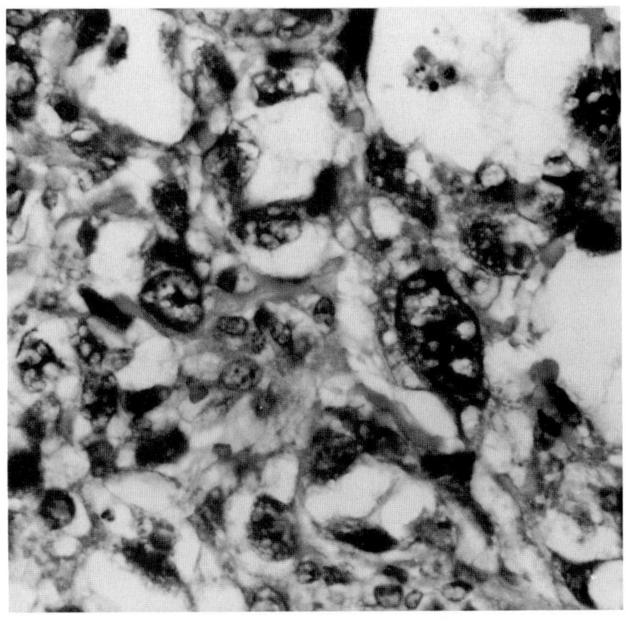

FIG. 34. Occasional yolk sac tumors have large bizarre nuclei as seen in this microcystic pattern.

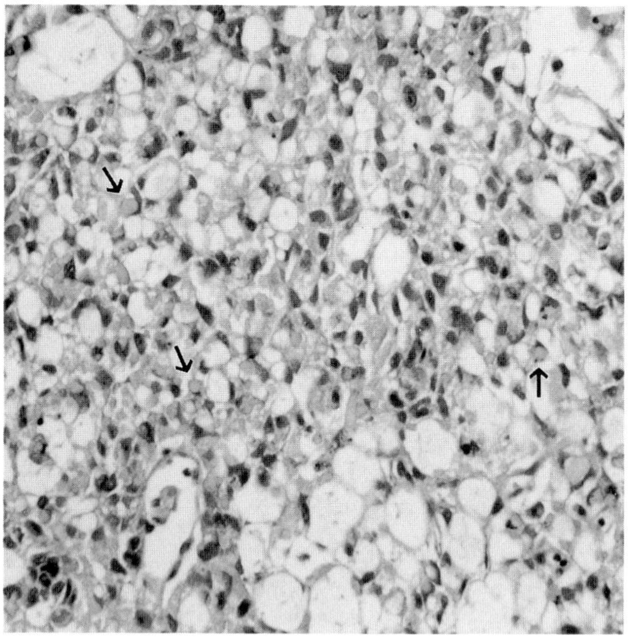

FIG. 35. A number of intracellular hyaline globules are present in this yolk sac tumor. A few representative globules are identified with the arrows.

tern. The intracytoplasmic inclusions (Fig. 35), which are often periodic acid–Schiff (PAS)–positive and diastase-resistant, may be positive by immunohistochemical stains for AFP or α_1-antitrypsin (AAT), but are more likely to be negative for both reactants (95,201,232,234). These inclusions can be useful in the separation of yolk sac tumor from embryonal carcinoma and germinoma. The inter- and intracellular strands (Fig. 36) are also PAS-positive and diastase-resistant and resemble basement membrane material in their immunohistochemical and electron microscopic appearances. They are frequently positive for laminin and appear as irregularly shaped masses arrayed in a linear arrangement along cell membranes or as membrane-limited, inhomogeneous electron-dense material in close association with cisternae of rough endoplasmic reticulum (179,234). When these latter deposits are present, the tumor is said to be exhibiting parietal yolk sac differentiation. This type of differentiation is common in yolk sac tumors, is seen most often in association with the microcystic or solid patterns, and may be useful in separating yolk sac tumors from other forms of malignancy (234,237). It has been reported that this is another pattern that seems to remain if chemotherapy is ineffective (235,237). Additional evidence for these strands being basement membrane–like material was demonstrated by Barsky et al. by placing a yolk sac tumor into a nude mouse, resulting in production of large amounts of laminin and type IV collagen (18).

The solid pattern is found in small foci in some yolk sac tumors and may have a wide variety of appearances. It is the pattern that is most often confused with embryonal carcinoma or germinoma, but careful microscopic studies usually will separate the two types of tumor. Yolk sac tumor cells in the solid pattern are smaller and less pleomorphic than similar cells in the solid portions of an embryonal carcinoma (Fig. 37) and tend to have less prominent nucleoli than either germinoma or embryonal carcinoma (95). The tendency for small microcysts to occur, the frequent presence of hyaline globules or strands in this pattern of yolk sac tumor, and the almost universal presence of focal AFP positivity in yolk sac tumors are additional findings that are useful in separating the two tumor types (234,237). Care must be taken, however, to differentiate hyaline globules and strands from the individually necrotic cells and fibrin that are often present in embryonal carcinomas (95,237).

Another solid pattern found in a number of yolk sac tumors is the so-called hepatoid pattern (201,234). This pattern is composed of cells with abundant eosinophilic cytoplasm that may occasionally have vacuoles suggestive of fat and nuclei with a single moderately prominent, round nucleolus. It resembles fetal or adult liver (Fig. 38) and has the immunohistochemical characteristics of true hepatic differentiation with positive staining for AFP, AAT, albumin, and the third and fourth components of complement (171,237).

The polyvesicular vitelline pattern is characterized by small, empty cystic structures lined by a single layer of malignant cells that merge from cuboidal to flat. These cells are often embedded in a loose, frequently myxoid stroma (Fig. 39) (95,229). It has been suggested that this pattern, either diffuse or focal, tends to be associated with a better prognosis (96,178), but the numbers of tumors

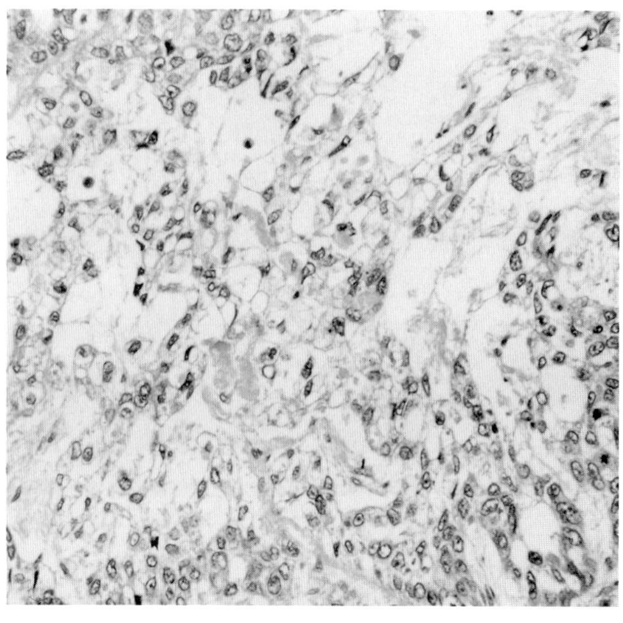

FIG. 36. This yolk sac tumor has large numbers of inter- and intracellular hyaline strands throughout the field.

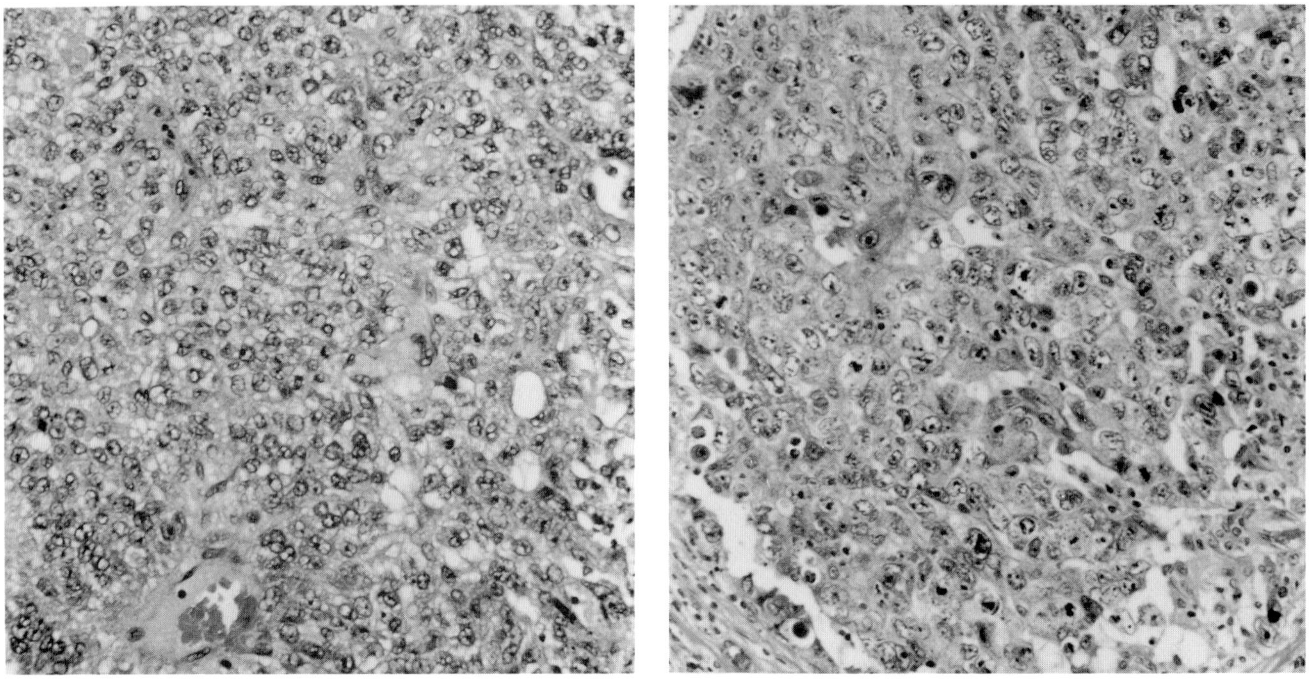

FIG. 37. **A**. The solid pattern of yolk sac tumor has small cells, moderately regular nuclei, and modest nucleoli. **B**. The embryonal carcinoma has sheets of cells with large, overlapping nuclei and very large, prominent nucleoli. Individual cell necrosis is also much more prominent.

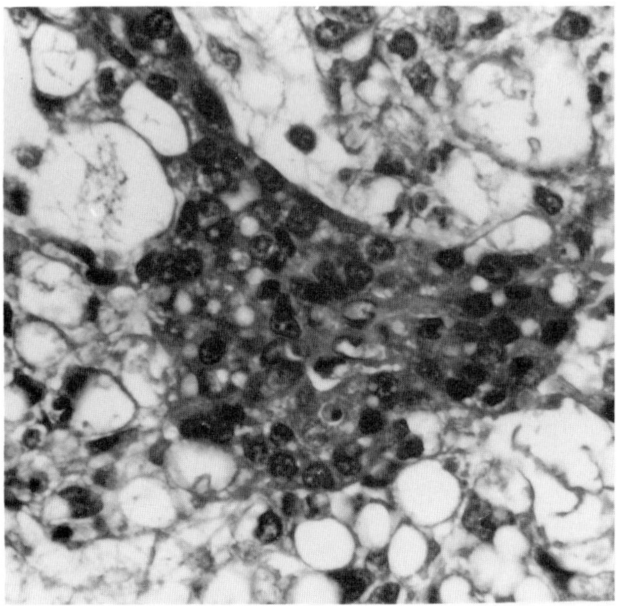

FIG. 38. Nest of cells with abundant eosinophilic cytoplasm and apparent intracytoplasmic lipid inclusions (hepatoid pattern) are present in this sacrococcygeal yolk sac tumor.

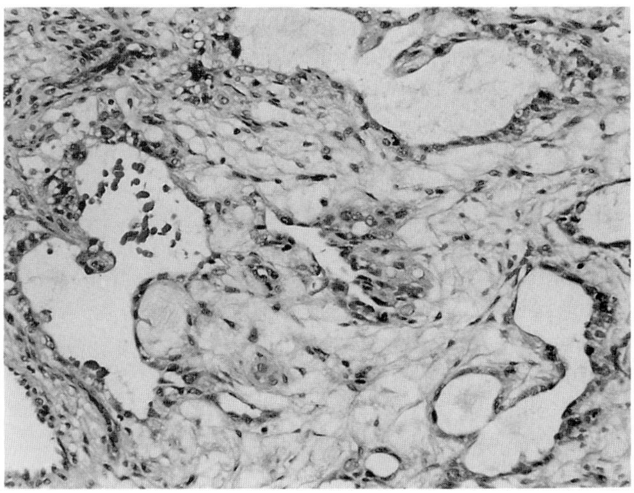

FIG. 39. The polyvesicular vitelline pattern has cystic spaces lined by flattened cells that merge with cuboidal to columnar cells. These cysts are present in a loose, myxoid stroma.

examined in these studies are small and may not be statistically valid. The loose, myxoid stroma is not limited to the polyvesicular vitelline pattern and may be seen in a wide variety of patterns (Fig. 40)

A number of yolk sac tumors have a glandular component that resembles the fetal human gut. This enteric component is characterized by cords of cells forming glandular structures that are intimately associated with the more usual patterns of yolk sac tumor (Fig. 41). The glands are lined by cuboidal to columnar cells that may have a recognizable brush border, stain positively for AFP and carcinoembryonic antigen (CEA), and by electron microscopy have a brush border with glycocalyx, glycocalyceal bodies, and microvilli with long filamentous rootlets (237). Freeze-fracture examination of some of these areas has also shown a close resemblance to normal intestine (42). A few tumors composed of a pure enteric component have also been described (229,237).

Modest numbers of yolk sac tumors are reported to have a pure, or focal, endometrioid pattern. This pattern is characterized by a prominent glandular component. The glands vary from small and round to elongated and tubular. They are lined by cuboidal cells that frequently have both sub- and supranuclear cytoplasmic vacuoles (Fig. 42). The cells exhibit AFP, AAT, and CEA positivity (41,237). It has been suggested that this pattern is actually a variant of the more commonly encountered enteric pattern (41). This latter suggestion seems reasonable, as the glandular structures frequently mimic those found in the early stages of fetal intestinal development (Fig. 42) (63).

Glandular structures similar to the enteric and endometrioid patterns may be seen in immature teratomas

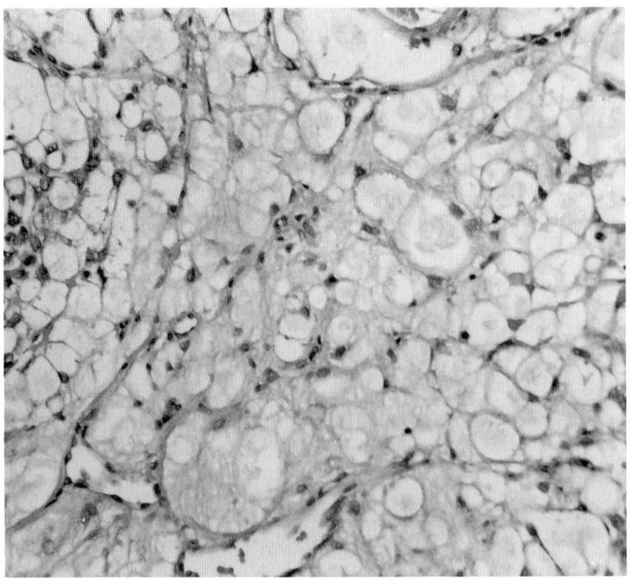

FIG. 40. This microcystic pattern of yolk sac tumor has a myxoid stroma.

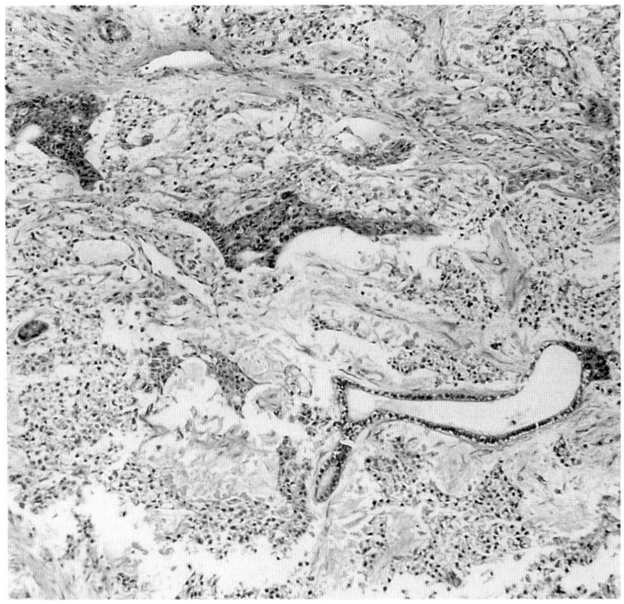

FIG. 41. Glandular structures lined by cells with hyperchromatic nuclei and basophilic (darker) cytoplasm characteristic of the "enteric" pattern are present in this yolk sac tumor.

(Fig. 17). At present, it is unclear as to whether these structures represent foci of yolk sac tumor or are simply extremely immature fetal tissue, as suggested by Perrone et al. (196). Because these structures may be associated with foci of unequivocal yolk sac tumor elsewhere in the tumor, they may at least serve to alert the examiner to search more diligently.

Finally, there is a loose, angioblastic stromal component, the mesenchymelike pattern, that is seen in a number of yolk sac tumors and is often the only component remaining in posttherapeutic specimens (Fig. 43) (55, 162,235). This component stains positively for cytokeratin and vimentin and is negative for AFP (55). It has been suggested that this component is relatively resistant to chemotherapy and may be the source of posttherapy sarcomas seen in some patients whose original tumor was a yolk sac tumor (187,235). The mesenchymelike component has also been suggested as the source of the hematopoietic malignancies that are associated primarily with mediastinal tumors (187).

Ultrastructurally, yolk sac tumor cells have irregular nuclei with prominent nucleoli and dispersed chromatin. The cytoplasm may contain glycogen, lipid inclusions, multivesicular bodies, and one of two types of intracytoplasmic material labeled type 1 and type 2 by Ulbright et al. (237). Type 1 material consists of uniformly electron-dense, nonmembrane-bound, spheroidal inclusions that correspond to the eosinophilic hyaline globules seen by light microscopy (Fig. 44). Type 2 material is present in membrane-limited spaces in close approximation to rough endoplasmic reticulum and

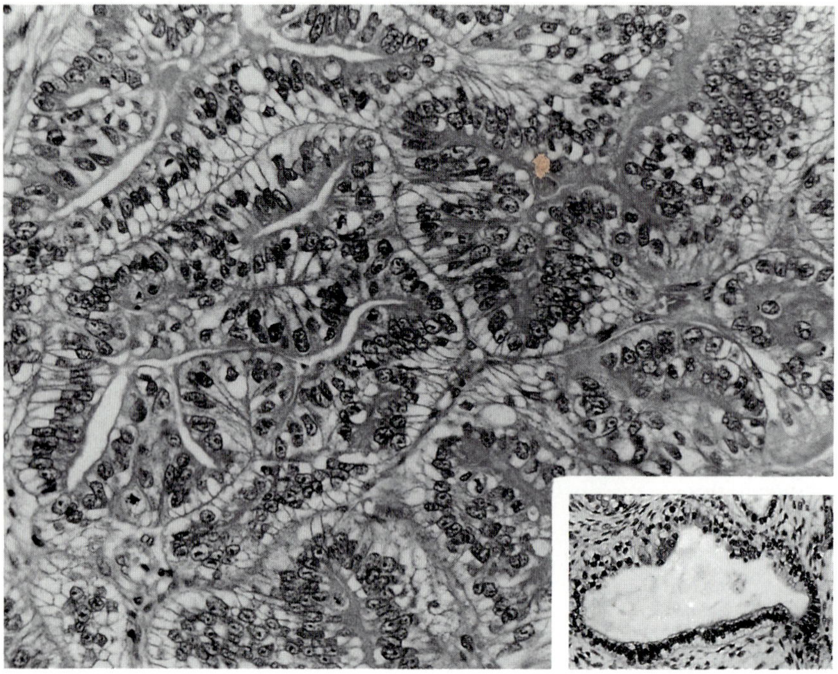

FIG. 42. The endometrioid pattern of yolk sac tumor has both sub- and supranuclear vacuoles and resembles endometrium or early fetal intestine. **Inset:** Glandular structure in an immature teratoma resembling early fetal intestine.

consists of irregular aggregates of variably electron-dense material (Fig. 44). Similar material in irregular aggregates or in poorly defined linear arrangements is present in the extracellular spaces and corresponds to the eosinophilic strandlike material seen by light microscopy in the areas of parietal differentiation (Fig. 45). The cells may have short microvilli on the free surfaces and cell junctions varying from well-formed desmosomes to interdigitating cell membranes (Fig. 46) (70,98,237).

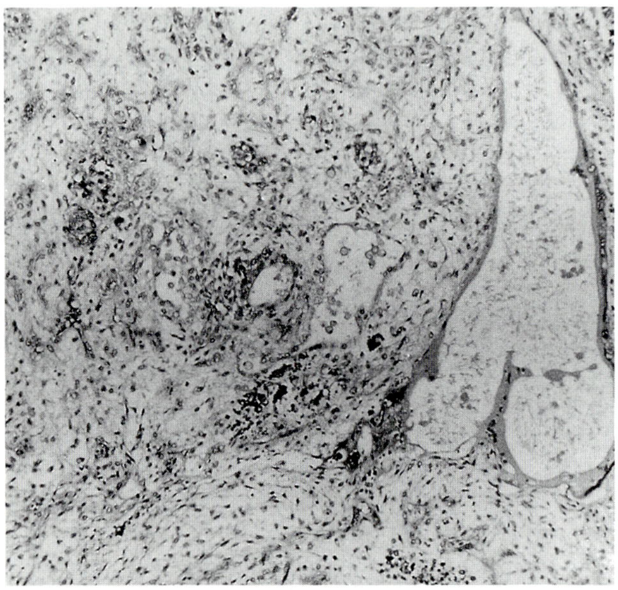

FIG. 43. This area of yolk sac tumor has loose mesenchyme in which numerous small capillaries are interspersed between a few cystic spaces lined by identifiable yolk sac tumor cells. Slender strands of eosinophilic hyaline material are present throughout the extracellular spaces.

Embryonal Carcinoma

Yolk sac tumors formerly were called "infantile" embryonal carcinomas to distinguish them from the "adult" embryonal carcinomas that are rarely seen in early childhood (58,95,164,229). Embryonal carcinomas in children seldom occur in pure form but are often a major component of the mixed malignant germ cell tumors of the testis and mediastinum in adolescents. They are less likely to be a component of adolescent ovarian germ cell tumors (229). These adult tumors have a gross appearance similar to that of yolk sac tumors, but microscopically they have some differences. The cells are generally larger than those of either yolk sac tumors or germinomas, and the nuclei have very large, round nucleoli and tend to overlap. The major pattern is epithelial and consists of large nests of cells with varying amounts of central necrosis. Individual cell necrosis is also a prominent feature (Fig. 47). Pseudotubular and papillary patterns that may be confused with yolk sac tumor are not uncommon (Fig. 48) but embryonal carcinomas do not have AFP-positive cells and lack the eosinophilic intercellular strandlike material characteristic of parietal differentiation in yolk sac tumors (234,237). Eosinophilic hyaline globules are also much less common in embryonal carcinomas. Care must be taken, however, not to mistake fibrin in areas of necrosis for this

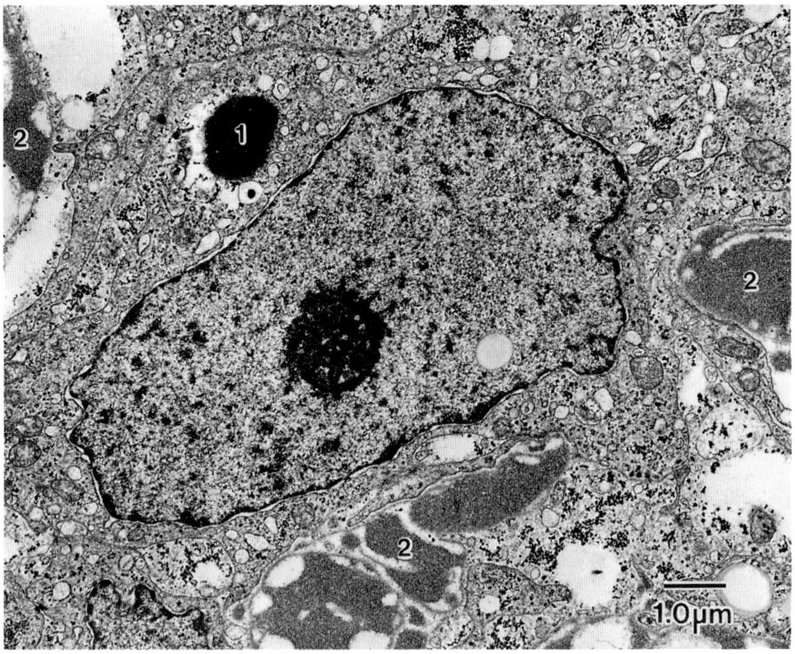

FIG. 44. A non-membrane bound, electron-dense spheroidal inclusion **(#1)** corresponds to the hyaline globules seen by light microscopy. The lighter, membrane-bound material **(#2)** corresponds to the Type 2 material described by Ulbright et al.

eosinophilic material or to mistake individually necrotic cells for intracellular hyaline inclusions (237). Ultrastructurally, the nuclei are irregularly shaped with clumped chromatin (heterochromatin) and nucleolonema forming skeinlike patterns. The free surfaces have focal stubby microvilli along acinar spaces, and there are some poorly formed intercellular junctional complexes that become more complex in the more differentiated cells. The cytoplasm has numerous organelles and occasional intermediate filaments and microtubules. Cytokeratin filaments, desmosomes, and true lumens are present in the more differentiated areas of tumor (70,98,104).

Choriocarcinomas

Choriocarcinoma is a very rare childhood tumor that may be pure in infants (7,20,77); but in older children, it usually occurs as a component of a mixed germ cell tumor (58,95,229). When it occurs in infants, it virtually always represents a maternal or placental metastasis and

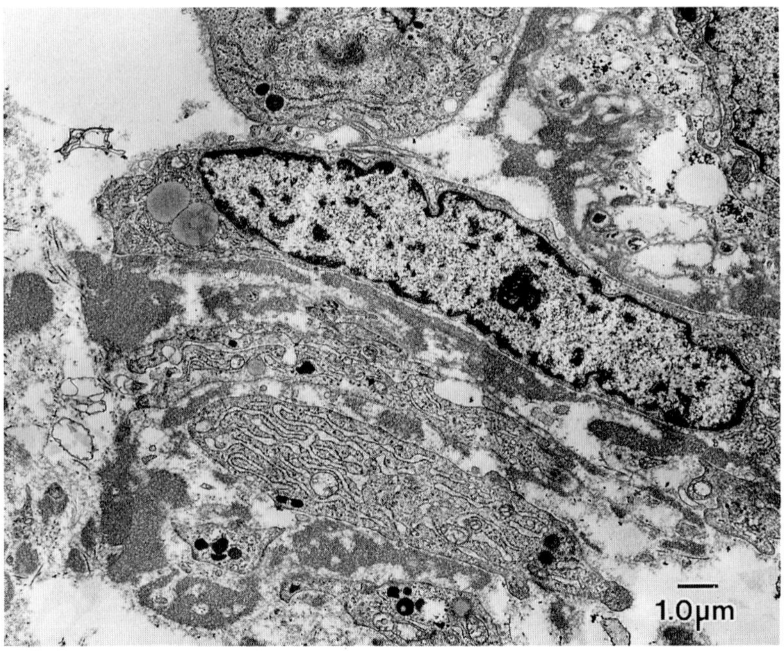

FIG. 45. Type 2 material is also found in extracellular strands and resembling basement membrane.

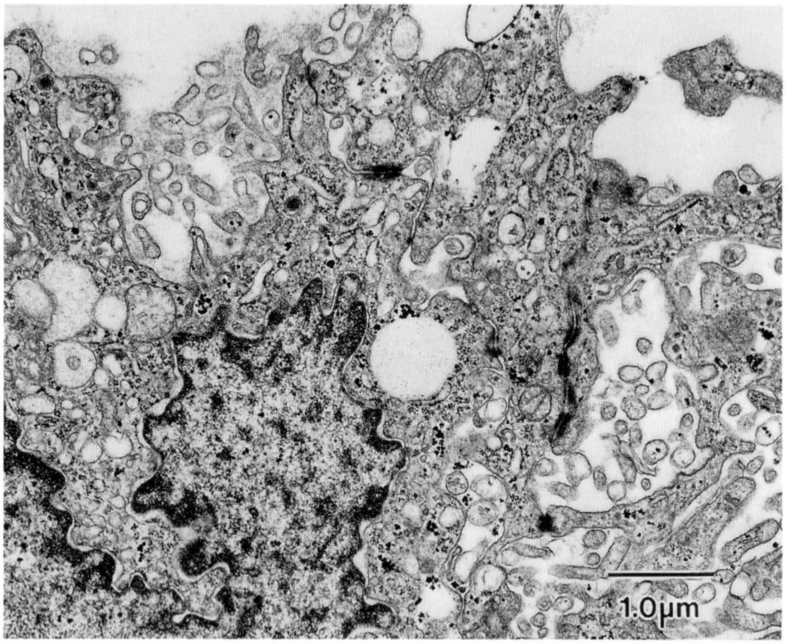

FIG. 46. The yolk sac cells in this field have short microvilli on the surface and prominent, well-formed desmosomes.

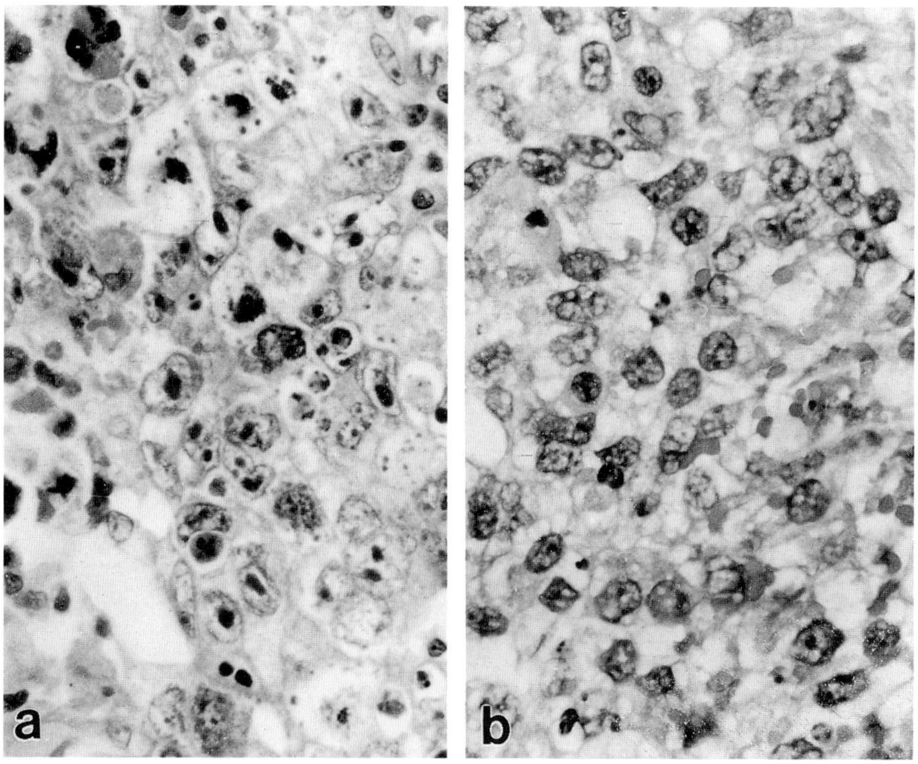

FIG. 47. An embryonal carcinoma with large, overlapping nuclei, large nucleoi and individual cell necrosis is shown in **(a).** In contrast, the solid pattern of yolk sac tumor with slightly smaller, more uniform nuclei and inconspicuous nucleoli is shown in **(b).**

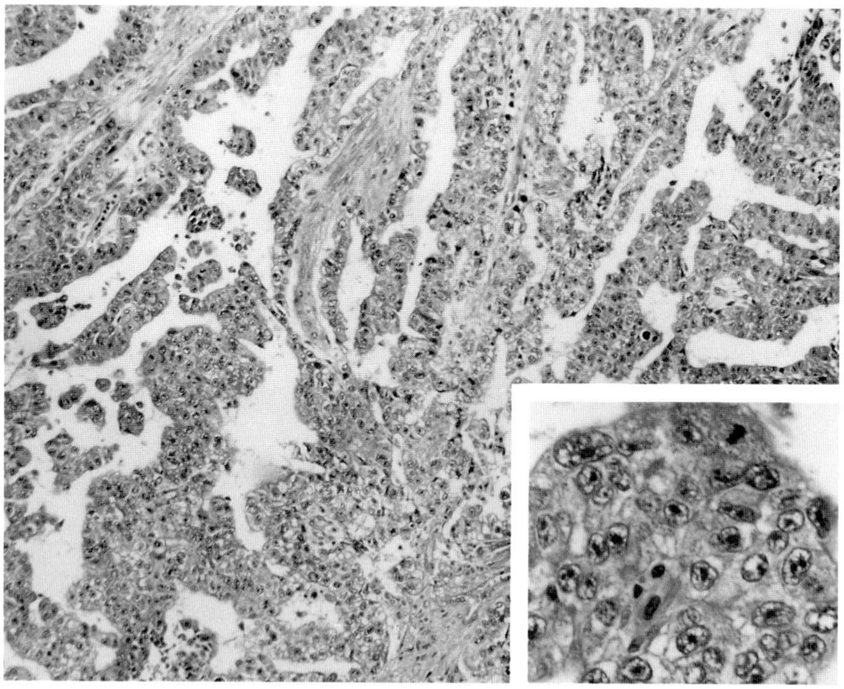

FIG. 48. This embryonal carcinoma has a pseudopapillary pattern reminiscent of that seen in yolk sac tumor, but the cell nuclei (**inset**) are those of an embryonal carcinoma.

thus is actually a gestational trophoblastic tumor rather than a germ cell tumor (20).

Grossly, the choriocarcinoma arising from a malignant germ cell is often so friable, hemorrhagic, and necrotic that the underlying gray–white tumor tissue cannot be identified macroscopically. Microscopically, the tumor is composed of two cell types—cytotrophoblasts and syncytiotrophoblasts—that must both be present. Cytotrophoblasts classically appear as closely packed nests of relatively uniform, medium-sized cells having clear, PAS-positive cytoplasm, distinct cell margins, and vesicular nuclei. Unfortunately, in practice, these cells may be more pleomorphic, less cohesive, and have less clear cytoplasm than the classic description, but they can usually be separated from other types of germ cells by the syncytiotrophoblastic pattern of association (Fig. 49). These latter cells when present by themselves in other types of germ cell tumors usually appear distinct from the surrounding cells (Fig. 50). When they are present in choriocarcinomas, they tend to develop syncytia and cover nests of cytotrophoblasts as they do in the normally developing chorionic villus (Fig. 49). Ultrastructural examination confirms the presence of syncytial and multinucleated cells. The nuclei are bizarre with finely dispersed chromatin and multiple nucleoli. The cells have many microvilli at the cell borders and within the cytoplasm. Desmosomes are plentiful, and the cytoplasm contains phagocytized erythrocytes and secondary lysosomes (70,104). Immunohistochemical staining for β-hCG is sometimes helpful in identifying the sourcc of metastatic lesions.

Mixed Malignant Germ Cell Tumors

In younger children, the usual type of mixed malignant germ cell tumor is the teratoma with malignant elements. A yolk sac tumor component is the most common malignant element in these teratomas and confers its usual malignant behavior upon the tumor. Germinoma is the second most common malignant element. Other types of malignant cells are unusual in this age group, although an occasional tumor will have a truly malignant, as opposed to immature, neural component (127,130). In postpubertal children, on the other hand, the malignant elements are frequently mixtures of one or more malignant germ cell tumor components: embryonal carcinoma, yolk sac tumor, germinoma, and choriocarcinoma with or without mature or immature teratomatous components. Nonneural malignant epithelial components are virtually never seen in childhood germ cell tumors, but sarcomatous elements may occasionally be present, most often in mediastinal tumors (56,65,95,152,238). Rarely, these latter tumors have also been associated with endocrine secretions such as testosterone and insulin (121).

In some germ cell tumors, embryoid bodies (peculiar structures said to resemble the mammalian blastocyst) (Fig. 51) are admixed with yolk sac or embryonal carcinomatous components (172). Rarely, an entire tumor is composed of these structures. It is then called a polyembryoma. There is disagreement as to the exact origin of embryoid bodies, ranging from parthenogenesis of primitive germ cells to differentiation of multipotential ma-

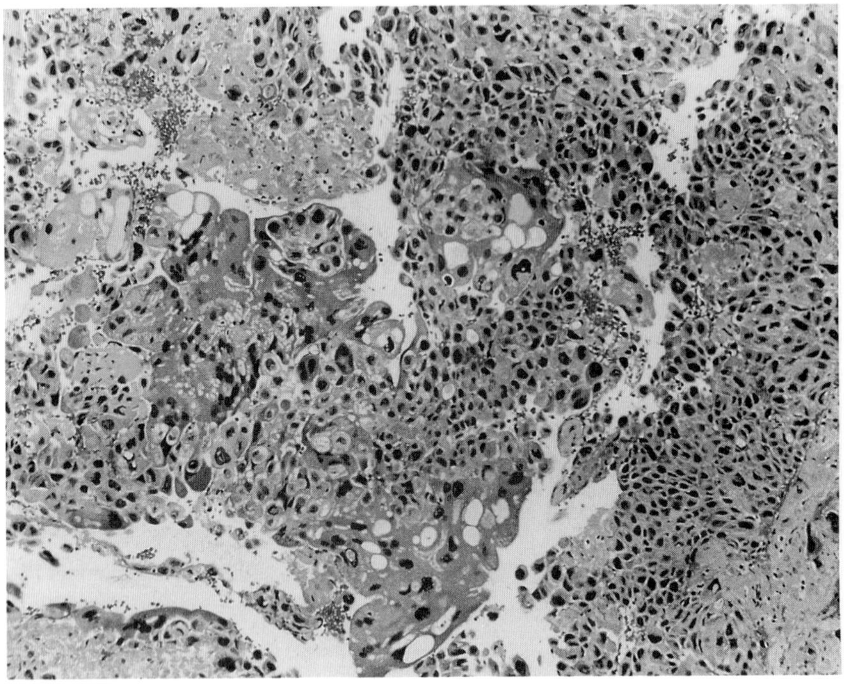

FIG. 49. In this choriocarcinoma, large syncytiotrophoblasts are in intimate contact with nests of small cytotrophoblasts. As is often true, the cytotrophoblasts in this field lack the classic clear cytoplasm.

lignant embryonal cells (229). Recently, Nakashima et al. made careful serial sections through three tumors containing a number of these bodies and determined that they appeared to be in continuity with intestinal and hepatic structures and thus were not real or teratomatous embryos (172). Their presence as isolated structures within a mixed malignant germ cell tumor does not alter the behavior of the tumor. Pure polyembryomas have been considered highly malignant tumors (229), but the response to present-day therapeutic regimens is the same as that of other germ cell tumors (172).

Tumors Postchemotherapy

Modern multidrug chemotherapeutic regimens incorporating a platinum-based agent have markedly improved the outcome for all children with malignant germ cell tumors. However, there are still children whose tumors recur or do not respond initially. In the younger children, the resistant component is almost always yolk sac tumor. The pattern of the residual or recurrent tumor tends to be less pleomorphic and is most likely to be pseudopapillary or mesenchymelike (122,124,162,235,

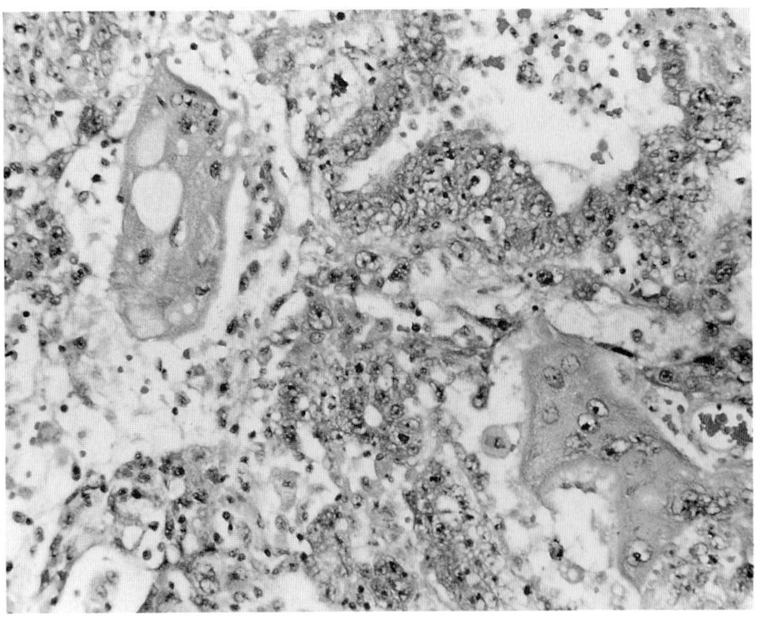

FIG. 50. Individual syncytiotrophoblasts may be seen in association with other germ cell tumors such as this embryonal carcinoma. Compare with the syncytia they form in a choriocarcinoma in Figure 50.

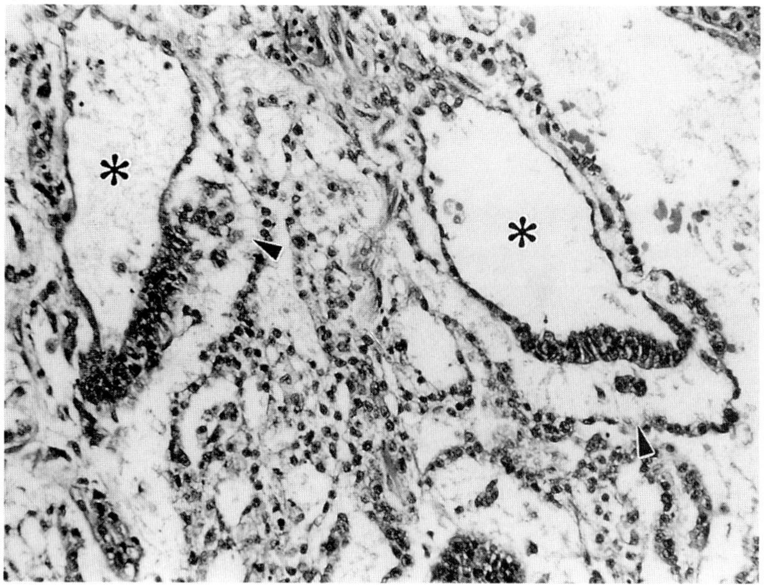

FIG. 51. Two "embryoid bodies" are present in this area of yolk sac tumor. The so-called amniotic sac *(asterisks)* is above the epithelial body and portions of the yolk sac *(arrowheads)* are below.

237). This latter pattern could be overlooked as it resembles reactive angiofibroblastic proliferations. In older children with mixed germ cell tumors, the only tumor tissue remaining may be mature teratoma admixed with areas of necrosis, calcification, foamy cells, and occasional bizarre nuclei. However, these children also may have areas of residual mesenchymelike or spindle cell tumor that need to be identified (162).

AIDS TO DIAGNOSIS

Immunohistochemistry

Malignant germ cell tumors can usually be diagnosed and classified by their light microscopic appearance. Some, however, are less distinctive. In these tumors, immunohistochemical markers may be useful. AFP, hCG and PLAP have traditionally been the most helpful of these markers. AFP-positive cells will be found focally in virtually 100% of pure yolk sac tumors, and the presence of such cells is strongly suggestive of the presence of yolk sac tumor (57,95,149,234,237). Occasional reports state that AFP is found in other tissues (73,99,108,196,243), but at least some of the structures stained appear to represent less well-recognized patterns of yolk sac tumor rather than other tissues. Thus, positive AFP staining remains relatively specific for yolk sac tumor, but it is not very sensitive. The exception to the specificity for yolk sac tumor of positive AFP staining is the presence of true hepatic tissue in teratomas (201,234). As stated earlier, double staining with Con A has been shown in one study to separate this type of tissue from the hepatoid pattern of yolk sac tumor (183). PLAP stains virtually all germinomas, but has also been found in lesser amounts and lesser intensity in embryonal carcinomas, some yolk sac tumors, and the syncytiotrophoblasts of choriocarcinomas. The pattern of staining in germinomas tends to be strongly membrane associated as well as cytoplasmic, whereas the staining in the remaining types of tumors is more likely to be cytoplasmic. PLAP is also strongly positive in ITGCN and negative in normal testicular germ cells (15,30,31,57,223). Syncytiotrophoblasts and intermediate trophoblasts are strongly positive for hCG (95,237). A combination of PLAP and cytokeratin stains may be helpful in separating germinomas from other germ cell tumors, as the majority of germinomas, other than those from the brain, stain weakly or not at all for cytokeratin, whereas yolk sac tumors, embryonal carcinomas, and choriocarcinomas (142,242) are generally strongly positive. Germinomas in the brain, however, are reported to be consistently positive for cytokeratin (57,73,142,170,223,237,242). Recently, investigators have found that CD30 (Ki-1) is present in the majority of embryonal carcinomas and absent in all other types of germ cell tumors (76,191). These five immunohistochemical stains, AFP, PLAP, hCG, cytokeratin, and CD30 (Ki-1), may be quite useful in identifying residual tumor in patients who have undergone chemotherapy (Table 2). Many other immunohistochemical stains have been applied to germ cell tumors (57,108,139,170), but at the present time these do not offer significant help in differentiating the various tumor types.

Serologic Markers

Serum concentrations of AFP, primarily produced by yolk sac tumor cells, and hCG, produced by syncytiotrophoblasts, have been proven to be reliable and useful markers of the presence of these tumor cells in the primary tumor and in recurrences (42,102,119,123,155,

TABLE 2. *Immunohistochemical staining patterns in germ cell tumors*

Tumor/cell type	AFP	hCG	PLAP C	PLAP M	CytoK	CD30
Yolk sac tumor	++	−	++	−	++	−
Embryonal carcinoma	−	−	+	−	++	++
Germinoma	−	−	++	++	±	−
Choriocarcinoma	−	++	+	−	++	−
ITGCN	−	−	++	++	−	−
Normal germ cells	−	−	−	−	−	−

Abbreviations: C, cytoplasm; M, membrane; AFP, α fetoprotein; hCG, human chrionic gonadotrophin; PLAP, placental alkaline phosphatase; CytoK, cytokeratin; ITGCN, intratubular germ cell neoplasia.

160,237,249). In young children whose markers return to normal after therapy, there is no need for second-look surgery (155). However, in adolescents with mixed testicular germ cell tumors, second-look surgery is still necessary because embryonal carcinoma and nongerm cell malignancies may be present (33,64). Some investigators suggest that AFP concentrations may be elevated in pure immature teratomas. In the majority of instances, this elevation is probably related to missed foci of yolk sac tumor or hepatic cells. However, one Japanese study suggests that low concentrations of AFP (below 1000 ng/dL) represent immature teratoma and higher concentrations represent yolk sac tumor (123).

In newborn infants, particularly if they are premature, serum AFP concentrations are normally high (250). In these children, it is often difficult to determine whether the AFP is from the normal tissues or from tumor. And, unfortunately, in this age group, the separation of Con A binding AFP from nonbinding AFP is least helpful (see above) (140).

Other serum components that have been suggested to be possible markers of germ cell tumor presence are PLAP and lactate dehydrogenase (LDH). Serum concentrations of PLAP have been reported to be elevated in patients with seminomas (251), but this component of serum has not been measured routinely in children with germ cell tumors. The total serum concentration of LDH has not proven very useful, but recent reports suggest that the LDH-1 fraction may be increased in children with yolk sac tumors and may rise again with recurrence of tumor (1,106).

The demonstration of any of these markers—AFP, hCG, PLAP, LDH-1—in cerebrospinal or tumor cyst fluid can also be helpful in diagnosing and differentiating germ cell tumors.

Fine-Needle Aspiration

The technique of fine-needle aspiration has been applied to the diagnosis of germ cell tumors in adults by a few investigators (2,17,206). Yolk sac tumor cells are described as having vacuolated cytoplasm and occasional hyaline globules and are arranged in tubulovesicular and papillary structures. Balslev and coworkers separated the five types of germ cell tumors on the basis of cytologic characteristics as follows: seminoma (germinoma) cells were monomorphic and dissociated with a thin rim of blue cytoplasm, a large nucleus, a prominent nucleolus, and a "tiger-striped" background; embryonal carcinoma cells tended to be arranged in epithelial clumps, were pleomorphic, and did not have a tiger-striped background; yolk sac tumor cells were also in tight epithelial clumps that sometimes formed spherical cell clusters but had vacuolated cytoplasm; choriocarcinomas had loose clusters of cells with indistinct cytoplasmic borders admixed with large, pleomorphic multinucleated cells; and teratomas had a mixture of epithelial and mesenchymal cells of varying degrees of maturation. These authors reported that they were able to identify 26 of 30 components in 3 pure and 10 mixed germ cell tumors (17).

In children, fine-needle aspiration may be a useful adjunct in the diagnosis of recurrent tumors and, occasionally, in the diagnosis of the primary tumor. However, the importance of increasing our understanding of the biology of these tumors and the need to determine those tumors that can be treated less aggressively require that more tissue than can be obtained by fine-needle aspiration be provided. In addition, studies have not yet shown that there is no advantage to debulking germ cell tumors prior to the administration of chemo- and radiotherapy, and at least one study has found that in yolk sac tumors of the ovary, debulking is an important prognostic feature (124).

CONCLUSIONS

Over 50% of germ cell tumors in children occur in extragonadal locations, and mature teratomas account for over half of these tumors in both gonadal and extragonadal locations. Of the malignant germ cell tumors, yolk sac tumors compose the majority in the young age group and are often one of the malignant components in the mixed germ cell tumors of adolescence. Germinomas occasionally occur in the ovary and in the central nervous system, but seminomas virtually never occur in the prepubertal male. Embryonal carcinomas are uncommon in early childhood but are a significant component of the mixed germ cell tumors of adolescence. Choriocarcinomas occur in early infancy, but these tumors are probably gestational trophoblastic tumors rather than germ cell tumors. After infancy, choriocarcinomas are not found until adolescence when they occur as a component of mixed germ cell tumors. Immature teratomas, in the absence of elevations of serum AFP and/or the demonstration of a true malignant component, behave in a benign fashion. When the latter component is identified, the teratoma should be classified as a teratoma with malignant elements rather than immature teratoma. The designation "immature teratoma" should be reserved for teratomas with immature, but not clearly malignant, tissue. Since the advent of multiagent platinum-containing chemotherapy, the prognosis for children with malignant gonadal germ cell tumors is very good and that for children with extragonadal tumors is markedly improved. The present and future advances in the understanding of the molecular biologic behavior of these tumors may help to tailor the therapy to the tumor type and improve the prognosis even more.

REFERENCES

1. Akang E, Odunfa A, Aghadiuno P. Childhood teratomas in Ibadan, Nigeria. *Hum Pathol* 1992;23:449–453.
2. Akhtar M, Ali M, Sackey K, Jackson D, Bakry M. Fine-needle aspiration biopsy diagnosis of endodermal sinus tumor: histologic and ultrastructural correlations. *Diagn Cytopathol* 1990;6:184–192.
3. Albrechtsen R, Wewer U, Wimberley P. Immunohistochemical demonstration of a hitherto undescribed localization of hemoglobin A and F in endodermal cells of normal human yolk sac and endodermal sinus tumor. *Acta Pathol Microbiol Scand* 1980;88: 175–178.
4. Almon E, Goldfinger N, Kapon A, Schwartz D, Levine AJ, Rotter V. Testicular tissue-specific expression of the p53 suppressor gene. *Oncogene* 1993;156:107–116.
5. Alter AD, Cove JK. Congenital nasopharyngeal teratoma: report of a case and review of the literature. *J Pediatr Surg* 1987;22:179–181.
6. Altman RP, Randolph JG, Lilly JR. Sacrococcygeal teratoma: American Academy of Pediatrics surgical section survey—1973. *J Pediatr Surg* 1974;9:389–394.
7. Aozasa K, Ito H, Kohro T, Ha K, Nakamura M, Okada A. Choriocarcinoma in infant and mother. *Acta Pathol Jpn* 1981;31: 317–322.
8. Arens R, Marcus D, Engelberg S. Cerebral germinomas and Klinefelter's syndrome: a review. *Cancer* 1988;61:1228–1231.
9. Arshadi S, Watson D. Teratocarcinoma of the heart. Case report and review of primary cardiac malignancies in children. *Am J Dis Child* 1966;112:87–91.
10. Atkin NB, Baker MC. i(12p): specific chromosomal marker in seminoma and malignant teratoma of the testis? *Cancer Genet Cytogenet* 1983;10:199–204.
11. Atkin NB, Baker MC. Chromosome analysis of three seminomas. *Cancer Genet Cytogenet* 1985;17:315–323.
12. Atkin NB, Baker MC. Abnormal chromosomes including small metacentrics in 14 ovarian cancers. *Cancer Genet Cytogenet* 1987;26:355–361.
13. Atkin NB, Baker MD. X-chromatin, sex chromosomes, and ploidy in 37 germ cell tumors of the testis. *Cancer Genet Cytogenet* 1992;59:54–56.
14. Bahari CM, Lurie M, Schoenfeld A, Joel-Cohen SJ. Ovarian teratoma with peritoneal gliomatosis and elevated serum alphafetoprotein. *Am J Clin Pathol* 1980;73:603–607.
15. Bailey D, Marks A, Stratis M, Baumal R. Immunohistochemical staining of germ cell tumors and intratubular malignant germ cells of the testis using antibody to placental alkaline phosphatase and a monoclonal anti-seminoma antibody. *Mod Pathol* 1991;4: 167–171.
16. Bale PM. Sacrococcygeal developmental abnormalities and tumors in children. *Perspect Pediatr Pathol* 1984;1:9–56.
17. Balslev E, Francis D, Jacobsen G. Testicular germ cell tumors. *Acta Cytol* 1990;34:690–694.
18. Barsky S, Layfield L, Varki N, Bhuta S. Two human tumors with high basement-membrane-producing potential. *Cancer* 1988;61: 1798–1806.
19. Beckwith JB. Wilms' tumor and other renal tumors of childhood. In: Finegold MJ, ed. *Pathology of Neoplasia in Children and Adolescents.* Philadelphia: WB Saunders; 1986:313–332.
20. Belchis D, Mowry J, Davis J. Infantile choriocarcinoma. *Cancer* 1993;72:2028–2032.
21. Berkovitz GD, Fechner PY, Zacur HW, et al. Clinical and pathologic spectrum of 46,XY gonadal dysgenesis: its relevance to the understanding of sex differentiation. *Medicine* 1991;70:375–383.
22. Bhalla S, Masih K, Rana R. Teratomas of rare sites: a review of ten cases. *J Indian Med Assoc* 1991;89:291–294.
23. Bjorkholm E, Lundell M, Gyftodimos A, Silfversward C. Dysgerminoma. The Radiumhemmet series 1927–1984. *Cancer* 1988;62:740–748.
24. Bosl GJ, Dmitrovsky E, Reuter VE, et al. Isochromosome of chromosome 12: clinically useful marker for male germ cell tumors. *JNCI* 1989;81:1874–1878.
25. Bratthauer G, Fanning T. Line-1 retrotransposon expression in pediatric germ cell tumors. *Cancer* 1993;71:2383–2386.
26. Brewer J, Tank E. Yolk sac tumors and alpha-fetoprotein in first year of life. *Urology* 1993;42:79–80.
27. Brodeur GM, Howarth CB, Pratt CB. Malignant germ cell tumors in 57 children and adolescents. *Cancer* 1981;48:1890–1898.
28. Brodsky G. Pathology of testicular germ cell tumors. *Hematol Oncol Clin North Am* 1991;5:1095–1126.
29. Brumback RA, Brown BS, di-Sant Agnese PA. Unique findings of prostatic tissue in a benign cystic ovarian teratoma. *Arch Pathol Lab Med* 1985;109:675–677.
30. Burke A, Mostofi F. Placental alkaline phosphatase immunohistochemistry of intratubular malignant germ cells and associated testicular germ cell tumors. *Hum Pathol* 1988;19:663–670.
31. Burke A, Mostofi F. Intratubular malignant germ cells in testicular biopsies: clinical course and identification by staining for placental alkaline phosphatase. *Mod Pathol* 1988;1:475–479.
32. Byard R, Smith C, Chan H. Endodermal sinus tumor of the nasopharynx and previous mature congenital teratoma. *Pediatr Pathol* 1991;11:297–302.
33. Carter G, Lieskovsky G, Skinner D, Daniels J. Reassessment of the role of adjunctive surgical therapy in the treatment of advanced germ cell tumors. *J Urol* 1987;138:1397–1401.
34. Casalone R, Righi R, Granata P, et al. Cerebral germ cell tumor and XXY karyotype. *Cancer Genet Cytogenet* 1994;74:25–29.
35. Castedo SM, de Jong B, Oosterhuis JW, et al. Chromosomal changes in mature residual teratomas following polychemotherapy. *Cancer Res* 1989;49:673–676.
36. Castedo SM, de Jong B, Oosterhuis JW, et al. Chromosomal changes in human primary testicular nonseminomatous germ cell tumors. *Cancer Res* 1989;49:5696–5701.
37. Castedo SM, de Jong B, Oosterjius JW, Seruca R, Idenburg VJ, Buist J. i(12p)-negative testicular germ cell tumors—a different group? *Cancer Genet Cytogenet* 1988;35:171–178.
38. Chaganti R, Ladanyi M, Samaniego F, et al. Leukemic differentiation of a mediastinal germ cell tumor. *Genes Chrom Cancer* 1989;1:83–87.
39. Chariot P, Monnet I, Gaulard P, Abd-Alsamad I, Ruffie P, De Cremoux H. Systemic mastocytosis following mediastinal germ cell tumor: an association confirmed. *Hum Pathol* 1993;24:111–112.

40. Cho K, De-Armond S, Barnwell S, Edwards M, Hoshino T. Proliferative characteristics of intracranial and spinal tumors of developmental origin. *Cancer* 1988;62:740–748.
41. Clement B, Young R, Scully R. Endometrioid-like variant of ovarian yolk sac tumor. *Am J Surg Pathol* 1987;11:767–778.
42. Cohen M, Friend D, Molnar J. Gonadal endodermal sinus (yolk sac) tumor with pure intestinal differentiation: a new histologic type. *Pathol Res Pract* 1987;182:609–616.
43. Conrad R, Gribbin D, Walker N, Ong T. Combined cystic teratoma and hepatoblastoma of the liver. *Cancer* 1993;72:2910–2913.
44. Copeland LJ, Sneige N, Ordonez NG. Endodermal sinus tumor of the vagina and cervix. *Cancer* 1985;55:2558–2565.
45. Corfman PA, Richardt RM. Chromosome number and morphology of benign ovarian cystic teratomas. *N Engl J Med* 1975;271: 1241–1244.
46. Costas C, Williams RL, Fortune RL. Intracardiac teratoma in an infant. *Pediatr Cardiol* 1986;7:179–181.
47. Coulson W. Peritoneal gliomatosis from gastric teratoma. *Am J Clin Pathol* 1990;94:87–89.
48. Cox L, Donald J, Machin G, Popkin J, Zacks D. Intraabdominal testis with yolk sac tumor in a 2 year-old child. *J Pediatr Surg* 1988;23:775–776.
49. Cox JN, Friedli B, Mechmeche R. Teratoma of the heart: a case report and review of the literature. *Virchows Arch A Histopathol Anat* 1983;402:163–174.
50. dal Cin P, Drochmans A, Moerman P, Van Den Berghe H. Isochromosome 12p in mediastinal germ cell tumor. *Cancer Genet Cytogenet* 1989;42:243–251.
51. Damjanov I. Is seminoma a relative or a precursor of embryonal carcinoma? *Lab Invest* 1989;60:1–3.
52. de Bruin TW, Slater RM, Defferrari R, et al. Isochromosome 12p-positive pineal germ cell tumor. *Cancer Res* 1994;54:1542–1544.
53. De Graaff W, Oosterhuis W, De Jong B, et al. Ploidy of testicular carcinoma in situ. *Lab Invest* 1992;66:166–168.
54. De Jong B, Oosterhuis W, Castedo S, Vos A, te Meerman G. Pathogenesis of adult testicular germ cell tumors: a cytogenetic model. *Cancer Genet Cytogenet* 1990;48:143–167.
55. Dehner L. Yet another face on the yolk sac tumor. *Arch Pathol Lab Med* 1989;113:1113–1114.
56. Dehner L. Germ cell tumors of the mediastinum. *Semin Diagn Pathol* 1990;7:266–284.
57. Dehner L, Mills A, Talerman A, Billman G, Krous H, Platz C. Germ cell neoplasms of head and neck soft tissues: a pathologic spectrum of teratomatous and endodermal sinus tumors. *Hum Pathol* 1990;21:309–318.
58. Dehner LP. Gonadal and extragonadal germ cell neoplasms; teratomas in childhood. In: Finegold MJ, ed. *Pathology of Neoplasia in Children and Adolescents.* Philadelphia: WB Saunders;1986: 282
59. DeLozier-Blanchet C, Walt H, Engel E, Vuagnat P. Cytogenetic studies of human testicular germ cell tumors. *Int J Androl* 1987;10:69–77.
60. Delozier-Blanchet CD, Walt H, Engel e, Vuagnat P. Cytogenetic studies of human testicular germ cell tumors. *Int J Androl* 1987;10:69–77.
61. deMent SH. Association between mediastinal germ cell tumors and hematologic malignancies: an update. *Hum Pathol* 1990;21: 699–703.
62. DiCostanzo D, Lele K, Chen Q, et al. Specific chromosomal abnormality in human male germ cell tumors (meeting abstract). *Proc Annu Meet Am Assoc Cancer Res* 1988;29:A107.
63. Dimmick JE, Hardwick DF. Gastrointestinal system and exocrine pancreas. In: Dimmick JE, Kalousek DK, eds. *Developmental Pathology of the Embryo and Fetus.* Philadelphia: JB Lippincott; 1992:511.
64. Donohue J, Roth L, Zachary J, Rowland R, Einhorn L, Williams S. Cytoreductive surgery for metastatic testis cancer: tissue analysis of retroperitoneal masses after chemotherapy. *J Urol* 1981; 127:1111–1114.
65. Dulmet E, Macchiarini P, Suc B, Verley J. Germ cell tumors of the mediastinum. *Cancer* 1993;72:1894–1901.
66. Dunn PJ. Pancreatic endocrine tissue in benign mediastinal teratoma. *J Clin Pathol* 1984;37:1105–1109.
67. Einhorn LH. Chemotherapy of disseminated germ cell tumors. *Cancer* 1987;60:570–573.
68. El Naggar AK, Ro JY, McLemore D, Ayala AG, Batsakis JG. DNA ploidy in testicular germ cell neoplasms. *Am J Surg Pathol* 1992;16:611–618.
69. Eng H, Chuang J, Lee T, Chen W. Fetus in fetu: a case report and review of the literature. *J Pediatr Surg* 1989;24:296–299.
70. Erlandson R. *Diagnostic Transmission Electron Microscopy of Tumors with Clinicopathological, Immunohistochemical, and Cytogenetic Correlations.* New York: Raven Press; 1994:327–349.
71. Esterhay R, Shapiro H, Sutterland J, McIntire R, Wiernik P. Serum alpha-fetoprotein concentration and tumor growth dissociation in a patient with ovarian teratocarcinoma. *Cancer* 1973;31: 835–839.
72. Falin LI. The development of genital glands and the origin of germ cells in human embryogenesis. *Acta Anat* 1969;72:195–232.
73. Felix I, Becker L. Intracranial germ cell tumors in children: An immunohistochemical and electron microscopic study. *Pediatr Neurosurg* 1990;16:156–162.
74. Fenoglio CM, Tlamsa G, Habif DV. Pituitary-containing benign cystic teratoma of the ovary in a patient with metastatic breast cancer: a case report. *Diag Histopathol* 1982;5:143–150.
75. Fernandes E, Etcubanas E, Rao B, Kumar M, Thompson E, Jenkins J. Two decades of experience with testicular tumors in children at St. Jude Children's Research Hospital. *J Pediatr Surg* 1989;24:677–682.
76. Ferreiro J. Ber-H2 expression in testicular germ cell tumors. *Hum Pathol* 1994;25:522–524.
77. Flam F, Lundstrom V, Silfversward C. Choriocarcinoma in mother and child. Case report. *Br J Obstet Gynaecol* 1989;96: 241–244.
78. Fleischhacker M, Strohmeyer T, Imai Y, Slamon DJ, Koeffler H. Mutations of the p53 gene are not detectable in human testicular tumors. *Mod Pathol* 1994;7:435–439.
79. Fujimoto Y, Monden Y, Nakahara K, Kawashima Y. Benign mediastinal teratoma associated with Klinefelter's syndrome. *Jpn J Surg* 1985;15:221–224.
80. Germa J, Llanos M, Tabernero J, Mora J. False elevations of alpha-fetoprotein associated with liver dysfunction in germ cell tumors. *Cancer* 1993;72:2491–2494.
81. Gibas Z, Prout GR, Pontes JE, Sandberg AA. Chromosome changes in germ cell tumors of the testis. *Cancer Genet Cytogenet* 1986;19:245–252.
82. Gibas Z, Prout GR, Sandberg AA. Malignant teratoma of the testis with an isochromosome no.12, (12p), as the sole structural cytogenetic abnormality. *J Urol* 1984;131:762–763.
83. Gibas Z, Talerman A, Faruqi S, Carlson J, Noumoff J. Cytogenetic analysis of an immature teratoma of the ovary and its metastasis after chemotherapy-induced maturation. *Int J Gynecol Pathol* 1993;12:276–280.
84. Giwercman A, Andrews P, Jorgensen N, Muller J, Graem N, Skakkebaek N. Immunohistochemical expression of embryonal marker TRA-1-60 in carcinoma in situ and germ cell tumors of the testis. *Cancer* 1993;72:1308–1314.
85. Giwercman A, Lindenberg S, Kimber S, Andersson T, Muller J, Skakkebaek N. Monoclonal antibody 43-9F as a sensitive immunohistochemical marker of carcinoma in situ of human testis. *Cancer* 1990;65:1135–1142.
86. Gonzalez-Crussi F. *Extragonadal Teratomas.* Second series. Washington, D.C.: Armed Forces Institute of Pathology; 1984.
87. Gonzalez-Crussi F, Winkler RF, Mirkin DL. Sacrococcygeal teratomas in infants and children, relationship of histology and prognosis in 40 cases. *Arch Pathol Lab Med* 1978;102:420–425.
88. Govindarajan S, Fong T, Ashcavai M. Concanavalin A affinity of alpha-fetoprotein. *Am J Clin Pathol* 1987;88:722–724.
89. Halme A, Kellokumpu-Lehtinen P, Teppo L. Morphology of testicular germ cell tumours in treated and untreated cryptorchidism. *Br J Urol* 1989;64:78-83.
90. Hamers A, de Jong B, Suijkerbuijk RF, et al. A 46,XY female with mixed gonadal dysgenesis and a 48,XY, -7, - i(12p) chromosome pattern in a primary gonadal tumor. *Cancer Genet Cytogenet* 1991;57:219–224.
91. Harms D, Janig U, Gobel U. Gliomatosis peritonei in childhood

and adolescence: clinicopathological study of 13 cases including immunohistochemical findings. *Pathol Res Pract* 1989;184:422–430.
92. Harms D, Janig U. Germ cell tumors of childhood: report of 170 cases including 59 pure and partial yolk-sac tumors. *Virchows Arch A Pathol Anat* 1986;409:233–239.
93. Hart WR, Burkonas DM. Germ cell neoplasms arising in gonadoblastomas. *Cancer* 1979;43:669–678.
94. Hartwick W, Ro J, Ordonez N, Ayala A. Testicular germ cell tumors under age 5. Does intratubular germ cell neoplasia exist? *Lab Invest* 1990;62:43A (abstract).
95. Hawkins EP. Pathology of germ cell tumors in children. *Crit Rev Oncol Hematol* 1990;10:165–179.
96. Hawkins E, Finegold M, Hawkins H, Krischer J, Starling K, Weinberg A. Nongerminomatous malignant germ cell tumors in children, a review of 89 cases from the Pediatric Oncology Group, 1971–1984. *Cancer* 1986;58:2579–2584.
97. Hawkins E, Isaacs H, Cushing B, Rogers P. Occult malignancy in neonatal sacroccygeal teratomas. A combined POG and CCG study. *Pediatr Hematol Oncol* 1993;15:406–409.
98. Henderson D, Papadimitriou J. *Ultrastructural Appearances of Tumours: A Diagnostic Atlas.* New York: Churchill Livingstone; 1982:318–330.
99. Ho DM, Liu H. Primary intracranial germ cell tumor. *Cancer* 1992;70:1577–1584.
100. Hoffner L, Deka R, Chakravarti A. Cytogenetics and origins of pediatric germ cell tumors. *Cancer Genet Cytogenet* 1994;74:54–58.
101. Hoffner L, Shen-Schwarz S, Deka R, Chakravarti A. Cytogenetics and origins of malignant ovarian germ cell tumors. *Cancer Genet Cytogenet* 1992;62:58–65.
102. Huddart S, Mann J, Gornall P, et al. The UK Children's Cancer Study Group: testicular malignant germ cell tumours 1979–1988. *J Pediatr Surg* 1990;25:406–410.
103. Ikarashi T. Immature teratoma of the ovary. Correlation between serum alpha-fetoprotein value and immunohistochemical analysis. *Asia Oceania J Obstet Gynaecol* 1984;10:523–530.
104. Inoue H, Naganuma H, Ono N. Pathobiology of intracranial germ-cell tumors: immunochemical, immunohistochemical, and electron microscopic investigations. *J Neurooncol* 1987;5:105–115.
105. Ishiguro T, Takahashi Y. Serum alpha-fetoprotein subfractions identified by Ricinus communis agglutinin I in hepatic malignancies, yolk sac tumor, benigh hepatic disease, and fetal stage. *Dis Markers* 1989;7:239–245.
106. Ito M, Taki T, Mitsuoka A, Miyake M. Lactate dehydrogenase isoenzyme-1 in the mediastinal yolk sac tumor. *Jpn J Surg* 1988;18:419–422.
107. Jacobsen G, Henriques U. A fetal testis with intratubular germ cell neoplasia (ITGCN). *Mod Pathol* 1992;5:547–549.
108. Jacobsen G, Jacobsen N, Clausen P. Distribution of tumor-associated antigens in the various histologic components of germ cell tumors of the testis. *Am J Surg Pathol* 1981;5:257–266.
109. Jacobsen GK, Henriksen OB, der Maase HV. Carcinoma in situ of testicular tissue adjacent to malignant germ-cell tumors: a study of 105 cases. *Cancer* 1981;47:2660–2662.
110. Jenkyn DJ, McCartney AJ. A chromosome study of three ovarian tumors. *Cancer Genet Cytogenet* 1987;26:327–337.
111. Jirasek J. Disorders of sexual differentiation. In: Simpson J, ed. *Principles of Reproductive Embryology.* New York: Academic Press; 1976:51–110.
112. Jones M, Clement P, Young R. Primary yolk sac tumors of the mesentery. *Am J Clin Pathol* 1994;101:42–47.
113. Jordan R, Gauderer M. Cervical teratomas: an analysis, literature review and proposed classification. *J Pediatr Surg* 1988;23:583–591.
114. Joshi VJ. *Common Problems in Pediatric Pathology.* New York: Igaku-Shoin; 1994.
115. Kallis P, Treasure T, Holmes S, Griffiths M. Exocrine pancreatic function in mediastinal teratomata: an aid to preoperative diagnosis? *Ann Thorac Surg* 1992;54:741–743.
116. Kang YK, Suh Y, Kim CW, Chi JG. Fetus in fetu: a case with complete umbilical cord and fetal sac. *Pediatr Pathol* 1994;14:411–419.
117. Kaplan C, Askin F, Benirschke K. Cytogenetics of extragonadal tumors. *Teratology* 1979;19:261–266.
118. Kaplan S, Bornstein S, Christopherson W, Surti U. Associated leukemia and mixed gem cell tumor in a patient with gonadal dysgenesis. *Int J Gynecol* 1991;35:83–88.
119. Kaplan G, Cromie W, Kelalis P, Silber I, Tank E, Jr. Prepubertal yolk sac testicular tumors: report of the Testicular Tumor Registry. *J Urol* 1988;140:1109–1112.
120. Kashiwagi A, Nagamori S, Toyota K, Maeno K, Koyanagi T. DNA ploidy of testicular germ cell tumors in childhood: Difference from adult testicular tumors. *Nippon Hinyokika Gakkai Zasshi* 1993;84:1655–1659.
121. Kaul T, Bakran A. Endocrine secreting malignant mediastinal teratoma. *Thorac Cardiovasc Surg* 1990;38:251–253.
122. Kawai M, Kano T, Furuhashi Y, et al. Immature teratoma of the ovary. *Gynecol Oncol* 1991;40:133–137.
123. Kawai M, Kano T, Kikkawa F, et al. Seven tumor markers in benign and malignant germ cell tumors of the ovary. *Gynecol Oncol* 1992;45:248–253.
124. Kawai M, Kano T, Furuhashi Y, et al. Prognostic factors in yolk sac tumors of the ovary, a clinicopathologic analysis of 29 cases. *Cancer* 1991;67:184–192.
125. Kelley JL, Naus GJ, Christopherson WA. Endodermal sinus tumor of the ovary: A case series with flow cytometric DNA content analysis. *Gynecol Oncol* 1991;42:34–38.
126. King M, DiGiovanni L, Yung J, Clarke-Pearson D. Immature teratoma of the ovary grade 3, with karyotype analysis. *Int J Gynecol Pathol* 1990;9:178–184.
127. King M, Micha J, Allen S, Mouradian J, Chaganti R. Immature teratoma of the ovary with predominant malignant retinal anlage component. *Am J Surg Pathol* 1985;9:221–231.
128. Kiss F, Juhasz J. Testicular germ cell tumours: current problems of histogenesis and classification. *Int Urol Nephrol* 1985;17:85–95.
129. Klein FA, Melamed MR, Whitmore WF, Jr. Intra-tubular malignant germ cells (carcinoma in situ) accompanying invasive testicular germ cell tumors. *J Urol* 1985;133:413–415.
130. Kleinman G, Young R, Scully R. Primary neuroectodermal tumors of the ovary. *Am J Surg Pathol* 1993;17:764–778.
131. Koide O, Iwai S, Baba K. Identification of testicular atypical germ cells by an immunohistochemical technique for placental alkaline phosphatase. *Cancer* 1987;60:1325–1330.
132. Kommoss F, Bibbo M, Talerman A. Nuclear deoxyribonucleic acid content (ploidy) of endodermal sinus (yolk sac) tumor. *Lab Invest* 1990;62:223–231.
133. Kooijman C. Immature teratomas in children. *Histopathology* 1988;12:491–502.
134. Koulos J, Hoffman J, Steinhoff M. Immature teratoma of the ovary. *Gynecol Oncol* 1989;34:46–49.
135. Kurman R, Norris H. Endodermal sinus tumor of the ovary, a clinical and pathologic analysis of 71 cases. *Cancer* 1976;38:2404–2419.
136. Lachman MF, Kim K, Koo B. Mediastinal teratoma associated with Klinefelter's syndrome. *Arch Pathol Lab Med* 1986;110:1067–1071.
137. Lack E, Weinstein H, Welch K. Mediastinal germ cell tumors in childhood. *J Thorac Cardiovasc Surg* 1985;89:826–835.
138. Ladanyi M, Samaniego F, Reuter VE, Motzer RJ, Jhanwar SC, Bosl GJ. Cytogenetic and immunohistochemical evidence for the germ cell origin of a subset of acute leukemias associated with mediastinal germ cell tumors. *JNCI* 1990;82:221–227.
139. Lahdenne P, Heikinheimo M, Perkkio M, Rapola J, Miettinen M. Cell differentiation in sacrococcygeal teratomas. *Pathol Res Pract* 1990;186:336–343.
140. Lahdenne P, Kuusela P, Siimes M, Ronnholm K, Salmenpera L, Heikinheimo M. Biphasic reduction and concanavalin A binding properties of serum alpha-fetoprotein in preterm and term infants. *J Pediatr* 1991;118:272–276.
141. Levasseur P, Regnard J, Paquet J, Dartevelle P. Autoimmune hemolytic anemia and mediastinal mature teratoma in a 6-year-old child: excision and cure of the anemia. *Ann Chir* 1988;42:170–172.
142. Lifschitz MB, Fogel M, Moll R, et al. Intermediate filament protein profiles of human testicular non-seminomatous germ cell tu-

mors: correlation of cytokeratin synthesis to cell differentiation. *Differentiation* 1991;48:191–198.
143. Linder D, McCaw BK, Hecht F. Human benign ovarian teratomas. *N Engl J Med* 1975;292:63–66.
144. Livingston RR, Sarembock LA. Testicular tumors in children. *S Afr Med J* 1986;70:168–169.
145. Looijena LH, Gillis JM, Van Putten WL, Oosterhuis JW. In situ numeric analysis of centromeric regions of chromosomes 1,12, and 15 of seminomas, nonseminomatous germ cell tumors, and carcinoma in situ of human testis. *Lab Invest* 1993;68:211–219.
146. Looijenga L, Gillis A, Van Putten W, Oosterhuis J. In situ numeric analysis of centromeric regions of chromosomes 1, 12, and 15 of seminomas, nonseminomatous germ cell tumors, and carcinoma in situ of human testis. *Lab Invest* 1993;68:211–218.
147. Luciano Z, Upadhyay S. Germ cell differentiation in mouse adrenal glands. *J Exp Zool* 1983;228:173–193.
148. Malogolowkin M, Ortega J, Krailo M, et al. Immature teratomas: identification of patients at risk for malignant recurrence. *JNCI* 1989;81:870–874.
149. Manivel J. Transformation of seminoma to yolk sac tumor. *Am J Clin Pathol* 1992;97:463–465.
150. Manivel J, Reinberg Y, Niehans G, Fraley E. Intratubular germ cell neoplasia in testicular teratomas and epidermoid cysts. *Cancer* 1989;64:715–720.
151. Manivel J, Simonton S, Wold L, Dehner L. Absence of intratubular germ cell neoplasia in testicular yolk sac tumors in children. *Arch Pathol Lab Med* 1988;112:641–645.
152. Manivel C, Wick MR, Abenoza P. The occurrence of sarcomatous components in primary mediastinal germ cell tumors. *Am J Surg Pathol* 1986;10:711–717.
153. Mann J, Pearson D, Barrett A, Raafat F, Barnes J, Wallendszus K. Results of the United Kingdom Children's Cancer Study Group's malignant germ cell tumor studies. *Cancer* 1989;63: 1657–1667.
154. Mann BD, Sparkes RS, Kern DH, Mortno DL. Chromosomal abnormalities of a mediastinal embryonal cell carcinoma in a patient with 47,XXY Klinefelter syndrome: evidence for the premeiotic origin of a germ cell tumor. *Cancer Genet Cytogenet* 1983;8:191–196.
155. Marina N, Rao B, Etcubanas E, Jenkins J, Kun L, Thompson E. The role of second-look surgery in the management of advanced germ cell malignancies. *Cancer* 1991;68:309–315.
156. Marina N, Fontanesi H, Kun L, et al. Treatment of childhood germ cell tumors. Review of the St. Jude experience from 1979 to 1988. *Cancer* 1992;70:2568–2575.
157. Marrink J, Sleijfer D, de Vries E, Koops H. Alpha-fetoprotein-lectin binding as a marker of tumour activity of liver damage. *Eur J Cancer* 1990;26:969–972.
158. Marsden HB, Birch HM, Swindell R. Germ cell tumours of childhood: a review of 137 cases. *J Clin Pathol* 1981;34:879–883.
159. McHenry C, Reynolds M, Raffensperger J. Vaginal neoplasms in infancy: the combined role of chemotherapy and conservative surgical resection. *J Pediatr Surg* 1988;23:842–845.
160. McKendrick J, Theaker J, Mead G. Nonseminomatous germ cell tumor with very high serum human chorionic gonadotropin. *Cancer* 1991;67:684–689.
161. McNeil MM, Leong AS, Sage RE. Primary mediastinal embryonal carcinoma in association with Klinefelter's syndrome. *Cancer* 1981;47:343–345.
162. Michael H, Ulbright TM, Brodhecker CA. The pluripotential nature of the mesenchyme-like component of yolk sac tumor. *Arch Pathol Lab Med* 1989;113:1115–1119.
163. Min K, Scheithauer B. Pineal germinomas and testicular seminoma: a comparative ultrastructural study with special references to early carcinomatous transformation. *Ultrastruct Pathol* 1990;14:483–496.
164. Mostofi FK, Price JB. *Tumors of the Male Genital System.* 2nd series. Washington, D.C.: Armed Forces Institute of Pathology; 1973:40–52.
165. Mostofi FK, Sesterhenn IA. Pathology of germ cell tumors of testes. *Prog Clin Biol Res* 1985;203:1–34.
166. Motzer R, Reuter V, Cordon-Cardo C, Bosl G. Blood group–related antigens in human germ cell tumors. *Cancer Res* 1988;48: 5342–5347.
167. Mukherjee AB, Murty VV, Rodriquez E, Reuter V, Bosl GJ, Chaganti RS. Detection and analysis of origin of i(12p), a diagnostic marker of human male germ cell tumors, by fluorescence in situ hybridization. *Genes Chrom Cancer* 1991;3:300–307.
168. Muller J, Skakkebaek NE, Nielson OH. Cryptorchidism and testis cancer: atypical infantile germ cells followed by carcinoma in situ and invasive carcinoma in adulthood. *Cancer* 1984;54:629–634.
169. Muller J, Skakkebaek NE, Ritzen M. Carcinoma in situ of the testis in children with 45,X/46,XY gonadal dysgenesis. *J Pediatr* 1985;106:431–436.
170. Nakagawa Y, Perentes E, Ross G, Ross A, Rubinstein L. Immunohistochemical differences between intracranial germinomas and their gonadal equivalents. An immunoperoxidase study of germ cell tumours with epithelial membrane antigen, cytokeratin, and vimentin. *J Pathol* 1988;156:67–72.
171. Nakashima N, Fukatsu T, Nagasaka T, Sobue M, Takeuchi J. The frequency and histology of hepatic tissue in germ cell tumors. *Am J Surg Pathol* 1987;11:682–692.
172. Nakashima N, Murakami S, Fukatsu T, et al. Characteristics of "embryoid body" in human gonadal germ cell tumors. *Hum Pathol* 1988;19:1144–1154.
173. Nakayama D, Killian A, Hill L, et al. The newborn with hydrops and sacrococcygeal teratoma. *J Pediatr Surg* 1991;26:1435–1438.
174. Nanda A, Schut L, Sutton L. Congenital forms of intracranial teratoma. *Childs Nerv Syst* 1991;7:112–114.
175. Neilson K, Taylor S. Quantitative DNA analysis of germ cell tumors in children. *Mod Pathol* 1989;2:5P.
176. Nichols C, Roth B, Heerema N, Griep J, Tricot G. Hematologic neoplasia associated with primary mediastinal germ cell tumors. *N Engl J Med* 1990;322:1425–1429.
177. Nielsen SN, Scheithauer BW, Gaffey TA. Gliomatosis peritonei. *Cancer* 1985;56:2499–2503.
178. Nogales FF, Mantilla A, Nogales-Ortiz F. Yolk sac tumors with pure and mixed polyvesicular vitelline patterns. *Hum Pathol* 1978;9:553–566.
179. Nogales-Fernandez F, Silverberg SG, Bloustein PA. Yolk sac carcinoma (endodermal sinus tumor), ultrastructure and histogenesis of gonadal and extragonadal tumors in comparison with normal human yolk sac. *Cancer* 1977;39:1462–1474.
180. Norris HJ, Jensen RD. Relative frequency of ovarian neoplasms in children and adolescents. *Cancer* 1972;30:713–719.
181. Odell J, Allen J, Badura R, Weinberger E. Massive congenital intracranial teratoma: a report of two cases. *Pediatr Pathol* 1987;7:333–340.
182. Ohama K, Nomura K, Okamoto E, Fukuda Y, Ihara T, Fujiwara A. Origin of immature teratoma of the ovary. *Am J Ostet Gynecol* 1985;152:896–900.
183. Okamota T, Hirabayashi K, Ishiguro T. Immunohistochemical type distinction of α-fetoprotein in various α-fetoprotein-secreting tumors. *Jpn J Cancer Res* 1993;84:360–364.
184. Oosterhuis J, Castedo S, De Jong B, et al. Ploidy of primary germ cell tumors of the testis. *Lab Invest* 1989;60:14–21.
185. Oosterhuis JW, Castedo SM, de Jong B, et al. Karyotyping and DNA flow cytometry of an orchidoblastoma. *Cancer Genet Cytogenet* 1988;36:7–11.
186. Oosterhuis JW, de Jong B, Cornelisse CJ, et al. Karyotyping and DNA flow cytometry of mature residual teratoma after intensive chemotherapy of disseminated nonseminomatous germ cell tumors of the testis: a report of two cases. *Cancer Genet Cytogenet* 1986;22:149–157.
187. Orazi A, Neiman R, Ulbright T, Heerema N, John K, Nichols C. Hematopoietic precursor cells within the yolk sac tumor component are the source of secondary hematopoietic malignancies in patients with mediastinal germ cell tumors. *Cancer* 1993;71: 3873–3881.
188. O'Riodain D, O'Connell P, Kirwan W. Hereditary sacral agenesis with presacral mass and anorectal stenosis: the Currarino triad. *Br J Surg* 1991;78:536–538.
189. Owen D, Hill A, Argent S. Origin of extragonadal teratomas and endodermal sinus tumors. *Nature* 1975;254:597–599.
190. Page DC. Hypothesis: A Y-chromosomal gene causes gonadoblastoma in dysgenetic gonads. *Dev Suppl* 1987;101:151–155.

191. Pallesen G, Hamilton-Dutoit S. Ki-1 (CD30) antigen is regularly expressed by tumor cells of embryonal carcinoma. *Am J Pathol* 1988;133:446–450.
192. Parrington JM, West LF, Povey S. The origin of ovarian teratomas. *J Med Genet* 1984;21:4–12.
193. Peng HQ, Hogg D, Malkin D, et al. Mutations of the p53 gene do not occur in testis cancer. *Cancer Res* 1993;53:3574–3578.
194. Perlman EJ, Cushing B, Hawkins E, Griffin CA. Cytogenetic analysis of childhood endodermal sinus tumors: a Pediatric Oncology Group study. *Pediatr Pathol* 1994;14:695–708.
195. Perlman EJ, Henneberry J, Hawkins E, Griffin CA. Cytogenetic and ploidy analysis of endodermal sinus tumors (EST) in infants. *Lab Invest* 1993;68:7P (abstract).
196. Perrone T, Steeper T, Dehner L. Alpha-fetoprotein localization in pure ovarian teratoma. *Am J Clin Pathol* 1987;88:713–717.
197. Perrone T, Steiner M, Dehner LP. Nodal gliomatosis and α-fetoprotein production: two unusual facets of grade I ovarian teratoma. *Arch Pathol Lab Med* 1986;110:975–977.
198. Peterson C, Strickler J, Gonzalez R, Dehner L. Uterus-like mass of the small intestine. Heterotopia or monodermal teratoma? *Am J Surg Pathol* 1990;12:390–394.
199. Pinkerton C, Broadbent V, Horwich A, et al. 'JEB': a carboplatin based regimen for malignant germ cell tumours in children. *Br J Cancer* 1990;62:257–262.
200. Pinkerton CR, Pritchard J, Spitz L. High complete response rate in children with advanced germ cell tumours using cisplatin-containing combination chemotherapy. *J Clin Oncol* 1986;4: 194–199.
201. Prat J, Bhan AK, Dickersin GR. Hepatoid yolk sac tumor of the ovary (endodermal sinus tumor with hepatoid differentiation): a light microscopic, ultrastructural and immunohistochemical study of seven cases. *Cancer* 1982;50:2355–2368.
202. Raju U, Kini R, Warrier R. An unusual embryonal tumor of the nasal cavity in a neonate: a nasal blastoma?: a clinical, histologic, and ultrastructural study. *Mod Pathol* 1989;2:681–686.
203. Renedo DE, Trainer TD. Intratubular germ cell neoplasia (ITGCN) with p53 and PCNA expression and adjacent mature teratoma in an infant testis. An immunohistochemical and morphologic study with a review of the literature. *Am J Surg Pathol* 1994;18:947–952.
204. Rodin AE, Singla P. Teratomas of the tongue present at birth. *Pediatr Pathol* 1985;3:291–298.
205. Rodriquez E, Mathew S, Mukherjee AB, Reuter VE, Bosl GJ, Chaganti RS. Analysis of chromosome 12 aneuploidy in interphase cells from human male germ cell tumors by fluorescence in situ hybridization. *Genes Chrom Cancer* 1992;5:21–29.
206. Ronacalli M, Gribaudi G, Simoncelli D, Servida E. Cytology of yolk-sac tumor of the ovary in ascitic fluid: report of a case. *Acta Cytol* 1988;32:113–116.
207. Rueda-Pedraza ME, Heifetz SA, Sesterhenn IA. Primary intracranial germ cell tumors in the first two decades of life. *Perspect Pediatr Pathol* 1987;10:160–186.
208. Rutgers J, Young R, Scully R. Ovarian yolk sac tumor arising from an endometrioid carcinoma. *Hum Pathol* 1987;18:1296–1299.
209. Samaniego F, Rodriquez E, Houldsworth J, et al. Cytogenetic and molecular analysis of human male germ cell tumors: chromosome 12 abnormalities and gene amplification. *Genes Chrom Cancer* 1990;1:289–300.
210. Schropp K, Lobe T, Rao B, et al. Sacrococcygeal teratoma: the experience of four decades. *J Pediatr Surg* 1992;27:1075–1079.
211. Schwartz D, Goldfinger N, Rotter V. Expression of p53 protein in spermatogenesis is confined to the tetraploid pachytene primary spermatocytes. *Oncogene* 1993;8:1487–1494.
212. Scully RE. Gonadoblastoma: a review of 74 cases. *Cancer* 1970;25:1340–1356.
213. Senocak M, Kale G, Buyukpamukcu N, Hicsonmez A, Caglar M. Gastric teratoma in children including the third reported female case. *J Pediatr Surg* 1990;25:681–684.
214. Shafie M, Furay RW, Chablani LV. Ovarian teratoma with peritoneal and lymph node metastases of mature "glial" tissue: a benign condition. *J Surg Oncol* 1984;27:18–22.
215. Shebib S, Sabbah R, Sackey K, Akhtar M, Aur R. Endodermal Sinus (yolk sac) tumor in infants and children, a clinical and pathologic study: an 11 year review. *Am J Pediatr Hematol Oncol* 1989;11:36–39.
216. Shuin T, Misaki H, Kubota Y, Yao M, Hosaka M. Differential expression of protooncogenes in human germ cell tumors of the testis. *Cancer* 1994;73:1721–1727.
217. Silver SA, Wiley JM, Perlman EJ. DNA ploidy analysis of pediatric germ cell tumors. *Mod Pathol* 1994;7:951–956.
218. Simpson I, Campbell P. Mediastinal masses in childhood: a review from a paediatric pathologist's point of view. *Prog Pediatr Surg* 1991;27:92–126.
219. Sinke RJ, Suijkerbuijk RF, de Jong B, Oosterhuis JW, van Kessell AG. Uniparental origin of i(12p) in human germ cell tumors. *Genes Chrom Cancer* 1993;6:161–165.
220. Skakkeback NE, Berthelsen JC. Carcinoma-in-situ of the testis and invasive growth of different types of germ cell tumours. A revised germ cell theory. *Int J Androl* 1981;4:26.
221. Sliver SA, Hawkins E, Cushing B, Perlman EJ. Intrinsic multidrug resistance gene expression in childhood endodermal sinus tumors: correlation with treatment outcome. *Lab Invest* 1994;70: 9P (abstract).
222. Sonnino R, Chou S, Guttman F. Hereditary sacrococcygeal teratomas. *J Pediatr Surg* 1989;24:1074–1075.
223. Soosay G, Bobrow L, Happerfield L, Parkinson M. Morphology and immunohistochemistry of carcinoma in situ adjacent to testicular germ cell tumours in adults and children: implications for histogenesis. *Histopathology* 1991;19:537–544.
224. Speleman F, DePotter C, dal Cin P, et al. i(12p) in a malignant ovarian tumor. *Cancer Genet Cytogenet* 1990;45:49–53.
225. Stephenson JA, Mayland DM, Kun LE, Etcubanas E, Thompson EI, Gross CW. Malignant germ cell tumors of the head and neck in childhood. *Laryngoscope* 1989;99:732–735.
226. Strohmeyer T, Peter S, Hartmann M, et al. Expression of the hist-1 and c-kit protooncogenes in human testicular germ cell tumors. *Cancer Res* 1991;51:1811–1816.
227. Surti U, Hoffner L, Chakravarti A, Ferrell R. Genetics and biology of human ovarian teratomas. 1. Cytogenetic analysis and mechanism of origin. *Am J Hum Genet* 1990;47:635–643.
228. Talerman A. Gonadoblastoma associated with embryonal carcinoma. *Obstet Gynecol* 1974;43:138–142.
229. Talerman A. Germ cell tumors of the ovary. In: Kurman RJ, ed. *Blaustein's Pathology of the Female Genital Tract.* 3rd ed. New York: Springer-Verlag; 1987:659–721.
230. Teilum G. Endodermal sinus tumors of the ovary and testis: comparative morphogenesis of the so-called mesonephroma ovarii (Schiller) and extraembryonic (yolk sac-allantoic) structures of the rat's placenta. *Cancer* 1959;12:1092–1105.
231. Thurlbeck WM, Scully RE. Solid teratoma of the ovary: a clinicopathological analysis of 9 cases. *Cancer* 1960;13:804–811.
232. Truong LD, Harris L, Mattioli C, et al. Endodermal sinus tumor of the mediastinum; a report of seven cases and review of the literature. *Cancer* 1986;58:730–739.
233. Truong LD, Jurco SI, McGavran MH. Gliomatosis peritonei: report of two cases and review of the literature. *Am J Surg Pathol* 1982;6:443–449.
234. Ulbright T, Roth L, Brodhecker BS. Yolk sac differentiation in germ cell tumors, a morphologic study of 50 cases with emphasis on hepatic, enteric and parietal yolk sac features. *Am J Surg Pathol* 1986;10:151–164.
235. Ulbright T, Michael H, Loehrer P, Donohue J. Spindle cell tumors resected from male patients with germ cell tumors: a clinicopathologic study of 14 cases. *Cancer* 1990;65:148–156.
236. Ulbright T, Orazi A, de Riese W, et al. The correlation of P53 protein expression with proliferative activity and occult metastases in clinical stage I non-seminomatous germ cell tumors of the testis. *Mod Pathol* 1994;7:64–68.
237. Ulbright T, Roth L. Recent developments in the pathology of germ cell tumors. *Semin Diagn Pathol* 1987;4:304–319.
238. Ulbright TM, Clark SA, Einhorn LH. Angiosarcoma associated with germ cell tumors. *Hum Pathol* 1985;16:268–272.
239. Upadhyay S, Zamboni L. Ectopic germ cells: Natural model for the study of germ cell sexual differentiation. *Proc Natl Acad Sci USA* 1982;79:6584–6588.
240. Valente A, Grant C, Orr J, Brereton R. Neonatal tonsillar teratoma. *J Pediatr Surg* 1988;23:364–366.

241. van Kessell AG, van Drunen E, de Jong B, Oosterhuis JW, Langeveld A, Mulder MP. Chromosome 12q heterozygosity is retained in i(12p)-positive testicular germ cell tumor cells. *Cancer Genet Cytogenet* 1989;40:129–134.

242. Verstuyf A, Sobis H, Goebels J, Fonteyn E, Cassiman JJ, Vandeputte M. Establishment and characterization of a continuous in vitro line from a rat choriocarcinoma. *Int J Cancer* 1990;45:752–756.

243. Wagener C, Menzel B, Breuer H, et al. Immunohistochemical localisation of alpha-fetoprotein (AFP) in germ cell tumours: evidence for AFP production by tissues different from endodermal sinus tumour. *Oncology* 1981;38:236–239.

244. Wakely J , Krummel T, Johnson D. Yolk sac tumor of the liver. *Mod Pathol* 1991;4:121–125.

245. Walt H, Arrenbrecht S, DeLozier-Blanchet C, Keller P, Nauer R, Hedinger C. A human testicular germ cell tumor with borderline histology between seminoma and embryonal carcinoma secreted beta-human chorionic gonadotropin and alpha-fetoprotein only as a xenograft. *Cancer* 1986;58:139–146.

246. Walt H, Emmerich P, Cremer T, Hofmann M, Bannwart F. Supernumerary chromosome 1 in interphase nuclei of atypical germ cells in paraffin-embedded human seminiferous tubules. *Lab Invest* 1989;61:527–531.

247. Watanatittan S, Othersen J , Hughson M. Cervical teratomas in children. *Prog Pediatr Surg* 1981;14:225–239.

248. Weinberg AG, Finegold MJ. Primary hepatic tumors in childhood. In: Finegold MJ, ed. *Pathology of Neoplasia in Children and Adolescents.* Philadelphia: WB Saunders; 1986:313–332.

249. Wollner N, Ghavimi F, Wachtel A, Luks E, Exelby P, Woodruff J. Germ cell tumors in children: gonadal and extragonadal. *Med Pediatr Oncol* 1991;19:228–239.

250. Wu J, Book L, Sudar K. Serum alpha fetoprotein (AFP) levels in normal infants. *Pediatr Res* 1981;15:50–52.

251. Yamamoto H, Ruden U, Esposti P, et al. Profiles of epitope defined markers in sera from patients with testicular germ cell tumors. *Urol Res* 1988;16:31–36.

252. Yang-Feng TL, Katz SN, Cancang ML, Schwartz PE. Cytogenetic analysis of ependymoma and teratoma of the ovary. *Cancer Genet Cytogenet* 1988;35:83–89.

253. Yu IT, Griffin CA, Phillips PC, Strauss LC, Perlman EJ. Numerical sex chromosomal abnormalities in pineal teratomas by cytogenetic analysis and fluorescence in situ hybridization. *Lab Invest* 1995;72:419–423.

Pediatric Neoplasia: Morphology and Biology, edited by David M. Parham.
Lippincott-Raven Publishers, Philadelphia © 1996.

CHAPTER 11

Liver Tumors and Tumorlike Masses

Kathleen Patterson

INTRODUCTION

Liver tumors of infancy and childhood include a broad spectrum of benign and malignant lesions as outlined in Table 1. Table 2 summarizes the relative incidence of these tumor types as compiled from three comprehensive reviews published in 1978 (67), 1986 (357), and 1992 (39). Some broad generalizations help put the relative import of these various tumors into perspective:

1. Malignant tumors outnumber benign ones by 2.5:1.
2. Malignant liver tumors account for 1–2% of all childhood malignancies (220,300).
3. Tumor type varies significantly with age.
   a. Hemangioendotheliomas typically occur in the first 6 months of life, accounting for 50–60% of liver tumors in this group (39,133).
   b. Hepatoblastoma typically occurs before 5 years of life.
   c. Hepatocellular carcinoma typically occurs in the second decade.

The following detailed discussion of these lesions focuses first on the benign followed by the malignant diseases.

BENIGN EPITHELIAL TUMORS

Focal Nodular Hyperplasia

Clinical Features

Focal nodular hyperplasia, a tumor that occurs most commonly in young adult women, accounts for approximately 4–10% of benign childhood liver tumors and <2% of childhood liver tumors overall (71,370). The female predominance noted in adults holds true in childhood as well with a female-to-male (F/M) ratio of >3:1 (190,246,317). In the Armed Forces Institute of Pathology (AFIP) files, approximately 8% of focal nodular hyperplasia cases occurred under 16 years of age (317), with a median age in the pediatric population of 6 years (190,246,317). Focal nodular hyperplasia in the first year of life is unusual, with only two reported cases (317). Presenting most commonly as an asymptomatic mass in an otherwise normal child, it has also been associated with a variety of clinical conditions and syndromes including hemihypertrophy (85), VACTERAL syndrome (42), biliary atresia following portoenterostomy (240), sickle cell anemia (140,207), intra- and extrahepatic vascular malformations (85,193,262,353), brain tumors (84,353, 354), congenital cardiovascular anomalies (283,354), and glycogen storage disease type I (246,257). Suggestions that oral contraceptives play a role in its pathogenesis appear invalid, although oral contraceptive use may induce growth or hemorrhage within a preexisting focal nodular hyperplasia (173). Recent studies suggest anomalous arterial supply with or without secondary thrombosis as a pathogenetic mechanism for these apparently nonneoplastic tumors (354).

Pathologic Features

Focal nodular hyperplasia occurs as a single or, less commonly, multifocal, circumscribed but nonencapsulated mass. Multifocal focal nodular hyperplasia occurs more often in association with an underlying condition (85,246,262). In adults, the mass is right-sided in two thirds of cases; whereas in children, 60% are on the left, 30% on the right, and 10% bilateral (317). Although usually subcapsular in location, more deeply situated or occasionally pedunculated masses occur (283). On cut surface, a highly characteristic central stellate scar, present

K. Patterson: Department of Pathology, University of Washington/Children's Hospital and Medical Center, Seattle, Washington 98105.

TABLE 1. *Tumor and tumorlike lesions of the liver*

Benign	Malignant
Epithelial	
Focal nodular hyperplasia	Hepatoblastoma
Hepatocellular adenoma	Hepatocellular carcinoma
Nodular regenerative hyperplasia	Fibrolamellar carcinoma
Mixed hamartoma	
Developmental cysts	
Mesenchymal	
Infantile hemangioendothelioma	Undifferentiated (embryonal) sarcoma
Mesenchymal hamartoma	Angiosarcoma
Cavernous hemangioma	Rhabdomyosarcoma
Inflammatory pseudotumor	Rhabdoid tumor
Germ cell neoplasia	
Teratoma	Endodermal sinus tumor

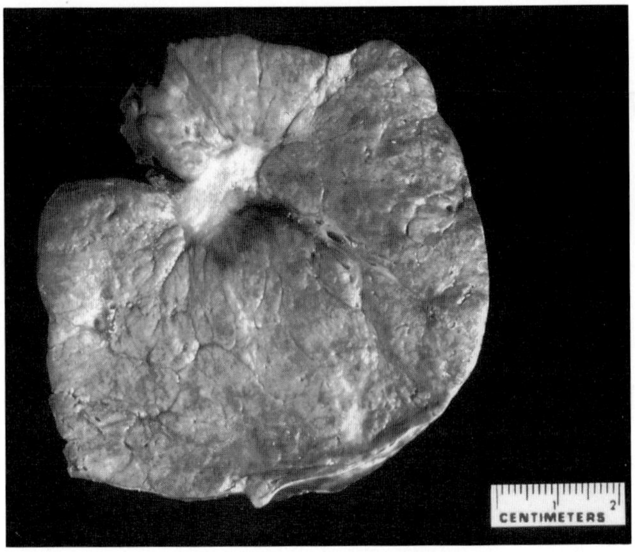

FIG. 1. The cut surface of this liver mass resected from a 6-year-old girl demonstrates the central scar characteristic of focal nodular hyperplasia. A thin rim of residual liver can be seen at the lower right corner of the mass.

in at least 50% of cases, particularly when >1 cm in diameter, distinguishes focal nodular hyperplasia from other liver masses (Fig. 1). Fibrous tissue radiating from the central scar subdivides the remainder of the mass into smaller nodules. The hepatic parenchyma is without bile staining and rarely shows hemorrhage or necrosis.

Microscopically, the central scar contains thick-walled vessels with marked fibromuscular hyperplasia and/or myxoid change. The smaller septa also contain vessels that may be thick-walled. These septa are without a central bile duct but show prominent ductular proliferation at the interface between the fibrous tissue and hepatocytes (Fig. 2). Variable numbers of acute and chronic inflammatory cells infiltrate the septa. Cords of hepatocytes, two to three cells thick, with associated sinusoids but without central veins comprise the parenchyma. Clusters of metaplastic ductules may also be scattered within the hepatic parenchyma, but well-formed portal triads are not present. The hepatocytes often contain fat and may show cholestasis but are without pleomorphism, mitotic activity, nuclear enlargement, or prominent nucleoli.

TABLE 2. *Hepatic tumors of childhood: relative incidence*

Tumor type	% Total
Hemangioendothelioma	13–27
Mesenchymal hamartoma	6
Focal nodular hyperplasia	2–7
Adenoma	2–5
Hepatoblastoma	28–43
Hepatocellular carcinoma	15–23
Embryonal sarcoma	6–8

Diagnostic and Prognostic Considerations

As focal nodular hyperplasia does not carry the risk of hemorrhage associated with benign adenomas and is not known to undergo malignant degeneration, resection is not always necessary and treatment can be individualized (153,173,190,246). This approach, however, depends on accurately distinguishing focal nodular hyperplasia from hepatocellular adenoma and carcinoma. With a resected specimen in hand, distinguishing focal nodular hyperplasia from an adenoma is straightforward, based on the gross and microscopic features described above. However, the distinction in biopsy tissue depends on the inclusion of bile ducts or the characteristic thick-wall vessels in the biopsy material (173). Fine-needle aspirate diagnosis based on the finding of epithelial cells forming tight clusters of ducts has also been reported (274). It should also be noted in passing that there are occasional reports of patients with multiple tumors, some showing features of focal nodular hyperplasia and some of hepatic adenoma (44,170). Distinguishing focal nodular hyperplasia from hepatocellular carcinoma on biopsy or fine needle aspirate material depends largely on the cytologic features of malignancy, which have been described for both the standard and the fibrolamellar variant (49,62).

Correlating the histopathologic findings with imaging studies is useful, as modern radiologic techniques, in particular magnetic resonance imaging (MRI) and color Doppler ultrasound can suggest a diagnosis of focal nodular hyperplasia with a fair degree of accuracy (113,203,332). However, there is significant overlap in

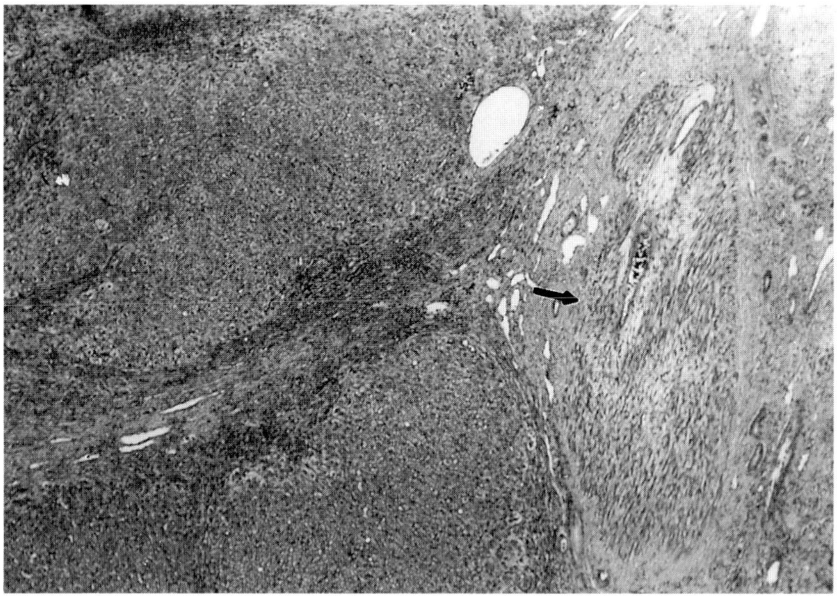

FIG. 2. Focal nodular hyperplasia. The nodules of benign hepatocytes are intersected by fibrous tracts with ductular proliferation at the interface. On the right a vein has been largely occluded by myointimal proliferation *(arrow)*.

the MRI features of the fibrolamellar variant of hepatocellular carcinoma (131), and when resection is not possible liver biopsy to exclude a malignant process is recommended. As an additional caveat, focal nodular hyperplasia occasionally accompanies fibrolamellar carcinoma (282,284), and biopsy taken through the focal nodular hyperplasia region could result in a false sense of security (265). This reported association of focal nodular hyperplasia with fibrolamellar carcinoma of course raises concerns of potential malignancy arising within incompletely resected focal nodular hyperplasia. However, even with incomplete excision or diagnosis by biopsy only, outcome seems to be excellent, with no reported progression or malignant degeneration after up to 15 years of follow-up (173,181,190,246).

Hepatocellular Adenoma

Clinical Features

Hepatocellular adenoma is a rare tumor, accounting for an estimated 4–6% of all benign liver masses in childhood (33,81) and occurring less commonly than focal nodular hyperplasia by a ratio of approximately 2.5:1 (33,71,81,190,370). These tumors span the full age spectrum, being occasionally diagnosed in utero (208). The tumors of early childhood occur almost exclusively in children without underlying disease (spontaneous). Those in the second decade occur with or without associated disease in about equal frequency (Fig. 3). In adults, there is a striking (>4:1) female predominance

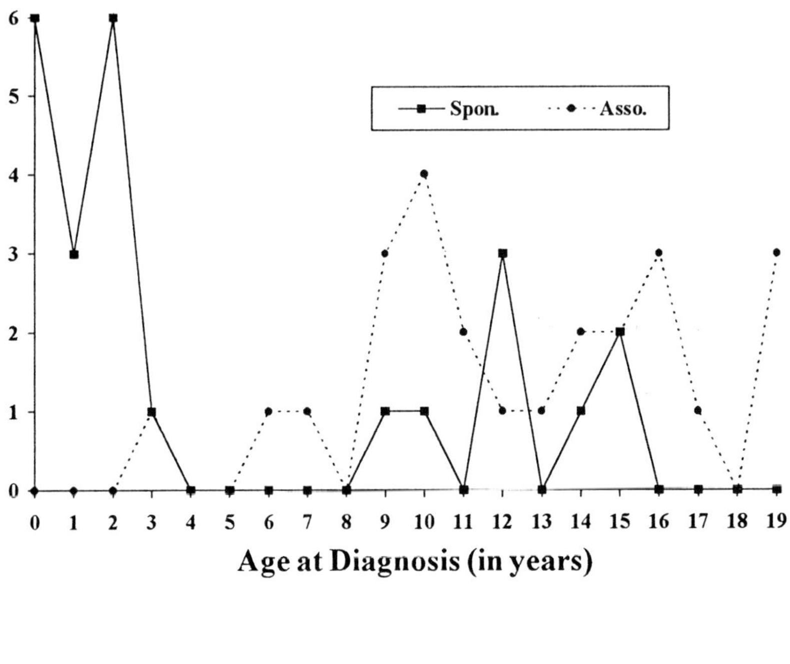

FIG. 3. Hepatic adenomas in children without an underlying inherited or metabolic disorder *(solid line)* show a bimodal age distribution with a prominant peak in the first 2 years of life (56,363), whereas children with adenomas and underlying glycogen storage disease or Fanconi's anemia *(dotted line)* are largely over 5 years old (26,38,194,224,295,333,374).

due largely to the association of hepatic adenoma with oral contraceptive usage (160,173). The average lag of more than 5 years between starting oral contraceptives and diagnosis of hepatic adenoma (56,214) takes most patients with oral contraceptive–associated tumors out of the pediatric age group. Thus, in children, there is a nearly equal number of affected boys and girls (Table 3). Unlike the typically incidental discovery of focal nodular hyperplasia, hepatic adenomas present as large masses, often with associated pain and fever (71,190,363). In adult women taking oral contraceptives, acute hemorrhage or rupture causes dramatic symptoms in up to 40% of cases (160,173,214), but this potentially fatal complication is less common in children. In over 50% of reported cases, childhood hepatic adenoma is associated with glycogen storage disease (GSD) I or Fanconi's anemia (Table 3). In the latter patients, androgen therapy seems to be the inciting factor, as similar tumors are seen in patients on androgens for other reasons (38,215,361), and approximately 50% of tumors regress with withdrawal of androgens (215,333). Less common associated conditions include GSD IV (3), Klinefelter's syndrome (25), type I diabetes mellitus (96), and β-thalassemia (38).

Pathologic Features

Typically, hepatic adenoma appears as a single, large (>10 cm), circumscribed, bulging, yellow–tan mass in the right hepatic lobe with or without central hemorrhage and necrosis (56). In adults, multifocal adenomas occur in approximately 1/3 of cases (160,173). In children with spontaneous tumors unassociated with underlying disease, solitary adenomas also predominate (363); however the majority (2/3 or more) of GSD or Fanconi's anemia patients have multiple tumors (26,38). The name adenomatosis has been sometimes applied to the livers with multiple (>4–10) adenomas (93).

The histopathology in nonandrogen-associated tumors is clearly benign, as the tumor is composed of well-differentiated hepatocytes arranged in 2- to 3-cell thick cords, or (less frequently) in sheets. These hepatocytes differ from the hepatocytes of the adjacent normal liver largely in the character of their cytoplasm, which may be acidophilic or vacuolated with or without cholestasis or steatosis. Mallory's hyaline with associated neutrophilic infiltrates and focal lamellar fibrosis has been described, particularly in association with GSD and oral contraceptive usage (26,56). Bile ducts are not present, and Kupffer cells line the sinusoids. Arteries and veins, without significant intimal thickening, course through the tumor. Although multinucleated cells may be present, tumor nuclei are uniform without an increased nuclear/cytoplasmic ratio, mitotic activity, or anaplasia. On the other hand, androgen-associated adenomas often contain large cells with marked nuclear hyperchromasia and acinus formation that fulfill the diagnostic criteria of well-differentiated hepatocellular carcinoma (38,224,295, 333). Peliosis, a recognized complication of androgen therapy, is seen in the adjacent liver parenchyma in approximately 50% of androgen-associated hepatic adenoma cases (38,224,295,333).

Diagnostic and Prognostic Considerations

The differential diagnosis includes focal nodular hyperplasia, hepatocellular carcinoma, and hepatoblastoma. With a resection specimen, differentiating hepatic adenoma from focal nodular hyperplasia is relatively straightforward (see above); distinguishing hepatic adenoma from well-differentiated hepatocellular carcinoma or hepatoblastoma in the younger children can be more problematic. Benign cytologic features and a nonaggressive growth pattern allow a confident diagnosis of adenoma (56,363). With biopsy or fine-needle aspiration material, cytologic features become paramount for diagnosis, thankfully with the errors more frequent on the side of overcalling benign lesions than undercalling malignancy (49,129,298,348). Most tumors removed from patients on androgen therapy demonstrate malignant features, but metastatic spread occurs rarely (36,223), and these tumors are currently classified as adenomas despite their histology (295,333).

The prognosis for children with hepatic adenomas varies, depending on associated conditions. Fanconi's anemia patients have a guarded prognosis, largely due to complications of their aplastic anemia rather than the hepatic tumors (333). Completely resected adenomas have a uniformly good prognosis (363). With incom-

TABLE 3. *Hepatic adenomas of childhood*

Associated conditions	No.	Age range	M/F	Ref.
Spontaneous	22	Newborn–15 yr	2:7	38, 56, 71, 190, 363
GSD I	18	3–19 yr	12:6	26
Fanconi's	7	9–14 yr	5:2	38, 194, 224, 295, 333
Other[a]	7	11 mo–19 yr	4:3	3, 38, 363

Abbreviations: M, male; F, female; GSD I, glycogen storage disease type I.

[a] Polyposis coli (1), β-thalassemia (2), portal vein thrombosis (1), renal transplant (1), glycogen storage disease IV (1), androgen therapy for aplastic anemia (1).

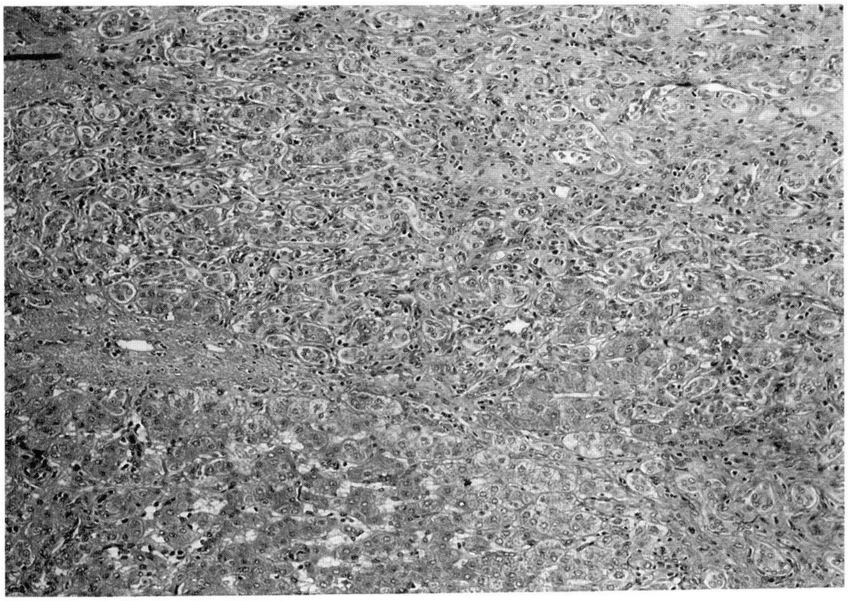

FIG. 4. The tumor illustrated grossly in Fig. 1 and composed microscopically in most areas by typical focal nodular hyperplasia show in this region extensive ductular transformation of hepatocytes resulting in broad fields composed predominantly of ductules *(upper two thirds)*.

pletely resected or multiple tumors, a small but real potential for malignant degeneration exists, signaled in at least some cases by increasing serum α-fetoprotein levels (163,189,358).

Other Benign Epithelial Tumors

Nodular Regenerative Hyperplasia

Nodular regenerative hyperplasia consists of small but widely distributed nodules of hepatocytes without associated fibrosis. The nodules are small, varying from 0.1 to 4 cm in size (321). Microscopically the nodules are composed of benign but hyperplastic hepatocytes that distort but do not replace the hepatic architecture. Nodules smaller than the hepatic lobules are disposed in a periportal distribution; larger nodules incorporate the portal triad. Hepatocytes within the nodules may show nuclear unrest and binucleation. Sinusoidal dilatation, arteriolar thickening, and portal venule thrombosis may also be seen (321). Portal hypertension, the most common complication, occurs in approximately 50% of adult cases, with many cases identified incidentally at autopsy (321,352). Nodular regenerative hyperplasia occurs in association with a wide variety of disease processes, probably as a result of abnormal hepatic blood flow (321). In the largest reported series in children, hepatosplenomegaly or suspected intra-abdominal tumor was the most common clinical presentation (225).

Mixed Hamartoma

Although its name suggests a similarity to the mesenchymal hamartoma, the mixed hamartoma more closely resembles focal nodular hyperplasia. Described rarely, the mixed hamartoma seems to differ from focal nodular hyperplasia largely in its relatively greater degree of ductular transformation within the fibrotic septa that subdivide the hepatocellular nodules (56,68,267). One tumor studied by the author that in most areas fulfills criteria for a diagnosis of focal nodular hyperplasia also included foci showing extensive ductular transformation like that described in the mixed hamartoma, suggesting that the latter lesion simply represents an unusual manifestation of the former (Fig. 4).

Developmental Cysts

Developmental cysts in the liver include a variety of lesions, including those associated with polycystic renal disease or extrahepatic choledochal cysts (56). Primary hepatic cysts occur rarely in childhood and include the solitary or simple cyst (32,277), epidermoid cyst (289), ciliated hepatic foregut cyst (362), and hepatobiliary cystadenoma (75).

BENIGN MESENCHYMAL TUMORS

Infantile Hemangioendothelioma

Clinical Features

Infantile hemangioendothelioma or hemangioma, the most common liver tumor in infancy (39,133), occurs as a single or multicentric liver mass in early childhood; 85–90% of patients are <6 months of age at presentation (66,144,217,313). As with hemangiomas elsewhere, there seems to be a female predominance, which is most prominent (approaching 2:1) with multicentric disease (18,155,217). Approximately 50% of cases present with otherwise asymptomatic hepatomegaly (18,144,217, 313). However, the vascular nature of the lesion, particularly when multicentric, can result in a more dramatic clinical presentation. Intratumoral arteriovenous shunts result in congestive heart failure (18,144,217,313). Sequestration of blood elements leads to thrombocytopenia with consumptive coagulopathy (Kasabach–Merritt syndrome) and even microangiopathic anemia (144,313,372). Heart failure and anemia in utero may result in nonimmune hydrops (301). In this age of routine prenatal ultrasound, in utero diagnosis of hepatic hemangioendotheliomas, occasionally with associated hydrops, is becoming more common (114,294,297). Rupture with hemoperitoneum is a rare complication (81). Up to 40% of all patients (70% of those with multicentric lesions) have hemangiomas elsewhere in the body, particularly on the skin (18,144, 217,313). Other associated anomalies are not common, though hepatic hemangioendotheliomas have been described in Beckwith–Wiedemann syndrome (79), Cornelia-de Lange syndrome (211), and an interstitial deletion of chromosome 6q (158).

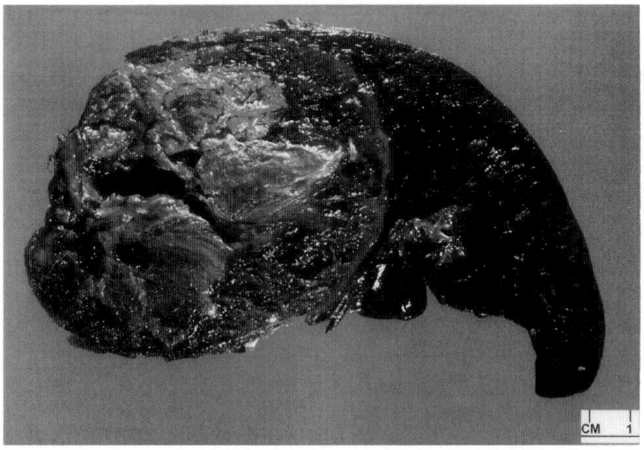

FIG. 6. The large infantile hemangioendothelioma replacing the right lobe of liver from this newborn infant resulted in thrombocytopenia and congestive heart failure resistant to medical therapy. Ligation of the hepatic artery resulted in partial necrosis of the tumor *(pale solid regions)*, but residual cavernous hemangioma persists at the interface of the tumor with the normal liver.

Gross Pathologic Features

The lesions, especially when small, may appear solid, belying their vascular nature (Fig. 5). However, larger lesions often include dilated, blood-filled spaces with associated calcification and fibrosis, particularly in the central regions (Fig. 6). Individual lesions appear circumscribed but nonencapsulated. When single the two lobes of liver are involved equally with infantile hemangioendothelioma; when multifocal, the lesions are commonly scattered throughout all lobes of liver (18,66,313).

Histopathologic Features

Two histologic patterns, designated by Dehner and Ishak as types I and II (66), continue to be recognized. Type I, comprising >80% of cases, is composed of small, often empty vascular spaces lined by uniform flat to plump benign endothelial cells and intermingled with scattered bile ducts and islands of extramedullary hematopoietic cells (Fig. 7). Plates of liver cells may also be

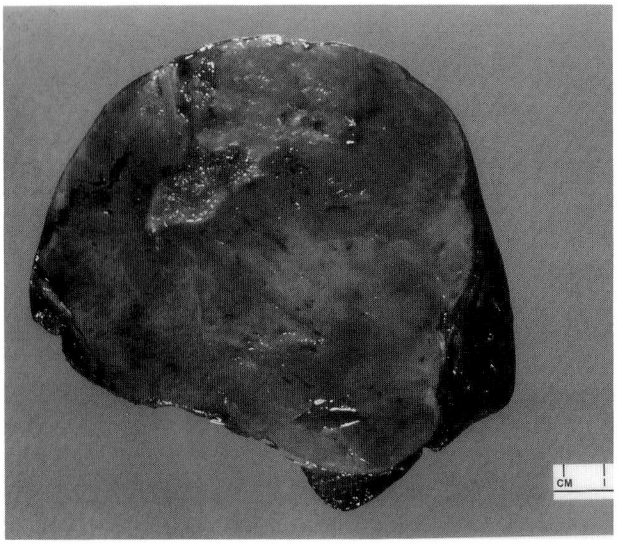

FIG. 5. The solid appearance of this infantile hemangioendothelioma belies its vascular nature. A focal area of necrosis is present superiorly.

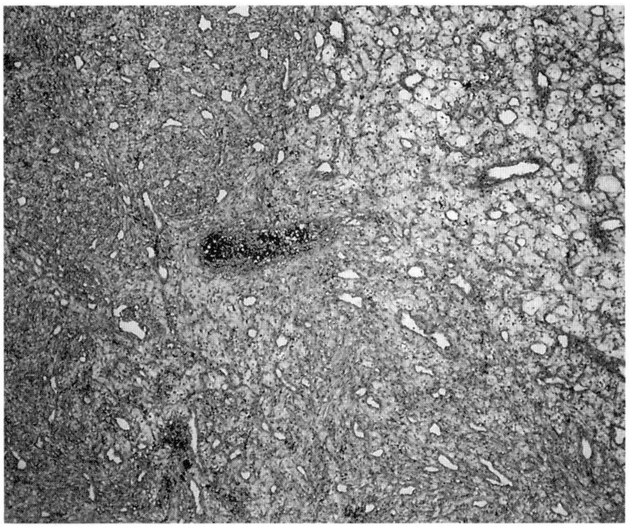

FIG. 7. Infantile hemangioendothelioma. Largely empty endothelial lined vascular channels are embedded within a loose myxoid stroma.

present, particularly at the periphery of the lesion. The intervening stroma varies from inconspicuous to abundant and is myxoid in character. Where this myxoid stroma predominates, histologic overlap with the mesenchymal hamartoma can lead to diagnostic confusion, particularly in a biopsy sample. Cavernous hemangiomalike areas are frequently present (Fig. 8). Mast cells, commonly seen in cutaneous hemangiomas (112), have not been noted to date. Type II histology differs from type I in the character of the endothelial cell proliferation. In type II lesions irregular budding and branching of plump, more pleomorphic endothelial cells with scattered mitoses can raise the spector of malignancy. These type II lesions invariably contain areas with type I histology but do not include areas with solid fibrosarcomatous features or extensive sinusoidal permeation as seen in adult-type angiosarcoma.

Electron Microscopy

The handful of published electron microscopic studies most commonly report endothelial cells without supporting pericytes (91,293). However, a study of two multicentric infantile hemangioendotheliomas identified pericytes (13,375) similar to those in studies of cutaneous hemangiomas (118).

Immunohistochemistry

Tumor endothelial cells reportedly stain uniformly with factor VIII–related antigen and more variably with *Ulex europaeus* I lectin and von Willebrand's factor (293,371). An immunohistochemical study in skin hemangiomas demonstrated an evolving pattern of reaction, with proliferating cell nuclear antigen, vascular endothelial growth factor, and type IV collagenase marking the proliferative phase and smooth muscle actin, tissue metalloproteinase inhibitors, and increased numbers of mast cells marking the involuting phase (328). Similar studies on the much less common hepatic hemangioendothelioma have not thus far been reported.

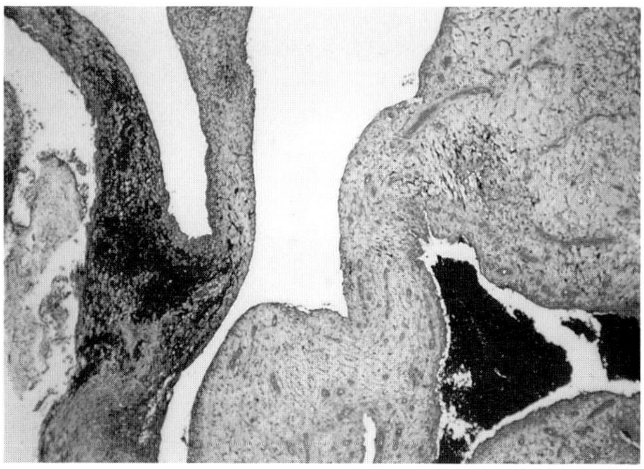

FIG. 8. Dilated blood-filled endothelial-lined spaces comprise the cavernous component of the infantile hemangioendothelioma illustrated grossly in Fig. 6.

Prognostic Considerations

The natural history of hepatic hemangioendotheliomas, like those located elsewhere in the body, follows a biphasic pattern of proliferation followed by spontaneous involution (92,249). Imaging studies can usually confidently enable the diagnosis, allowing for a conservative watch-and-wait approach in many cases (60,174). When symptomatic, attempted control of hepatic infantile hemangioendotheliomas by steroids, α-interferon, radiation, embolization, hepatic artery ligation, laser coagulation, and surgical resection have all been reported (19,297,313,349). Although the outcome for infants with solitary and asymptomatic masses is good, mortality in the face of uncontrollable heart failure and multifocal lesions remains high (15–40%) (81,293,313). Malignant degeneration to angiosarcoma is rare but has been documented in three reports (180,236,320).

Mesenchymal Hamartoma

Clinical Features

Mesenchymal hamartoma, the second most common benign hepatic tumor in childhood, presents most commonly and with equal sex frequency in infancy as a slowly enlarging liver mass (67,74,81,187,202,370). Although cases have been occasionally reported in adults (41,78,121,346), >80% of patients are under 2 years of age at diagnosis (187,318). Ten to twenty percent are present at birth, and prenatal ultrasound diagnosis has been documented (143). Although most cases are in patients without a malformation syndrome, mesenchymal hamartoma has been reported in association with adrenal cytomegaly, diffuse endocrinopathy, left ventricular endocardial fibroelastosis, and biliary atresia (187,318). An occasional report of mesenchymal hamartoma-associated heart failure (302) illustrates the clinical overlap with the infantile hemangioendothelioma.

Pathologic Features

This usually unifocal mass shows a striking right-sided preference; 75–80% occur in the right lobe, with 15–30% protruding as a pedunculated mass from the inferior border (187). The nonencapsulated mass can reach massive size (up to 25 cm and 6,800 g). Cystic change, present in 85%, can be single or multifocal, with the cysts contain-

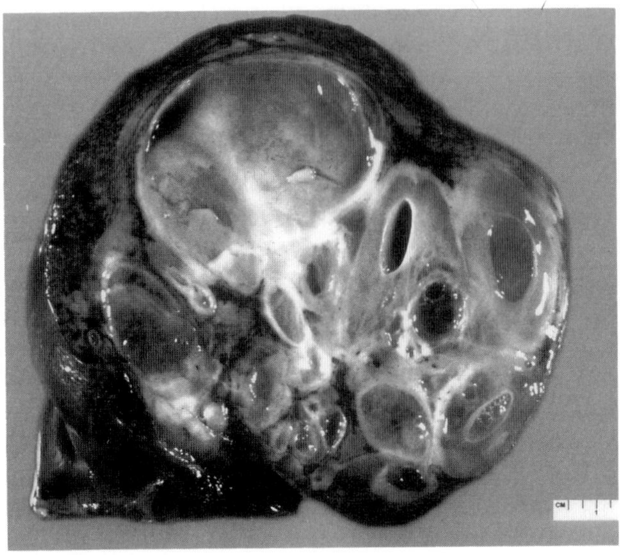

FIG. 9. Multiple cysts dominate the cut surface of the mesenchymal hamartoma. The blurred interface between hamartoma and liver are best appreciated on the left and lower aspects of the specimen.

ing an ultrafiltrate of plasma (Fig. 9). The pale white nodular mass merges irregularly with the adjacent liver, with islands of brown residual liver parenchyma frequently intermixed with the tumor, particularly at the periphery. By light microscopy, myxoid or fibrous stroma surrounds irregular distorted bile ducts and occasional islands of bland hepatocytes (Fig. 10). However, normal hepatic architecture is not present. Thin-walled vascular channels may be focally prominent, suggesting the possibility of a vascular tumor. The cystic spaces are lined by flattened cells of indeterminate type or may be without lining. As with other liver tumors in infancy, foci of extramedullary hematopoiesis are frequently seen. At the periphery of the tumor, the myxoid stroma appears to extend along or possibly arise from portal tracts, compressing the intervening liver parenchyma.

Diagnostic and Prognostic Considerations

Infantile hemangioendothelioma is the major consideration in the differential diagnosis of mesenchymal hamartoma. Radiologic features, though usually fairly characteristic, may overlap with those of infantile hemangioendothelioma (168). Biopsy findings may also be indistinguishable in these two lesions due to focal myxoid change in infantile hemangioendothelioma or focal vascular prominence in mesenchymal hamartoma. With the entire specimen for examination, this distinction is usually easily resolved.

In the past, most reports have referred to mesenchymal hamartoma as a developmental lesion rather than a neoplasm, with suggested pathogenetic mechanisms including aberrant development of portal mesenchyme (69), bile duct obstruction (241), and ischemic injury perhaps related to an anomalous solitary vascular supply (195). However, two recent reports of a specific translocation involving the long arm of chromosome 19 (213,312) and an additional report of aneuploid DNA content in a subset of mesenchymal hamartomas (244) suggest the possibility that some cases may be neoplastic in nature. Mesenchymal hamartoma behaves in a benign manner, with low recurrence risk after resection and until recently no documented malignant transformation (74,187,318). However, a 1994 report of embryonal sarcoma of the liver arising in conjunction with a mesenchymal hamartoma (63) challenges this commonly held belief that mesenchymal hamartoma harbors no malignant potential.

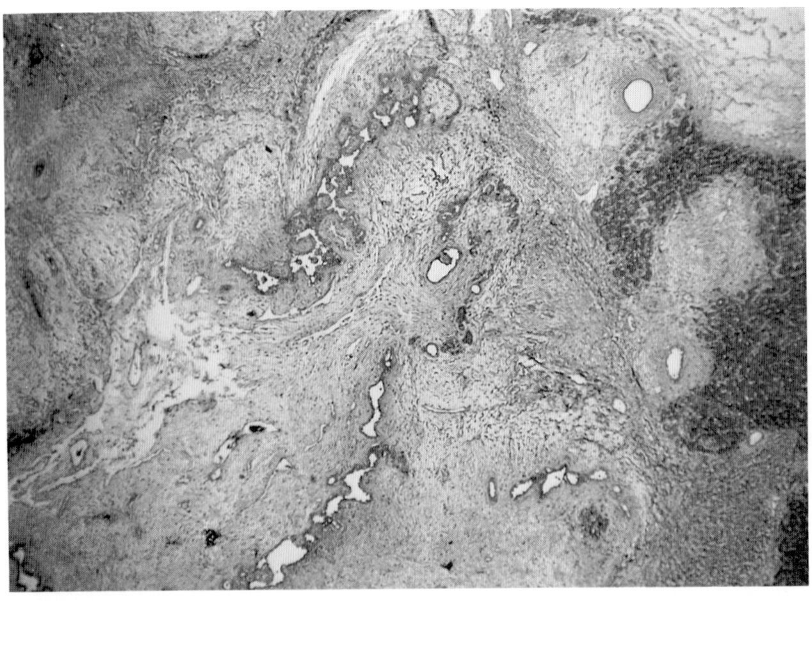

FIG. 10. Mesenchymal hamartoma. Loose connective tissue surrounds irregular tortuous bile ducts centrally. At the right, nodules of fibrous tissue partially isolate a tongue of hepatocytes.

Other Benign Mesenchymal Tumors

Cavernous Hemangioma

Although in adults the cavernous hemangioma is the most common benign tumor in the liver and is present in approximately 1% of all autopsies, it is usually small (<5 cm), unifocal, and asymptomatic (53). In children, pure cavernous hemangiomas also occur most often as incidental findings at autopsy (66). They appear grossly as soft, deep red, well-circumscribed, blood-filled masses that on cut surface may have a meshlike appearance. Areas of thrombosis, calcification, or fibrosis may also be present. The characteristic histopathology includes irregular large vascular spaces lined by flattened endothelial cells and separated by a paucicellular or myxoid stroma. Cavernous hemangiomas tend to be stable over time, without the proliferative and involuting phases characteristic of the infantile hemangioendothelioma (102).

Inflammatory Pseudotumor

Since the first report in 1964 (128), more than 50 cases of hepatic inflammatory pseudotumor, or inflammatory myofibroblastic tumor, have been described (7,147,296). The liver is the second most common site for this enigmatic lesion (6). Reported cases span a spectrum of ages from 10 months to 75 years, with approximately 20% of cases occurring in children. Whereas in adults there is a striking male predominance (M/F 4:1), in children the reported cases have a more equal sex distribution. Inflammatory pseudotumor, also called inflammatory myofibroblastic tumor, frequently presents with systemic symptoms including fever, hypergammaglobulinemia, leukocytosis, and weight loss (7). When centered at the porta hepatis, obstructive jaundice dominates the picture (142,258). The clinical and radiologic picture in many cases leads to a preoperative diagnosis of malignancy; two such reported cases were in patients with earlier Wilms' tumor (138,231,345).

As elsewhere in the body, inflammatory pseudotumor in the liver is a poorly circumscribed mass composed of a variety of cells in varying proportions, including reactive spindle cells (myofibroblasts), lymphocytes, plasma cells, macrophages, foam cells, and occasional scattered neutrophils and eosinophils. Immunocytochemical studies confirm the polyclonal nature of the lymphocytes (29,156). The spindle cell component in some areas may predominate and include mitotic figures, raising a suspicion of malignancy (296). Venous invasion frequently occurs and may result in portal and/or hepatic vein thrombosis (29,43,142,304). In the liver cholangitis is also often noted (120,228,229,296). The right lobe is slightly preferred over the left by solitary tumors, with approximately 10% centering in the porta hepatis and approximately 20% being multifocal (7,147,296). Despite the aggressive appearance, many examples of regression after incomplete resection have been reported (29,43,156,162).

On biopsy of a liver mass, diagnosis depends on finding a benign spindle cell proliferation combined with the mixed inflammatory infiltrate. The benign, though often reactive, nuclear cytology distinguishes inflammatory pseudotumor from the recently described inflammatory fibrosarcoma which mimics many of the clinical and histologic features of inflammatory pseudotumor but includes frank nuclear atypia (218). The inflammatory fibrosarcomas tend to recur locally and may metastasize distally. For discussion of similar pseudosarcomatous lesions at other sites, consult Chapters 8 and 14.

MALIGNANT EPITHELIAL TUMORS

Hepatoblastoma

Clinical Features

Though uncommon in the overall spectrum of abdominal masses, hepatoblastoma is the most common primary hepatic tumor in childhood, accounting for nearly 40% of all hepatic tumors (39,67,356) and approximately 55% of malignant tumors (33,39,110,125, 287,356). As is true of the other embryonic tumors, hepatoblastoma's peak incidence occurs in the first 2 years of life, with 80–90% of cases presenting before 5 years of age (33,39,110,119,125,287,356). Hepatoblastoma has been occasionally reported as a cause of fetal death (21,243) and as a source of placental metastases (269). Hepatoblastoma shows a 1.6:1 preference for boys and no racial or geographic differences (86,119,125,154,188, 287). It presents as an enlarging mass that may be associated with anorexia and weight loss (125,154,188). In 80–90% of cases, a dramatically elevated serum α-fetoprotein (AFP) level serves as a tumor marker, aiding not only in the initial diagnosis but also in the routine follow-up for disease progression or recurrence (86,110,186, 188,287). Cystathionuria, occurring in 40–70% of patients (105,106) and once touted as a useful tumor marker, has since proven to be of limited diagnostic value (141).

A variety of paraneoplastic syndromes may also color the clinical picture. Human chorionic gonadotropin (hCG) (227,230) or, rarely, testosterone production (100) by the tumor cells results in precocious puberty in 6% of the boys (125,188,287). Thrombocytosis, with platelet counts as high as 1 million, occurs in 25–65% of cases (106,125,186,188). This thrombocytosis seems not to be due to production of interleukin-6 by the tumor cells, as has been described in other malignancies, but rather to the inexplicable induction of interleukin-6 production in tumor-associated endothelial cells and fibroblasts (344). Osteoporosis, evident on imaging studies in 20–30% of patients, may be complicated by pathologic fracture (188).

Hepatoblastoma occurs in association with a variety of genetic and environmental risk factors (Table 4). In contrast to childhood hepatocellular carcinoma, prior hepatitis B infection (239,261) or cirrhosis due to chronic hepatitis or metabolic disease (30,64,99) are not significant risk factors for hepatoblastoma. Familial polyposis coli was first identified as a possible risk factor in 1983 (178), with subsequent reports confirming the original observation (103,111,151,159,268). Familial polyposis is now known to be associated with mutation or microdeletion at chromosome 5q21 (123,179), a region not yet reported as abnormal in cytogenetic studies of hepatoblastoma (see below). Hemihypertrophy carries an increased risk for abdominal tumors, particularly Wilms' tumor and adrenal cortical tumors (22,97,98, 307), with numerous reports also documenting an association with hepatoblastoma (99,105,106,154,188). The Beckwith–Wiedemann syndrome, comprising a variety of congenital malformations and overgrowths including hemihypertrophy, is associated with a similar spectrum of tumors (209,310,366). This phenomenon is particularly evident when hemihypertrophy is also present (308,309), suggesting an as-yet-unclear pathogenetic relationship between the two (307,308). Evidence linking the Beckwith–Wiedemann syndrome to abnormalities on the short arm of chromosome 11 includes cytogenetic studies demonstrating a variety of 11p abnormalities in individual patients (127,253,336,355) and restriction fragment–linked polymorphism analysis in carrier families narrowing linkage to 11p15 (182,256) (see Chapter 3).

TABLE 4. *Hepatoblastoma: associations and risk factors*

Genetic/congenital risk factors	Ref.
Familial colonic polyposis	See text
Beckwith–Wiedemann syndrome	See text
Hemihypertrophy	See text
Synchronous Wilms' tumor	99, 188
Occasional genetic/chromosomal associations	
Trisomy 21	119
Trisomy 18	204
Prader–Willi syndrome	136
Glycogen storage disease 1a	157
Other associations	
Fetal alcohol syndrome	104, 175, 287
Maternal oral contraceptive use	245
Genitourinary anomalies	119
Human immunodeficiency virus infection	10

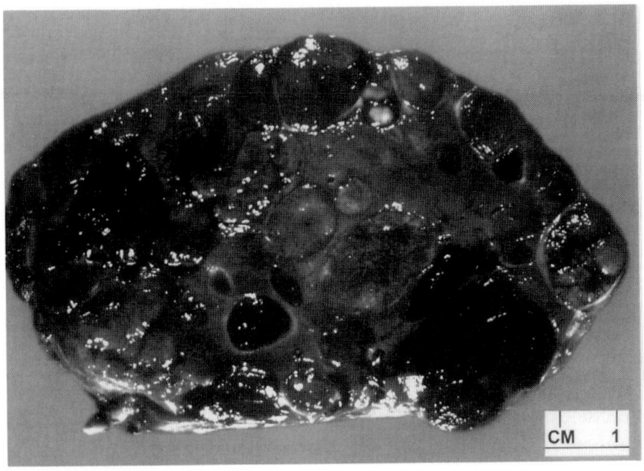

FIG. 11. Multiple variegated nodules compose the cut surface of this previously untreated hepatoblastoma.

Gross Pathologic Features

Hepatoblastoma shows a preference for the right (55–60%) vs. left (15%) lobe of the liver, with 25–30% of cases extending into both lobes (154,188,221). The size ranges from 5.5 to 17 cm and 180 to 1300 g. (154,188). On cut surface it appears lobulated due to fibrous septa intersecting the variegated tan–brown, green, and black tumor nodules that often include areas of hemorrhage and necrosis (Fig. 11). The interface with adjacent normal liver may appear either distinct or blurred (154,188) (Fig. 12). Although usually solitary, 15% of tumors are multifocal at presentation, with a large primary mass associated with smaller satellite nodules (104,154).

Light Microscopic Features

As the embryonic tumor of the liver, hepatoblastoma exhibits, like its counterparts in the pancreas and kidney, an astounding range of histologic patterns that include both epithelial and mesenchymal elements. The epithelial components exhibit a range of differentiation including (a) small primitive "anaplastic" cells, (b) poorly differentiated "embryonal" cells, (c) well-differentiated "fetal" hepatocytes, and (d) larger atypical hepatocytes that are similar to cells seen in a hepatocellular carcinoma and are associated with the macrotrabecular growth pattern. Pathologic subclassification of hepatoblastoma depends on the mixture of the above components present in a given tumor (Table 5).

The fetal and embryonal patterns are seen most frequently, with most tumors including a mixture of these two elements. The fetal epithelium is composed of obvious hepatocytes, which are slightly smaller than hepatocytes in adjacent normal liver and are arranged in distinctive cords composed of two- to three-cell layers and separated by well-formed sinusoids (Fig. 13). These fetal hepatocytes may have condensed eosinophilic cyto-

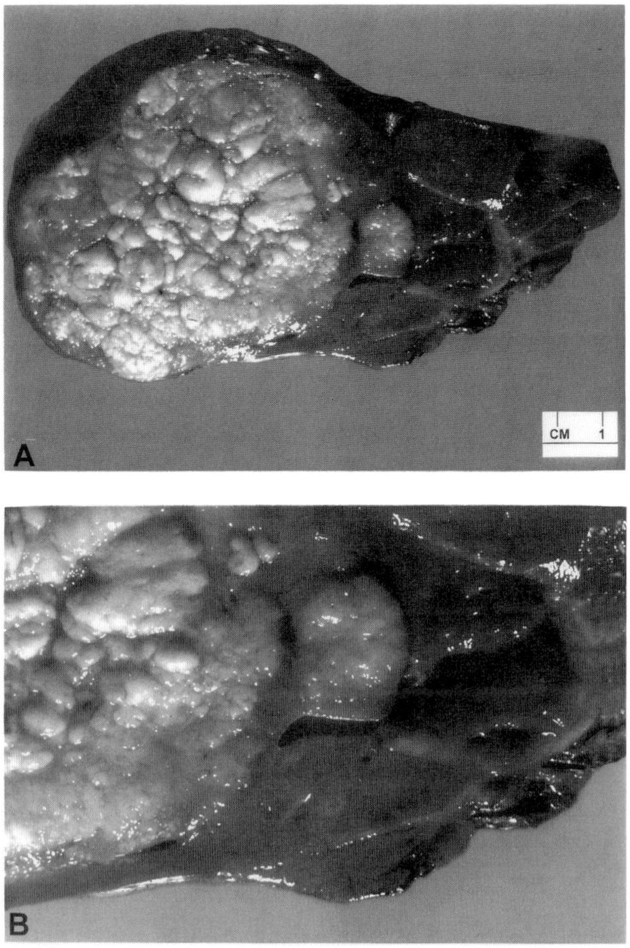

FIG. 12. This pure fetal hepatoblastoma lacks the variegated appearance of the combined fetal and embryonal tumor illustrated in Fig. 11. The irregular interface between tumor and liver with small satellite nodules present in **A** can be seen to better advantage in the close up **B**.

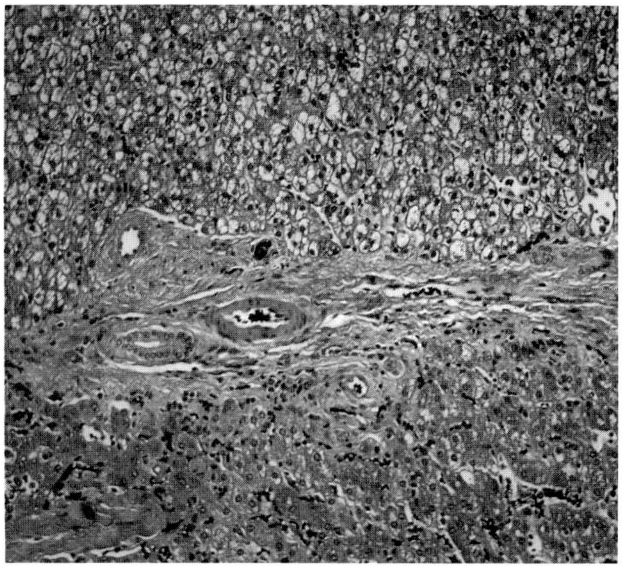

FIG. 13. The difficulty in distinguishing between normal hepatocytes *(lower half)* and the slightly smaller but otherwise very well differentiated fetal hepatoblasts *(upper half)* is readily apparent here.

plasm or clear lipid and glycogen-rich cytoplasm, producing the mixed "dark and light cell" appearance classically described (154) (Fig. 14). The sinusoids of untreated fetal hepatoblastoma virtually always contain hematopoietic cells. Intracellular bile may be present but bile ducts are not a feature. The embryonal hepatocytes contain larger, more hyperchromatic nuclei with less abundant cytoplasm than their fetal counterpart (Fig. 15). Multinucleated giant cells may also be present, particularly in hCG-producing tumors, where they can be stained with anti-hCG antibody (226,227). The embryonal cells grow as sheets interrupted by primitive tubular differentiation or rosette formation (119). Occasionally, the embryonal cells grow in a papillary pattern mimicking the Schiller–Duval bodies seen in endodermal sinus tumors (188) (see Chapter 10).

The much less common macrotrabecular and anaplastic patterns may be present in combination with the

TABLE 5. *Hepatoblastoma: histopathologic classification (1, 51, 119, 154, 188, 356)*

Histologic subtype	% Total
Epithelial	50–60
Pure fetal	27
Fetal and embryonal	17–30
Macrotrabecular	
Undifferentiated small cell (anaplastic)	
Mixed epithelial and mesenchymal	35–40
Without teratoid features	
With teratoid features	
Nonclassifiable	9

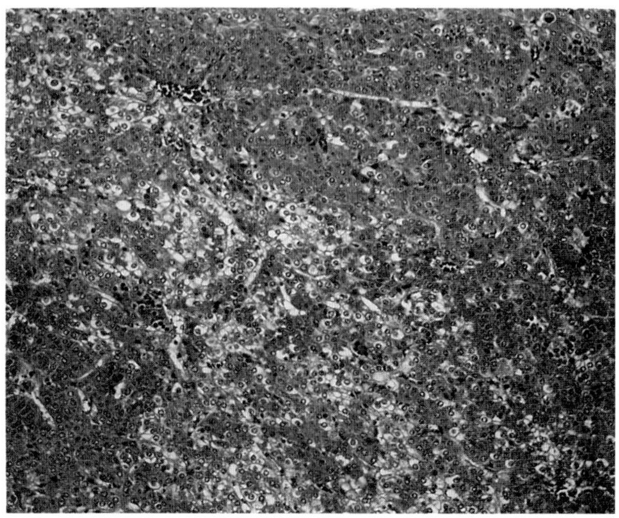

FIG. 14. Fetal hepatoblastoma. Sinusoids separating the two- to three-cell-thick cords of dark and light fetal hepatoblasts contain scattered clusters of small dark hematopoietic cells.

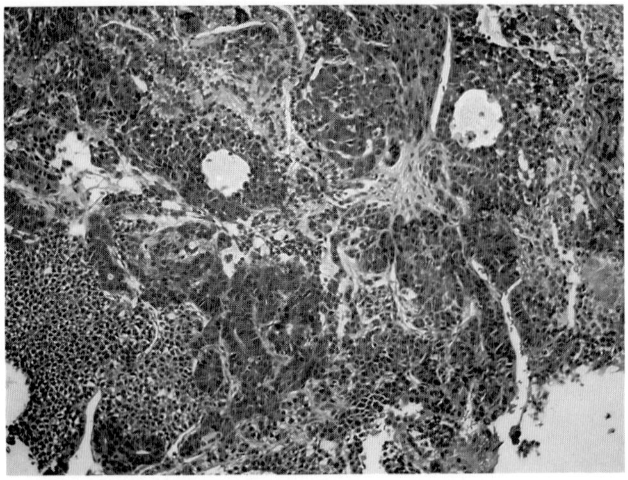

FIG. 15. Hepatoblastoma. Embryonal hepatoblasts forming irregular trabecular and glandlike spaces are mixed with more primitive anaplastic cells.

more common patterns described above or may occasionally be the dominant tumor pattern. Macrotrabecular foci, identified by 5- to 10-cell thick trabeculae, may include fetal, embryonal, or large epithelial cells. The large cells with abundant eosinophilic cytoplasm, large vesicular nuclei, and prominent nucleoli closely mimic cells from well-differentiated hepatocellular carcinoma. In contrast, anaplastic foci are composed of small cells with round dense nuclei and minimal cytoplasm, growing as sheets without evidence of epithelial differentiation (Figs. 16 and 17). These cells may be embedded in a mucoid ground substance (34,164).

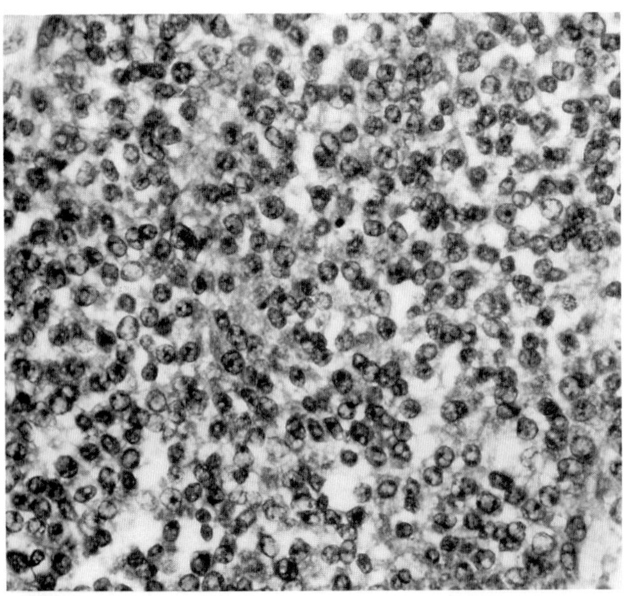

FIG. 16. Anaplastic hepatoblastoma. Sheets of primitive round cells with scant cytoplasm and no differentiation features by light microscopic examination characterize the anaplastic hepatoblasts.

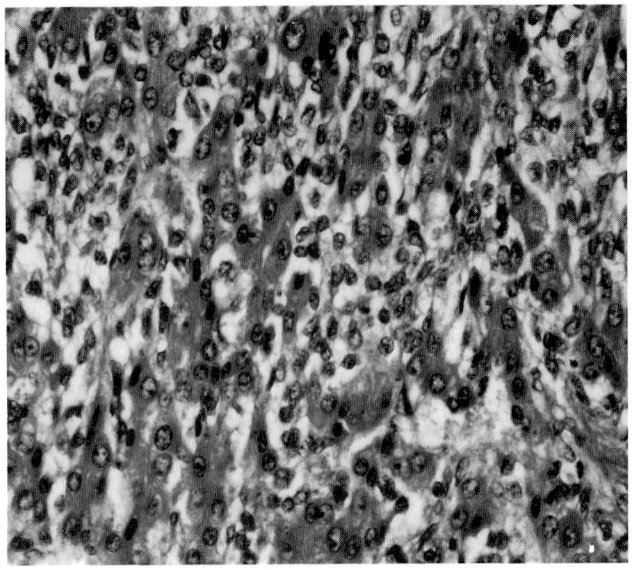

FIG. 17. The primitive small round blue cells of anaplastic hepatoblastoma infiltrate the sinusoids of adjacent liver in a fashion mimicking metastatic neuroblastoma.

When present, the mesenchymal component most often includes foci of eosinophilic "osteoid"-appearing matrix (Fig. 18) with cartilage seen less frequently and skeletal muscle only rarely (51,67,119,154,188). Divergent epithelial differentiation in these mixed tumors yields squamous pearls and mucus-secreting glands (154,188). Rare cases also demonstrate immunohistochemical evidence of neuroepithelial differentiation, melanin production, and even formation of ganglion cells (206,271,272). Though these multiple forms of divergent differentiation raise the diagnostic possibility of teratoma, a more accurate designation is teratoid hepatoblastoma (51,206). We reserve the appellation teratoma for tumors with organoid differentiation.

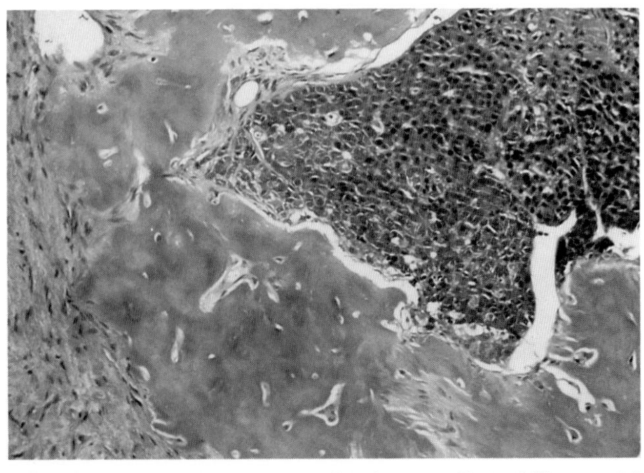

FIG. 18. Hepatoblastoma, mixed type. Osteoidlike matrix partially surrounds the embryonal hepatoblasts present at the right of the photo.

Immunohistochemical Features

As expected, the fetal and embryonal components of hepatoblastoma stain with a variety of epithelial markers (Table 6). Perhaps more surprisingly, the cells embedded within the osteoidlike matrix of the mesenchymal component also mark with epithelial antibodies. When studied using monoclonal antibodies specific for hepatocyte-type and bile duct–type cytokeratins, the embryonal, fetal, and osteoid-associated cells marked for both types (340).

Electron Microscopic Features

The ultrastructural features of hepatoblastoma parallel the light microscopic features of hepatocellular differentiation (1,146,348). The cytoplasm of hepatocytes in the fetal regions contain abundant organelles, including rough and smooth endoplasmic reticulum, numerous mitochondria, and scattered bundles of filaments. Well-developed junctions and canalicular formation with microvilli further define the cells as hepatocytes. The embryonal cell cytoplasm contains fewer organelles with less well-developed junctions and fewer microvilli. The osteoid-associated cells also show features of hepatocellular differentiation, including formation of cell junctions and intercellular lumen containing microvilli. The anaplastic cells have not been as well studied, but in at least one instance they did show occasional cell junctions and microvillus formation, helping to distinguish them from those of the other small round blue cell tumors of childhood (117).

Cytogenetic and Molecular Diagnostic Features

Unlike some of the other childhood malignancies, no single chromosomal translocation or deletion characterizes hepatoblastoma. Of the variety of structural cytogenetic abnormalities identified in hepatoblastoma cells, the most frequently recurring are trisomy 20 and trisomy 2q, one or both of which are seen in two thirds of studied cases (5,14,16,94,127,132,212,243,270,311). It can be noted in passing that trisomy 2 has also been described as a recurring genetic abnormality in embryonal rhabdomyosarcomas (351). Structural abnormalities of chromosome 11 occur occasionally (127), with loss of heterozygosity in the chromosome 11p15 region reported more frequently (31,183,199). This latter observation serves as an additional link with embryonal rhabdomyosarcoma (291), Wilms' tumor, adrenal cortical tumors, and the Beckwith–Wiedemann syndrome (31,183).

There is also no evidence to date of a role for oncogene activation or *p53* gene mutation in the pathogenesis of hepatoblastoma. Searches for amplification of c-*erbB-2*, c-*myc*, N-*myc*, and *ras* oncogenes have been largely fruitless (107,326,335) except for a single case demonstrating a k-*ras* point mutation by an allele-specific polymerase chain reaction (PCR) amplification technique (319). Strong evidence of *p53* gene alterations also elude documentation. Although positive immunocytochemical staining for the *p53* product has been demonstrated in many hepatoblastomas (67% in one study) (172,273), loss of heterozygosity at the *p53* locus or mutation of the *p53* gene can be demonstrated in very few (65,166,172). This discrepancy between positive p53 immunocytochemical staining and the lack of an associated gene mutation can occur due to a variety of cellular protein interactions that stabilize the *p53* product (130).

TABLE 6. *Hepatoblastoma: immunohistochemical staining of cell types (1, 271)*

	Epithelial[a]	Anaplastic	Osteoid-associated
Cytokeratin	+	+	+
EMA	−	−	+
CEA	+	−	+/−
Vimentin	−	+	+
AFP	+	−	+/−

Abbreviations: EMA, epithelial membrane antigen; CEA, carcinoembryonic antigen; AFP, α-fetoprotein.
[a] Includes fetal and embryonal types.

Diagnostic Considerations

The differential diagnosis of hepatoblastoma depends in part on the pathologic subtype of tumor present. With pure epithelial tumors, the major point of differential diagnosis is from other hepatocellular neoplasms, in particular hepatocellular carcinoma. Features that are particularly helpful in this differential include (a) the small size of fetal hepatocytes compared to adjacent normal liver in contrast with the larger size of tumor cells in hepatocellular carcinoma, (b) foci of hematopoiesis and, (c) presence of dark and light cells (154). Foci of Schiller–Duval-like structures in hepatoblastoma may cause confusion with a primary endodermal sinus tumor of the liver. When the macrotrabecular pattern of growth predominates, differentiation from hepatocellular carcinoma may become more difficult. A search for fields of more typical fetal or embryonal hepatoblastoma will usually point to the correct diagnosis. A predominantly small cell (anaplastic) hepatoblastoma raises the possibility of the spectrum of small round cell tumors. The small cells in hepatoblastoma are low molecular weight cytokeratin-positive and are negative for lymphoid and neural markers. With mixed hepatoblastoma, particularly with multiple forms of differentiation, the question of a primary teratoma becomes the primary consideration. The lack of organoid structure and the presence of otherwise typical hepatoblastoma resolve the issue in most cases (see also the discussion of teratomas later in this chapter).

TABLE 7. *Hepatoblastoma: fine-needle aspiration cytology (34, 73, 303, 348)*

Characteristic	Fetal/embryonal	Anaplastic
Smear character	Cohesive 3-D cell clumps	Loose cell clumps
Nuclear features	Finely granular chromatin, single nucleolus, N/C ratio 1:2–1:3; few mitoses	Finely granular chromatin, single nucleolus, N/C ratio 1:1, many mitoses
Cytoplasm	Well-defined cell border; granular, clear vacuoles	Ill-defined cytoplasm
Stroma	EMH, +/− osteoid-like matrix, +/− mucoid matrix	None

N/C, nuclear/cytoplasmic; EMH, extramedullary hematopoiesis, 3-D, three-dimensional.

The current trend toward preoperative chemotherapy dictates that diagnosis must be made more frequently on small fragments of aspirate or biopsy tissue, compounding the problems of differential diagnosis. The reported fine-needle aspiration cytologic features of the histologic subtypes of hepatoblastoma mirror the histologic patterns (303). Table 7 outlines the most salient reported fine-needle aspirate characteristics. With only small fragments of tissue, immunocytochemical and ultrastructural studies as outlined above may take on greater significance (73,237,348).

Prognostic Features

Complete surgical resection is the most important prognostic factor in hepatoblastoma (51,70,126,188), and the staging of hepatoblastoma (Table 8) centers on this historical fact. Preoperative chemotherapy of unresectable tumors leads in many cases to shrinkage of the tumor and enables subsequent complete resection (254,266) and more favorable outcome (177). The serum AFP level at diagnosis shows no correlation with outcome, but failure of AFP levels to fall to normal after tumor resection correlates with residual active disease (177) and bodes ill for the patient. Attempts to correlate histologic subtype with clinical outcome have met with variable success. Although there is a suggestion that predominantly fetal tumors do better, this observation is not demonstrated in all studies (51,70,126,167,356). The presence of mesenchymal tissue seems to have little bearing on outcome. A predominantly macrotrabecular growth pattern seems to be associated with poorer outcome (70,119). The small cell (anaplastic) tumors show a uniformly poor outcome (70,167,188).

Tumor DNA content and proliferation indices likewise have an equivocal effect on survival. Flow and image cytometry on paraffin-embedded tumor demonstrates aneuploid DNA content in approximately 35% of studied cases (51,137,288), with statistically poorer outcome for aneuploid tumors documented in one study (137). A tendency to better outcome with lower proliferation indices was noted in one study but did not reach statistical significance (288).

Preoperative chemotherapy induces the expected tumor necrosis without apparent preference for cell type (95,285) (Fig. 19). Increased prominence of the mesenchymal component, particularly the osteoidlike material, is also described (285); and it is possible that preop-

TABLE 8. *Hepatoblastoma: clinicopathologic staging (51, 177)*

Stage	Indications
I	Complete resection
II	Microscopic residual tumor Negative lymph nodes No tumor spill
III	Gross residual tumor *OR* Positive lymph nodes *OR* Tumor spill
IV	Metastatic disease

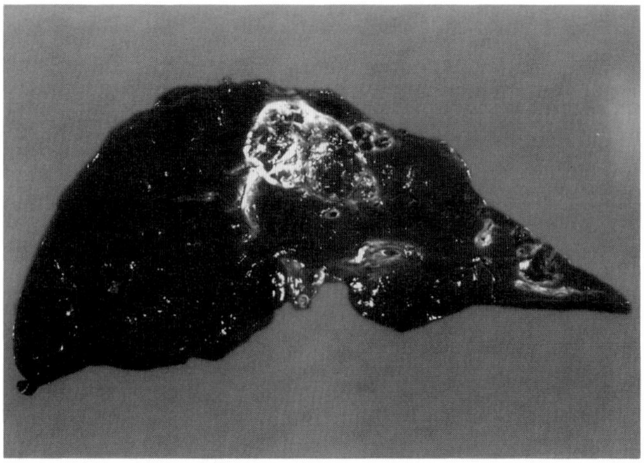

FIG. 19. Preoperative chemotherapy resulted in dramatic shrinkage of this multifocal hepatoblastoma. Tumor present centrally as well as in the left lobe shows extensive necrosis with a thick sclerotic border. Despite a dramatic response to therapy, this tumor because of its central location remained unresectable, so that the patient underwent hepatectomy and liver transplantation.

TABLE 9. *Hepatocellular carcinoma vs. hepatoblastoma: relative number of cases*

	HCC	HBL	Ref.
Age:			45, 154, 167, 200, 287
<5 yr	7	163	
≥5 yr	94	6	
Geography:			
AFIP	12	35	154
USA	98	129	86
Germany	14	24	287
Texas	33	43	356
Boston	32	54	189
Japan	13	57	167
Japan	21	16	200
Taiwan	30	10	45

Abbreviations: HCC, hepatocellular carcinoma; HBL, hepatoblastoma; AFIP, Armed Forces Institute of Pathology.

erative treatment might induce or unmask teratoid features in some tumors (95,206). The extent of posttherapy necrosis relative to outcome has not been studied to date.

Hepatocellular Carcinoma

Clinical Features

Only 0.5–1% of all hepatocellular carcinomas occur before 20 years of age (35,200), and they account for a similar percentage of pediatric solid tumors (37,220, 300). Among pediatric hepatic tumors, the relative incidence of hepatocellular carcinoma varies with age and, to some extent, with geography (Table 9). The geographic differences relate to the relative incidence of hepatitis B infection as discussed below. Hepatocellular carcinoma in young patients can be usefully divided in two distinct clinicopathologic subtypes: "usual" hepatocellular carcinoma and the fibrolamellar variant covered in the following section.

The usual hepatocellular carcinoma occurs at all ages, with a mean age of 12–14 years and few cases occurring under the age of 5 years. Most patients present with an abdominal mass, often with associated abdominal pain and anorexia and less often with fever, weight loss, jaundice, and elevated liver enzymes. Forty to sixty percent of cases have serum AFP elevation, which serves as a useful tumor marker (86,90,154,189,234,287,356). Paraneoplastic syndromes are less common with hepatocellular carcinoma than with hepatoblastoma. In addition to age, differences in sex distribution and associated liver disease distinguish the disease in adults from that in childhood (Table 10). On a global basis, the single largest risk factor for developing hepatocellular carcinoma in childhood is clearly hepatitis B infection (40,45,201, 329), often acquired perinatally (17,40,45,329). In countries with low endemic rates for hepatitis B infection, other causes of chronic liver disease, often metabolic (Table 11), take on a greater relative importance. Hepatocellular carcinoma associated with chronic hepatitis C infection occurs in adults but has thus far not been documented in childhood (108).

Pathologic Features

Hepatocellular carcinoma occasionally occurs as a solitary circumscribed mass in one liver lobe, most often the right, but more often multiple nodules or a diffusely infiltrating mass involve both lobes of the liver, rendering the tumor unresectable (45,86,189,234) (Fig. 20). The cut surface of hepatocellular carcinoma, unlike that of hepatoblastoma, is often bile-stained and more frequently shows areas of hemorrhage and necrosis. In adults, macroscopic features that aid in predicting an increased risk of local recurrence include tumor size >5 cm, presence of multiple nodules, and presence of grossly visible venous invasion (11,161,200,281,373).

Microscopic features of hepatocellular carcinoma in children are similar to those seen in the adult form of the disease (57,90,154,189,281). Well-differentiated areas contain large cells with moderately pleomorphic nuclei, often prominent nucleoli, and abundant eosinophilic cytoplasm with distinct cell borders (Fig. 21). These form trabeculae of few to many cells widely separated by sinusoidal spaces (the trabecular pattern). In other areas similar hepatocytelike cells may be arranged as sheets without well-formed sinusoids (solid pattern) or form pseudoglandular structures representing dilated bile canaliculi that may be filled with bile or eosinophilic, hyaline, PAS-positive diastase-resistant material (acinar pattern) (Fig. 22). Clear cells, focally present in occasional tumors, may mimic the clear cells seen in fetal hepa-

TABLE 10. *Hepatocellular carcinoma: adults vs. children (28, 57, 90, 154, 167, 189, 287, 300, 356)*

	Adults	Childhood
M/F ratio	3:1	3:2
Cirrhosis	70–80%	20–35%
Associated liver disease	Chronic HB infection, alcoholic cirrhosis	Chronic HB infection, biliary cirrhosis, metabolic cirrhosis

Abbreviations: M, male; F, female; HB, hepatitis B.

TABLE 11. *Hepatocellular carcinoma in childhood: associated conditions*

	Comment	Ref.
	Well-recognized associations	
Biliary atresia	With biliary cirrhosis	90, 242
Familial cholestatic cirrhosis	Byler's syndrome included	61, 337
Tyrosinemia	35% incidence HCC if survive >2 yr	72, 279, 358
Idiopathic cirrhosis		87, 216
Alagille's syndrome	With/without cirrhosis; usually adults	12, 46, 169, 263, 290
Ataxia-telangiectasia		185, 360
α_1-Antitrypsin deficiency	Usually adults	82, 198, 259
	Rare associations of uncertain significance	
Congenital hepatic fibrosis		205
Chronic TPN		342
Methotrexate-induced fibrosis		275
Neurofibromatosis		83
Cerebral gigantism		322
Prior radiation therapy		189
Cystinosis		39
Galactosemia		39
Osteogenesis imperfecta		39
Wilson's disease	Usually adults	39
	Overlap associations	
Familial polyposis	Usually hepatoblastoma	359, 376
Glycogen storage disease	Usually adenoma	26, 149, 374
Fanconi's anemia	Usually adenoma	90, 194

Abbreviations: HCC, hepatocellular carcinoma; TPN, total parenteral nutrition.

toblastoma, but the larger overall cell size and lack of extramedullary hematopoiesis in hepatocellular carcinoma aids in distinguishing between these tumors. Poorly differentiated tumors, composed of spindle cells with or without tumor giant cells, may suggest a primary (or metastatic) sarcoma. Osteoclastlike giant cells associated with focal ossification, a pattern that could easily suggest hepatoblastoma, has been described in hepatocellular carcinoma (281).

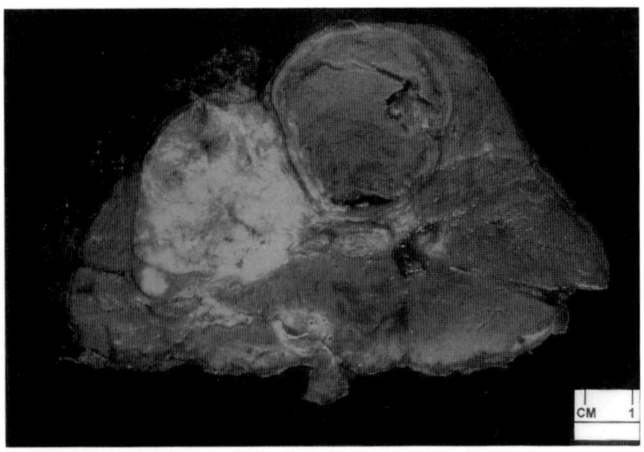

FIG. 20. Hepatocellular carcinoma. This multinodular tumor includes a largely necrotic dark-colored well-circumscribed nodule on the right and a lighter colored poorly circumscribed nodule on the left.

Immunohistochemical Staining

Normal hepatocytes express only cytokeratins 8 and 18, making differential cytokeratin staining useful in diagnosis. However, some hepatocellular carcinomas, particularly less differentiated tumors, exhibit aberrant staining for other forms of cytokeratin (260,341). A canalicular pattern of polyclonal carcinoembryonic antigen (CEA) staining is touted as being specific for hepatocellular carcinoma (48,281,369). Albumin, a protein produced in hepatocytes, would be an attractive immunocytochemical marker were there not such high quantities of the protein in serum, resulting in nonspecific staining reactions. In situ hybridization for albumin mRNA yields much more specific results (247). Neuroendocrine differentiation as demonstrated by immunocytochemical staining may occur in hepatocellular carcinoma (150,378). Poorly differentiated spindle (sarcomatoid) cells may stain with both vimentin and cytokeratin (165,238).

Cytogenetic and Molecular Biologic Considerations

The extant reports of cytogenetic and molecular biologic studies on hepatocellular carcinoma include virtually no tumors from childhood. No tumor-specific cytogenetic aberrations have surfaced; loss of chromosome

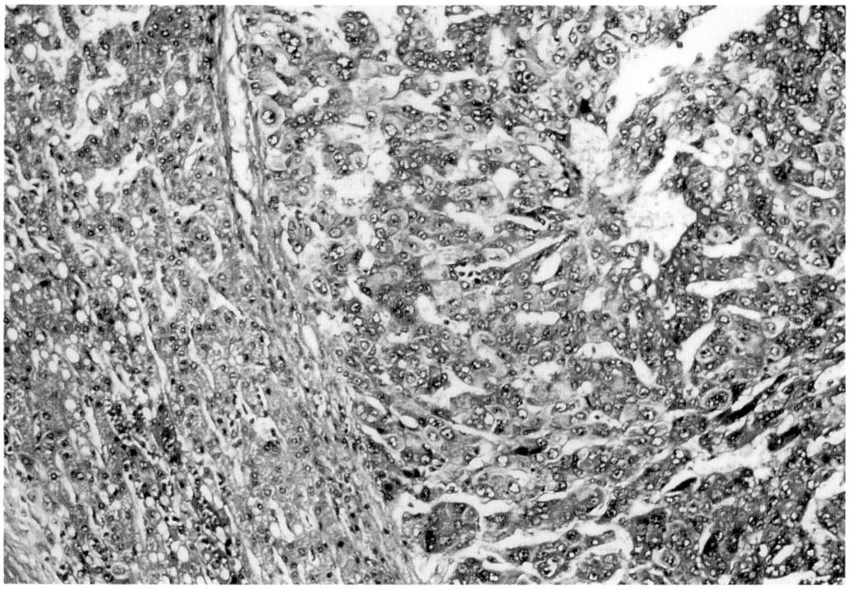

FIG. 21. The normal hepatocytes on the left contrast with the larger more pleomorphic cells on the right which form distinct trabeculae in this well differentiated hepatocellular carcinoma.

1p, 6q, and 16 material have been suggested as significant findings (15,299). Table 12 catalogs reported tumor suppressor gene alterations and oncogene and growth factor overexpression.

Diagnostic and Prognostic Considerations

The differential diagnosis of hepatocellular carcinoma in children most conspicuously includes hepatoblastoma, with metastatic carcinoma being a much less likely consideration. Features favoring hepatocellular carcinoma over hepatoblastoma include (a) large tumor cell size relative to normal hepatocytes (Fig. 21), (b) lack of hematopoiesis, (c) lack of a mesenchymal component, and (d) presence of bile in tumors cells (154). In poorly differentiated tumors, primary or metastatic sarcoma may also become a major issue. With a resection specimen, extensive sampling will usually yield areas of diagnostic tumor. However, when faced with a needle or fine-needle aspirate biopsy, accurate distinction of hepatocellular carcinoma from a benign adenoma or focal nodular hyperplasia, on the one hand, and from hepatoblastoma or sarcoma, on the other, may be problematic. Features that aid in distinguishing well-differentiated hepatocellular carcinoma from benign tumors include high nuclear/cytoplasmic ratio, atypical naked hepatocytic nuclei, and the hepatocellular carcinomalike trabecular growth pattern (56,280). With poorly differentiated tumors immunohistochemical staining (see above) and ultrastructural examination may help.

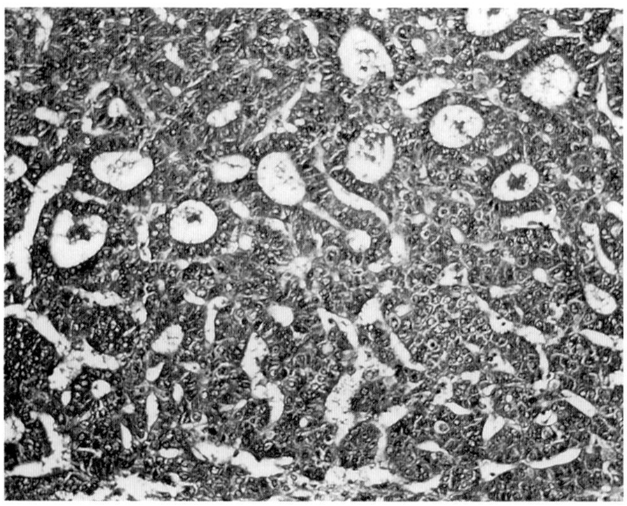

FIG. 22. The cells of this poorly differentiated hepatocellular carcinoma are arranged in a mixed trabecular and acinar pattern.

TABLE 12. *Hepatocellular carcinoma in adults: tumor suppressor gene and oncogene function*

	Ref.
Tumor suppressor genes:	
p53 point mutations	109, 233, 278, 343
17p (*p53* locus) allele loss	76
13q (*RB* locus) LOH	377
Oncogene overexpression:	
c-myc	9, 278
c-fos	9
c-met	323
cyclin D1	235
k-ras	319, 326
n-ras	325
Growth factor overexpression:	
Transforming growth factor α	286, 325
Insulin-like growth factor II	325

Abbreviations: RB, retinoblastoma; LOH, loss of heterozygosity.

Cure of hepatocellular carcinoma currently depends on surgical resectability. Unfortunately, at best approximately one third of cases are resectable, and another one third are amenable to hepatectomy and transplantation (90,189,234,356). Survival rates of 17–29% with a multimodality approach (177,327) show limited improvement over prior reported mortality rates of 90% (189,234) and compare unfavorably with similarly treated hepatoblastoma survival rates of 63–67% (177,327).

Fibrolamellar Variant of Hepatocellular Carcinoma

Clinical Features

Accounting for <10% of all hepatocellular carcinoma (57,80,248) but 30% of hepatocellular carcinoma in patients <20 years of age (90,110,126,189,196,248, 287,356), fibrolamellar carcinoma occurs almost exclusively in adolescents and young adults without sex preference and without underlying cirrhosis, fibrosis, viral infection, or metabolic abnormality (23,24,58,90,305). It also presents as an abdominal mass, often with associated acute or chronic pain but with infrequent jaundice and minimal elevations of liver enzymes or AFP. A specific abnormality of vitamin B_{12}–binding protein has been described in fibrolamellar carcinoma, with elevated levels of the unsaturated binding protein serving as a tumor marker (248,364).

Pathologic Features

The fibrolamellar variant occurs most commonly as a single well-circumscribed mass with a predilection for the left lobe (24,58,90). On cut surface examination, fibrolamellar carcinoma is firm with radiating septae that may grossly mimic the appearance of focal nodular hyperplasia (Fig. 23). The tumors are tan–white or brown with only focal bile staining; hemorrhage and necrosis are infrequently present. Capsular and vascular invasion, common features of the usual hepatocellular carcinoma, are also infrequent in fibrolamellar carcinoma.

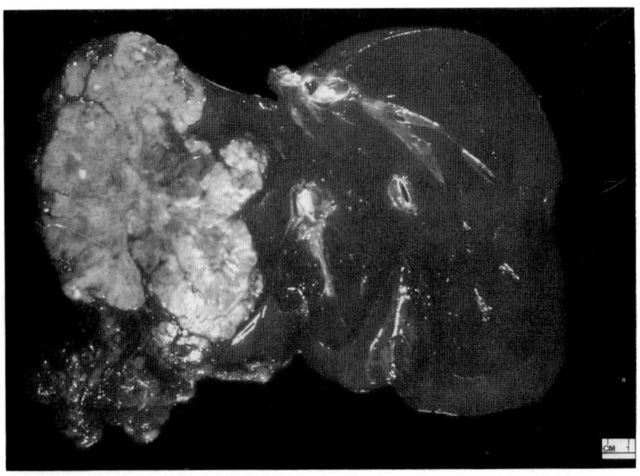

FIG. 23. The sclerotic appearance of this liver tumor is characteristic of the fibrolamellar carcinoma. The irregular margins are unusual, however, for this usually well-circumscribed tumor.

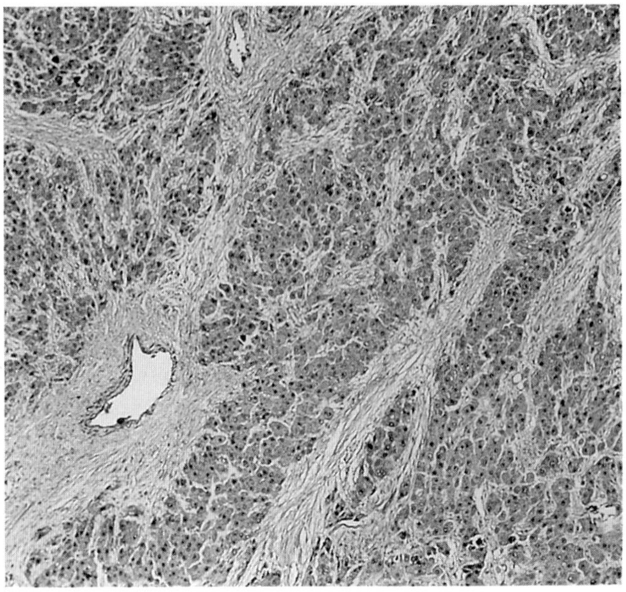

FIG. 24. Cords of well-differentiated hepatocytes separated by dense fibrous tissue characterize the histology of the fibrolamellar carcinoma.

The distinctive histopathology of fibrolamellar carcinoma comprises parallel hyalinized bands of paucicellular collagen separating nests and columns of neoplastic hepatocytes that contain abundant deeply eosinophilic cytoplasm (Figs. 24 and 25). Electron microscopic examination demonstrates abundant mitochondria within the tumor cells, resulting in their "oncocytic" appearance (58,89). Although the fibrolamellar pattern of tumor growth defines this hepatocellular carcinoma variant, these neoplasms may include foci of more conventional hepatocellular carcinoma (24,57,58). The adjacent liver may show features of focal nodular hyperplasia, perhaps as a reaction to the tumor (see also the discussion of focal nodular hyperplasia) (23,24,282).

Immunohistochemical Features

The hepatocytes in fibrolamellar carcinoma show an aberrant cytokeratin phenotype similar to that of usual hepatocellular carcinoma (339), but differing in that fewer cells stain with AFP (23). In fibrolamellar carcinoma, the hepatocytes characteristically stain for copper and copper-binding proteins (23), whereas usual hepatocellular carcinoma less frequently demonstrates copper positivity (124).

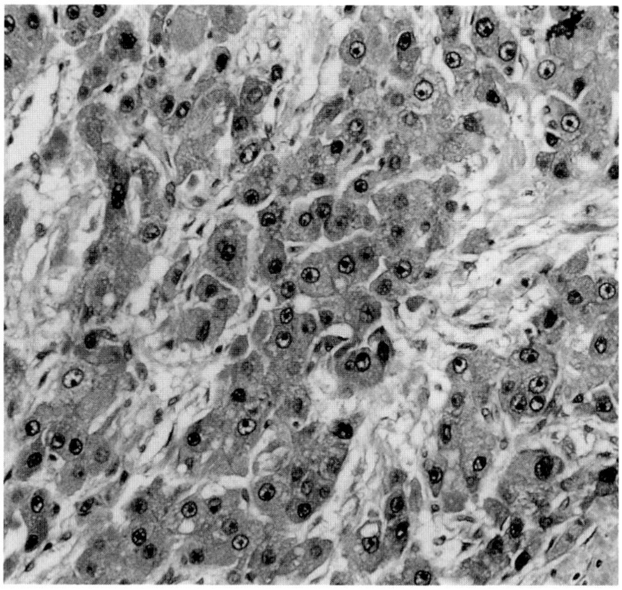

FIG. 25. Fibrolamellar carcinoma. At higher magnification, the abundant granular oncocytic cytoplasm of the fibrolamellar carcinoma cells can be appreciated.

Diagnostic and Prognostic Considerations

The distinctive histologic features make diagnosis of resected fibrolamellar carcinoma cases straightforward. The large oncocytic cells and associated stromal features may yield characteristic features with needle biopsy or aspiration material (62). However, a significant risk for sampling error exists, given the radiologic overlap of the neoplasm with focal nodular hyperplasia (131) and the known propensity for fibrolamellar carcinoma to be associated with focal nodular hyperplasialike changes in the adjacent liver (23,24,282).

Due to its comparatively indolent course, fibrolamellar carcinoma carries a reputation for having a better prognosis than the usual hepatocellular carcinoma. This indolent nature manifests itself in several ways (see Table 13). The better prognosis enjoyed by fibrolamellar carcinoma patients depends, however, on stage; with unresectable or metastatic disease, the outcome for fibrolamellar carcinoma does not differ significantly from that of usual hepatocellular carcinoma (126).

TABLE 13. *Fibrolamellar vs. usual hepatocellular carcinoma (%)*

	FLC	HCC	Ref.
5-yr survival	62	30	24
1.5- to 8-yr-survival	50	0	90
Multifocal disease	20	64	90
Advanced disease at diagnosis	10–50	60–70	90, 122
Surgically resectable	60	10	90, 189

Abbreviations: FLC, fibrolamellar carcinoma; HCC, hepatocellular carcinoma.

Undifferentiated (Embryonal) Sarcoma of Liver

Clinical Features

Undifferentiated (embryonal) sarcoma, also called malignant mesenchymoma, accounts for 5–10% of all liver tumors (39,67,356). Although cases have been reported in infancy and adults, the peak incidence based on three series of more than ten cases seems to be in the second half of the first decade without sex predilection (192,250,316). Children commonly present with abdominal pain or mass that may progress to an acute abdomen after tumor rupture (148,316). Jaundice is rare and serum AFP levels normal. The tumor's propensity to invade the hepatic vein with extension into the inferior vena cava and right atrium (8,192) may result in presentation as an intracardiac mass (101). Among the >100 cases reported, only occasional hints of predisposing factors or associated anomalies have been noted (Table 14).

Gross Pathology

A single mass is present on the right in 75% of cases and involving both liver lobes in an additional 15%. It usually appears well circumscribed (8,192,197,316) and in up to one fourth of cases is pedunculated (192). These usually large (>10 cm, >1,000 g) tumors not infrequently invade locally into the diaphragm or omentum (148,171,192,197,219,314,316,350). The cut surfaces appear tan-white with a gelatinous appearance and often central cyst formation, mimicking the benign mesenchymal hamartoma except for extensive areas of hemorrhage and necrosis (192,316,350) (Fig. 26). The cystic component may dominate the radiologic picture, resulting in its misinterpretation as infectious (334).

Microscopic Pathology

The undifferentiated (embryonal) sarcoma is primarily composed of undifferentiated spindled cells with hyperchromatic coarsely granular nuclei and poorly defined cytoplasmic processes that lie within a myxoid stroma. The variable numbers of larger pleomorphic and even multinucleated cells and abundant often atypical

TABLE 14. *Undifferentiated (embryonal) sarcoma: associated conditions and anomalies*

Condition	Ref.
Li–Fraumeni syndrome	192
Phenytoin embryopathy	27
Benign hemangioma	250
Ovarian teratoma	250
Bifid ribs	250

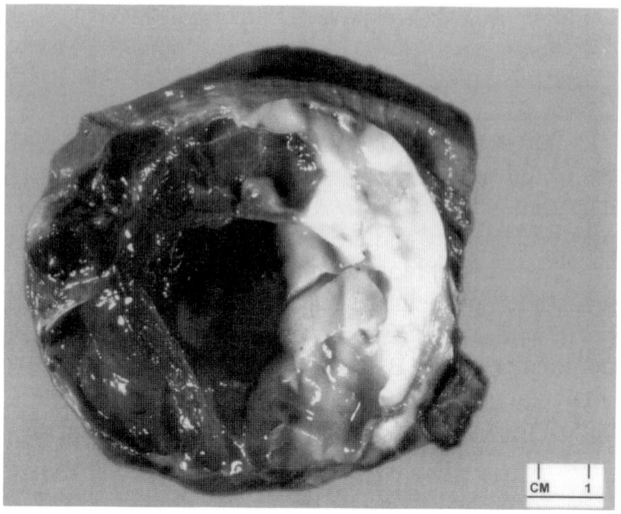

FIG. 26. The mixed cystic and solid appearance of this undifferentiated (embryonal) sarcoma mimics the gross appearance of a mesenchymal hamartoma.

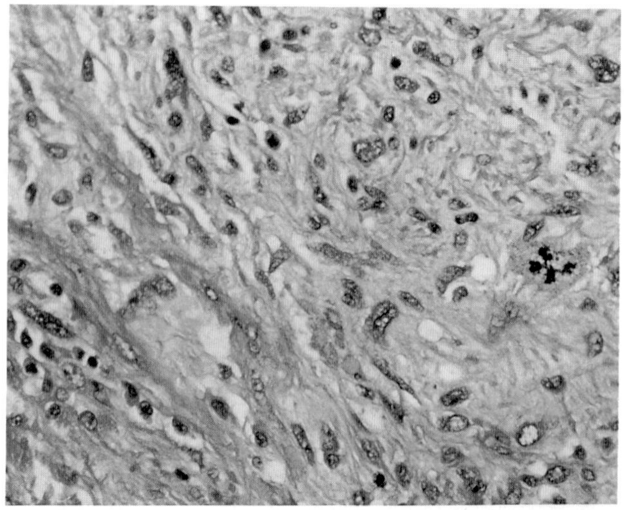

FIG. 27. Microscopic examination of the stromal cells in undifferentiated (embryonal) sarcoma reveals markedly pleomorphic nuclei with numerous and atypical mitotic figures, distinguishing this tumor from the mesenchymal hamartoma.

mitoses clearly define the tumor as malignant (Fig. 27). Focally, a more compact spindle cell component may grow as fascicles (250) or in a storiform pattern (8,192). The tumor border may be demarcated by a thin fibrous band. Entrapped hepatocytes and often cystically dilated bile ducts characteristically occur in this fibrous rim as well as intermingled with the tumor (8,192,316) (Fig. 28). The benign-appearing bile ducts, though largely limited to the periphery, occasionally occur more diffusely throughout the tumor (350) and have at least twice been identified within tumor infiltrating outside the liver (101,316). Periductal tumor condensation to form the cambium layer characteristic of botryoid rhabdomyosarcoma has been described in these areas only rarely (8), and some would argue that this pattern should change the diagnosis to rhabdomyosarcoma (148). PAS-positive, diastase-resistant hyaline globules frequent the tumor cells as well as the intervening stroma (8,250,350). Venous invasion is common but carries uncertain prognostic significance. The stroma contains nests of hematopoietic cells in approximately one half of cases (192).

Immunocytochemical Features

Immunohistochemical studies have yielded a variety of results (Table 15). The α_1-antitrypsin staining is largely cytoplasmic with only some of the PAS-positive globules marking. The divergent positive staining for histiocytic (α_1-antitrypsin, α_1-antichymotrypsin), muscle

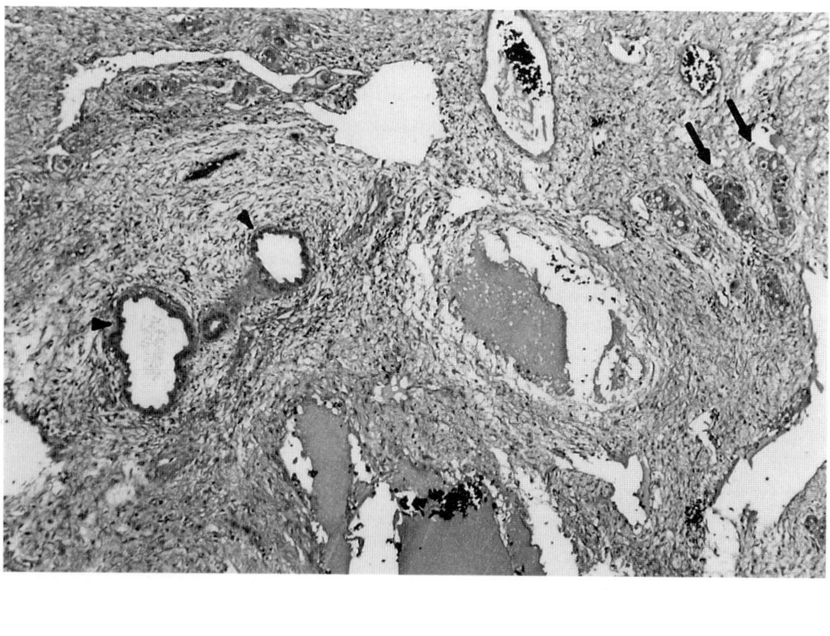

FIG. 28. The large irregular cystic spaces in this undifferentiated (embryonal) sarcoma are degenerative in nature without distinct lining cells. Smaller cysts lined by benign bile duct epithelial are seen at the left *(arrowheads)*; small islands of residual hepatocytes are present on the right *(arrows)*.

TABLE 15. *Undifferentiation (embryonal) sarcoma: immunocytochemical staining*

Antibody	Ref.[a]			
	250	192	8	197
α_1-Antitrypsin	8/12	8/8	5/6	2/8
α_1-Antichymotrypsin	10/12	ND	6/6	0/6
α-Fetoprotein	0/12	0/5	0/3	0/6
Vimentin	10/12	8/11	6/6	8/8
Desmin	6/12	1/8	4/6	5/8
Muscle-specific actin	5/12	0/6	3/6	0/6
Cytokeratin	4/12	3/11	0/5	5/8
Myoglobin	0/12	ND	ND	0/7
S-100 protein	0/11	0/10	3/6	0/6

[a] Results reported here as number positive/total stained.
Abbreviations: ND, not done.

TABLE 16. *Undifferentiated (embryonal) sarcoma: electron microscopic features*

Feature	Ref.
Cytoplasmic microvillus processes	8
Large electron-dense lysosomal bodies	171, 192, 219, 250
Myofibroblastic features	8, 250, 350
Cytoplasmic filaments, NOS	171, 192, 250, 315
With leiomyomatous features	8, 116
Rhabdomyoblastic features	8, 101
Tonofilamentous bundles	219
Abundant cytoplasmic lipid	52, 101, 250
Cell junctions	219, 250
Basal lamina	8, 116, 219, 250

Abbreviations: NOS, not otherwise specified.

(desmin and muscle-specific actin), and epithelial (cytokeratin) markers suggests that this undifferentiated tumor arises from a very primitive precursor cell.

Electron Microscopic Features

Ultrastructural studies also reveal divergent differentiation features, as noted in Table 16, similar to what might be anticipated from light microscopy and immunocytochemical features.

Diagnosis and Prognostic Features

Differential diagnostic considerations revolve predominantly around mesenchymal hamartoma and rhabdomyosarcoma. Although grossly mesenchymal hamartoma and undifferentiated (embryonal) sarcoma may resemble each other, the blatant malignant changes in the stromal cells of undifferentiated (embryonal) sarcoma usually readily exclude a benign diagnosis or microscopic exam. A recent report of undifferentiated (embryonal) sarcoma arising adjacent to a mesenchymal hamartoma (63) raises the possibility of a histogenetic link, which has not been further substantiated to date.

Distinguishing undifferentiated (embryonal) sarcoma from hepatic rhabdomyosarcoma can be much more difficult, with the histopathologic differential hinging on the light microscopic finding of convincing rhabdomyoblasts (148,250). The clinical features of the usual undifferentiated (embryonal) sarcoma and hepatic rhabdomyosarcoma differ significantly (Table 17), supporting the concept of two distinct clinicopathologic diseases. However, histologic evidence of rhabdoblastic differentiation does not clearly discriminate between these two groups. Overlap cases include intrahepatic tumors with rhabdomyoblastic differentiation without involvement of the biliary tract (148) and common bile duct tumors without rhabdomyoblastic differentiation (116). To add further confusion, Dehner describes a single case of anaplastic hepatoblastoma demonstrating extensive rhabdomyoblastic differentiation after treatment (68). The histologic overlap between these two clinicopathologic entities suggests the need for further tumor biology studies to better define these diseases.

Although historically this highly malignant tumor carries an 80% mortality rate (316), it is responsive to chemotherapy (134) and shows improved survival using a multimodality approach (232,338). Needle biopsy findings have been reported once (255); this mode of diagnosis will undoubtedly become more common in the future. The scanty flow cytometry studies to date show aneuploidy in some cases, with a uniformly high proliferation index (47,197).

Other Malignant Mesenchymal Tumors

Angiosarcoma

Hepatic angiosarcoma, an uncommon tumor in adults, is even rarer in childhood, with less than 30 ac-

TABLE 17. *UES vs. RMS: clinical comparison*

Feature	UES	RMS
Age	6–10 yr	<5 yr
Presenting symptoms	Abd. pain, mass	Jaundice
Site of involvement	Right lobe	Common bile duct, porta hepatis

Abbreviations: UES, undifferentiated (embryonal) sarcoma; RMS, rhabdomyosarcoma; Abd., abdominal.

ceptable reported cases (4,88,180,236,292,320,356). Comparing the reported cases in childhood with an adult series (54) reveals some significant differences:

1. In adults, there is a striking 3:1 male predominance; in children, the M/F ratio is closer to equal.
2. In adults, approximately 40% of cases are secondary to known environmental toxins including Thoratrast, arsenic, and vinyl chloride; in children, only one case with arsenic exposure is documented (88).
3. In adults, there is no evidence for a preexisting benign vascular malformation; in children, multiple examples demonstrate a relationship between benign infantile hemangioendothelioma and angiosarcoma.

Two reports document regression of an infantile hemangioendothelioma followed by frankly malignant progression (180,320). One case with initial histologic features of type 2 hemangioendothelioma followed a rapidly progressive clinical course with concomitant histologic progression to a more mitotically active and cytologically atypical tumor (236).

Two major patterns of malignant tumor growth allow the diagnosis of angiosarcoma (88,292). In the first, dilated sinusoidal spaces lined by one or more layers of pleomorphic atypical endothelial cells envelop trabeculae containing entrapped hepatocytes or fibrous tissue. More solid nodules composed of mitotically active large pleomorphic spindle cells occur as fascicles or distinct whorls surrounding a central fibrotic region that often contains an artery (292). PAS-positive, diastase-resistant, intracytoplasmic and extracellular globules are commonly present and stain variably positive for α_1-antitrypsin and α_1-antichymotrypsin and negative for AFP (292). Most tumors also include areas with features of infantile hemangioendothelioma or cavernous hemangioma. Fibrous septa containing residual bile ducts often transect the tumor. Immunohistochemical and lectin staining for endothelial markers (factor VIII–related antigen, *Ulex europaeus*) is variably positive in the tumor cells (292).

Rhabdomyosarcoma

Rhabdomyosarcomas of the liver account for <1% of all rhabdomyosarcomas (276). The mean age of 3–4 years and equal sex distribution (191,276) are similar to the demographics of embryonal rhabdomyosarcoma elsewhere in the body. Two types of hepatic rhabdomyosarcoma have been described. In the more common form, tumor arises within the extrahepatic biliary tree with secondary infiltration of the liver. This involvement of the biliary tree results in obstructive jaundice, the usual presenting symptom (191,210,276). The growth of rhabdomyosarcoma into the lumen of the biliary tree results in a botryoid growth pattern similar to intraluminal rhabdomyosarcomatous growth elsewhere in the body. The histologic features also closely resemble embryonal rhabdomyosarcoma at other sites.

The second type arises as a primary intrahepatic tumor, similar in location and appearance to the undifferentiated (embryonal) sarcoma (148). The histologic distinction between undifferentiated (embryonal) sarcoma and this intrahepatic form of rhabdomyosarcoma hinges on the finding of convincing light microscopic features of rhabdomyoblasts or a cambium layer in association with a bile duct (148). Given the immunocytochemical and ultrastructural evidence for rhabdomyoblastic differentiation in some tumors otherwise classified as undifferentiated (embryonal) sarcoma (see previous section), it can be questioned as to whether these two tumors may in fact represent two points on the spectrum of a single entity (250). Molecular biologic studies, as yet undone, might help to elucidate this relationship.

Rhabdoid Tumor

Although the rhabdoid tumor is best characterized in the kidney, tumors with identical histologic features occur in multiple other sites, including soft tissue, brain, and liver (115,152,251,252,306). The histologic features of this tumor in the liver are similar to those elsewhere and will not be further detailed here. It is important to remember, however, that many tumors can show foci with the rhabdoid phenotype, with the diagnosis of rhabdoid tumor being one of exclusion. A propos of this observation, one liver tumor originally diagnosed as rhabdoid tumor was recategorized as hepatocellular carcinoma on review (252).

GERM CELL TUMORS

Germ cell tumors primary in the liver occur rarely in one of three forms: teratoma, yolk sac tumor, or choriocarcinoma. Hepatic teratoma, the most common of the three, is nonetheless rare, accounting for <1% of all teratomas (330) and <1% of all liver tumors (67) in childhood. Of the fewer than 20 examples reported in the literature, 80% occurred in infants under 1 year of age; 30% were documented in utero or in the newborn (77,184,264,331,367,368). As with teratomas at other sites, there is a 3:1 female predominance. A unique case of a fetus-in-fetu present in the right lobe of the liver was differentiated from a teratoma by virtue of a vertebral axis and limb buds (2). The best-documented teratomas may include immature as well as mature elements but behave in a benign fashion without documented metastases (368). The one case reported as a malignant teratoma (222) probably in fact represented a teratoid hepatoblastoma (51,206). To qualify as a hepatic teratoma, a tumor should fulfill criteria similar to those laid out for kidney tumors (20), i.e., (a) the tumor unequivocally arises from the liver, without teratomas at remote sites as possible source of metastases, and (b) the tumor unequivocally attempts heterotopic organogenesis, as distinct from exhibiting divergent differentiation without organoid formation.

Since the first report in 1975 (135), only a handful of cases of yolk sac tumor arising in the liver have been reported (55,324,347,365). Diagnosis of most of the more recent cases solely by biopsy raises a question of accuracy, given the histologic overlap between yolk sac tumor and hepatoblastoma.

Hepatic choriocarcinoma occurs rarely, usually as a metastasis from occult placental choriocarcinoma (176). Primary hepatic choriocarcinoma occurs even more rarely (139,145,176). Distinguishing choriocarcinoma from hCG-producing hepatoblastoma hinges on finding the typical syncytio- and cytotrophoblastic cells without features typical of the latter tumor.

To further muddy the water, classic teratoma or endodermal sinus tumor occasionally arises juxtaposed to classic hepatoblastoma (50,59). This not only raises nosologic issues but also poses intriguing questions as to the histogenesis of these germ cell neoplasms.

REFERENCES

1. Abenoza P, Manivel JC, Wick MR, Hagen K, Dehner LP. Hepatoblastoma: an immunohistochemical and ultrastructural study. *Hum Pathol* 1987;18:1025–1035.
2. al-Baghdadi R. Fetus in fetu in the liver: case report and review of the literature. *J Pediatr Surg* 1992;27:1491–1492.
3. Alshak NS, Cocjin J, Podesta L, et al. Hepatocellular adenoma in glycogen storage disease type IV. *Arch Pathol Lab Med* 1994;118: 88–91.
4. Alt B, Hafez GR, Trigg M, Shahidi NT, Gilbert EF. Angiosarcoma of the liver and spleen in an infant. *Pediatr Pathol* 1985;4: 331–339.
5. Annerén G, Nordlinder H, Hedborg F. Chromosome aberrations in an alpha-fetoprotein-producing hepatoblastoma. *Genes Chrom Cancer* 1992;4:99–100.
6. Anthony PP. Inflammatory pseudotumour (plasma cell granuloma) of lung, liver and other organs. *Histopathology* 1993;23: 501–503.
7. Anthony PP, Telesinghe PU. Inflammatory pseudotumour of the liver. *J Clin Pathol* 1986;39:761–768.
8. Aoyama C, Hachitanda Y, Sato JK, Said JW, Shimada H. Undifferentiated (embryonal) sarcoma of the liver. A tumor of uncertain histogenesis showing divergent differentiation. *Am J Surg Pathol* 1991;15:615–624.
9. Arbuthnot P, Kew M, Fitschen W. c-fos and c-myc oncoprotein expression in human hepatocellular carcinomas. *Anticancer Res* 1991;11:921–924.
10. Arico M, Caselli D, D'Argenio P, et al. Malignancies in children with human immunodeficiency virus type 1 infection. The Italian Multicenter Study on Human Immunodeficiency Virus Infection in Children. *Cancer* 1991;68:2473–2477.
11. Arii S, Tanaka J, Yamazoe Y, et al. Predictive factors for intrahepatic recurrence of hepatocellular carcinoma after partial hepatectomy. *Cancer* 1992;69:913–919.
12. Békássy AN, Garwicz S, Wiebe T, Hagerstrand I, Jensen OA. Hepatocellular carcinoma associated with arteriohepatic dysplasia in a 4-year-old girl. *Med Pediatr Oncol* 1992;20:78–83.
13. Balázs M, Dénes J, Lukács VF. Fine structure of multiple neonatal haemangioendothelioma of the liver. *Virchows Arch A Histopathol* 1978;379:157–168.
14. Bardi G, Johansson B, Pandis N, et al. i(8q) as the primary structural chromosome abnormality in hepatoblastoma. *Cancer Genet Cytogenet* 1991;51:281–283.
15. Bardi G, Johansson B, Pandis N, et al. Cytogenetic findings in three primary hepatocellular carcinomas. *Cancer Genet Cytogenet* 1992;58:191–195.
16. Bardi G, Johansson B, Pandis N, et al. Trisomy 2 as the sole chromosomal abnormality in a hepatoblastoma. *Genes Chrom Cancer* 1992;4:78–80.
17. Beasley RP, Shiao I-S, Wu T-C, Hwang L-Y. Hepatoma in a HBsAg carrier—seven years after perinatal infection. *J Pediatr* 1982;101:83–84.
18. Becker JM, Heitler MS. Hepatic hemangioendotheliomas in infancy. *Surg Gynecol Obstet* 1989;168:189–200.
19. Becker JM, Heitler MS. Hepatic hemangioendotheliomas in infancy. *Surg Gynecol Obstet* 1989;168:189–200.
20. Beckwith JB. Wilms' tumor and other renal tumors of childhood: a selective review from the National Wilms' Tumor Study Pathology Center. *Hum Pathol* 1983;14:481–492.
21. Benjamin E, Lendon M, Marsden HB. Hepatoblastoma as a cause of intrauterine fetal death. Case report. *Br J Obstet Gynecol* 1981;88:329–332.
22. Benson PF, Vuilamy DG, Taubman JO. Congenital hemihypertrophy and malignancy. *Lancet* 1963;1:468.
23. Berman MA, Burnham JA, Sheahan DG. Fibrolamellar carcinoma of the liver: an immunohistochemical study of nineteen cases and a review of the literature. *Hum Pathol* 1988;19:784–794.
24. Berman MM, Libbey NP, Foster JH. Hepatocellular carcinoma. Polygonal cell type with fibrous stroma—an atypical variant with a favorable prognosis. *Cancer* 1980;46:1448–1455.
25. Beuers U, Richter WO, Ritter MM, Wiebecke B, Schwandt P. Klinefelter's syndrome and liver adenoma. *J Clin Gastroenterol* 1991;13:214–216.
26. Bianchi L. Glycogen storage disease I and hepatocellular tumours. *Eur J Pediatr* 1993;152 Suppl 1:S63–S70.
27. Blattner WA, Henson DE, Young RC, Fraumeni JF,Jr.. Malignant mesenchymoma and birth defects. Prenatal exposure to phenytoin. *JAMA* 1977;238:334–335.
28. Boutron MC, Faivre J, Milan C, Bedenne L, Hillon P, Klepping C. Primary liver cancer in Cote d'Or (France). *Int J Epidemiol* 1988;17:21–26.
29. Broughan TA, Fischer WL, Tuthill RJ. Vascular invasion by hepatic inflammatory pseudotumor. A clinicopathologic study. *Cancer* 1993;71:2934–2940.
30. Buckley JD, Sather H, Ruccione K, et al. A case-control study of risk factors for hepatoblastoma: a report from the Children's Cancer Study Group. *Cancer* 31989;64:1169–1176.
31. Byrne JA, Simms LA, Little MH, Algar EM, Smith PJ. Three non-overlapping regions of chromosome arm 11p allele loss identified in infantile tumors of adrenal and liver. *Genes Chrom Cancer* 1993;8:104–111.
32. Byrne WJ, Fonkalsrud EW. Congenital solitary nonparasitic cyst of the liver: a rare cause of rapidly enlarging abdominal mass in infancy. *J Pediatr Surg* 1982;17:316–317.
33. Callea F, Bonetti M, Medicina D, Alberti D, Fabbretti G, Brisigotti M. Hepatic tumor and tumor-like lesions in childhood. *J Surg Oncol* Suppl 1993;3:170–172.
34. Cangiarella J, Greco MA, Waisman J. Hepatoblastoma. Report of a case with cytologic, histologic and ultrastructural findings. *Acta Cytol* 1994;38:455–458.
35. Carriaga MT, Henson DE. Liver, gallbladder, extrahepatic bile ducts, and pancreas. *Cancer* 1995;75:171–190.
36. Cattan D, Kalifat R, Wautier JL, Meignan S, Vesin P, Piet R. Maladie de Fanconi et cancer du foie. *Arch Fr Mal App Dig* 1974;63:41–48.
37. Caty MG, Shamberger RC. Abdominal tumors in infancy and childhood. *Pediatr Clin North Am* 1993;40:1253–1271.
38. Chandra RS, Kapur SP, Kelleher J, Luban N, Patterson K. Benign hepatocellular tumors in the young. A clinicopathologic spectrum. *Arch Pathol Lab Med* 1984;108:168–171.
39. Chandra RS, Stocker JT. The liver, gallbladder, and biliary tract.

In: Stocker JT, Dehner LP, eds. *Pediatric Pathology*. Philadelphia: JB Lippincott; 1992:703–789.
40. Chang M-H, Hsu H-C, Lee C-Y, Chen D-S, Lee C-H, Lin K-S. Fraternal hepatocellular carcinoma in young children in two families. *Cancer* 1984;53:1807–1810.
41. Chau KY, Ho JWC, Wu PC, Yuen WK. Mesenchymal hamartoma of liver in a man: comparison with cases in infants. *J Clin Pathol* 1994;47:864–866.
42. Chawla A, Kahn E, Becker J, et al. Focal nodular hyperplasia of the liver and hypercholesterolemia in a child with VACTERL syndrome. *J Pediatr Gastroenterol Nutr* 1993;17:434–437.
43. Chen KT. Inflammatory pseudotumor of the liver. *Hum Pathol* 1984;15:694–696.
44. Chen KT, Bocian JJ. Multiple hepatic adenomas. *Arch Pathol* Lab Med 1983;107:274–275.
45. Chen WJ, Lee JC, Hung WT. Primary malignant tumor of liver in infants and children in Taiwan. *J Pediatr Surg* 1988;23:457–461.
46. Chiaretti A, Zampino G, Botto L, Polidori G. Alagille syndrome and hepatocarcinoma: a case report. *Acta Paediatr* 1992;81:937.
47. Chou P, Mangkornkanok M, Gonzalez-Crussi F. Undifferentiated (embryonal) sarcoma of the liver: ultrastructure, immunohistochemistry, and DNA ploidy analysis of two cases. *Pediatr Pathol* 1990;10:549–622.
48. Christensen WN, Boitnott JK, Kuhajda FP. Immunoperoxidase staining as a diagnostic aid for hepatocellular carcinoma. *Mod Pathol* 1989;2:8–12.
49. Cohen MB, Haber MM, Holly EA, Ahn DK, Bottles K, Stoloff AC. Cytologic criteria to distinguish hepatocellular carcinoma from nonneoplastic liver. *Am J Clin Pathol* 1991;95:125–130.
50. Conrad RJ, Gribbin D, Walker NI, Ong TH. Combined cystic teratoma and hepatoblastoma of the liver: probable divergent differentiation of an uncommitted hepatic precursor cell. *Cancer* 1993;72:2910–2913.
51. Conran RM, Hitchcock CL, Waclawiw MA, Stocker JT, Ishak KG. Hepatoblastoma: the prognostic significance of histologic type. *Pediatr Pathol* 1992;12:167–183.
52. Cozzutto C, De Bernardi B, Comelli A, Soave F. Malignant mesenchymoma of the liver in children: a clinicopathologic and ultrastructural study. *Hum Pathol* 1981;12:481–485.
53. Craig JR, Peters RL, Edmondson HA. Benign mesenchymal tumors and tumor-like conditions. In: *Atlas of Tumor Pathology. Second Series, Fascicle 26. Tumors of the Liver and Intrahepatic Bile Ducts.* Washington, D.C.: Armed Forces Institute of Pathology; 1988:63–101.
54. Craig JR, Peters RL, Edmondson HA. Primary malignant mesenchymal tumors. In: *Atlas of Tumor Pathology. Second Series, Fascicle 26. Tumors of the Liver and Intrahepatic Bile Ducts.* Washington, D.C.: Armed Forces Institute of Pathology; 1988: 223–255.
55. Craig JR, Peters RL, Edmondson HA. Tumors of heterotopic tissue and uncertain origin. In: *Atlas of Tumor Pathology. Second Series, Fascicle 26. Tumors of the Liver and Intrahepatic Bile Ducts.* Washington, D.C.: Armed Forces Institute of Pathology; 1988:102–122.
56. Craig JR, Peters RL, Edmondson HA. Benign epithelial tumors and tumor-like conditions. In: *Atlas of Tumor Pathology. Second Series, Fascicle 26. Tumors of the Liver and Intrahepatic Bile Ducts.* Washington, D.C.: Armed Forces Institute of Pathology; 1988:8–62.
57. Craig JR, Peters RL, Edmondson HA. Primary malignant epithelial tumors. In: *Atlas of Tumor Pathology. Second Series, Fascicle 26. Tumors of the Liver and Intrahepatic Bile Ducts.* Washington, D.C.: Armed Forces Institute of Pathology; 1989:123–222.
58. Craig JR, Peters RL, Edmondson HA, Omata M. Fibrolamellar carcinoma of the liver: A tumor of adolescents and young adults with distinctive clinico-pathologic features. *Cancer* 1980;46:372–379.
59. Cross SS, Variend S. Combined hepatoblastoma and yolk sac tumor of the liver. *Cancer* 1992;69:1323–1326.
60. Dachman AH, Lichtenstein JE, Friedman AC, Hartman DS. Infantile hemangioendothelioma of the liver: a radiologic-pathologic-clinical correlation. *AJR* 1983;140:1091–1096.
61. Dahms BB. Hepatoma in familial cholestatic cirrhosis of childhood: its occurrence in twin brothers. *Arch Pathol Lab Med* 1979;103:30–33.
62. Davenport RD. Cytologic diagnosis of fibrolamellar carcinoma of the liver by fine-needle aspiration. *Diagn Cytopathol* 1990;6: 275–279.
63. de Chadarevian J-P, Pawel BR, Faerber EMN, Weintraub WH. Undifferentiated (embryonal) sarcoma arising in conjunction with mesenchymal hamartoma of the liver. *Mod Pathol* 1994;7: 490–493.
64. De Potter CR, Robberecht E, Laureys G, Cuvelier CA. Hepatitis B related childhood hepatocellular carcinoma. Childhood hepatic malignancies. *Cancer* 1987;60:414–418.
65. Debuire B, Paterlini P, Pontisso P, Basso G, May E. Analysis of the p53 gene in European hepatocellular carcinomas and hepatoblastomas. *Oncogene* 1993;8:2303–2306.
66. Dehner LP. Vascular tumors of the liver in infants and children. A study of 30 cases and review of the literature. *Arch Pathol Lab Med* 1971;92:101–111.
67. Dehner LP. Hepatic tumors in the pediatric age group: a distinctive clinicopathologic spectrum. *Perspect Pediatr Pathol* 1978;4: 217–268.
68. Dehner LP. Liver, gallbladder, and extrahepatic biliary tract. In: Dehner LP, ed. *Pediatric Surgical Pathology*, 2nd ed. Baltimore: Williams & Wilkins; 1987:433–523.
69. Dehner LP, Ewing SL, Sumner HW. Infantile mesenchymal hamartoma of the liver. Histologic and ultrastructural observations. *Arch Pathol* 1975;99:379–382.
70. Dehner LP, Manivel JC. Hepatoblastoma: an analysis of the relationship between morphologic subtypes and prognosis. *Am J Pediatr Hematol Oncol* 1988;10:301–307.
71. Dehner LP, Parker ME, Franciosi RA, Drake RM. Focal nodular hyperplasia and adenoma of the liver. A pediatric experience. *Am J Pediatr Hematol Oncol* 1979;1:85–93.
72. Dehner LP, Snover DC, Sharp HL, Ascher N, Nakhleh R, Day DL. Hereditary tyrosinemia type I (chronic form): pathologic findings in the liver. *Hum Pathol* 1989;20:149–158.
73. Dekmezian R, Sneige N, Popok S, Ordonez NG. Fine-needle aspiration cytology of pediatric patients with primary hepatic tumors: a comparative study of two hepatoblastomas and a liver-cell carcinoma. *Diagn Cytopathol* 1988;4:162–168.
74. DeMaioribus CA, Lally KP, Sim K, Isaacs H, Mahour GH. Mesenchymal hamartoma of the liver. A 35-year review. *Arch Surg* 1990;125:598–600.
75. Devaney K, Goodman ZD, Ishak KG. Hepatobiliary cystadenoma and cystadenocarcinoma. A light microscopic and immunohistochemical study of 70 patients. *Am J Surg Pathol* 1994;18: 1078–1091.
76. Ding SF, Jalleh RP, Dooley J, Wood CB, Habib NA. Chromosome 17 allele loss in hepatocellular carcinoma but not in synchronous liver adenoma. *Eur J Surg Oncol* 1993;19:195–197.
77. Dische MR, Gardner HA. Mixed teratoid tumors of the liver and neck in Trisomy 13. *Am J Clin Pathol* 1978;69:631–637.
78. Drachenberg CB, Papadimitriou JC, Rivero MA, Wood C. Distinctive case. Adult mesenchymal hamartoma of the liver: report of a case with light microscopic, FNA cytology, immunohistochemistry, and ultrastructural studies and review of the literature. *Mod Pathol* 1991;4:392–395.
79. Drut R, Drut RM, Toulouse JC. Hepatic hemangioendotheliomas, placental chorioangiomas, and dysmorphic kidneys in Beckwith–Wiedemann syndrome. *Pediatr Pathol* 1992;12:197–203.
80. Dunk AA, Spiliadis H, Sherlock S, et al. Hepatocellular carcinoma: clinical, aetiological and pathological features in British patients. *Int J Cancer* 1988;41:1723.
81. Ehren H, Mahour GH, Isaacs H, Jr. Benign liver tumors in infancy and childhood. Report of 48 cases. *Am J Surg* 1983;145: 325–329.
82. Eriksson S, Carlson J, Velez R. Risk of cirrhosis and primary liver cancer in alpha-1-antitrypsin deficiency. *N Engl J Med* 1986;314: 736–739.
83. Ettinger LJ, Freeman AI. Hepatoma in a child with neurofibromatosis. *Am J Dis Child* 1979;133:528–531.

84. Everson RB, Fraumeni JF,Jr. Familial glioblastoma with hepatic focal nodular hyperplasia. *Cancer* 1976;38:310–313.
85. Everson RB, Museles M, Henson DE, Grundy GW. Focal nodular hyperplasia of the liver in a child with hemihypertrophy. *J Pediatr* 1976;88:985–987.
86. Exelby PR, Filler RM, Grosfeld JL. Liver tumors in children in the particular reference to hepatoblastoma and hepatocellular carcinoma: American Academy of Pediatrics Surgical Section Survey—1974. *J Pediatr Surg* 1975;10:329–337.
87. Fajers C-M, Falkmer S, Frisell E, Pehrson M. Primary carcinoma of the liver and giant-cell hepatitis in infancy. *Acta Paediatr* 1960;49:96–110.
88. Falk H, Herbert JT, Edmonds L, Heath CW,Jr., Thomas LB, Popper H. Review of four cases of childhood hepatic angiosarcoma-elevated environmental arsenic exposure in one case. *Cancer* 1981;47:382–391.
89. Farhi DC. Ultrastructure of fibrolamellar oncocytic hepatoma. *Cancer* 1982;50:702–709.
90. Farhi DC, Shikes RH, Murari PJ, Silverberg SG. Hepatocellular carcinoma in young people. *Cancer* 1983;52:1516–1525.
91. Feldman PS, Shneidman D, Kaplan C. Ultrastructure of infantile hemangioendothelioma of the liver. *Cancer* 1978;42:521–527.
92. Fishman SJ, Mulliken JB. Hemangiomas and vascular malformations of infancy and childhood. *Pediatr Clin North Am* 1993;40:1177–1200.
93. Flejou J-F, Barge J, Menu Y, et al. Liver adenomatosis. An entity distinct from liver adenoma? *Gastroenterology* 1985;89:1132–1138.
94. Fletcher JA, Kozakewich HP, Pavelka K, et al. Consistent cytogenetic aberrations in hepatoblastoma: a common pathway of genetic alterations in embryonal liver and skeletal muscle malignancies? *Genes Chrom Cancer* 1991;3:37–43.
95. Forouhar FA, Quinn JJ, Cooke R, Foster JH. The effect of chemotherapy on hepatoblastoma. *Arch Pathol Lab Med* 1984;311:314.
96. Foster JH, Donohue TA, Berman MM. Familial liver-cell adenomas and diabetes mellitus. *N Engl J Med* 1978;299:239–241.
97. Fraumeni JF, Jr., Geiser CF, Manning MD. Wilms' tumor and congenital hemihypertrophy: report of five new cases and review of literature. *Pediatrics* 1967;40:886–899.
98. Fraumeni JF, Jr., Miller RW. Adrenocortical neoplasms with hemihypertrophy, brain tumors, and other disorders. *J Pediatr* 1967;70:129–138.
99. Fraumeni JF, Jr., Miller RW, Hill JA. Primary carcinoma of the liver in childhood: an epidemiologic study. *JNCI* 1968;40:1087–1099.
100. Galifer RB, Sultan C, Margueritte G, Barneon G. Testosterone-producing hepatoblastoma in a 3-year-old boy with precocious puberty. *J Pediatr Surg* 1985;20:713–714.
101. Gallivan MVE, Lack EE, Chun B, Ishak KG. Undifferentiated ("embryonal") sarcoma of the liver: ultrastructure of a case presenting as a primary intracardiac tumor. *Pediatr Pathol* 1983;1:291–300.
102. Gandolfi L, Leo P, Solmi L, Vitelli E, Verros G, Colecchia A. Natural history of hepatic haemangiomas: clinical and ultrasound study. *Gut* 1991;32:677–680.
103. Garber JE, Li FP, Kingston JE, et al. Hepatoblastoma and familial adenomatous polyposis. *JNCI* 1988;80:1626–1628.
104. Gauthier F, Valayer J, Thai BL, Sinico M, Kalifa C. Hepatoblastoma and hepatocarcinoma in children: analysis of a series of 29 cases. *J Pediatr Surg* 1986;21:424–429.
105. Geiser CF, Baez A, Schindler AM, Shih VE. Epithelial hepatoblastoma associated with congenital hemihypertrophy and cystathioninuria: presentation of a case. *Pediatrics* 1970;46:66–73.
106. Geiser CF, Shih VE. Cystathioninuria and its origin in children with hepatoblastoma. *J Pediatr* 1980;96:72–75.
107. George E, Niehans GA, Swanson PE, Strickler JG, Singleton TP. Overexpression of the c-erbB-2 oncogene in sarcomas and small round-cell tumors of childhood: an immunohistochemical investigation. *Arch Pathol Lab Med* 1992;116:1033–1035.
108. Gerber MA, Shieh YS, Shim KS, et al. Detection of replicative hepatitis C virus sequences in hepatocellular carcinoma. *Am J Pathol* 1992;141:1271–1277.
109. Gerbes AL, Caselmann WH. Point mutations of the P53 gene, human hepatocellular carcinoma and aflatoxins. *J Hepatol* 1993;19:312–315.
110. Giacomantonio M, Ein SH, Mancer K, Stephens CA. Thirty years of experience with pediatric primary malignant liver tumors. *J Pediatr Surg* 1984;19:523–526.
111. Giardiello FM, Offerhaus GJ, Krush AJ, et al. Risk of hepatoblastoma in familial adenomatous polyposis. *J Pediatr* 1991;119:766–768.
112. Glowacki J, Mulliken JB. Mast cells in hemangiomas and vascular malformations. *Pediatrics* 1982;70:48–51.
113. Golli M, Mathieu D, Anglade MC, Cherqui D, Vasile N, Rahmouni A. Focal nodular hyperplasia of the liver: value of color Doppler US in association with MR imaging. *Radiology* 1993;187:113–117.
114. Gonen R, Fong K, Chiasson DA. Prenatal sonographic diagnosis of hepatic hemangioendothelioma with secondary nonimmune hydrops fetalis. *Obstet Gynecol* 1989;73:485–487.
115. Gonzalez-Crussi F. Infantile sarcoma with intracytoplasmic filamentous inclusions. Distinctive tumor of possible histiocytic origin. *Cancer* 1982;49:2365–2375.
116. Gonzalez-Crussi F. Undifferentiated (embryonal) liver sarcoma of childhood: evidence of leiomyoblastic differentiation. *Pediatr Pathol* 1983;1:281–290.
117. Gonzalez-Crussi F. Undifferentiated small cell ("anaplastic") hepatoblastoma. *Pediatr Pathol* 1991;11:155–161.
118. Gonzalez-Crussi F, Reyes Mugica M. Cellular hemangiomas ("hemangioendotheliomas") in infants. Light microscopic, immunohistochemical, and ultrastructural observations. *Am J Surg Pathol* 1991;15:769–778.
119. Gonzalez-Crussi F, Upton MP, Maurer HS. Hepatoblastoma. Attempt at characterization of histologic subtypes. *Am J Surg Pathol* 1982;6:599–612.
120. Gough J, Chakrabarti S. Inflammatory pseudotumor of the liver in a patient with chronic sclerosing cholangitis. *Am J Gastroenterol* 1993;88:1452–1453.
121. Gramlich T L., Killough BW, Garvin AJ. Mesenchymal hamartoma of the liver: report of a case in a 28-year-old. *Hum Pathol* 1988;19:991–992.
122. Greenberg M, Miller RM. Hepatic tumors. In: Pizzo PA, Pooplack DG, eds. *Principles and Practice of Pediatric Oncology.* 2nd ed. Philadelphia: JB Lippincott; 1993:697–711.
123. Groden J, Thliveris A, Samowitz W, et al. Identification and characterization of the familial adenomatous polyposis coli gene. *Cell* 1991;66:589–600.
124. Guigui B, Mavier P, Lescs M-C, Pinaudeau Y, Dhumeaux D, Zafrani ES. Copper and copper-binding protein in liver tumors. *Cancer* 1988;61:1155–1158.
125. Gururangan S, O'Meara A, MacMahon C, et al. Primary hepatic tumours in children: a 26-year review. *J Surg Oncol* 1992;50:30–36.
126. Haas JE, Muczynski KA, Krailo M, et al. Histopathology and prognosis in childhood hepatoblastoma and hepatocarcinoma. *Cancer* 1989;64:1082–1095.
127. Haas OA, Zoubek A, Grumayer ER, Gadner H. Constitutional interstitial deletion of 11p11 and pericentric inversion of chromosome 9 in a patient with Wiedemann–Beckwith syndrome and hepatoblastoma. *Cancer Genet Cytogenet* 1986;23:95–104.
128. Haith EE, Kepes JJ, Holder TM. Inflammatory pseudotumor involving the common bile duct of a six-year-old boy: successful pancreatico-duodenectomy. *Surgery* 1964;56:436–441.
129. Hajdu SI, D'Ambrosio FG, Fields V, Lightdale CJ. Aspiration and brush cytology of the liver. *Semin Diagn Pathol* 1986;3:227–238.
130. Hall PA, Lane DP. p53 in tumour pathology: can we trust immunohistochemistry? Revisited. *J Pathol* 1994;172:1–4.
131. Hamrick-Turner JE, Shipkey FH, Cranston PE. Fibrolamellar hepatocellular carcinoma: MR appearance mimicking focal nodular hyperplasia. *J Comput Assist Tomogr* 1994;18:301–304.
132. Hansen K, Bagtas J, Mark HF, Homans A, Singer DB. Undifferentiated small cell hepatoblastoma with a unique chromosomal translocation: a case report. *Pediatr Pathol* 1992;12:457–462.
133. Harms D, Schmidt D, Leuschner I. Abdominal, retroperitoneal

and sacrococcygeal tumours of the newborn and the very young infant. Report from the Kiel Paediatric Tumour Registry. *Eur J Pediatr* 1989;148:720–728.

134. Harris MB, Shen S, Weiner MA, et al. Treatment of primary undifferentiated sarcoma of the liver with surgery and chemotherapy. *Cancer* 1984;54:2859–2862.
135. Hart WR. Primary endodermal sinus (yolk sac) tumor of the liver. First reported case. *Cancer* 1975;35:1453–1458.
136. Hashizume K, Nakajo T, Kawarasaki H, et al. Prader–Willi syndrome with del(15)(q11,q13) associated with hepatoblastoma. *Acta Paediatr Jpn* 1991;33:718–722.
137. Hata Y, Ishizu H, Ohmori K, et al. Flow cytometric analysis of the nuclear DNA content of hepatoblastoma. *Cancer* 1991;68: 2566–2570.
138. Hata Y, Sasaki F, Matuoka S, et al. Inflammatory pseudotumor of the liver in children: report of cases and review of the literature. *J Pediatr Surg* 1992;27:1549–1552.
139. Heaton GE, Matthews TH, Christopherson WM. Malignant trophoblastic tumors with massive hemorrhage presenting as liver primary. A report of two cases. *Am J Surg Pathol* 1986;10:342–347.
140. Heaton ND, Pain J, Cowan NC, Salisbury J, Howard ER. Focal nodular hyperplasia of the liver: a link with sickle cell disease? *Arch Dis Child* 1991;66:1073–1074.
141. Helson L, Peterson RHF, Schwartz MK. Cystathionine excess in children with hepatic cancer. *Cancer Res* 1973;33:1570–1573.
142. Hertzer NR, Hawk WA, Hermann RE. Inflammatory lesions of the liver which simulate tumor: report of two cases in children. *Surgery* 1971;69:839–846.
143. Hirata GI, Matsunaga ML, Medearis AL, Dixon P, Platt LD. Ultrasonographic diagnosis of a fetal abdominal mass: a case of a mesenchymal liver hamartoma and a review of the literature. *Prenat Diagn* 1990;10:507–512.
144. Holcomb GW,III, O'Neill JA,Jr., Mahboubi S, Bishop HC. Experience with hepatic hemangioendothelioma in infancy and childhood. *J Pediatr Surg* 1988;23:661–666.
145. Hongo T, Fujii Y, Fukuoka T, et al. Long-term treatment in infantile choriocarcinoma. *Acta Paediatr Jpn* 1992;34:52–59.
146. Horie A, Kotoo Y, Hayashi I. Ultrastructural comparison of hepatoblastoma and hepatocellular carcinoma. *Cancer* 1979;44: 2184–2193.
147. Horiuchi R, Uchida T, Kojima T, Shikata T. Inflammatory pseudotumor of the liver. Clinicopathologic study and review of the literature. *Cancer* 1990;65:1583–1590.
148. Horowitz ME, Etcubanas E, Webber BL, et al. Hepatic undifferentiated (embryonal) sarcoma and rhabdomyosarcoma in children. Results of therapy. *Cancer* 1987;59:396–402.
149. Howell RR, Stevenson RE, Ben Menachem Y, Phyliky RL, Berry DH. Hepatic adenomata with type 1 glycogen storage disease. *JAMA* 1976;236:1481–1484.
150. Hsueh C, Tan XD, Gonzalez-Crussi F. Primary hepatic neuroendocrine carcinoma in a child. Morphologic, immunocytochemical, and molecular biologic studies. *Cancer* 1993;71:2660–2665.
151. Hughes LJ, Michels VV. Risk of hepatoblastoma in familial adenomatous polyposis. *Am J Med Genet* 1992;43:1023–1025.
152. Hunt SJ, Anderson WD. Malignant rhabdoid tumor of the liver. A distinct clinicopathologic entity. *Am J Clin Pathol* 1990;94: 645–648.
153. Hutton KA, Spicer RD, Arthur RJ, Batcup G. Focal nodular hyperplasia of the liver in childhood. *Eur J Pediatr Surg* 1993;3: 370–372.
154. Ishak KG, Glunz PR. Hepatoblastoma and hepatocarcinoma in infancy and childhood. Report of 47 cases. *Cancer* 1967;20:396–422.
155. Ishak KG, Rabin L. Benign tumors of the liver. *Med Clin North Am* 1975;59:995–1013.
156. Isobe H, Nishi Y, Fukutomi T, et al. Inflammatory pseudotumor of the liver associated with acute myelomonocytic leukemia. *Am J Gastroenterol* 1991;86:238–240.
157. Ito E, Sato Y, Kawauchi K, et al. Type 1a glycogen storage disease with hepatoblastoma in siblings. *Cancer* 1987;59:1776–1780.
158. Ito H, Yamasaki T, Okamoto O, Tahara E. Infantile hemangioendothelioma of the liver in patient with interstitial deletion of chromosome 6q: report of an autopsy case. *Am J Med Genet* 1989;34:325–329.
159. Iwama T, Mishima Y. Mortality in young first-degree relatives of patients with familial adenomatous polyposis. *Cancer* 1994;73: 2065–2068.
160. Iwatsuki S, Todo S, Starzl TE. Excisional therapy for benign hepatic lesions. *Surg Gynecol Obstet* 1990;171:240–246.
161. Izumi R, Shimizu K, Ii T, et al. Prognostic factors of hepatocellular carcinoma in patients undergoing hepatic resection. *Gastroenterology* 1994;106:720–727.
162. Jackson RB, Gatling RR. Inflammatory pseudotumor of the liver. *Surgery* 1991;109:329–332.
163. Janes CH, McGill DB, Ludwig J, Krom RA. Liver cell adenoma at the age of 3 years and transplantation 19 years later after development of carcinoma: a case report. *Hepatology* 1993;17:583–585.
164. Joshi VV, Kaur P, Ryan B, Saad S, Walters TR. Mucoid anaplastic hepatoblastoma. A case report. *Cancer* 1984;54:2035–2039.
165. Kakizoe S, Kojiro M, Nakashima T. Hepatocellular carcinoma with sarcomatous change. Clinicopathologic and immunohistochemical studies of 14 autopsy cases. *Cancer* 1987;59:310–316.
166. Kar S, Jaffe R, Carr BI. Mutation at codon 249 of p53 gene in a human hepatoblastoma. *Hepatology* 1993;18:566–569.
167. Kasai M, Watanabe I. Histologic classification of liver-cell carcinoma in infancy and childhood and its clinical evaluation. A study of 70 cases collected in Japan. *Cancer* 1970;25:551–563.
168. Kaufman RA. Is cystic mesenchymal hamartoma of the liver similar to infantile hemangioendothelioma and cavernous hemangioma on dynamic computed tomography? *Pediatr Radiol* 1992;22:582–583.
169. Kaufman SS, Wood RP, Shaw BW,Jr., Markin RS, Gridelli B, Vanderhoof JA. Hepatocarcinoma in a child with the Alagille syndrome. *Am J Dis Child* 1987;141:698–700.
170. Kawakatsu M, Vilgrain V, Belghiti J, Flejou J-F, Nahum H. Association of multiple liver cell adenomas with spontaneous intrahepatic portohepatic shunt. *Abdom Imag* 1994;19:438–440.
171. Keating S, Taylor GP. Undifferentiated (embryonal) sarcoma of the liver: ultrastructural and immunohistochemical similarities with malignant fibrous histiocytoma. *Hum Pathol* 1985;16:693–699.
172. Kennedy SM, Macgeogh C, Jaffe R, Spurr NK. Overexpression of the oncoprotein p53 in primary hepatic tumors of childhood does not correlate with gene mutations. *Hum Pathol* 1994;25: 438–442.
173. Kerlin P, Davis GL, McGill DB, Weiland LH, Adson MA, Sheedy PF. Hepatic adenoma and focal nodular hyperplasia: clinical, pathologic, and radiologic features. *Gastroenterology* 1983;84:994–1002.
174. Keslar PJ, Buck JL, Selby DM. From the archives of the AFIP. Infantile hemangioendothelioma of the liver revisited. *Radiographics* 1993;13:657–670.
175. Khan A, Bader JL, Hoy GR, Sinks LF. Hepatoblastoma in child with fetal alcohol syndrome. *Lancet* 1979;1403–1404.
176. Kim SN, Chi JG, Kim YW, et al. Neonatal choriocarcinoma of liver. *Pediatr Pathol* 1993;13:723–730.
177. King DR, Ortega J, Campbell J, et al. The surgical management of children with incompletely resected hepatic cancer is facilitated by intensive chemotherapy. *J Pediatr Surg* 1991;26:1074–1080.
178. Kingston JE, Herbert A, Draper GJ, Mann JR. Association between hepatoblastoma and polyposis coli. *Arch Dis Child* 1983;58:959–962.
179. Kinzler KW, Nilbert MC, Su LK, et al. Identification of FAP locus genes from chromosome 5q21. *Science* 1991;253:661–665.
180. Kirchner SG, Heller RM, Kasselberg AG, Greene HL. Infantile hepatic hemangioendothelioma with subsequent malignant degeneration. *Pediatr Radiol* 1981;11:42–45.
181. Knowles DM, Wolff M. Focal nodular hyperplasia of the liver. A clinicopathologic study and review of the literature. *Hum Pathol* 1976;7:533–545.
182. Koufos A, Grundy P, Morgan K, et al. Familial Wiedemann–Beckwith syndrome and a second Wilms tumor locus both map to 11p15.5. *Am J Hum Genet* 1989;44:711–719.
183. Koufos A, Hansen MF, Copeland NG, Jenkins NA, Lampkin

BC, Cavenee WK. Loss of heterozygosity in three embryonal tumours suggests a common pathogenetic mechanism. *Nature* 1985;316:330–334.
184. Kraudel K, Williams CH. Ultrasound case report of hepatic teratoma in newborn. *J Clin Ultrasound* 1984;12:98–101.
185. Krishna Kumar G, Al Saadi A, Yang SS, McCaughey RS. Ataxia-telangiectasia and hepatocellular carcinoma. *Am J Med Sci* 1979;278:157–160.
186. Kuo CY, Liu HC, Chang MH, et al. Hepatoblastoma in infancy and childhood: a clinical and pathological study of 32 cases. *Acta Paediatr Sin* 1991;32:79–87.
187. Lack EE. Mesenchymal hamartoma of the liver. A clinical and pathologic study of nine cases. *Am J Pediatr Hematol Oncol* 1986;8:91–98.
188. Lack EE, Neave C, Vawter GF. Hepatoblastoma. A clinical and pathologic study of 54 cases. *Am J Surg Pathol* 1982;6:693–705.
189. Lack EE, Neave C, Vawter GF. Hepatocellular carcinoma. Review of 32 cases in childhood and adolescence. *Cancer* 1983;52:1510–1515.
190. Lack EE, Ornvold K. Focal nodular hyperplasia and hepatic adenoma: a review of eight cases in the pediatric age group. *J Surg Oncol* 1986;33:129–135.
191. Lack EE, Perez Atayde AR, Schuster SR. Botryoid rhabdomyosarcoma of the biliary tract. *Am J Surg Pathol* 1981;5:643–652.
192. Lack EE, Schloo BL, Azumi N, Travis WD, Grier HE. Undifferentiated (embryonal) sarcoma of the liver. Clinical and pathologic study of 16 cases with emphasis on immunohistochemical features. *Am J Surg Pathol* 1991;15:1–16.
193. Lalonde L, Van Beers B, Trigaux JP, Delos M, Melange M, Pringot J. Focal nodular hyperplasia in association with spontaneous intrahepatic portosystemic venous shunt. *Gastrointest Radiol* 1992;17:154–156.
194. LeBrun DP, Silver MM, Freedman MH, Phillips MJ. Fibrolamellar carcinoma of the liver in a patient with Fanconi anemia. *Hum Pathol* 1991;22:396–398.
195. Lennington WJ, Gray GF,Jr., Page DL. Mesenchymal hamartoma of liver. A regional ischemic lesion of a sequestered lobe. *Am J Dis Child* 1993;147:193–196.
196. Leuschner I, Harms D, Schmidt D. The association of hepatocellular carcinoma in childhood with hepatitis B virus infection. *Cancer* 1988;62:2363–2369.
197. Leuschner I, Schmidt D, Harms D. Undifferentiated sarcoma of the liver in childhood: morphology, flow cytometry, and literature review. *Hum Pathol* 1990;21:68–76.
198. Lieberman J, Silton RM, Agliozzo CM, McMahon J. Hepatocellular carcinoma and intermediate α1-antitrypsin deficiency (MZ phenotype). *Am J Clin Pathol* 1975;64:304–310.
199. Little MH, Thomson DB, Hayward NK, Smith PJ. Loss of alleles on the short arm of chromosome 11 in a hepatoblastoma from a child with Beckwith-Wiedemann syndrome. *Hum Genet* 1988;79:186–189.
200. Liver Cancer Study Group of Japan. Primary liver cancer in Japan. Clincopathologic features and results of surgical treatment. *Ann Surg* 1990;211:277–287.
201. Lok ASF, Lai Ching-Lung. Factors determining the development of hepatocellular carcinoma in hepatitis B surface antigen carriers. A comparison between families with clusters and solitary cases. *Cancer* 1988;61:1287–1291.
202. Luks FI, Yazbeck S, Brandt ML, Bensoussan AL, Brochu P, Blanchard H. Benign liver tumors in children: a 25-year experience. *J Pediatr Surg* 1991;26:1326–1330.
203. Mahfouz AE, Hamm B, Taupitz M, Wolf KJ. Hypervascular liver lesions: differentiation of focal nodular hyperplasia from malignant tumors with dynamic gadolinium-enhanced MR imaging. *Radiology* 1993;186:133–138.
204. Mamlok V, Nichols M, Lockhart L, Mamlok R. Trisomy 18 and hepatoblastoma. *Am J Med Genet* 1989;33:125–126.
205. Manes JL, Kissane JM, Valdes AJ. Congenital hepatic fibrosis, liver cell carcinoma and adult polycystic kidneys. *Cancer* 1977;39:2619–2623.
206. Manivel C, Wick MR, Abenoza P, Dehner LP. Teratoid hepatoblastoma. The nosologic dilemma of solid embryonic neoplasms of childhood. *Cancer* 1986;2168:2174.
207. Markowitz RI, Harcke HT, Ritchie WG, Huff DS. Focal nodular hyperplasia of the liver in a child with sickle cell anemia. *AJR* 1980;134:594–597.
208. Marks F, Thomas P, Lustig I, Greco MA, Raghavendra BN, Wasserman R. In utero sonographic description of a fetal liver adenoma. *J Ultrasound Med* 1990;9:119–122.
209. Martelli C, Blandamura S, Massaro S, Zulian M, Altavilla G, Piazza M. A case study of Beckwith-Wiedemann syndrome associated with hepatoblastoma. *Clin Exp Obstet Gynecol* 1993;20:82–87.
210. Martinez FLA, Haase GM, Koep LJ, Akers DR. Rhabdomyosarcoma of the biliary tree: the case for aggressive surgery. *J Pediatr Surg* 1982;17:508–511.
211. Maruiwa M, Nakamura Y, Motomura K, et al. Cornelia de Lange syndrome associated with Wilms' tumour and infantile haemangioendothelioma of the liver: report of two autopsy cases. *Virchows Arch A Histopathol Anat* 1988;413:463–468.
212. Mascarello JT, Jones MC, Kadota RP, Krous HF. Hepatoblastoma characterized by trisomy 20 and double minutes. *Cancer Genet Cytogenet* 1990;47:243–247.
213. Mascarello JT, Krous HF. Second report of a translocation involving 19q13.4 in a mesenchymal hamartoma of the liver. *Cancer Genet Cytogenet* 1992;58:141–142.
214. Mays ET, Christopherson W. Hepatic tumors induced by sex steroids. *Semin Liver Dis* 1984;4:147–157.
215. McCaughan GW, Bilous MJ, Gallagher ND. Long-term survival with tumor regression in androgen-induced liver tumors. *Cancer* 1985;56:2622–2626.
216. McGoldrick JP, Boston VE, Glasgow JF. Hepatocellular carcinoma associated with congenital macronodular cirrhosis in a neonate. *J Pediatr Surg* 1986;21:177–179.
217. McLean RH, Moller JH, Warwick WJ, Satran L, Lucas RV, Jr. Multinodular hemangiomatosis of the liver in infancy. *Pediatrics* 1972;49:563–573.
218. Meis JM, Enzinger FM. Inflammatory fibrosarcoma of the mesentery and retroperitoneum. A tumor closely simulating inflammatory pseudotumor. *Am J Surg Pathol* 1991;15:1146–1156.
219. Miettinen M, Kahlos T. Undifferentiated (embryonal) sarcoma of the liver. Epithelial features as shown by immunohistochemical analysis and electron microscopic examination. *Cancer* 1989;64:2096–2103.
220. Miller RW, Young JL Jr, Novakovic B. Childhood cancer. *Cancer* 1995;75:395–405.
221. Misugi K, Okajima H, Misugi N, Newton WA. Classification of primary malignant tumors of liver in infancy and childhood. *Cancer* 1967;20:1760–1771.
222. Misugi K, Reiner CB. A malignant true teratoma of liver in childhood. *Arch Pathol* 1965;80:409–412.
223. Mokrohisky ST, Ambruso DR, Hathaway WE. Fulminant hepatic neoplasia after androgen therapy. *N Engl J Med* 1977;296:1411–1412.
224. Moldvay J, Schaff Z, Lapis K. Hepatocellular carcinoma in Fanconi's anemia treated with androgen and corticosteroid. *Zentralbl Pathol* 1991;137:167–170.
225. Moran CA, Mullick FG, Ishak KG. Nodular regenerative hyperplasia of the liver in children. *Am J Surg Pathol* 1991;15:449–454.
226. Morinaga S, Yamaguchi M, Watanabe I, Kasai M, Ojima M, Sasano N. An immunohistochemical study of hepatoblastoma producing human chorionic gonadotropin. *Cancer* 1983;51:1647–1652.
227. Nakagawara A, Ikeda K, Tsuneyoshi M, et al. Hepatoblastoma producing both alpha-fetoprotein and human chorionic gonadotropin. Clinicopathologic analysis of four cases and a review of the literature. *Cancer* 1985;56:1636–1642.
228. Nakajima T, Sugano I, Matsuzaki O, et al. Hepatic inflammatory lesions manifested as a pseudotumor. Report of two cases with different characteristics. *Arch Pathol Lab Med* 1993;117:157–159.
229. Nakanuma Y, Tsuneyama K, Masuda S, Tomioka T. Hepatic inflammatory pseudotumor associated with chronic cholangitis: report of three cases. *Hum Pathol* 1994;25:86–91.

230. Navarro C, Corretger JM, Sancho A, Rovira J, Morales L. Paraneoplastic precocious puberty. Report of a new case with hepatoblastoma and review of the literature. *Cancer* 1985;56:1725–1729.
231. Newbould MJ, Kelsey A, Lendon M, Gururangan S. Inflammatory pseudotumor of the liver masquerading as a metastasis in a child treated for nephroblastoma. *Med Pediatr Oncol* 1992;20:172–175.
232. Newman KD, Schisgall R, Reaman G, Guzzetta PC. Malignant mesenchymoma of the liver in children. *J Pediatr Surg* 1989;24:781-783.
233. Ng IO, Chung LP, Tsang SW, et al. p53 gene mutation spectrum in hepatocellular carcinomas in Hong Kong Chinese. *Oncogene* 1994;9:985–990.
234. Ni Y-Hn, Chang M-H, Hsu H-Y, et al. Hepatocellular carcinoma in childhood. Clinical manifestations and prognosis. *Cancer* 1991;68:1737–1741.
235. Nishida N, Fukuda Y, Komeda T, et al. Amplification and overexpression of the cyclin D1 gene in aggressive human hepatocellular carcinoma. *Cancer Res* 1994;54:3107–3110.
236. Noronha R, Gonzalez-Crussi F. Hepatic angiosarcoma in childhood. A case report and review of the literature. *Am J Surg Pathol* 1984;8:863–871.
237. Obers VJ, Phillips JI. fine-needle aspiration of pediatric abdominal masses. Cytologic and electron microscopic diagnosis. *Acta Cytol* 1991;35:165–170.
238. Oda Y, Katsuda S, Nakanishi I. An autopsy case of hepatic sarcomatoid tumor: immunohistochemical comparison with a sarcomatous component of hepatocellular carcinoma. *Pathol Int* 1994;44:230–236.
239. Ohaki Y, Misugi K, Saski Y, Tsunoda A. Hepatitis B surface antigen positive hepatocellular carcinoma in children. Report of a case and review of the literature. *Cancer* 1983;51:822–828.
240. Ohtomo K, Itai Y, Hasizume K, Kosaka N, Iio M. CT and MR appearance of focal nodular hyperplasia of the liver in children with biliary atresia. *Clin Radiol* 1991;43:88–90.
241. Okeda R. Mesenchymal hamartoma of the liver—an autopsy case with serial sections and some comments on its pathogenesis. *Acta Pathol Jpn* 1976;26:229–236.
242. Okuyama K. Primary liver cell carcinoma associated with biliary cirrhosis due to congenital bile duct atresia. First report of a case. *J Pediatr* 1965;67:89–93.
243. Orozco-Florian R, McBride JA, Favara BE, Steele A, Brown SJ, Steele P. Congenital hepatoblastoma and Beckwith–Wiedemann syndrome: a case study including DNA ploidy profiles of tumor and adrenal cytomegaly. *Pediatr Pathol* 1991;11:131–142.
244. Otal TM, Hendricks JB, Pharis P, Donnelly WH. Mesenchymal hamartoma of the liver. DNA flow cytometric analysis of eight cases. *Cancer* 1994;74:1237–1242.
245. Otten J, Smets R, de Jager R, Gerard A, Maurus R. Hepatoblastoma in an infant after contraceptive intake during pregnancy. *N Engl J Med* 1977;222.
246. Pain JA, Gimson AE, Williams R, Howard ER. Focal nodular hyperplasia of the liver: results of treatment and options in management. *Gut* 1991;32:524–527.
247. Papotti M, Pacchioni D, Negro F, Bonino F, Bussolati G. Albumin gene expression in liver tumors: diagnostic interest in fine needle aspiration biopsies. *Mod Pathol* 1994;7:271–275.
248. Paradinas FJ, Mella WM, Wilkinson MI, et al. High serum vitamin B12 binding capacity as a marker of the fibrolamellar variant of hepatocellular carinoma. *Br Med J* 1982;285:840–842.
249. Pardes JG, Bryan PJ, Gauderer MW. Spontaneous regression of infantile hemangioendotheliomatosis of the liver: demonstration by ultrasound. *J Ultrasound Med* 1982;1:349–353.
250. Parham DM, Kelly DR, Donnelly WH, Douglass EC. Immunohistochemical and ultrastructural spectrum of hepatic sarcomas of childhood: evidence for a common histogenesis. *Mod Pathol* 1991;4:648–653.
251. Parham DM, Peiper SC, Robicheaux G, Ribeiro RC, Douglass EC. Malignant rhabdoid tumor of the liver. Evidence for epithelial differentiation. *Arch Pathol Lab Med* 1988;112:61–64.
252. Parham DM, Weeks DA, Beckwith JB. The clinicopathologic spectrum of putative extrarenal rhabdoid tumors. An analysis of 42 cases studied with immunohistochemistry or electron microscopy. *Am J Surg Pathol* 1994;18:1010–1029.
253. Pettenati MJ, Haines JL, Higgins RR, Wappner RS, Palmer CG, Weaver DD. Wiedemann–Beckwith syndrome: presentation of clinical and cytogenetic data on 22 new cases and review of the literature. *Hum Genet* 1986;74:143–154.
254. Pierro A, Langevin AM, Filler RM, Liu P, Phillips MJ, Greenberg ML. Preoperative chemotherapy in "unresectable" hepatoblastoma. *J Pediatr Surg* 1989;24:24–29.
255. Pieterse AS, Smith M, Smith LA, Smith P. Embryonal (undifferentiated) sarcoma of the liver. Fine-needle aspiration cytology and ultrastructural findings. *Arch Pathol Lab Med* 1985;109:677–680.
256. Ping AJ, Reeve AE, Law DJ, Young MR, Boehnke M, Feinberg AP. Genetic linkage of Beckwith–Wiedemann syndrome to 11p15. *Am J Hum Genet* 1989;44:720–723.
257. Pizzo CJ. Type I glycogen storage disease with focal nodular hyperplasia of the liver and vasoconstrictive pulmonary hypertension. *Pediatrics* 1980;65:341–343.
258. Pokorny CS, Painter DM, Waugh RC, McCaughan GW, Gallagher ND, Tattersall MH. Inflammatory pseudotumor of the liver causing biliary obstruction. Treatment by biliary stenting with 5-year follow-up. *J Clin Gastroenterol* 1991;13:338–341.
259. Poley JR. Malignant liver disease in alpha-1-antitrypsin deficiency. *Acta Paediatr Suppl* 1994;393:27–32.
260. Pontisso P, Barzon M, Basso G, Cecchetto G, Perilongo G, Alberti A. Cytokeratins patterns in childhood primary liver tumors. *Int J Clin Lab Res* 1993;23:225–227.
261. Pontisso P, Basso G, Perilongo G, et al. Does hepatitis B virus play a role in primary liver cancer in children of Western countries? *Cancer Detect Prev* 1991;15:363–368.
262. Portmann B, Stewart S, Higenbottam TW, Clayton PT, Lloyd JK, Williams R. Nodular transformation of the liver associated with portal and pulmonary arterial hypertension. *Gastroenterology* 1993;104:616–621.
263. Rabinovitz M, Imperial JC, Schade RR, Van Thiel DH. Hepatocellular carcinoma in Alagille's syndrome: a family study. *J Pediatr Gastroenterol Nutr* 1989;8:26–30.
264. Rao PL, Venkatesh A, Murthy VS. Cystic teratoma in the bare area of liver. *Indian J Pediatr* 1987;54:275–278.
265. Reuland P, Aicher KP, Brambs HJ, et al. Incidental finding of a hepatic lesion: differential diagnostic problems for fibrolamellar hepatic carcinoma. *J Nucl Med* 1994;35:1342–1346.
266. Reynolds M, Douglass EC, Finegold M, Cantor A, Glicksman A. Chemotherapy can convert unresectable hepatoblastoma. *J Pediatr Surg* 1992;27:1080–1083.
267. Rhodes RH, Marchildon MB, Luebke DC, Edmondson HA, Mikity VG. A mixed hamartoma of the liver: light and electron microscopy. *Hum Pathol* 1978;9:211–221.
268. Riikonen P, Tuominen L, Seppa A, Perkkio M. Simultaneous hepatoblastoma in identical male twins. *Cancer* 1990;66:2429–2431.
269. Robinson HB, Bolande RP. Fetal hepatoblastoma with placental metastases. *Pediatr Pathol* 1985;4:163–167.
270. Rodriguez E, Reuter VE, Mies C, Bosl GJ, Chaganti RS. Abnormalities of 2q: a common genetic link between rhabdomyosarcoma and hepatoblastoma? *Genes Chrom Cancer* 1991;3:122–127.
271. Ruck P, Harms D, Kaiserling E. Neuroendocrine differentiation in hepatoblastoma: an immunohistochemical investigation. *Am J Surg Pathol* 1990;14:847–855.
272. Ruck P, Kaiserling E. Melanin-containing hepatoblastoma with endocrine differentiation: an immunohistochemical and ultrastructural study. *Cancer* 1993;72:361–368.
273. Ruck P, Xiao JC, Kaiserling E. P53 protein expression in hepatoblastoma: an immunohistochemical investigation. *Pediatr Pathol* 1994;14:79–85.
274. Ruschenburg I, Droese M. Fine needle aspiration cytology of focal nodular hyperplasia of the liver. *Acta Cytol* 1989;33:857–860.
275. Ruymann FB, Mosijczuk AD, Sayers RJ. Hepatoma in a child with methotrexate-induced hepatic fibrosis. *JAMA* 1977;238:2631–2633.
276. Ruymann FB, Raney RB Jr, Crist WM, Lawrence W Jr, Lindberg

RD, Soule EH. Rhabdomyosarcoma of the biliary tree in childhood. A report from the Intergroup Rhabdomyosarcoma Study. *Cancer* 1985;56:575–581.

277. Rypens F, Avni EF, Houben JJ, Struyven J. Large solitary nonparasitic cyst of the liver. *J Belge Radiol* 1993;76:24–25.
278. Saegusa M, Takano Y, Kishimoto H, Wakabayashi G, Nohga K, Okudaira M. Comparative analysis of p53 and c-myc expression and cell proliferation in human hepatocellular carcinomas—an enhanced immunohistochemical approach. *J Cancer Res Clin Oncol* 1993;119:737–744.
279. Salt A, Barnes ND, Rolles K, Calne RY, Clayton PT, Leonard JV. Liver transplantation in tyrosinaemia type 1: the dilemma of timing the operation. *Acta Paediatr* 1992;81:449–452.
280. Sangalli G, Livraghi T, Giordano F. Fine needle biopsy of hepatocellular carcinoma: improvement in diagnosis by microhistology. *Gastroenterology* 1989;96:524–526.
281. Saul SH. Masses of the liver. In: Sternberg SS, Antonioli DA, eds. *Diagnostic Surgical Pathology*. 2nd ed. New York: Raven Press; 1994:1517–1580.
282. Saul SH, Titelbaum DS, Gansler TS, et al. The fibrolamellar variant of hepatocellular carcinoma. Its association with focal nodular hyperplasia. *Cancer* 1987;60:3049–3055.
283. Sawhney S, Jain R, Safaya R, Berry M. Pedunculated focal nodular hyperplasia. *Pediatr Radiol* 1992;22:231–232.
284. Saxena R, Humphreys S, Williams R, Portmann B. Nodular hyperplasia surrounding fibrolamellar carcinoma: a zone of arterialized liver parenchyma. *Histopathology* 1994;25:275–278.
285. Saxena R, Leake JL, Shafford EA, et al. Chemotherapy effects on hepatoblastoma: A histological study. *Am J Surg Pathol* 1993;17:1266–1271.
286. Schaff Z, Hsia CC, Sarosi I, Tabor E. Overexpression of transforming growth factor-alpha in hepatocellular carcinoma and focal nodular hyperplasia from European patients. *Hum Pathol* 1994;25:644–651.
287. Schmidt D, Harms D, Lang W. Primary malignant hepatic tumours in childhood. *Virchows Arch A Histopathol Anat* 1985;407:387–405.
288. Schmidt D, Wischmeyer P, Leuschner I, et al. DNA analysis of hepatoblastoma by flow and image cytometry. *Cancer* 1993;72:2914–2919.
289. Schullinger JN, Wigger HJ, Price JB, Benson M, Harris RC. Epidermoid cysts of the liver. *J Pediatr Surg* 1983;18:240–242.
290. Schwarzenberg SJ, Grothe RM, Sharp HL, Snover DC, Freese D. Long-term complications of arteriohepatic dysplasia. *Am J Med* 1992;93:171–176.
291. Scrable H, Cavenee W, Ghavimi F, Lovell M, Morgan K, Sapienza C. A model for embryonal rhabdomyosarcoma tumorigenesis that involves genome imprinting. *Proc Natl Acad Sci USA* 1989;86:7480–7484.
292. Selby DM, Stocker JT, Ishak KG. Angiosarcoma of the liver in childhood: a clinicopathologic and follow-up study of 10 cases. *Pediatr Pathol* 1992;12:485–498.
293. Selby DM, Stocker JT, Waclawiw MA, Hitchcock CL, Ishak KG. Infantile hemangioendothelioma of the liver. *Hepatology* 1994;20:39–45.
294. Sepúlveda WH, Donetch G, Giuliano A. Prenatal sonographic diagnosis of fetal hepatic hemangioma. *Eur J Obstet Gynecol Reprod Biol* 1993;48:73–76.
295. Shapiro P, Ikeda RM, Ruebner BJ, Conners MH, Halsted CC, Abildgaard CF. Multiple hepatic tumors and peliosis hepatis in Fanconi's anemia treated with androgens. *Am J Dis Child* 1994;131:1104–1106.
296. Shek TW, Ng IO, Chan KW. Inflammatory pseudotumor of the liver. Report of four cases and review of the literature. *Am J Surg Pathol* 1993;17:231–238.
297. Sheu BC, Shyu MK, Lin YF, et al. Prenatal diagnosis and corticosteroid treatment of diffuse neonatal hemangiomatosis: case report. *J Ultrasound Med* 1994;13:495–499.
298. Shimizu S, Takayama T, Kosuge T, et al. Benign tumors of the liver resected because of a diagnosis of malignancy. *Surg Gynecol Obstet* 1992;174:403–407.
299. Simon D, Knowles BB, Weith A. Abnormalities of chromosome 1 and loss of heterozygosity on 1p in primary hepatomas. *Oncogene* 1991;6:765–770.
300. Sinniah D, Campbell PE, Colebatch JH. Proceedings: Primary hepatic cancer in childhood. *Arch Dis Child* 1974;49:496.
301. Skopec LL, Lakatua DJ. Non-immune fetal hydrops with hepatic hemangioendothelioma and Kasabach-Merritt syndrome: a case report. *Pediatr Pathol* 1989;9:87–93.
302. Smith WL, Ballantine TVN, Gonzalez-Crussi F. Hepatic mesenchymal hamartoma causing heart failure in the neonate. *J Pediatr Surg* 1978;13:183–185.
303. Sola Pérez J, Pérez Guillermo M, Bas Bernal AB, Mercader JM. Hepatoblastoma. An attempt to apply histologic classification to aspirates obtained by fine needle aspiration cytology. *Acta Cytol* 1994;38:175–182.
304. Someren A. "Inflammatory pseudotumor" of liver with occlusive phlebitis: report of a case in a child and review of the literature. *Am J Clin Pathol* 1978;69:176–181.
305. Soreide O, Czemiak A, Bradpiece H, Bloom S, Slumgart L. Characteristics of fibrolamellar hepatocellular carcinoma. A study of nine cases and a review of the literature. *Am J Surg* 1986;151:518–523.
306. Sotelo-Avila C, Gonzalez Crussi F, deMello D, et al. Renal and extrarenal rhabdoid tumors in children: a clinicopathologic study of 14 patients. *Semin Diagn Pathol* 1986;3:151–163.
307. Sotelo-Avila C, Gonzalez-Crussi F. Congenital tumours. In: Wigglesworth JS, Singer DB, eds. *Textbook of Fetal and Perinatal Pathology*. Boston: Blackwell Scientific; 1991:455–497.
308. Sotelo-Avila C, Gonzalez-Crussi F, Fowler JW. Complete and incomplete forms of Beckwith-Wiedemann syndrome: their oncogenic potential. *J Pediatr* 1980;96:47–50.
309. Sotelo-Avila C, Gonzalez-Crussi F, Starling KA. Wilms' tumor in a patient with an incomplete form of Beckwith-Wiedemann syndrome. *Pediatrics* 1980;66:121–123.
310. Sotelo-Avila C, Gooch WM, III. Neoplasms associated with the Beckwith-Wiedemann syndrome. *Perspect Pediatr Pathol* 1976;3:255–272.
311. Soukup SW, Lampkin BL. Trisomy 2 and 20 in two hepatoblastomas. *Genes Chrom Cancer* 1991;3:231–234.
312. Speleman F, De Telder V, De Potter KR, et al. Cytogenetic analysis of a mesenchymal hamartoma of the liver. *Cancer Genet Cytogenet* 1989;40:29–32.
313. Stanley P, Geer GD, Miller JH, Gilsanz V, Landing BH, Boechat IM. Infantile hepatic hemangiomas. Clinical features, radiologic investigations, and treatment of 20 patients. *Cancer* 1989;64:936–939.
314. Stanley RJ, Dehner LP, Hesker AE. Primary malignant mesenchymal tumors (mesenchymoma) of the liver in childhood. An angiographic-pathologic study of three cases. *Cancer* 1973;32:973–984.
315. Steiner M, Bostrum B, Leonard AS, Dehner LP. Undifferentiated (embryonal) sarcoma of the liver. A clinicopathologic study of a survivor treated with combined technique therapy. *Cancer* 1989;64:1318–132.
316. Stocker JT, Ishak KG. Undifferentiated (embryonal) sarcoma of the liver. Report of 31 cases. *Cancer* 1978;42:336–348.
317. Stocker JT, Ishak KG. Focal nodular hyperplasia of the liver. A study of 21 pediatric cases. *Cancer* 1981;48:336–345.
318. Stocker JT, Ishak KG. Mesenchymal hamartoma of the liver: report of 30 cases and review of the literature. *Pediatr Pathol* 1983;1:245–267.
319. Stork P, Loda M, Bosari S, Wiley B, Poppenhusen K, Wolfe H. Detection of K-ras mutations in pancreatic and hepatic neoplasms by non-isotopic mismatched polymerase chain reaction. *Oncogene* 1991;6:857–862.
320. Strate SM, Rutledge JC, Weinberg AG. Delayed development of angiosarcoma in multinodular infantile hepatic hemangioendothelioma. *Arch Pathol Lab Med* 1984;108:943–944.
321. Stromeyer FW, Ishak KG. Nodular transformation (nodular "regenerative" hyperplasia) of the liver. A clinicopathologic study of 30 cases. *Hum Pathol* 1981;12:60–71.
322. Sugarman GI, Heuser ET, Reed WB. A case of cerebral gigantism and hepatocarcinoma. *Am J Dis Child* 1977;631:633.
323. Suzuki K, Hayashi N, Yamada Y, et al. Expression of the c-met

protooncogene in human hepatocellular carcinoma. *Hepatology* 1994;20:1231–1236.
324. Szucs RA, Narla LD. Primary endodermal sinus tumor of the liver detected by CT. *Pediatr Radiol* 1992;2:449–450.
325. Tabor E. Tumor suppressor genes, growth factor genes, and oncogenes in hepatitis B virus—associated hepatocellular carcinoma. *J Med Virol* 1994;42:357–365.
326. Tada M, Omata M, Ohto M. Analysis of ras gene mutations in human hepatic malignant tumors by polymerase chain reaction and direct sequencing. *Cancer Res* 1990;50:1121–1124.
327. Tagge EP, Tagge DU, Reyes J, et al. Resection, including transplantation, for hepatoblastoma and hepatocellular carcinoma: impact on survival. *J Pediatr Surg* 1992;27:292–296.
328. Takahashi K, Mulliken JB, Kozakewich HP, Rogers RA, Folkman J, Ezekowitz RA. Cellular markers that distinguish the phases of hemangioma during infancy and childhood. *J Clin Invest* 1994;93:2357–2364.
329. Tanaka T, Miyamoto H, Hino O, et al. Primary hepatocellular carcinoma with hepatitis B virus-DNA integration in a 4-year-old boy. *Hum Pathol* 1986;17:202–204.
330. Tapper D, Lack EE. Teratomas in infancy and childhood. A 54-year experience at the Children's Hospital Medical Center. *Ann Surg* 1983;198:398–410.
331. Todani T, Tabuchi K, Watanabe Y, Tsutsumi A. True hepatic teratoma with high alpha fetoprotein in serum. *J Pediatr Surg* 1977;12:591–592.
332. Toma P, Taccone A, Martinoli C. MRI of hepatic focal nodular hyperplasia: a report of two new cases in the pediatric age group. *Pediatr Radiol* 1990;20:267–269.
333. Touraine RL, Bertrand Y, Foray P, Gilly J, Philippe N. Hepatic tumours during androgen therapy in Fanconi anaemia. *Eur J Pediatr* 1993;152:691–693.
334. Tozzi MC, Tarani L, Di Nardo R, et al. The hepatic malignant mesenchymoma: a case report. *Eur J Pediatr* 1992;151:488–491.
335. Tsuda H, Shimosato Y, Upton MP, et al. Retrospective study on amplification of N-myc and c-myc genes in pediatric solid tumors and its association with prognosis and tumor differentiation. *Lab Invest* 1988;59:321–327.
336. Turleau C, de Grouchy J, Chavin Colin F, Martelli H, Voyer M, Charlas R. Trisomy 11p15 and Beckwith–Wiedemann syndrome. A report of two cases. *Hum Genet* 1984;67:219–221.
337. Ugarte N, Gonzalez Crussi F. Hepatoma in siblings with progressive familial cholestatic cirrhosis of childhood. *Am J Clin Pathol* 1981;76:172–177.
338. Urban CE, Mache CJ, Schwinger W, et al. Undifferentiated (embryonal) sarcoma of the liver in childhood. Successful combined-modality therapy in four patients. *Cancer* 1993;72:2511–2516.
339. Van Eyken P, Sciot R, Brock P, Casteels Van Daele M, Ramaekers FC, Desmet VJ. Abundant expression of cytokeratin 7 in fibrolamellar carcinoma of the liver. *Histopathology* 1990;17:101–107.
340. Van Eyken P, Sciot R, Callea F, Ramaekers F, Schaart G, Desmet VJ. A cytokeratin-immunohistochemical study of hepatoblastoma. *Hum Pathol* 1990;21:302–308.
341. Van Eyken P, Sciot R, Paterson A, Callea F, Kew MC, Desmet VJ. Cytokeratin expression in hepatocellular carcinoma: an immunohistochemical study. *Hum Pathol* 1988;19:562–568.
342. Vileisis RA, Sorensen K, Gonzalez-Crussi F. Liver malignancy after parenteral nutrition. *J Pediatr* 1982;100:88–90.
343. Volkmann M, Hofmann WJ, Muller M, et al. p53 overexpression is frequent in European hepatocellular carcinoma and largely independent of the codon 249 hot spot mutation. *Oncogene* 1994;9:195–204.
344. Von Schweinitz D, Hadam MR, Welte K, Mildenberger H, Pietsch T. Production of interleukin-1b and interleukin-6 in hepatoblastoma. *Int J Cancer* 1993;53:728–734.
345. Vujanic GM, Milovanovic D, Aleksandrovic S. Aggressive inflammatory pseudotumor of the abdomen 9 years after therapy for Wilms tumor. A complication, coincidence, or association? *Cancer* 1992;70:2362–2366.
346. Wada M, Ohashi E, Jin H, et al. Mesenchymal hamartoma of the liver: report of an adult case and review of the literature. *Intern Med* 1992;31:1370–1375.
347. Wakely PE, Jr., Krummel TM, Johnson DE. Yolk sac tumor of the liver. *Mod Pathol* 1991;4:121–125.
348. Wakely PE, Jr., Silverman JF, Geisinger KR, Frable WJ. Fine needle aspiration biopsy cytology of hepatoblastoma. *Mod Pathol* 1990;3:688–693.
349. Waldschmidt J, Schier F, Bein U, Soerensen M. The use of the laser in the treatment of arterio-venous malformations and vascular tumours of the liver. *Eur J Pediatr Surg* 1993;3:217–223.
350. Walker NI, Horn MJ, Strong RW, Lynch SV, Cohen J, Ong TH. Undifferentiated (embryonal) sarcoma of the liver. Pathologic findings and long-term survival after complete surgical resection. *Cancer* 1992;69:52–59.
351. Wang-Wuu S, Soukup S, Ballard E, Gotwals B, Lampkin B. Chromosomal analysis of sixteen human rhabdomyosarcomas. *Cancer Res* 1988;48:983–987.
352. Wanless IR. Micronodular transformation (nodular regenerative hyperplasia) of the liver: a report of 64 cases among 2,500 autopsies and a new classification of benign hepatocellular nodules. *Hepatology* 1990;11:787–797.
353. Wanless IR, Albrecht S, Bilbao J, et al. Multiple focal nodular hyperplasia of the liver associated with vascular malformations of various organs and neoplasia of the brain: a new syndrome. *Mod Pathol* 1989;2:456–462.
354. Wanless IR, Mawdsley C, Adams R. On the pathogenesis of focal nodular hyperplasia of the liver. *Hepatology* 1985;5:1194–1200.
355. Waziri M, Patil SR, Hanson JW, Bartley JA. Abnormality of chromosome 11 in patients with features of Beckwith–Wiedemann syndrome. *J Pediatr* 1983;102:873–876.
356. Weinberg AG, Finegold MJ. Primary hepatic tumors of childhood. *Hum Pathol* 1983;14:512–537.
357. Weinberg AG, Finegold MJ. Primary hepatic tumors in childhood. In: Finegold M, ed. *Pathology of Neoplasia in Children and Adolescents.* Philadelphia: WB Saunders; 1986:333–372.
358. Weinberg AG, Mize CE, Worthen HG. The occurrence of hepatoma in the chronic form of hereditary tyrosinemia. *J Pediatr* 1976;434:438.
359. Weinberger JM, Cohen Z, Berk T. Polyposis coli preceded by hepatocellular carcinoma: report of a case. *Dis Colon Rectum* 1981;24:296–300.
360. Weinstein S, Scottolini AG, Loo SY, Caldwell PC, Bhagavan NV. Ataxia telangiectasia with hepatocellular carcinoma in a 15-year-old girl and studies of her kindred. *Arch Pathol Lab Med* 1985;109:1000–1004.
361. Westaby D, Portmann B, Williams R. Androgen related primary hepatic tumors in non-Fanconi patients. *Cancer* 1983;51:1947–1952.
362. Wheeler DA, Edmondson HA. Ciliated hepatic foregut cyst. *Am J Surg Pathol* 1984;8:467–470.
363. Wheeler DA, Edmondson HA, Reynolds TB. Spontaneous liver cell adenoma in children. *Am J Clin Pathol* 1986;85:6–12.
364. Wheeler K, Pritchard J, Luck W, Rossiter M. Transcobalamin I as a "marker" for fibrolamellar hepatoma. *Med Pediatr Oncol* 1986;14:227–229.
365. Whelan JS, Stebbings W, Owen RA, Calne R, Clark PI. Successful treatment of a primary endodermal sinus tumor of the liver. *Cancer* 1992;70:2260–2262.
366. Wilfong AA, Parke JT, McCrary JA,III. Opsoclonus-myoclonus with Beckwith–Wiedemann syndrome and hepatoblastoma. *Pediatr Neurol* 1992;8:77–79.
367. Winter TC, 3d., Freeny P. Hepatic teratoma in an adult. Case report with a review of the literature. *J Clin Gastroenterol* 1993;17:308–310.
368. Witte DP, Kissane JM, Askin FB. Hepatic teratomas in children. *Pediatr Pathol* 1983;1:81–92.
369. Wolber RA, Greene CA, Dupuis BA. Polyclonal carcinoembryonic antigen staining in the cytologic differential diagnosis of primary and metastatic hepatic malignancies. *Acta Cytol* 1991;35:215–220.
370. Yandza T, Valayer J. Benign tumors of the liver in children: analysis of a series of 20 cases. *J Pediatr Surg* 1986;21:419–423.

371. Yasunaga C, Sueishi K, Ohgami H, Suita S, Kawanami T. Heterogenous expression of endothelial cell markers in infantile hemangioendothelioma. Immunohistochemical study of two solitary cases and one multiple one. *Am J Clin Pathol* 1989;91:673–681.
372. Yohannan MD, Abdulla AM, Patel PJ. Neonatal hepatic haemangioendothelioma: presentation with jaundice and microangiopathic haemolytic anaemia. *Eur J Pediatr* 1990; 149:804–805.
373. Yuki K, Hirohashi S, Sakamoto M, Kanai T, Shimosato Y. Growth and spread of hepatocellular carcinoma. A review of 240 consecutive autopsy cases. *Cancer* 1990;66:2174–2179.
374. Zangeneh F, Limbeck GA, Brown BI, et al. Hepatorenal glycogenosis (type I glycogenosis) and carcinoma of the liver. *J Pediatr* 1969;74:78–83.
375. Zerbini MC, Vianna MR, Ribeiro D, Ayoub AA, Porta G, Sesso A. Is there a role for pericytic cells in the vascular bed of infantile hemangioendothelioma of the liver? *J Submicrosc Cytol Pathol* 1991;23:141–145.
376. Zeze F, Ohsato K, Mitani H, Ohkuma R, Koide O. Hepatocellular carcinoma associated with familial polyposis of the colon. Report of case. *Dis Colon Rectum* 1983;26:465–468.
377. Zhang X, Xu HJ, Murakami Y, et al. Deletions of chromosome 13q, mutations in retinoblastoma 1, and retinoblastoma protein state in human hepatocellular carcinoma. *Cancer Res* 1994;54: 4177–4182.
378. Zhao M, Laissue JA, Zimmermann A. "Neuroendocrine" differentiation in hepatocellular carcinomas (hepatocellular carcinomas): immunohistochemical reactivity is related to distinct tumor cell types, but not to tumor grade. *Histol Histopathol* 1993;8: 617–626.

Pediatric Neoplasia: Morphology and Biology, edited by David M. Parham.
Lippincott-Raven Publishers, Philadelphia © 1996.

CHAPTER 12

Carcinomas, Adenomas, Precursor Lesions, and Second Malignancies

David M. Parham, M. Frederick Bugg, and Charles B. Pratt

INTRODUCTION

In this chapter, we will discuss lesions that are usually associated with adults but occur sporadically in children (275). As with adults, such lesions are treated primarily by surgical means. As a group, these entities are not particularly responsive to chemotherapy, although exceptions do occur. A number of these lesions occur as second malignancies following successfully treated childhood tumor. In some, this may be related to the effects of oncolytic therapy; and in others, it appears to be related to the effects of mutated cancer suppressor genes such as *p53*. Some tumors may arise by a combination of the two mechanisms, so that patients with constitutional tendencies to acquire tumors may be more susceptible to the oncogenic effects of chemotherapy and/or radiation therapy (26). Many of the "adult-type" tumors discussed in this section arise in patients having specific syndromes, such as the Li–Fraumeni syndrome or xeroderma pigmentosa, that are related to a constitutional genotypic lesion. Neoplastic transformation thus arises relatively early in life or is incited by comparatively less stimulation than with the general population. Because the morphologic features of adult tumors are more appropriately covered in standard surgical pathology texts, we do not cover the microscopic anatomy of these lesions in an exhaustive fashion but rather emphasize features that are relatively unique to children.

D. M. Parham: Department of Pathology, University of Arkansas for Medical Sciences; and Department of Pediatric Pathology, Arkansas Children's Hospital, Little Rock, Arkansas 72202.

M. F. Bugg: Department of Pathology, MidSouth Pathology Group, Inc., Baptist Memorial Hospital, Memphis, Tennessee 38146.

C. B. Pratt: Department of Hematology/Oncology, St. Jude Children's Research Hospital; and Department of Pediatrics, University of Tennessee, Memphis, Tennessee 38105.

THYROID

Thyroid lesions in particular have been associated with prior cancer treatment, primarily radiation therapy to the neck for leukemia, lymphoma, or Hodgkin's disease. A number of relatively large series have documented this association (69,91,102,107,133,135,288, 317,375,399). Nodular thyroid lesions arising in adolescents previously exposed to ionizing radiation, however, may represent nodular hyperplasia or adenoma rather than carcinoma, so that fine-needle aspiration is frequently employed for preliminary diagnosis (69,107). The frequency of carcinoma in solitary nodules occurring in patients below the age of 20 years is very high [said to be greater than 50% (299)], so that care is necessary in cytologic interpretation. Nuclear pleomorphism, which commonly occurs as a postirradiation change, adds significant potential for confusion and overdiagnosis (299).

In one large series (133), the actuarial risk for thyroid disease 20 years after treatment for Hodgkin's disease was 52%, and it increased to 67% at 26 years. Hypothyroidism was the most common lesion, occurring in almost one third of treated patients and requiring replacement therapy in 90% of affected individuals. The incidence of Graves' disease was also highly elevated as compared to normal subjects. Three percent of the irradiated patients developed single or multiple nodules, 59% of which were excised. These included 10 benign adenomas, 6 hyperplastic nodules, 4 multinodular goiters, and 6 cancers (3 papillary, 2 mixed papillary and follicular, and 1 follicular). This incidence yielded an actuarial risk of cancer of 1.7% beyond 19 years after neck irradiation, compared with an expected risk of 0.07 per cent in a matched control population (133).

Similar results were obtained in a retrospective survey of 298 St. Jude patients receiving neck irradiation for acute lymphoblastic leukemia, nasopharyngeal carcinoma, Hodgkin's disease, and other lesions (107). Again, varying degrees of hypothyroidism were the most common abnormality, occurring in 17 patients. Seven patients developed thyroid nodules; the five excised lesions were diagnosed as papillary or follicular carcinoma, follicular adenoma, and nodular hyperplasia. This article included a review of the literature on postirradiation thyroid neoplasia, which indicated a prevalence of 0–1.4% in childhood cancer patients. Radiation-associated pediatric thyroid cancers have arisen following radiotherapy for diverse benign conditions such as thymic enlargement and acne, as well as exposure to the atomic bombs that were detonated at Nagasaki and Hiroshima or the nuclear accident that occurred at the Chernobyl reactor (248). If one excludes series specifically composed of postirradiation patients, the overall percentage of thyroid neoplasms that occur in children is very low, ranging from 1% to 9% in several large series (41,111, 145,331).

Of interest is a report that thyroid neoplasms arise five times more frequently following treatment for neuroblastoma than for other childhood cancers. This epidemiologic observation was used to suggest that neuroblastoma and thyroid tumors may share a common mechanism of oncogenesis (77).

Morphologically, thyroid neoplasms are not significantly different from those occurring in adults (299). Papillary carcinoma is by far the most common lesion, followed by medullary carcinoma and oncocytic tumors

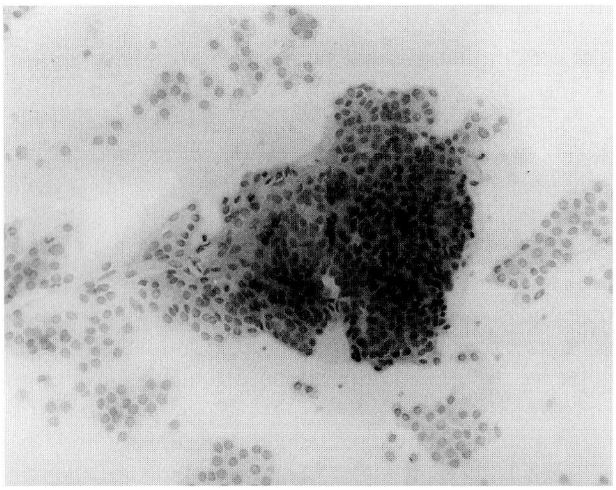

FIG. 1. Fine needle aspiration biopsy of papillary carcinoma arising in the thyroid gland of a patient previously treated for Hodgkin's disease. Note the papillary cluster. Papanicolaou's stain.

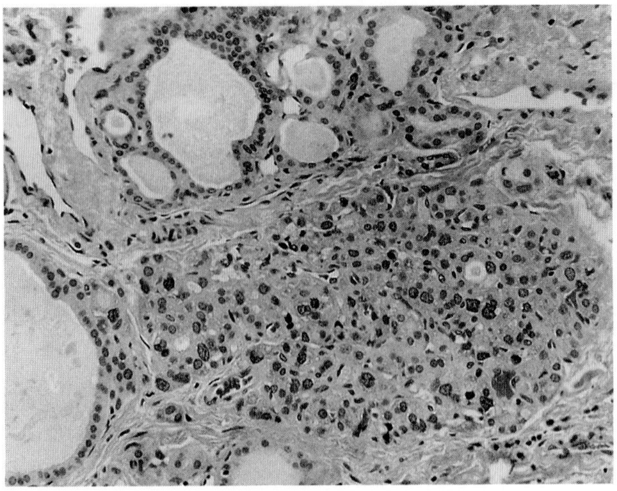

FIG. 2. Area of pleomorphism in multinodular hyperplastic goiter removed from patient previously treated for Hodgkin's disease. In spite of the severe cytologic atypia, the lesion was considered benign.

(299). A number of follicular carcinomas have been reported, but the true incidence of this neoplasm cannot be determined by a review of older literature because the occurrence of the follicular variant of papillary carcinoma (41,299) confounds the interpretation of previous studies. Childhood papillary carcinomas tend to have squamous or solid areas, but this does not affect their generally good prognosis (299).

At St. Jude and elsewhere (69,187,209,228,318,395), fine-needle aspiration has been used to evaluate nodular lesions occurring in the thyroid of childhood cancer patients. In general, the results of these studies have often been excellent, with false-negative findings ranging from 2.3% to 27% and false-positives ranging from 0 to 20% (131,162,187,201,228,395). Inadequate material is the most common source of diagnostic inaccuracy (131,162). Features that we rely on to make a diagnosis of papillary carcinoma include nuclear grooving, nuclear inclusions, psammoma bodies, and the occurrence of papillary structures ("minibiopsies") (Fig. 1). Pleomorphism occurs relatively frequently in the thyroid epithelium of our postirradiation patient population (Fig. 2) and should not be used as a sole diagnostic criterion for cancer. Features that in our experience favor nodular hyperplasia include fibrosis and siderophages. Interested readers may wish to refer to the excellent short review of thyroid cytology written by Willems and Lowhagen (395). One must be cognizant that a variety of lesions, both neoplasms and hyperplastic nodules, may coexist in multinodular thyroids, so that caution is indicated. We also routinely use frozen section interpretation to further guide excisional therapy, although diagnostic error may still lead to incorrect surgery (132).

Besides epithelial neoplasms and nodular hyperplasia,

causes of thyroid tumors include thyroiditis, which may occur after irradiation (107,288), and a variety of uncommon congenital and neoplastic entities. These include thyroglossal duct cysts, teratomas, lymphomas, and sarcomas. These entities are vanishingly rare in our experience, although benign cystic lesions of the neck are generally not referred to a tertiary care hospital. Lymphomas may arise after a history of thyroiditis (9,33) and are generally B-cell lesions of the large cell variety (9). One must also consider the occurrence of benign thyroid epithelium outside of the gland proper, sometimes leading to a mistaken diagnosis of metastatic carcinoma (298). With medullary carcinomas occurring in children, the possibility of a familial multiple endocrine neoplasia syndrome should be considered (see Chapter 6).

Cytogenetically, abnormalities involving chromosome 19q13, usually occurring as a balanced translocation, appear to be important in the development of some follicular adenomas (73). The majority of tested cases of these tumors have been diploid and karyotypically normal, but numerical abnormalities also occur (73).

ADRENAL CORTEX

Adrenal cortical neoplasms are infrequently encountered in all age groups and are particularly rare in the pediatric population. From 1973 to 1987, 21 cases of adrenal cortical carcinomas were reported in children less than 15 years of age by the National Cancer Institute's Surveillance, Epidemiology, End Results (SEER) program (229). This is a large epidemiologic study encompassing approximately 10% of the total population of the United States. In a 20-year review of 141 cases of pediatric adrenal tumors accrued at Manchester, England, 130 were neuroblastoma, 8 were adrenal cortical neoplasms, and 3 were pheochromocytomas (354). Adrenal cortical carcinomas account for only 0.2% of all pediatric malignancies (229). Retrospective studies have shown that approximately 25% of pediatric adrenal cortical neoplasms are benign adenomas (32,196,241). There is statistical evidence that indicates that adrenal cortical carcinomas of older pediatric patients tend to be more aggressive than those of the very young (196,313). These tumors usually cause a palpable abdominal mass. Most studies indicate a slight right-sided predominance (196,313,354).

Pediatric adrenal cortical neoplasms occur most commonly in the 0–5 year age group (202). The average age of diagnosis is 4.6 years (196,241). Most patients are Caucasian, and most are female (2–3:1 female-to-male ratio) (18,196,241). A bimodal distribution of the tumors occur in children, with a clustering of cases during early childhood and a more evenly distributed group occurring during adolescence (196). There seem to be geographic differences in the incidence of pediatric adrenal cortical neoplasia, as cases have been relatively numerous in southern Brazil (98,216,290) and extremely rare in Africa (75).

Adrenal cortical neoplasms have been associated with a strong family history of malignant tumors (183), occurrence in multiple siblings (212), and the possibly related sarcoma–breast cancer–lymphoma–adrenal cancer (SBLA) and Li-Fraumeni syndromes (196). They may also be associated with genitourinary anomalies, neurofibromatosis, pigmented nevi, brain tumors, cutaneous hemangiomas, isolated hemihypertrophy, and the Beckwith–Wiedemann syndrome (19,112,319,348). There have also been rare instances occurring in patients with congenital adrenal hyperplasia (138,261, 361,379). Multiple endocrine neoplasia (MEN) syndrome type I (Vermer–Morrison syndrome) has an association with both adrenal cortical hyperplasia and neoplasia (160,343). There may be a possible relationship between adrenal cortical neoplasia and the fetal alcohol syndrome (159).

Children with adrenal cortical neoplasia almost always have endocrinologic abnormalities. Virilization is the most common clinical presentation and causes pubic and axillary hair growth, clitoromegaly or phallomegaly, hirsutism, increased muscle mass, and acne. Ribeiro et al. (290) described 40 cases of pediatric adrenal cortical carcinomas, 39 of which were functional tumors, 37 causing virilization, 22 a mixture of Cushing's syndrome and virilization, and 2 pure Cushing's syndrome. Features of feminization have also been reported (313). Primary hyperaldosteronism (Conn's syndrome) is an extremely rare pediatric complication of these tumors and except for one case of adrenal cortical carcinoma (110) has only been reported in small adenomas (6). Data regarding the behavior of functioning tumors as compared to nonfunctioning ones are conflicting (155,185, 240,290).

Grossly, adrenal cortical neoplasms are pale to bright yellow, encapsulated, bulging lesions that may have areas of necrosis and hemorrhage (Fig. 3; see figure in color plate section). They must be weighed, measured, and examined carefully. Benign tumors generally weigh 100 g or less and are well encapsulated without grossly evident necrosis. However, there have been reported adrenal cortical carcinomas that were 40 g or smaller (118,290). Nevertheless, most tumors weighing less than 200 g do not metastasize, and tumors weighing more than 500 g are usually malignant (32,37,80). Likewise tumor volume of >200 cm^3 has been associated with malignancy (290). None of the adrenal cortical tumors <5 cm in greatest diameter in our study had disease recurrence after treatment (32).

The histologic features of adrenal cortical neoplasms vary considerably. Benign adenomas may greatly resemble the normal adrenal cortex and are composed of cells with round, regular nuclei and voluminous clear to light pink cytoplasm, arranged in a sinusoidal, trabecular, or solid pattern with a prominent vasculature (Fig. 4). Hyaline droplets or lipochrome pigment may be apparent. Often adrenal cortical neoplasms contain cells with considerable nuclear pleomorphism and bizarre appearances that at first glance may obscure the diagnosis (Fig. 5). Both apoptosis and confluent necrosis are common in carcinomas. Evidence of invasion into the tumor capsule, blood vessels, and/or sinusoids may occur and is an important feature to consider in diagnosis (32). Capsular invasion should not be confused with native adrenal cortical nodules entrapped in the peritumoral tissues.

A malignant adrenal cortical tumor reported by Molberg et al. (231) was called an adrenocortical blastoma because of its mixed content of primitive epithelium and mesenchyme. We have seen an adrenal tumor completely lacking epithelial elements and composed of a heterogeneous mixture of undifferentiated mesenchyme and primitive muscle and cartilage. Considering the mesodermal origin of the adrenal cortex (233), this primitive neoplasm may have resulted from a complete absence of epithelial cell induction and may be a related lesion.

Immunohistochemical studies of adrenal cortical neoplasms have consistently revealed decreased expression of cytokeratin and increased expression of vimentin relative to their degree of malignancy (149,240). The absence of cytokeratin staining and strong vimentin staining has been used to discriminate these tumors from renal cell carcinomas and other tumors (149,223,240, 393). A newly described monoclonal antibody, D11, detects a molecule present in the nuclei of adrenal cortex tumor cells and has been used as a tumor marker (363). Because it stains primarily well-differentiated tumors, its presence tends to connote benignancy and it is not detected in adrenomedullary tumors (363). Conversely, neural markers, particularly synaptophysin, may be present in adrenal cortical carcinomas (127,323). Some of these biphenotypic tumors also display neuroendocrine features by electron microscopy (226).

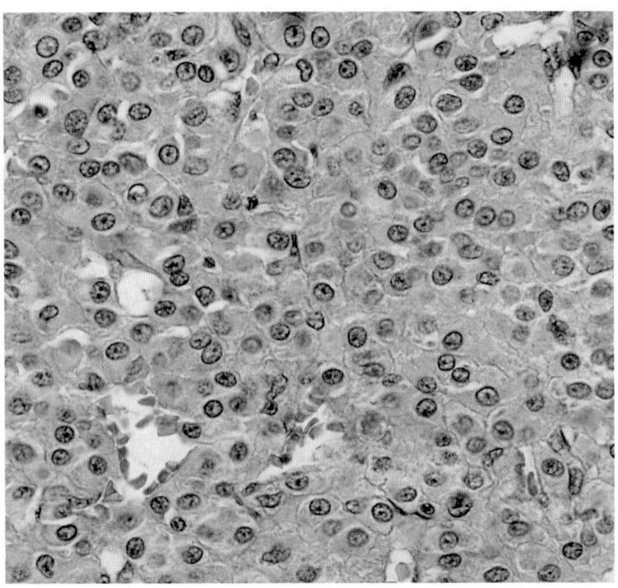

FIG. 4. Adrenal cortical adenoma. The tumor is well-differentiated, strongly resembling normal adrenal cortex, and contains no mitoses.

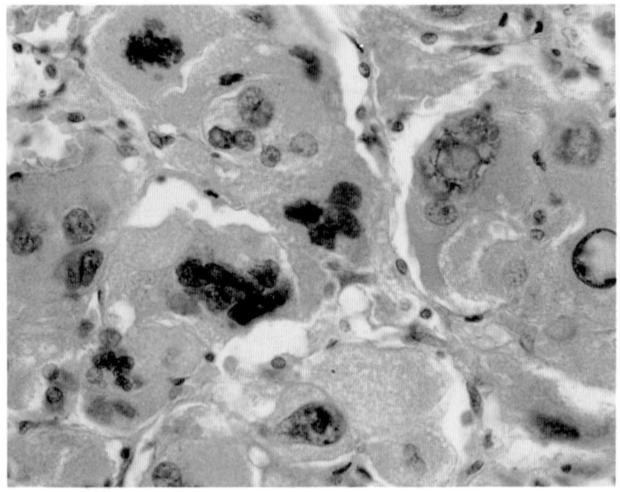

FIG. 5. Adrenal cortical carcinoma. There is marked cellular pleomorphism and mitotic activity.

Electron microscopy of adrenal cortical neoplasms typically reveals structures found in steroid-secreting cells and thus may assist in the diagnosis (99). These organelles include prominent smooth endoplasmic reticulum, stacked rough endoplasmic reticulum, and mitochondria with tubulovesicular or shelflike cristae (99,196). However, the ultrastructural features of these neoplasms are variable.

Unlike tumor size, the use of histology as a means of predicting behavior of pediatric adrenal cortical neoplasms has been hotly debated, although there is little doubt concerning its value in adult tumors (223,380, 390,391). Mitotic activity appears to be the single best predictor of outcome in adult adrenal cortical neoplasms (223). Histologic criteria for grading adrenal cortical tumors include those of Hough, Weiss, and Van Slooten. The system of Van Slooten et al. (380) uses a numeric value system combined with subjective criteria such as regressive changes and/or structural changes. The modified criteria of Weiss et al. is less subjective and is based on the presence of histologic criteria such as mitotic index, atypical mitoses, confluent necrosis, and venous, sinusoidal, or capsular invasion (391). In the authors' own study (32), adrenal cortical neoplasms were designated as benign, low-grade carcinoma, and high-grade carcinoma based on Weiss's criteria and were found to have a strong predictive value in pediatric lesions. With slight modification, the diagnoses were based on the mitotic index of 50 high-power fields: adenomas contained $\leq$ 5mitoses, low-grade carcinomas contained $>$5 but $\leq$20 mitoses, and carcinomas contained $>$20. Nuclear pleomorphism is not a reliable predictor of malignancy and can be misleading (32,80).

Using histologic criteria, tumor weight, and clinical criteria, Hough et al. (161) devised a system for predicting the biologic behavior of adrenal cortical neoplasms in adults. Numeric values are assigned for each criteria and are totaled to determine if whether a tumor is malignant, intermediate, or benign. In Ribeiro's series of 40 pediatric adrenal cortical tumors (290), all of the above three grading systems were tested. Only four tumors failed to meet the criteria for malignancy by all three systems. Cagle et al. (37) found size to be the single most important prognostic indicator for pediatric adrenal cortical neoplasms. Their study indicates that these tumors are more likely to be benign than previously thought and that morphologic criteria for predicting biologic behavior in adult neoplasms do not necessarily apply to pediatric ones. However, because endocrine symptoms often lead to early clinical recognition and resection, tumors that are clinically benign but histologically malignant may be low-grade carcinomas that are cured prior to metastasis. Some have cautioned against the sole use of tumor size as the sole predictor of malignancy (196). Among Ribeiro's cases (37), there was one carcinoma that weighed only 15 g but led to the demise of the patient. Gandour and Grizzle (118) encountered a similar lesion.

Ploidy, proliferative indices, and argyrophilic nucleolar organizer region (AgNOR) number also have been tested as means of predicting behavior of adrenal cortical neoplasms. There are contradictory data regarding ploidy. Some studies (8,38) have shown no correlation between outcome and aneuploidy or heterogeneous DNA content. In other studies (86,360), including one with pediatric tumors (367), an abnormal DNA content predicted metastatic potential. In our own study (32), ploidy was inconclusive because of the common occurrence of aneuploid cells. Similarly, our studies of proliferative index using anti-PCNA immunohistochemistry failed to reveal a significant predictive value, although there was a trend toward more aggressive behavior with tumors having a proliferative index of 10%. AgNOR numbers also appear to have little prognostic value (320).

Similar to many other pediatric tumors, adrenal cortical neoplasms express insulinlike growth factor (IGF), insulinlike growth factor receptor, and insulin receptors and thus show evidence of an autocrine growth loop (176). Cytogenetic studies also suggest an IGF-2 abnormality, as a locus on chromosome 11p15 appears to be misfunctioning in these lesions (223). Transforming growth factor–α may also play a role in tumorigenesis (89), and *p53* mutations and *Rb* overexpression are seen in tumors associated with the Li–Fraumeni syndrome (223). Similarly, loss of heterozygosity may be seen at chromosome 17p, the site of the *p53* gene (404).

GASTROINTESTINAL TRACT

Colon carcinoma, in spite of its stature as the second leading cause of cancer-related demise in adults, is a rare lesion in children. It is estimated to affect 1 per 1 million individuals under the age of 20 per year (276), compared to 60 per 1 million adults per year (372). Nevertheless, colon carcinoma is a well-recognized pediatric neoplasm, but because of its rarity it is often not diagnosed at an early stage (87,96,167,230,286,353). In addition, colon carcinoma is associated with a number of premalignant colonic lesions that may appear in childhood and often coexist with hamartomatous or neoplastic lesions of other organs. In general, these multitumor syndromes present in the colon as polypoid lesions that have a tendency for malignant transformation. These syndromes are listed in Table 1. In general, they have an autosomal dominant pattern of inheritance. Close inspection of this table will show a number of recurring themes in the associated lesions, indicating that they derive from a similar set of genetic lesions, typically affecting tumor suppressor genes, with comparable multiorgan consequences.

Roughly stated, there are three modes of colon carcinoma development: sporadic, familial, and hereditary. Lynch et al. (211) defined these operational terms as follows: sporadic tumors occur in patients with no similarly affected first-degree relative and no evidence of hereditary disease; familial tumors occur in patients with at least one similarly affected first-degree relative and no hereditary disease in the family history; and hereditary disease is defined as occurring in a family grouping associated with autosomal dominant inheritance and well-defined phenotypic features as outlined in Table 1. This admittedly operational definition has the advantages of predicting outcome and planning patient management, but because of the high frequency of colon carcinoma in the general population, it is sometimes difficult to apply in individual circumstances.

Of primary interest to pediatric pathologists is the fact that hereditary forms of colon cancer may become manifest during childhood. In some syndromes listed on Table 1, such as the flat adenoma or the hereditary nonpolyposis syndromes, the lesions predominate in the right side of the colon (211). Conversely, with other conditions such as the familial polyposis syndrome, lesions usually first appear in the left colon. This dyssynchrony probably results from the separate embryogenesis of the two sides of the large bowel, which is also evidenced by a number of other biologic and phenotypic features of this organ. Another factor to consider is variable penetrance of the genetic abnormality, so that the number of polyps may vary from few to many, causing the colon to resemble a lush pile carpet (Fig. 6). This multiplicity of lesions may be manifest in a synchronous or metachronous fashion, so that routinely scheduled colonoscopy is man-

tion. This complication is prone to occur after viral infections (232). Gastrointestinal lymphoid hyperplasia may also be seen in human immunodeficiency virus (HIV)-infected patients (308).

PANCREAS

Similar to colon carcinoma, the rarity of pancreatic carcinoma in children belies its frequency in adults. In general, only isolated case reports of the usual adult-type carcinoma are available in the literature (365). Some are associated with heritable cancer syndromes (71). Acinar cell carcinomas appear to make up a relatively large proportion of these lesions (195,365). At times, childhood pancreatic cancers assume an adenoid cystic configuration (365). One of the largest series of pediatric exocrine pancreatic carcinoma is that of Lack et al. (195), who describe eight cases, only three of which were the usual adult duct cell type. In the large series of 406 cases of exocrine pancreatic cancers accumulated by Cubilla and Fitzgerald (70), only one case occurred in a child. Aside from the occasional example of adult-type ductal or acinic adenocarcinoma, primary pancreatic lesions in children and adolescents are usually pancreatoblastomas or papillary cystic tumors.

Pancreatoblastoma is an embryonal neoplasm analogous to hepatoblastoma and Wilms' tumor. The basic component of these tumors is a small cell population common to most embryonal tumors, admixed with varying numbers of more differentiated glandular cells (186). Eosinophilic cells with zymogen-type granules may be present, and similar to Wilms' tumor and hepatoblastoma, there may be teratoid differentiation into cartilage, bone, osteoid, spindle cells, and squamous cells. The squamous, glandular, and undifferentiated elements may be intermingled in an organoid fashion (Fig. 9) (65,157). Zymogen granules may be seen with electron microscopy as well as light microscopy (65,340). Smaller, neurosecretory-type granules have also been reported (340), but the endocrine function of these organelles has not been conclusively proven.

Both histochemistry (65) and immunohistochemistry (157,234,340) have been used to support the diagnosis of pancreatoblastoma. In particular, α_1-antitrypsin is strongly positive by immunohistochemistry (157), and activity of glucose-6-phosphatase, acid phosphatase, esterase, and esteroprotease may be demonstrated by histochemistry (65). Positive immunohistochemical staining for cytokeratin, CA19-9, neuron-specific enolase, carcinoembryonic antigen, pancreatic enzymes, and α-fetoprotein (AFP) have also been reported (168,234, 340). Occasional examples also may appear to show endocrine differentiation by immunohistochemistry (31).

Pancreatoblastoma usually occurs in younger children with an average age of 5 years (157). There is an equal sex ratio, and serum AFP levels may be elevated (157, 168,234,256). Adrenocorticotropic hormone (ACTH)–associated Cushing's syndrome has also been described (265). These tumors are clinically aggressive and should be treated as high-grade malignancies. However, spread can be slow, and they are often cured by excision alone (186). An association with Beckwith–Wiedemann syndrome has been reported (90,189). Adjuvant chemotherapy has evoked "maturation" of pancreatoblastoma into well-differentiated ductal and acinar adenocarcinoma (256).

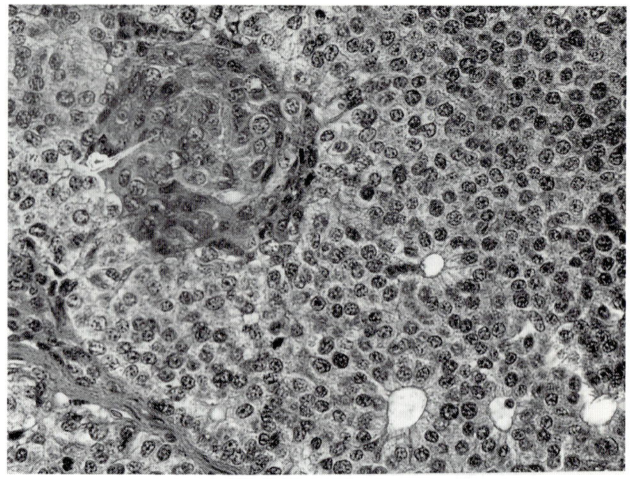

FIG. 9. Pancreatoblastoma containing mixture of small cell, glandular, and squamous cell elements.

Papillary cystic (also known as solid and cystic) tumors of the pancreas clinically differ from pancreatoblastomas in that they occur in older patients, predominantly females, and are typically associated with a good prognosis (157,186). These tumors grossly display cystic, necrotic, and hemorrhagic foci imparting a variegated appearance. There may be associated pancreatic inflammation (76) or pseudocyst formation (238). Histologically, the tumor cells are arranged into well-formed papillae surrounded by red blood cells. The cytologic features of the tumor cells are typically bland, with smooth nuclear membranes, oval nuclei, inconspicuous nucleoli, finely dispersed chromatin, and rare mitoses (Fig. 10). The tumor cell cytoplasm is eosinophilic, sometimes with prominent periodic acid–Schiff (PAS)–positive granules. Areas of myxoid degeneration, similar to myxopapillary ependymoma or pleomorphic adenoma, may be apparent (70). Perivascular sclerosis may be associated with tumor necrosis. Solid foci of foamy histiocytes, cholesterol clefts, and giant cells are also typical (357).

Ultrastructural study of papillary cystic tumors discloses abundant rough endoplasmic reticulum and mitochondria and relatively large numbers of annulate lamellae (271). As with light microscopy, cytoplasmic granules of varying diameter may be present (357).

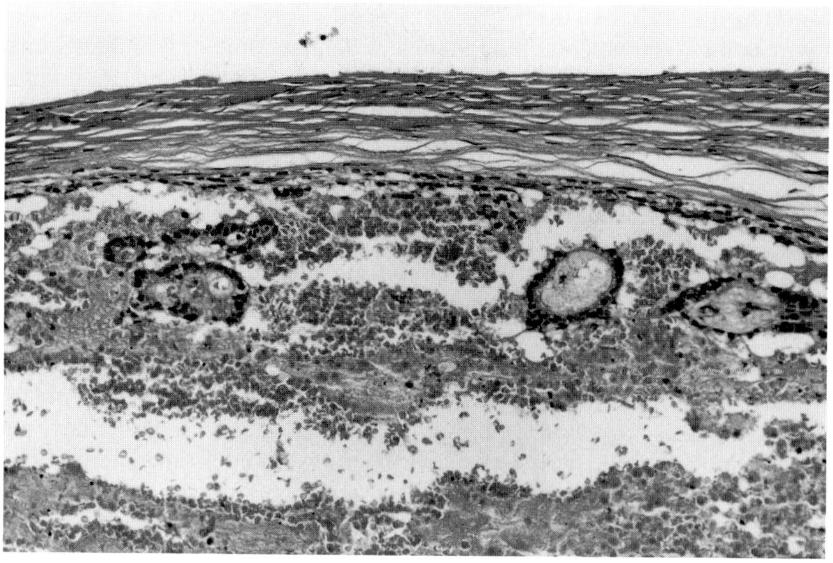

FIG. 10. Papillary cystic tumor of pancreas of adolescent female. The tumor is composed of papillae lined by bland epithelial cells. There is abundant necrosis and hemorrhage, surrounded by a fibrous capsule.

Immunohistochemical analysis reveals α_1-antitrypsin and α_1-antichymotrypsin positivity. The presence of neuron-specific enolase and synaptophysin staining was interpreted as evidence of endocrine differentiation in one report, but S-100, pancreatic hormone, or chromogranin positivity was not seen (357). However, occasional chromogranin and S-100 staining was seen in another series (249). Miettenen et al. (227) also demonstrated clusters of cells with hormone immunoreactivity. There are a number of reports further indicating that papillary cystic tumors are derived from pluripotent cells capable of differentiating along both exocrine and endocrine pathways (217,235); others have shown no definitive evidence of either type of differentiation (271). Occasional lesions may appear predominately endocrine (402). There are also discrepant results using immunostains for estrogen receptors (227,403), perhaps related to the specificity of pancreas-related estrogen receptors (40). Progesterone receptors have also been demonstrated in these tumors by both chemical and immunohistochemical methods (250).

Metastases from papillary cystic tumors are rare; Cubilla and Fitzgerald (71) quote Oertel as seeing metastases in only 2 of 52 patients. Nishihara et al. (249) analyzed the histologic, flow cytometric, and immunohistochemical features of 22 examples to find features predictive of dissemination. In their series, venous invasion, a higher nuclear grade, and prominent necrobiotic nests were associated with hepatic, peritoneal, and/or nodal metastases in three patients. One of these lesions was also aneuploid. Aneuploidy has been demonstrated in other metastasizing papillary cystic tumors as well (39), but differences in immunohistochemical staining have not been apparent.

Similar to pancreatic exocrine tumors, islet cell tumors are rare in childhood (146). These may arise as a dominant nodule in infants with nesidioblastosis, an abnormal diffuse proliferation of islet cells that may occur sporadically or as part of a growth abnormality (422). Thus, infantile lesions compose a large proportion of pediatric islet cell tumors. Prompt diagnosis of islet cell tumors in infancy is critical, as severe mental retardation secondary to hypoglycemia is an ominous sequela of a delay in therapy (42). Heitz (146) reported a combined gastrinoma-insulinoma in a 12-year-old patient; the tumor contained large amounts of extravascular amyloid substance similar to that seen in medullary carcinoma of the thyroid. Multihormonal secretion by these neoplasms is not unusual (237,381).

Islet cell tumors may also be associated with MEN I (114), which can be diagnosed in childhood. This tendency to multiple endocrine tumors is inherited in autosomal dominant fashion and is associated with tumors of the thyroid, parathyroids, adrenal cortex, and pancreatic islets (321) (see Chapter 6). We have encountered an insulin-secreting islet cell carcinoma in a 14-year-old. This patient died of multiple metabolic derangements due to massive abdominal metastases despite a heroic attempt at cure via hepatoduodenopancreatic transplantation. It should be noted that vasoactive intestinal peptide production with associated symptoms (watery diarrhea, abdominal distension, hypokalemia) is often due to ganglioneuromatous tumors rather that islet cell tumors (see Chapter 6) (282,347).

Although islet cell carcinomas may bear some resemblance to primitive neuroectodermal tumors of children, immunohistochemistry and electron microscopy can be of great assistance in rendering a secure diagnosis. To compound the potential for diagnostic dilemma, it has been our observation that neuroblastomas arising in the celiac plexus may infiltrate the pancreas. Nevertheless, immunohistochemical stains for hormonal production can be of great value in diagnosis (237), and tumor cytoarchitecture (237) and ultrastructure (125) may also further indicate the type of endocrine function of the tumor. Conversely to the endocrine differentiation reported in pancreatoblastomas and papillary cystic carcinomas, exocrine differentiation may be observed in pediatric islet cell tumors (43).

SALIVARY GLAND

Salivary gland neoplasms in children compose less than 5% of the total population of cases (371). Malignancy is relatively common in epithelial lesions and is seen in approximately half of pediatric salivary gland neoplasms (325,337). These lesion fall within two uncommon but well-recognized groups: those affecting infants and those affecting older children. The tumors of older children are basically the same lesions that occur in adults but with a differing predominance of histologic types, whereas infantile lesions are often congenital and are distinct histologic entities. As with adults, most salivary gland neoplasms in children occur in the parotid gland (13,337). Despite the high incidence of malignancy, the morbidity and mortality of these tumors in children is low (53,324).

Mucoepidermoid carcinoma is the most common histologic variant of juvenile salivary gland neoplasia and is usually a low-grade lesion that tends to recur rather than metastasize (337). It has been reported as a second malignancy (179,210). Identification of the mucinous elements in these tumors may be enhanced with mucin stains such as mucicarmine. Parotid gland lesions occur most commonly, followed by submandibular tumors. Grading of mucoepidermoid tumors is important in predicting subsequent tumor behavior and is dependent on the relative amount of mucinous vs. epidermoid cells, relative cellularity vs. cystic composition, and pattern of invasion of adjacent tissue (4,101). Thus, tumors with a greater degree of epidermoid composition, minimal cyst formation, or permeative tumor margins tend to be more aggressive (4,101).

The most frequent benign pediatric salivary gland neoplasm is the pleomorphic adenoma, which again generally displays histologic and clinical features similar to those of adults. Pediatric carcinoma ex pleomorphic adenoma has occurred as an exceedingly rare event (45). Finally, adenoid cystic carcinomas, acinic cell carcinomas, and ductal adenocarcinomas compose the remainder of the catalog of adult-type pediatric epithelial neoplasia. Adenoid cystic carcinoma was relatively common in one series (13). However, it should be noted that some reported examples of adenoid cystic carcinoma arising in infants may have been misdiagnosed (164). Acinic cell carcinoma is relatively common in children, in contrast to its rarity in adults (192).

In the newborn, most salivary gland tumors are benign vascular lesions such as hemangioma or lymphangioma (164,192). Epithelial salivary gland lesions in infants usually occur as parotid tumors but may arise as intraoral or nasopharyngeal neoplasms (81). One infantile tumor, the sialoblastoma (164), has been reported under a variety of synonyms such as adenoid cystic carcinoma, monomorphic adenoma, and embryoma. As noted above, this lesion most often occurs in the parotid gland, but we have seen an example arising in the minor salivary glands of the palate. Sialoblastoma has a distinctive histology composed of nests of primitive epidermoid cells embedded in a fibrous stroma (Fig. 11). The epidermoid nests may contain ductal elements, particularly on the periphery. A peripheral basaloid arrangement of the nests creates a similarity to adenoid cystic carcinoma or monomorphic adenoma. Immunohistochemical staining reveals positivity for cytokeratin, vimentin, actin, and S-100, with predominance of S-100- and vimentin-positive cells in the solid portion of the nests. This diversity suggests a maturation sequence, and indeed these tumors are architecturally similar to the embryonic salivary gland. Clinically they have a propensity for local recurrence if incompletely excised but seldom if ever metastasize. To date, they have not been associated with a tumor-related death (164).

A similar but histologically distinct tumor is the salivary gland anlage tumor described by Dehner et al. (81). Like sialoblastoma, these lesions are frequently congenital, but they typically arise from the midline of the nasopharynx as peduculated masses. Because of this location, the affected children often present with respiratory distress in the immediate postnatal period. Salivary gland anlage tumors have the general architectural features of sialoblastomas but differ in that masses of primitive mesenchyme rather than epithelioid cells form the nests embedded in a fibrous stroma. Ductular and epidermoid

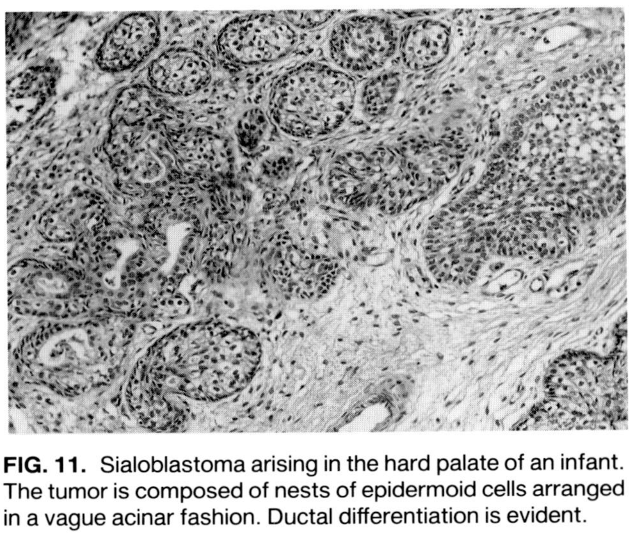

FIG. 11. Sialoblastoma arising in the hard palate of an infant. The tumor is composed of nests of epidermoid cells arranged in a vague acinar fashion. Ductal differentiation is evident.

elements are peripherally intermingled with these primitive cells. The mesenchymal cells have bland cytologic features and may be disposed into an organoid pattern resembling craniopharyngioma. Immunohistochemical reactivity for anticytokeratin and antiepithelial membrane antigen characterizes the periphery of the nests, whereas the solid component shows positivity for vimentin, cytokeratin, and muscle-specific actin. Both regions display positivity for salivary gland amylase. Architectural and epidemiologic similarities between sialoblastomas and salivary anlage tumors may tempt the "lumpers" to speculate on the interrelatedness of the two lesions, but they differ in the cytologic composition of the cellular nests, the usual primary site, and the pattern of S-100 staining. Like sialoblastomas, salivary gland anlage tumors behave in a benign fashion following excision, and they are likewise strongly reminiscent of the developing salivary gland, possibly being hamartomas rather than true neoplasms (81).

No discussion of salivary gland lesions in children would be complete without mention of embryonal rhabdomyosarcoma, which not uncommonly occurs in the parotid-masseteric region (297) (see Chapter 5). Inflammatory lesions and benign cysts also occur and in fact constitute the majority of salivary gland enlargements in children (192). Lymphomas, particularly Burkitt's lymphoma (Chapter 16), are also a diagnostic consideration. We have also seen peripheral neuroepitheliomas and primitive ectomesenchymomas (Chapter 4) arise from the cheek.

NONSALIVARY GLAND HEAD AND NECK TUMORS

In our experience at St. Jude Children's Research Hospital, the most common nonlymphoid neoplasms arising in the extracranial head and neck region have been rhabdomyosarcoma and nasopharyngeal carcinoma. There is a higher proportion of alveolar rhabdomyosarcomas in the sinonasal region than is generally appreciated; spindle cell rhabdomyosarcomas often arise in the orbital area (unpublished observations). Other mesenchymal lesions, particularly fibromatoses, hemangiomas, lymphangiomas, fibrosarcomas, granular cell tumors, and myofibrosarcomas, also arise in the head and neck. Considerations in the nasal region include chordomas, esthesioneuroblastomas, and nasal gliomas, which are outgrowths of heterotopic gliomatous tissue (266). Paragangliomas may occur in the cervical and auditory regions. Malformative developmental cystic lesions such as teratomas and thyroglossal duct cysts compose a large portion of lesions in the head and neck of children and may give rise to carcinomas (25). Finally, a rare but well-characterized craniofacial neoplasm is the melanotic neuroectodermal tumor, which because of its similarity to peripheral neuroectodermal tumors is discussed in Chapter 4. These exclusions leave two primary groups of tumors—nasopharyngeal carcinomas and odontogenic lesions—for further consideration.

NASOPHARYNGEAL CARCINOMA

Nasopharyngeal carcinoma has been the subject of extensive biologic and epidemiologic investigations because of its unique geographic and racial distribution and its association with Epstein–Barr virus (EBV) (52). The geographic distribution of nasopharyngeal carcinoma has been a fascinating subject to epidemiologists, as it has revealed a high incidence of the disease in widely diverse populations, including native Chinese (166), Alaskan and Greenland Eskimos (225), Tunisians (20), Maghrebians (172), Singaporians (203,333), and Sudanese (152). Because of the obvious racial susceptibility patterns, studies into associated markers such as human leukocyte antigen (HLA) genetic loci have been performed. These reveal some apparent associations but there are discrepancies (20). A familial susceptibility pattern has also been reported (59). However, present evidence generally favors environmental factors rather than inherent genetic susceptibility as the major risks for contracting the disease, as high-risk populations moving into areas of decreased prevalence, such as the United States or France, show a gradual decline in incidence through succeeding generations. Conversely, people from low-incidence areas moving into high-incidence regions appear to suffer an increased risk of contracting the disease (172). Nevertheless, a combination of genetic, environmental, and biologic factors is probably operative (52,392).

In the United States, a racial pattern is also apparent, with blacks having a greater risk of acquiring nasopharyngeal carcinoma than whites. Again, this has been theorized to be associated with environmental rather than racial factors (124). The age incidence of African-Americans is also of interest, as a peak appears in the adolescent age group (124). A similar association with age has been noted in the Sudan (152), where nasopharyngeal carcinoma is the commonest pediatric cancer, and in Bombay (14); this contrasts with the relatively higher median age of incidence among Chinese (35).

The primary apparent cause of pediatric nasopharyngeal carcinoma in these diverse groups is EBV. The association of EBV with the tumor cells of nasopharyngeal carcinoma has been proven by a variety of methods, using serologic, genetic, electron microscopic, cell culture, and immunohistochemical techniques (52,141,247, 355,373). It appears that affected children are infected by a large dose of the virus at a young age or have repeated exposures (117). Serologic studies form the primary basis for these observations. In particular, serum titers of viral capsid antigen (VCA), the diffuse (D) component of the early antigen (EA) complex, and EBV-associated nuclear antigen (EBNA) are usually elevated in affected patients. Typically, the IgG titers of VCA and D-EA rise and wane with disease activity, sometimes prior to clinical evidence of remission or recurrence (148,239). As a result, serologic testing for EBV should be incorporated into both diagnostic and follow-up studies (206,242).

Clinically, nasopharyngeal carcinoma often presents with metastatic disease, particularly in the cervical lymph nodes, prior to discovery of the primary tumor. Blind biopsy of the nasopharynx has occasionally been necessary for proof of primary disease. Metastatic disease also may be found in the bone, bone marrow, liver, lungs, and other sites. The tumor has a peculiar tendency to occasionally spread to the mediastinum (262). Paraneoplastic syndromes may also occur and are absent during periods of remission; these conditions include fever of unknown origin, leukemoid reaction, and hypertrophic osteoarthropathy (72,351). Clinical outcome is primarily dependent on the extent of the primary disease rather than the presence of cervical node metastasis, but patients with disseminated disease at presentation or relapse usually have poor survival rates (141,173). The disease is typically more aggressive in children than adults; but paradoxically, the survival rates of affected teenagers appear to be increasing, thanks to the responsiveness of these tumors to chemotherapy and radiation (35).

By the World Health Organization (WHO) classification (163,334), nasopharyngeal carcinomas comprise three main varieties: keratinizing squamous cell carcinoma, nonkeratinizing squamous cell carcinoma, and undifferentiated carcinoma. The keratinizing carcinomas are rare in children. These are adult-type squamous cell carcinomas composed of epidermoid cells with varying degrees of squamous differentiation, so that one encounters squamous eddies, keratin pearls, and so forth. This may be transformed into spindle cell carcinoma or carcinosarcoma, considerations in spindle cell malignancies that appear to arise from the mucosal surfaces (394); however, these lesions are vanishingly rare in children. Pediatric epidermoid cancers of this type are often associated with papillomavirus infection (described in Chapter 14), and patients typically do not show elevated serum EBNA (105).

Undifferentiated carcinomas often occur as the variety known as lymphoepithelioma, a name derived from the intense plasmalymphocytic infiltration that abuts the epithelial element, at times to the point of obscuring it. Undifferentiated carcinomas are the lesions most closely associated with EBV infection and have a high incidence in certain pediatric populations. Tumors of this type may arise in a variety of areas besides the nasopharynx, particularly the thymus (336,401). However, the nasopharynx is by far the most common primary site. Histologically, undifferentiated carcinoma is characterized by the occurrence of cohesive groups of primitive epithelial cells nestled among the aforementioned inflammatory elements, typically mature lymphocytes and plasma cells. These neoplastic epithelial cells have large nuclei with characteristically prominent eosinophilic nucleoli and modest amounts of amphophilic cytoplasm (Fig. 12A). Usually, there is no overt squamous differentiation, but careful microscopic inspection may reveal the "baseball stitch" appearance of desmosomal junctions attenuated by fixation.

Cohesiveness of the cell clusters is usually evident with routine stains and contrasts with the usual lack of consolidation of lymphomas. However, problem cases may

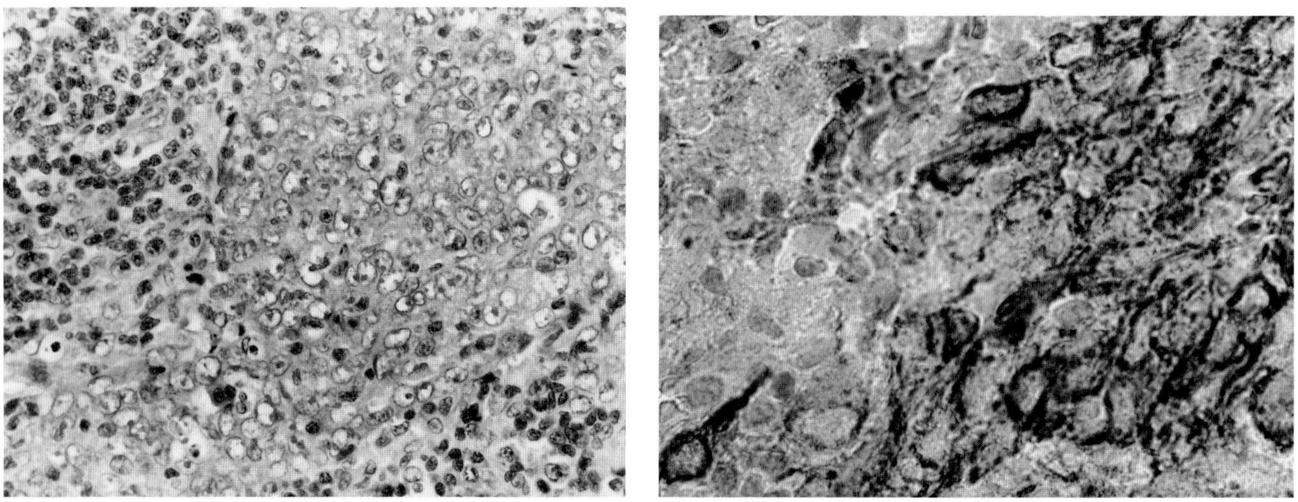

A B

FIG. 12. Undifferentiated nasopharyngeal carcinoma, metastatic to a cervical lymph node. There is a large cohesive nest of cells with large oval nuclei and prominent nucleoli **(A)**. The cells are strongly cytokeratin-positive **(B)**. Inmunofluorescence of an imprint reveals the presence of EBNA (see figure in color plate section) **(C)**. **A:** H&E; **B:** ABC technique; **C:** indirect immunofluorescence with anti-EBNA. (Part **C** courtesy of Dr. John Sixbey, St. Jude Children's Research Hospital.)

be encountered, so that ancillary studies can be of great assistance in diagnosis. In particular, cytokeratin staining (Fig. 12B) usually reveals the epidermal nature of these primitive cells (175,366), although one must remember that cytokeratin positivity has been reported in rare lymphomas (113). Epithelial membrane antigen is a useful but not extremely reliable marker because of its frequent presence in anaplastic large cell lymphomas (115). On the other hand, the usual CD45 positivity of lymphoma has not been recorded to date in undifferentiated carcinoma, although CD30 staining may be seen with primitive epithelial neoplasms (49). Electron microscopy may also be of benefit in demonstrating the ultrastructural features that characterize the epithelial phenotype, i.e., desmosomes and tonofilaments (99). Although intercellular junctions are traditionally used to exclude the possibility of lymphoid malignancy, certain lymphoid neoplasms, particularly those of dendritic cells, may also possess them (48,103). Nevertheless, exceptions to the keratin and intercellular junction negativity of lymphomas are extremely uncommon, so that these features are generally of value in the diagnosis of undifferentiated carcinoma. Studies of EBV and immunoglobulin genomes via genetic probes can also be diagnostic (385).

As noted above, biologic studies of nasopharyngeal carcinoma have given much insight into its association with EBV. EBV is secreted by the nasal epithelium during an active infection, and it persists in the nuclei of these cells in a latent form in nasopharyngeal carcinoma (Fig. 12C) (341). The EBV antigen EBNA is now recognized as a complex of several different proteins. The production of one of these proteins, EBNA-1, appears to be critical for the maintenance of the virus in a latent state. Another EBV protein, latent membrane antigen 1 (LMP1), is found in the plasma membrane of tumors cells and can be demonstrated by immunohistochemistry (355). Transfection of the LMP1-associated gene into various normal and neoplastic cell lines causes phenotypic transformation and tumorigenicity, suggesting a role in tumor production (247). The analogous production of this protein in nasopharyngeal carcinoma cells has been hypothesized to be the cause of the undifferentiated phenotype commonly seen with this tumor. On the other hand, evidence of EBV infection is not found in the inflammatory cells that infiltrate this lesion (141). Polymeric IgA specific for EBV may promote entrance of the virus into epithelial cells and also neutralize its infectivity for B cells (342).

Other proteins and oncogenes have been studied in nasopharyngeal carcinoma cells. Grossly abnormal chromosomes may be seen in cytogenetic studies (106,207). Although the c-*myc* gene is not amplified or rearranged, it may be overexpressed (207). The retinoblastoma gene and *p53* may be similarly overexpressed (207,246). An association of the overexpression of tumor suppressor genes with EBV-encoded proteins is speculated but unproven at present. The cancer cells also release the soluble form of CD23, which may be used clinically as a tumor marker (309).

LESIONS OF THE JAWS

Lesions of the jaws of infants, children, and adolescents are noteworthy for their vast diversity, which encompasses both the epithelial and mesenchymal components of the tooth-forming organ. These range from common normal variants (dental lamina cysts or "Epstein's pearls") through rare and aggressive carcinomas and sarcomas. Discussion of the purely mesenchymal nonodontogenic lesions of the jaw, which tend to be more common in children (79), is found in Chapter 9. The following brief dissertation on these pediatric lesions will be limited to a consideration of the cystic, hamartomatous, and neoplastic odontogenic tumors that occur in patients less than 20 years of age. These are listed in Table 2. First, of note is that certain of these lesions may be associated with constitutional genetic disorders, as with the basal cell nevus syndrome, or with progressive transformation into a malignant state, as with the dentigerous cyst-ameloblastoma sequence. Second, although not discussed in this text, inflammatory lesions such as periapical cysts constitute the vast bulk of oral tumors, so that it behooves the surgical pathologist to be competent in the diagnosis of nonneoplastic cysts and granulomas of the jaw. Another group of lesions to consider in the diagnosis of oral cysts consists of the developmental cysts, such as the palatal cysts, which arise

TABLE 2. *Odontogenic lesions of the jaw in children*

Primordial cyst[a]
Odontogenic keratocyst
Calcifying odontogenic cyst
Dentigerous cyst–eruption cyst[b]
Dental lamina cyst of the newborn (Epstein's pearls)
Globulomaxillary cyst
Ameloblastoma
Calcifying epithelial odontogenic tumor
Adenomatoid odontogenic tumor
Ameloblastic fibroma
Ameloblastic fibro-odontoma
Odontoameloblastoma
Odontoma
Odontogenic myxoma
Odontogenic fibroma
Dentinoma
Cementoblastoma
Cementifying fibroma
Odontogenic carcinoma
Ameloblastic fibrosarcoma

[a] Considered by the World Health Organization to be a variant of the odontogenic keratocyst.

[b] Dentigerous cysts arise in bone; eruption cysts are identical tumors that arise in the soft tissue of the gingiva.

of myogenesis. They should also not be confused with a normal developing tooth, which may present histologically similar features but has sharp, even, convex margins with eosinophilic condensation. The potential for this mistake is commonplace because of the practice of removal of unerupted permanent teeth as part of pediatric oral or maxillofacial surgery. Other lesions in the category of predominantly mesenchymal odontogenic tumors include those with a more mature collagenous and vascular stroma (odontogenic fibroma), dentin production (dentinoma), cementum production (periapical cemental dysplasia and cementoblastoma), and resemblance to ossifying fibroma (cementifying fibroma).

SKIN

As with other lesions discussed in this chapter, malignant epithelial tumors of skin are relatively rare in children, especially when compared to their abundance in adults. However, benign hamartomatous melanocytic lesions arise almost universally in Caucasian children, and malignant melanomas are the second most common pediatric adult-type cancer, following thyroid carcinoma (285). Another facet comparable to pediatric epithelial malignancies of other sites is the existence of inherited conditions, such as xeroderma pigmentosa, basal cell nevus syndrome, neurofibromatosis type 1, Cowden's disease, and the familial atypical mole-melanoma (FAMM) syndrome, that predispose to tumor development at an early age.

As noted above, acquired and congenital melanocytic nevi are arguably the most common neoplasms/hamartomas occurring in children. Acquired melanocytic nevi progress through a predictable series of morphologic configurations, beginning with the intraepidermal junctional phase with its propensity for expansion and ending with the intradermal phase with its tendency to steady involution (55). This series of steps is analogous to the biologic progression of malignant melanoma, which commonly begins as an in situ epidermal lesion and progresses through horizontal and vertical expansion phases. The primary difference between the two lesions is the usual failure of the melanoma to involute but rather to gradually acquire genotypic and phenotypic characteristics related to tumor growth and spread (55). Melanomas may also arise secondarily from initially benign nevi that misprogram the sequence of steps leading to involution. These carcinogenic moles are usually junctional lesions, but melanomas may rarely develop in intradermal nevi (54,55). The sequence of steps in de novo carcinogenesis and malignant transformation of moles may be observed grossly (55), forming the primary strategy of successful treatment: excision of tumors at an early stage of development prior to lymphatic invasion. Nevertheless, caution is necessary in histologic assessment of childhood nevi, for they often look worse that they act. For example, pagetoid spread and mitotic activity do not always portend malignancy, particularly in infants (224). On the other hand, true melanomas occurring in children do not de facto exhibit a less aggressive behavior than those arising in adults (224). In fact, some authors have noted that children more often have nodular melanomas, which bypass the easily curable early stages of superficial spreading tumors (224).

During the development of a malignant melanoma, a preexisting nevus may assume a series of morphologic alterations analogous to those seen in the uterine cervix during carcinogenesis. Nevi with these features are termed "dysplastic nevi" or "nevi with atypical features" and are characterized by the following cytohistologic features: melanocytic nuclear pleomorphism and hyperchromatism, proliferation of irregularly oriented, basally situated melanocytes, elongation of affected rete ridges (termed "lentiginous dysplasia"), failure to form discrete nevus cell aggregates (or "theques"), and adjacent inflammation and fibrosis particularly seen next to elongated rete ridges (Fig. 16) (16,23,58,95,289). Mitotic activity, a feature of frank malignancy, should be minimal. Dysplastic nevi also have characteristic gross features that may be observed clinically (123). They arise as sporadically occurring lesions or as part of the FAMM syndrome. In the latter condition, patients typically present at an early age with large numbers of premalignant moles that can progress to malignant melanoma. Usually, FAMM patients have similarly affected family members, with some dying from metastatic melanoma (95). Dysplastic nevi have also been associated with neurofibromatosis (356) and Hodgkin's disease (377). The latter condition conversely may exacerbate the tendency to develop melanomas because of its associated deficiency in

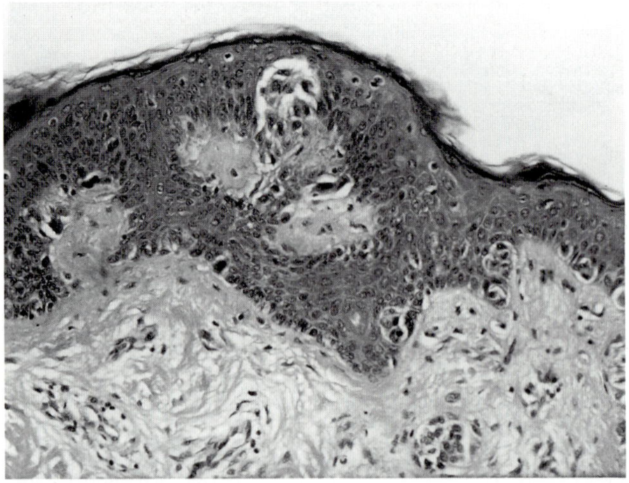

FIG. 16. Dysplastic nevus arising in familial atypical mole-melanoma (FAMM) patient previously treated for Hodgkin's disease. There are pleomorphic cells in irregular theques, associated with dermal fibrosis.

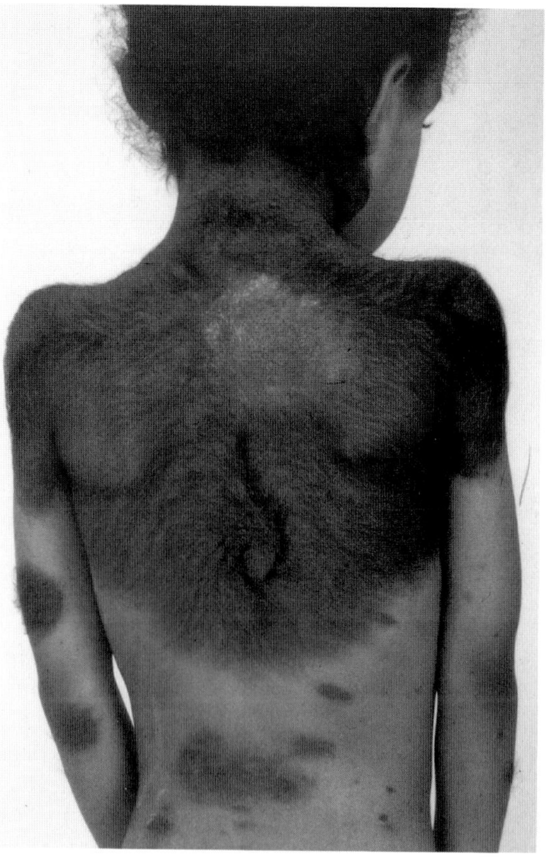

FIG. 17. Young girl with large, disfiguring, hairy, congenital nevus covering the upper back. (Courtesy of Dr. Alberto Pappo, St. Jude Children's Research Hospital.)

immune surveillance. Although the FAMM syndrome may be diagnosed in children and adolescents, the malignant lesions typically occur in older individuals, so that affected patients form only a small percentage of the melanomas seen in the juvenile age range (224). Nevertheless, the onset of puberty frequently heralds the development of dysplastic nevi in predisposed patients, suggesting a hormonal effect (123).

Malignant transformation of congenital nevi accounts for many examples of melanoma in pediatric series. Congenital nevi are often large, disfiguring hamartomatous lesions that cover a large proportion of the body surface. The term "bathing trunk" nevus is applied to those tumors circumferentially affecting the pelvis, back, upper thighs, and abdomen (Fig. 17). Affected patients may have multiple nevi over other portions of the body. Generally, about 1% of infants are born with a few small melanocytic nevi of uncertain malignant potential (396). The large bathing trunk lesions not only cause severe disfigurement but also may be sources of melanoma. Melanocytic overgrowth may also occur in the meninges as part of the neurocutaneous melanosis syndrome; these meningeal lesions also can develop as tumors (224) (see Chapter 7). A caveat worth remembering is that benign nevus cells may migrate to or arise in lymph nodes in affected patients and should not be mistaken for metastatic deposits (134,291). The premalignant status of small congenital nevi is controversial, but some recommend excision at an early age (396).

Microscopically, congenital nevi have a characteristic diffuse pattern of cellular distribution composed of small, dark nevus cells scattered throughout the dermis and organized into discrete subepidermal theques (Fig. 18). There may be a distinct association of congenital nevus cells with peripheral nerve twigs, and in fact these terminal neural ramifications may constitute the primordium from whence the lesional cells arise (68). This hypothesis is supported by the frequent observation of neural (or "neuroid") differentiation in portions of congenital nevi and by the hamartomatous melange of tissues often found in the deeper portions of these lesions (Fig. 19). These heterologous components may display

A

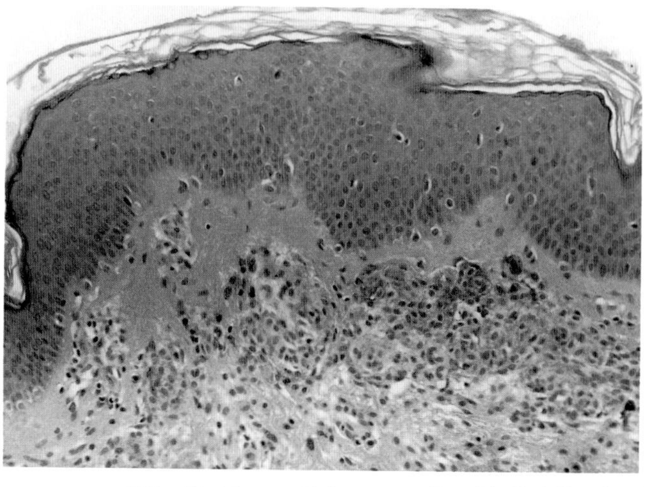

B

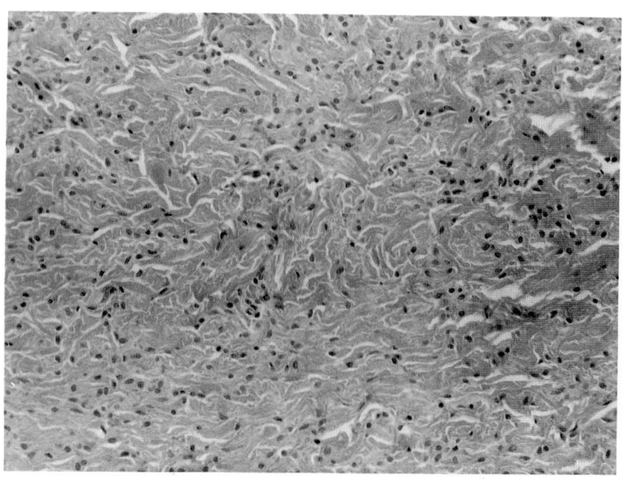

FIG. 18. Congenital nevus with with ill-defined subepidermal theques **(A)** and diffuse array of dermal melanocytes **(B)**.

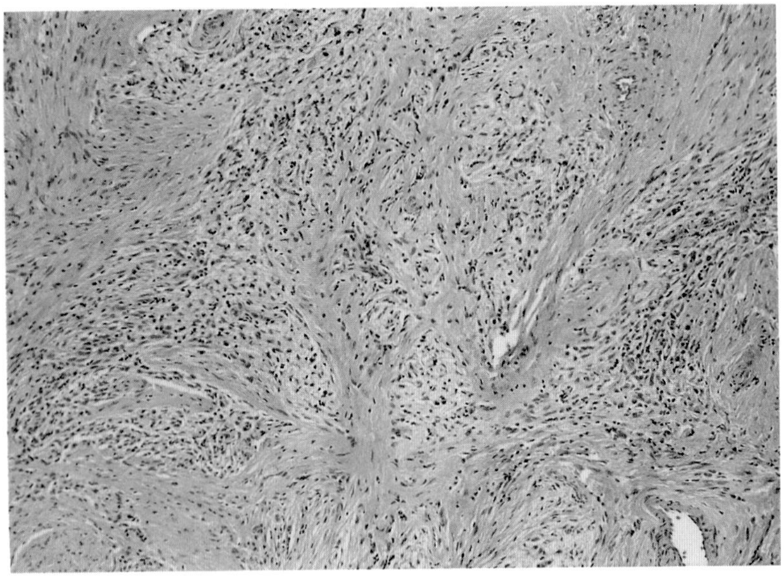

FIG. 19. Neuroectodermal hamartoma arising in the deep portion of a congenital nevus.

features of glia, Schwann cells, tactile corpuscles, neuroepithelium, and even cartilage and muscle (147).

From the primordium of a congenital nevus may arise dominant nodules and areas of increased pigmentation and rapid growth. These lesions are often biopsied to rule out evidence of malignant melanomatous transformation. Some of these nodules are truly malignant and give rise to metastases striking the death knell of the unfortunate patients, who are characteristically difficult to manage because of the wide shadow cast by their hamartomatous expanse. However, nodules that show nuclear pleomorphism and epidermal invasion may be clinically and biologically benign (Fig. 20) (214). These hyperplastic melanoma simulants typically do not show a discrete margination from the adjacent inactive nevus, and nodules that arise in the neonatal period do not appear to have the malignant potential of ones occurring in older patients (214).

Perhaps the most diagnostically perplexing pediatric melanocytic lesion is the spindle cell or Spitz nevus. This entity was established as a pathologic entity in 1948 by Dr. Sophie Spitz (350), who recognized that it histologically simulated melanoma but usually did not metastasize. These "juvenile melanomas," as they were initially called (the name was changed for obvious reasons), have a characteristic histologic pattern typified by spindle cell cytology, abutment to a hyperplastic epidermis, and maturation to more typical rounded melanocytes at the base (Fig. 21). The histologic architecture of these spindle cell lesions has been likened to a torrent of rain falling

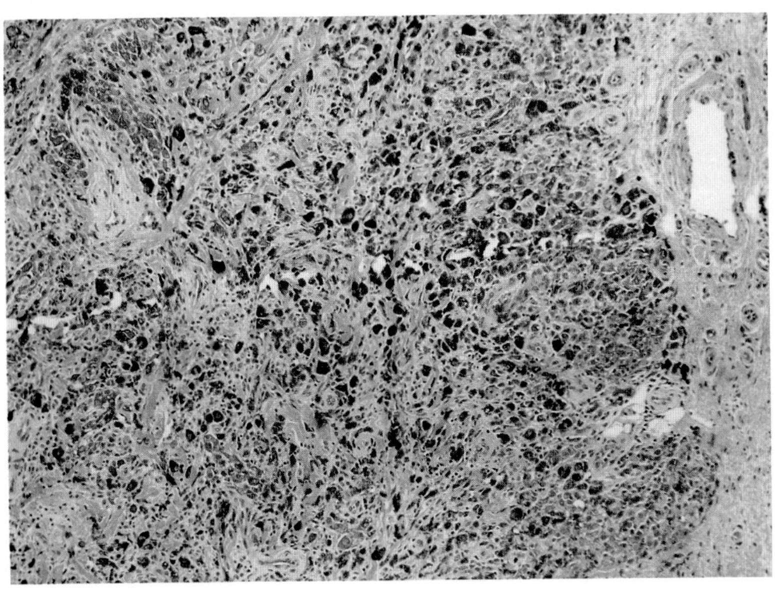

FIG. 20. Area of melanocytic hyperplasia in nodule arising in large congenital nevus. In spite of the marked pleomorphism and cellularity, the patient has suffered no recurrences.

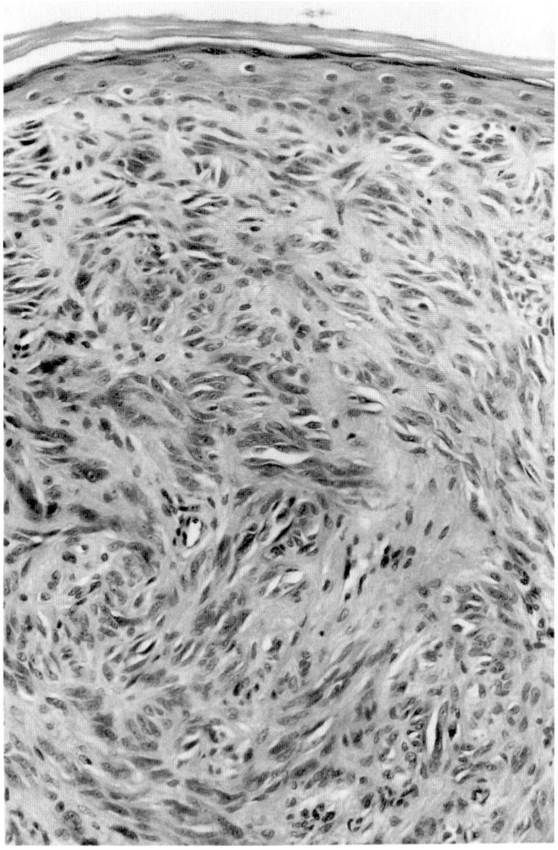

FIG. 21. Spitz nevus, with spindle cell melanocytes closely abutting the basal epidermis.

from the lower epidermis. Clinically they are usually non-pigmented pink papules similar to pyogenic granulomas (287), but pigmented variants also occur (15,314).

After Spitz's description of this lesion, it became apparent that the tumor cells could be epithelioid as well as spindle shaped and that some of these neoplasms behaved in a malignant fashion; in fact, one of the original cases subsequently metastasized. As a result, a disproportionately large number of studies have been published in an attempt to discern histologic features of spindle cell nevi that connote malignancy (15,270,314,344,388). These observations have been summarized in Table 3. In spite of all attempts at prognostication, the sad fact remains that a small percentage will metastasize in spite of their "benign" morphology, even following the assurances of pathology consultants. It has been stated that these "malignant" Spitz nevi only metastasize locally (344), but we have seen a fatal example with disseminated spread. Atypical heterogeneous immunohistochemical staining with HMB45 and S-100 is also a feature of Spitz nevi, as well as congenital and dysplastic nevi, but is not a marker of malignancy per se (260). Some cases of Spitz nevi display features of dysplastic nevi (15).

Biologic investigations of melanocytic tumors have often been as confusing as morphologic studies. For example, a vast of array of cytogenetic features have been described, but there are no universally recurring genetic anomalies. Nevertheless, genes on chromosomes 1, 6, 7, and 9 have been strongly incriminated in melanoma etiology (109). In particular, nonrandom rearrangements on 1p, 6p, 6q, and 7q (67) and the formation of marker chromosomes (267) are common events. Hyperdiploidy occurs in melanoma arising in giant congenital nevi (259). Naturally, the FAMM syndrome has been a prime target for genotypic analysis, but the results thus far indicate involvement of two separate loci on chromosomes 9p21 and 1p (188). The 9p21 gene is termed *MLM* and is also involved in the evolution of nonhereditary melanomas (188). The 9q21 location is also altered in other neoplasms such as brain tumors and leukemia, but the exact gene locus is currently unidentified (188). On the other hand, a number of other biologic indicators of malignant transformation have been well characterized. These include alterations of cell surface adhesion molecules such as integrins (74), which are affected as part of the sequence of events leading to loss of contact inhibition and acquisition of migratorial capability. The melanocytic cytoskeletal system also undergoes metamorphosis, with altered expression of intermediate filaments (11,22). Finally, melanomas undergoing malignant transformation are characterized by the usual disarray of growth factors, growth factor receptors, proto-oncogenes, and tumor suppressor genes (7,129,191) that affects tumor cells of other organs (62,389).

In contrast to melanomas, cutaneous basal cell and squamous cell carcinomas are very unusual in children, and their appearance always indicates the presence of an underlying genetic predisposition. In particular, xeroderma pigmentosa is typified by a tendency for the development of cutaneous malignancy, with melanomas occurring as well as epithelial cancer (60). These unfortunate patients are grossly disfigured by the multiplicity of the lesions, which occur as a result of a heightened sensitivity to the actinic rays of the sun (Fig. 22). The biologic basis for this condition has been well studied

TABLE 3. *Features of potential malignancy in Spitz nevi*

High mitotic rate
Lack of basal maturation
Increased cellularity
Loss of cellular cohesion
Large size
Ulceration
Plasma cells
Infiltrative lateral margins
High degree of pagetoid spread
Prominent epithelioid component
Marked pleomorphism and nuclear atypia
Atypical mitoses
Destruction of dermal collagen

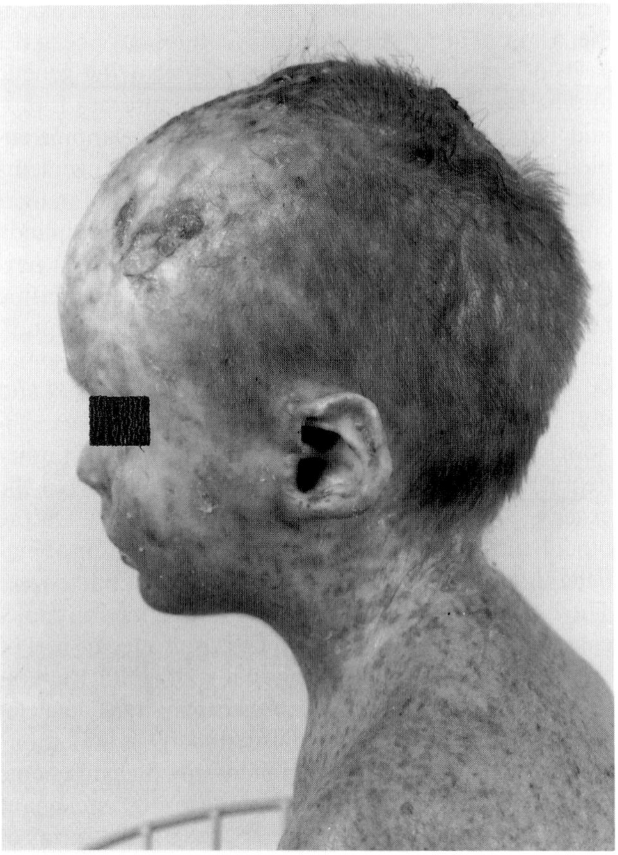

FIG. 22. Patient with xerodermal pigmentosa. There are myriads of actinic keratoses, and disfigurement from previously excised skin cancers is apparent.

(57,84,180,310,359) and is due to lack of repair enzymes that normally maintain the integrity of DNA strands adversely affected by electromagnetic radiation. Without these genetic handymen, abnormal strands of DNA arise from which critical tumor suppressor information has been deleted, resulting in tumorigenesis.

Basal cell nevus (Gorlin's) syndrome and Cowden's syndrome are also characterized by a predisposition for skin tumors. Basal cell nevus syndrome, as noted above, is associated with bony abnormalities, calcification of the falx cerebri, palmar pits, and odontogenic keratocysts as well as other tumors (170,349). The basal cell carcinomas seen in this condition are similar to those that arise in adults. They typically occur in crops on the face, neck, and back, but also commonly arise in nonexposed areas (170). There is a well-documented association with medulloblastoma (349), which is often diagnosed before the syndrome is recognized. Patients subsequently treated with craniospinal radiation give rise to crops of rapidly growing new skin lesions in port sites (Fig. 23; see figure in color plate section) (188). Using linkage analysis, a gene on chromosome 9q31 has been incriminated in the etiology of this disfiguring syndrome. Loss of heterozygosity for 9q is also common in these patients (188).

Facial trichilemmomas, tumors of the hair shaft apparatus, are a primary facet of Cowden's disease, which is also associated with a markedly increased risk of early onset breast carcinoma (30). These lesions typically appear on the face of adolescent females affected with the disorder (30). Desmoplastic trichoepitheliomas, similar benign tumors of the hair shaft, also show a peak incidence in adolescents and young adults (29). Again, most lesions appear on the face of young women, suggesting a relationship to Cowden's disease. Desmoplastic trichoepitheliomas have a morphealike appearance but should not be confused with basal cell carcinoma.

Cowden's disease is a rare autosomal dominant syndrome characterized by the occurrence of hamartomatous lesions in multiple organ sites (51,126,316,383). These widely diverse tumors are composed of tissues derived from ectodermal, mesodermal, and endodermal layers and are listed in Table 4. To date, investigations into a possible genetic or viral etiology for these lesions have proven unfruitful (352). On the other hand, immunologic studies have uncovered characteristic abnormalities in T-cell function (130). However, the relation of the immune system to the etiology of the disease is unknown at present.

TABLE 4. *Lesions reported in Cowden's disease*

Organ	Lesion
Skin	Fibromas, melanocytic lesions, keratoses, tricholemmomas
Soft tissues	Fibromas, lipomas, angiomyomas, lymphangiomas
Oral cavity	Papillomatosis, squamous hyperplasia
Gastrointestinal tract	Hyperplastic polyps, lipomas, angiomas, leiomyomas, fibromas
Brain	Cerebellar hypertrophy (Lhermitte–Duclos disease), meningiomas
Thyroid gland	Multinodular goiter, adenoma
Breast	Fibrocystic disease, carcinoma
Ovary	Cysts
Eye	Retinal gliomas, lens drusens, choroidal hamartomas, conjunctival papillomas
Kidney	Adenoangiomyolipoma, carcinoma
Skeleton	Craniomegaly, pathologic fracture
Lung	Hamartoma

BREAST

Although breast diseases are considered to be unusual diseases in children and adolescents, they occur more frequently than is commonly realized. However, most mammary gland problems encountered in juveniles are physiologic rather than neoplastic, so that relatively few specimens are seen by pathologists (12). Breast tumors reported in children are listed in Table 5. Fibroadenomas are by far the most common neoplasms in adolescent girls [>90% (12,253)] and are characterized by their sharply circumscribed margins and intermingling of benign-appearing ductal and fibrous elements. Seemingly from time immortal, medical students have been asked to memorize the pericanalicular and intracanalicular patterns of this histology, but in fact this distinction totally lacks clinical relevance (304). Of more importance is the amount of stroma relative to the epithelial tissue and the degree of atypia in the mesenchymal component, for these features distinguish fibroadenoma from the cystosarcoma phyllodes, a potentially malignant lesion. Fibroadenomas also frequently contain fibrocystic elements such as sclerosing adenosis, and it is also important not to confuse these features with invasive carcinoma, particularly on frozen section (304). Rarely, an in situ lesion such as intraductal or intralobular carcinoma may arise in these tumors (82), but this phenomenon usually occurs in adults. Squamous metaplasia and smooth muscle cells may also be noted, and infarction is not an uncommon event in pregnancy, when lactational changes may radically alter the morphology of fibroadenomas.

In occasional cases of fibroadenomas occurring in young girls, one may see rapid growth and even multiple tumors, particularly in blacks (304). These "juvenile fibroadenomas" present a worrisome microscopic appearance, with intraductal hyperplasia and epithelial atypia resembling in situ carcinoma. However, the stromal cell element should be benign-appearing and does not overwhelm the epithelial element as in cystosarcoma, and the tumor should maintain its sharp circumscription. It is important not to overdiagnose these cases and to preserve as much breast tissue as possible at surgery.

TABLE 5. *Breast tumors in children*

Fibroadenoma
Juvenile
Giant
Juvenile papillomatosis
Ductal papilloma/papillary duct hyperplasia
Cystosarcoma phylloides
Benign
Malignant
Secretory carcinoma
Malignant lymphoma
Inflammatory carcinoma
Poorly differentiated adenocarcinoma
Capillary hemangioma
Rhabdomyosarcoma
Angiosarcoma

When examining rapidly growing breast masses, one should also consider the possibility of cystosarcoma phyllodes. Grossly the epithelial component of these often huge tumors typically produces clefts and polypoid areas with a leaflike pattern; hence the name "phyllodes" (Greek for "leaflike"). Microscopically there is overgrowth of the stromal tissues, which show varying degrees of atypia and increased cellularity and mitotic activity as compared to fibroadenomas (Fig. 24). Production of heterologous elements such as bone, cartilage, and skeletal muscle is not uncommon; these tissues may predominate in metastases, which are typically pulmonary and rarely lymphatic. Cystosarcomas have been graded by a variety of features, including mitotic index, cellularity, nuclear atypia, peripheral stromal overgrowth, necrosis, and amount of heterologous elements (12,304). However, even apparently low-grade tumors may metastasize. Determination of ploidy and S-phase analysis is of doubtful prognostic significance (181). These tumors are rare in pediatrics; of overriding importance is not to confuse them with "giant" fibroadenomas, with which they have been lumped in several publications (12).

Breast carcinomas are very rare in children (386). As noted above, they may be associated with familial cancer syndromes such as the Lynch syndrome, the Li–Fraumeni syndrome, and Cowden's disease. One of the first studies of pediatric breast cancer was that of McDivitt and Stewart at Memorial Hospital (218). The most remarkable histologic feature of the lesions was the large amount of PAS- and mucin-positive material contained within the cytoplasm and lumina of the tumor cells (Fig. 25). This material at times gave the tumors the appearance of clear cell carcinomas such as occur in the kidney. Also, there was an excellent clinical outcome; only one patient suffered nodal metastasis and none expired in spite of often limited resections. These tumors were initially named "juvenile carcinomas," but it later became apparent that similar lesions arose more often in adults (254); hence the current term "secretory carcinoma." Histologically these lesions are basically intraductal carcinomas with invasive elements; by electron microscopy the clear cell appearance is created by large intracytoplasmic vacuoles lined by microvilli (304). Apocrine differentiation may also be seen. The tumors are curable by limited excision, with sparing of normal developing breast tissue.

Another breast lesion that is typically encountered in adolescents is juvenile papillomatosis (301,302). This uncommon lesion is characterized by the formation of a prominent multicystic component that is grossly evi-

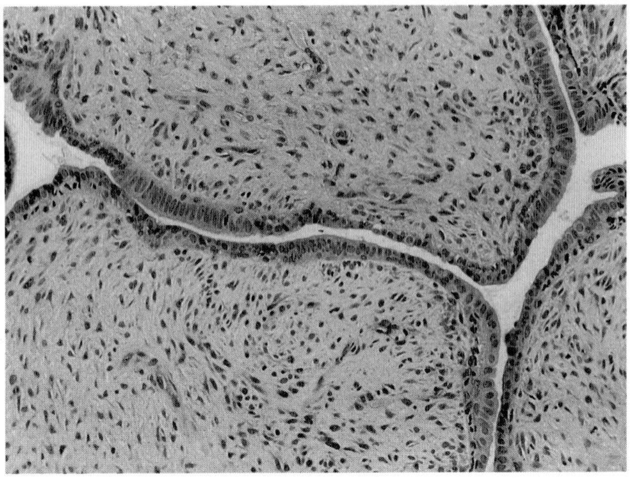
A

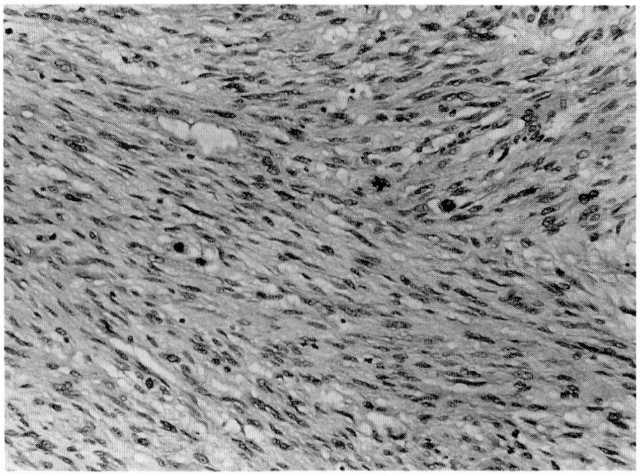
B

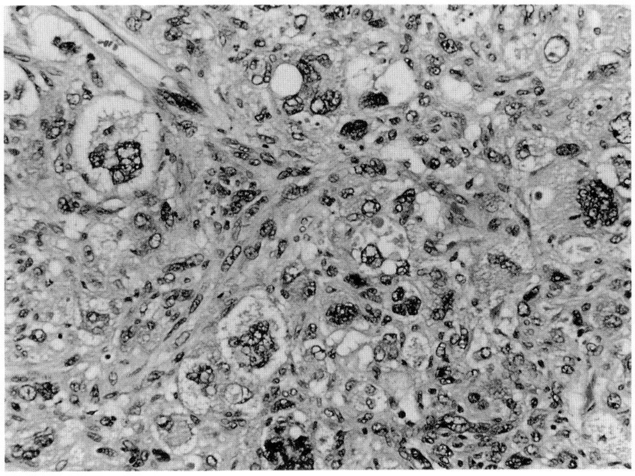
C

FIG. 24. Malignant cystosarcoma phyllodes arising in the breast of an adolescent female. There are areas containing intermingled epithelial and stromal elements **(A)** and areas resembling fibrosarcoma **(B)** and high-grade pleomorphic-storiform malignant fibrous histiocytoma **(C)**.

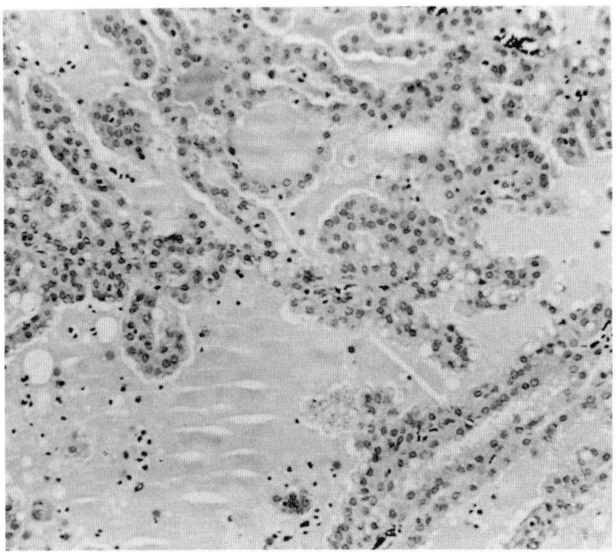

FIG. 25. Secretory carcinoma of breast. Tumor cells form papillary clusters separated by abundant extracellular secretions. A "bubbly" cytoplasm is apparent. (From Rosen PP, Cranor ML. *Arch Pathol Lab Med* 1991;115:141–145. Permission granted by the American Medical Association and the senior author.)

dent; hence the synonym "Swiss cheese disease" (Fig. 26). Microscopically, epithelial hyperplasia is present in a combination of papillomatosis, sclerosing adenosis, and apocrine metaplasia, with associated duct stasis. Severe epithelial atypia and necrosis may cause the microscopist to consider a diagnosis of cancer, but these are benign lesions that are usually cured by limited excision. However, there is a high incidence of familial breast carcinoma in affected patients, and a number of these women have also had coexisting or subsequent malignancy (303). As a result, it behooves the clinician to prepare the patient for long-term clinical follow-up, but preventive mastectomy or psychologic devastation is unwarranted. Epithelial hyperplasia and papillomatosis of the usual type also may occur in juveniles, but these lesions do not carry the same premalignant significance (300).

Besides juvenile papillomatosis and Cowden's disease, a familial risk for early onset breast carcinoma is associated with alterations in the tumor suppressor gene *p53* and the associated Li–Fraumeni syndrome (61,338) (see Chapter 5). The protein product of this gene appears to bind with the protein produced by the *MDM2* (murine

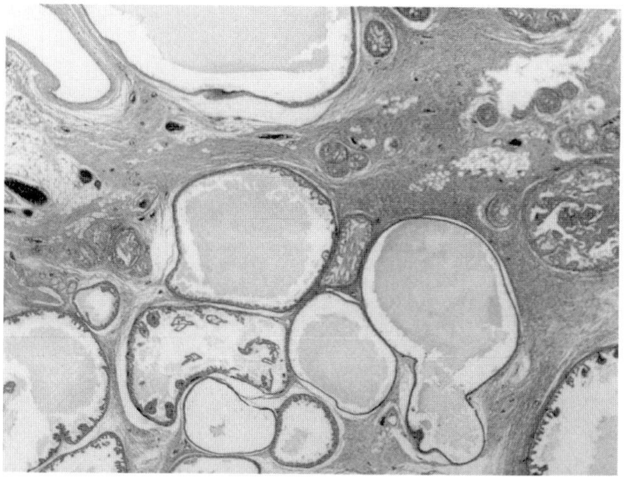

FIG. 26. Juvenile papillomatosis of the breast. There is marked ductular dilatation, creating a low-power resemblance to Swiss cheese. (Courtesy of Dr. Peter Rosen, Memorial Sloan-Kettering Cancer Center, New York, NY)

double- minute 2) gene in a negative regulatory fashion (335). *MDM2* expression is in turn modulated by estrogen, which thus may orchestrate its growth stimulatory effects on breast carcinoma cells by indirectly inactivating p53 (335). *p53* mutations also frequently occur in sporadic breast carcinomas (61) but do not account for all cases of familial tumors (279). Nevertheless, overexpression of *p53* is associated with high-grade, aggressive breast tumors and decreased patient survival (169). *p53* mutations most commonly occur in breast carcinomas with a medullary histology (215); this tumor type is also more frequent in younger (<40 years) familial breast cancer patients (56).

GENITOURINARY TRACT

Ovaries

Pediatric ovarian neoplasms are rare. There were only 43 ovarian neoplasms identified in the 220,934 admissions to the Children's Hospital of Michigan from 1947 to 1973. Of these, only 8 were malignant (5). Lindfors (208) reported an incidence of pediatric ovarian neoplasms in Finland and Sweden of only 2.6 cases per 100,000 per year. The relative frequency of malignancy of pediatric ovarian neoplasms is estimated to range from about 20% to 67%, but the average figure is considered to be about 35% (27). The frequency of malignancy is significantly higher in solid ovarian neoplasms.

Not surprisingly, the incidence of pediatric ovarian neoplasms increases with age. Norris and Jensen (252) reported that the incidence of pediatric ovarian neoplasms doubles every 5 years from birth to 19 years of age: 5% of childhood ovarian tumors occur at 0–4 years, 10% at 5–9 years, 23% at 10–14 years, and 62% at 15–19 years. Malignant pediatric ovarian neoplasms have a similar incidence with age: 14% at 0–4 years, 25% at 5–9 years, and 61% at 10–15 years. In the National Cancer Institute's SEER program (229), there were less than 62 primary pediatric ovarian carcinomas reported from 1973 to 1982. This corresponds to a rate of about 1.3 per 1 million population.

Surface epithelial ovarian neoplasms are extremely uncommon in the very young and are more likely to be benign than overtly malignant. The combined results of five clinical studies of pediatric/adolescent ovarian neoplasms and cysts show that of 191 tabulated cases there were only 12 surface epithelial neoplasms. Six of these tumors were malignant. Conversely, there were 152 germ cell tumors, 23 of which were malignant (283). There is a well-known relationship between age and types of pediatric ovarian neoplasms: germ cell tumors are especially more common in the prepubertal age group, whereas surface epithelial tumors are much more frequent in postpubertal patients, accounting for almost one third of the pediatric ovarian neoplasms in the 15- to 19-year-old age group (252).

Surface Epithelial Tumors

The recent WHO classification of ovarian neoplasms divides surface epithelial neoplasms of the ovary into serous, mucinous, transitional, endometrial, and clear cell types. These tumors can be further classified into benign, borderline, and malignant (328). The benign tumors generally display little or no epithelial proliferation, stratification, mitotic activity, or nuclear pleomorphism. If a noninvasive surface epithelial tumor unequivocally displays at least two of these criteria, then it is best designated a borderline neoplasm (311). Overt stromal invasion by the tumor cells places the lesion into the carcinoma category. Mucinous and serous carcinomas are essentially unheard of before the age of 9 years (198), although one serous carcinoma has been reported in a 4-year-old (156). It is important for the pathologist to carefully and extensively section borderline surface epithelial tumors so that a correct diagnosis can be made and to not overinterpret benign intrusion (so-called pseudoinvasion) (312). Borderline serous and mucinous surface epithelial tumors are more frequently seen in children and rarely may be associated with peritoneal implants (120,198). Endometrial, clear cell, and transitional tumors are even rarer in children than serous and mucinous tumors. There have been rare pediatric examples of these neoplasms.

Juvenile Granulosa Cell Tumors

Sex cord stromal tumors account for about 13–14% of all pediatric ovarian neoplasms (5). One half or more are associated with endocrine hormone production (5). Juvenile granulosa cell tumors account for almost half of the sex cord stromal tumors of the pediatric/adolescent age group. They differ from adult granulosa cell tumors not only by virtue of their occurrence before puberty but also by their histologic features. A large study of juvenile granulosa cell tumors showed that 97% of these tumors occurred in the first three decades and usually resulted in isosexual pseudoprecocity, with prepubertal breast development, axillary hair growth, clitoral enlargement, stimulation and enlargement of other external and internal secondary sex organs, vaginal discharge, and irregular uterine bleeding. Galactorrhea is a rare endocrine manifestation. Accelerated bone or somatic growth may be an associated finding (197,406). Other associations include Ollier's disease, Maffucci's syndrome, infantile dysmorphism, and ambiguous genitalia (198).

Juvenile granulosa cell tumors are usually large neoplasms, averaging about 12 cm (21,197,406), so that they are typically palpable on examination and may also cause abdominal distension, pain, or ascites. A few cases have ruptured before or during surgery (198). Grossly, juvenile granulosa cell tumors may be solid and/or cystic and are bilateral in 2% of affected patients (406). The cut surface is mostly gray or gray–tan, and there usually is a well-developed capsule. Parenchymal hemorrhage, both remote and/or recent, may be present (Fig. 27).

Histologically, juvenile granulosa cell tumors generally exhibit a solid diffuse growth pattern with a lesser follicular component. However, uniformly solid or follicular microscopic patterns may be seen (Fig. 28) (406). The follicles are usually anisomorphic and pleomorphic but may be regular and round (405). The lumina contain eosinophilic or basophilic material that is usually mucin-positive. The follicles are lined by granulosa cells that occasionally may be encompassed by theca cells (405). Solid areas may be punctuated with nodules of granulosa cells with intervening theca cells (198). Rarely theca cells predominate over granulosa cells in the solid diffuse areas. Juvenile granulosa cell tumors have cytologic characteristics not shared by their adult counterparts, as they usually do not exhibit nuclear grooves and have luteinized features, with large amounts of lipid-rich or eosinophilic cytoplasm and nuclear hyperchromasia. The theca cell component is also luteinized with lipid-rich cytoplasm. Juvenile granulosa cell tumors may display nuclear atypia with increased mitoses, sometimes >3 per 10 high-power fields (406). They may simulate small cell carcinoma, clear cell carcinoma, undifferentiated carcinoma, and metastatic neoplasms (especially malignant melanoma) (405). Clinical history, microscopic features, special stains (eg, mucicarmine), immunohistochemistry, and electron microscopy can usually resolve the diagnosis.

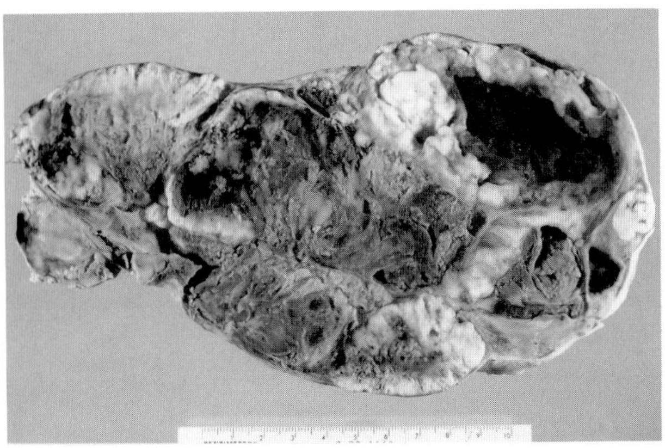

FIG. 27. Juvenile granulosa cell tumor of the ovary. A large, lobulated, well-encapsulated mass contains broad areas of hemorrhage and necrosis.

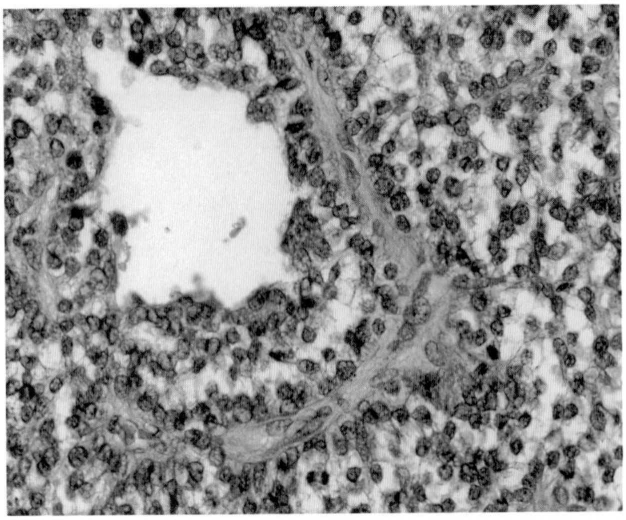

FIG. 28. Juvenile granulosa cell tumor of the ovary. Both solid and cystic areas are apparent and are composed of tumor cells with clear cytoplasm.

Ultrastructurally, juvenile granulosa cell tumors show luteinized features, especially in cells in the periphery of the microscopic nodules. Their cytoplasm is replete with smooth endoplasmic reticulum, mitochondria with tubular cristae, and large lipid droplets suggesting steroidogenesis (21). Another study has shown features of luteinization in rare cells intermediate between granulosa cell and theca cells in juvenile granulosa cell tumors but a paucity of luteinizing features in well-defined granulosa and theca cells (307).

In spite of the sometimes ominous histologic features of juvenile granulosa cell tumors, the majority behave in a benign fashion. Usually the tumors are stage I at the time of diagnosis and are cured by unilateral salpingo-oophorectomy (197). Conversely, Sifversward's study (339) indicated that although 91% of 192 patients had stage I disease at presentation, 25% (42 patients) died from tumor progression. However, juvenile granulosa cell tumors present an excellent prognosis in most studies (21,197,406).

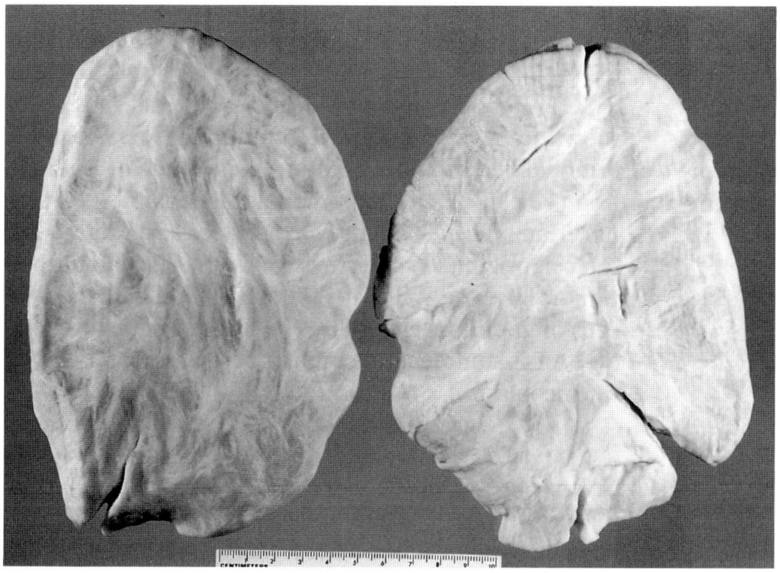

FIG. 29. Fibroma of ovary of adolescent female. There is a firm, fibrous-appearing, homogeneous cut surface.

Juvenile granulosa cell tumors have a characteristic karyotypic abnormality, i.e., trisomy 12. This chromosomal aberration has been identified in other stromal cell tumors such as fibromas, thecomas, fibrothecomas, and adult granulosa cell tumors (108,322).

Fibromas and Thecomas

Ovarian fibromas and thecomas are much more common in adults than in children. The exception is luteinized thecomas, which have conspicuous rather than occasional foci of luteinized cells, occur in nonpregnant females, and are more common in the younger age group than typical thecomas or fibromas (420).

Ovarian fibromas are closely associated with basal cell nevus syndrome (122). Many and possibly all of these female subjects have ovarian fibromas that are usually multinodular and calcified (34). This syndrome has a well-known proclivity for many different types of benign and malignant neoplasms in both the pediatric and adult populations (see above). Pediatric ovarian fibromas may also occur sporadically and in one instance have been inherited through four successive generations (92).

The distinction between fibromas and thecomas may be nebulous. Fibromas are usually solid, well circumscribed, and firm with a gray–white external and cut surface (Fig. 29). Histologically, the tumor usually has a fascicular pattern bestowed by constituent spindle cells arrayed in bundles. There may be small foci of luteinized cells. Ovarian myxomas and massive ovarian edema (Fig. 30) may be difficult to distinguish from a fibroma that is edematous and has a myxoid stroma (93,177, 370). Some of these tumors may be more cellular with increased mitoses. Prat and Scully (273) found that cellular fibromas usually behave in a benign fashion if the mitotic index is <3 mitoses per 10 high-power fields, whereas those with a higher count usually have a malignant course and should be called fibrosarcomas. Of note is that of the 17 cases studied by Prat and Scully, the 3 adolescent patients had cellular fibromas with no evidence of recurrent disease, whereas 6 of 14 adults had ovarian fibrosarcomas. Most of the fibrosarcomas exhibited marked cellular and nuclear pleomorphism.

Most thecomas differ from fibromas by the fact that they usually contain lipid that imparts a focally to diffusely yellow to orange cut surface. Again, there are interlacing bundles of spindle cells giving a fascicular appearance. However, it may be impossible to differentiate

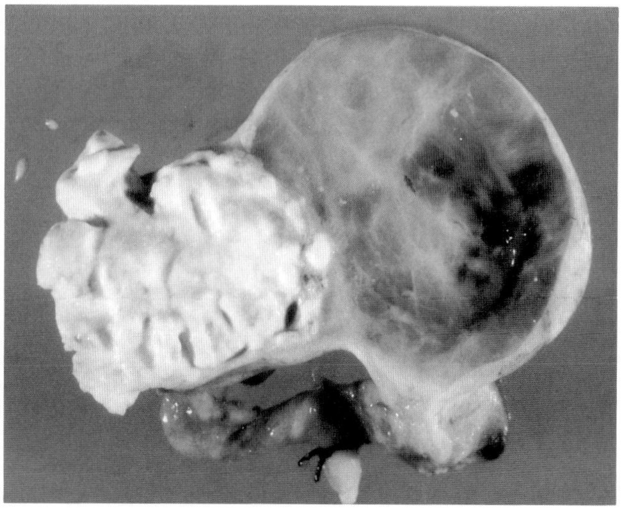

FIG. 30. Massive ovarian edema. This lesion was excised because it appeared as a pelvic mass evident several weeks following oophexy. The apparent cause was lymphatic obstruction. There is a large corpus luteum on the left side of the photograph.

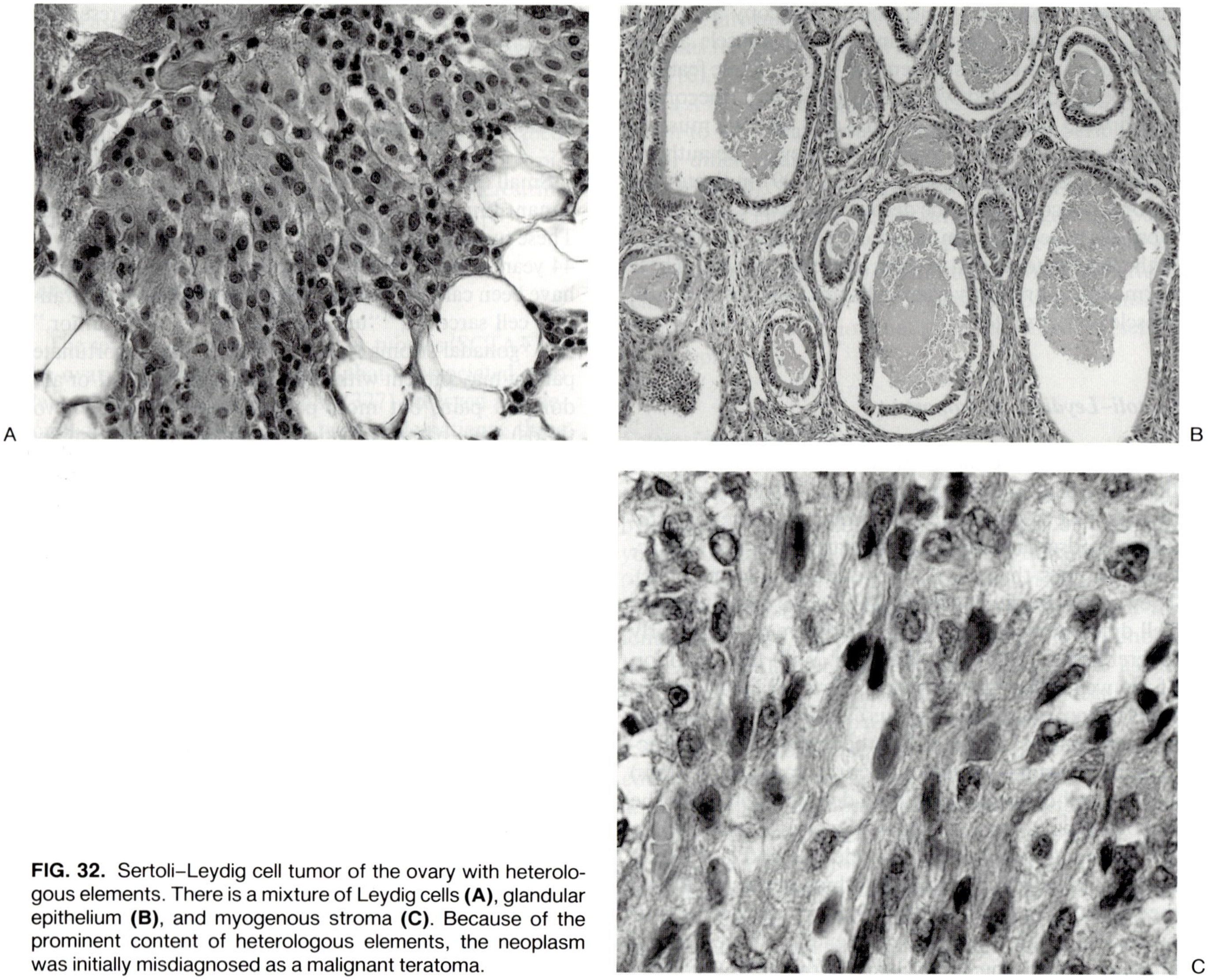

FIG. 32. Sertoli–Leydig cell tumor of the ovary with heterologous elements. There is a mixture of Leydig cells **(A)**, glandular epithelium **(B)**, and myogenous stroma **(C)**. Because of the prominent content of heterologous elements, the neoplasm was initially misdiagnosed as a malignant teratoma.

Immunohistochemistry has been utilized not only to aid in identification of ovarian small cell carcinoma but also to ascertain its histogenesis. Most tumors display reactivity for various cytokeratins, supporting an epithelial origin. Many stain for vimentin but not as profoundly as for cytokeratin. Epithelial membrane antigen staining has also been reported (198,329). Generally immunostaining for parahormone-related peptide is negative, but positive staining has been rarely reported (329). Even though extensive ultrastructural and immunocytochemical studies have been done, the histogenesis of this lesion remains an enigma.

Equally frustrating has been the prognosis of ovarian small cell carcinoma. Even early stage tumors have a dismal prognosis. Ironically, DNA studies have demonstrated diploidy and no aneuploidy (329). The survival rate is approximately 30% for stage 1A tumors and only about 10% overall. The tumors may be radiosensitive and/or chemosensitive (329). Combination radiation therapy/chemotherapy has occasionally succeeded in producing a partial or complete response (198). Scully (329) suggests that treatment with newer chemotherapeutic agents and radiation may improve clinical outcome.

These lesions should not be confused with other small cell tumors that occur in the ovary, namely, dysgerminoma, lymphoma/leukemia (46,258), metastatic alveolar rhabdomyosarcoma (413), or desmoplastic small cell tumor (407).

Cervix and Vagina

Epidermoid carcinoma of the cervix usually results from sexual activity and generally arises from a slowly progressive intraepithelial lesion that passes through a well-defined series of cytologic stages. As such this tumor is essentially unheard of in children, but an in situ lesion

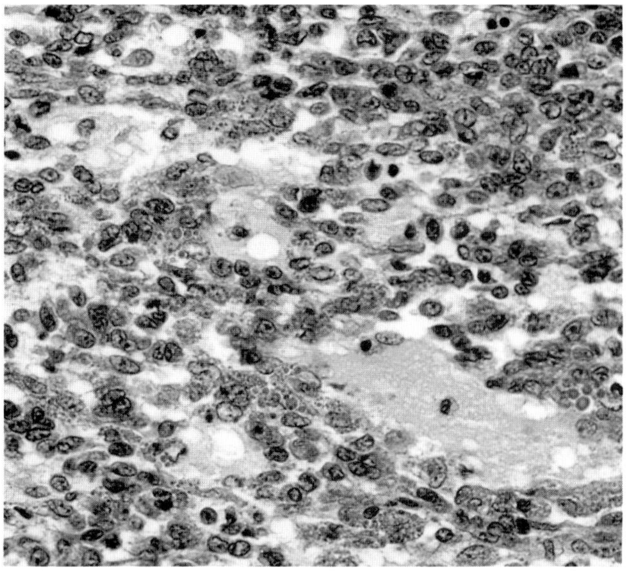

FIG. 33. Small cell carcinoma arising in the ovary of an adolescent female with hypercalcemia. The tumor is composed of primitive cells with vague epithelial features. There are scattered hyaline droplets.

in a 15-year-old girl was reported by Hadju et al. in 1968 (128). Of far more importance in pediatrics is the recognition of the botryoid rhabdomyosarcoma, a malignant lesion of young children, and its congener, the genital rhabdomyoma, a benign tumor that can occur in adolescents (see Chapter 5). These neoplasms aside, the most important pediatric neoplasm of the vagina and cervix is the clear cell adenocarcinoma, which is associated with maternal exposure to diethylstilbestrol (153) and which usually occurs between the ages of 14 and 25 years (294).

The primary effect of diethylstilbestrol ingestion in pregnant females occurs in the developing vagina of the female conceptus (153). This teratogenic stimulus is manifested in a number of minor congenital anomalies that includes vaginal and cervical erosion, ridges, hoods, and coxscombs. Of note is that clear cell adenocarcinomas unassociated with maternal steroid ingestion may also be accompanied by congenital anomalies such as double uterus and vagina or unilateral renal agenesis (251). This association indicates that a variety of untoward influences on Müllerian development may precipitate both vaginal anomalies and neoplasms.

The second teratogenic effect of maternal diethylstilbestrol use is the inappropriate occurrence of tuboendometrial glands in the cervix and vagina, histopathologic lesions known as cervical ectropion and vaginal adenosis, respectively. These misplaced glandular elements are the soil from whence arises clear cell adenocarcinoma, as adenosis exhibits a progressive glandular atypia that is associated with the development of these neoplasms (295).

Grossly, clear cell carcinomas are generally exophytic,

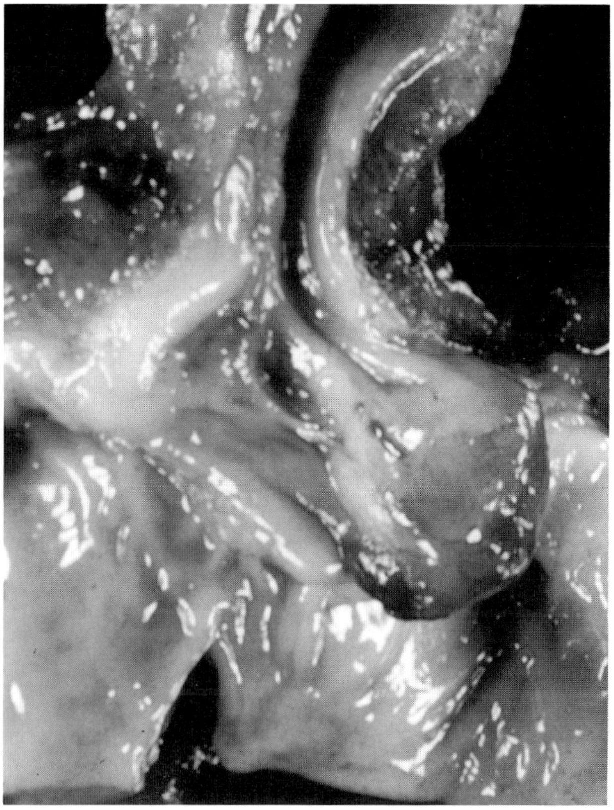

FIG. 34. Clear cell adenocarcinoma of the uterine cervix. A glistening polypoid mass protrudes from the cervical os.

friable lesions that project from the cervix or vagina (Fig. 34); rare examples may be endophytic (251). Histologically these neoplasms are composed of large, polyhedral, clear cells that line papillae, microcysts, and tubules (Fig. 35). The cells lining the papillae typically project outward in a "hobnail" fashion. Psammoma bodies or endometrioid features may be present (251). Adjacent to

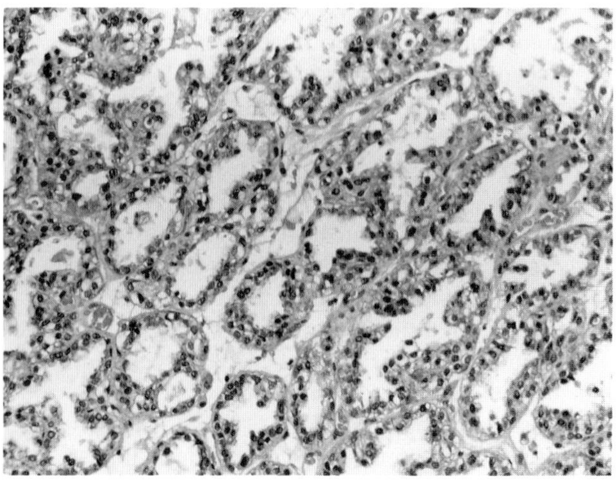

FIG. 35. Clear cell adenocarcinoma of the uterine cervix. The tumor is composed of glands lined by cells with clear cytoplasm.

the adenocarcinoma one typically finds vaginal adenosis that often presents atypical cytologic features (295).

Clear cell adenocarcinoma is locally invasive and capable of lymphatic and vascular metastasis. Pelvic lymph node metastases may be found in approximately one sixth of patients, and recurrences often occur in the lungs or supraclavicular lymph nodes (294). Fortunately, most tumors are discovered early, so that the overall 5-year survival rate is high, particularly with stage I lesions. However, late recurrences are well recognized, so that long-term follow-up is necessary (294).

Two cervicovaginal lesions may easily be confused with clear cell adenocarcinoma; these are microglandular hyperplasia and yolk sac tumor. Microglandular hyperplasia is a benign, tumorlike condition that like clear cell adenocarcinoma may be associated with maternal diethylstilbestrol ingestion, but more commonly it is seen in patients on long-term contraceptive use or during pregnancy. Histologically, microglandular hyperplasia differs from clear cell carcinoma in that the glandular elements are lined by mucinous epithelium, sometimes with squamous metaplasia that may be cytologically misleading (294,414).

Yolk sac tumor rarely occurs in the vagina and cervix (66). It typically arises in young females less than 3 years of age, in contradistinction to the usual appearance of clear cell carcinoma during adolescence. The histologic features of this tumor are described in Chapter 10. Because it is often composed of glandlike spaces, yolk sac carcinoma can resemble clear cell carcinoma. Immunohistochemistry using antibodies against α-fetoprotein and CD15 (Leu M1) have been utilized to make the distinction (421), but both tumors may react with both markers, leading to additional confusion.

Testes

As with the ovaries, the great majority of pediatric testicular neoplasms are germ cell tumors. However, tumors of gonadal stroma are relatively frequent in infants and children and constitute about 19% of their testicular neoplasms (236). They present histologic and clinical features that are entirely analogous to the ovarian neoplasms discussed in the preceding section of this chapter. Even surface epithelial neoplasms such as cystadenomas and cystadenocarcinomas have been reported in the testes of children (412). Juvenile granulosa cell tumors may occur in the infantile testes (200) and may be associated with sexual ambiguity (284,408). Leydig cell tumors occur in an older age group and cause macrogenitosomia and isosexual pseudoprecocity (184,236); these tumors constitute the most common group of testicular sex cord stromal tumors (415). Other stromal tumors may cause gynecomastia or occur as part of the Peutz–Jeghers syndrome (184,236). Leydig cell tumor–like masses may occur in patients with adrenogenital syndromes (415). Other masses occurring in the testes of children and adolescents include epidermoid cysts (332), cystic dysplasia (415), and inflammatory lesions. Hematologic neoplasms are the most common type of primary testicular cancer in older men but are almost always secondary lesions in children (415). Metastases from pediatric tumors such as neuroblastoma or retinoblastoma can also involve the testes (140).

Of particular note is a distinctive Sertoli cell tumor of the testes that predominately occurs in pediatric patients. This lesion is called the "large cell calcifying Sertoli cell tumor" (278,387) because of the presence of variable amounts of intratumoral calcification and the size of the constituent cells. Calcification can be massive and may occur in laminated masses. The tumor cells contain abundant, finely granular, eosinophilic cytoplasm and superficially resemble Leydig cells. However, they occur within adjacent seminiferous tubules as well as the main tumor, and they do not contain Reinke crystals. The cells form nests, cords, and trabeculae separated by a myxomatous to collagenous stroma. Charcot–Böttcher crystalloids, typical of Sertoli cells, have been observed with electron microscopy (387). Large cell calcifying Sertoli cell tumors may be bilateral or multifocal and can occur as a component of a complex endocrine disorder or as familial tumors associated with cardiac myxoma (278).

Urinary Tract

By 1989 fewer than 125 cases of malignant urothelial tumors had been reported to affect the urinary bladders of children. Typically they were solitary, low-grade, low-stage lesions with a low rate of recurrence (326). Conversely, the pediatric bladder cancer reported by Scott et al. (326) was a high-grade, aggressive neoplasm. Genetic analysis of this lesion surprisingly showed a diploid chromosome number by flow cytometry and a reciprocal t(17;22) and a nonreciprocal t(18;22) by karyotyping. This tumor type could conceivably be the source of putative extrarenal rhabdoid tumors reported in the renal pelvis, prostate, and bladder (94,137,158,193).

SECOND MALIGNANCIES

The American Cancer Society has indicated that the 5-year relative survival rates for all childhood cancers under the age of 15 has increased dramatically between 1960 and 1990, the percentages ranging from 28% in 1960–1963 to 68% in 1990–1993 (397). During this 30-year period there have been dramatic increases in the proportion of patients surviving with acute lymphoblastic leukemia (from 4% to approximately 73%), acute myeloid leukemia (3–28%), Wilms' tumor (38–88%), brain tumors (35–60%), neuroblastoma (25–57%), bone and joint tumors (20–59%), Hodgkin's disease (52–90%), and non-Hodgkin's lymphomas (18–70%). Approximately 1,600 cancer-related deaths in children aged 1–14 continue to occur per annum and represent 10% of all deaths in this group. Comparatively, accidents account for approximately 40% of all childhood deaths.

Besides prolonging survival and yielding higher cure rates, the continued improvement in the treatment of childhood cancer has increased our awareness of the late effects of therapy. These late effects may not appear for a decade or more after the completion of cancer treatment (255). The most serious side effects have been the development of second malignant neoplasms, which may be attributed to the effects of radiation, antineoplastic drugs, or both (143). Specific gene mutations, some inherited in an autosomal dominant manner, greatly increase the risk of second malignancies (50,204).

Estimating the risk of secondary cancers after successful treatment of primary neoplasms has become the subject of numerous publications (136). Tucker (374) reviewed the risk of development of bone sarcomas related to prior radiation and chemotherapy for childhood cancer and noted a 2.74-fold risk in patients receiving prior irradiation, with a sharp dose–response reaching a 40-fold risk after doses of more than 6,000 rad. In the late 1960s the Late Effects Study Group (LESG) was organized to evaluate the effects of oncotherapy on cancer survivors. This group and others (257,368) have provided useful information on the incidence and characteristics of second malignant neoplasms. Most of their reports have categorized second malignancies that have followed retinoblastoma and Hodgkin's disease (220). Adequate second-tumor treatment particularly has been limited by prior treatment of the primary neoplasms. At present little specific information has been published related to the outcome of second malignancies following pediatric cancer.

For patients with primary acute lymphoblastic leukemia or solid tumors, the risk of secondary acute nonlymphoblastic leukemia has been directly proportional to the dosage of alkylating agents (376), epipodophyllotoxins (243), and radiation (243). Pederson–Bjergaard (268) reported that the incidence of secondary neoplasms increased relative to patient age at the time of primary tumor diagnosis. Tucker (376) reported that both radiation therapy and alkylating agent chemotherapy increased the risk of second malignant neoplasms. The risk of development of acute nonlymphoblastic leukemia following in acute lymphoblastic leukemia is increased relative to the intensity of epipodophyllotoxin therapy (144,281, 346,398). With primary malignant solid tumors or Hodgkin's disease, increased risk of subsequent acute nonlymphoblastic leukemia has been associated with recurrence of the primary disease, combined radiotherapy and alkylating agent chemotherapy, or age greater than 12 years at the time of primary tumor diagnosis (17,280). A higher proportion of secondary malignancies has also occurred in females treated for Hodgkin's disease as compared to males (362). The LESG reported that the probability for developing leukemia or lymphoma after treatment for Hodgkin's disease was 1% at 5 years, 3% at 10 years, and 4% at 15 and 20 years. The overall risk of developing secondary hematopoietic neoplasms, however, appears to decrease after 10 years (222). For the development of the solid tumors, cumulative probability was less than 1% at 5 years, 2% at 10 years, 6% at 15 years, and 16% at 20 years (222). The LESG found that most second malignant neoplasms in children were associated with prior irradiation. Most secondary tumors linked to radiation were soft tissue and bony sarcomas, leukemia, or lymphomas (221,244). As higher dosages of radiation are being delivered using hyperfractionation techniques, it is hoped that there will be fewer effects on normal tissues and a decreased incidence of radiation-associated second malignant neoplasms.

Secondary cancers also have been reported in organ recipients, including patients receiving bone marrow transplantation for leukemia and aplastic anemia (400). These transplantation-related cancers primarily include non-Hodgkin's lymphoma, leukemia, and solid tumors such as melanoma, glioblastoma, and squamous cell carcinoma. There is a declining rate of secondary cancers 1 year after transplantation, yet the age-adjusted incidence of secondary cancer is 6.69 times higher than that of the primary cancer for the general population. Bone marrow transplant recipients have a low but significant risk of a secondary cancer, primarily non-Hodgkin's lymphoma (400). In our own leukemia population we have encountered one patient with secondary osteosarcoma following syngeneic transplantation and another with non-Hodgkin's lymphoma of the brain following allogeneic transplantation.

Roughly equal numbers of survivors of childhood acute lymphoblastic leukemia have developed secondary acute nonlymphoblastic leukemia or solid tumors. The solid neoplasms that have occurred after acute lymphoblastic leukemia have primarily been neural crest tumors or carcinomas (78,142,243,419). Other secondary tumors have included chronic myelogenous leukemia, non-Hodgkin's lymphoma, and Hodgkin's disease. Secondary tumors of neural crest origin following acute lymphoblastic leukemia include high-grade gliomas and infiltrative meningiomas (243,292). The spectrum of carcinomas following acute lymphoblastic leukemia comprises those of basal cell, hepatocellular, thyroidal, pancreatic, cervical, breast, and parotid origin. Secondary sarcomas are very unusual in patients with primary acute lymphoblastic leukemia. Secondary neural crest tumors have exceeded secondary carcinomas in our own patient population and have occurred with a frequency similar to that reported by Neglia et al. (243).

Conversely, acute lymphoblastic leukemia rarely occurs as a second malignancy and represents 5–10% of secondary leukemias in both adults and children. Cases have appeared following neuroblastoma, Wilms' tumor, retinoblastoma, and Hodgkin's disease (165,277). Pui et al. (280) studied secondary leukemias in 3,259 consecutive children or adolescents and found a cumulative risk of this complication of 1.3% at 10 years for pediatric patients with Hodgkin's disease, non-Hodgkin's lymphoma, or neuroblastoma. The incidence of secondary leukemia was increased in Hodgkin's disease patients who were older that 12 years at primary diagnosis or who received additional treatment for recurrence or a combination of radiation and alkylating agent therapy.

There has been considerable interest in the incidence of second malignant neoplasms following retinoblastoma, beginning in 1976 with the report by Abramson et al. (3). This report and a follow-up article (2) indicated that among 2,302 survivors of retinoblastoma, 80 developed 84 nonocular tumors. Among these 80 patients, 78 had bilateral retinoblastoma. Fifty-seven of the second neoplasms developed within the field of radiation therapy, following an average latent period of 11.4 years. Nineteen of these radiation-associated tumors were osteosarcomas. Three of the 80 patients who developed second malignancies had received no radiation therapy; the others developed tumors outside of the involved field. Additional study on 215 patients with bilateral retinoblastoma studied at the Armed Forces Institute of Pathology indicated a cumulative incidence of second neoplasms of 4.4% during the first 10 years of follow-up, 18.3% after 20 years, and 26.1% after 30 years. A 30-year cumulative incidence of 35.1% was reported for the 130 patients who received radiation therapy, compared to 5.8% in 78 patients who were not so treated. The studies of Roarty et al. (293) and Eng et al. (97) indicate that while approximately 60% of retinoblastomas are unilateral, 98% of the secondary malignancies occur in patients with bilateral disease or in the 15% of patients with unilateral retinoblastoma that harbor a constitutional *RB* mutation. The spectrum of malignant neoplasms that have followed retinoblastoma includes osteosarcoma, fibrosarcoma, carcinomas, melanomas, rhabdomyosarcomas, acute lymphoblastic leukemia, and Ewing's sarcoma. In the series reported by Draper et al. (88), the cumulative incidence rates of second tumors in the whole series of retinoblastoma patients were 2.0% at 12 years and 4.2% at 18 years after diagnosis. For patients with a genetic form of retinoblastoma, the cumulative incidence rate after 18 years was 8.4% for all second neoplasms and 6.0% for osteosarcoma alone. These authors suggested that patients with retinoblastoma might be particularly sensitive to the carcinogenic effects of irradiation and that patients with hereditary retinoblastoma may have an increased risk. Patients with bilateral retinoblastoma infrequently develop a histologically similar malignancy, pineoblastoma, following cyclophosphamide therapy (see Chapter 9).

Many reports have related the frequency of secondary neoplasms in long-term survivors of childhood and adult Hodgkin's disease and compared their incidence after treatment with nitrogen mustard–vincristine–prednisone–procarbazine or doxorubicin–adriamycin–bleomycin–vinblastine–dacarbazine (10,24,116,171,174, 369,378). Meadows et al. (222) reported that most solid tumors that follow childhood Hodgkin's disease develop within irradiated tissue and are not associated with alkylating agent therapy, splenectomy, or recurrence. Survivors of childhood or adult onset Hodgkin's disease have also developed non-Hodgkin's lymphoma as a secondary neoplasm (17,378). In both children and adults, the excessive risk of nonlymphocytic leukemia and non-Hodgkin's lymphoma appears to reach a plateau at 10 years. Tucker (376) indicated that the risk of leukemia appeared to reach a plateau of 3.3 ± 0.6% at 10 years, whereas non-Hodgkin's lymphoma continued to increase to 1.6 ± 0.7% at the end of this follow-up period. The risk of the leukemia was thought to be elevated after radiation therapy but was much higher after either adjuvant chemotherapy or chemotherapy alone, suggesting that the risk of having a solid tumor after therapy for Hodgkin's disease continues to increase with time.

The incidence and risk factors involved in the development of second malignant neoplasms after treatment of primary rhabdomyosarcoma were evaluated for patients enrolled in the Intergroup Rhabdomyosarcoma Studies I and II (150). Along the 1,770 patients treated between 1972 and 1982, 22 second malignant neoplasms were reported through 1991. The most common types of second malignancies were bone sarcomas and acute nonlymphoblastic leukemias that developed between 1 and 16 years and reached a 10-year cumulative incidence rate of 1.7%. It was thought that a combination of chemotherapy with an alkylating agent and radiation therapy played significant roles in the development of these second malignancies, as compared to therapy with only one of these modalities. The types of second malignancies encountered in this group included acute nonlymphoblastic leukemia (151), osteosarcoma and its variants, and carcinomas of the larynx and lung.

Recent reports from the National Wilms' Tumor Study Committee indicate that 7% of the survivors of Wilms' tumor have developed benign tumors and 1% a second malignant neoplasm (28,100). The types of tumors that have followed Wilms' tumor have included carcinomas of the skin, thyroid, parotid, and liver; leukemias of lymphoblastic and myeloid types; and various sarcomas, particularly osteosarcoma.

The second malignant neoplasms that have followed Ewing's sarcoma have primarily been sarcomas. Strong et al. (358) indicated that the cumulative risk over 10 years for irradiated patients was 35% ± 15.1%, with intensive chemotherapy seeming to exert an enhancing effect. Most of these second malignancies were osteosarcomas or malignant fibrous histiocytomas (194, 345,358).

Myelodysplastic syndromes and acute lymphoblastic leukemia have been noted to follow treatment of osteosarcoma (178,263). Among our osteosarcoma patients, two have developed colorectal carcinoma. Other second malignancies in osteosarcoma survivors treated at our institution have included glioblastoma multiforme and malignant fibrous histiocytoma.

Secondary cancers have been recorded in children with primary adrenal cortical carcinoma and include medulloblastoma and lymphocytic lymphoma (205).

As more patients survive pediatric brain tumors, it may be expected that there will be an increased incidence of other tumors, benign and malignant (104). Ghim et al. (121) have reviewed the English language literature related to the development of intracranial meningiomas after high-dose irradiation and observed that most of these meningeal tumors are calvarial in location, rarely multiple, and mostly benign in histologic type. Complete removal is possible for most patients. Osteosarcoma of the skull has been reported following treatment for cerebellar astrocytoma (44,182).

Another second malignant neoplasm related to prior chemotherapy is bladder carcinoma, which occurs after cyclophosphamide treatment (269). One of our St. Jude patients developed transitional cell carcinoma of the bladder 16 years after the diagnosis of acute lymphoblastic leukemia, during which time he received multiple agent chemotherapy that included at least 85 g/m^2 of cyclophosphamide delivered over a 9-year period. This patient later developed medulloblastoma following two courses of cranial irradiation for recurrent central nervous system leukemia.

Nichols et al. (245) report hematologic neoplasia developing in patients with nonseminomatous mediastinal germ cell tumors, especially those with serologic or histologic evidence of a yolk sac component (see Chapter 10). The effect of cisplatin-based chemotherapy on the development of these secondary neoplasms is speculative, as these patients have also received epipodophyllotoxins.

As greater numbers of children survive treatment of childhood leukemia and malignant solid tumors, more information will become available about the patterns of secondary malignant neoplasms and their relation to prior therapy, including chemotherapy, radiation therapy, or a combination thereof. Additional valuable information is accumulating regarding genetic predisposition to cancers, especially in individuals with *p53* gene abnormalities (213). Presently, it is recognized that chemotherapy with alkylating agents and topoisomerase inhibitors are major contributors to the development of secondary myeloid leukemia and that alkylating agents, especially cyclophosphamide, have an important role in the development of secondary bladder carcinomas. Radiation therapy given in moderate to high doses has been demonstrated to have a significant effect on the development of secondary brain tumors and osteosarcoma. Among the second malignant neoplasms that follow both leukemia and solid tumors, the median time to development of secondary leukemias and lymphomas is shorter than that for neural crest tumors, carcinomas, and sarcomas, with the carcinomas and sarcomas occurring at a median of about 10 years following diagnosis. With recognition of the time–risk relations for development of second neoplasms, it may be possible to evaluate patients more carefully for specific tumors, depending on the time from initial treatment of the primary cancer.

ACKNOWLEDGMENT

Supported by National Cancer Institute (NCI) Center Support Grant P30 CA217657, NCI Grant CA23099, and American Lebanese Syrian Associated Charities (ALSAC).

REFERENCES

1. Abeler V, Kjorstad KE, Nesland JM, Kjrstad KE. Small cell carcinoma of the ovary. A report of six cases. *Int J Gynecol Pathol* 1988;7:315–329.
2. Abramson DH, Ellsworth RM, Kitchin FD, Tung G. Second nonocular tumors in retinoblastoma survivors. Are they radiation-induced? *Ophthalmology* 1984;91:1351–1355.
3. Abramson DH, Ellsworth RM, Zimmerman LE. Nonocular cancer in retinoblastoma survivors. *Trans Am Acad Ophthalmol Otolaryngol* 1976;81:454–457.
4. Accetta PA, Gray GF, Jr., Hunter RM, Rosenfeld L. Mucoepidermoid carcinoma of salivary glands. *Arch Pathol Lab Med* 1984;108:321–325.
5. Adelman S, Benson CD, Hertzler JH. Surgical lesions of the ovary in infancy and childhood. *Surg Gynecol Obstet* 1975;141:219–226.
6. Agarwala S, Mitra DK, Bhatnagar V, Menon PS, Gupta AK. Aldosteronoma in childhood: a review of clinical features and management. *J Pediatr Surg* 1994;29:1388–1391.
7. Albino AP, Fountain JW. Molecular genetics of human malignant melanoma. *Cancer Treat Res* 1993;65:201–255.
8. Amberson JB, Vaughan ED, Jr., Gray GF, Naus GJ. Flow cytometric analysis of nuclear DNA from adrenocortical neoplasms. A retrospective study using paraffin-embedded tissue. *Cancer* 1987;59:2091–2095.
9. Aozasa K, Inoue A, Tajima K, Miyauchi A, Matsuzuka F, Kuma K. Malignant lymphomas of the thyroid gland. Analysis of 79 patients with emphasis on histologic prognostic factors. *Cancer* 1986;58:100–104.
10. Arseneau JC, Sponzo RW, Levin DL, et al. Nonlymphomatous malignant tumors complicating Hodgkin's disease. Possible association with intensive therapy. *N Engl J Med* 1972;287:1119–1122.
11. Azumi N, Battifora H. The distribution of vimentin and keratin in epithelial and nonepithelial neoplasms. A comprehensive immunohistochemical study on formalin- and alcohol-fixed tumors. *Am J Clin Pathol* 1987;88:286–296.
12. Azzopardi JG. *Problems in Breast Pathology*. London: WB Saunders; 1979:318–322.
13. Baker SR, Malone B. Salivary gland malignancies in children. *Cancer* 1985;55:1730–1736.

14. Balakrishnan U. An additional younger-age peak for cancer of the nasopharynx. *Int J Cancer* 1975;15:651–657.
15. Barnhill RL, Barnhill MA, Berwick M, Mihm MC, Jr. The histologic spectrum of pigmented spindle cell nevus: a review of 120 cases with emphasis on atypical variants. *Hum Pathol* 1991;22: 52–58.
16. Barnhill RL, Roush GC, Duray PH. Correlation of histologic architectural and cytoplasmic features with nuclear atypia in atypical (dysplastic) nevomelanocytic nevi. *Hum Pathol* 1990;21:51–58.
17. Beaty O, Hudson MM, Greenwald C, et al. Subsequent malignancies in children and adolescents after treatment for Hodgkin's disease. *J Clin Oncol.* 1995;13:603–609.
18. Benaily M, Schweisguth O, Job JC. Les tumeurs cortico-surrenales de l'infant. *Arch Fr Pediatr* 1975;32:441–453.
19. Benson PF, Vulliamy DG, Taubman JO. Congenital hemihypertrophy and malignancy. *Lancet* 1963;1:468–469.
20. Betuel H, Camoun M, Colombani J, Day NE, Ellouz R, de-The G. The relationship between nasopharyngeal carcinoma and the HL-A system among Tunisians. *Int J Cancer* 1975;16:249–254.
21. Biscotti CV, Hart WR. Juvenile granulosa cell tumors of the ovary. *Arch Pathol Lab Med* 1989;113:40–46.
22. Bishop PW, Menasce LP, Yates AJ, Win NA, Banerjee SS. An immunophenotypic survey of malignant melanomas. *Histopathology* 1993;23:159–166.
23. Black WC, Hunt WC. Histologic correlations with the clinical diagnosis of dysplastic nevus. *Am J Surg Pathol* 1990;14:44–52.
24. Blayney DW, Longo DL, Young RC, et al. Decreasing risk of leukemia with prolonged follow-up after chemotherapy and radiotherapy for Hodgkin's disease. *N Engl J Med* 1987;316:710–714.
25. Bosch JLHR, Kummer EW, Hohmann FR. Carcinoma of the thyroglossal duct. *Netherlands J Surg* 1986;38:36–40.
26. Brachman DG, Hallahan DE, Beckett MA, Yandell DW, Weichselbaum RR. p53 gene mutations and abnormal retinoblastoma protein in radiation-induced human sarcomas. *Cancer Res* 1991;51:6393–6396.
27. Breen JL, Maxson WS. Ovarian tumors in children and adolescents. *Clin Obstet Gynecol* 1977;20:607–623.
28. Breslow NE, Norkool PA, Olshan A, Evans A, D'Angio GJ. Second malignant neoplasms in survivors of Wilms' tumor: a report from the National Wilms' Tumor Study. *JNCI* 1988;80:592–595.
29. Brownstein MH, Shapiro L. Desmoplastic trichoepithelioma. *Cancer* 1977;40:2979–2986.
30. Brownstein MH, Wolf M, Bikowski JB. Cowden's disease: a cutaneous marker of breast cancer. *Cancer* 1978;41:2393–2398.
31. Buchino JJ, Castello FM, Nagaraj HS. Pancreatoblastoma. A histochemical and ultrastructural analysis. *Cancer* 1984;53:963–969.
32. Bugg MF, Ribeiro RC, Roberson PK, et al. Correlation of pathologic features with clinical outcome in pediatric adrenocortical neoplasia. A study of a Brazilian population. Brazilian Group for Treatment of Childhood Adrenocortical Tumors. *Am J Clin Pathol* 1994;101:625–629.
33. Burke JS, Butler JJ, Fuller LM. Malignant lymphomas of the thyroid: a clinical pathologic study of 35 patients including ultrastructural observations. *Cancer* 1977;39:1587–1602.
34. Burket RL, Rauh JL. Gorlin's syndrome: ovarian fibromas at adolescence. *Obstet Gynecol* 1976;47:43S–46S.
35. Burt RD, Vaughan TL, McKnight B. Descriptive epidemiology and survival analysis of nasopharyngeal carcinoma in the United States. *Int J Cancer* 1992;52:549–556.
36. Bychkov V, Kijek M. Massive ovarian edema. Four cases and some pathogenetic considerations. *Acta Obstet Gynecol Scand* 1987;66:397–399.
37. Cagle PT, Hough AJ, Pysher J, et al. Comparison of adrenal cortical tumors in children and adults. *Cancer* 1986;57:2235–2237.
38. Camuto P, Schinella R, Gilchrist K, Citrin D, Fredrickson G. Adrenal cortical carcinoma: flow cytometric study of 22 cases, an ECOG study. *Urology* 1991;37:380–384.
39. Cappellari JO, Geisinger KR, Albertson DA, Wolfman NT, Kute TE. Malignant papillary cystic tumor of the pancreas. *Cancer* 1990;66:193–198.
40. Carbone A, Ranelletti FO, Rinelli A, Vecchio FM, Lauriola L, Piantelli M, Capelli A. Type II estrogen receptors in the papillary cystic tumor of the pancreas. *Am J Clin Pathol* 1989;92:572–576.
41. Carcangiu ML, Zampi G, Pupi A, Castagnoli A, Rosai J. Papillary carcinoma of the thyroid. A clinicopathologic study of 241 cases treated at the University of Florence, Italy. *Cancer* 1985;55:805–828.
42. Carcassonne M, Delarue A, LeTourneau JN. Surgical treatment of organic pancreatic hypoglycemia in the pediatric age. *J Pediatr Surg* 1983;18:75–79.
43. Casanova P, Guidon J, Laffargue P. Les insulinomes de l'enfant. Etude histologique et ultrastructurale (A propos de deux cas). *Ann Anat Pathol* (Paris) 1975;20:489–503.
44. Casentini L, Visona A, Colombo F, Pansa VS, Pozza F, Benedetti A. Osteogenic osteosarcoma of the calvaria following radiotherapy for cerebellar astrocytoma: report of a case in childhood. *Tumori* 1985;71:391–396.
45. Castro EB, Huvos AG, Strong EW, Foote FW Jr. Tumors of the major salivary glands in children. *Cancer* 1972;29:312–317.
46. Cecalupo AJ, Frankel LS, Sullivan MP. Pelvic and ovarian extramedullary leukemic relapse in young girls: a report of four cases and review of the literature. *Cancer* 1982;50:587–593.
47. Chalvardjian A, Scully RE. Sclerosing stromal tumors of the ovary. *Cancer* 1973;31:664–670.
48. Chan JKC, Tsang WYW, Ng CS, Tang SK, Yu HC, Lee AWM. Follicular dendritic cell tumors of the oral cavity. *Am J Surg Pathol* 1994;18:148–157.
49. Chang KL, Arber DA, Weiss LM. CD30: a review. *Appl Immunohistochem* 1993;1:244–255.
50. Chen PL, Chen YM, Bookstein R, Lee WH. Genetic mechanisms of tumor suppression by the human p53 gene. *Science* 1990;250: 1576–1580.
51. Chen YM, Ott DJ, Wu WC, Gelfand DW. Cowden's disease: a case report and literature review. *Gastrointest Radiol* 1987;12: 325–329.
52. Choi PH, Suen MW, Huang DP, Lo KW, Lee JC. Nasopharyngeal carcinoma: genetic changes, Epstein–Barr virus infection, or both. A clinical and molecular study of 36 patients. *Cancer* 1993;72:2873–2878.
53. Chong GC, Beahrs OH, Chen ML, Hayles AB. Management of parotid gland tumors in infants and children. *Mayo Clin Proc* 1975;50:279–283.
54. Clark WH, Jr., Ainsworth AM, Bernardino EA, Yang CH, Mihm CM, Jr., Reed RJ. The developmental biology of primary human malignant melanomas. *Semin Oncol* 1975;2:83–103.
55. Clark WH, Jr., Elder DE, Guerry D, Epstein MN, Greene MH, Van Horn M. A study of tumor progression: the precursor lesions of superficial spreading and nodular melanoma. *Hum Pathol* 1984;15:1147–1165.
56. Claus EB, Risch N, Thompson WD, Carter D. Relationship between breast histopathology and family history of breast cancer. *Cancer* 1993;71:147–153.
57. Cleaver JE. Do we know the cause of xeroderma pigmentosum? *Carcinogenesis* 1990;11:875–882.
58. Clemente C, Cochran AJ, Elder DE, et al. Histopathologic diagnosis of dysplastic nevi: concordance among pathologists convened by the World Health Organization Melanoma Programme. *Hum Pathol* 1991;22:313–319.
59. Coffin CM, Rich SS, Dehner LP. Familial aggregation of nasopharyngeal carcinoma and other malignancies. A clinicopathologic description. *Cancer* 1991;68:1323–1328.
60. Cohen MM, Levy HP. Chromosome instability syndromes. *Adv Hum Genet* 1989;18:43–149, 365–71.
61. Coles C, Condie A, Chetty U, Steel CM, Evans HJ, Prosser J. p53 mutations in breast cancer. *Cancer Res* 1992;52:5291–5298.
62. Collins VP, James CD. Gene and chromosomal alterations associated with the development of human gliomas. *FASEB J* 1993;7: 926–930.
63. Connelly JH, Robey-Cafferty SS, Cleary KR. Mucinous carcinomas of the colon and rectum: an analysis of 62 stage B and C lesions. *Arch Pathol Lab Med* 1991;115:1022–1025.

64. Cooper HS. Intestinal neoplasms. In: Sternberg SS, ed. *Diagnostic Surgical Pathology*. New York: Raven Press; 1989:1015–1057.
65. Cooper JE, Lake BD. Use of enzyme histochemistry in the diagnosis of pancreatoblastoma. *Histopathology* 1989;15:407–414.
66. Copeland LJ, Sneige N, Ordonez NG, Hancock KC, Gershenson DM, Saul PB, Kavanagh JJ. Endodermal sinus tumor of the vagina and cervix. *Cancer* 1985;55:2558–2565.
67. Cowan JM, Halaban R, Lane AT, Francke U. The involvement of 6p in melanoma. *Cancer Genet Cytogenet* 1986;20:255–261.
68. Cramer SF. The origin of epidermal melanocytes: Implications for the histogenesis of nevi and melanomas. *Arch Pathol Lab Med* 1991;115:115–119.
69. Crile G, Jr., Esselstyn CB, Jr., Hawk WA. Needle biopsy in the diagnosis of thyroid nodules appearing after radiation [editorial]. *N Engl J Med* 1979;301:997–999.
70. Cubilla AL, Fitzgerald PJ. Cancer of the pancreas (nonendocrine): a suggested morphologic classification. *Semin Oncol* 1979;6:285–297.
71. Cubilla AL, Fitzgerald PJ. *Tumors of the Exocrine Pancreas*. Fascicle 19. Washington, D.C.: Armed Forces Institute of Pathology; 1984.
72. Cvitkovic E, Bachouchi M, Boussen H, et al. Leukemoid reaction, bone marrow invasion, fever of unknown origin, and metastatic pattern in the natural history of advanced undifferentiated carcinoma of nasopharyngeal type: a review of 255 consecutive cases. *J Clin Oncol* 1993;11:2434–2442.
73. Dal Cin P, Sneyers W, Aly MS, Segers A, Ostijn F, Van Damme B, Van Den Berghe H. Involvement of 19q13 in follicular thyroid adenoma. *Cancer Genet Cytogenet* 1992;60:99–101.
74. Danen EH, van Muijen GN, ten Berge PJ, Ruiter DJ. Integrins and melanoma progression. *Recent Results Cancer Res* 1993;128:119–132.
75. Davies JN. International comparisons of childhood neoplasms. *Clin Pediatr (Phila)* 1967;6:567–569.
76. de Agustin JC, Rivilla F, Santana A, Utrilla JG. Papillary cystic tumor of the pancreas. *Z Kinderchir* 1989;44:379–381.
77. De Vathaire F, François P, Schlumberger M, et al. Epidemiological evidence for a common mechanism for neuroblastoma and differentiated thyroid tumour. *Br J Cancer* 1992;65:425–428.
78. De Vathaire F, Schweisguth O, Rodary C, et al. Long-term risk of second malignant neoplasm after a cancer in childhood. *Br J Cancer* 1989;59:448–452.
79. Dehner LP. Tumors of the mandible and maxilla in children. I. Clinicopathologic study of 46 histologically benign lesions. *Cancer* 1973;31:364–384.
80. Dehner LP. Neoplasms of the adrenal cortex. Preoccupation bordering on obsession. *Am J Clin Pathol* 1994;101:557–558.
81. Dehner LP, Valbuena L, Perez-Atayde A, Reddick RL, Askin FB, Rosai J. Salivary gland anlage tumor ("congenital pleomorphic adenoma"): a clinicopathologic, immunohistochemical and ultrastructural study of nine cases. *Am J Surg Pathol* 1994;18:25–36.
82. Diaz NM, Palmer JO, McDivitt RW. Carcinoma arising within fibroadenomas of the breast. A clinicopathologic study of 105 patients. *Am J Clin Pathol* 1991;95:614–622.
83. Dickersin GR, Kline IW, Scully RE. Small cell carcinoma of the ovary with hypercalcemia: a report of eleven cases. *Cancer* 1982;49:188–197.
84. Digweed M. Human genetic instability syndromes: single gene defects with increased risk of cancer. *Toxicol Lett* 1993;67:259–281.
85. DiSaia PJ. Ovarian neoplasms. In: Scott JR, DiSaia PJ, Hammond CB, Spellacy W, eds. *Danforth's Obstetrics and Gynecology*. Philadelphia: J. Lippincott; 1994:969–1018.
86. Díaz-Cano S, González-Cámpora R, Ríos-Martín JJ, et al. Nuclear DNA patterns in adrenal cortex proliferative lesions. *Virchows Arch A Histopathol Anat* 1993;423:323–328.
87. Donaldson MH, Taylor P, Rawitscher R, Sewell JB Jr. Colon carcinoma in childhood. *Pediatrics* 1971;48:307–312.
88. Draper GJ, Sanders BM, Kingston JE. Second primary neoplasms in patients with retinoblastoma. *Br J Cancer* 1986;53:661–671.
89. Driman DK, Kobrin MS, Kudlow JE, Asa SL. Transforming growth factor-α in normal and neoplastic human endocrine tissues. *Hum Pathol* 1992;23:1360–1365.
90. Drut R, Jones MC. Congenital pancreatoblastoma in Beckwith–Wiedemann syndrome: an emerging association. *Pediatr Pathol* 1988;8:331–339.
91. Duffy BJ, Fitzgerald PJ. Thyroid cancer in childhood and adolescence: a report on twenty-eight cases. *Cancer* 1950;3:1018–1032.
92. Dumont-Herskowitz RA, Safaii HS, Senior B. Ovarian fibromata in four successive generations. *J Pediatr* 1978;93:621–624.
93. Eichhorn JH, Scully RE. Ovarian myxoma: clinicopathologic and immunocytologic analysis of five cases and a review of the literature. *Int J Gynecol Pathol* 1991;10:156–169.
94. Ekfors TO, Aho HJ, Kekomaki M. Malignant rhabdoid tumor of the prostatic region. Immunohistological and ultrastructural evidence for epithelial origin. *Virchows Arch A Histopathol Anat* 1985;406:381–388.
95. Elder DE, Goldman LI, Goldman SC, Greene MH, Clark WH, Jr. Dysplastic nevus syndrome: a phenotypic association of sporadic cutaneous melanoma. *Cancer* 1980;46:1787–1794.
96. Elliot MS, Steven DM. Carcinoma of the colon and rectum in patients under 30 years of age. *South Afr Med J* 1984;66:129–131.
97. Eng C, Li FP, Abramson DH, et al. Mortality from second tumors among long-term survivors of retinoblastoma. *JNCI* 1993;85:1121–1128.
98. Epelman S, Gorender EF, Spindola-Castro A, Bianchi A. High incidence of adrenocortical carcinomas in Sao Paulo (abstract). *Proc Annu Meet Am Soc Clin Oncol* 1991;10:A1109.
99. Erlandson RA. *Diagnostic Transmission Electron Microscopy of Tumors, with Clinicopathological, Immunohistochemical, and Cytogenetic Correlations*. New York: Raven Press; 1994.
100. Evans AE, Norkool P, Evans I, Breslow N, D'Angio GJ. Late effects of treatment for Wilms' tumor. A report from the National Wilms' Tumor Study Group. *Cancer* 1991;67:331–336.
101. Evans HL. Mucoepidermoid carcinoma of salivary glands: a study of 69 cases with special attention to histologic grading. *Am J Clin Pathol* 1984;81:696–701.
102. Exelby PE, Frazell EL. Carcinoma of the thyroid in children. *Surg Clin North Am* 1969;49:249–259.
103. Eyden BP, Harris M. An immunohistochemically defined non-Hodgkin's lymphoma showing intercellular junctions. A case report. *Virchows Arch A Histopathol Anat* 1989;415:297–300.
104. Farwell J, Flannery JT. Second primaries in children with central nervous system tumors. *J Neuro-oncol* 1984;2:371–375.
105. Fernandez CH, Cangir A, Samaan NA, Rivera R. Nasopharyngeal carcinoma in children. *Cancer* 1976;37:2787–2791.
106. Finerty S, Jarvis JE, Epstein MA, Trumper PA, Ball G, Giovanella BC. Cytogenetics of malignant epithelial cells and lymphoblastoid cell lines from nasopharyngeal carcinoma. *Br J Cancer* 1978;37:231–239.
107. Fleming ID, Black TL, Thompson EI, Pratt C, Rao B, Hustu O. Thyroid dysfunction and neoplasia in children receiving neck irradiation for cancer. *Cancer* 1985;55:1190–1194.
108. Fletcher JA, Gibas Z, Donovan K, Perez-Atayde A, Genest D, Morton CC, Lage JM. Ovarian granulosa-stromal cell tumors are characterized by trisomy 12. *Am J Pathol* 1991;138:515–520.
109. Fountain JW, Bale SJ, Housman DE, Dracopoli NC. Genetics of melanoma. *Cancer Surv* 1990;9:645–671.
110. Frasch W, Gnekow A, Bolkenius M, Wagner T, Dhom G, Dorr HG, Knorr D. Nebennierenrinden-karzinom. Eine seltene Ursache eines Conn-Syndroms im Kindesalter. *Monatsschr Kinderheilkd* 1992;140:95–101.
111. Frauenhoffer CM, Patchefsky AS, Cobanoglu A. Thyroid carcinoma: a clinical and pathologic study of 125 cases. *Cancer* 1979;43:2414–2421.
112. Fraumeni JF, Jr., Miller RW. Adrenocortical neoplasms with hemihypertrophy, brain tumors, and other disorders. *J Pediatr* 1967;70:129–138.
113. Frierson HF, Bellafiore FJ, Gaffey MJ, McCary WS, Innes Jr, Williams ME. Cytokeratin in anaplastic large cell lymphoma. *Mod Pathol* 1994;7:317–321.
114. Friesen SR. Tumors of the endocrine pancreas. *N Engl J Med* 1982;306:580–590.

115. Frizzera G. The distinction of Hodgkin's disease from anaplastic large cell lymphoma. *Semin Diag Pathol* 1992;9:291–296.
116. Fryer CJ, Hutchinson RJ, Krailo M, et al. Efficacy and toxicity of 12 courses of ABVD chemotherapy followed by low-dose regional radiation in advanced Hodgkin's disease in children: a report from the Children's Cancer Study Group. *J Clin Oncol* 1990;8: 1971–1980.
117. Gaffey MJ, Weiss LM. Association of Epstein–Barr virus with human neoplasia. *Pathol Annu* 1992;27 Pt 1:55–74.
118. Gandour MJ, Grizzle WE. A small adrenocortical carcinoma with aggressive behavior. An evaluation of criteria for malignancy. *Arch Pathol Lab Med* 1986;110:1076–1079.
119. Gardner DG. Plexiform unicystic ameloblastoma: a diagnostic problem in dentigerous cysts. *Cancer* 1981;47:1358–1363.
120. Gershenson DM, Silva EG. Serous ovarian tumors of low malignant potential with peritoneal implants. *Cancer* 1990;65:578–585.
121. Ghim TT, Seo JJ, O'Brien M, Meacham L, Crocker I, Krawiecki N. Childhood intracranial meningiomas after high-dose irradiation. *Cancer* 1993;71:4091–4095.
122. Gorlin RJ. Nevoid basal-cell carcinoma syndrome. *Medicine (Baltimore)* 1987;66:98–113.
123. Greene MH, Clark WH, Jr., Tucker MA, et al. Acquired precursors of cutaneous malignant melanoma. The familial dysplastic nevus syndrome. *N Engl J Med* 1985;312:91–97.
124. Greene MH, Fraumeni JF, Hoover R. Nasopharyngeal cancer among young people in the United States: racial variations by cell type. *JNCI* 1977;58:1267–1270.
125. Greider MH, Bencosme SA, Lechago J. The human pancreatic islet cells and their tumors. I. The normal pancreatic islets. *Lab Invest* 1970;22:344–354.
126. Guerin V, Bene MC, Judlin P, Beurey J, Landes P, Faure G. Cowden disease in a young girl: gynecologic and immunologic overview in a case and in the literature. *Obstet Gynecol* 1989;73:890–892.
127. Haak HR, Fleuren G. Neuroendocrine differentiation of adrenocortical tumors. *Cancer* 1995;75:860–864.
128. Hajdu SI, So-Bosita J, Little AB. Epidermoid carcinoma in situ of the cervix in a young girl. *Am J Obstet Gynecol* 1968;100: 1154–1155.
129. Halaban R, Moellmann G. Proliferation and malignant transformation of melanocytes. *Crit Rev Oncog* 1991;2:247–258.
130. Halevy S, Sandbank M, Pick AI, Feuerman EJ. Cowden's disease in three siblings: electron-microscope and immunological studies. *Acta Derm Venereol (Stockh)* 1985;65:126–131.
131. Hall TL, Layfield LJ, Philippe A, Rosenthal DL. Sources of diagnostic error in fine-needle aspiration of the thyroid. *Cancer* 1989;63:718–725.
132. Hamburger JI, Husain M, Nishiyama R, Nunez C, Solomon D. Increasing the accuracy of fine-needle biopsy for thyroid nodules. *Arch Pathol Lab Med* 1989;113:1035–1041.
133. Hancock SL, Cox RS, McDougall IR. Thyroid diseases after treatment of Hodgkin's disease. *N Engl J Med* 1991;325:599–605.
134. Hara K. Melanocytic lesions in lymph nodes associated with congenital naevus. *Histopathology* 1993;23:445–451.
135. Harness JK, Thompson NW, Nishiyama RH. Childhood thyroid carcinoma. *Arch Surg* 1971;102:278–284.
136. Harris JR, Coleman CN. Estimating the risk of second primary tumors following cancer treatment [editorial]. *J Clin Oncol* 1989;7:5–6.
137. Harris M, Eyden BP, Joglekar VM. Rhabdoid tumour of the bladder: a histological, ultrastructural and immunohistochemical study. *Histopathology* 1987;11:1083–1092.
138. Harrison JH, Jenkins D, Bennett AH. Hyperplasia and tumors of the adrenal cortex. *Urol Int* 1972;27:81–117.
139. Hart WR, Kumar N, Crissman JD. Ovarian neoplasms resembling sex cord tumors with annular tubules. *Cancer* 1980;45: 2352–2363.
140. Haupt HM, Mann RB, Trump DL, Abeloff MD. Metastatic carcinoma involving the testis: clinical and pathologic distinction from primary testicular neoplasms. *Cancer* 1984;54:709–714.
141. Hawkins EP, Krischer JP, Smith BE, Hawkins HK, Finegold MJ. Nasopharyngeal carcinoma in children—a retrospective review and demonstration of Epstein-Barr viral genomes in tumor cell cytoplasm: a report of the Pediatric Oncology Group. *Hum Pathol* 1990;21:805–810.
142. Hawkins MM. Second primary tumors following radiotherapy for childhood cancer. *Int J Radiat Oncol Biol Phys* 1990;19: 1297–1301.
143. Hawkins MM, Draper GJ, Kingston JE. Incidence of second primary tumours among childhood cancer survivors. *Br J Cancer* 1987;56:339–347.
144. Hawkins MM, Wilson LM, Stovall MA, Marsden HB, Potok MH, Kingston JE, Chessells JM. Epipodophyllotoxins, alkylating agents, and radiation and risk of secondary leukaemia after childhood cancer. *BMJ* 1992;304:951–958.
145. Heitz P, Moser H, Staub JJ. Thyroid cancer: a study of 573 thyroid tumors and 161 autopsy cases observed over a thirty-year period. *Cancer* 1976;37:2329–2337.
146. Heitz P, Steiner H, Halter F, Egli F, Kapp JP. Multihormonal, amyloid-producing tumour of the islets of Langerhans in a twelve year old boy: clinical, morphological, and biochemical data and review of the literature. *Virchows Arch A Histopathol Anat* 1971;353:312–324.
147. Hendrickson MR, Ross JC. Neoplasms arising in congenital giant nevi: morphologic study of seven cases and a review of the literature. *Am J Surg Pathol* 1981;5:109–135.
148. Henle W, Ho JH, Henle G, Chau JC, Kwan HC. Nasopharyngeal carcinoma: significance of changes in Epstein-Barr virus–related antibody patterns following therapy. *Int J Cancer* 1977;20:663–672.
149. Henzen-Logmans SC, Stel HV, van Muijen GN, Mullink H, Meijer CJ. Expression of intermediate filament proteins in adrenal cortex and related tumours. *Histopathology* 1988;12:359–372.
150. Heyn R, Haeberlen V, Newton WA, et al. Second malignant neoplasms in children treated for rhabdomyosarcoma. Intergroup Rhabdomyosarcoma Study Committee. *J Clin Oncol* 1993;11: 262–270.
151. Heyn R, Khan F, Ensign LG, et al. Acute myeloid leukemia in patients treated for rhabdomyosarcoma with cyclophosphamide and low-dose etoposide on Intergroup Rhabdomyosarcoma Study III: an interim report. *Med Pediatr Oncol* 1994;23:99–106.
152. Hidayatalla A, Malik MO, El Hadi AE, Osman AA, Hutt MS. Studies on nasopharyngeal carcinoma in the Sudan—I. Epidemiology and aetiology. *Eur J Cancer Clin Oncol* 1983;19:705–710.
153. Hilgers RD. Prenatal oncogenesis and the development of malignant tumors in the infant and adolescent vagina—a review and hypothesis. *Gynecol Oncol* 1977;5:262–272.
154. Hoffman S, Jacoway JR, Krolls SO. *Atlas of Tumor Pathology. Second Series, Fascicle 24. Intraosseous and Parosteal Tumors of the Jaws.* Washington, D.C.: Armed Forces Institute of Pathology; 1987.
155. Hogan TF, Gilchrist KW, Westring DW, Citrin DL. A clinical and pathological study of adrenocortical carcinoma: therapeutic implications. *Cancer* 1980;45:2880–2883.
156. Hong SJ, Lurain JR, Tsukada Y, Piver MS, Humbert JR, Freeman AI. Cystadenocarcinoma of the ovary in a 4-year-old: benign transformation during therapy. *Cancer* 1980;45:2227–2230.
157. Horie A, Haratake J, Jimi A, Matsumoto M, Ishii N, Tsutsumi Y. Pancreatoblastoma in Japan, with differential diagnosis from papillary cystic tumor (ductuloacinar adenoma) of the pancreas. *Acta Pathol Jpn* 1987;37:47–63.
158. Horie H, Etoh T, Maie M. Cytogenetic characteristics of a malignant rhabdoid tumor arising from the paravertebral region. A case report. *Acta Pathol Jpn* 1992;42:460–465.
159. Hornstein L, Crowe C, Gruppo R. Adrenal carcinoma in child with history of fetal alcohol syndrome [letter]. *Lancet* 1977;2: 1292–1293.
160. Houdelette P, Chagnon A, Dumotier J, Marthan E. Corticosurrenalome malin dans le cadre d'un syndrome de Wermer. A propos d'une observation. *J Chir (Paris)* 1989;126:385–387.
161. Hough AJ, Hollifield JW, Page DL, Hartmann WH. Prognostic factors in adrenal cortical tumors: a mathematical analysis of clinical and morphologic data. *Am J Clin Pathol* 1979;72:390–399.
162. Hsu C, Boey J. Diagnostic pitfalls in the fine needle aspiration of

thyroid nodules. A study of 555 cases in Chinese patients. *Acta Cytol* 1987;31:699–704.

163. Hsu HC, Chen CL, Hsu MM, Lynn TC, Tu SM, Huang SC. Pathology of nasopharyngeal carcinoma. Proposal of a new histologic classification correlated with prognosis. *Cancer* 1987;59:945–951.
164. Hsueh C, Gonzalez-Crussi F. Sialoblastoma: a case report and review of the literature on congenital epithelial tumors of salivary gland origin. *Pediatr Pathol* 1992;12:205–214.
165. Hunger SP, Sklar J, Link MP. Acute lymphoblastic leukemia occurring as a second malignant neoplasm in childhood: report of three cases and review of the literature. *J Clin Oncol* 1992;10:156–163.
166. Hwang HN. Nasopharyngeal carcinoma in the people's Republic of China: incidence, treatment, and survival rates. *Radiology* 1983;149:305–309.
167. Ibrahim NK, Abdul-Karim FW. Colorectal adenocarcinoma in young Lebanese adults. The American University of Beirut-Medical Center experience with 32 patients. *Cancer* 1986;58:816–820.
168. Iseki M, Suzuki T, Koizumi Y, Hirose M, Laskin WB, Nakazawa S, Ohaki Y. Alpha-fetoprotein-producing pancreatoblastoma. A case report. *Cancer* 1986;57:1833–1835.
169. Isola J, Visakorpi T, Holli K, Kallioniemi OP. Association of overexpression of tumor suppressor protein p53 with rapid cell proliferation and poor prognosis in node-negative breast cancer patients. *JNCI* 1992;84:1109–1114.
170. Jackson R, Gardere S. Nevoid basal cell carcinoma syndrome. *Can Med Assoc J* 1971;105:850–860.
171. Jacquillat C, Khayat D, Desprez-Curely JP, et al. Non-Hodgkin's lymphoma occurring after Hodgkin's disease. Four new cases and a review of the literature. *Cancer* 1984;53:459–462.
172. Jeannel D, Ghnassia M, Hubert A, Sancho-Garnier H, Eschwege F, Crognier E, de-The G. Increased risk of nasopharyngeal carcinoma among males of French origin born in Maghreb (north Africa). *Int J Cancer* 1993;54:536–539.
173. Jenkin RD, Anderson JR, Jereb B, Thompson JC, Pyesmany A, Wara WM, Hammond D. Nasopharyngeal carcinoma—a retrospective review of patients less than thirty years of age: a report of Children's Cancer Study Group. *Cancer* 1981;47:360–366.
174. Kaldor JM, Day NE, Clarke EA, et al. Leukemia following Hodgkin's disease. *N Engl J Med* 1990;322:7–13.
175. Kamino H, Huang SJ, Fu YS. Keratin and involucrin immunohistochemistry of nasopharyngeal carcinoma. *Cancer* 1988;61:1142–1148.
176. Kamio T, Shigematsu K, Kawai K, Tsuchiyama H. Immunoreactivity and receptor expression of insulinlike growth factor I and insulin in human adrenal tumors: An immunohistochemical study of 94 cases. *Am J Pathol* 1991;138:83–91.
177. Kanbour AI, Salazar H, Tobon H. Massive ovarian edema: a non-neoplastic pelvic mass of young women. *Arch Pathol Lab Med* 1979;103:42–45.
178. Kapelushnik J, Dube I, Wilson P, Greenberg M. Acute lymphoblastic leukemia with t(4;11) translocation after osteogenic sarcoma. *Cancer* 1991;67:2887–2889.
179. Kaste SC, Hedlund G, Pratt CB. Malignant parotid tumors in patients previously treated for childhood cancer: clinical and imaging findings in 8 cases. *Am J Radiol* 1994;162:665–659.
180. Kaufmann WK. In vitro complementation of xeroderma pigmentosum. *Mutagenesis* 1988;3:373–380.
181. Keelan PA, Myers JL, Wold LE, Katzmann JA, Gibney DJ. Phyllodes tumor: Clinicopathologic review of 60 patients and flow cytometric analysis in 30 patients. *Hum Pathol* 1992;23:1048–1054.
182. Kellie SJ, Hutchison RE, Robertson JT, Pratt CB. Successful treatment of a radiation-associated extradural osteosarcoma with chemotherapy in an adolescent girl. *Med Pediatr Oncol* 1989;17:514–519.
183. Kenny FM, Hashida Y, Askari HA, Sieber WH, Fetterman GH. Virilizing tumors of the adrenal cortex. *Am J Dis Child* 1968;115:445–458.
184. Kim I, Young RH, Scully RE. Leydig cell tumors of the testis. A clinicopathological analysis of 40 cases and review of the literature. *Am J Surg Pathol* 1985;9:177–192.
185. King DR, Lack EE. Adrenal cortical carcinoma: a clinical and pathologic study of 49 cases. *Cancer* 1979;44:239–244.
186. Kissane JM. Pancreatoblastoma and solid and cystic papillary tumor: two tumors related to pancreatic ontogeny. *Semin Diag Pathol* 1994;11:152–164.
187. Klemi PJ, Joensuu H, Nylamo E. Fine needle aspiration biopsy in the diagnosis of thyroid nodules. *Acta Cytol* 1991;35:434–438.
188. Knudson AG. Antioncogenes and human cancer. *Proc Natl Acad Sci USA* 1993;90:10914–10921.
189. Koh TH, Cooper JE, Newman CL, Walker TM, Kiely EM, Hoffmann EB. Pancreatoblastoma in a neonate with Wiedemann–Beckwith syndrome. *Eur J Pediatr* 1986;145:435–438.
190. Kramer IR, Pindborg JJ, Shear M. The WHO Histological Typing of Odontogenic Tumours. A commentary on the Second Edition. *Cancer* 1992;70:2988–2994.
191. Krasagakis K, Garbe C, Orfanos CE. Cytokines in human melanoma cells: synthesis, autocrine stimulation and regulatory functions–an overview. *Melanoma Res* 1993;3:425–433.
192. Krolls SO, Trodahl JN, Boyers RC. Salivary gland lesions in children. A survey of 430 cases. *Cancer* 1972;30:459–469.
193. Kumar S, Kumar D, Cowan DF. Transitional cell carcinoma with rhabdoid features. *Am J Surg Pathol* 1992;16:515–521.
194. Kuttesch JF, Wexler LH, Marcus RB, Fairclough D, Weaver-McClure L, White M, Mao L, et al. Second malignant neoplasms after Ewing sarcoma: relationships between radiation dose and incidence of second sarcomas. *Med Pediatr Oncol* 1994;23:239(Abstract).
195. Lack EE, Cassady JR, Levey R, Vawter GF. Tumors of the exocrine pancreas in children and adolescents. A clinical and pathologic study of eight cases. *Am J Surg Pathol* 1983;7:319–327.
196. Lack EE, Mulvihill JJ, Travis WD, Kozakewich HPW. Adrenal cortical neoplasms in the pediatric and adolescent age group: clinicopathologic study with emphasis on epidemiological and prognostic factors. *Pathol Annu* 1992;27 (Pt. 1):1–53.
197. Lack EE, Perez-Atayde AR, Murthy ASK, Goldstein DP, Crigler JF, Vawter GF. Granulosa theca cell tumors in premenarchal girls: a clinical and pathologic study of ten cases. *Cancer* 1981;48:1846–1854.
198. Lack EE, Young RH, Scully RE. Pathology of ovarian neoplasms in childhood and adolescence. *Pathol Annu* 1992;27 Pt 2:281–356.
199. Lastarria D, Sachdev RK, Babury RA, Yu HM, Nuovo GJ. Immunohistochemical analysis for desmin in normal and neoplastic ovarian stromal tissue. *Arch Pathol Lab Med* 1990;114:502–505.
200. Lawrence WD, Young RH, Scully RE. Juvenile granulosa cell tumor of the infantile testis. A report of 14 cases. *Am J Surg Pathol* 1985;9:87–94.
201. Layfield LJ, Mohrmann RL, Kopald KH, Giuliano AE. Use of aspiration cytology and frozen section examination for management of benign and malignant thyroid nodules. *Cancer* 1991;68:130–134.
202. Lee PD, Winter RJ, Green OC. Virilizing adrenocortical tumors in childhood: eight cases and a review of the literature. *Pediatrics* 1985;76:437–444.
203. Lee YS, Chong SM. Pathology of the 5 most common cancers in Singapore. *Ann Acad Med Singapore* 1990;19:186–200.
204. Levine AJ, Momand J. Tumor suppressor genes: the p53 and retinoblastoma sensitivity genes and gene products. *Biochim Biophys Acta* 1990;1032:119–136.
205. Levine GW. Adrenocortical carcinoma in two children with subsequent primary tumors. *Am J Dis Child* 1978;132:238–240.
206. Levine PH. Immunologic markers for Epstein–Barr virus in the control of nasopharyngeal carcinoma and Burkitt lymphoma. *Cancer Detect Prev Suppl* 1987;1:217–223.
207. Lin C-T, Chan W-Y, Chen W, et al. Characterization of seven newly established nasopharyngeal carcinoma cell lines. *Lab Invest* 1993;68:716–727.
208. Lindfors O. Primary ovarian neoplasms in infants and children. A study of 81 cases diagnosed in Finland and Sweden. *Ann Chir Gynaecol Fenn Suppl* 1971;177:1–66.
209. Lowhagen T, Sprenger E. Cytologic presentation of thyroid tumors in aspiration biopsy smear. A review of 60 cases. *Acta Cytol* 1974;18:192–197.
210. Loy TS, McLaughlin R, Odom LF, Dehner LP. Mucoepidermoid

carcinoma of the parotid as a second malignant neoplasm in children. *Cancer* 1989;64:2174–2177.
211. Lynch HT, Watson P, Smyrk TC, et al. Colon cancer genetics. *Cancer* 1992;70:1300–1312.
212. Mahloudji M, Ronaghy H, Dutz W. Virilizing adrenal carcinoma in two sibs. *J Med Genet* 1971;8:160–163.
213. Malkin D, Li FP, Strong LC, et al. Germ line p53 mutations in a familial syndrome of breast cancer, sarcomas, and other neoplasms. *Science* 1990;250:1233–1238.
214. Mancianti ML, Clark WH, Hayes FA, Herlyn M. Malignant melanoma simulants arising in congenital melanocytic nevi do not show experimental evidence for a malignant phenotype. *Am J Pathol* 1990;136:817–829.
215. Marchetti A, Buttitta F, Pellegrini S, et al. p53 mutations and histological type of invasive breast carcinoma. *Cancer Res* 1993;53:4665–4669.
216. Marigo C, Muller H, Davies JN. Survey of cancer in children admitted to a Brazilian charity hospital. *JNCI* 1969;43:1231–1240.
217. Matsunou H, Konishi F. Papillary-cystic neoplasm of the pancreas. A clinicopathologic study concerning the tumor aging and malignancy of nine cases. *Cancer* 1990;65:283–291.
218. McDivitt RW, Stewart FW. Breast carcinoma in children. *JAMA* 1966;195:388–390.
219. McMahon JT, Hart WR. Ultrastructural analysis of small cell carcinomas of the ovary. *Am J Clin Pathol* 1988;90:523–529.
220. Meadows AT. Risk factors for second malignant neoplasms: report from the Late Effects Study Group. *Bull Cancer (Paris)* 1988;75:125–130.
221. Meadows AT, Baum E, Fossati-Bellani F, et al. Second malignant neoplasms in children: an update from the Late Effects Study Group. *J Clin Oncol* 1985;3:532–538.
222. Meadows AT, Obringer AC, Marrero O, et al. Second malignant neoplasms following childhood Hodgkin's disease: treatment and splenectomy as risk factors. *Med Pediatr Oncol* 1989;17:477–484.
223. Medeiros LJ, Weiss LM. New developments in the pathologic diagnosis of adrenal cortical neoplasms. A review. *Am J Clin Pathol* 1992;97:73–83.
224. Mehregan AH, Mehregan DA. Malignant melanoma in childhood. *Cancer* 1993;71:4096–4103.
225. Melbye M, Ebbesen P, Levine PH, Bennike T. Early primary infection and high Epstein–Barr virus antibody titers in Greenland Eskimos at high risk for nasopharyngeal carcinoma. *Int J Cancer* 1984;34:619–623.
226. Miettinen M. Neuroendocrine differentiation in adrenocortical carcinoma: new immunohistochemical findings supported by electron microscopy. *Lab Invest* 1992;66:169–174.
227. Miettinen M, Partanen S, Fraki O, Kivilaakso E. Papillary cystic tumor of the pancreas. An analysis of cellular differentiation by electron microscopy and immunohistochemistry. *Am J Surg Pathol* 1987;11:855–865.
228. Miller JM, Hamburger JI, Kini S. Diagnosis of thyroid nodules. Use of fine-needle aspiration and needle biopsy. *JAMA* 1979;241: 481–484.
229. Miller RW, Young JL, Novakovic B. Childhood cancer. *Cancer* 1995;75:395–405.
230. Mills SE, Allen MS Jr. Colorectal carcinoma in the first three decades of life. *Am J Surg Pathol* 1979;3:443–448.
231. Molberg K, Vuitch F, Stewart D, Albores-Saavedra J. Adrenocortical blastoma. *Hum Pathol* 1992;23:1187–1190.
232. Montgomery EA, Popek EJ. Intussusception, adenovirus, and children: a brief reaffirmation. *Hum Pathol* 1994;25:169–174.
233. Moore KL. *The Developing Human: Clinically Oriented Embryology*. 4th ed. Philadelphia: WB Saunders; 1988:364–401.
234. Morohoshi T, Kanda M, Horie A, Chott A, Dreyer T, Kloppel G, Heitz PU. Immunocytochemical markers of uncommon pancreatic tumors. Acinar cell carcinoma, pancreatoblastoma, and solid cystic (papillary-cystic) tumor. *Cancer* 1987;59:739–747.
235. Morrison DM, Jewell LD, McCaughey WT, Danyluk J, Shnitka TK, Manickavel V. Papillary cystic tumor of the pancreas. *Arch Pathol Lab Med* 1984;108:723–727.
236. Mostofi FK. *Tumors of the Male Genital System*. Fascicle 8. Bethesda: Armed Forces Institute of Pathology; 1973.
237. Mukai K, Grotting JC, Greider MH, Rosai J. Retrospective study of 77 pancreatic endocrine tumors using the immunoperoxidase method. *Am J Surg Pathol* 1982;6:387–399.
238. Munoz NA, Takehara H, Komi N, Hirose T. Papillary and cystic tumor of the pancreas possibly concealed within a pseudocyst. *Acta Paediatr Jpn* 1992;34:316–323.
239. Naegele RF, Champion J, Murphy S, Henle G, Henle W. Nasopharyngeal carcinoma in American Children: Epstein–Barr virus–specific antibody titers and prognosis. *Int J Cancer* 1982;29:209–212.
240. Nakano M. Adrenal cortical carcinoma. A clinicopathological and immunohistochemical study of 91 autopsy cases. *Acta Pathol Jpn* 1988;38:163–180.
241. Neblett WW, Frexes-Steed M, Scott HW Jr. Experience with adrenocortical neoplasms in childhood. *Am Surg* 1987;53:117–125.
242. Neel HB, Pearson GR, Weiland LH, et al. Application of Epstein–Barr virus serology to the diagnosis and staging of North American patients with nasopharyngeal carcinoma. *Otolaryngol Head Neck Surg* 1983;91:255–262.
243. Neglia JP, Meadows AT, Robison LL, et al. Second neoplasms after acute lymphoblastic leukemia in childhood. *N Engl J Med* 1991;325:1330–1336.
244. Newton WA, Jr., Meadows AT, Shimada H, Bunin GR, Vawter GF. Bone sarcomas as second malignant neoplasms following childhood cancer. *Cancer* 1991;67:193–201.
245. Nichols CR, Roth BJ, Heerema N, Griep J, Tricot G. Hematologic neoplasia associated with primary mediastinal germ-cell tumors. *N Engl J Med* 1990;322:1425–1429.
246. Niedobitek G, Agathanggelou A, Barber P, Smallman LA, Jones EL, Young LS. P53 overexpression and Epstein–Barr virus infection in undifferentiated and squamous cell nasopharyngeal carcinomas. *J Pathol* 1993;170:457–461.
247. Niedobitek G, Young LS, Sam CK, Brooks L, Prasad U, Rickinson AB. Expression of Epstein–Barr virus genes and of lymphocyte activation molecules in undifferentiated nasopharyngeal carcinomas. *Am J Pathol* 1992;140:879–887.
248. Nikiforov Y, Gnepp DR. Pediatric thyroid cancer after the Chernobyl disaster: pathomorphologic study of 84 cases (1991–1992) from the Republic of Belarus. *Cancer* 1994;74:748–766.
249. Nishihara K, Nagoshi M, Tsuneyoshi M, Yamaguchi K, Hayashi I. Papillary cystic tumors of the pancreas. Assessment of their malignant potential. *Cancer* 1993;71:82–92.
250. Nishihara K, Tsuneyoshi M, Ohshima A, Yamaguchi K. Papillary cystic tumor of the pancreas. Is it a hormone-dependent neoplasm? *Pathol Res Pract* 1993;189:521–526.
251. Nordqvist SR, Fidler WJ, Jr., Woodruff JM, Lewis JL, Jr. Clear cell adenocarcinoma of the cervix and vagina. A clinicopathologic study of 21 cases with and without a history of maternal ingestion of estrogens. *Cancer* 1976;37:858–871.
252. Norris HJ, Jensen RD. Relative frequency of ovarian neoplasms in children and adolescents. *Cancer* 1972;30:713–719.
253. Oberman HA. Breast lesions in the adolescent female. *Pathol Annu* 1979;14:175–201.
254. Oberman HA. Secretory carcinoma of the breast in adults. *Am J Surg Pathol* 1980;4:465–470.
255. Ochs J, Mulhern RK. Late effects of antileukemic treatment. *Pediatr Clin North Am* 1988;35:815–833.
256. Ohaki Y, Misugi K, Sasaki Y, Okudaira M. Pancreatic carcinoma in childhood. Report of an autopsy case and a review of the literature. *Acta Pathol Jpn* 1985;35:1543–1554.
257. Olsen JH. Risk of second cancer after cancer in childhood. *Cancer* 1986;57:2250–2254.
258. Osborne BM, Robboy SJ. Lymphomas or leukemia presenting as ovarian tumors. An analysis of 42 cases. *Cancer* 1983;52:1933–1943.
259. Padilla RS, McConnell TS, Gribble JT, Smoot C. Malignant melanoma arising in a giant congenital melanocytic nevus. A case report with cytogenetic and histopathologic analyses. *Cancer* 1988;62:2589–2594.
260. Palazzo J, Duray PH. Typical, dysplastic, congenital, and Spitz nevi: a comparative immunohistochemical study. *Hum Pathol* 1989;20:341–346.
261. Pang S, Becker D, Cotelingam J, Foley TP, Jr., Drash AL. Adre-

nocortical tumor in a patient with congenital adrenal hyperplasia due to 21-hydroxylase deficiency. *Pediatrics* 1981;68:242–246.
262. Papavasiliou C, Pavlatou M, Pappas J. Nasopharyngeal cancer in patients under the age of thirty years. *Cancer* 1977;40:2312–2316.
263. Pappo A, Schneider NR, Sanders JM, Buchanan GR. Secondary myelodysplastic syndrome complicating therapy for osteogenic sarcoma. *Cancer* 1991;68:1373–1375.
264. Parham DM, Webber B, Holt H, Williams WK, Maurer HM. Immunohistochemical study of childhood rhabdomyosarcomas and related neoplasms: results of an Intergroup Rhabdomyosarcoma Study project. *Cancer* 1991;67:3072–3080.
265. Passmore SJ, Berry PJ, Oakhill A. Recurrent pancreatoblastoma with inappropriate adrenocorticotrophic hormone secretion. *Arch Dis Child* 1988;63:1494–1496.
266. Patterson K, Kapur S, Chandra RS. "Nasal gliomas" and related brain heterotopias: a pathologist's perspective. *Pediatr Pathol* 1986;5:353–362.
267. Pedersen MI, Bennett JW, Wang N. Nonrandom chromosome structural aberrations and oncogene loci in human malignant melanoma. *Cancer Genet Cytogenet* 1986;20:11–27.
268. Pedersen-Bjergaard J, Daugaard G, Hansen SW, Philip P, Larsen SO, Rorth M. Increased risk of myelodysplasia and leukaemia after etoposide, cisplatin, and bleomycin for germ-cell tumours. *Lancet* 1991;338:359–363.
269. Pedersen-Bjergaard J, Ersboll J, Hansen VL, et al. Carcinoma of the urinary bladder after treatment with cyclophosphamide for non-Hodgkin's lymphoma. *N Engl J Med* 1988;318:1028–1032.
270. Peters MS, Goellner JR. Spitz naevi and malignant melanomas of childhood and adolescence. *Histopathology* 1986;10:1289–1302.
271. Pettinato G, Manivel JC, Ravetto C, et al. Papillary cystic tumor of the pancreas. A clinicopathologic study of 20 cases with cytologic, immunohistochemical, ultrastructural, and flow cytometric observations, and a review of the literature. *Am J Clin Pathol* 1992;98:478–488.
272. Piver MS. Management of children with unilateral ovarian malignancies. *Pediatr Annu* 1981;10:46–52.
273. Prat J, Scully RE. Cellular fibromas and fibrosarcomas of the ovary: a comparative clinicopathologic analysis of seventeen cases. *Cancer* 1981;47:2663–2670.
274. Prat J, Young RH, Scully RE. Ovarian Sertoli-Leydig cell tumors with heterologous elements. II. Cartilage and skeletal muscle: a clinicopathologic analysis of twelve cases. *Cancer* 1982;50:2465–2475.
275. Pratt CB, George SL, Green AA, Fields LA, Dodge RK. Carcinomas in children: clinical and demographic characteristics. *Cancer* 1988;61:1046–1050.
276. Pratt CB, Parham DM, Rao BN, Fleming ID, Dilawari R. Multiple colorectal carcinomas, polyposis coli, and neurofibromatosis. *JNCI* 1988;80:1170–1172.
277. Pratt CB, Pui CH. Secondary acute lymphoblastic leukemia in childhood [letter]. *J Clin Oncol* 1992;10:866
278. Proppe KH, Scully RE. Large-cell calcifying Sertoli cell tumor of the testis. *Am J Clin Pathol* 1980;74:607–619.
279. Prosser J, Elder PA, Condie A, MacFadyen I, Steel CM, Evans HJ. Mutations in p53 do not account for heritable breast cancer: a study in five affected families. *Br J Cancer* 1991;63:181–184.
280. Pui CH, Hancock ML, Raimondi SC, et al. Myeloid neoplasia in children treated for solid tumours. *Lancet* 1990;336:417–421.
281. Pui CH, Ribeiro RC, Hancock ML, et al. Acute myeloid leukemia in children treated with epipodophyllotoxins for acute lymphoblastic leukemia. *N Engl J Med* 1991;325:1682–1687.
282. Quak SH, Prabhakaran K, Kwok R, O'Reilly AP. Vasoactive intestinal peptide secreting tumours in children: a case report with literature review. *Aust Paediatr J* 1988;24:55–58.
283. Raffensperger JG. Ovarian tumors. In: Raffensperger JG, ed. *Swenson's Pediatric Surgery.* Norwalk, CT: Appleton and Lange; 1990:393–397.
284. Raju U, Fine G, Warrier R, Kini R, Weiss L. Congenital testicular juvenile granulosa cell tumor in a neonate with X/XY mosaicism. *Am J Surg Pathol* 1986;10:577–583.
285. Rao BN, Hayes FA, Pratt CB, et al. Malignant melanoma in children: its management and prognosis. *J Pediatr Surg* 1990;25:198–203.
286. Rao BN, Pratt CB, Fleming ID, Dilawari RA, Green AA, Austin BA. Colon carcinoma in children and adolescents. A review of 30 cases. *Cancer* 1985;55:1322–1326.
287. Reed RJ, Ichinose H, Clark WH, Jr., Mihm MC, Jr. Common and uncommon melanocytic nevi and borderline melanomas. *Semin Oncol* 1975;2:119–147.
288. Refetoff S, Harrison J, Karanfilski BT, Kaplan EL, De Groot LJ, Bekerman C. Continuing occurrence of thyroid carcinoma after radiation to the neck in infancy and childhood. *N Engl J Med* 1975;292:171–175.
289. Rhodes AR, Mihm MC, Jr., Weinstock MA. Dysplastic melanocytic nevi: a reproducible histologic definition emphasizing cellular morphology. *Mod Pathol* 1989;2:306–319.
290. Ribeiro RC, Neto RS, Schell MJ, Lacerdo L, Sambaio GA, Cat I. Adrenocortical carcinoma in children: a study of 40 cases. *J Clin Oncol* 1990;8:67–74.
291. Ridolfi RL, Rosen PP, Thaler H. Nevus cell aggregates associated with lymph nodes: estimated frequency and clinical significance. *Cancer* 1977;39:164–171.
292. Rimm IJ, Li FC, Tarbell NJ, Winston KR, Sallan SE. Brain tumors after cranial irradiation for childhood acute lymphoblastic leukemia. A 13-year experience from the Dana-Farber Cancer Institute and the Children's Hospital. *Cancer* 1987;59:1506–1508.
293. Roarty JD, McLean IW, Zimmerman LE. Incidence of second neoplasms in patients with bilateral retinoblastoma. *Ophthalmology* 1988;95:1583–1587.
294. Robboy SJ, Welch WR. Selected topics in the pathology of the vagina. *Hum Pathol* 1991;22:868–876.
295. Robboy SJ, Young RH, Welch WR, Truslow GY, Prat J, Herbst AL, Scully RE. Atypical vaginal adenosis and cervical ectropion. Association with clear cell adenocarcinoma in diethylstilbestrol-exposed offspring. *Cancer* 1984;54:869–875.
296. Robinson L, Martinez MG. Unicystic ameloblastoma: a prognostically distinct entity. *Cancer* 1977;40:2278–2285.
297. Rogers DA, Rao BN, Bowman L, Marina N, Fleming ID, Schropp KP, Lobe TE. Primary malignancy of the salivary gland in children. *J Pediatr Surg* 1994;29:44–47.
298. Rosai J, Carcangiu ML. Pitfalls in the diagnosis of thyroid neoplasms. *Pathol Res Pract* 1987;182:169–179.
299. Rosai J, Carcangiu ML, DeLellis RA. *Atlas of Tumor Pathology. Third Series, Fascicle 5. Tumors of the Thyroid Gland.* Washington, D.C.: Armed Forces Institute of Pathology; 1992.
300. Rosen PP. Papillary duct hyperplasia of the breast in children and young adults. *Cancer* 1985;56:1611–1617.
301. Rosen PP, Cantrell B, Mullen DL, DePalo A. Juvenile papillomatosis (Swiss cheese disease) of the breast. *Am J Surg Pathol* 1980;4:3–12.
302. Rosen PP, Kimmel M. Juvenile papillomatosis of the breast. A follow-up study of 41 patients having biopsies before 1979. *Am J Clin Pathol* 1990;93:599–603.
303. Rosen PP, Lyngholm B, Kinne DW, Beattie EJ, Jr. Juvenile papillomatosis of the breast and family history of breast carcinoma. *Cancer* 1982;49:2591–2595.
304. Rosen PP, Oberman HA. *Atlas of Tumor Pathology. Third Series, Fascicle 7. Tumors of the Mammary Gland.* Washington, D.C.: Armed Forces Institute of Pathology; 1994.
305. Roth LM, Anderson MC, Govan AD, Langley FA, Gowing NF, Woodcock AS. Sertoli–Leydig cell tumors: a clinicopathologic study of 34 cases. *Cancer* 1981;48:187–197.
306. Roth LM, Deaton RL, Sternberg WH. Massive ovarian edema. A clinicopathologic study of five cases including ultrastructural observations and review of the literature. *Am J Surg Pathol* 1979;3:11–21.
307. Roth LM, Nicholas TR, Ehrlich CE. Juvenile granulosa cell tumor: a clinicopathologic study of three cases with ultrastructural observations. *Cancer* 1979;44:2194–2205.
308. Rotterdam H, Tsang P. Gastrointestinal disease in the immunocompromised patient. *Hum Pathol* 1994;25:1123–1140.
309. Rousselet G, Bachouchi M, Busson P, et al. Clinical implications of the serum level of CD23 in patients with undifferentiated nasopharyngeal carcinoma. *J Clin Oncol* 1993;11:2143–2149.
310. Rubin JS. The molecular genetics of the incision step in the DNA excision repair process. *Int J Radiat Biol* 1988;54:309–365.
311. Russell P. The pathological assessment of ovarian neoplasms. I:

Introduction to the common "epithelial" tumours and analysis of benign 'epithelial' tumours. *Pathology* 1979;11:5–26.

312. Russell P. Surface epithelial–stromal tumors of the ovary. In: Kurman RJ, ed. *Blaustein's Pathology of the Female Genital Tract*. New York: Springer-Verlag; 1994:705–782.
313. Sabbaga CC, Avilla SG, Schulz C, Garbers JC, Blucher D. Adrenocortical carcinoma in children: clinical aspects and prognosis. *J Pediatr Surg* 1993;28:841–843.
314. Sagebiel RW, Chinn EK, Egbert BM. Pigmented spindle cell nevus. Clinical and histologic review of 90 cases. *Am J Surg Pathol* 1984;8:645–653.
315. Saitoh A, Tsutsumi Y, Osamura RY, Watanabe K. Sclerosing stromal tumor of the ovary. Immunohistochemical and electron-microscopic demonstration of smooth-muscle differentiation. *Arch Pathol Lab Med* 1989;113:372–376.
316. Salem OS, Steck WD. Cowden's disease (multiple hamartoma and neoplasia syndrome). A case report and review of the English literature. *J Am Acad Dermatol* 1983;8:686–696.
317. Samuel AM, Sharma SM. Differentiated thyroid carcinomas in children and adolescents. *Cancer* 1991;67:2186–2190.
318. Santana VM, Boulden T, Jenkins J, Parham D, Behm F. Percutaneous fine needle aspiration in children. *Proc Am Assoc Cancer Res* 1988;29:223(Abstract).
319. Sartori P, Symons JC, Taylor NF, Grant DB. Adrenal cortical adenoma in a 13-year-old girl with neurofibromatosis. Case report and review of the literature. *Acta Paediatr Scand* 1989;78: 476–478.
320. Sasano H, Saito Y, Sato I, Sasano N, Nagura H. Nucleolar organizer regions in human adrenocortical disorders. *Mod Pathol* 1990;3:591–595.
321. Schimke RN. The multiple endocrine neoplasia syndromes. *Cancer Treat Res* 1983;17:249–264.
322. Schofield DE, Fletcher JA. Trisomy 12 in pediatric granulosa-stromal cell tumors: demonstration by a modified method of fluorescence in situ hybridization on paraffin-embedded material. *Am J Pathol* 1992;141:1265–1269.
323. Schroder S, Padberg BC, Achilles E, Lauritzen I, Dralle H, Kloppel G. Histologie, Immunocytochemie und DNA-Cytophotometrie bei Nebennierenrinden-(NNR)-Tumoren—eine morphologischklinische Untersuchung an 72 Tumoren. *Verh Dtsch Ges Pathol* 1990;74:284–288.
324. Schuller DE, McCabe BF. Salivary gland neoplasms in children. *Otolaryngol Clin North Am* 1977;10:399–412.
325. Schuller DE, McCabe BF. The firm salivary mass in children. *Laryngoscope* 1977;87:1891–1898.
326. Scott AA, Stanley W, Worsham GF, Kirkland TA, Gansler T, Garvin AJ. Aggressive bladder carcinoma in an adolescent: report of a case with immunohistochemical, cytogenetic, and flow cytometric characterization. *Am J Surg Pathol* 1989;13:1057–1063.
327. Scully RE. Sex cord tumor with annular tubules: a distinctive ovarian tumor of the Peutz–Jeghers syndrome. *Cancer* 1970;25: 1107–1121.
328. Scully RE. World Health Organization classification and nomenclature of ovarian cancer. *Natl Cancer Inst Monogr* 1975;42:5–7.
329. Scully RE. Small cell carcinoma of hypercalcemic type. *Int J Gynecol Pathol* 1993;12:148–152.
330. Seidman JD, Patterson JA, Bitterman P. Sertoli–Leydig cell tumor associated with a mature cystic teratoma in a single ovary. *Mod Pathol* 1989;2:687–692.
331. Selzer G, Kahn LB, Albertyn L. Primary malignant tumors of the thyroid gland: a clinicopathologic study of 254 cases. *Cancer* 1977;40:1501–1510.
332. Shah KH, Maxted WC, Chun B. Epidermoid cysts of the testis: a report of three cases and an analysis of 141 cases from the world literature. *Cancer* 1981;47:577–582.
333. Shanmugaratnam K, Chan SH, de-The G, Goh JE, Khor TH, Simons MJ, Tye CY. Histopathology of nasopharyngeal carcinoma: correlations with epidemiology, survival rates and other biological characteristics. *Cancer* 1979;44:1029–1044.
334. Shanmugaratnam K, Sobin L. *Histological Typing of Upper Respiratory Tract Tumors*. Geneva: World Health Organization; 1978.
335. Sheikh MS, Shao ZM, Hussain A, Fontana JA. The p53-binding protein MDM2 gene is differentially expressed in human breast carcinoma. *Cancer Res* 1993;53:3226–3228.
336. Shibata D, Tokunaga M, Uemura Y, Sato E, Tanaka S, Weiss LM. Association of Epstein–Barr virus with undifferentiated gastric carcinomas with intense lymphoid infiltration: Lymphoepithelioma-like carcinoma. *Am J Pathol* 1991;139:469–474.
337. Shikhani AH, Johns ME. Tumors of the major salivary glands in children. *Head Neck Surg* 1988;10:257–263.
338. Sidransky D, Tokino T, Helzlsouer K, et al. Inherited p53 gene mutations in breast cancer. *Cancer Res* 1992;52:2984–2986.
339. Silfversward C. Prognostic factors in granulosa-cell tumors. *Gynecol Oncol* 1981;11:261–274.
340. Silverman JF, Holbrook CT, Pories WJ, Kodroff MB, Joshi VV. Fine needle aspiration cytology of pancreatoblastoma with immunocytochemical and ultrastructural studies. *Acta Cytol* 1990;34:632–640.
341. Sixbey JW. Epstein–Barr virus and epithelial cells. *Adv Viral Oncol* 1989;8:187–202.
342. Sixbey JW, Yao QY. Immunoglobulin A–induced shift of Epstein–Barr virus tissue tropism. *Science* 1992;255:1578–1580.
343. Skogseid B, Larsson C, Lindgren P, et al. Clinical and genetic featrues of adrenocortical lesions in multiple endocrine neoplasia type 1. *J Clin Endocrinol Metab* 1992;75:76–81.
344. Smith KJ, Barrett TL, Skelton HG, Lupton GP, Graham JH. Spindle cell and epithelioid cell nevi with atypia and metastasis (malignant Spitz nevus). *Am J Surg Pathol* 1989;13:931–939.
345. Smith LM, Cox RS, Donaldson SS. Second cancers in long-term survivors of Ewing's sarcoma. *Clin Orthop* 1992;275–281.
346. Smith MA, Rubinstein L, Ungerleider RS. Therapy-related acute myeloid leukemia following treatment with epipodophyllotoxins: estimating the risks. *Med Pediatr Oncol* 1994;23:86–98.
347. Socha J, Dobrzanska A, Rowecka K, et al. Chronic diarrhea due to VIPoma in two children. *J Pediatr Gastroenterol Nutr* 1984;3: 143–148.
348. Sotelo-Avila C, Gooch WM. Neoplasms associated with the Beckwith–Wiedemann syndrome. *Perspect Pediatr Pathol* 1976; 3:255–272.
349. Southwick GJ, Schwartz RA. The basal cell nevus syndrome: disasters occurring among a series of 36 patients. *Cancer* 1979;44: 2294–2305.
350. Spitz S. Melanomas of childhood. *Am J Pathol* 1948;24:591–609.
351. Staalman CR, Umans U. Hypertrophic osteoarthropathy in childhood malignancy. *Med Pediatr Oncol* 1993;21:676–679.
352. Starink TM, van der Veen JP, Arwert F, de Waal LP, de Lange GG, Gille JJ, Eriksson AW. The Cowden syndrome: a clinical and genetic study in 21 patients. *Clin Genet* 1986;29:222–233.
353. Steinberg JB, Tuggle DW, Postier RG. Adenocarcinoma of the colon in adolescents. *Am J Surg* 1988;156:460–462.
354. Stewart DR, Jones PH, Jolleys A. Carcinoma of the adrenal gland in children. *J Pediatr Surg* 1974;9:59–67.
355. Stewart JP, Arrand JR. Expression of the Epstein–Barr virus latent membrane protein in nasopharyngeal carcinoma biopsy specimens. *Hum Pathol* 1993;24:239–242.
356. Stokkel MP, Kroon BB, van der Sande JJ, Neering H. Malignant cutaneous melanoma associated with neurofibromatosis in two sisters from a family with familial atypical multiple mole melanoma syndrome. Case reports and review of the literature. *Cancer* 1993;72:2370–2375.
357. Stommer P, Kraus J, Stolte M, Giedl J. Solid and cystic pancreatic tumors. Clinical, histochemical, and electron microscopic features in ten cases. *Cancer* 1991;67:1635–1641.
358. Strong LC, Herson J, Osborne BM, Sutow WW. Risk of radiation-related subsequent malignant tumors in survivors of Ewing's sarcoma. *JNCI* 1979;62:1401–1406.
359. Suarez HG. Activated oncogenes in human tumors. *Anticancer Res* 1989;9:1331–1343.
360. Suzuki T, Sassano H, Nisikawa T, Rhame J, Wilkinson DS, Nagura H. Discerning malignancy in human adrenocortical neoplasms: utility of DNA flow cytometry and immunohistochemistry. *Mod Pathol* 1992;5:224–231.
361. Takayama K, Ohashi M, Haji M, Matsumoto T, Mihara Y, Kumazawa J, Kato K. Adrenocortical tumor in a patient with untreated congenital adrenocortical hyperplasia owing to 21-

hydroxylase deficiency: characterization of steroidogenic lesions. *J Urol* 1988;140:803–805.

362. Tarbell NJ, Gelber RD, Weinstein HJ, Mauch P. Sex differences in risk of second malignant tumours after Hodgkin's disease in childhood. *Lancet* 1993;341:1428–1432.
363. Tartour E, Caillou B, Tenenbaum F, Schroder S, Luciani S, Talbot M, Schlumberger M. Immunohistochemical study of adrenocortical carcinoma. Predictive value of the D11 monoclonal antibody. *Cancer* 1993;72:3296–3303.
364. Tavassoli FA, Norris HJ. Sertoli tumors of the ovary. A clinicopathologic study of 28 cases with ultrastructural observations. *Cancer* 1980;46:2281–2297.
365. Taxy JB. Adenocarcinoma of the pancreas in childhood. Report of a case and a review of the English language literature. *Cancer* 1976;37:1508–1518.
366. Taxy JB, Hidvegi DF, Battifora H. Nasopharyngeal carcinoma: antikeratin immunohistochemistry and electron microscopy. *Am J Clin Pathol* 1985;83:320–325.
367. Taylor SR, Roederer M, Murphy RF. Flow cytometric DNA analysis of adrenocortical tumors in children. *Cancer* 1987;59: 2059–2063.
368. Terracini B, Pastore G, Zurlo MG, et al. Late deaths and second primary malignancies among long-term survivors of childhood cancer: an Italian multicentre study. *Eur J Cancer Clin Oncol* 1987;23:499–504.
369. Tester WJ, Kinsella TJ, Waller B, et al. Second malignant neoplasms complicating Hodgkin's disease: the National Cancer Institute experience. *J Clin Oncol* 1984;2:762–769.
370. Tetu B, Bonenfant JL. Ovarian myxoma. A study of two cases with long-term follow-up. *Am J Clin Pathol* 1991;95:340–346.
371. Thackray AC, Lucas RB. *Atlas of Tumor Pathology. Second Series, Fascicle 10. Tumors of the Major Salivary Glands.* Washington, D.C.: Armed Forces Institute of Pathology; 1974.
372. Thomas RM, Sobin LH. Gastrointestinal cancer. *Cancer* 1995;75:154–170.
373. Trumper PA, Epstein MA, Giovanella BC, Finerty S. Isolation of infectious EB virus from the epithelial tumour cells of nasopharyngeal carcinoma. *Int J Cancer* 1977;20:655–662.
374. Tucker MA, D'Angio GJ, Boice JD, Jr., et al. Bone sarcomas linked to radiotherapy and chemotherapy in children. *N Engl J Med* 1987;317:588–593.
375. Tucker MA, Jones PH, Boice JD, Jr., et al. Therapeutic radiation at a young age is linked to secondary thyroid cancer. The Late Effects Study Group. *Cancer Res* 1991;51:2885–2888.
376. Tucker MA, Meadows AT, Boice JD, Jr., et al. Leukemia after therapy with alkylating agents for childhood cancer. *JNCI* 1987;78:459–464.
377. Tucker MA, Misfeldt D, Coleman CN, Clark WH, Jr., Rosenberg SA. Cutaneous malignant melanoma after Hodgkin's disease. *Ann Intern Med* 1985;102:37–41.
378. Valagussa P, Santoro A, Fossati-Bellani F, Banfi A, Bonadonna G. Second acute leukemia and other malignancies following treatment for Hodgkin's disease. *J Clin Oncol* 1986;4:830–837.
379. van Seters AP, van Aalderen W, Moolenaar AJ, Gorsiro MC, van Roon F, Backer ET. Adrenocortical tumour in untreated congenital adrenocortical hyperplasia associated with inadequate ACTH suppressibility. *Clin Endocrinol (Oxf)* 1981;14:325–334.
380. van Slooten H, Schaberg A, Smeenk D, Moolenaar AJ. Morphologic characteristics of benign and malignant adrenocortical tumors. *Cancer* 1985;55:766–773.
381. Venkatesh S, Ordonez NG, Ajani J, Schultz PN, Hickey RC, Johnston DA, Samaan NA. Islet cell carcinoma of the pancreas. A study of 98 patients. *Cancer* 1990;65:354–357.
382. Vickers RA, Gorlin RJ. Ameloblastoma: delineation of early histopathologic features of neoplasia. *Cancer* 1970;26:699–710.
383. Vinchon M, Blond S, Lejeune JP, Krivosik I, Fossati P, Assaker R, Christiaens JL. Association of Lhermitte–Duclos and Cowden disease: report of a new case and review of the literature. *J Neurol Neurosurg Psychiatry* 1994;57:699–704.
384. Vogelstein B, Fearon ER, Hamilton SR, Kern SE, Preisinger AC, Leppert M. Genetic alteration during colorectal tumor development. *N Engl J Med* 1988;319:525–532.
385. Vonsover A, Rechavi G, Kesler A, et al. EBV genome and immunoglobulin gene rearrangement in the differential diagnosis of nasopharyngeal carcinoma and lymphoma. *Med Pediatr Oncol* 1991;19:246–252.
386. Wallgren A, Silfversward C, Hultborn A. Carcinoma of the breast in women under 30 years of age: a clinical and histopathological study of all cases reported as carcinoma to the Swedish Cancer Registry, 1958–1968. *Cancer* 1977;40:916–923.
387. Waxman M, Damjanov I, Khapra A, Landau SJ. Large cell calcifying Sertoli tumor of the testis. Light microscopic and ultrastructural study. *Cancer* 1984;54:1574–1581.
388. Weedon D, Little JH. Spindle and epithelioid cell nevi in children and adults. A review of 211 cases of the Spitz nevus. *Cancer* 1977;40:217–225.
389. Weinberg RA. Oncogenes and tumor suppressor genes. *CA Cancer J Clin* 1994;44:160–170.
390. Weiss LM. Comparative histologic study of 43 metastasizing and nonmetastasizing adrenocortical tumors. *Am J Surg Pathol* 1984;8:163–169.
391. Weiss LM, Medeiros LJ, Vickery AL, Jr. Pathologic features of prognostic significance in adrenocortical carcinoma. *Am J Surg Pathol* 1989;13:202–206.
392. West S, Hildesheim A, Dosemeci M. Non-viral risk factors for nasopharyngeal carcinoma in the Philippines: results from a case-control study. *Int J Cancer* 1993;55:722–727.
393. Wick MR, Cherwitz DL, McGlennen RC, Dehner LP. Adrenocortical carcinoma. An immunohistochemical comparison with renal cell carcinoma. *Am J Pathol* 1986;122:343–352.
394. Wick MR, Swanson PE. Carcinosarcomas: current perspectives and an historical review of nosological concepts. *Semin Diagn Pathol* 1993;10:118–127.
395. Willems JS, Lowhagen T. Fine-needle aspiration cytology in thyroid disease. *Clin Endocrinol Metab* 1981;10:247–266.
396. Williams ML, Pennella R. Melanoma, melanocytic nevi, and other melanoma risk factors in children. *J Pediatr* 1994;124:833–845.
397. Wingo PA, Tong T, Bolden S. Cancer statistics. *CA Cancer J Clin* 1995;45:8–30.
398. Winick NJ, McKenna RW, Shuster JJ, et al. Secondary acute myeloid leukemia in children with acute lymphoblastic leukemia treated with etoposide. *J Clin Oncol* 1993;11:209–217.
399. Winship T, Rosvoll RV. A study of thyroid cancer in children. *Am J Surg* 1961;102:747–752.
400. Witherspoon RP, Fisher LD, Schoch G, et al. Secondary cancers after bone marrow transplantation for leukemia or aplastic anemia. *N Engl J Med* 1989;321:784–789.
401. Wu T-C, Kuo T-T. Study of Epstein–Barr virus early RNA1 (EBER1) expression by in situ hybridization in thymic epithelial tumors of Chinese patients in Taiwan. *Hum Pathol* 1993;24:235–238.
402. Yagihashi S, Sato I, Kaimori M, Matsumoto J, Nagai K. Papillary and cystic tumor of the pancreas. Two cases indistinguishable from islet cell tumor. *Cancer* 1988;61:1241–1247.
403. Yamaguchi K, Miyagahara T, Tsuneyoshi M, et al. Papillary cystic tumor of the pancreas: an immunohistochemical and ultrastructural study of 14 patients. *Jpn J Clin Oncol* 1989;19:102–111.
404. Yano T, Linehan M, Anglard P, et al. Genetic changes in human adrenocortical carcinomas. *JNCI* 1989;81:518–523.
405. Young RH. Ovarian tumors other than those of surface epithelial-stromal type. *Hum Pathol* 1991;22:763–775.
406. Young RH, Dickersin GR, Scully RE. Juvenile granulosa cell tumor of the ovary. A clinicopathological analysis of 125 cases. *Am J Surg Pathol* 1984;8:575–596.
407. Young RH, Eichhorn JH, Dickersin GR, Scully RE. Ovarian involvement by the intra-abdominal desmoplastic small round cell tumor with divergent differentiation: A report of three cases. *Hum Pathol* 1992;23:454–464.
408. Young RH, Lawrence WD, Scully RE. Juvenile granulosa cell tumor—another neoplasm associated with abnormal chromosomes and ambiguous genitalia. A report of three cases. *Am J Surg Pathol* 1985;9:737–743.
409. Young RH, Prat J, Scully RE. Ovarian Sertoli–Leydig cell tumors with heterologous elements. I. Gastrointestinal epithelium and

carcinoid: a clinicopathologic analysis of thirty-six cases. *Cancer* 1982;50:2448–2456.

410. Young RH, Scully RE. Ovarian sex cord-stromal tumors: recent progress. *Int J Gynecol Pathol* 1982;1:101–123.
411. Young RH, Scully RE. Ovarian Sertoli cell tumors: a report of 10 cases. *Int J Gynecol Pathol* 1984;2:349–363.
412. Young RH, Scully RE. Testicular and paratesticular tumors and tumor-like lesions of ovarian common epithelial and mullerian types. A report of four cases and review of the literature. *Am J Clin Pathol* 1986;86:146–152.
413. Young RH, Scully RE. Alveolar rhabdomyosarcoma metastatic to the ovary: a report of two cases and a discussion of the differential diagnosis of small cell malignant tumors of the ovary. *Cancer* 1989;64:899–904.
414. Young RH, Scully RE. Atypical forms of microglandular hyperplasia of the cervix simulating carcinoma. A report of five cases and review of the literature. *Am J Surg Pathol* 1989;13:50–56.
415. Young RH, Talerman A. Testicular tumors other than germ cell tumors. *Semin Diagn Pathol* 1987;4:342–360.
416. Young RH, Welch WR, Dickersin GR, Scully RE. Ovarian sex cord tumor with annular tubules: review of 74 cases including 27 with Peutz–Jeghers syndrome and four with adenoma malignum of the cervix. *Cancer* 1982;50:1384–1402.
417. Young S, Gooneratne S, Straus FH, Zeller WP, Bulun SE, Rosenthal IM. Feminizing Sertoli cell tumors in boys with Peutz–Jeghers syndrome. *Am J Surg Pathol* 1995;19:50–58.
418. Zaloudek C, Norris HJ. Sertoli–Leydig tumors of the ovary. A clinicopathologic study of 64 intermediate and poorly differentiated neoplasms. *Am J Surg Pathol* 1984;8:405–418.
419. Zarrabi MH, Rosner F, Grunwald HW. Second neoplasms in acute lymphoblastic leukemia. *Cancer* 1983;52:1712–1719.
420. Zhang J, Young RH, Arseneau J, Scully RE. Ovarian stromal tumors containing lutein or Leydig cells (luteinized thecomas and stromal Leydig cell tumors)—a clinicopathological analysis of fifty cases. *Int J Gynecol Pathol* 1982;1:270–285.
421. Zirker TA, Silva EG, Morris M, Ordonez NG. Immunohistochemical differentiation of clear-cell carcinoma of the female genital tract and endodermal sinus tumor with the use of alphafetoprotein and Leu-M1. *Am J Clin Pathol* 1989;91:511–514.
422. Zuppinger K. Disorders of the endocrine pancreas. *Prog Pediatr Surg* 1983;16:51–61.

Pediatric Neoplasia: Morphology and Biology, edited by David M. Parham.
Lippincott-Raven Publishers, Philadelphia © 1996.

CHAPTER 13

Eye Tumors

Ming X. Wang, Jesse J. Jenkins III, Andrew B. Cu-Unjieng, David Meyer, and Larry A. Donoso

INTRODUCTION

Retinoblastoma is the most frequent malignant neoplasm of the eye in childhood, occurring in approximately 1 of 14,000 live births. It is the third most common intraocular malignancy in all ages, following malignant melanoma of the choroid and metastatic carcinoma. Other primary neoplasms of the eye in childhood are very rare and include medulloepithelioma (dictyoma), hemangiomas as part of von Hippel–Lindau disease, and hamartomas as part of type I neurofibromatosis. Because of the importance of early diagnosis and proper staging in the successful treatment of retinoblastoma, confounding lesions simulating retinoblastoma will also be discussed.

The last few years has seen a rapid development in the molecular genetics of ocular disorders, particularly pediatric ocular neoplasia. As of 1994, chromosomal linkages have been reported in many conditions with ophthalmic manifestations (Table 1), and in a few instances the gene defects have been identified at the molecular level. Because many of the pediatric ocular tumors can now be effectively treated and in some instances cured, the appropriate diagnosis and management of these diseases is an important aspect of current ophthalmic practice. In addition, the unique developmental and genetic features of these diseases have long attracted the attention of clinicians and molecular biologists alike, resulting in some of the most exciting discoveries in molecular oncology in the past few decades. Herein we describe recent advances in pediatric ocular neoplasia, emphasizing the clinical and molecular genetics relevant to these discoveries. We begin with a description of the histopathology and differential diagnosis of the common and uncommon eye tumors and end by describing the general approaches used in the molecular characterization of these tumors.

M. X. Wang, and L. A. Donoso: Research Division, Wills Eye Hospital, Philadelphia, Pennsylvania 19107.

A. B. Cu-Unjieng: Department of Ophthalmology and Visual Sciences, University of Louisville, Louisville, Kentucky 40206.

J. J. Jenkins: Department of Pathology and Laboratory Medicine, St. Jude Children's Research Hospital, Memphis, Tennessee 38105.

D. Meyer: Vitreoretinal Foundation, Memphis, Tennessee 38119.

HISTOPATHOLOGY OF EYE TUMORS

Retinoblastoma

Retinoblastoma is the prototypic pediatric eye tumor and has played a critical role in our understanding of the molecular mechanisms of tumorigenesis in the past decade. It is the most common intraocular tumor of childhood and has both familial and sporadic varieties (59). Clinically, patients often present at a young age (usually less than 5 years) with a white pupillary reflex or leukocoria (Fig. 1), often first noted by the parents. Although this clinical presentation may resemble a cataract, it is important to note that the lens in patients with retinoblastoma is almost always clear. Other childhood conditions that can present with leukocoria and simulate retinoblastoma include persistent hyperplastic primary vitreous (PHPV), Coats' disease, and toxocariasis. It is important to differentiate between these simulating lesions, as retinoblastoma requires prompt diagnosis, accurate pathologic staging, and initiation of treatment to prevent the virtually certain fatality of metastatic disease. Retinoblastomas occur sporadically in 94% of cases, whereas the remaining 6% occur in individuals with a family history of retinoblastoma (59). Among the sporadic cases, approximately 30% are due to new germ line mutations, whereas 70% are the result of somatic

TABLE 1. *Mapped eye diseases*

Disease	Map location
Adenomatous polyposis of the colon	5q22-q23
Aicardi's syndrome	Xp22
Aland's eye disease	Xp11.4-q21
Aland's eye disease (Forsius–Erikson)	Xp21.3-p21.1
Albinism, ocular, Nettleship–Falls type	Xp22.3
Albinism, oculocutaneous 2, tyrosinase-positive	2q31.2 or 4q31.22
Albinism oculocutaneous, tyrosinase-negative	11q14-q21
Aniridia, isolated 1	2p1
Aniridia, isolated 2	11p13
Aniridia	2p25
WAGR (aniridia with Wilms' tumor)	11p13
Anophthalmos, X-linked	Xq27-q28
Anterior segment mesenchymal dysgenesis	4q
Arthroophthalmopathy, Stickler's syndrome	12q14.3
Ataxia telangiectasia	11q22-q23
Blepharophimosis	3q23
Blue cone monochromacy (red/green)	Xq28
Blue cone pigment (Tritan color blindness)	7q22-qter
Cataract, Coppock-like	2q33-q35
Cataract, posterior, polar	16
Cataract, pulverulent, zonular, coppock type	1q21-q25
Cataract, Mariner type	16
Cataract, anterior, polar	2p25 or 14q24
Cataract, congenital, total	Xp
Cerebrotendinous xanthomatosis	2q33-qter2,3
CHARGE association	6cen/8cen2,3
Choroideremia	Xq21.2
Coats' syndrome	3p21 or 3q28
Cokayne's syndrome	2q21
Collagen, type II, α_1 chain (Stickler's)	12q13.1-q13.3
Collagen I, α_1 chain (Marfan's syndrome)	17q21.3-q22.05
Coloboma of iris	2pter-p25.1
Color blindness, blue cone monochromacy	Xq28
Color blindness, deutan (green cone pigment)	Xq28
Color blindness, protan (red cone pigment)	Xq28
Cone dystrophy	1Xp21.1-p11.3
Cone dystrophy 2/defect of red cone pigment	Xq28
Cone dystrophy 3	6q27
Cone-rod dystrophy	18q21.1-q22.2
Congenital hypertrophy of RPE	15q21-q22
Congenital stationary night blindess	Xp11.4-p11.23
Dermoids of cornea	Xp
Dystrophia myotonia	19p13.3-q13.1
Galactosemia, type II	17q23-q25
Goldenhar's syndrome (conjunctival dermoids)	7p
Green–blue eye color	19
Homocystinuria	21q22.3
Leber hereditary optic neuropathy	Xp1
Leber's hereditary optic neuropathy	mitoDNA
Macular dystrophy, atypical vitteliform	8q24
Macular dystrophy, vitteliform, Best type	11q13-qter
Marfan's syndrome, type I α	7q21.3-q22
Marfan's syndrome	15q15-q21.3
Megalocornea, X-linked	Xq12-q26
Microphthalmia	Xp22
Moebius's syndrome	13q2
Myopia 1, X-linked, Bornholm's eye disease	Xq
Nance–Horan syndrome	Xp22.3-p21.1
Neurofibromatosis 1	17q11.2
Neurofibromatosis 2	22q11-q12.2
Niemann–Pick disease	17
Niemann–Pick, type A/ sphingomyelinase	11p15.4-p15.1
Norrie's disease	Xp11.4-p11.3
Ocular albinism	Xp22
Optic atrophy	18
Optic atrophy, polyneuropathy, and deafness	Xqdistal
Pelizaeus–Merzbacher	Xq21.3-q22
Peripherin-retinal degeneration slow protein	6p
Retinitis pigmentosa 1	8p11-q21
Retinitis pigmentosa 2	Xp11.4-p11.23
Retinitis pigmentosa 3	Xp21.1
Retinitis pigmentosa 4/rhodopsin	3q21-q24
Retinitis pigmentosa 5	3q21-q22
Retinitis pigmentosa 6/peripherin	6p
Retinoblastoma	13q14.1-q14.2
Retinoschisis	Xp22.3-p22.1
Reiger's syndrome	4q22.2-q25
Rod cGMP phosphodiesterase β	4p16
Rod outer segment protein 1	11p13
S-antigen	2q24-q37
Oculocerebrorenal syndrome, Lowe	Xq25-q26.1
Tapetochoroidal dystrophy	Xp21.1-q21.2
Tritanopia	7q22-qter
Tuberous sclerosis 1	19q34
Tuberous sclerosis 2	11q22-q23
Tuberous sclerosis 3	12q22-q24.1
Usher's syndrome 1	14q
Usher's syndrome 2	1q
Vitelliform dystrophy	8q
von Hippel–Lindau disease	3p26-p24
Waardenburg's syndrome	2q37
Werner's syndrome	8
Wieacker–Wolff	Xq11-q12
Wilson's disease	13q14-q21
Wolf–Hirshhorn syndrome	4pter-p16.3

Abbreviations: RPE, retinal pigment epithelium.
(Adapted from refs. 20 and 45.)

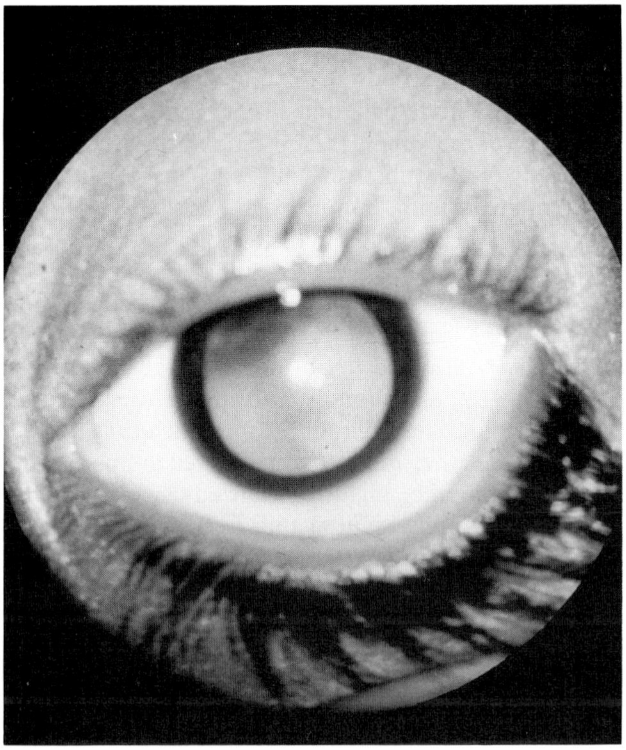

FIG. 1. White pupillary reflex (leukocoria) in a child with retinoblastoma.

mutations. If a child is born with bilateral retinoblastoma, the disease is considered to be hereditary (due either to an inherited mutation or a new germ line mutation). If, however, a child has unilateral retinoblastoma, there is still a 20% chance that the disease is hereditary (new or old germ mutations).

Careful orientation, dissection, and staging of the tumor-bearing globe or orbital exenteration specimen after formalin fixation is important for the subsequent planning of the chemo- and radiotherapy of retinoblastoma. Detailed dissection guides for these specimens have been published in several locations (53,57). In most instances, review of the ultrasound and magnetic resonance imaging as well as transillumination for location of the internal tumor mass will be of value in deciding whether or not to open the globe in the usual horizontal meridian. Other meridians may be chosen as long as the axis is carefully recorded and the central slice contains the pupil and optic nerve. A complete evaluation will include anteroposterior, horizontal, and vertical dimensions of the globe; horizontal and vertical dimensions of the cornea and pupil; length and diameter of the optic nerve stump; location of transillumination shadows marked on the scleral surface with indelible ink; identification of the optic nerve resection margin; identification of other appropriate resection margins if an orbital exenteration has been done; and of course careful description and measurement of the tumor. The tumor cut surfaces (Fig. 2) are very soft and friable and vary from translucent gray–white when viable through opaque yellow–white when necrotic to opaque chalky white when dystrophically calcified. Necrosis and dystrophic calcification are common, lending the cut surfaces a characteristic punctate appearance composed of small islands of viable tumor around small vessels surrounded by a sea of necrosis and calcification. Foci of old or recent hemorrhage are often noted. Choroidal invasion can sometimes be seen grossly as discontinuities in the very thin, black retinal pigment epithelium, particularly if the observer is aided by a hand lens or inverted microscope ocular. Dissemination within the eye is grossly recognized by usually small, white nodules floating in the vitreous humor or by identical nodules on the usually detached retina. Multicentric primaries have an identical gross appearance in the retina to disseminated tumor.

The microscopic appearance of any given retinoblas-

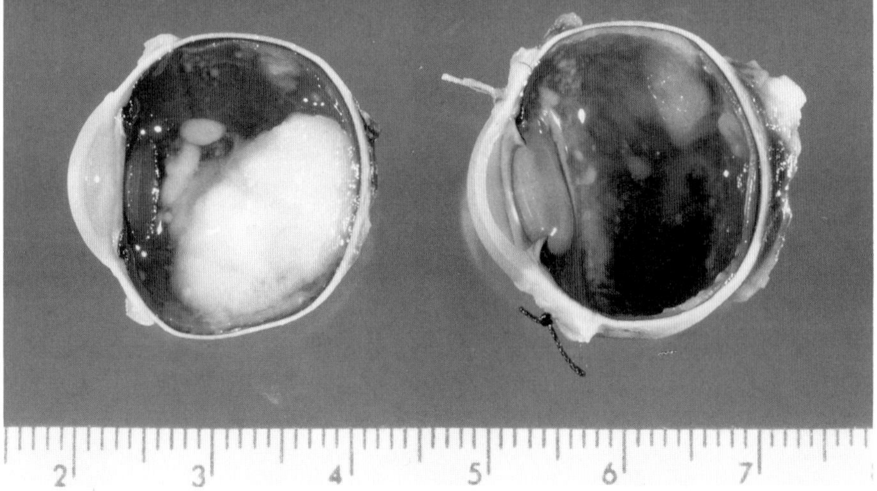

FIG. 2. Retinoblastoma with extensive vitreous seeding as well as multicentric primary tumor sites.

toma depends on its degree of differentiation. Undifferentiated retinoblastomas are composed of small undifferentiated cells with little visible cytoplasm, high nucleocytoplasmic ratio, and nuclei with coarsely granular chromatin and irregular nuclear membranes. Necrosis is common, with relative survival of tumor cells near blood vessels. Dystrophic calcification in the necrotic zones provides the chalky gross appearance in many tumors. Particularly around the regions of necrosis, it is not unusual to see DNA encrustation of blood vessels (the so-called Azzopardi phenomenon) (18, 46,55,81). Hemosiderin is often seen locally, suggesting remote hemorrhage. Visually pleasing and distinctive arrangements of tumor cells in retinoblastomas are traditional indicators of differentiation and include Homer–Wright rosettes, Flexner–Wintersteiner rosettes, and fleurettes (9,55,56,81). The Homer–Wright rosette, more often seen in neuroblastoma and medulloblastoma and infrequently seen in retinoblastoma, is composed of an irregular circlet of tumor cell nuclei arranged around a lightly eosinophilic, variably sized tangle of cell processes with no lumen. The Flexner–Wintersteiner rosette (Fig. 3), for all practical purposes seen only in retinoblastoma and rarely pineoblastoma, is composed of a circlet of tumor nuclei displaced away from a central lumen that is sharply bounded by an eosinophilic membrane analogous to the outer limiting membrane of the normal retina. The lumen contains an acid mucopolysaccharide similar to that found around normal rods and cones (55,56,67,79) and may be nearly obliterated by cell processes if very small. Flexner–Wintersteiner rosettes are seen in approximately 70% of retinoblastomas. The fleurette (Fig. 4), first described in 1970 by Ts'o and colleagues (68), is less often seen than the Flexner–Wintersteiner rosette and is another manifestation of photosensory differentiation. It is composed of larger cells whose abundant eosinophilic cytoplasm is arranged in a distinctive fleur-de-lis. Especially well-differentiated tumors composed almost entirely of fleurettes have been called retinomas or retinocytomas (41,68,69).

The histogenesis of retinoblastoma has been controversial (60). Reports appeared as early as 1864 by Virchow who considered the tumor to be glial in origin. Flexner in 1891 and Wintersteiner in 1897 described the classic histologic features of the tumor including rosettes (Fig. 3), which they believed to be related to photoreceptor cells (Fig. 5), i.e., highly specialized sensory neurons. Based on these observations they considered the tumor to be neural rather than glial in origin, a concept held by most ophthalmic pathologists today. Many subsequent immunohistochemical and electron micrographic studies have emphasized the neural and/or neuronal components of these tumors, where ultrastructurally retinoblastoma cells resemble primitive photoreceptor cells. In such cases, neurofilament triplet proteins are immunohistochemically associated with tumor cells (Fig. 6; see figure in color plate section) (50). Of particular note is the presence of photoreceptor cell–associated proteins such as rhodopsin, rhodopsin kinase, S antigen, and transducin, all involved in the visual phototransductive pathway. Of these antigens, S antigen has been the most well-characterized with respect to retinoblastoma. S antigen is a 48-kd protein that is intimately involved in the

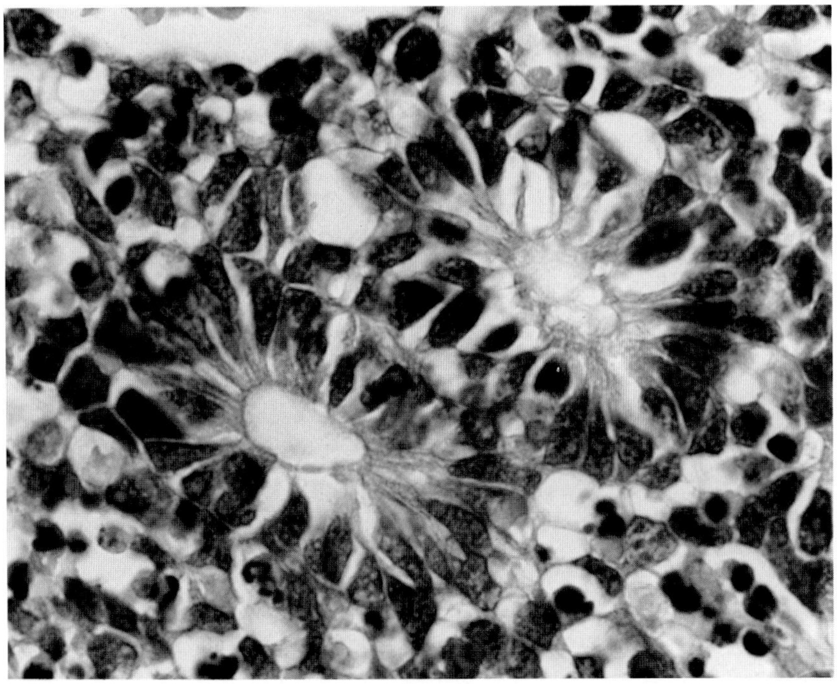

FIG. 3. Flexner–Wintersteiner rosettes in a well-differentiated retinoblastoma.

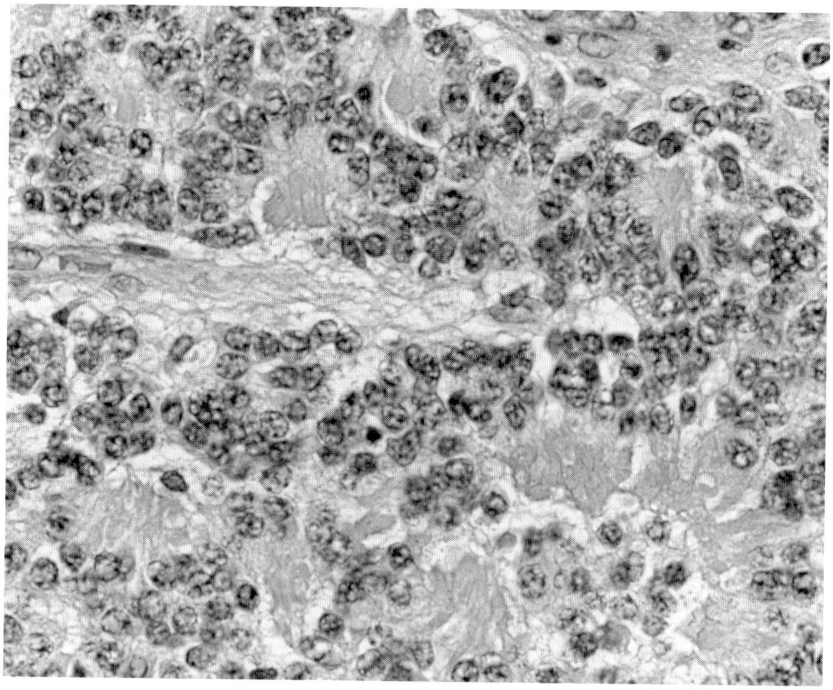

FIG. 4. Fleurettes in a well-differentiated retinoblastoma.

visual process, by binding to photoexcited rhodopsin and thereby quenching or arresting light-induced cyclic guanosine monophosphate phosphodiesterase activity. In the normal retina, S antigen has been shown to completely surround the photoreceptor cells (Fig. 7). In retinoblastomas, S-antigen immunoreactivity is has been localized to tumor cells, particularly those tumors with well-defined Flexner–Wintersteiner rosettes or fleurettes (Fig. 8). Occasionally, disorganized normal retina may be entrapped within a retinoblastoma and the resultant immunohistochemical staining may be mistaken for tumor cell positivity (Fig. 9).

Although retinoblastomas appear to be neuronal in origin, some tumors contain small groups or individual cells that stain positively for the glial immunohistochemical markers, glial fibrillary acidic protein, S-100 protein,

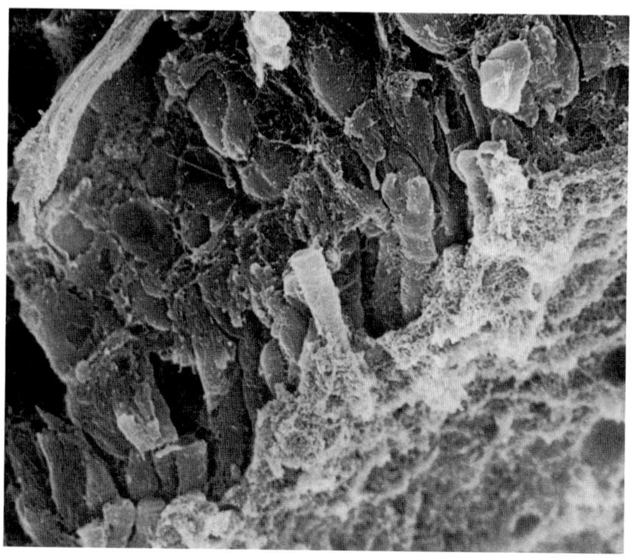

FIG. 5. Scanning electron photomicrograph of normal human retina showing rodlike projections corresponding to photoreceptor cells.

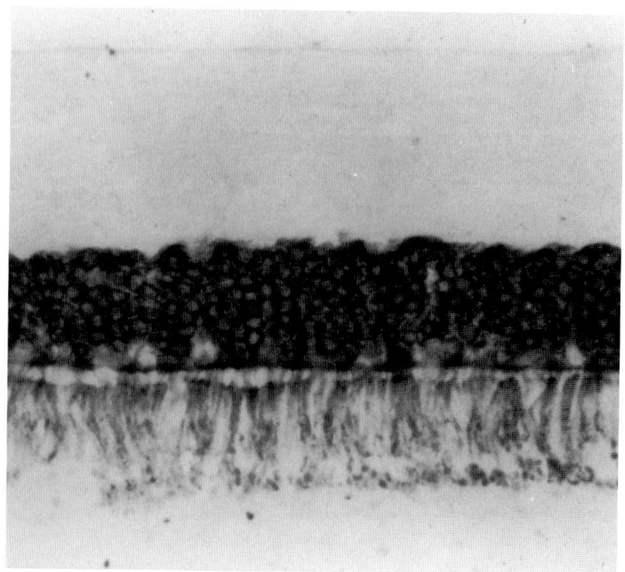

FIG. 7. Indirect immunoperoxidase stain of normal human retina showing S-antigen immunoreactivity completely surrounding the photoreceptor cell. (Used by permission. *Invest Ophthalmol Vis Sci* 1985;26:561–567.)

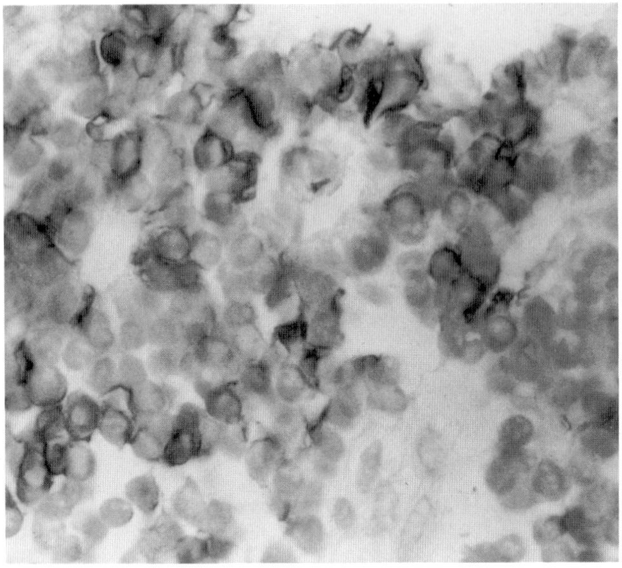

FIG. 8. S-Antigen immunoreactivity in a well-differentiated retinoblastoma.

vimentin, or Leu 7; however, this staining pattern has been mainly ascribed to the presence of reactive glial element entrapped by the tumor (Fig. 10; see figure in color plate section) and is usually traceable in multiple sections to adjacent disorganized retina (31,50,55). In contrast, however, several observers have identified neoplastic glial cells in their material by either ultrastructural or immunohistochemical study (17,45,63,66).

Ultrastructurally, retinoblastoma cells also demonstrate photoreceptor differentiation with the presence of the distinctive rosettes described above, cilia with the 9-0 microtubule doublet pattern, abundant cytoplasmic microtubules, synaptic ribbons, and neurosecretory granules (1,55).

Despite retinoblastoma having a specific, well-documented chromosomal defect, the chromosomal abnormalities that involve the long arm of chromosome 13 (13q) are not detectable by routine methods in most cases. However, in a small number of patients with retinoblastoma a deletion of the long arm of chromosome 13 is detectable: this combination is called the D-deletion syndrome (32,70). With special techniques that expand the chromosome lengths, other patients with 13q deletions are detected (76).

Trilateral Retinoblastoma

There is a significant incidence of pineoblastomas and other midline intracranial tumors (see Chapter 7) in patients with hereditary retinoblastoma (80). The term "trilateral" retinoblastoma refers to this condition (4,5,8). From an embryologic standpoint, this association is not surprising. In lower vertebrates, the pineal gland is structurally and functionally a photoreceptive organ (Fig. 11), and the mammalian pineal gland has a phylogenetic and ontologic relationship to photoreception (74,75,78). This relationship is further illustrated by the immunohistochemical localization of several retinal photoreceptor cell–associated proteins, including S antigen (16,19,20,28,33), interphotoreceptor retinol-binding protein (IRBP) (12), and rhodopsin kinase (62), to the pineocytes of the pineal gland (Fig. 12). In addition, S-antigen and IRBP gene probes that specifically hybridize to the retinal m-RNA isolated have also been shown to bind to pineal m-RNA.

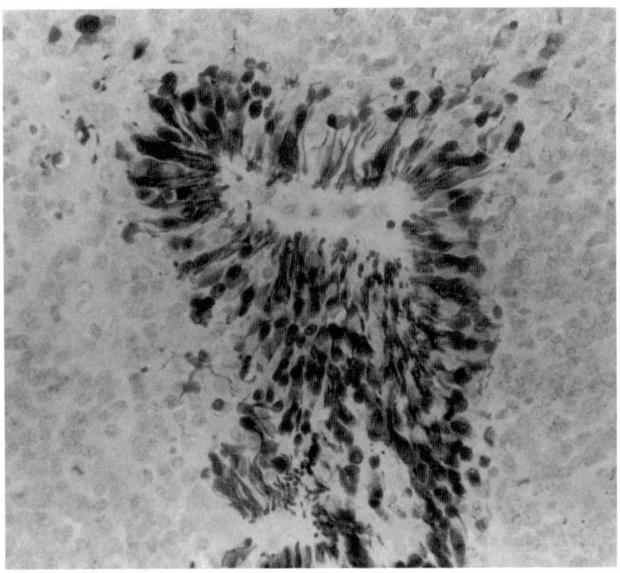

FIG. 9. Disorganized retina entrapped within retinoblastoma with positive staining for S-antigen.

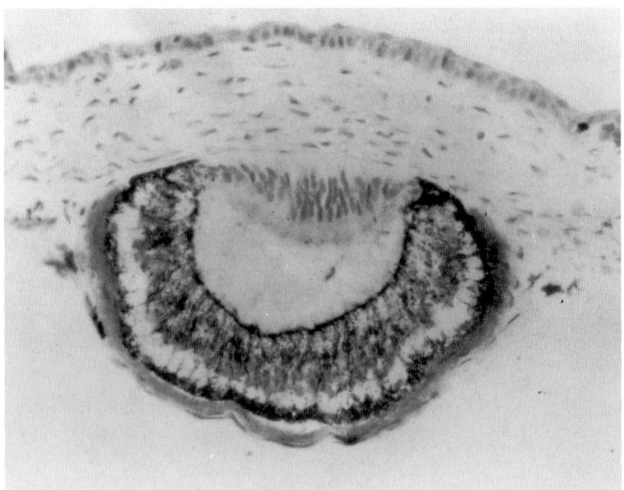

FIG. 11. Parietal eye of lizard. Note remarkable similarity to normal human eye, including cornea, lens, vitreous, and retina. (Photomicrograph provided by Gustav Engbretson.)

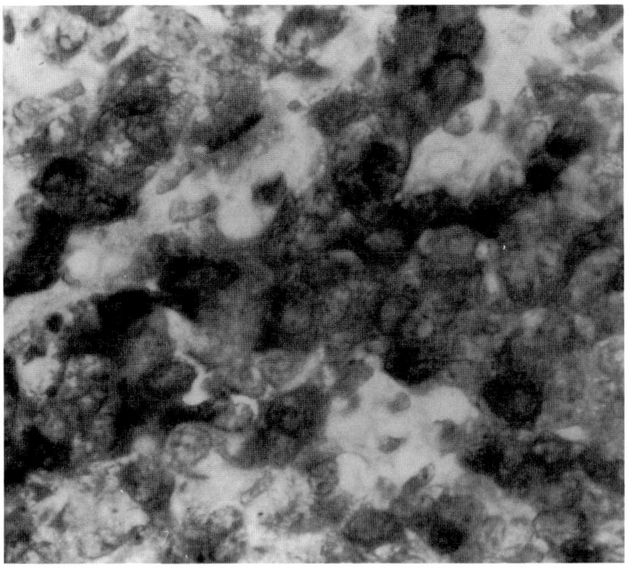

FIG. 12. S-antigen immunoreactivity in normal pineal gland.

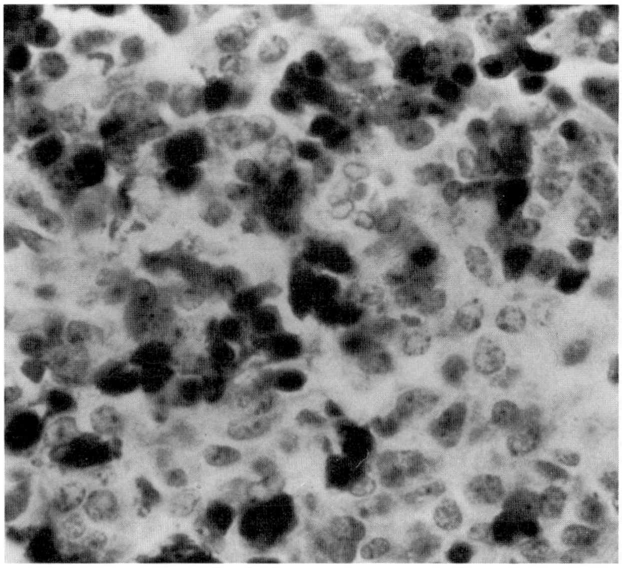

FIG. 14. S-antigen immunoreactivity in pineal tumor of child with trilateral retinoblastoma.

In patients with trilateral retinoblastoma, clinical documentation of the intracranial tumor (Fig. 13) may precede the discovery of the eye tumor. Histopathologically in most cases, the brain tumor resembles undifferentiated retinoblastoma but with the more frequent formation of Homer–Wright rosettes, as described above. In addition, they may occasionally have Flexner–Wintersteiner rosettes, fleurettes, or stain positively for photoreceptor cell–specific antigens such as rhodopsin or S antigen (Fig. 14), further illustrating the close relationship between the retina and pineal gland.

Additional new support for the close biochemical, immunologic, and genetic linkage between these two photoreceptor organs was provided by the production of a murine transgenic trilateral retinoblastoma model system (26) in which transgenic mice expressed the SV40 T-antigen oncogene specifically in photoreceptor cells. All mice developed retinoblastomas and pineoblastomas with 100% penetrance, representing a heritable model for human trilateral retinoblastomas. The possibility of pineoblastoma should be considered in the genetic counseling of patients with the hereditary form of retinoblastoma because most cases of trilateral retinoblastoma are fatal.

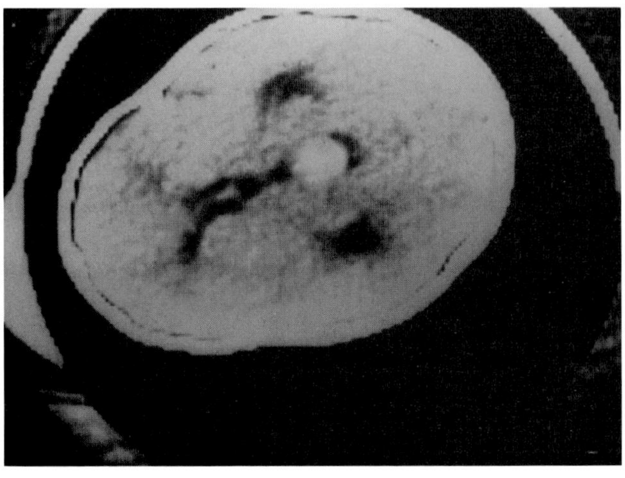

FIG. 13. Computed tomography of brain showing pineal tumor in patient with trilateral retinoblastoma.

Medulloepithelioma

Medulloepithelioma is a very rare tumor of the infant or young child and closely resembles primitive medullary epithelium or the primitive nonpigmented epithelium of the ciliary body derived from the inner layer of the optic cup. It usually arises in the ciliary body, but cases have been reported in the retina and optic nerve (6,7). This entity was first described as a teratoneuroma in 1904 by Verhoeff, as distinct from retinoblastoma (71). It is composed of convoluted ribbons of cuboidal cells producing tubular and papillary structures aligned on an eosinophilic material (Fig. 15). This substance resembles vitreous on one side and contains junctional complexes resembling the outer limiting membrane of the retina on the other. A vague netlike arrangement of cells, particularly at the periphery of these tumors, has lead to the alternate name dictyoma (from the Greek word for "netlike"). These tumors may occasionally express photoreceptor cell proteins such as S antigen and rhodopsin (Fig. 16). In roughly half of cases, heterotopic differentiation in the form of cartilage, striated muscle, or glia has lead to the designation "teratoid medulloepithelioma" (6,7). Foci of undifferentiated retinoblastoma

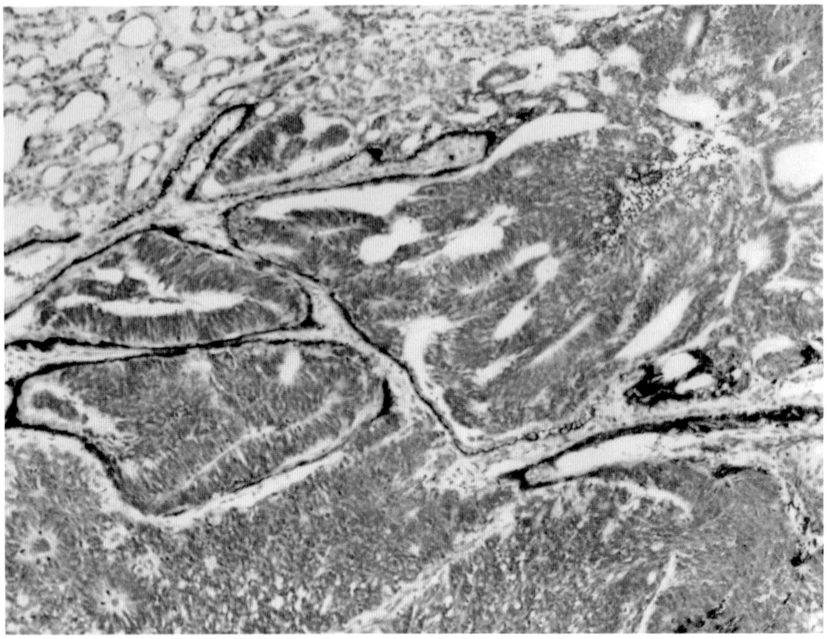

FIG. 15. Medulloepithelioma with ribbons of tumor cells arranged as tubules. Dark line is entrapped retinal pigment epithelium.

in these tumors has also been described (3). The biologic behavior of these tumors has been variable, with about two thirds of the cases reported by Broughton and Zimmerman being malignant as based on cytologic criteria and histologic evidence of invasion (6). These authors also found that most of the teratoid variety are malignant, whereas the nonteratoid variety are equally divided between benign and malignant. Alternatively, those cases reported by Andersen were mostly considered benign (3). Because patients with this condition may also present with leukocoria, such lesions must be distinguished from retinoblastoma and other similar lesions.

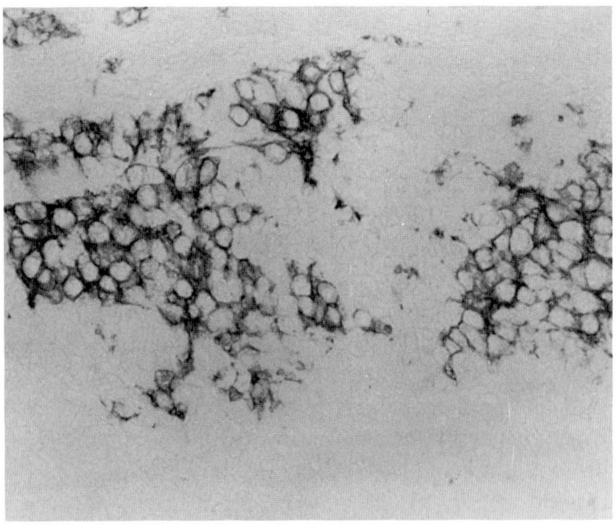

FIG. 16. Rhodopsin immunoreactivity in nonteratoid medulloepithelioma arising from the nonpigmented ciliary epithelium. (Used by permission. *Arch Ophthalmol* 1990;108:481–482. Copyright 1990, American Medical Association.)

Phakomatoses

The phakomatoses (mother spots) compose a group of disorders that primarily involve the eyes, skin, and central nervous system. Clinically, these are important conditions to be recognized because many of these patients will be previously undiagnosed at the time of discovery of an ocular lesion.

von Hippel–Lindau Disease

von Hippel–Lindau disease (VHL), or retinocerebellar capillary hemangiomatosis, is an autosomal dominant phacoma characterized in part by retinal capillary hemangiomas, which may be multiple or bilateral with similar lesions in the cerebellum (Fig. 17). Histologically, the capillary hemangioma consists of a series of proliferating retinal capillaries that may replace the full thickness of the retina. This disease is an autosomal dominantly inherited cancer syndrome that predisposes affected individuals to a variety of tumors, including central nervous system hemangioblastoma, renal cell carcinoma, and pheochromocytoma (see Chapters 3 and 7).

Much progress has been made recently with regard to the molecular biology of this condition. The syndrome has been shown to be caused by a tumor suppressor gene (*VHL*) that was recently cloned (34) using positional cloning techniques. The *VHL* gene is located on human chromosome 3p25-p26. A restriction fragment encompassing the gene showed rearrangements in 28 of 221 VHL kindreds. Eighteen of these rearrangements were due to deletions in the *VHL* gene. The *VHL* gene is evolutionarily conserved and encodes two transcripts of approximately 6 and 6.5 kilobases (kb). The partial sequence of the inferred gene product shows no homology

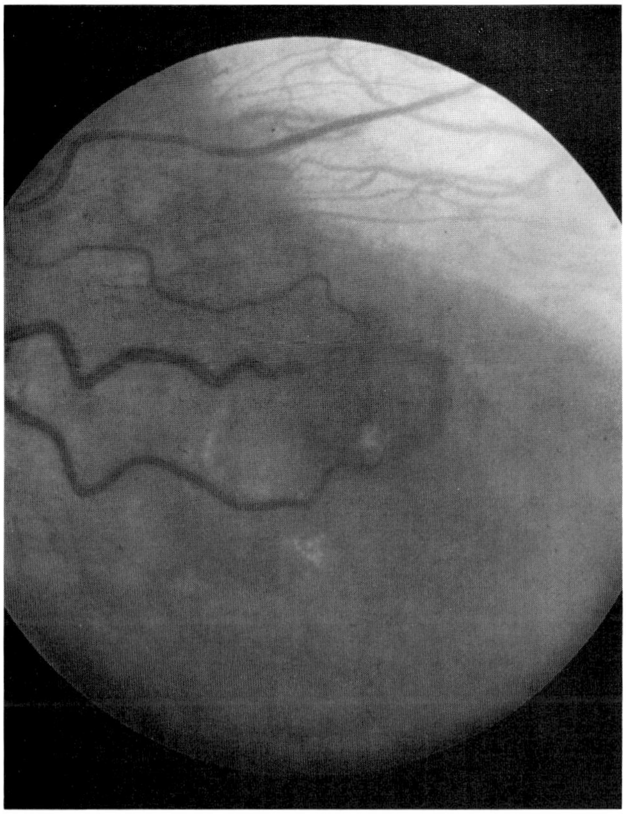

FIG. 17. Fundus photomicrograph of peripheral retina showing capillary hemangioma.

to other proteins, except for an acidic repeat domain found in the procyclic surface membrane glycoprotein of *Trypanosoma brucei*. Intragenic and flanking DNA markers are useful for the presymptomatic diagnosis of VHL disease. Maher et al. (38) studied 14 families containing 23 asymptomatic subjects at a 50% prior risk of VHL disease. By combining age-related and DNA-based risk information, the carrier risk for 11 of those 23 subjects was reduced to <2%.

Neurofibromatosis

Neurofibromatosis is another of the phacomatoses (see Chapter 8). There are several types of neurofibromatosis, which is a neuro-oculocutaneous syndrome. Neurofibromatosis type 1 (NF1) is also referred to as peripheral neurofibromatosis or von Recklinghausen's disease and has typical clinical features such as neurofibromas, cafe-au-lait spots, and Lisch nodules of the iris. There are many associated ocular findings in patients with NF1, including iris, choroidal, and retinal hamartomas; optic nerve glioma and meningioma; and retinal astrocytic hamartomas. The *NF1* gene (see Chapter 8) is located on human chromosome 17q11.2, spanning 350 kb of DNA. The gene consists of 51 exons and encodes for a messenger RNA (mRNA) of 11–13 kb (11,40,72). The coding region of the *NF1* gene specifies a protein of 2,818 amino acids and a molecular weight of 327 kd. *NF1* is thought to be another example of tumor suppressor gene. A normal individual has two copies of the *NF1* gene, whereas an NF1 patient contains only one functional copy of the *NF1* gene in every cell, and the disruption of this one remaining *NF1* gene presumably leads to tumorigenesis. Currently, the diagnosis of NF1 is still largely based on clinical criteria (see Chapter 8).

In contrast to NF1, NF2 is mainly associated with the development of central nervous system tumors such as schwannomas, meningiomas, and ependymomas (see Chapter 7). NF2 represents a disease genetically distinct from NF1. Whereas the *NF1* gene has been mapped to chromosome 17, the putative *NF2* gene is located on chromosome 22. Recently, a candidate gene has been identified that encodes a putative membrane-organization protein (54,65). The identification of the *NF2* gene is based on the experimental evidence that constitutional intragenic mutations are present in the gene in NF2 patients. The *NF2* gene may also be a tumor suppressor gene because tumors containing mutations in the *NF2* gene show loss of the normal allele (54,65). Presymptomatic diagnosis of NF2 based on detection of deletions and point mutations in the *NF2* gene may soon become available.

Tuberous Sclerosis

Tuberous sclerosis, or Bourneville disease, is characterized by multiple hamartomas present in the skin, cerebral cortex, kidney, and eye. The classic ocular findings include astrocytic hamartomas of the retina. These benign lesions may take on a characteristic "mulberrylike" appearance. Histologically, the lesions are composed of well-differentiated astrocytes of varying size. Both the ocular and brain lesions may become calcified, giving rise to "brain stones" on skull X-ray films. Its inheritance pattern is autosomal dominant. To date, several genetic loci have been described for tuberous sclerosis. Haines et al. (25) reported linkage of tuberous sclerosis to chromosome 9q32-9q34. Kandt et al. (29) described the locus for tuberous sclerosis at chromosome 16p13, with a high LOD score of 9.50. The LOD score is the logorithm to base 10 of the odds in favor of linkage. For example, a LOD score of 3 (odds of 1000:1 in favor) is taken as a proof of linkage. Linkage to chromosomes 11q22-23 (27) and 11q14-q23 (61) has also been reported. Based on these findings, tuberous sclerosis is likely a heterogeneous group of diseases involving several genes.

Ocular Manifestations of Systemic Neoplasia

Leukemia and Lymphoma

Other systemic neoplasms that affect the eye include the leukemias and lymphomas. Burkitt's lymphoma pa-

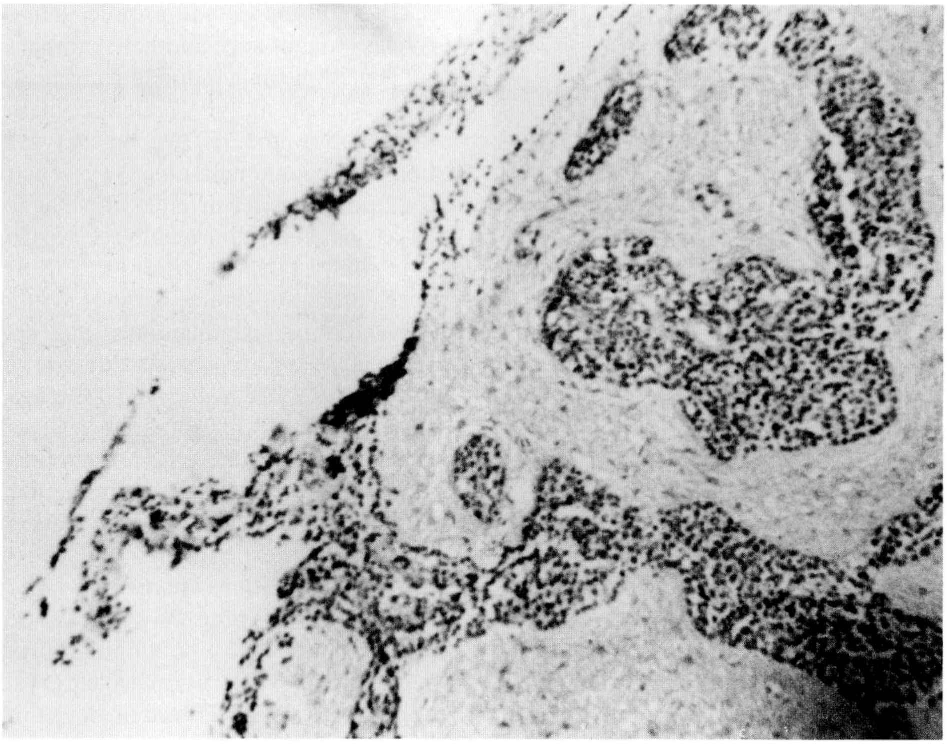

FIG. 18. Lymphomatous optic neuropathy in patient with Burkitt's lymphoma. Note invasion of tumor cells into the optic nerve. (Used by permission. *Pediatr Ophthalmol* 1981;18:48–50.)

tients often present clinically with involvement of abdominal and pelvic sites; these tumors contain small round cells with hyperchromic nuclei interspersed with large, tingible body macrophages giving a "starry sky" appearance (see Chapter 16). Although central nervous system involvement is fairly common, intraocular involvement is relatively rare and usually involves the optic nerves (Fig. 18), which clinically can produce a dramatic papilledema (Fig. 19).

Other Tumors

Pediatric sarcomas, particularly rhabdomyosarcomas and neuroblastomas, may arise in the orbit or eyelid and give rise to ocular symptoms (see Chapter 5). Other relatively rare ocular tumors that can involve the pediatric population include fibrous dysplasia and atrial myxoma. In fibrous dysplasia, the bone marrow of the orbit may be replaced by fibro-osseous tissue, giving rise to ocular manifestations. Visual loss can result from compression of the optic nerve (Fig. 20). In such cases, optic nerve decompression may be successful in preventing further visual loss (Fig. 21). Ophthalmologists should be aware of this condition when confronted with a patient with visual disturbances, osseous abnormalities, pigmented cutaneous lesions, and endocrine dysfunction (McCune–Albright syndrome) (see Chapter 9) (2,42).

Atrial myxoma is another relatively rare tumor that may occasionally involve the eye. In these cases the eye may become secondarily involved from tumor emboli arising primarily from the left atrium. These tumors are largely composed of loosely arranged cells within an amorphous mucoid matrix (Fig. 22).

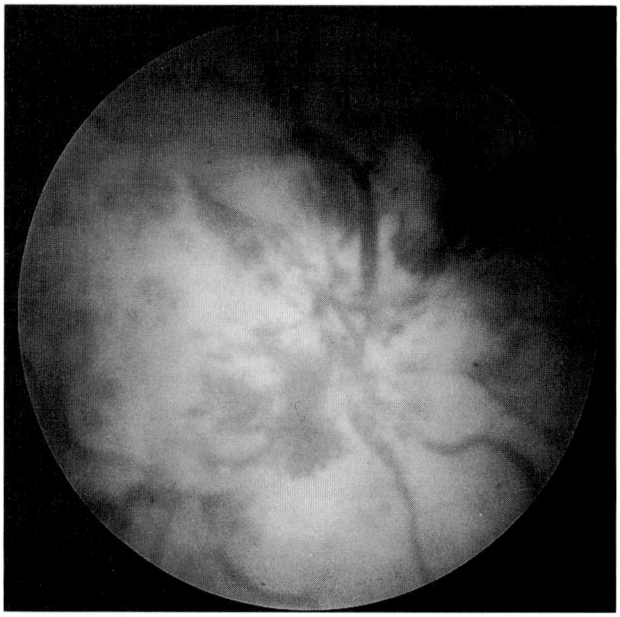

FIG. 19. Gross papilledema of right eye secondary to Burkitt's lymphoma. (Used by permission. *Pediatr Ophthalmol* 1981;18:48–50.)

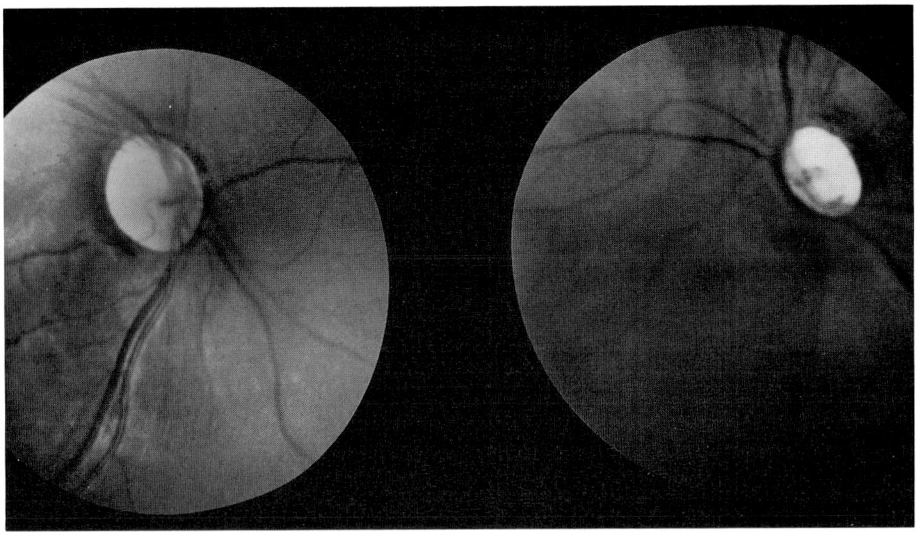

FIG. 20. Optic atrophy secondary to compression of optic nerve in patient with fibrous dysplasia. Note extreme pallor of optic nerve head.

Pseudotumors

Occasionally, eyes are enucleated for a clinical suspicion of retinoblastoma. With the possible exception of medulloepithelioma, these same entities are not easily confused with retinoblastoma on histopathologic examination. Persistent hyperplastic primary vitreous, Coats' disease, and *Toxocara* endophthalmitis account for about 60% of these pseudoretinoblastomas (58) and for that reason are discussed in this chapter.

Persistent Hyperplastic Primary Vitreous

Persistent hyperplastic primary vitreous (PHPV) is a developmental defect that results from the abnormal persistence of the embryonic hyaloid vascular system (hyaloid artery, primary vitreous, and tunica vasculosa lentis) with concurrent hyperplasia of embryonic connective tissue in the developing eye. It was first recognized and described as a full-spectrum entity by Reese in 1955 (51,52). These children present in the perinatal

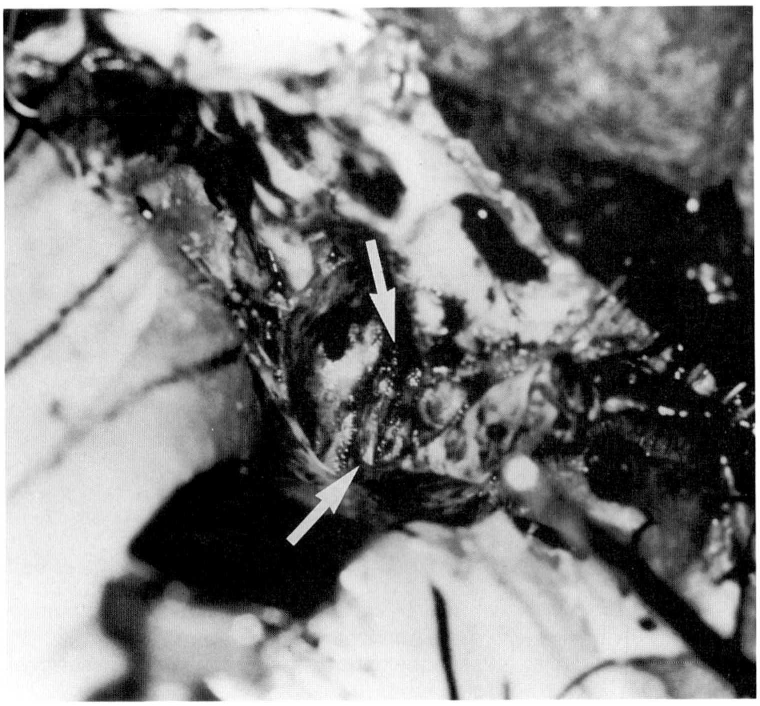

FIG. 21. Decompression of greater wing of sphenoid bone in patient with fibrous dysplasia. Note optic nerve *(arrows)*.

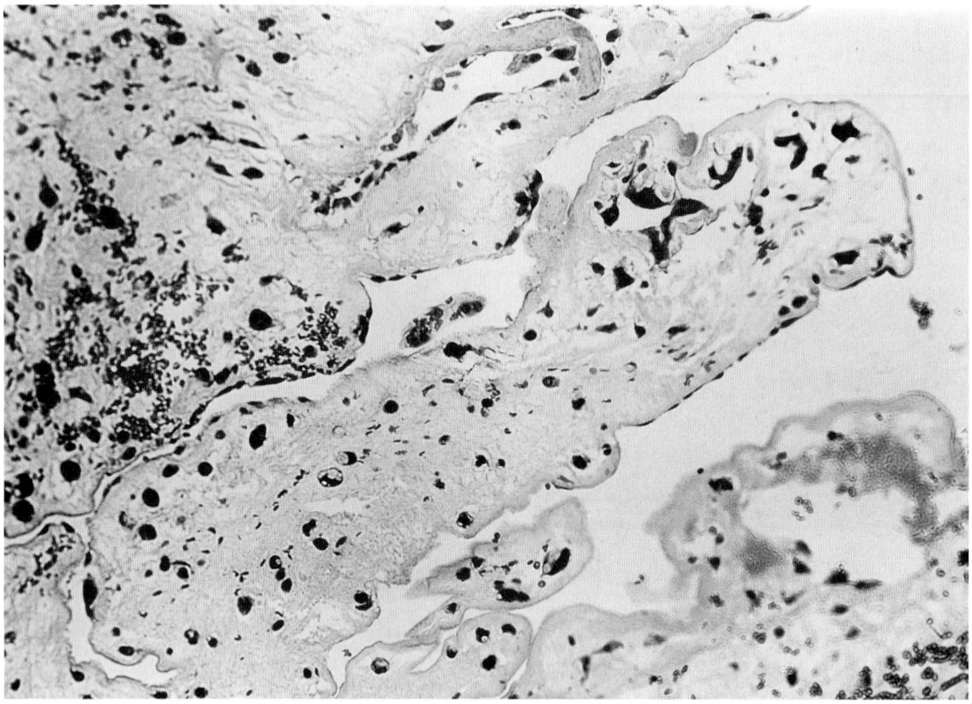

FIG. 22. Atrial myxoma consisting of loosely arranged tumor cells within an amorphous mucoid matrix. (Published with permission from *Neuro-Ophthalmology* 1981;2:59–65. Copyright by Æolus Press.)

period with leukocoria, microphthalmia, and cataract and are usually examined for possible retinoblastoma. After the eye is sectioned, a loose, fibrous mass is found to be broadly attached to the posterior surface of the lens, which may be small or even absent. This retrolental mass often displaces the lens forward into a small anterior chamber and is attached to the optic disk by a strand of connective tissue and glia containing the persistent hyaloid artery (Fig. 23). The range of histopathologic features are exhaustively described and illustrated by Haddad and colleagues (24). The pathology and imaging findings are well correlated and illustrated by Kaste et al. (30). There is persistence of the posterior portion of the vascular tunica of the lens and the hyaloid system with hyperplasia of the surrounding mesoderm, forming a loose mesenchymal, retrolental mass into which the hyaloid artery arising from the optic disk is inserted (24).

Coats' Disease

Coats' disease is a unilateral, nonfamilial, exudative retinopathy that usually affects males under the age of 21. It was first described in 1908 by Coats (15). These patients characteristically present with leukocoria that, particularly in the younger patient, may result in enucleation for a diagnosis of retinoblastoma. Detached retina is pushed forward by a firm subretinal exudate in which glittering cholesterol crystals are usually grossly visible (Fig. 24). Microscopically, there is retinal telangiectatic change, particularly in the periphery of the retina where there is usually saccular and fusiform aneurysm formation. Ultrastructurally, gaps between endothelial cells with the accumulation of a proteinaceous exudate in the vessel walls has been demonstrated (37,43), and some investigators postulate that the primary abnormality is a change in endothelial permeability (64). This exudate extends into the retina and the subretinal space with de-

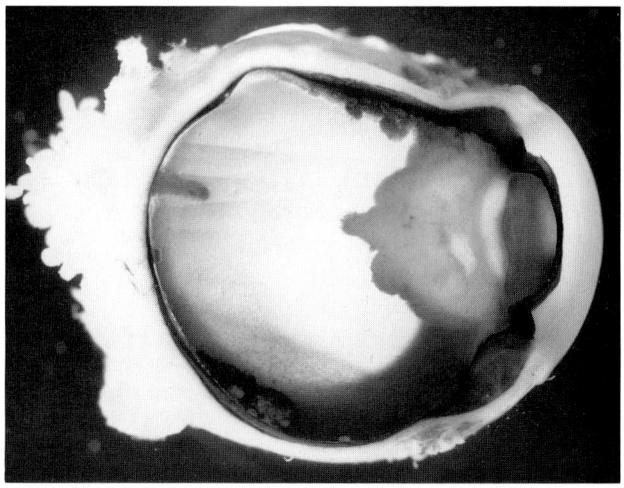

FIG. 23. Incomplete form of persistent hyperplastic primary vitreous where the connective tissue strand connecting the retrolental mass to the optic disk is discontinuous. The specimen is transilluminated.

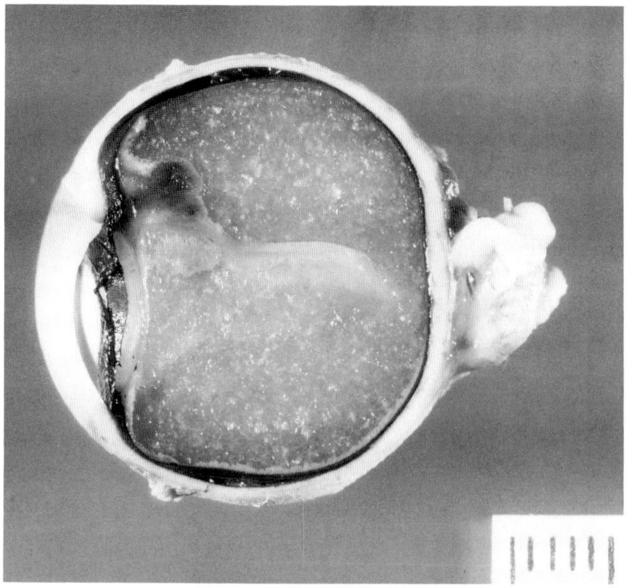

FIG. 24. Coats' disease. Numerous small cholesterol crystals are present in the subretinal exudate.

tachment of the retina. The exudate includes plasma, degenerating retinal components, large numbers of macrophages and ghost cells, cholesterol crystals, and a reactive granulomatous response. The retina also shows disorganization and gliosis with foci of recent and old hemorrhage. Inflammation is not usually a prominent part of the disease process (13,37).

Toxocara canis Endophthalmitis

A retrolental inflammatory fibrous mass caused by the migratory larva of *Toxocara canis*, or less commonly *Toxocara cati*, presents as painless leukocoria. It is the end result of an inflammatory and fibrous reaction to the dead larva that produces a white to yellow–white vitreous mass with traction detachment of the retina. Histologically, the fibrotic reaction is accompanied by a well-localized, mixed inflammatory reaction with many plasma cells and eosinophils. The organisms are small (20 by 400 μM) and are easily missed on routine sections. When found, the larvae are frequently surrounded by a cuticle of antigen–antibody complexes known as the Splendore–Hoeppli phenomenon (48). Particularly nice gross photographs and light micrographs of this disease are found a publication by McLean et al. (44).

Congenital Retinal Macrovessels

An unusual vascular anomaly termed congenital retinal macrovessels is characterized clinically by large retinal vessels that are noted to supply or drain the macula area (Fig. 25). The eyes may show abnormal areas of capillary nonperfusion and perifoveolar arteriovenous communications. Often, the visual acuity in these eyes is excellent, so that the vascular abnormalities are discovered during a routine eye examination on an asymptomatic patient.

Cancer-Causing Genes

There are two types of cancer-causing genes—oncogenes and tumor suppressor genes—which have opposite effects in carcinogenesis (see Chapter 1). Oncogenes, when activated, facilitate malignant transformation, whereas tumor suppressor genes normally inhibit tumor development. Most oncogenes are mutated forms of the normal genes (proto-oncogenes). The mutation and activation of certain proto-oncogenes in human cancer has been in some cases linked to a viral etiology. Several oncogenes involved in pediatric tumors include the *myc* oncogene in Burkitt's lymphoma and *BCR-abl* in acute lymphoblastic leukemia (see Chapters 15 and 16).

A highly important recent discovery was the identification of the gene predisposing patients to the development of retinoblastoma as a tumor suppressor gene (10,22,23,36). In the inherited form of the disease, the patient is born with a mutant copy of the tumor suppressor gene, and the subsequent loss or inactivation of the remaining normal copy leads to tumorigenesis. Several additional tumor suppressor genes of ophthalmic interest have also been identified. These genes include the neurofibromatosis type 1 gene, the *p53* gene, and the von Hippel–Lindau disease gene (Table 1). Studies of genetic alterations in these tumor suppressor genes have signifi-

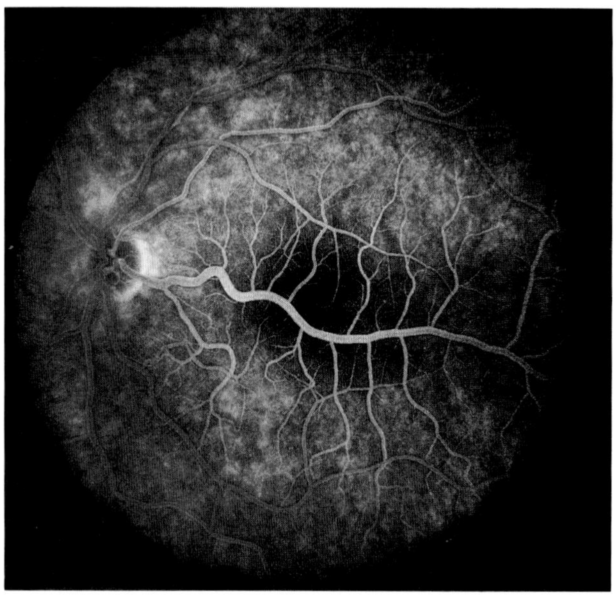

FIG. 25. Fundus photograph demonstrating anomalous retinal macrovessels.

cantly improved our understanding of the pathogenesis of pediatric ocular tumors.

Methods of Identification

Genetic Linkage Studies

Chromosomal linkage studies offer a powerful tool for gene localization, particularly when cytogenetic findings are either absent or inconsistent or the resolution in chromosomal distance is limited. Recent developments in the human genome project and the availability of second- and third-generation human genome markers, with the resolution of 2 centimorgans or less, has created an unprecedented new frontier for gene tracking in human diseases. In chromosomal linkage studies, the goal is to establish linkage between a known chromosome marker and a disease gene locus. Often, a chromosome marker is chosen because of its various alternative forms within that chromosome locus (DNA polymorphism). Using pedigrees, statistical analysis is performed to determine the probability of cosegregation of the testing markers and the individuals affected with the disease. The closer in chromosomal distance between a DNA marker and a disease gene, the more likely that the marker will travel together with the disease gene in chromosomal recombination events. An LOD score ("logarithm of the odds favoring linkage") is established to assay the gene distance and represents the logarithm to base 10 of the odds in favor of linkage. An LOD score of 3 represents a probability of 1000:1 that the observation did not occur by chance and is often taken as the minimal LOD value for presumptive evidence of linkage. In the past few years, DNA markers located within several genes (intragenic markers) associated with pediatric ocular tumors have been identified. These markers proved to be very useful in genetic diagnosis because they cosegregate with the disease genes.

Gene Mapping

The identification of the gene defect causing a specific disease is the final and often most difficult step in gene tracking. Two major approaches are used today, namely, functional cloning and positional cloning. In functional cloning, or the candidate gene approach, the biochemical defect associated with a clinical disease is known or assumed, and the genes encoding for the diseased protein are examined for mutations. In pediatric ocular tumors, this approach has not often been used because in most cases little is known about the biochemical defect. The second approach is termed positional cloning in which one has no prior knowledge concerning the nature of the biochemical defects and genes involved. From chromosomal linkage studies, one approaches the disease gene locus by successively analyzing different sets of DNA markers until one identifies one or a few markers that cosegregate with the disease. The identification of the genes involved in retinoblastoma, neurofibromatosis, and Wilms' tumor were accomplished by the positional cloning approach. Today, molecular biologists are using a combination of functional and positional cloning techniques in gene tracking. The final step in gene tracking involves the specific identification of the genetic defect at the molecular level.

Mutation Detection

For detecting gross deletions or DNA alterations many techniques are available, such as Southern blot analysis and allele-specific hybridization, competitive oligonucleotide priming, amplification refractory mutation system, and oligonucleotide ligation assay (21,47). On the other hand, there has been rapid progress in the development of techniques for efficiently identifying small DNA alterations or single-base-pair mutations. These techniques include single-strand DNA conformational polymorphism (SSCP), RNase protection assay, denaturing gradient gel electrophoresis (DGGE), constant denaturing gel electrophoresis, primer-specified restriction map modification, and detection of mutations with hydroxylamine and osmium tetroxide (21,47). The ability to rapidly detect small alterations in genes has significantly accelerated the progress in elucidating molecular mechanisms involved in tumorigenesis.

Molecular Characterization of Pediatric Ocular Tumors

The identification and characterization of the retinoblastoma gene on chromosome 13q14 and the spectrum of mutations in the retinoblastoma gene has been at the forefront of molecular biology research (22,23,36). As shown in Fig. 26, more than 40 types of mutations or deletions have been identified to date. Notably, more than one third of the mutations occur in the noncoding regions of the gene (73,77). These mutations give rise to grossly altered retinoblastoma proteins by affecting RNA splicing. There appears to be no obvious "hot spot" or preferred region for mutations within the 27 exons of the retinoblastoma gene. This is particularly relevant to clinical studies because it may be necessary in many cases to screen all exons and adjacent introns for oncogenic mutations, an expensive and labor-intensive task.

The characterization of the biologic function of the retinoblastoma protein, ppRB110, is one of the most intensive research areas in molecular oncology. This protein appears to be involved in the control of cell cycle progression by interacting with other proteins involved in cellular proliferation. ppRB110 has been shown to be

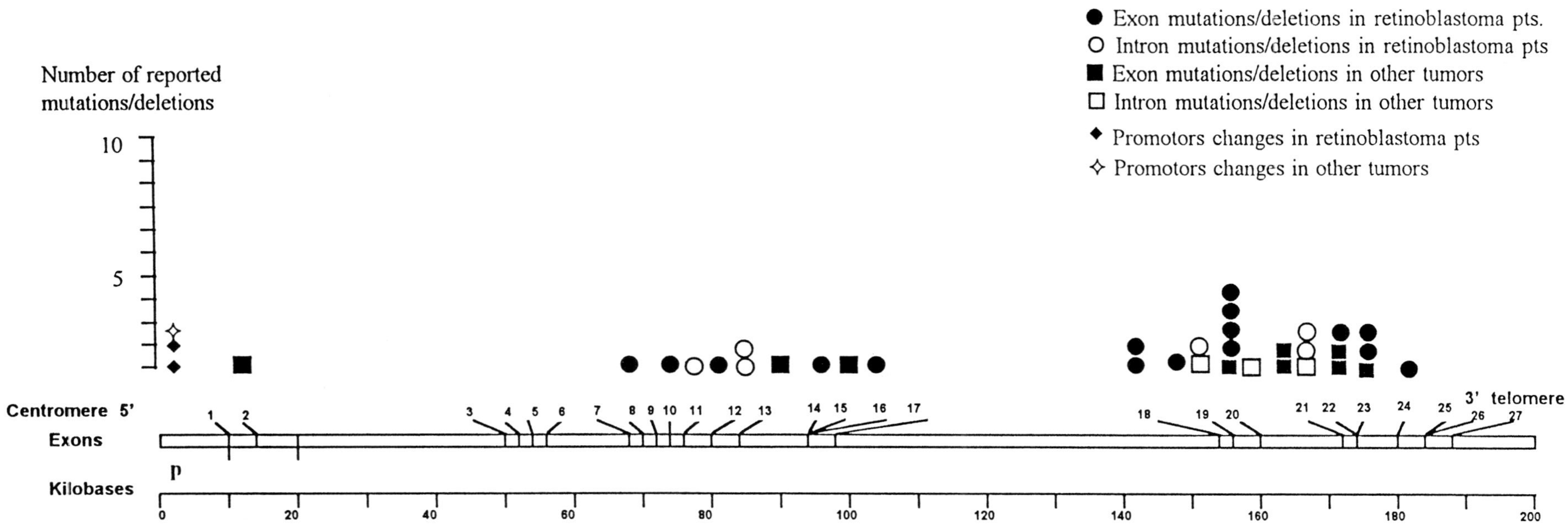

FIG. 26. Spectrum of mutations/deletions in the retinoblastoma gene.

a intranuclear protein (Fig. 27) and to interact with transcriptional factor E2F (14,77). It has been hypothesized that the retinoblastoma protein exerts its tumor-suppressive activity through binding to and inactivation of oncogenic proteins such as E2F. Events that disrupt this interaction release and activate E2F, leading to tumorigenesis. Active research is being pursued to characterize the role of the ppRB110 in DNA replication and binding to cyclin, a protein involved in cell cycle regulation. Although initial studies of the retinoblastoma gene primarily indicated a role in the development of retinoblastoma, more recent studies indicate that it may be involved in the pathogenesis of nonocular cancers involving organs such as breast, prostate, and urinary bladder (35).

Genetic Counseling

Because many ocular tumors have an inherited basis, genetic counseling is an important aspect of an ophthalmic oncology practice. The goal of genetic counseling is to convey medical and genetic facts to an affected or potentially affected family and to explain the options that may be available. This is particularly important for families of children with ocular tumors because many of the neoplasms are autosomal dominantly transmitted. There are many settings in which genetic counseling plays an important role. For example, if a child is born with retinoblastoma, the family may be concerned with the well-being of future children. Individuals with a family history of retinoblastoma may want to know if they harbor a potentially harmful gene and if an unborn child carries the dominant gene mutations. In general, genetic counseling includes the following steps (39):

1. *Medical diagnosis.* This is particularly important because a number of conditions may have multiple causes. The clinician may want to examine other members of the family or possibly family photos in addition to the patient. Laboratory studies can include karyotyping, as well as biochemical and molecular analysis of blood and tumor samples.
2. *Pedigree analysis.* Ideally, a complete three- to four-generation family pedigree should be obtained with special attention paid to such important clues as miscarriage, stillbirths, or mildly affected relatives (e.g., regressed retinoblastoma).
3. *Determination of future risks.* One needs to address the question, how likely is it that a given pediatric ocular tumor will recur in a subsequent birth? With the advent of recombinant DNA technologies and the cloning of disease genes such as retinoblastoma, genetic defects can now be detected prenatally by analyzing fetal cells obtained through amniocentesis or chorionic villus sampling. Often the predictions of risk depend on genetic linkage of a particular set of DNA markers to the disease locus or by direct detection of the causative DNA mutations.
4. *Options.* If the genetic prognosis is unfavorable, a couple may decide to refrain from childbearing or risk a defective birth. The degree of risk that parents are willing to accept is highly subjective and depends on their personality, experience, religious background, moral convictions, and especially on the burden of care imposed by the condition.
5. *Follow-up and supportive services.* Families should be informed of promising new research and allowed the opportunity of participating in research protocols. For example, ongoing investigations are improv-

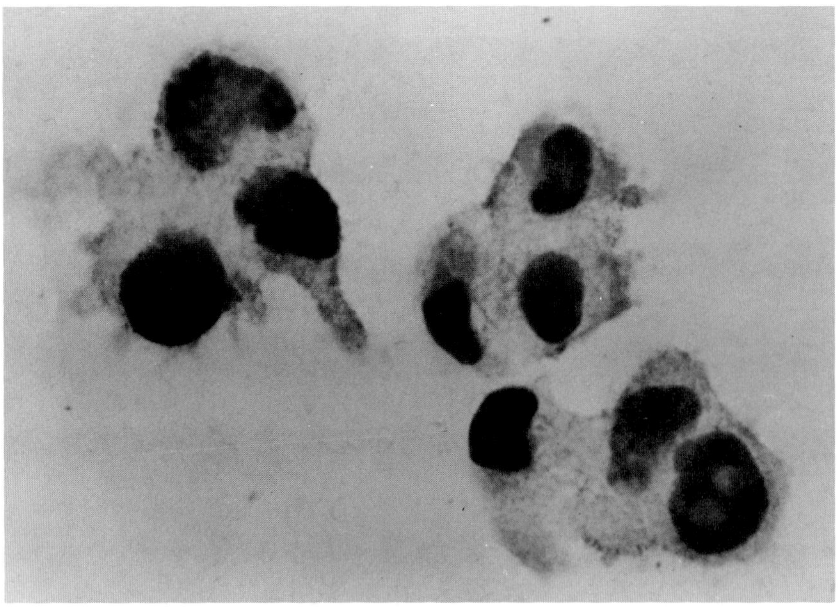

FIG. 27. Intranuclear staining corresponding to ppRB110 in normal human cells. Indirect immunoperoxidase stain.

ing the accuracy of diagnostic tests for hereditary retinoblastoma.

The success of the genetic diagnosis for retinoblastoma was demonstrated by the recent report by Onadim et al. (49), who carried out a presymptomatic blood testing of retinoblastoma gene carrier status in ten individuals with a family history of retinoblastoma. Samples for analysis were obtained prenatally by chorionic villus sampling, from cord blood samples, or from venipuncture of neonates. One child was shown to carry the mutant retinoblastoma gene and subsequently developed bilateral tumors. Six other children who do not carry the mutant gene copy are disease-free. Earlier detection of individuals with retinoblastoma will significantly improve their visual prognosis by allowing clinicians to treat the tumors while small and also will likely lead to improved systemic prognosis. The role of such genetic tests in clinical management is currently being evaluated.

ACKNOWLEDGMENT

Supported in part by the Eye Research Institute, Bernard Kant Estate; the Elizabeth C. King Trust; the Bertha Lambert Estate; the Harry B. Wright Estate; the Robert Beckman Foundation; the estate of Bessie Case Winter; Cancer Center Support CORE Grant, P30 CA21765; and the American Lebanese Syrian Associated Charities (ALSAC). The authors thank Ralph Sando, MD; Richard Goldberg, MD; Richard Lanning, MD; Thomas Pheasant, MD; Charles B. Pratt, MD; and Jerry A. Shields, MD for their support.

REFERENCES

1. Albert DM. Tumors of the retina. In: Garner A, Klintworth GK, eds. *Pathobiology of Ocular Disease.* New York: Marcel Dekker; 1982:705–740.
2. Albright F, Butler AM, Hampton AO, Smith P. Syndrome characterized by osteitis fibrosis disseminata, areas of pigmentation and endocrine dysfunction, with precocious puberty in females. *N Engl J Med* 1937;216:727–746.
3. Andersen SR. Medulloepithelioma of the retina. *Int Ophthalmol Clin* 1962;2:483–506.
4. Bader JL, Meadows AT, Zimmerman LE, et al. Bilateral retinoblastoma and ectopic intracranial retinoblastoma. Trilateral retinoblastoma. *Cancer Genet Cytogenet* 1982;5:203–213.
5. Bader JL, Miller RW, Meadows AT, Zimmerman LE, Champion LA, Voute PA. Trilateral retinoblastoma. *Lancet* 1980;2:582–583.
6. Broughton WL, Zimmerman LE. A clinicopathologic study of 56 cases of intraocular medulloepitheliomas. *Am J Ophthalmol* 1978;85:407–418.
7. Brownstein S, Barsoum-Homsy M, Conway VH, Sales C, Condon G. Nonteratoid medulloepithelioma of the ciliary body. *Ophthalmology* 1984;91:1118–1122.
8. Brownstein S, de Chadare´vian J-P, Little JM. Trilateral retinoblastoma. Report of two cases. *Arch Ophthalmol* 1984;102:257–262.
9. Burger PC, Scheithauer BW. *Atlas of Tumor Pathology. Tumors of the Central Nervous System.* Washington, D.C.: Armed Forces Institute of Pathology; 1994.
10. Cavenee WK, Dryja TP, Phillips RA, et al. Expression of recessive alleles by chromosomal mechanisms in retinoblastoma. *Nature* 1983;305:779–784.
11. Cawthon RM, Weiss R, Xu GF, et al. A major segment of the neurofibromatosis type I gene: cDNA sequence, genomic structure, and point mutations. *Cell* 1990;62:193–201.
12. Chader GJ, Wiggert B, Lai YI, Lee L, Fletcher RT. Interphotoreceptor retinol-binding protein: a possible role in retinoid transport to the retina. In: Osborne NN, Chader GJ, eds. *Progress in Retinal Research.* New York: Pergamon Press; 1983:163–189.
13. Chang MM, McLean IW, Merritt JC. Coats' disease: a study of 62 histologically confirmed cases. *J Pediatr Ophthalmol Strabismus* 1984;21:163–168.
14. Chellappan SP, Hiebert S, Mudryj M, Horowitz JM, Nevins JR. The E2F transcription factor is a cellular target for the RB protein. *Cell* 1991;65:1053–1061.
15. Coats G. Forms of retinal disease with massive exudation. *Roy London Ophthal Hosp Rep* 1908;17:440–525.
16. Craft CM, Stein P, Klein DC, Gery I, Shinohara T. Isolation of cDNA clones for S-antigen. *Invest Ophthalmol Vis Sci* 1985;26:28 (Abstract).
17. Craft JL, Sang DN, Dryja TP, Brockhurst RJ, Robinson NL, Albert DM. Glial cell component in retinoblastoma. *Exp Eye Res* 1985;40:647–659.
18. Datta BN. DNA coating of blood vessels in retinoblastoma. *Am J Clin Pathol* 1974;62:94–96.
19. Donoso LA, Merryman CF, Edelberg KE, Naids R, Kalsaw C. S-antigen in the developing retina and pineal gland: a monoclonal antibody study. *Invest Ophthalmol Vis Sci* 1985;26:561–567.
20. Donoso LA, Shields CL, Lee EY. Immunohistochemistry of retinoblastoma. A review. *Ophthalmic Paediatr Genet* 1989;10:3–32.
21. Frezal J, Kaplan J, Dollfus H. Mapping the eye diseases. *Ophthalmic Paediatr Genet* 1992;13:37–47.
22. Friend SH, Bernards R, Rogelj S, et al. A human DNA segment with properties of the gene that predisposes to retinoblastoma and osteosarcoma. *Nature* 1986;323:643–646.
23. Fung YK, Murphree AL, T'Ang A. Structural evidence for the authenticity of the human retinoblastoma gene. *Science* 1987;236:1657–1661.
24. Haddad R, Font RL, Reeser F. Persistent hyperplastic primary vitreous. A clinicopathologic study of 62 cases and review of the literature. *Surv Ophthalmol* 1978;23:123–134.
25. Haines JL, Short MP, Kwiatkowski DJ, et al. Localization of one gene for tuberous sclerosis within 9q32-9q34, and further evidence for heterogeneity. *Am J Hum Genet* 1991;49:764–772.
26. Howes KA, Lasudry JGH, Albert DM, Windle JJ. Photoreceptor cell tumors in transgenic mice. *Invest Ophthalmol Vis Sci* 1994;35:342–351.
27. Jannsen LA, Povey S, Altwood J. A comparative study of genetic heterogeneity in tuberous sclerosis: evidence for one gene on 9q34 and a second gene on 11q22-23. *Ann NY Acad Sci* 1991;615:306–315.
28. Kalsow CM, Wacker WB. Pineal reactivity of anti-retina sera. *Invest Ophthalmol Vis Sci* 1977;16:181–184.
29. Kandt RS, Haines JL, Smith M. Linkage of an important gene locus for tuberous sclerosis to a chromosome 16 marker for polycystic kidney disease. *Nature Genet* 1992;2:37–41.
30. Kaste SC, Jenkins JJ, Meyer D, Fontanesi J, Pratt CB. Persistent hyperplastic primary vitreous of the eye: imaging findings with pathologic correlation. *AJR* 1994;162:437–440.
31. Kivela¨ T, Tarkkanen A, Virtanen I. Intermediate filaments in the human retina and retinoblastoma. An immunohistochemical study of vimentin, glial fibrillary acidic protein, and neurofilaments. *Invest Ophthalmol Vis Sci* 1986;27:1075–1084.
32. Knudson AG, Jr., Meadows AT, Nichols WW, Hill R. Chromosomal deletion and retinoblastoma. *N Engl J Med* 1976;295:1120–1123.
33. Korf HW, Moller M, Gery I. Immunohistochemical demonstration of retinal S-antigen in the pineal organ of four mammalian species. *Cell Tissue Res* 1985;239:81–85.
34. Latif F, Kalman T, Gnarra J. Identification of the von Hippel-Lindau disease tumor suppressor gene. *Science* 1993;260:1317–1320.
35. Lee EY-H, Huang S, Shew J-Y, Donoso LA, Lee W-H. Diverse mutations lead to inactivation of the retinoblastoma gene. In:

Chader G, ed. *Molecular Biology of the Retina: Basic and Clinically Relevant Studies.* New York: Wiley-Liss; 1991:221–240.
36. Lee W-H, Bookstein R, Hong F. Human retinoblastoma susceptibility gene: cloning, identification, and sequence. *Science* 1987;235:1394–1399.
37. Lucas DR. *Greer's Ocular Pathology.* Boston: Blackwell Scientific; 1989.
38. Maher ER, Bentley E, Payne SJ. Presymptomatic diagnosis of von Hippel–Landau disease with flanking DNA markers. *J Med Genet* 1992;29:902–905.
39. Mange AP, Mange EJ. *Genetics: Human Aspects.* Sunderland, MA: Sinauer Associates; 1990.
40. Marchuk DA, Saulino AM, Tavakkol R. cDNA cloning of the type 1 neurofibromatosis gene: complete sequence of the NF1 gene product. *Genomics* 1991;11:931–940.
41. Margo C, Hidayat A, Kopelman J, Zimmerman LE. Retinocytoma: a benign variety of retinoblastoma. *Arch Ophthalmol* 1983;101:1519–1531.
42. McCune DJ. Osteitis fibrosis cystica: the case of a nine year old girl who also exhibits precocious puberty, multiple pigmentation of the skin, and hyperthyroidism. *Am J Dis Child* 1936;52:740–745.
43. McGettrick PM, Loeffler KU. Bilateral Coats' disease in an infant (a clinical, angiographic, light and electron microscopic study). *Eye* 1987;1:136–145.
44. McLean IW, Burnier MN, Zimmerman LE, Jakobiec FA. *Atlas of Tumor Pathology. Tumors of the Eye and Ocular Adenexa.* Washington, D.C.: Armed Forces Institute of Pathology; 1994.
45. Molnar ML, Stefansson K, Marton LS, Tripathi RS, Molnar GK. Immunohistochemistry of retinoblastomas in humans. *Am J Ophthalmol* 1984;97:301–307.
46. Mullaney J. DNA in retinoblastoma. *Lancet* 1968;2:918.
47. Musarella MA. Gene mapping of ocular diseases. *Surv Ophthalmol* 1992;36:285–312.
48. Neafie RC, Connor DH. Viceral larva migrans. In: Binford CH, Connor DH, ed. *Pathology of Tropical and Extraordinary Diseases. An Atlas.* Washington, D.C.: Armed Forces Institute of Pathology; 1976:433–436.
49. Onadim Z, Hungerford J, Cowell JK. Follow-up retinoblastoma patients having prenatal and perinatal predictions for mutant gene carrier status using intragenic probes from the RB1 gene. *Br J Cancer* 1992;65:711–716.
50. Perentes E, Herbort CP, Rubinstein LJ, et al. Immunohistochemical characterization of human retinoblastoma in situ with multiple markers. *Am J Ophthalmol* 1987;103:647–658.
51. Reese AB. Persistent hyperplastic primary vitreous. *Am J Ophthalmol* 1955;40:317–331.
52. Reese AB. Persistent hyperplastic primary vitreous. Jackson Memorial Lecture. *Trans Am Acad Ophthalmol Otolaryngol* 1955;59: 271–286.
53. Rosai J. *Manual of Surgical Pathology Gross Room Procedures.* Minneapolis: University of Minnesota Press; 1981.
54. Rouleau GA, Merel P, Lutchman M, et al. Alteration in a new gene encoding a putative membrane-organizing protein causes neurofibromatosis type 2. *Nature* 1993;363:515–521.
55. Russell DS, Rubinstein LJ. *Pathology of Tumours of the Nervous System.* Baltimore: Williams and Wilkins; 1989.
56. Sang DN, Albert DM. Retinoblastoma: clinical and histopathologic features. *Hum Pathol* 1982;13:133–147.
57. Schmidt WA. *Principles and Techniques of Surgical Pathology.* Menlo Park, CA: Addison-Wesley; 1983.
58. Shields JA. *Diagnosis and Management of Intraocular Tumors.* St. Louis: CV Mosby; 1983.
59. Shields JA, Shields CL. Genetics of retinoblastoma. In: Shields JA, Shields CL, eds. *Intraocular Tumors. A Text and Atlas.* Philadelphia: WB Saunders; 1992:333–339.
60. Shields JA, Shields CL. Retinoblastoma: Clinical and pathologic features. In: Shields JA, Shields CL, eds. *Intraocular Tumors: A Text and Atlas.* Philadelphia: WB Saunders; 1992:305–332.
61. Smith M, Smalley S, Cantor R, et al. Mapping of a gene determining tuberous sclerosis to human chromosome 11q14-11q23. *Genomics* 1990;6:105–114.
62. Stein PJ, Rasenick MM, Bitensky MW. Biochemistry of the cyclic nucleotide-related enzymes in rod photoreceptors. In: Osborn NN, Chader GJ, eds. *Progress in Retinal Research VI.* New York: Pergamon Press; 1982:227–243.
63. Terenghi G, Polak JM, Ballesta J, et al. Immunocytochemistry of neuronal and glial markers in retinoblastoma. *Virchows Arch A Histopathol Anat* 1984;404:61–73.
64. Tripathi R, Ashton N. Electron microscopical study of Coats' disease. *Br J Ophthalmol* 1971;55:289–301.
65. Trofatter JA, MacCollin MM, Rutter JL, et al. A novel moesin-, ezrin-, radixin-like gene is a candidate for the neurofibromatosis 2 tumor suppressor. *Cell* 1993;72:791–800.
66. Ts'o MOM. Clues to the cells of origin in retinoblastoma. *Int Ophthalmol Clin* 1980;20:191–210.
67. Ts'o MOM, Fine BS, Zimmerman LE. The Flexner–Wintersteiner rosettes in retinoblastoma. *Arch Pathol* 1969;88:664–671.
68. Ts'o MOM, Fine BS, Zimmerman LE. The nature of retinoblastoma. II. Photoreceptor differentiation: an electron microscopic study. *Am J Ophthalmol* 1970;69:350–359.
69. Ts'o MOM, Zimmerman LE, Fine BS. The nature of retinoblastoma. I. Photoreceptor differentiation: a clinical and histopathologic study. *Am J Ophthalmol* 1970;69:339–349.
70. Turleau C, de Grouchy J, Chavin-Colin F, et al. Cytogenetic forms of retinoblastoma: their incidence in a survey of 66 patients. *Cancer Genet Cytogenet* 1985;16:321–334.
71. Verhoeff FH. A rare tumor arising from the pars ciliaris retinae (teratoneuroma), of a nature hitherto unrecognized and its relation to the so-called glioma retinae. *Trans Am Ophthalmol Soc* 1904;10:351–377.
72. Wallace MR, Andersen LB, Saulino AM. A de novo insertion mutation causing neurofibromatosis type 1. *Nature* 1991;353:864–866.
73. Wang MX, Donoso LA. Gene research and the eye. *Curr Opin Ophthalmol* 1991;353:864–866.
74. Wurtman RJ, Axelrod J, Kelley DE. *The Pineal Gland.* New York: Academic Press, 1968.
75. Wurtman RJ, Moskowitz MA. The pineal organ. *N Engl J Med* 1977;296:1329–1333.
76. Yunis JJ, Ramsay N. Retinoblastoma and subband deletion of chromosome 13. *Am J Dis Child* 1978;132:161–163.
77. Zhang K, Wang MX, Munier F. Molecular genetics of retinoblastoma. *Int Ophthalmol Clin* 1993;33:53–65.
78. Zimmerman BL, Ts'o MOM. Morphologic evidence of photoreceptor differentiation of pinealocytes in the neonatal rat. *J Cell Biol* 1975;66:60–75.
79. Zimmerman LE. Applications of histochemical methods for the demonstration of acid mucopolysaccharides to ophthalmic pathology. *Trans Am Acad Ophthalmol Otolaryngol* 1958;62:697–703.
80. Zimmerman LE. Trilateral retinoblastoma. In: Blodi FC, ed. *Retinoblastoma.* New York: Churchill Livingstone; 1985:185–210.
81. Zimmerman LE, Sobin LH. *Histological Typing of Tumours of the Eye and Its Adenexa.* Geneva: World Health Organization; 1980.

Pediatric Neoplasia: Morphology and Biology, edited by David M. Parham.
Lippincott-Raven Publishers, Philadelphia © 1996.

CHAPTER 14

Respiratory Tract and Serosal Tumors

Alfredo Pinto, Geoffrey A. Machin, and Cynthia L. Trevenen

INTRODUCTION

Tumors of the upper and lower respiratory tract are uncommon in children and may pose diagnostic problems for the surgical pathologist. Most reported cases have been discovered coincidentally in chest radiographs in asymptomatic children or in children who have had a history of an unresponsive upper respiratory tract infection. Other cases have presented as endobronchial masses, which may cause hemoptysis or lead to distal inflammatory changes (34,104). Because of the nonspecificity of clinical and radiologic findings, the diagnosis may be delayed resulting in an adverse outcome.

Malignant lung tumors in children have been reported in preexisting cysts (76,181) or simultaneously recognized in cystic adenomatoid disease of the lung (17, 34,170,172), mesenchymal cystic hamartomas (16,22, 47,71,110), and pulmonary hamartomas (91) (Table 1). Recently, Dehner (42b,42c) postulated that some of these cases may correspond to type I pleuropulmonary blastomas. In some cases the cyst antedated the resection of the tumor by periods of 1–7 years (17,76,91,157), and in other cases the cystic lesions were discovered at the time of the resection of the tumor. An association of congenital cystic malformations with 4% (71) and 8.6% (70) of malignant and 4.3% of benign lung tumors has been reported. Bove (22) postulates that the subepithelial mesenchyme in mesenchymal cystic hamartomas in children is a precursor of mesenchymal neoplasms.

In our experience, pulmonary metastases from extrathoracic sites are by far the most common intrathoracic malignant neoplasms in children. The data from four published series of tumors from the pediatric respiratory tract are summarized in Table 2.

Most pulmonary tumors reported in children have a histologic equivalent in adults; however, the biology of the pediatric form may be different (34). The purpose of this chapter is to review the pathology of the more common tumors of the respiratory tract in children with emphasis on new biologic concepts as they relate to light and, electron microscopy, immunocytochemistry, molecular studies, and cytogenetics.

JUVENILE LARYNGOTRACHEOBRONCHIAL PAPILLOMATOSIS

Laryngeal papillomas (106), the most common tumor of the upper respiratory tract in children (50), are caused by human papilloma viruses (HPVs), which have a specific tropism for squamous epithelial cells and induce cellular proliferation or dysplasia (26). It is presumed that this condition results from exposure of the infant to HPV during its passage through the birth canal. The natural history of uncomplicated laryngeal papillomatosis is spontaneous regression at puberty. Recurrence and distal spread of the papillomas into the pulmonary parenchyma may occasionally occur (75,93). Dissemination and subsequent growth of the benign squamous epithelium may cause pneumothorax (7) or may be extensive enough to produce respiratory insufficiency and rarely death (5). The development of squamous cell carcinoma in association with juvenile laryngotracheobronchial papillomatosis (JLP) has been reported in patients who have had radiation therapy (134) and in both children (31,114) and adults (74) without a history of radiation therapy. Malignant transformation seems to depend on HPV-induced epithelial proliferation and the specific HPV subtype causing the infection.

A. Pinto, and C. L. Trevenen: Department of Pathology, University of Calgary and Alberta Children's Hospital, Calgary, Alberta, Canada T2T 5C7.

G. A. Machin: Department of Pathology, University of Alberta Hospital, Calgary, Alberta, Canada T2T 5C7.

TABLE 1. *Malignant lung tumors in children associated with cystic and hamartomatous lesions*

Age (yr)	Sex	Malignant tumor	Association	Ref.
11	M	Adenocarcinoma	Hamartoma	91
4	M	Blastoma	Pneumatocele	76
$2\frac{1}{2}$	M	Blastoma	BPD	181
19	M	Bronchiooalveolar ca.	CCAM	17
3	M	Blastoma	Mesothelial cyst	172
4	F	Blastoma	Mesothelial cyst	172
$2\frac{1}{2}$	F	RMS	CCAM	170
2	F	Blastoma	Multiloculated cyst	112
$1\frac{1}{2}$	F	Sarcoma	Mesenchymal cystic hamartoma	22
4	F	Blastoma	Congenital multiloculated cyst	157
2	M	Sarcoma	Mesenchymal cystic hamartoma	16
2	F	RMS	Bronchogenic cyst	94
3	M	Malignant mesenchymoma	Unilocular cyst	180
2	F	Myxosarcoma	Cystic hamartoma	155

Abbreviations: BPD, bronchopulmonary dysplasia; CCAM, congenital cystic adenomatoid malformation; RMS, rhabdomyosarcoma; ca, carcinoma.

More than 60 varieties of HPV have been identified by DNA probes (41). Papillomatous laryngeal disease has been associated with HPV-11 (62) and HPV-6 types (63). Four subtypes of HPV-6 have been identified in biopsy specimens, and one subtype, HPV-6C, is associated with more extensive spread of the disease (123). The oncogenic potential of HPV types 6 and 11 is small; in contrast, HPV types 16 and 18 have a high malignant potential (41,133). HPV-DNA is extrachromosomal in benign tissue but is integrated into the host DNA in malignant tissue (98,186). Byrne et al. (26) described the association of HPV-11 with a squamous cell carcinoma of the lung in a young patient with chronic JLP. DiLorenzo et al. (45) described a HPV type 6a DNA in the lung carci-

TABLE 2. *Respiratory tract tumors in children: review of four published series*

Tumor	Hartman (71) (1983)	Stocker (156) (1989)	Cohen (34) (1992)	Hanock (70) (1993)
	Benign			
Inflammatory pseudotumor of lung	45	52	3	3
Hamartoma	15	3		
Neurogenic tumor	9			
Leiomyoma	6	2		
Mucous gland adenoma	2			
Granular cell myoblastoma	2	3		
Hemangioma			1	
Teratoma		1		
Bronchial chondroma		1		
Total	79	62	4	3
	Malignant			
Metastasis			35	
Carcinoid	49	35		3
Mucoepidermoid carcinoma	12	9	1	1
Adenoid cystic carcinoma	4	2		
Bronchogenic carcinoma	47	27		
Pulmonary blastoma	14	6	2	
Leiomyosarcoma	9	6		
Rhabdomyosarcoma	6	7		1
Hemangiopericytoma	3			
Lymphoma	3			
Teratoma	2			
Plasmacytoma	1			
Myxosarcoma	1			
Fibrosarcoma		8	1	1
Total	151	104	39	6

noma of a patient with recurrent laryngeal papillomatosis. In the rare cases when HPV-6 or HPV-11 genomes have been detected in malignant lesions, they were found to have undergone mutations, insertions, and/or duplications in regulatory sequences, suggesting that such molecular changes are necessary to confer malignant potential (21,45,134). The mere presence and expression of the viral DNA appears not to be sufficient to produce malignant transformation, so that other factors appear to be involved. Byrne et al. (26) speculated that the viral DNA serves as a mutagen by integrating into a chromosome at a critical locus and inducing chromosomal rearrangement. The role of other HPV types such as 31, 33, and 35 in carcinogenesis remains unclear. Brachman et al. (23) reported that HPV infections can produce alteration of *p53* tumor suppressor gene function.

Hoarseness and inspiratory stridor are the commonest clinical presentations. Within the larynx and trachea, the lesions grow as papillary or sessile structures along the mucosal surfaces. Microscopically, stratified squamous epithelium with orderly maturation from the basal layers and koilocytotic atypia in the superficial layers are the classic histologic features (Fig. 1A). In tissue sections, HPV can be detected using immunostains with specific antibodies or in situ hybridization with specific DNA probes (Fig. 1B). The most sensitive diagnostic technique appears to be DNA hybridization (Southern blot), which detects both viral presence and type. More recently, polymerase chain reaction and dot-blot hybridization have been used.

Local resection with external beam radiation, photodynamic therapy, and interferon have been attempted with variable succcss (81,89).

HAMARTOMA

A hamartoma is a benign tumor or tumorlike malformation that consists of an abnormal mixture of the tissues normally present within a given organ. A pulmonary hamartoma is usually composed of epithelial and connective tissues, the latter being regarded as the essential element by some investigators (71). Pulmonary hamartoma is an unusual tumor that can occur in both children and adults as part of a variety of syndromes

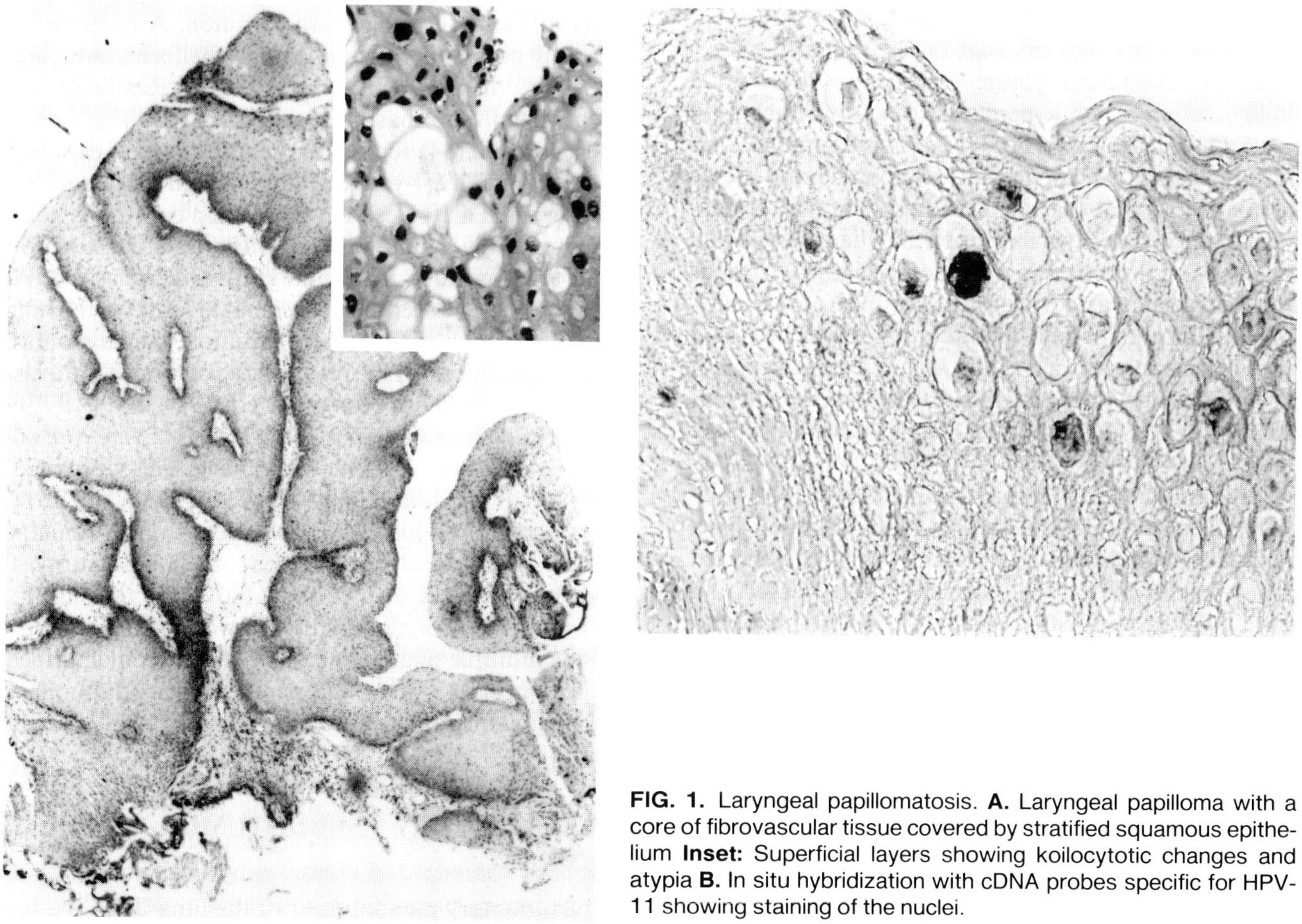

A

B

FIG. 1. Laryngeal papillomatosis. **A.** Laryngeal papilloma with a core of fibrovascular tissue covered by stratified squamous epithelium **Inset:** Superficial layers showing koilocytotic changes and atypia **B.** In situ hybridization with cDNA probes specific for HPV-11 showing staining of the nuclei.

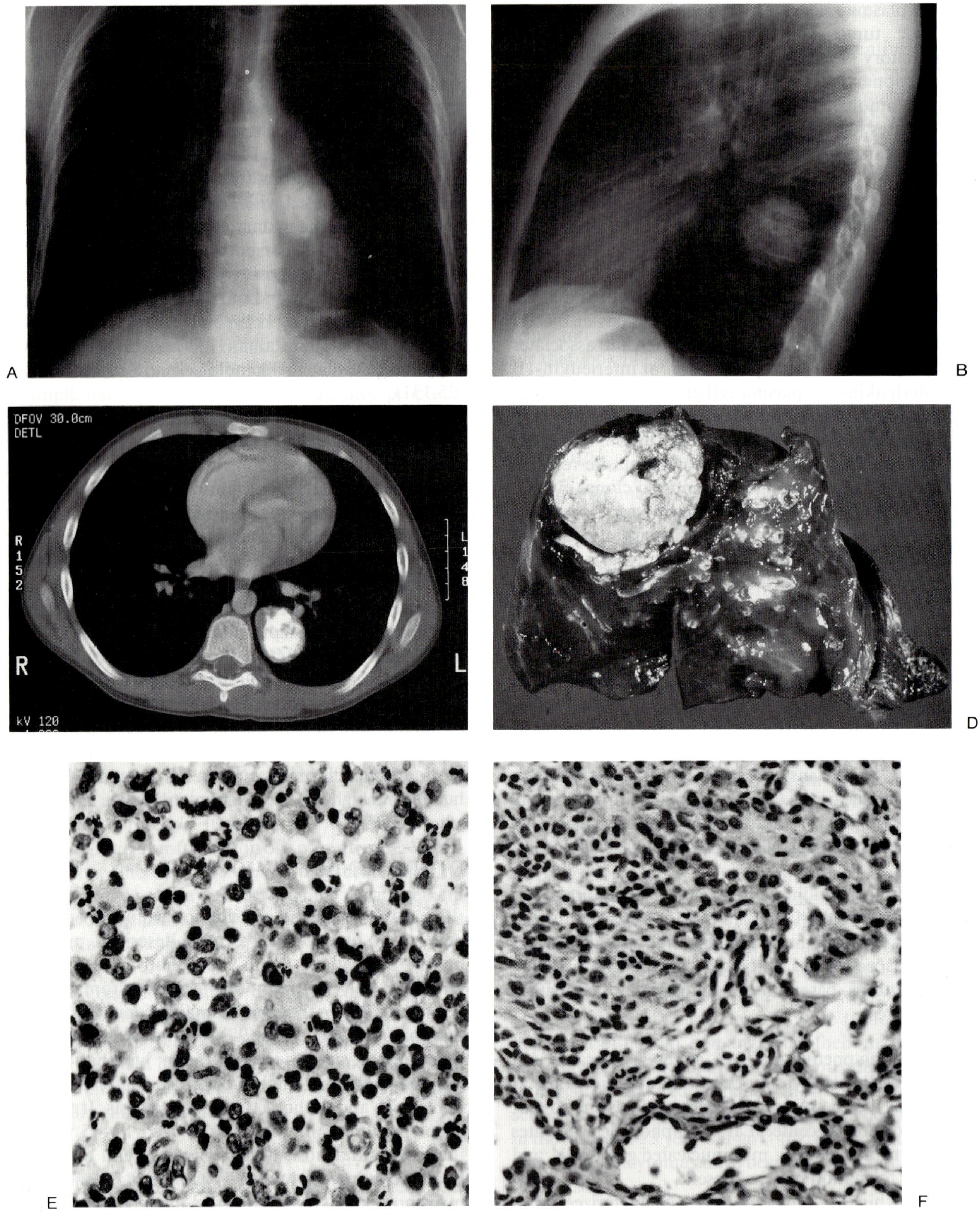

FIG. 2. Inflammatory pseudotumor of the lung. Chest AP **(A)** and lateral radiographs **(B)** showing a rounded lesion in the left lower lobe. **C.** Unenhanced axial computed tomography section showing calcification within the pulmonary mass. **D.** Pneumonectomy specimen showing a well-circumscribed pale-gray lesion with areas of calcification. **E.** Histologic examination showing an inflammatory infiltrate with lymphocytes, plasma cells, and vacuolated histocytes. **F.** Areas showing a more fibrous background with extension into the adjacent lung.

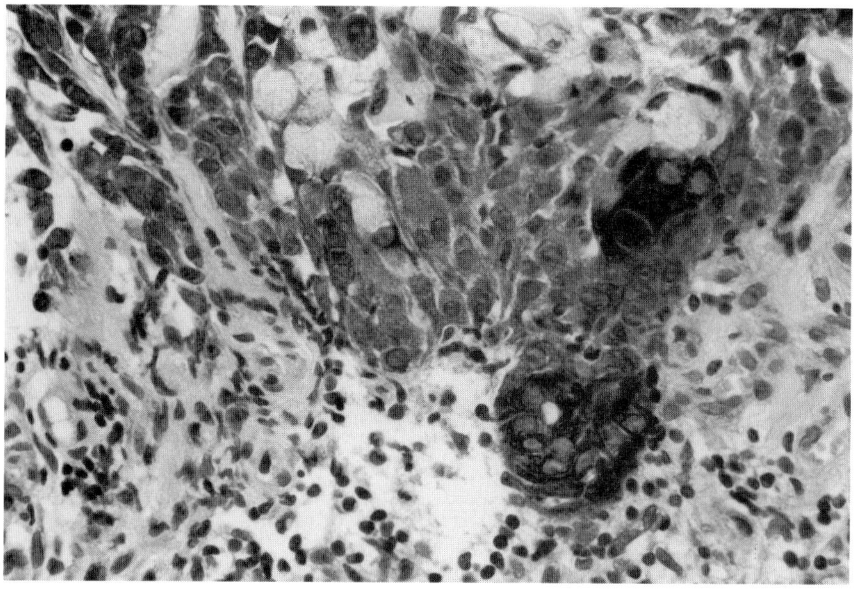

FIG. 3. Mucoepidermoid carcinoma. The tumor is composed of squamous, transitional, and mucous cells.

BRONCHIAL GLAND TUMORS

Submucosal glands in the tracheobronchial system are the counterpart to the minor salivary gland system and are subject to most of the tumors that involve the salivary glands of the head and neck (see Chapter 12). Historically, the term bronchial adenoma, which is no longer in use, has been used to designate the tumors known as bronchial carcinoid, mucoepidermoid carcinoma, and adenoid cystic carcinoma, which account for 45% of the primary malignant pediatric tumors of the lung (156).

Adenoid cystic carcinomas account for 20–35% of all tracheal tumors (111), resemble those seen in the salivary gland, and present with clinical and endoscopic findings similar to the other bronchial gland tumors. They have a tendency to grow in linear fashion along the tracheobronchial wall. Ahel et al. (1) described a bronchial adenoid cystic carcinoma in a 13-year-old girl with recurrent pneumonia and saccular bronchiectasis.

Mucoepidermoid carcinomas are rare tumors that tend to occur more commonly in the central bronchi than in the trachea (39,121) (Fig. 3). A mucoepidermoid carcinoma of the larynx in a 13-year-old boy was reported (122). Occasionally, they may present as a persistent unilateral hyperlucent lung (4). Most of the reported mucoepidermoid carcinomas in children are low grade (8,73,124) with few exceptions (146). Low-grade tumors may evolve into high-grade tumors (43).

Other rare bronchial gland tumors described in children include mucous gland adenoma (44,64,182), acinic cell tumor (87), pleomorphic adenoma (27b,72a), bronchial adenocarcinoma, and clara cell adenoma (153) (Table 4).

BRONCHIAL CARCINOID

Bronchial carcinoid (BC) is the most common intrabronchial primary tumor in children (71,97). BC is exceedingly rare under the age of 12 years and has a slight predominance in females (97). BCs are neuroendocrine tumors of endodermal origin. They arise from the Kulschitzky cells (187) that are normally found in the basal layer of bronchial epithelium.

BC usually presents as a slowly growing solitary polypoid intrabronchial mass that may obstruct a distal bronchus and cause recurrent pulmonary infections (Fig. 4A). Because of the vascularity of the tumor, hemoptysis can be the presenting symptom. BCs are usually biochemically quiescent. Occasionally, they have been reported to secrete biologically active agents including gastrin, insulin, calcitonin, vasoactive intestinal polypeptide, and corticotropin (154). Symptoms of glucocorticoid excess or hypersomatotropic gigantism have led to the detection of a corticotropin- (12) or ectopic growth hormone–releasing hormone BC (101). Rarely, typical

TABLE 4. *Tracheobronchial tumors*

Tumor	Ref.
Bronchial carcinoid	71,97
Mucoepidermoid carcinoma	39,121
Adenoid cystic carcinoma	1
Mucous gland adenomas	44,64,182
Acinic cell tumor	87
Pleomorphic adenoma	72a
Clara cell adenoma	153
Granular cell tumor	97
Endobronchial fibrosarcoma	34

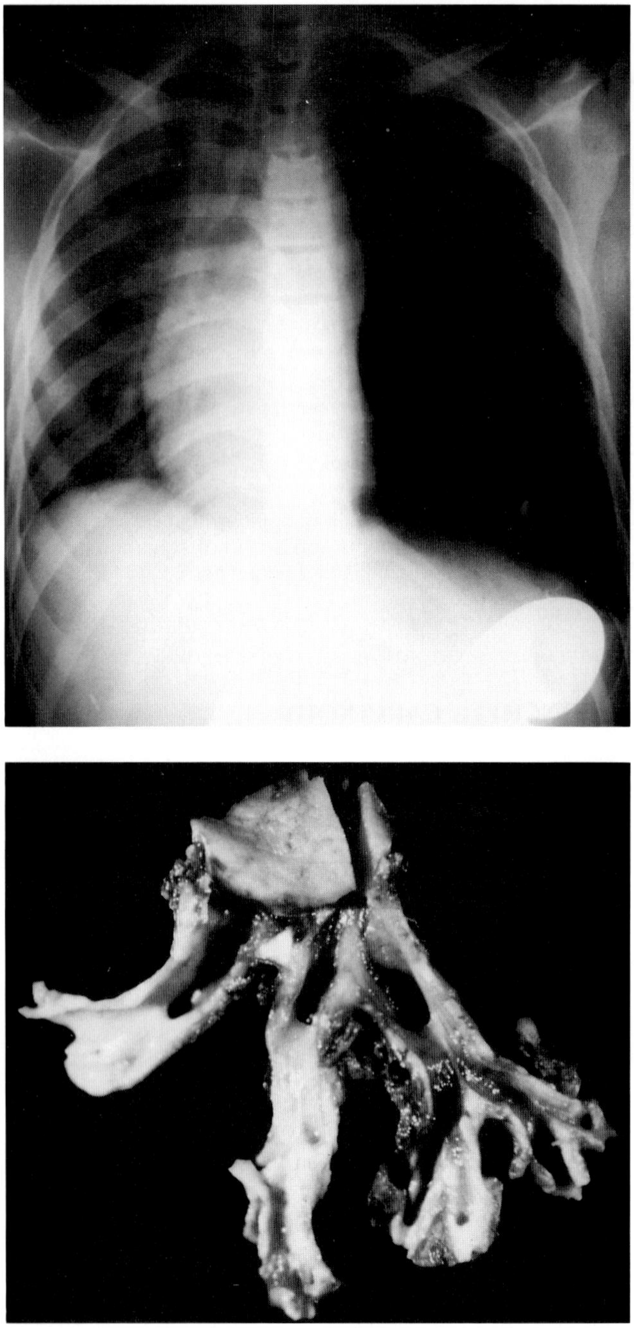

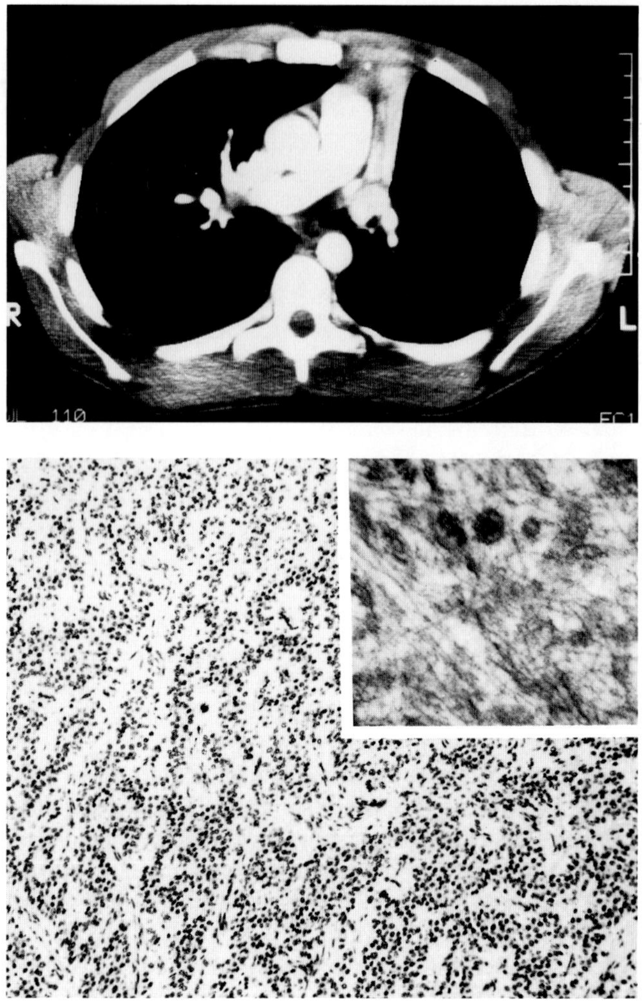

A B C D

FIG. 4. Bronchial carcinoid. **A.** Forced expiratory AP chest radiograph showing hyperinflation of the left lung indicating an endobronchial lesion. **B.** Enhanced computed tomography section showing a mass within the left lower lobe bronchus. **C.** Left lower lobe bronchial tree showing a partial obstruction of the main bronchus by a well-circumscribed tumor. **D.** Microscopic examination showing the classical carcinoid appearance. **Inset:** Neurosecretory granules in a background of intermediate filaments (×2,500).

carcinoid syndrome (97) and elevated 5-HIAA in the urine has been documented. In some cases the tumor has been found to secrete 5-hydroxytryptophan instead of serotonin (139). Occasionally, BC may be associated with endocrine tumors in other sites (49) and with multiple endocrine adenomatosis (184).

With few exceptions, BC in children arises in the main, lobar, or segmental bronchi at regions of bronchial bifurcation (Fig. 4B, C). Eighty percent are visible bronchoscopically as polypoid vascular tumors covered by bronchial mucosa, which is rarely ulcerated. The cut surface is firm and has a homogeneous tan color; occasionally, focal areas of hemorrhage may be noted. Peripheral carcinoid tumors of the lung are very rare in children.

The most common histologic type is the classical carcinoid, composed of small, uniformly stained clear cells arranged either in festoons or poorly developed trabecula (Fig. 4D). The cells display round central nuclei, rare mitoses, and moderate amounts of finely granular cytoplasm. The trabecula or clumps have an organoid appearance and are surrounded by a thin layer of stroma. The stroma of the tumor is very vascular as in the counterpart in the bowel. BC can form acini and secrete mucus. Histologic variants (atypical and spindle) are rare in children. Ultrastructurally, BC have abundant dense-core granules measuring up to 500 μm (Fig. 4D) with obvious desmosomes and even tonofilaments (105). Some variability in the granules has led to the suggestion that BC involves at least two different endocrine cell types (28). There is no apparent correlation between granule caliber and secretory product.

Argyrophilia (as demonstrated by the Grimelius–Sevier–Munger or Bodian techniques) is easily demonstrated in BC. On the other hand, argentaffin cells (as demonstrated by the Fontana Masson technique) are generally not found. There is variable immunohistochemical staining for keratin, serotonin, neuron-specific enolase, chromogranin, synaptophysin, opioid peptides, Leu 7, and neurofilaments (11,100,138). Immunohistochemistry with specific antibodies has shown that the following hormones, alone or in combination, can be detected in individual tumors: 5-hydroxytryptamine (serotonin), a gastrinlike substance, and adrenocorticotropinlike substance (ACTH), an antidiureticlike hormone (ADH), an inhibitor of antigrowth hormone–releasing factor, melanin-stimulating hormone, bombesin, somatostatin, calcitonin, substance P, and vasoactive intestinal polypeptide (VIP) (138,140,154,178). BC may show paranuclear fibrillary inclusions that stain with anticytokeratins and antivimentin antibodies, suggesting a derangement in the metabolism and synthesis of intermediate filaments (11) and leading to a diagnostic consideration of extrarenal rhabdoid tumor. Sustentacular cells in BC have been reported to stain positively with S-100 protein (11).

BCs are low-grade malignant tumors that rarely metastasize beyond the thorax. In children, most of these tumors are cured with complete resection. Endobronchial resection is not recommended and should be reserved for patients who cannot tolerate thoracotomy and lobar or pulmonary resection. The combination of tumor size and mean nuclear area may be predictive of regional lymph node metastases (164). Late local recurrences have been reported (97), and staining with carcinoembryonic antigen has been associated with a more aggressive behavior (18).

Numeric and structural abnormalities in chromosomes have been reported in BC (85). Trisomy 7 is the most frequent abnormality found in typical carcinoids, and complex structural chromosomal abnormalities are found in atypical carcinoids. Because genes involved in cell proliferation, cell recognition, and chromatin function are located in chromosome 7, it is speculated that this chromosome may be selectively engaged in various malignant and premalignant tumors and may be an indicator of aggressiveness in borderline neoplasms (162,163). It has also been suggested that carcinoid tumors may resemble other tumor types in that the more malignant tumors display more complex karyotypes. DNA flow cytometric analysis has shown diploidy and aneuploidy in both typical and atypical carcinoids, but aneuploidy was more common in tumors with the most malignant histologic features (86) and in those secreting biogenic amines (95).

PLEUROPULMONARY BLASTOMA (PULMONARY BLASTOMA OF CHILDHOOD)

Pulmonary blastoma (PB) is a rare malignant tumor of the lung described by Barnard (13,14) as "embryoma" and further investigated and classified by Spencer (151). PB has been reported mainly in adults (92) and occasionally in children (35,76,92,108,172), including neonates (130). Lesions histopathologically similar to PB have been reported in the upper respiratory tract (48).

Manivel and associates (108) proposed the term "pleuropulmonary blastoma" (PPB) for the childhood variant of PB. PPB appears to constitute a distinct clinicopathologic entity different from the adult-type pulmonary blastoma (42b,42c,67a).

The pathogenesis of PB is controversial (9). Early theories, to the effect that PB arises from a single cell line, were based on the concept of Waddel (176) that peripheral parts of the lung, both epithelial and mesenchymal, develop from pluripotential mesoderm ("blastema") analogous to the development of the kidney and thus to Wilms' tumor. More recent studies (56,116) argue against this interpretation but indicate instead that interstitial tissues of the lung derive from mesoderm whereas epithelial structures are of endodermal origin. Ultrastructural (56,116) and immunohistochemical studies (185,189) have revealed that the tumor cells in PB recapitulate early embryologic lung development before the fourth gestational month (56,116). Tamai et al. (159) suggests an endodermal origin of PB based on an ultrastructural study of a tumor transplanted into nude mice. On the other hand, Manivel and associates (108) propose that childhood PPB arises from the thoracic splanchnopleural or somatopleural mesoderm.

PPB has been reported with preexisting (76,181) or simultaneously recognized cystic adenomatoid disease of the lung (35,170,172), cysts associated with bronchopulmonary dysplasia (181), mesothelial cysts (172), congenital cysts (157), and pneumatocele (76). It is not clear as to whether preexisting lung cysts have a role in the pathogenesis of malignant mesenchymal tumors of the lung. Ueda et al. (170) suggest that certain malformations are intrinsically susceptible to carcinogenesis; Bove (22) similarly indicates that mesenchymal cystic hamartoma is a pulmonary malformation containing unstable myofibrogenic mesenchyme with a substantial neoplastic potential.

Children with PPB usually present with a history of an

unresponsive upper respiratory tract infection that persists despite medical therapy. The radiologic findings are nonspecific and may show a tumor mass at the periphery of the lung, pneumothorax, pleural effusion, partial or total opacification of the hemithorax with mediastinal deviation, or multiloculated cyst.

PPBs are generally bulky solid or multiloculated cystic tumors that vary in size from 3 to 18 cm. At the time of surgery, PPB may be found to be extrapulmonary (involving the mediastinum or the pleural surface), intrapulmonary, or diffusely infiltrating the lung and pleura or mediastinum (108). Characteristically, the tumor is located peripherally in the lung (pleural-based mass). Dehner et al. (42b, 42c) classify PPB as follows: type 1 is a multicystic lesion with smooth glistening lining; type III is a solid lesion with a variegated appearance that includes areas of hemorrhage and necrosis; and type II is an intermediate lesion with solid and cystic areas.

PPB is composed of blastemal and mesenchymal elements that resemble embryonic lung at the pseudoglandular stage of development (185,189) and lack malignant epithelial elements. A variety of patterns of differentiation have been described. Most of the malignant mesenchymal cells are undifferentiated cells with hyperchromatic spindle nuclei and scanty cytoplasm with areas showing chondrosarcomatous, osteosarcomatous, rhabdomyosarcomatous, or fibrosarcomatous differentiation. The blastematous areas are composed of primitive cells with frequent mitoses and cells suggestive of myogenic differentiation. Immature and sarcomatous cartilage, myxoid change, and intra- and extracytoplasmic eosinophilic inclusions can also be present (Fig. 5A, B). No malignant epithelial component was identified in 38 cases of PPB in children between the ages of 15 and 144 months, and metastases lacked epithelial elements (42b,42c,108). However, Koss et al. (92) reported two cases of PB in children with biphasic pattern, with both cases having typical foci of endometroid glands and malignant stroma. These cases may represent the adult variant of pulmonary blastoma which may occur very infrequently in children. Manning et al. (109) described a pulmonary endodermal tumor resembling fetal lung in a 12-year-old boy. Dehner et al. (42b,42c) described type I PPB as pulmonary cysts resembling bronchogenic cysts or congenital cystic adenomatoid malformations with a sarcoma botryoides pattern of primitive cells and rhabdomyoblastic differentiation beneath the surface epithelium that lines the cysts. Type II PPB is composed of solid areas and type III has solid areas with blastomatous and sarcomatous elements.

Ultrastructural examination reveals primitive undifferentiated mesenchymal cells with fibroblastlike features. Rhabdomyoblastic differentiation may be predominant (108), leading to confusion with rhabdomyosarcoma. Siegel (150) reported the presence of a yolk sac pattern positive for α-fetoprotein.

Childhood PPBs are generally devoid of cytokeratin positivity and had immunophenotypic diversity in the mesenchymal cells with frequent coexpression of intermediate filaments (35,67a). The coexpression of intermediate filaments has also been reported in fetal tissue, including fetal lung (174).

The histogenesis of and relationship between PB and PPB are controversial. Based on the premise that peripheral lung develops from both mesodermal and endodermal elements (56,116), it may be possible that a spectrum of differentiation encompassing pure mesodermal forms (PPB), mesodermal and endodermal forms (adult variant of PB), and pure endodermal forms (fetal lung adenocarcinoma) may occur (Table 5). Also histologic features may be related to age at diagnosis. Cohen et al. (35) suggested that PB, malignant mesenchymoma of the lung, and primary pulmonary rhabdomyosarcoma may have a common pathogenetic origin. However, Dehner et al. (42b,42c) propose that PB and PPB are distinctive clinicopathologic entities that are not histogenetically related.

Early surgery with complete excision appears to offer the best chance of a cure. This should be supplemented by radiation and chemotherapy if the resection is incomplete. A histologic grading system for PB has been proposed to assess prognosis (92). Dehner et al. (42c) speculate that in their classification type 1 PPB may have a more favorable outcome than type 2 and type 3 PPB.

An association between PPB and cystic nephroma (CN) of the kidney in siblings (42d,42c) led to the hypothesis that an inherent germ cell line mutation predisposes to either tumor and that a second mutation may determine the specific type (42d). Recently, other neoplasms have been reported either as second neoplasms in already affected PPB patients or a first neoplasm in first- and second-degree relatives (42b,42c). It is postulated that PPB may serve as a marker of predisposition for childhood neoplasms in other family members (42b,42c).

RHABDOMYOSARCOMA

Primary pulmonary rhabdomyosarcoma (PPRMS) has been associated with cystic lesions of the lung (3,170). Some of these cases have subsequently been reclassified as PPB type I (42b). PPRMS tends to occur in older children, and disease is usually advanced at presentation (38). The authors recently saw a case of pleural rhabdomyosarcoma in a 12-year-old girl who presented with opacification of the left hemithorax (Fig. 6A). Originally, the tumor was thought to be a small, noncleaved cell lymphoma in a cytologic preparation from pleural fluid aspiration (Fig. 6B). Subsequently, a biopsy confirmed a small round cell undifferentiated tumor that had a translocation t(2;13) (Fig. 6C). The patient did not

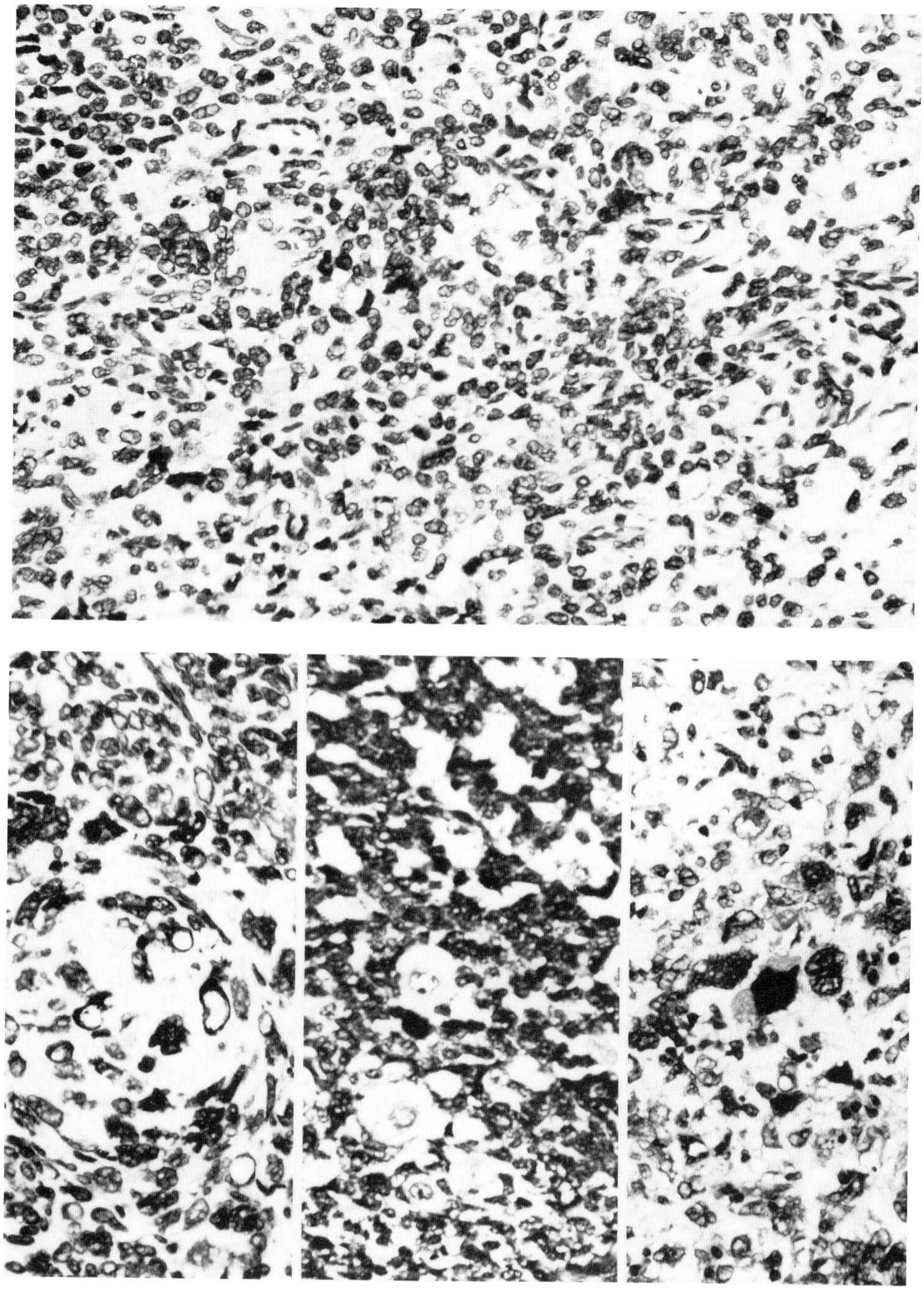

A

B

FIG. 5. Pulmonary blastoma. **A.** Low power reveals a cellular undifferentiated anaplastic tumor (Hematoxylin and eosin ×100). **B.** Areas of the tumor showing chondroid, rhabdoid, and anaplastic components.

TABLE 5. *Variants of pulmonary blastoma*

Pure mesodermal:	Pleuropulmonary blastoma
Endodermal and mesodermal:	Adult variant PB
Pure endodermal:	Pulmonary endodermal tumor (tubular adenocarcinoma)

respond to therapy and died of widespread disseminated disease. Postmortem examination of the tumor revealed widespread disseminated small undifferentiated tumor with unequivocal areas of alveolar RMS (Fig. 6D). It is presumed that chemotherapy induced differentiation of the tumor. This phenomenon is discussed in more detail in Chapter 5.

FIBROSARCOMA/LEIOMYOSARCOMA

Primary bronchopulmonary fibrosarcoma (PBPF) in children and adolescents is an uncommon but well-recognized entity (34,61,71,136). Pettinato and associates (132) reported five new cases of PBPF and reviewed an additional 21 cases from the literature. They proposed that PBPF is the counterpart of congenital-infantile fibrosarcoma of soft tissues. Jimenez et al. (84) described a bronchopulmonary leiomyosarcoma (LMS) in childhood causing nonimmune hydrops fetalis; this case was subsequently reclassified as PBPF (132). Recently, a nonrandom relationship between pediatric human immunodeficiency virus (HIV) infection and spindle cell tumors of muscle origin mainly involving the lungs and gastrointestinal tract was reported (30,113,173). Pediat-

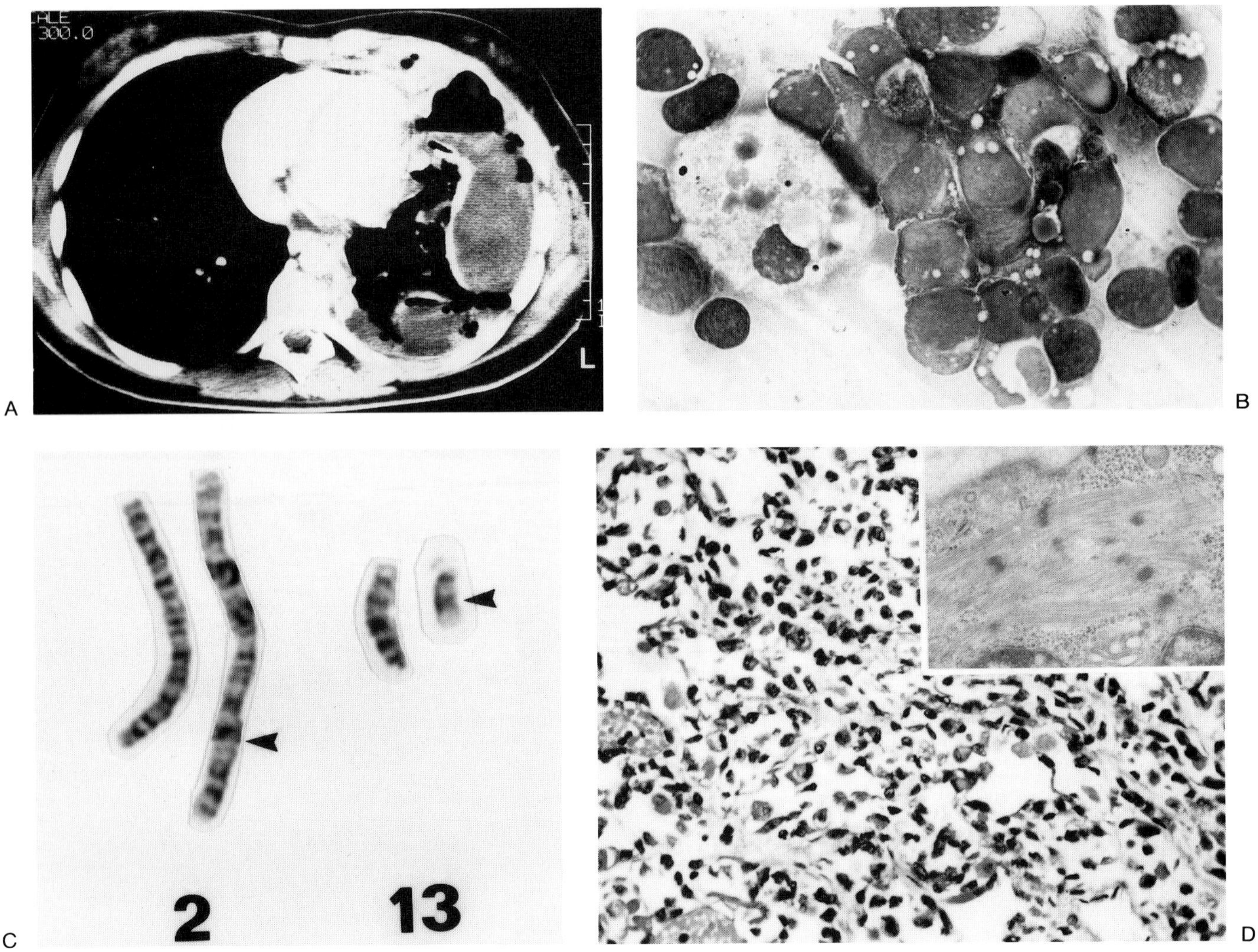

FIG. 6. Rhabdomyosarcoma. **A.** Enhanced computed tomography section showing a left large pleural mass. **B.** At diagnosis, cytology of the pleural fluid showed an undifferentiated small round cell tumor with small cytoplasmic vacuoles. **C.** Chromosomes 2 and 13 showing the typical 2;13 reciprocal translocation with break points at 2q35 and 13q14. **D.** After therapy, the tumor was consistent with alveolar rhabdomyosarcoma. **Inset:** electron photomicrograph showing Z-band formation.

ric LMS has also been associated with immunosuppression during renal transplantation (177), liver transplantation (165), and chemotherapy for leukemia (149). The importance of diagnosing LMS relates to the clinical nature of this tumor. The accurate diagnosis of childhood LMS depends in large part on ultrastructural evaluation. Immunohistochemical study is of less use because lesions with ultrastructural features of LMS may not uniformly express desmin or actin (158). Recently, McGinnis and associates (119) reported congenital peribronchial tumor associated with nonimmune hydrops fetalis and composed primarily of myofibroblasts; they proposed the term "congenital pulmonary myofibroblastic tumor" to encompass the terms bronchopulmonary leiomyosarcoma, bronchopulmonary fibrosarcoma, congenital fibroleiomyosarcoma, and massive congenital mesenchymal malformation of the lung. Analysis of fetal lung and these lesions using immunocytochemical, ultrastructural, and flow cytometric data demonstrates that they arise from the condensed mesenchyme that surrounds those respiratory ducts that progress to form large bronchi (119).

These tumors are grossly well-circumscribed masses that may occupy most of the involved lobe and may be peribronchial. Upon sectioning they reveal a fleshy, yellowish tan to gray appearance and are distinctly trabeculated (84,119,132). Microscopically, the tumor consists of broad interlacing cords of spindle cells with uniform elongated nuclei and scant cytoplasm. The mitotic index is usually low.

BRONCHOGENIC CARCINOMAS

Primary pulmonary carcinomas are rare in children. In 1951, Cailey et al. (27) reviewed the literature and described 15 histologically proven cases of primary carcinoma of the lung in children. Four of the cases were adenocarcinomas, three anaplastic, three epithelioid, and two small cell/oat cell carcinoma. Three additional pediatric cases were reported in a series of 102 cases by Kyriakos and Webber (96), and other sporadic examples have been described (148,161). Bronchioloalveolar carcinoma of the lung in children has been reported as a second malignancy (167) and associated with congenital cystic adenomatoid malformation (17). Benjamin (17) speculates that the latter disease may predispose to development of epithelial malignancies of the lung, whereas mesenchymal hamartomas are usually associated with nonepithelial neoplasms. Hartman and Schochat (71) reported two cases—one squamous cell carcinoma and one adenocarcinoma—arising in congenital cystic malformations in children. A case of pulmonary adenocarcinoma was reported in an 11-year-old boy and was antedated by a pulmonary hamartoma by at least 8 years (91). As mentioned earlier, laryngotracheal papillomatosis can also evolve into squamous cell carcinoma.

LYMPHOPROLIFERATIVE DISORDERS

Infiltration of the lung by Hodgkin's and non-Hodgkin's lymphoma is rare. Over the past decade lymphoid tissues associated with normal mucosal surfaces have been found to have distinctive characteristics and are referred to as mucosal-associated lymphoid tissue (MALT). In the bronchial-associated lymphoid tissue (BALT) the lymphomas described are usually low grade (82). In our experience, these lymphomas are very rare in children.

A spectrum of pulmonary lymphoid proliferations, including pulmonary lymphoid hyperplasia (PLH), lymphoid interstitial pneumonitis (LIP), complex PLH/LIP, polyclonal polymorphic B-cell lymphoproliferative disorders (PBLPD), and malignant lymphomas, has been described in children with acquired immunodeficiency syndrome (AIDS) (84a, 84b) (Table 6). LIP is characterized by a massive interstitial pulmonary infiltrate of plasma cell, lymphocytes, immunoblasts, and scattered histiocytes (84a). PBLPD is characterized by a polymorphic lymphoid infiltrate and is considered to be an intermediate form between benign and malignant lymphoproliferative disorder because of the overlapping features (84b).

Ebstein–Barr virus (EBV) DNA has been found in lymphoproliferative disorders of children with AIDS (7a). EBV by itself or in synergism with HIV may be related to the pathogenesis of lymphoproliferative disorders in children with AIDS.

LANGERHANS CELL HISTIOCYTOSIS (HISTIOCYTOSIS X)

Pulmonary Langerhans cell histiocytosis (PLCH) is a distinctive form of interstitial lung disease characterized by a diffuse reticulonodular radiographic appearance (nodules 0.5–1.5 cm diameter); honeycomb fibrosis is observed in 10–15% of cases at the time of diagnosis (Fig. 7A). Lung involvement can occur in 23–50% of children with disseminated LCH but it is not clear as to whether

TABLE 6. *Pulmonary lymphoid proliferations in children with AIDS*

Pulmonary lymphoid hyperplasia (PLH)
Lymphoid interstitial pneumonitis (LIP)
Complex PLH/LIP
Polyclonal polymorphic B cell lymphoproliferative disorders
Malignant lymphomas

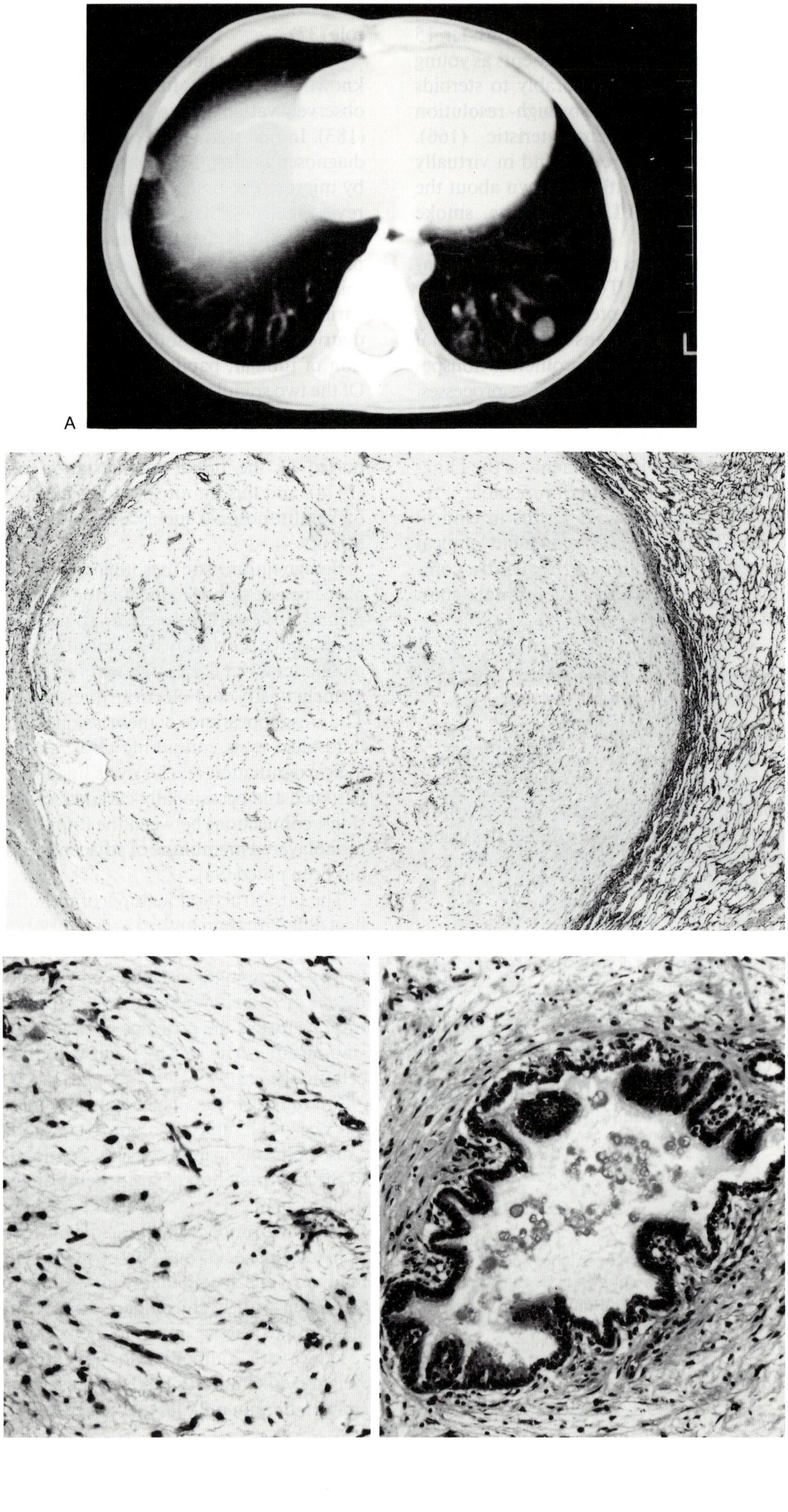

A

B

C

mentin. Most do not express carcinoembryonic antigen (CEA) (69). Sarcomatoid mesotheliomas coexpress CK and vimentin. Fibrous mesotheliomas express vimentin but not CK (69). Leu M1 antigen is expressed in most pulmonary adenocarcinomas but not in mesothelioma (147). New monoclonal antibodies are being developed that may be relatively mesothelioma-specific.

METASTASES

The differential diagnosis of pulmonary infiltrates in children with malignant tumors is difficult and important for future therapeutic decisions. Cohen and associates (36) reported 90 children with malignant tumors, 41% of whom developed pulmonary nodules after diagnosis. In 67% of these patients the nodules were metastases, but in 33% they were benign lesions. Pathologic evaluation of the benign lesions showed histoplasmosis, pneumonia, atelectasis, inflammatory pseudotumor, hamartoma, and radiation pneumonitis.

Pulmonary metastases may be present at diagnosis or develop later in the course of illness in about half of the children with Wilms' tumor (WT). Therapy can induce maturation of WT pulmonary metastases to benign fibromas (2) or to benign lesions with ganglion cell differentiation (10). Postchemotherapy metastatic pulmonary nodules may persist as masses detectable by diagnostic imaging studies. We have seen a case of persistent pulmonary nodules after chemotherapy in a 5-year-old boy with bilateral WT (Fig. 8A). The nodules were resected on two occasions. Microscopic examination revealed fibrous nodules with benign ductal structures resembling a hamartomatous lesion and with no malignant potential (Fig. 8B, 8C).

Pulmonary metastases from osteosarcoma (OS) are very common. An aggressive surgical approach combined with chemotherapy may be curative. Nodular lesions mimicking metastases have been described secondary to bleomycin toxicity (141,144). Santrach et al. (141) reported three patients with OS in whom pulmonary nodules developed during a course of multiagent, bleomycin-containing therapy. The predominant histopathologic pattern was bronchiolitis obliterans organizing pneumonia (BOOP). Nodular pulmonary toxicity from bleomycin has also been reported in germ cell tumors of the testis (46). Helton and associates (74a) reported BOOP in four children after nonbleomycin-containing chemotherapy. In the present authors' institution, we have seen a patient with OS with persistent pulmonary nodules that were interpreted radiologically as metastases (Fig. 9A). The pulmonary nodules were biopsied and revealed fibrosis with changes indicative of BOOP (Fig. 9B).

FIG. 8. A. Enhanced computed tomography section of the chest in a patient with metastatic Wilms' tumor showing peripheral nodules in both lung bases. **B.** Histologic examination after chemotherapy revealed fibrous nodules surrounded by normal lung parenchyma. **C.** Detail of the fibrous nodules showing myxoid fibrous tissue and benign ductal structures.

DESMOPLASTIC SMALL ROUND CELL TUMOR

Desmoplastic small round cell tumor (DSRCT) is a recently recognized neoplasm predominantly affecting young adult men. This tumor diffusely involves the peritoneum and pursues an aggressive clinical course (59,60,65,127,128). Abdominal distension and pain are the usual complaints. An abdominal mass can be palpated in most instances, sometimes in association with ascites. At laparotomy, a large intra-abdominal mass associated with smaller peritoneal implants of similar appearance is the usual finding (59). An intrascrotal mass due to involvement of the tunica albuginea is another presentation (133a). Gonzales-Crussi et al. (65) reported two patients who presented with the clinical picture of acute appendicitis. Recently, Parkash and associates (130a) reported three cases with primary pleural involvement and Tison et al. (165b), one intracranial case. DSRCT has been classified under the category of small round cell tumors of infancy and childhood, but its unique topographic, morphologic, immunohistochemical, and genetic features indicate that this tumor represents a distinctive clinicopathologic entity.

Gross examination usually reveals multinodular, firm, bulky tumors with smooth bosselated surfaces. The cut surface is gray–white, occasionally myxoid, and sometimes exhibits sharply outlined necrotic foci. Direct invasion of the wall of the bladder, small bowel, large bowel, stomach, and outer portions of the pancreas or spleen is apparent at surgery or autopsy (59).

The most conspicuous feature at low magnification is the presence of sharply demarcated islands of small round cells within a dense fibrous or fibromyxoid stroma (Fig. 10A). Foci of central necrosis in the nests of tumor cells are also frequently reported. The tumor cells are largely undifferentiated, having small round to oval hyperchromatic nuclei with inconspicuous nucleoli and scant to moderate pale-staining cytoplasm (Fig. 10B). Occasional tumor cells show eosinophilic cytoplasm that displaces the nucleus laterally to produce a rhabdoid appearance (59,60). Areas exhibiting gland formation (188), Homer–Wright rosettes (59,127), a carcinoidlike appearance (59), signet ring forms (125), lumen formation within solid areas (65,127,128), and areas resembling transitional cell carcinoma (127) may be present. The stroma in some areas may be reminiscent of nodular fasciitis (59). The pattern of growth is invasive with a generally pushing nature. Permeation of lymph vessels and tumor thrombi within blood vessels are frequent.

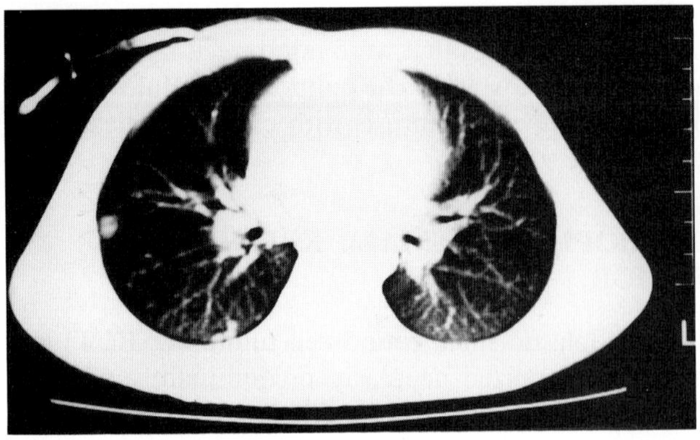

A

FIG. 9. **A.** Enhanced computed tomography section of the chest of a patient with osteosarcoma revealing multiple peripheral nodules. **B.** Histologic examination showing foci of fibrosis with obliteration of terminal bronchiole and alveolar duct consistent with bronchiolitis obliterans-organizing pneumonia (BOOP). Note also some atypical cells probably related to chemotherapy.

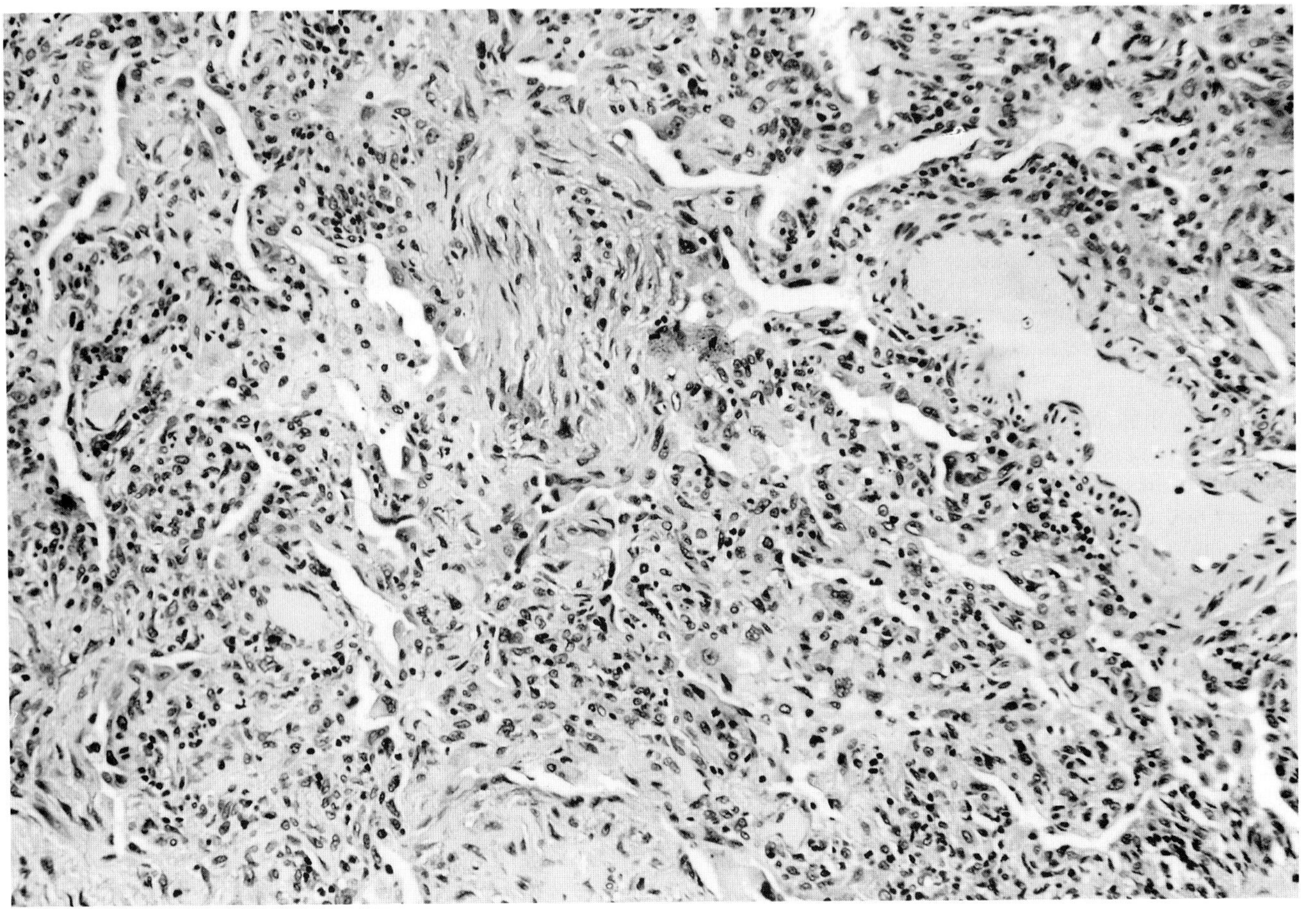

B

Ultrastructural examination revealed cells with a primitive appearance displaying irregularly shaped nuclei and scanty nondescript cytoplasm containing numerous ribosomes, scattered mitochondria, profiles of granular endoplasmic reticulum (59), prominent Golgi apparatus, and distended profiles of rough endoplasmic reticulum (65). A consistent finding is the presence of haphazardly arranged cytoplasmic filaments of intermediate sizes packed in perinuclear bundles and whorls, sometimes entrapping mitochondria and other organelles (59,125,128). Cytoplasmic membrane–bound electron-dense granules have been found in a few cells (59,175). Cell junctions are easily found, as are small desmosomes with tonofilaments (128) and desmosomelike intercellular junctions (125,175). Other reported features include an acinar configuration, with microvilli protruding into the lumen and tight junctions between adjacent cells at the luminal border. Ordonez et al. (128,129) reported small lumens into which irregular microvilli projected; the number and size of microvilli varied but they never contained microfilament cores. These were considered to be indicative of glandular

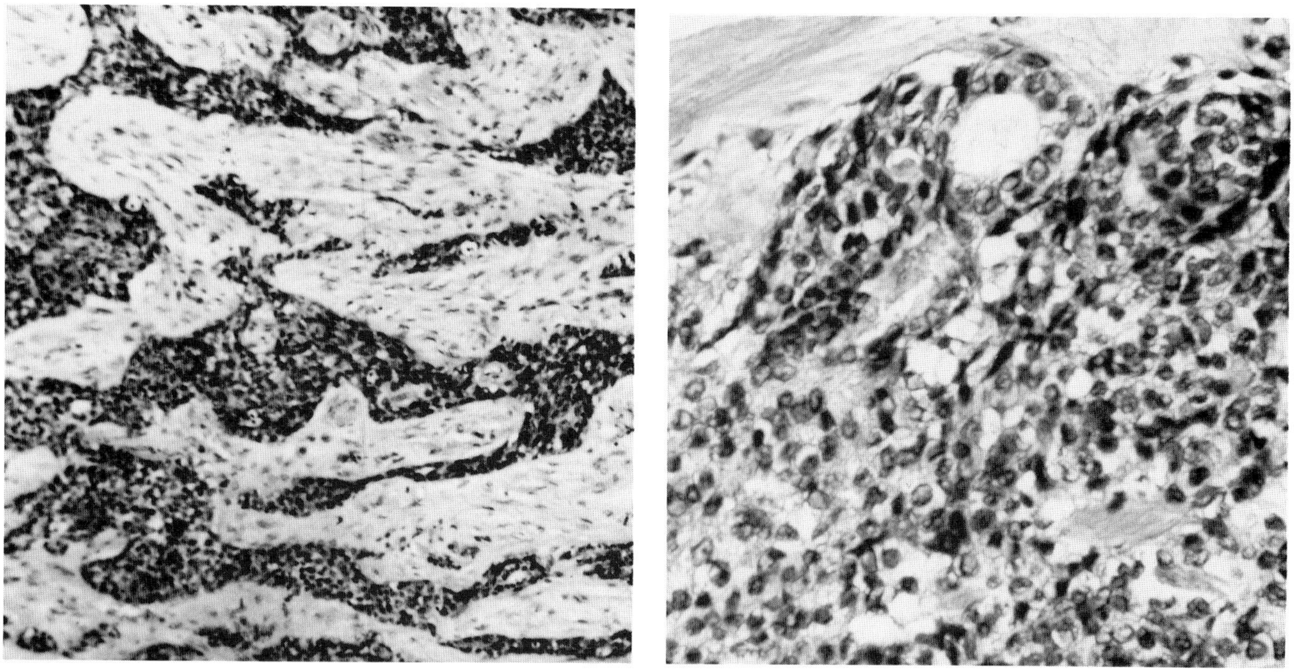

FIG. 10. Desmoplastic small round cell tumor. **A.** Low magnification showing variably sized and shaped tumor cell nests separated by a desmoplastic stroma (Hematoxylin and eosin ×100). **B.** High magnification showing primitive tumor cells with round nuclei and scanty cytoplasm. Note focal tubular formation (Hematoxylin and eosin ×400).

differentiation (175). The bushy appearance described for mesothelioma is not seen (65,175). A discontinuous basal lamina may be identified around the tumor nests (59).

The immunophenotype of DSRCT has been extensively studied (59,65,128) (Table 7). Reactivity for epithelial (CK and EMA), mesenchymal (vimentin), and muscle markers (desmin) is often coexpressed by the tumor cells (59,128). Low molecular weight CK is widely expressed in tumor cells either throughout the cytoplasm or in the perinuclear area (125). High molecular weight CK is detected in only 20–25% of neoplastic cells, where it stains mainly the perinuclear cytoplasm (125). Strong EMA reactivity has a diffuse cytoplasmic quality (59). Immunoreactivity with keratin, vimentin, and desmin has shown differences in intensity and pattern of staining, pattern of staining for desmin and vimentin being reported as diffuse or paranuclear dot positivity (65, 99,125,128,188). Variable reactivity with neural markers (neuron-specific enolase, chromogranin, Leu 7, synaptophysin) has also been reported (59,65,99,127). Consistently, no staining with neurofilament and S-100 protein antibodies has been reported (99,128).

DSRCT appears to be an embryonal tumor with divergent differentiation. The histogenesis is controversial. Because of the massive involvement of the peritoneal cavity, an origin from mesothelium or submesothelial mesenchymal cells has been postulated (59,129,145, 130a); however, the immunohistochemical and ultrastructural studies are not entirely supportive of this concept. Gonzales-Crussi et al. (65) postulate that DSRCT may originate from cellular elements present within the serosal mantle of the abdominal cavity. Others postulate that DSRCT may represent blastomas arising from primitive cells formed in the splanchnophrenic intraembryonic mesoderm or intraembryonic coelom (99); this may explain the range of features resembling the expression of some fetal qualities (128). Definitive diagnosis is generally made by exclusion. Nephroblastoma, metastatic Wilms' tumor, metastatic carcinoma, neuroendocrine tumors, mesothelioma, rhabdoid tumors, and Ewing's sarcoma must be ruled out (60,99). High serum neuron-specific enolase and negative catecholamine excretion may be of diagnostic value (145).

This tumor behaves aggressively with massive intraabdominal spread, distant metastases, and poor response to chemotherapy and radiation therapy. Sixteen of 22 patients died of widespread metastases 8–50 months following diagnosis (128). Occasional response to combined therapy has been reported (65).

The translocation t(11;22)(p13;q12) appears to be a recurrent translocation in DSRCT (17a,97a,136a,143). The chromosomal band 11p13 is the locus for several putative or definitive transcription factors: Wilms' tumor zinc finger gene *WT*1 (27a), the aniridia paired box and homebox gene *AN2 PAX6* (165a), and a LIM do-

TABLE 7. *Immunohistochemical staining of DSRCT*

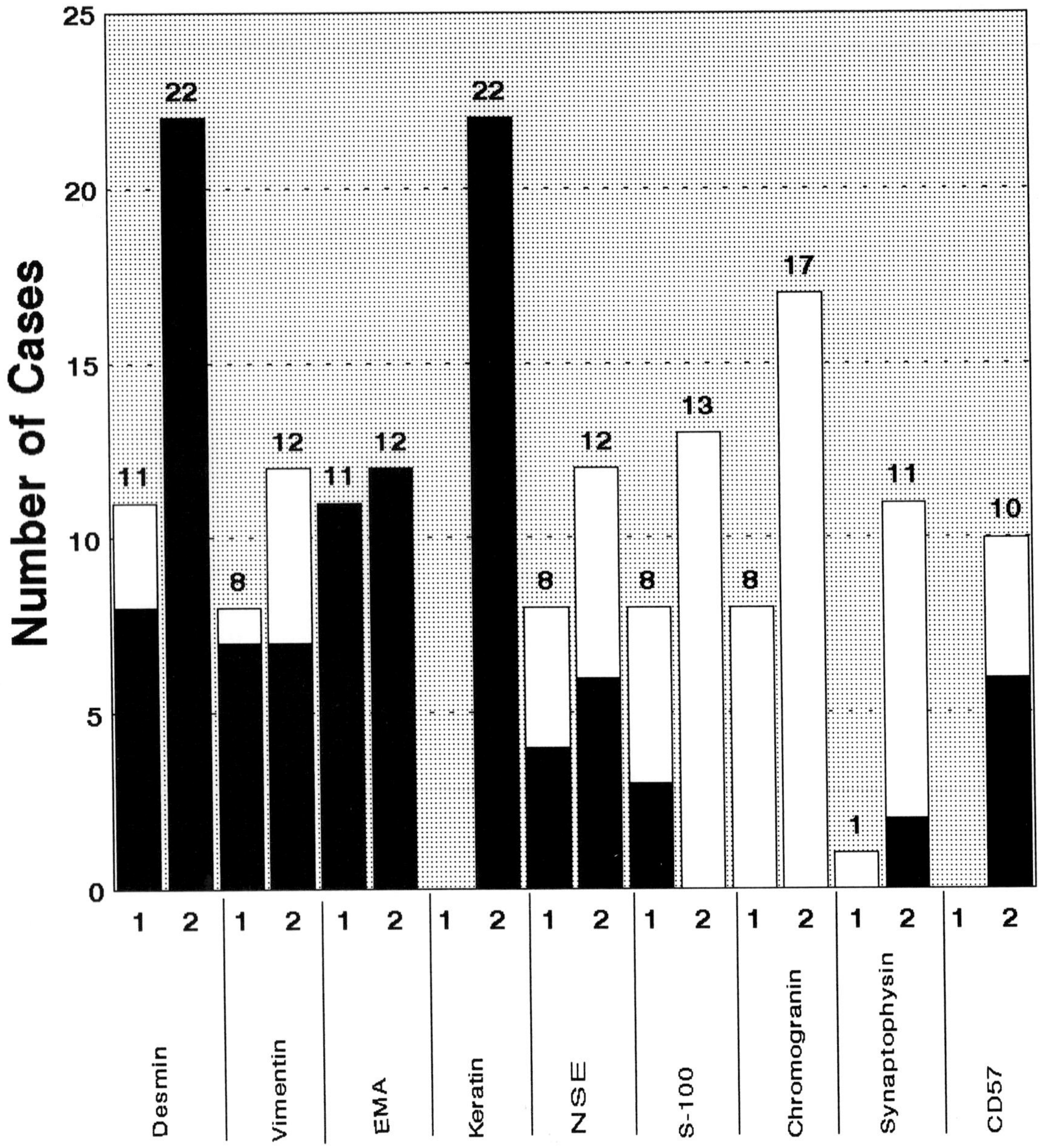

□ Negative; ■positive.
Column 1—from ref. 128; column 2—from ref. 59.

main oncogene (19a). The chromosomal band 22q12 is the site for the *EWS* gene, which is involved in sarcoma-associated translocations (see Chapter 4) (42a,150a,190). Recently, Ladanyi and Gerald (97a) reported the fusion of *EWS* and *WT*1 genes and the presence of chimeric messenger RNA in DSRCT. They postulate that different translocation partners of the *EWS* gene may be responsible for the biologic differences between ES, clear cell sarcoma, and DSRCT.

Eleven DSRCTs were analyzed by flow cytometry; nine tumors were diploid, one tetraploid, and one aneuploid. The DNA pattern and proliferative fraction did not correlate with the histologic pattern, mitotic rate, extent of necrosis, or longer survival (128).

REFERENCES

1. Ahel V, Zubovic I, Rozmanic V. Bronchial adenoid cystic carcinoma with saccular bronchiectasis as a cause of recurrent pneumonia in children. *Pediatr Pulmonol* 1992;12:260–262.
2. Alvarez-Silvan AM, Gonzalez del Castillo J, Martinez Caro A, et al. Maturation of Wilms tumor pulmonary metastases to benign fibromas after therapy. *Med Pediatr Oncol* 1984;12:218–220.
3. Allan BT, Day DB, Dehner LP. Primary pulmonary rhabdomyosarcoma of the lung in children. Report of two cases presenting with spontaneous pneumothorax. *Cancer* 1987;59:100–1011.

4. Allen ED, McCoy KS. Presentation of bronchial mucoepidermoid carcinoma as unilateral hyperlucent lung. *Pediatr Pulmonol* 1990;8:294–297.
5. Al-Saleem T, Peale AR, Norris CM. Multiple papillomatosis of the lower respiratory tract. Clinical and pathologic study of eleven cases. *Cancer* 1968;22:1173–1184.
6. Anderson KA, Hurley WC, Hyrley BT, Ohrt DW. Malignant pleural mesothelioma following radiotherapy in a 16 year old boy. *Cancer* 1985;56:273–276.
7. Anderson KC, Roy TM, Fields CL, Collins LC. Juvenile laryngeal papillomatosis: a new complication. *South Med J* 1993;86: 447–449.
7a. Andiman WA, Eastman R, Martin K, et al. Opportunistic lymphoproliferation associated with Ebstein–Barr viral DNA in infants and children with AIDS. *Lancet* 1985;2:1390–1393.
8. Archer RL, Grogg SE, Sanders SP. Mucoepidermoid bronchial adenoma in a 6 year old girl. A case report and review of the literature. *J Thorac Cardiovasc Surg* 1987;94:452–453.
8a. Armstrong GR, Raafat F, Ingram L, Mann JR. Malignant peritoneal mesothelioma in childhood. *Arch Pathol Lab Med* 1988;112:1159–1162
9. Ashworth TG. Pulmonary blastoma, a true congenital neoplasm. *Histopathology* 1983;7:585–594.
9a. Ball NJ, Urbanski SJ, Green FHY, Kieser T. Pleural multicystic mesothelial proliferation. The so-called multicystic mesothelioma. *Am J Surg Pathol* 1990;14:375–378.
10. Bannayan GA, Huvos AG, D'Angio GJ. Effect of irradiation on the maturation of Wilms' tumor. *Cancer* 1971;4:812–818.
11. Barbareschi M, Frigo B, Cristina S, Valentini L, Leonardi L, Mosca L. Bronchial carcinoid with paranuclear fibrillary inclusions related to cytokeratins and vimentin. *Virch Arch A Histopathol Anat* 1989;415:31–46.
12. Barbareschi M, Ferrero S, Frigo B, Mariscotti C, Mosca L. Bronchial carcinoid with S-100 positive sustentacular cells. *Tumori* 1988;74:705–711.
13. Barnard WG. Embryoma of lung. *Thorax* 1952;7:299–301.
14. Barret NR, Barnard WG. Some unusual thoracic tumors. *Br J Surg* 1945;32:447–457.
15. Bateson EM, Hayes JA, Woo-Ming M. Endobronchial teratoma associated with bronchiectasis and bronchiolectasis. *Thorax* 1968;23:69.
16. Becroft DMO, Japush MF. Pulmonary sarcomas arising in mesenchymal cystic hamartomas. *Pediatr Pathol* 1987;7:478 (Abstr).
17. Benjamin DR, Cahill JL. Bronchioloalveolar carcinoma of the lung and congenital cystic adenomatoid malformation. *Am J Clin Pathol* 1991;95:889–892.
17a. Biegel JA, Conard K, Brooks JJ. Translocation (11;22)(p13:q12): primary change in intra-abdominal desmoplastic small round cell tumor. *Genes Chrom Cancer* 1993;7:119–121.
18. Bishopric GA Jr, Ordonez NG. Carcinoembryonic antigen in primary carcinoid tumors of the lung. *Cancer* 1986;58:1316–1320.
19. Blobel GA, Moll R, Franke WW, Kayser KW, Gould VE. The intermediate filament cytoskeleton of malignant mesotheliomas and its diagnostic significance. *Am J Pathol* 1985;121:235–247.
19a. Boehm T, Foroni L, Kaneko Y, Perutz MF, Rabbits TH. The rhombotin family of cyteine-rich LIM-domain oncogenes: distinct members are involved in T-cell translocations to human chromosomes 11p15 and 11p13. *Proc Natl Acad Sci USA* 1991;88:4367–4371.
20. Bolen Jw, Hammar SP, McNutt MA. Reactive and neoplastic serosal tissue: a light microscopic, ultrastructural and immunocytochemical study. *Am J Surg Pathol* 1986;10:34–47.
21. Boshart M, zur Hasen H. Human papillomaviruses in Buschke-Lowenstein tumors: physical state of the DNA and identification of a tandem duplication in the noncoding region of a human papillomavirus 6 subtype. *J Virol* 1986;58:963–966.
22. Bove KE. Case 6. Sarcoma arising in pulmonary mesenchymal hamartoma. *Pediatr Pathol* 1989;9:785–792.
23. Brachman DG, Graves D, Yokes E, et al. Occurence of p53 gene deletion and human papilloma virus infection in human head and neck cancer. *Cancer Res* 1992;53:4832–36.
24. Brenner J, Sordillo P, Magill B. Malignant mesothelioma in children: report of seven cases and review of the literature. *Med Pediatr Oncol* 1981;9:367–373.
25. Buell R, Wang N-S, Seemayer TA, Ahmed MN. Endobronchial plasma cell granuloma (xanthomatous pseudotumor). A light and electron microscopic study. *Hum Pathol* 1976;7:411–426.
26. Byrne JC, Tsao MS, Fraser RS, Howley PM. Human papilloma virus-11 DNA in a patient with chronic laryngotracheobronchial papillomatosis and metastatic squamous cell carcinoma of the lung. *N Engl J Med* 1987;317:873–878.
27. Cailey CK, Caez HJ, Mersheimer W. Primary bronchogenic carcinoma of the lung in children. *Am J Dis Child* 1951;82:49–60.
27a. Call KM, Glaser T, Ito CY, et al. Isolation and characterization of a zinc finger polypeptide gene at the human chromosome 11 Wilm's tumor locus. *Cell* 1990;60:509–520.
27b. Can Basaklar A, Sonmez K, Memis L, Kale N. Pleomorphic adenoma of the main bronchus. *J Pediatr Surg* 1994;29:1550
28. Capella C, Gabrielli M, Polak JM, Buffa R, Solcia E, Bordi C. Ultrastructural and histologic study of 11 bronchial carcinoids. Evidence for different types. *Virch OWS Arch A Histopathol Anat* 1979;381:313–329.
29. Carney JA. The triad of gastric epithelioid leiomyosarcoma, pulmonary chondroma and functioning extraadrenal paraganglioma. A five year review. *Medicine (Baltimore)* 1983;62:159–169.
30. Chadwick EG, Connor EJ, Hanson C, et al. Tumors of smooth-muscle origin in HIV-infected children. *JAMA* 1990;263:3182–3184.
31. Chaput M, Ninane J, Gosseye S, et al. Juvenile laryngeal papillomatosis and epidermoid carcinoma. *J Pediatr* 1989;114:269–272.
32. Cin PD, Kools P, Jonge ID, Moerman P, Van de ven W, Van den Berghe H. Rearrangement of 12q14-15 in pulmonary chondroid hamartoma. *Genes Chrom Cancer* 1993;8:131–133.
33. Coffin CM, Dehner LP. Mesothelial and related neoplasms in children and adolescents: a clinicopathologic and immunohistochemical analysis of eight cases. *Pediatr Pathol* 1992;12:333–348.
34. Cohen C, Kaschula ROC. Primary pulmonary tumors in childhood: a review of 31 years experience and the literature. *Pediatr Pulmonol* 1992;140:222–232.
35. Cohen M, Emms M, Kaschula ROC. Childhood pulmonary blastoma: a pleuropulmonary variant of the adult-type pulmonary blastoma. *Pediatr Pathol* 1991;11:737–749.
36. Cohen M, Smith WL, Weetman R, et al. Pulmonary pseudometastases in children with malignant tumors. *Radiology* 1981;141: 371–374.
37. Cooper SP, Fraire AE, Buffler PA, Greenberg SD, Langston C. Epidemiologic aspects of childhood mesothelioma. *Pathol Immunopathol Res* 1989;8:276–286.
38. Crist WM, Raney RB, Newton W, Lawrence W Jr, Teft M, Foulkes MA. Intrathoracic soft tissue sarcomas in children. *Cancer* 1982;50:598–604.
39. Dail DH. Uncommon lung tumors. In: Dail DH, Hammar SP, eds. *Pulmonary Pathology*. New York: Springer-Verlag; 1988: 847–972.
40. Dail DH, Liebow AA, Gmelich JT, et al. Intravascular bronchiolar and alveolar tumor of the lung (IVBAT): an analysis of twenty cases of a peculiar sclerosing endothelial tumor. *Cancer* 1983;51: 452–464.
41. Davis AJ, Emans SJ. Human papilloma virus infection in the pediatric and adolescent patient. *J Pediatr* 1989;115:1–9.
42. Day DW, Taylor SA. Pulmonary teratoma associated with thymic tissue. *Thorax* 1960;23:69–70.
42a. Delattre O, Zucman J, Plougastel B, et al. Gene fusion with an ETS DNA-binding domain caused by chromosome translocation in human tumours. *Nature (Lond)* 1992;359:162–165.
42b. Dehner LP. Pleuropulmonary blastoma is the pulmonary blastoma of childhood. *Semin Diagn Pathol* 1994;11:141–151.
42c. Dehner LP, Watterson J, Priest J. Pleuropulmonary blastoma: a unique intrathoracic-pulmonary neoplasm of childhood. In: Askin FB, Langston C, Rosenberg HS, Bernstein J, eds. *Pulmonary Disease. (Perspectives in Pediatric Pathology*, vol 18). Basel: Karger; 1995:214–226.
42d. Delahunt B, Thomson KJ, Ferguson AF, Neale TJ, Meffan PJ, Nacey JN. Familial cystic nephroma and pleuropulmonary blastoma. *Cancer* 1993;71:1338–1342.
43. de Paredes CG, Pierce WS, Groff DS, Waldhausen JA. Bronchogenic tumors in children. *Arch Surg* 1970;100:574–576.

44. Dickstein PJ, Amaral SMM, Silva AMLF, Saltro PA, Ferreira AJ, Alex A. Bronchial mucous gland adenomas presenting as bronchogenic cyst. *Pediatr Pulmonol* 1993;16:370–374.
45. DiLorenzo TP, Tamsen A, Abramson AL, Steinberg BM. Human papillomavirus type 6a DNA in the lung carcinoma of a patient with recurrent laryngeal papillomatosis is characterized by a partial duplication. *J Gen Virol* 1992;73:423–428.
46. Dincen MK, Englander LS, Huben RP. Bleomycin-induced nodular pulmonary fibrosis masquerading as metastatic testicular cancer. *J Urol* 1986;136:473–475.
47. Domizio P, Liesner RJ, Dicks-Mireaux C, Risdon RA. Malignant mesenchymoma associated with a congenital lung cyst in a child. *Pediatr Pathol* 1990;10:785–797.
48. Eble JN, Hull MT, Bojrab D. Laryngeal blastoma. A light and electron microscopic study of a novel entity analogous to pulmonary blastoma. *Am J Clin Pathol* 1985;84:378–385.
49. Eusebi V, Pileri S, Usellini L, Grassigli A, Capella C. Primary carcinoid of the parotid gland associated with a lung carcinoid. A possible new association. *J Clin Pathol* 1982;35:611–616.
50. Fearon B, MacRae D. Laryngeal papillomatosis in children. *J Otolaryngol* 1976:5:493–496.
51. Fisher JE, Khan AR, Jewett TC, Allen J, Afshani E. Childhood pneumoblastoma (pulmonary blastoma) and adult chondroid hamartoma of the lung. A unifying concept. *Pediatr Pathol* 1986;5:94–95 (abstr).
52. Fletcher JA, Pinkus GS, Donovan K, et al. Clonal rearrangement of chromosome band 9p21 in the mesenchymal component of pulmonary chondroid hamartoma. *Cancer Res* 1992;52:6224–6228.
53. Fletcher JA, Pinkus GS, Weidner N, Morton CC. Lineage restricted clonality in biphasic solid tumors. *Am J Pathol* 1991;138: 1199–1207.
53a. Fletcher JA, Longtine J, Wallace K, Mentzer SJ, Sugarbaker DJ. Cytogenetic and histologic findings in 17 pulmonary chondroid hamartomas: Evidence for a pathogenetic relationship with lipomas and leiomyomas. *Genes Chrom Cancer* 1995;12:220–223.
54. Fraire AE, Cooper S, Greenberg SD, Buffler P, Langston C. Mesothelioma of childhood. *Cancer* 1988;62:838–847.
55. Fukuda T, Machinami R, Joshita T, Nagashima K. Benign clear cell tumor of the lung in an 8-year-old girl. *Arch Pathol Lab Med* 1986;110:664–666.
56. Fung CH, Lo JW, Yonan T, et al. Pulmonary blastoma. An ultrastructural study with a brief review of the literature and a discussion of pathogenesis. *Cancer* 1977;39:153–163.
57. Gabrail NY, Zara BY. Pulmonary hamartoma syndrome. *Chest* 1990;97:962–65.
58. Galliani CA, Beatty JF, Grosfeld JL. Cavernous hemangioma of the lung in an infant. *Pediatr Pathol* 1992;12:105–111.
59. Gerald WL, Miller HK, Battifora H, Miettinen M, Silva EG, Rosai J. Intraabdominal desmoplastic small-round cell tumor: report of 19 cases of a distinctive type of high-grade polyphenotypic malignancy affecting young individuals. *Am J Surg Pathol* 1991;15:499–513.
60. Gerald WL, Rosai J. Desmoplastic small cell tumor with divergent differentiation. *Pediatr Pathol* 1989;9:177–183.
61. Gerbasi FS, Margileth AM, Kibler RS. Primary fibrosarcoma of the lung in a young child. A case treated by lobectomy and cobalt therapy. *J Pediatr* 1959;54:488.
62. Gissmann L, Diehl V, Schultz-Coulon HJ, zur Hausen H. Molecular cloning and characterization of human papilloma virus DNA derived from a laryngeal papilloma. *J Virol* 1982;44:393–400.
63. Gissmann L, Wolnik L, Ikenberg H, Koldovsky U, Schnurch HG, Hausen H. Human papillomavirus types 6 and 11 DNA sequences in genital and laryngeal papillomas and in some cervical cancers. *Proc Natl Acad Sci USA* 1983;80:560–3.
64. Goldman A, Conner CL. Benign tumors of lungs with special reference to adenomatous bronchial tumors. *Dis Chest* 1950;17: 644–648.
65. Gonzalez-Crussi F, Crawford SE, Sun C-C J. Intraabdominal desmoplastic small-cell tumors with divergent differentiation. Observations on three cases of childhood. *Am J Surg Pathol* 1990; 14:633–642.
66. Grundy GW, Miller RW. Malignant mesothelioma in childhood. *Cancer* 1972;30:1216–1218.
67. Ha SJ, Helms P, Fletcher M, Broadbent V, Pritchard J. Lung involvement in Langerhans cell histiocytosis: prevalence, clinical features and outcome. *Pediatrics* 1992;89:466–9.
67a. Hachitanda Y, Aoyama C, Sato JK, Shimada H. Pleuropulmonary blastoma in childhood. A tumor of divergent differentiation. *Am J Surg Pathol* 1993;17:382–391.
68. Hague AK, Kanz MF. Asbestos bodies in children's lungs. An association with sudden infant death syndrome and bronchopulmonary dysplasia. *Arch Pathol Lab Med* 1988;112:514–518.
68a. Haibach H, Burns TW, Carlson HE, Burman KD, Deftos LJ. Multiple hamartoma syndrome (Cowden's disease) associated with renal cell carcinoma and primary neuroendocrine carcinoma of the skin (merkel cell carcinoma). *Am J Clin Pathol* 1992;97:705–712.
69. Hammar SP, Bolen JW. Pleural neoplasms. In: Dail DH, Hammar SP, eds. *Pulmonary Pathology*. New York: Springer-Verlag; 1988;973–1028.
70. Hanock BJ, Di Lorenzo M, Youssef S, Yazbeck S, Marcotte JE, Collin PP. Childhood primary pulmonary neoplasms. *J Pediatr Surg* 1993;28:1133–1136.
71. Hartman GE, Schochat SJ. Primary pulmonary neoplasms of childhood: a review. *Ann Thorac Surg* 1983;36:108–119.
72. Hedlund GL, Bisset III GS, Bove KE. Malignant neoplasms arising in cystic hamartoma of the lung in childhood. *Radiol* 1989;173:77–79.
72a. Heifetz SA, Collins B, Matt BH. Pleomorphic adenoma (benign mixed tumor) of the trachea. *Pediatr Pathol* 1992;12:563–574.
73. Helin I, Tedgard U, Dejmek A, Lindgren S. Muco-epidermoid tumor of the bronchus. *Int J Pediatr Otorhinolaryngol* 1984;7: 289–295.
74. Helmut RA, Strate RW. Squamous carcinoma of the lung in a nonirradiated, nonsmoking patient with juvenile laryngeal papillomatosis. *Am J Surg Pathol* 1987;11:643–640.
74a. Helton KJ, Kuhn JP, Fletcher BD, Jenkins III JJ, Parham DM. Broncholitis obliterous-organizing pneumonia (BOOP) in children with malignant disease. *Pediatr Radiol* 1992;22:270–274.
75. Hitz HB, Oesterlin E. A case of multiple papillomata of the larynx with aerial metastases to the lungs. *Am J Pathol* 1932;8:333–338.
76. Holland-Moritz RM, Heyn RM. Pulmonary blastoma associated with cystic lesions in children. *Med Pediatr Oncol* 1984;12:85–88.
77. Hull MT, Gonzalez-Crussi F, Grosfield J. Multiple fibroleiomyomatous hamartomas in childhood. *J Pediatr Surg* 1979;14: 428–431.
78. Hurvitz CH, Greenberg SH, Song CH, Gans SL. Hemangiomatosis of the pleura with hemorrhage and disseminated intravascular coagulation. *J Pediatr Surg* 1982;17:73–75.
79. Igbal UA, Callahan R. Prognostic significance of genetic alteration in human breast carcinoma. In: Cossman J, ed. *Molecular Genetics in Cancer Diagnosis*. New York: Elsevier; 1990:289–301.
80. Imperato JP, Folkman J, Sagerman RH, Cassady JR. Treatment of plasma cell granuloma of the lung with radiation therapy: a report of two cases and a review of the literature. *Cancer* 1986;57: 2127–2129.
81. Irwin BC, Hendricks WR, Pincott JR, Bailey CM, Evans JNG. Juvenile laryngeal papillomatosis. *J Laryngol Otol* 1986;100:435.
82. Isaacson PG, Wright DH. Malignant lymphoma of mucosa-associated lymphoid tissue. *Histopathol* 1987;11:445–462.
83. Jeresaty RM, Knight HF, Hart WE. Pulmonary arteriovenous fistulas in children. *Am J Dis Child* 1966;111:256–261.
84. Jimenez JF, Uthman EO, Townsend JW, Gloster ES, Seibert JJ. Primary bronchopulmonary leiomyosarcoma in childhood. *Arch Pathol Lab Med* 1986;110:348–351.
84a. Joshi VV, Oleske JM, Minnetor AB, et al. Pathologic pulmonary findings in children with the acquired immunodeficiency syndrome: a study of ten cases. *Hum Pathol* 1985;16:241–246.
84b. Joshi VV, Kauffman S, Oleske JM, et al. Polyclonal polymorphic B-cell lymphoproliferative disorder with prominent pulmonary involvement with children with acquired immunodeficiency syndrome. *Cancer* 1987;59:1455–1492.

84c. Joshi VV, Beckwith JB. Multilocular cyst of the kidney (cystic nephroma) and cystic, partially differentiated nephroblastoma. Terminology and criteria for diagnosis. *Cancer* 1989;64:466–479.
85. Johansson M, Heim S, Mandahl N, Hambraeus G, Johansson L, Mitelman F. Cytogenetic analysis of six bronchial carcinoids. *Cancer Genet Cytogenet* 1993;66:33–38.
86. Jones DJ, Hasleton PS, Moore M. DNA ploidy in bronchopulmonary carcinoids. *Thorax* 1988;43:195–199.
87. Katz DR, Bubis JJ. Acinic cell tumor of the bronchus. *Cancer* 1976;38:830–832.
88. Kaufman SL, Stout AP. Mesothelioma in children. *Cancer* 1964;14:539–544.
89. Kavuru MS, Mehta AC, Eliachar I. Effect of photodynamic therapy and external beam radiation therapy on juvenile laryngotracheobronchial papillomatosis. *Annu Rev Respir Dis* 1990;141:509–510.
90. Kellett HS, Lipphard D, Willis RA. Two unusual examples of heteroplasia in the lung. *J Pathol Bacteriol* 1962;84:421–425.
91. Kojima R, Mizuguchi M, Beesho F, et al. Pulmonary carcinoma associated with hamartoma in an 11 year-old boy. *Am J Pediatr Hematol-Oncol* 1993;15:364–369.
92. Koss MN, Hochholzer L, O'Leary T. Pulmonary blastoma. *Cancer* 1991;67:2368–2381.
93. Kramer SS, Wehunr WD, Stocker JT, Kashema H. Pulmonary manifestations of juvenile laryngeal papillomatosis. *AJR* 1985;144:687.
94. Krous HF, Sexauer CL. Embryonal rhabdomyosarcoma arising within a congenital bronchogenic cyst in a child. *J Pediatr Surg* 1981;16:506–508.
95. Kujari H. A flow cytometric analysis of 23 carcinoid tumors. *Cancer* 1988;61:2513–2520.
96. Kyriakos M. Webber B. Cancer of the lung in young men. *J Thorac Cardiovasc Surg* 1974;67:634–648.
97. Lack EE, Clifton-Harris GB, Eralkis EJ, Vawter GF. Primary bronchial tumors in childhood. A clinicopathologic study of six cases. *Cancer* 1983;51:492–497.
97a. Ladanyi M, Gerald W. Fusion of the EWS and WT1 genes in the desmoplastic small round cell tumors. *Cancer Res* 1994;54:2837–2840.
98. Lancaster WD, Castellano C, Santos C, Delgado G, Kurman RJ, Jenson AB. Human papillomavirus deoxyribonucleic acid in cervical carcinoma from primary and metastatic sites. *Am J Obstet Gynecol* 1986;154:115–9.
99. Layfield LJ, Lenarsky C. Desmoplastic small cell tumors of the peritoneum coexpressing mesenchymal and epithelial markers. *Am J Clin Pathol* 1991;96:536–543.
99a. Ledet SC, Brown RW, Cagle PT. p53 immunostaining in the differentiation of inflammatory pseudotumor from sarcoma involving the lung. *Mod Pathol* 1995;8:282–286.
100. Letho V-P, Miettinen M, Dahl D, Virtanen J. A dual expression of cytokeratin and neurofilaments in bronchial carcinoid cells. *Int J Cancer* 1985;35:421–425.
101. Levenston S, McKeel DW, Buckley PJ, et al. Acromegaly and Cushing's syndrome associated with foregut carcinoid tumor. *J Clin Endocrinol Metab* 1981;53:682–689.
102. Liebow AA, Hubbell DS. Sclerosing hemangioma (histiocytoma, xanthoma) of the lung. *Cancer* 1956;9:53–75.
103. Lin-Chu M, Lee JY, Ho MY. Malignant mesothelioma in infancy. *Arch Pathol Lab Med* 1989;113:409–411.
104. Lund C, Sorensen IM, Axelsen F, Larsen K. Pulmonary histiocytomas. *Eur J Respir Dis* 1983;64:141–149.
105. Mackay B, Osborne BM, Wilson RA. Ultrastructure of lung neoplasms. In: Straus MJ, ed. *Lung Cancer*. New York: Grune and Stratton; 1977:71–84.
106. Mackenzie M. *Essays in Growth in the Larynx with Report of an Analysis of 100 Consecutive Cases Treated by the Author*. London: J and A Churchill; 1871.
107. Maier HC, Sommers SC. Recurrent and metastatic pulmonary fibrous histiocytoma/plasma cell granuloma in a child. *Cancer* 1987;60:1073–1076.
108. Manivel JC, Priest JR, Watterson J, et al. Pleuropulmonary blastoma. The so-called pulmonary blastoma of childhood. *Cancer* 1988;62:1516–1526.
109. Manning JT, Ordonez NG, Rosenberg HS, Walker WE. Pulmonary endodermal tumor resembling fetal lung. *Arch Pathol Lab Med* 1985;109:48–50.
110. Mark EJ. Mesenchymal cystic hamartoma of the lung. *N Engl J Med* 1983;315:1255–1259.
111. Markel SF, Abell MR, Haight C, French AJ. Neoplasms of bronchus commonly designated as adenomas. *Cancer* 1964;17:590–608.
112. Martinez JC, Pecero FC, de la Pena GG, et al. Pulmonary blastoma: report of a case. *J Pediatr Surg* 1978;13:93–94.
113. Martinez S, Young R, Moll B, et al. Simultaneous leiomyosarcoma and leiomyoma in pediatric HIV infection (abstr). *Ann Allergy* 1990;64:89.
114. Matsuba HM, Thawley SE, Maurey M, Spector GJ, Pikul FJ. Laryngeal epidermoid carcinoma associated with juvenile laryngeal papillomatosis. *Laryngoscope* 1985;95:1264–6.
115. Matsubara O, Tan-Liu NS, Kenney RM, Mark EJ. Inflammatory pseudotumors of the lung. Progression from organising pneumonia to fibrous histiocytoma or to plasma cell granuloma in 32 cases. *Hum Pathol* 1988;19:807–814.
116. McCann MP, Fu YS, Kay S. Pulmonary blastoma. *Cancer* 1976;38:789.
117. McCue CM, Hartenberg M, Nance WE. Pulmonary arteriovenous malformations related to Rendu–Osler–Weber syndrome. *Am J Med Genet* 1984;19:19–27.
118. McDowell HP, Macfarlane PI, Martin J. Isolated pulmonary histiocytosis. *Arch Dis Child* 1988;63:423–426.
119. McGinnis M, Jacobs G, El-Naggar A, Redline RW. Congenital peribronchial myofibroblastic tumor (so-called "congenital leiomyosarcoma"). A distinctive neonatal lung lesion associated with nonimmune hydrops fetalis. *Mod Pathol* 1993;6:487–492.
120. Meade JB, Whitwell F, Bickford BJ, Waddington JKB. Primary hemangiopericytoma of lung. *Thorax* 1974;29:1.
120a. Mennemeyer R, Smith H. Multicystic peritoneal mesothelioma: a case report with electron microscopy of a case mimicking intraabdominal cystic hygroma (lymphangioma). *Cancer* 1979;44:692–698.
121. Michael P. *Tumors of Infancy and Childhood*. Philadelphia: JB Lippincott; 1964:253–257.
122. Mitchell DB, Humphreys S, Kearns DB. Mucoepidermoid carcinoma of the larynx in a child. *Int J Pediatr Otorhinolaryngol* 1988;15:211–215.
123. Mounts P, Kashima H. Association of human papillomavirus subtype and clinical course in respiratory papillomatosis. *Laryngoscope* 1984;94:28–33.
124. Nakagwara A, Ikeda K, Fukuoka HO. Mucoepidermoid tumor of the bronchus in an infant. *J Pediatr Surg* 1979;14:608–609.
125. Nikolaou I, Barbatis C, Laopodis V, Bekir S, Fletcher CDM. Intraabdominal desmoplastic small-cell tumors with divergent differentiation. Report of two cases and review of the literature. *Pathol Res Pract* 1992;188:981–988.
126. Nondahl SR, Finlay JL, Farrel PM, Warner TF, Hong RA. A case report and literature review of primary pulmonary histiocytosis X of childhood. *Med Pediatr Oncol* 1986;14:57–62.
127. Norton J, Monaghan P, Carter RL. Intra-abdominal desmoplastic small cell tumor with divergent differentiation. *Histopathology* 1991;19:560–562.
128. Ordonez NG, El-Naggar AD, Ro JY, Silva EG, Mackay B. Intraabdominal desmoplastic small cell tumor: a light microscopic, immunocytochemical, ultrastructural and flow cytometric study. *Hum Pathol* 1993;24:850–865.
129. Ordonez NG, Zirkin R, Bloom RE. Malignant small-cell epithelial tumor of the peritoneum coexpressing mesenchymal-type intermediate filaments. *Am J Surg Pathol* 1989;13:413–421.
130. Pacharee P, Parichatikanond P. Pulmonary blastoma. A case review in an infant and review of the literature. *J Med Assoc Thai* 1972;55:43.
130a. Parkash V, Gerald WL, Parma A, Miettinen M, Rosai J. Desmoplastic small round cell tumor of the pleura. *Am J Surg Pathol* 1995;19:659–665.
131. Pettinato G, Manivel JC, de Rosa N, Dehner LP. Inflammatory

myofibroblastic tumor (plasma cell granuloma). Clinicopathologic study of 20 cases with immunohistochemical and ultrastructural observations. *Am J Clin Pathol* 1990;94:538–546.

132. Pettinato G, Manivel JC, Saldana MJ, Peyser J, Dehner LP. Primary bronchopulmonary fibrosarcoma of childhood and adolescence: reassessment of a low-grade malignancy. Clinicopathologic study of five cases and review of the literature. *Hum Pathol* 1989;20:463–471.
133. Popper HH, Wirnsgerber C, Juttner-Smolle FM, Pongratz MG, Sommersgutter M. The predictive value of human papilloma virus (HPV) typing in the prognosis of bronchial squamous papillomas. *Histopathololog*y 1992;21:323-330.
133a. Prat J, Matias-Guiu X, Algaban F. Desmoplastic small round cell tumor. *Am J Surg Pathol* 1992;16: 306–307.
133b. Priest J, Watterson J, Dehner L et al. Childhood pleuropulmonary blastoma (PPB) as a unique marker for familial childhood neoplasm. *Proc ASCO* 1994;13:186.
134. Rabbett WF. Juvenile laryngeal papillomatosis: the relation of irradiation to malignant degeneration in this disease. *Ann Otol Rhinol Laryngol* 1965;74:1149–1163.
135. Rando RF, Groff DE, Chirikjian JG, Lancaster WD. Isolation and characterization of a novel human papillomavirus type 6 DNA from an invasive vulvar carcinoma. *J Virol* 1986;57:353–356.
136. Robb D. A case of neonatal fibrosarcoma of lung. *Br J Surg* 1958;46:173.
136a. Rodriguez E, Sreekantaiah C, Gerald W, Reuter VE, Motzer RJ, Chaganti RSK. A recurring translocation t(11;22)(p13;11.2), characterizes intra-abdominal desmoplastic small round cell tumors. *Cancer Genet Cytogenet* 1993;69:17–21.
137. Roggli VL, Kim HS, Hawkins E. Congenital generalized fibromatosis with visceral involvement: a case report. *Cancer* 1980;45: 954–960.
137a. Rohrlich P, Peuchmaur M, de Napoli Cocci S, Durand Gasselin I, Garel C, Aigrain Y, Galanaud P, Vilmer E, Emile D. Interleukin-6 and interleukin-1 production in a pediatric plasma cell granuloma of the lung. *Am J Surg Pathol* 1995;19:590–595.
138. Said JW, Vimadal S, Nash G, et al. Immunoreactive neuron specific enolase, bombesin and chromogranin as markers for neuroendocrine lung tumors. *Hum Pathol* 1985;16:236–240.
138a. Sanchez-Jimenez J, Ballister-Martinez A, Lodo-Besse J, Huguet-Redecilla P, Martinez-Gonzalez S, Cobos-Barroso N. Papillary adenoma of type 2 pneumocytes. *Pediatr Pulmonol* 1994;17: 396–400.
139. Sandler M, Scheuer PJ, Watt PJ. 5-Hydroxytryptophan-secreting bronchial carcinoid tumor. *Lancet* 1961;2:1067–1069.
140. Sano T, Saito H, Yamasaki R, et al. Immunoreactive somatostatin and calcitonin in pulmonary neuroendocrine tumors. *Cancer* 1986;57:64–68.
141. Santrach PJ, Askin FB, Wells RJ, Azizkhan RG, Mierten DF. Nodular form of bleomycin-related pulmonary injury in patients with osteogenic sarcoma. *Cancer* 1989;64:806–811.
142. Saruk M, Stern H, Tronic BS, Neumann RD, Livolsi VA. Intrapulmonary benign cystic teratoma. *Connecticut Med* 1980;44: 687.
143. Sawyer JR, Tryka AF, Lewis JM. A novel reciprocal chromosomal translocation t(11;22)(p13;q12) in an intrabdominal desmoplastic small round-cell tumor. *Am J Surg Pathol* 1992;16: 411–416.
144. Scharstein R, Johnson JF, Cook BA, et al. Bleomycin nodules mimicking metastatic osteogenic sarcoma. *Am J Pediatr Hematol-Oncol* 1987;9:219–221.
145. Schroder S, Padberg BC. Desmoplastic small-cell tumor of the peritoneum with divergent differentiation: immunocytochemical and biochemical findings. *Am J Clin Pathol* 1993;99:353–355.
146. Seo IN, Warren J, Mirkin D, Weisman SJ, Grosfeld JL. Mucoepidermoid carcinoma of the bronchus in a 4-year-old child. A high grade variant with lymph node metastasis. *Cancer* 1984;53: 1600–1604.
147. Sheibani K, Battifora H, Burke JS. Antigenic phenotype of malignant mesotheliomas and pulmonary adenocarcinomas: an immunohistologic analysis demonstrating the value of Leu M1 antigen. *Am J Pathol* 1986;123:211–219.
148. Shelly BE, Lorenzo RL. Primary squamous cell carcinoma of the lung in childhood. *Pediatr Radiol* 1983;13:92–94.
149. Shen SC, Yunis EJ. Leiomyosarcoma developing in a child during remission of leukemia. *J Pediatr* 1976;89:780–782.
150. Siegel RJ, Bueso-Ramos C, Cohen C, Ross M. Pulmonary blastoma with germ cell (yolk sac) differentiation: report of two cases. *Mod Pathol* 1991;4:566–570.
150a. Sorensen PHB, Lessnick SL, Lopez-Terrada D, Liu XF, Triche TJ, Denny CT. A second Ewing's sarcoma translocation t(21;22), fuses the EWS gene to another ETS-family transcription factor, ERF. *Nat Genet* 1994;6:146–151.
150b. Snyder CS, Dell'Aquila M, Haghighi P, Baergen RN, Suh YK, Yi ES. Clonal changes in inflammatory pseudotumor of the lung. *Cancer* 1995;76:1545–1549.
151. Spencer H. Pulmonary blastomas. *J Pathol Bacteriol* 1961;82: 161–165.
152. Spencer H. The pulmonary plasma cell/histiocytoma complex. *Histopathology* 1984;8:903–916.
153. Spencer H, Dail DH, Arneaud J. Non-invasive bronchial epithelial papillary tumors. *Cancer* 1980;45:1486–1497.
154. Spencer H. *Pathology of the Lung*. 4th ed. Oxford: Pergamon Press; 1985.
155. Stephanopoulos C, Catsaras H. Myxosarcoma complicating a cystic hamartoma of the lung. *Thorax* 1963;18:144–145.
156. Stocker TJ. The respiratory tract. In: Stocker JT, Dehner LP, eds. *Pediatric Pathology*. Philadelphia: JB Lippincott; 1992:549–574.
157. Sumner TE, Phelps CR II, Crowe JE, Poolos SP, Shaffner JB. Pulmonary blastoma in a child. *AJR* 1979;133:147–148.
157a. Sussman J, Rosai J. Lymph node metastases as the initial manifestation of malignant mesothelioma. Report of six cases. *Am J Surg Pathol* 1990;14:819–828.
158. Swanson PE, Wick MR, Dehner LP. Leiomyosarcoma of somatic soft tissues in childhood. An immunohistochemical analysis of six cases with ultrastructural correlation. *Hum Pathol* 1991;22: 569–577.
158a. Talerman A, Chilcote RR, Montero JR, Okagaki T. Diffuse malignant peritoneal mesothelioma in a 13 year old girl. Report of a case and review of the literature. *Am J Surg Pathol* 1985:73–80.
159. Tamai S, Kameya Y, Shimosato Y, Tsumuraya M, Wada T. Pulmonary blastoma: an ultrastructural study of a case and its transplanted tumor in athymic nude mice. *Cancer* 1980;46:1389–1396.
159a. Tang TT, Segura A, Oechler HW, et al. Inflammatory myofibrohistiocytic proliferation simulating sarcoma in children. *Cancer* 1990;65:1626–1634.
160. Teplick JG, Teplick SK, Haskim ME. Granular cell myoblastoma of the lung. *AJR Radium Ther Nucl Med* 1975;125:890–894.
161. Tepperman BS, Feld R, Fosse RG. Squamous cell carcinoma of the bronchus associated with hypercalcemia in a twenty year old. *Cancer* 1981;47:2690–2695.
162. Teyssier JR, Adnett JJ, Pigeon F, Bajolle F. Cytogenetic changes in an ovarian granulosa cell tumor. Similarity with carcinoma. *Cancer Genet Cytogenet* 1985;14:147–152.
163. Teyssier JR, Sadrin R, Nou JM, et al. Trisomy 7 in a lung carcinoid tumor: precocious index of malignant transformation. *Cancer Genet Cytogenet* 1985;15:277–282.
164. Thunnissen FBJM, Van Ejik J, Baak JPA, et al. Bronchopulmonary carcinoids and regional lymph node metastases: a quantitative pathologic investigation. *Am J Pathol* 1988;132:119–122.
165. Timmons CF, Richards S, Katz JA, Andrews WS. Hepatic leiomyosarcoma of donor genotype in a liver transplant recipient. *Mod Pathol* 1993;6:9, Abstract no. 51.
165a. Ton CC, Hirvonen H, Miwa H, et al. Positional cloning and characterization of a paired box- and homeobox-containing gene from the aniridia region. *Cell* 1991;67:1059–1074.
165b. Tison V, Cerasoli S, Morisi F, Ladanyi M, Gerald WL, Rosai J. Intracranial desmoplastic small-cell tumor. Report of a case. *Am J Surg Pathol* 1996;20:112–117.
166. Travis WD, Borok Z, Roum JH, et al. Pulmonary Langerhans cell granulomatosis (Histiocytosis X). A clinicopathologic study of 48 cases. *Am J Surg Pathol* 1993;17:971–986.

167. Travis WD, Linnoila RI, Horowitz M, et al. Pulmonary nodules resembling bronchioloalveolar carcinoma in adolescent cancer patients. *Mod Pathol* 1988;1:372–377.
168. Trivedi SA, Mehta KN, Nanavaty JM. Teratoma of the lung. Report of a case. *Br J Dis Chest* 1966;60:156.
169. Tuman KJ, Chicote RR, Berkow RI, Moohr JW. Mesothelioma in a child with prenatal exposure to isoniazid. *Lancet* 1980;2:362.
170. Ueda K, Gruppo R, Unger F, Martin C, Bove K. Rhabdomyosarcoma of lung arising in congenital cystic adenomatoid malformation. *Cancer* 1977;40:383–388.
171. Unger PD, Geller SA, Anderson PJ. Pulmonary lesion in a patient with neurofibromatosis. *Arch Pathol Lab Med* 1984;108:654–657.
172. Valderrama E, Saluja G, Shende A, Lanzkowisky P, Berkman J. Pulmonary blastoma. Report of two cases in children. *Am J Surg Pathol* 1978;2:415–422.
173. van Hoeven KH, Factor SM, Kress Y, Woodruff JM. Visceral myogenic tumors. A manifestation of HIV infection in children. *Am J Surg Pathol* 1993;17:1176–1181.
174. van Muijen GNP, Ruiter DJ, Warnaar SO. Coexpression of intermediate filament polypeptides in human fetal and adult tissues. *Lab Invest* 1987;57:359–369.
175. Variend S, Gerrard M, Norris PD, Goepel JR. Intra-abdominal neuroectodermal tumor of childhood with divergent differentiation. *Histopathology* 1991;18:45–51.
176. Waddel WR. Organoid differentiation of the fetal lung. A histologic study of the differentiation of mammalian fetal lung in utero and in transplants. *Arch Pathol* 1949;47:227–247.
177. Walker D, Gill TJ III, Corson JM. Leiomyosarcoma in a renal allograft recipient treated with immunosuppressive drugs. *JAMA* 1971;215:2084–2086.
178. Warren WH, Memoli VA, Gould VE. Immunohistochemical and ultrastructural analysis of bronchopulmonary neuroendocrine neoplasms. I. Carcinoids. *Ultrastruct Pathol* 1984;6:15–27.
179. Warter A, Statge D, Roescin N. Angio-invasive plasma cell granulomas of the lung. *Cancer* 1987;59:435–443.
180. Weinberg AG, Currarino G, Moore GC, Votreler TP. Mesenchymal neoplasia and congenital pulmonary cysts. *Pediatr Radiol* 1980;9:179–182.
181. Weinblatt ME, Siegel SE, Isaacs H. Pulmonary blastoma associated with cystic lung disease. *Cancer* 1982;49:669–671.
182. Wellons HA, Eggleston P, Golden G, Allen S. Bronchial adenomas in childhood. *Am J Dis Child* 1976;130:301–304.
183. Whitaker D, Shilkin KB. Diagnosis of pleural malignant mesothelioma in life—a practical approach. *J Pathol* 1984;143:147–75.
184. Williams ED, Celestin LR. The association of bronchial carcinoid and pluriglandular adenomatosis. *Thorax* 1962;17:120–127.
185. Yasawa T, Ogata T, Kamma H, Shibagaki T, Iijima T, Horiguchi H. Pulmonary blastoma with a topographic transition from blastic to more differentiated areas. *Virch Arch A Histopathol Anat* 1991;419:513–518.
186. Yee C, Krishnan-Hewlett I, Baker CC, Schlegel R, Howley PM. Presence and expression of human papillomavirus sequences in human cervical carcinoma cell lines. *Am J Pathol* 1985;119:361–366.
187. Yesner R. Small cell tumors of the lung. *Am J Surg Pathol* 1983;7:775–785.
188. Young RH, Eichorn JH, Dickersin GR, Scully RE. Ovarian involvement by the intra-abdominal desmoplastic small round cell tumor with divergent differentiation. A report of three cases. *Hum Pathol* 1992;23:454–464.
189. Yousem SA, Wick MR, Randhawa P, Manivel JC. Pulmonary blastoma. An immunohistochemical analysis with comparison with fetal lung in pseudoglandular stage. *Am J Clin Pathol* 1990;93:167–175.
190. Zucman J, Delattre O, Desmaze C, et al. EWS and ATF-1 gene fusion induced by t(12;22) translocation in malignant melanoma of soft parts. *Nat Genet* 1993;4:341–345.

Pediatric Neoplasia: Morphology and Biology, edited by David M. Parham. Lippincott-Raven Publishers, Philadelphia © 1996.

CHAPTER 15

Malignancies of the Bone Marrow

Frederick G. Behm

INTRODUCTION

Leukemia is the most common type of childhood cancer, accounting for about one third of all pediatric malignancies in the United States. Each year 2,500 children are diagnosed with leukemia. The frequency of leukemia rapidly increases after birth, peaks at 4–5 years of age, and then declines (186). Acute lymphoblastic leukemia (ALL) accounts for the early peak, whereas the incidence of acute myeloid leukemia (AML) remains constant. The incidence rates in the United States per 100,000 children per year are 12.9 for whites and 9.8 for blacks (405,603). The incidence of leukemia in white children is higher than in black children due to the lower incidence of ALL in the latter population (405). Like many other childhood cancers, leukemia occurs more often in males than females. Approximately 85% of acute leukemias are lymphoblastic. Acute myeloid leukemias account for approximately 15% of pediatric leukemias. About 10% of children with AML are less than 1 year of age, and most infants less than 4 weeks of age with congenital leukemia have AML. Chronic myelocytic (myelogenous, granulocytic) leukemia and myelodysplastic syndromes account for 2–5% of pediatric bone marrow malignancies. Chronic lymphocytic leukemia, HTLV-1-associated leukemia/lymphoma, T-gamma lymphoproliferative disorders, and plasma cell myeloma are rare in children.

ETIOLOGY

Genetic, inherited, immunologic, and environmental factors are all linked to leukemogenesis (202,216,387, 479,480). The higher incidence rates for acute leukemia in Down and Klinefelter's syndromes, which have extra chromosomes, point to a relationship between genetic abnormalities and leukemia (181,386,431,466). Bloom's syndrome and Fanconi's anemia, characterized by abnormalities of DNA repair, also have higher incidence rates for acute leukemia (54,216,373,386). An increased incidence of leukemia is observed in children with primary immune deficiency diseases such as Wiskott–Aldrich syndrome and ataxia telangiectasia (314,408, 609). Support for inherited factors for leukemogenesis is largely confined to the high concordance rate of infant leukemia in identical twins. The risk of developing leukemia before age 6 years in the identical twin of a patient with leukemia, usually acute myelomonocytic or monoblastic and chronic myelomonocytic leukemias, is 20% (285,377). However, more recent evidence suggests that transplacental dissemination of leukemic blasts from one twin to the other and not necessarily hereditary factors is responsible for these concordant rates (340). Genomic imprinting was suggested as being involved in the formation of the reciprocal translocation t(9:22)(q34: q11) that characterizes chronic myelogenous leukemia. Initial studies pointed to the translocated chromosome 22q- and the 9q- derivatives as being derived from maternal and paternal chromosomes, respectively (212). This would imply that the fusion *BCR/ABL* gene on the Philadelphia (Ph^1) chromosome of chronic myelogenous leukemia is derived from *BCR* sequences of maternal and *ABL* sequences of paternal origins. If this were true then a predisposition to some leukemias might be inherited. However, subsequent studies have provided evidence that normally functioning *BCR* and *ABL* genes can be of either maternal or paternal origin (177,363).

Exposure to radiation, solvents, chemicals, pesticides, drugs, and electromagnetic fields has been linked with leukemia. Young survivors of the atomic bomb in Japan and children exposed to diagnostic irradiation in utero have shown an increased incidence of ALL (241,255, 338,386). Exposure to benzene, pesticides, and herbi-

F. G. Behm: Department of Pathology and Laboratory Medicine, St. Jude Children's Research Hospital, Memphis, Tennessee 38105.

cides is associated with development of leukemia in adults, but this association is less clear in children. A leukemogenic potential for chemotherapy agents, particularly alkylating agents and epipodophyllotoxins, also exists (420,563). Studies of residential electromagnetic field exposure and childhood malignancy suggest a possible leukemic risk, but studies of adults and electromagnetic exposure show no leukemic risk (20,484).

With the exception of human T-cell leukemia virus (HTLV-1), viral infections do not appear to have a direct role in the causation of childhood leukemia. The contribution of Epstein–Barr virus to the development of Burkitt's lymphoma and its leukemic phase is uncertain at present (159,203,283,610) (see Chapter 16).

The majority of hematopoietic malignancies have identifiable, acquired cytogenetic defects, and it is widely accepted although not proven that human hematopoietic malignancies are the result of these chromosomal abnormalities. Indeed, only a small number of leukemias can be attributed to the risk factors mentioned in the previous paragraphs, but all of these factors appear to contribute to the development of cytogenetic abnormalities. The major cytogenetic abnormalities consist of total or partial chromosomal deletions or duplications and chromosomal translocations or inversions. The mechanisms leading to these chromosomal abnormalities are unclear, but most of these chromosome aberrations result in deregulation of tumor suppressor genes, activation of oncogenes, or the production of novel fusion proteins having potential transcriptional activity (444,445). Like most other types of childhood cancer, pediatric leukemias are predominantly "embryonic" in type and evolve from malignant transformation of developing hematopoietic cells. Thus, an understanding of leukemogenesis awaits elucidation of the roles that oncogenes and transcriptional factors play in normal cellular differentiation, growth, and death.

ACUTE LEUKEMIA

Childhood acute leukemias are broadly divided into lymphoblastic (ALL) and myeloid (AML) types. The presence of 30% or more blasts in the bone marrow smear is, by arbitrary definition, acute leukemia (33,34). The bone marrow of most children with ALL usually has more than 85% of the marrow cells composed of lymphoblasts, whereas marrow harboring AML frequently contains fewer than 80% blasts. Lymphoblastic and Burkitt's (or small noncleaved follicular center cell) lymphomas may also involve the marrow and present with cytologic and immunologic features that are indistinguishable from lymphoblastic leukemia. If cells of these two types of lymphoma compose 25% of more of the marrow cellularity, the process is generally considered acute leukemia for treatment purposes.

The diagnosis and classification of acute leukemias rests on the recognition of leukemic blasts and determination of the malignant cell's lineage. Herein lies the diagnostic challenge for the pathologist and hematologist. In the myeloid leukemias the leukemic blast may be of several types. Type I blasts lack cytoplasmic granules and have a low nucleocytoplasmic ratio, fine or lacy chromatin, and usually one or more distinct nucleoli (34,103) (Fig. 1; see figure in color plate section). These blasts usually have detectable myeloperoxidase. Type II blasts usually have more cytoplasm than type I blasts and contain a small number of azurophilic granules that contain myeloperoxidase (34,103) (Fig. 2; see figure in color plate section). Some subtypes of AML consist predominantly of leukemic cells corresponding to the promyelocytic or later stages of myeloid and monocytic development. The majority of lymphoblastic leukemias are composed of blasts that resemble type I myeloblasts but are often smaller, usually lack cytoplasmic granules, have high nucleocytoplasmic ratios, and display condensed nuclear chromatin with vague or small nucleoli. Lymphoblasts uniformly lack cytochemical evidence of myeloperoxidase.

Auer rods are pathognomonic of an acute myeloid leukemia. These cytoplasmic, crystalline inclusions are distinct rod- or needle-shaped bodies that stain pink to red with Giemsa and Wright stains (Fig. 3; see figure in color plate section) (187). They contain acid phosphatase, myeloperoxidase, and myeloid-associated esterases that suggest a derivation from the incorporation of primary granules of early myeloid cells into autophagic vacuoles. Auer rods are usually found in leukemic myeloblasts but on careful searching can be detected in maturing myeloid cells and segmented neutrophils derived from the leukemic clone. Although common to most acute myeloid types of leukemia, Auer rods also may be seen in blasts of the acute monocytic leukemias and the transforming stage of myelodysplastic syndrome (32,464). The ultrastructure of Auer rods of acute promyelocytic leukemia differs from those of the other subtypes of acute myeloid leukemias (564). Auer rods in acute promyelocytic leukemia consist of tubules in a hexagonal array with a periodicity of 25 nm, whereas in the other myeloid leukemias the internal rod structure is either homogeneous or lamellar with periodicities between 6 nm and 13 nm (67,188). Rarely, cases of acute myeloid leukemia will contain a small number of blasts with myeloperoxidase-positive Auer rods but no chemically detectable myeloperoxidase activity in the remaining blasts. Crystalline inclusions mimicking Auer rods may be observed in rare cases of adult chronic lymphocytic and prolymphocytic leukemias but have not been described in lymphoproliferative processes in children (261).

LABORATORY STUDIES OF ACUTE LEUKEMIA

Most childhood myeloid leukemias are readily identified by morphologic and cytochemical studies. The presence of myeloperoxidase-positive granules or Auer rods is sufficient to make a diagnosis of AML. However, small myeloblasts without significant cytoplasmic granulation and no or little myeloperoxidase may be confused with lymphoblasts. Similarly, large lymphoblasts with copious amounts of cytoplasm or azurophilic granules may be mistaken for leukemic myeloblasts. Because a correct diagnosis of ALL or AML is crucial for appropriate therapy and relaying prognosis, the lineage of all acute leukemias without demonstrable myeloperoxidase or Auer rods must be confirmed by immunologic, ultrastructural, or molecular analysis.

Cytochemical Stains

Prior to the availability of dependable immunologic reagents, cell lineage assignment was largely based on the patterns of blast reaction with a panel of enzymatic reactions that included myeloperoxidase, Sudan black B, esterases, acid phosphatase, and periodic acid–Schiff (PAS) (Table 1). With the exception of myeloperoxidase, Sudan black B, and the α-naphthylbutyrate esterase reactions, these assays have been largely replaced by immunologic studies and contribute little to the management of childhood acute leukemias.

Myeloperoxidase and Sudan Black B

Myeloperoxidase (MPO) and Sudan black B (SBB), which react with peroxidase and phospholipids, respectively, give parallel staining reactions with myelocytic and monocytic granules [Fig. 4 (see figure in color plate section) Table 1]. The SBB stain is often preferred because it avoids the carcinogenic reagents used in the MPO method. The SBB stain is also considered a more sensitive assay than MPO, but at the price of decreased specificity (223). Well-documented SBB-positive cases of ALL that were negative for MPO have been described (100,238,482,528,557). The MPO stain may therefore be a more specific stain and should be performed in all SBB-positive leukemias for which the morphology is suggestive of ALL or when confirmatory immunologic marker studies are not available. Myeloperoxidase activity declines with time after aspirate smears have been prepared. The SBB reaction, which recognizes sudanophilic lipids, is more stable and may be preferred for cytologic preparations more than 5 days old. Some cases of myeloblastic leukemia will have very little MPO that can only be detected with the electron microscope (157). Not infrequently, marrows harboring lymphoblastic disease also retain residual normal myeloblasts that may be difficult to distinguish from the leukemic blasts. This difficulty is particularly evident with marrows that are partially involved by T-lineage lymphoblastic lymphoma.

A newer approach for the detection of MPO is the use of immunofluorescence or immunohistochemical assays with monoclonal antibodies to the MPO protein (76,372,532). Although the cytochemical test for peroxidase requires the presence of functional enzyme, the antibody test needs only the intact protein. Myeloperoxidase enzymatic activity decays with time, but peroxidase proteins in old cytologic preparations appear to retain sufficient antigenic sites for antimyeloperoxidase antibody binding. The monoclonal antibody test therefore may be more sensitive than the cytochemical assay for MPO. Several small subsets of patients with MPO-negative acute leukemia have tested positive with use of antimyeloperoxidase antibody assays (76,248,249, 250,532,569,570). This may be due to reactions with proenzyme forms or nonfunctional MPO. Not all investigators agree that the anti-MPO method is more sensitive than the classic cytochemical MPO reaction (141).

TABLE 1. *Cytochemical reaction patterns of acute lymphoid and myeloid leukemias*

	ALL		AML (FAB subtype)							
Cytochemical test	B-lineage	T-lineage	M0	M1	M2	M3	M4	M5	M6	M7
MPO (myeloperoxidase)	0	0	0	1–2+	1–3+	3+	2+	0–2+	1+	0
SBB (Sudan black B)	0[a]	0	0	1–2+	1–3+	3+	2+	0–2+	1+	0
CAE (chloroacetate esterase)	0[a]	0	0	0–1+	1–3+	3+	1–2+	0–1+	0–1+	0
ANB (α-naphthyl butyrate esterase)	0[b]	0–1+[c]	0	0	0	0[b]	1–3+[d]	3+[d]	0	0
ANA (α-naphthyl acetate esterase)	0	0–1+[c]	0–1+	0–1+	0–1+	0–1+	2+[d]	3+[d]	0–1+	1–3+[d,e]
ANA-NaF (ANA with NaF inhibition)	0	0–1+[c]	0–1+	0–1+	0–1+	0–1+	0	0	0–1+	1–2+[d,e]

Abbreviations: ALL, acute lymphoblastic leukemia; AML, acute myeloid leukemia; FAB, French–American–British classification; NaF, sodium fluoride; 0 = no staining; 1+ = weak staining; 2+ = moderate staining; 3+ = strong staining.

[a] Rare positive reaction.

[b] Occasional positive reaction.

[c] Punctate cytoplasmic pattern.

[d] Diffuse cytoplasmic pattern.

[e] Granular cytoplasmic pattern.

Thus larger prospective studies of acute leukemia are necessary to more fully assess the value of monoclonal antibody testing in leukemia.

Chloracetate Esterase

The naphthol AS-D chloracetate esterase (CAE) reaction is primarily used to distinguish myeloid from monocytic lineages. This reaction probably detects a group of enzymes that includes elastase and chymotrypsinlike enzyme. The CAE reaction is of limited value in differentiating acute leukemias because many forms of acute nonlymphocytic leukemia, including FAB-M0, -M6, -M7, and most -M1 subtypes, give negative CAE reactions (Table 1). Blasts of monoblastic leukemias (FAB-M5a) may give a diffuse weak and rarely a strong reaction with CAE (223,468). A case of ALL with CAE-positive blasts and unusual immunologic findings has been reported (277). Unlike myeloperoxidase, chloroacetate esterases are very stable and can be detected in old cytologic material. The activity of esterases detected by the CAE reaction is not destroyed by formalin fixatives and paraffin embedding, providing a limited but useful stain for assaying bone marrow biopsy material (309).

Nonspecific Esterases

The nonspecific esterases (NSEs), using α-naphthylbutyrate (ANB), α-naphthylacetate (ANA), or α-naphthyl AS-D acetate as substrates, primarily document monocytic lineage when used in conjunction with sodium fluoride (NaF) inhibition (Fig. 5; see figure in color plate section) (223). The enzymes detected by these assays are found in various proportions in most cell lineages (Table 1). With careful control of pH and substrate conditions, these enzymes can be demonstrated selectively. Enzymatic activity is demonstrable in both myeloid and monocytic cells using ANA at a neutral pH. Using ANB at an acidic pH will result in reactions in monocytes and T lymphocytes but not myeloid lineage cells. The NSE reactivity with monoblasts and monocytes is inhibited by exposure to NaF, whereas blasts of most other lineages are relatively resistant to this treatment. A focal paranuclear staining pattern with ANA, which is variably inhibited by NaF, is frequently detected in normal T cells and lymphoblasts of T lineage (36,223). Other studies have demonstrated focal reaction patterns with ANA and ANB in non-T ALL blasts (124,604). Leukemic megakaryoblasts usually show a diffuse granular reaction with ANA but little or no reactivity to ANB.

Other Cytochemical Reactions

The PAS, alkaline phosphatase (ALP), and oil red O (ORO) reactions played prominent roles in the assessment of leukemias in the past but have largely been replaced by other laboratory studies. The Schiff reagent reacts with carbohydrate-containing molecules to form a bright red reaction product. Glycogen often accumulates in leukemic blasts, probably as a result of disordered cell metabolism. Blasts of most ALLs contain large blocks or globules of PAS-positive material in the cytoplasm. Although this block pattern of reactivity is characteristic of ALL, the same pattern may be seen in nonlymphoid leukemias and nonhematopoietic small cell tumors. The presence and number of PAS-positive blasts in ALL have no independent prognostic significance, but their presence is associated with good prognostic factors including young age, low WBC counts, CD10 (CALLA)–positive blasts, and chromosomal hyperdiploidy (265, 317,320,366).

A positive ALP reaction is largely confined to mature neutrophils and eosinophils. The content of ALP varies among neutrophils, and the collective neutrophil ALP activity is influenced by many disease processes. Enzymatic activity (the leukocyte alkaline phosphatase [LAP] score) is increased in bacterial infections, normal in viral infections, and decreased in sickle cell anemia (275). The markedly decreased LAP score associated with chronic granulocytic leukemia lacks the specificity of cytogenetic detection of the Ph^1 chromosome and the sensitivity of detecting chimeric *BCR/ABL* fusion genes by molecular methods.

Neutral fat-containing vacuoles of leukemias with L3 cytology typically stain positive with ORO, which at one time was a confirmatory test for this type of leukemia (223). However, not all L3 leukemias contain detectable cytoplasmic lipids and some L1 and L2 leukemias may be ORO-positive (92).

Platelet Peroxidase

The demonstration of platelet peroxidase (PPO) in blasts by electron microscopy is one method of confirming a diagnosis of acute megakaryoblastic leukemia (68,69,70,72) (Fig. 6). The method requires fixative concentrations and buffers that differ from those used in routine ultrastructural studies. Lymphoid leukemias give no reaction with PPO, but the morphologist needs to be fully aware of the similarities and small differences in the reaction patterns of myeloid, monocytic, erythroid, and megakaryoblastic leukemias (Table 2). Optimal studies of PPO incorporate immunoelectron microscopy to ensure that only leukemic blasts are being scored (70). Because of cost considerations and a long turnaround testing time, the PPO assay has been replaced by immunologic procedures that use antibodies to platelet and megakaryocyte antigens.

Terminal Deoxynucleotidyltransferase

Terminal deoxynucleotidyltransferase (TDT) is an intranuclear DNA polymerase involved in the addition of

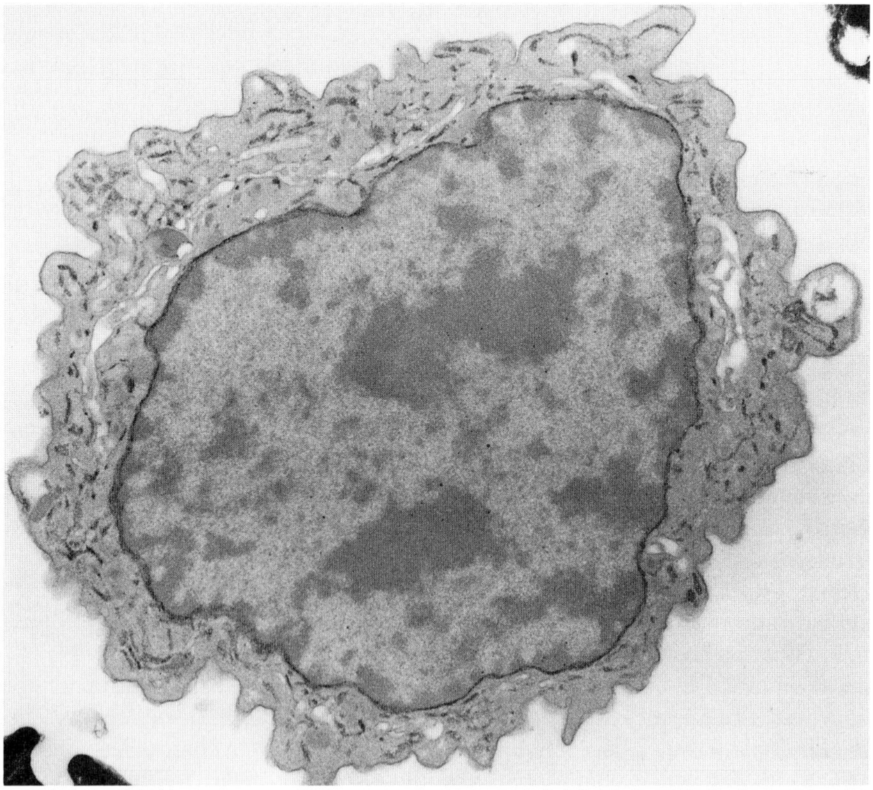

FIG. 6. Acute megakaryocytic leukemia, AML-M7. The platelet peroxidase (PPO) reaction produces fine electron-dense deposits that partially outline the nucleus and line the endoplasmic reticulum. (Electron microscopy with PPO reaction.)

nucleotides to the N regions of immunoglobulin and T-cell receptor genes undergoing rearrangement (137, 196,290). Thus, TDT is normally detected in the nuclei of immature B and T lymphocytes and disappears with lymphocyte maturation (58,353,505). In healthy individuals, cells bearing TDT are found only in the bone marrow and thymus. TDT can be detected with a biochemical assay or with immunofluorescence and immunohistochemical techniques using cell smears, touch preparations, cytospin smears, or frozen tissue sections. All of these tissue preparations rapidly lose TDT if left at room temperature for more than 24 hours. Formalin fixation of bone marrow and other tissues renders the TDT protein unreactive with anti-TDT antibodies, but immunologic reactivity can be restored by microwave or by other antigen retrieval techniques prior to immunohistochemical studies (397).

The blasts of more than 90% of B- and T-lineage lymphoblastic leukemias and lymphomas contain abundant TDT (257,297,378), whereas the cells of almost all non-lymphoblastic lymphomas lack detectable levels (21,65). Sensitive immunohistochemical assays will reveal TDT in up to 45% of acute myeloid leukemias (151,163,523). The blasts of chronic myelogenous leukemias in lymphoid blast crisis express TDT (344). Although TDT assays are not useful for determining the lineage of a malignant process, they are helpful in several diagnostic situations. The presence of TDT-positive cells in spinal, pleural, or peritoneal fluid, testicular biopsies, or other nonthymic extramedullary tissues is indicative of lymphoblastic malignancy. The TDT assays are also helpful in distinguishing lymphoblastic lymphoma from Burkitt's and large cell lymphomas. Dual immunofluorescence techniques with anti-TDT and anti-CD3 can be

TABLE 2. *Ultrastructural patterns with the myeloperoxidase (MPO) and platelet peroxidase (PPO) reactions*

Type of leukemia	MPO	PPO
Acute lymphoblastic leukemia (FAB-L1,-L2)	No reaction	No reaction
Acute myeloid leukemia (FAB-M0)	No reaction, or positive Golgi or membrane-bound granules	No reaction or weak positive nuclear envelope
Acute monoblastic leukemia (FAB-M5)	Positive granules, endoplasmic reticulum, and Golgi	Positive (weak) endoplasmic reticulum or nuclear envelope
Acute erythroblastic leukemia (FAB-M6), blastic variant	No positive granules	Positive endoplasmic reticulum and nuclear envelope
Acute megakaryoblastic leukemia (FAB-M7)	No positive granules	Positive endoplasmic reticulum and nuclear envelope

used to detect minimal residual disease in the bone marrow of patients with T-lineage ALL (81).

Immunologic Marker Studies

Immunophenotyping, or antibody-directed study of cellular antigen expression, began in the 1970s with the development of polyclonal antisera against human hematopoietic cells. The earliest immunophenotyping panels included tests with antisera to T lymphocytes, immunoglobulin heavy and light chains, common acute lymphoblastic leukemia antigen (CALLA), HLA-DR molecules, and TDT. The interesting phenomenon of "rosetting" of lymphocytes by sheep erythrocytes was also used to identify normal and malignant T cells. By the end of the 1970s it became possible to identify the cell lineage of the majority of acute leukemias by using these assays together with cytochemical studies.

With the establishment of monoclonal antibody (MoAb) technology and the commercial distribution of these reagents, immunophenotyping quickly became an important tool in the diagnosis and classification of acute leukemia. The efforts of the International Workshops on Leukocyte Differentiation Antigens has culminated in the assignment of several hundred MoAbs to clusters of differentiation (CDs) (39,284,360,458,486). The MoAbs within each CD group recognize the same antigen, although not necessarily the identical epitope and not always with similar reactivity patterns within the tissue being studied. With the conclusion of the Fifth International Workshop, 130 CD groups had been defined (486). The CD groups and examples of MoAbs within these clusters important in the study of acute leukemias are presented in Table 3.

B-Cell Development and Antigen Expression

The earliest bone marrow cells of B-lineage, pre-B or early pre-B (EPB) cells, express CD10, CD19, CD24, CD34, HLA-DR, and TDT (83,329) (Fig. 7). CD22 is expressed in the cytoplasm but only weakly on the surface of EPB cells. Immunoglobulins are not detectable, although the immunoglobulin μ heavy genes have already undergone rearrangements. CD45, or the common leukocyte antigen, is weakly expressed on EPB cells but increases in intensity with cell maturation (78). Subsequent to the EPB stage, immunoglobulin μ heavy chains appear in the cytoplasm but not on the surface of pre-B (PB) cells. The late PB cell loses TDT and CD10 and expresses surface CD20, CD22, CD37, CD19, and CD24.

During the late stages of PB cell maturation or the transitional pre-B (TPB) stage, lymphocytes express surface μ but not immunoglobulin light chains. The μ heavy chains are thought to be transported to the cell surface in the company of several pseudo-λ or surrogate immunoglobulin light chains (ψ LC) (77,467). These pseudolight chains, also referred to as ω and ι ψ LCs, resemble the variable and constant regions of normal immunoglobulin λ light chains (Fig. 8). The ω and ι ψ LCs are encoded

TABLE 3. *Clusters of differentiation (CD) antigens useful in the immunologic classification of acute leukemias*

	Monoclonal antibodies[a]					
Group	B-D[b]	Coulter[c]	I-T[d]	DAKO[e]	Identity	Normal distribution
CD1a	Leu 6	T6	BL6	NA1/34	48-kD glycoprotein/binds β_2-microglobulin	Thymic T cells, subset of B cells, Langerhan cells
CD2	Leu 5b	T11	GF10.3	MT910	50-kD transmembrane glycoprotein; LFA-3 ligand, LFA-2 receptor, E-rosette receptor	All T cells, most NK cells
CD3	Leu 4	T3	UCHT1	UCHT1	Composed of five chains: γ, δ, ϵ, ζ, and η; binds to α/β and γ/δ	Thymic and mature T cells
CD4	Leu 3a	T4	BL4	MT310	59-kD transmembrane glycoprotein; MHC class II receptor	Some thymic T cells, inducer T cells, monocytes, macrophages
CD5	Leu 1	T1	BL1a	DK23	67-kD glycoprotein	Thymic and mature T cells, subset of B cells
CD7	Leu 9	3A1	8H8	DK24	40-kD protein	All T cells, NK cells
CD8	Leu 2a	T8	B9.2	DK25	32-kD protein composed of chains (α-α or α-β-heterodimers); MHC class I receptor	Subset of thymic T cells, suppressor/cytotoxic T cells, subset of NK cells

TABLE 3. *Continued.*

	Monoclonal antibodies[a]					
Group	B-D[b]	Coulter[c]	I-T[d]	DAKO[e]	Identity	Normal distribution
CD10	CALLA	J5	ALB1	SS2/36	100-kD protein; neutral endopeptidase	Precursor-B and germinal center B cells; some thymic T cells; PMN
CD13	Leu M7	MY7	SJ1D1	WM47	150-kD glycoprotein; aminopeptidase	Myeloid cells
CD14	Leu M3	MY4	RMO52	TÜK4	55-kD phosphoinositol-linked glycoprotein	Mature monocytes; weakly present on some B cells
CD15	Leu M1		80H5	CD3-1	X-hapten; Lewis-X (Le^x); phagocytosis	Monocytic and myelocytic cells
CD19	Leu 12	B4	J4.119	HD37	90 k D glycoprotein; associates with CD21; activation; proliferation	Precursor and mature B cells
CD20	Leu 16	B1	BLy-1	B-Ly1	35-kD phosphoprotein; cellular activation	Late precursor and mature B cells
CD21	CR2	B2	BL13	1F8	140-kD glycoprotein; C3d and EBV receptor	Mature B; some thymic T cells; follicular dendritic cells
CD22	Leu 14	B3	SJ10.1H11	To15	135-kD glycoprotein; adhesion and activation	Precursor and mature B cells
CD33	Leu M9	MY9	P3HL60	WM54	67-kD transmembrane protein	Myeloid and monocytic cells
CD34	HPCA1		QBEND10		105- to 120-kD transmembrane glycoprotein	Early lymphoblasts and myeloblasts
CD36			FA6.152		Platelet gpIV; thrombospondin receptor	Subset of monocytes; megakaryocytes and platelets; erythroblasts
CD41a		Plt-1	P2	5B12	Platelet gp IIb/IIIa; receptor for fibronectin, fibrinogen, and von Willebrand's factor	Megakaryocytes and platelets
CD42b			SZ22		Platelet gp IIb, which forms a complex with gp IX (CD42a); receptor for von Willebrand's factor–ristocetin	Megakaryocytes and platelets
CD45	HLE-1	KC56	J33	T29/33	180- to 220-kD glycoprotein; tyrosine phosphatase	Leukocytes; early erythroblasts
CD56	Leu 19	NKH-1	T199	T199	140-kD isform of N-CAM; cellular adhesion	NK cells; cytotoxic T cells
CD61			SZ21	Y2/51	Integrin β3 chain of vitronectin receptor and gp IIb/IIIa	Megakaryocytes and platelets
CD65			88H7		Cerimide (dodecasaccharide 4c)	Myeloid and monocytic cells
CD72			J3.109		43/39-kD heterodimeric glycoprotein; ligand for CD5	Precursor and mature B cells
CD79α				HM57	Mb-1; associates with CD75β; signal transduction from surface Ig to cytoplasm	Precursor and mature B cells
CD79β[f]					B29; associates with CD79α; signal transduction from surface Ig to cytoplasm	Precursor and mature B cells

Abbreviations: MoAb, monoclonal antibody; EBV, Epstein–Barr virus; NK, natural killer; PMN, polymorphonuclear cells (neutrophils); N-CAM, neural cell adhesion molecule.

[a] Monoclonal antibodies listed by clone or commercial name.

[b] Becton–Dickinson, San Jose, CA.

[c] Coulter, Hialeah, FL.

[d] Immunotech International, Westbrook, ME.

[e] DAKO Corporation, Carpinteria, CA.

[f] Recognized by MoAb SN8 (Ref. 486).

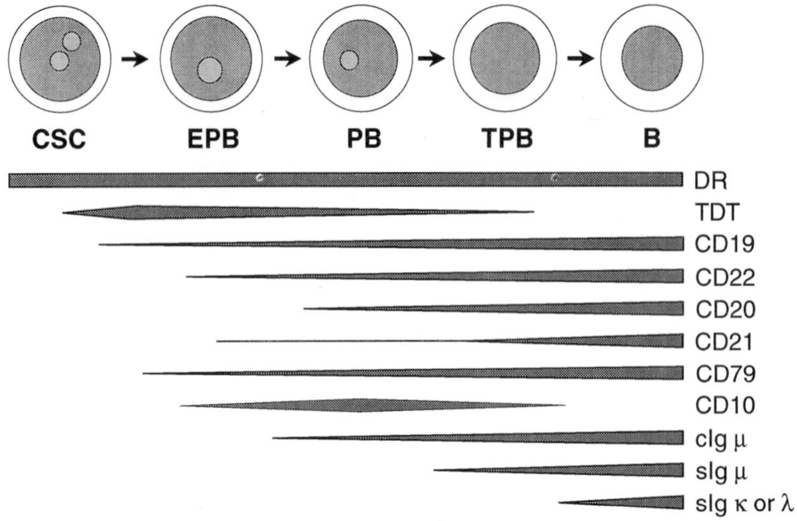

FIG. 7. Schematic of normal B-cell development and expression of B-lymphoid-associated antigens. Stages of B-lymphocyte development: CSC, committed stem cell; EPB, early pre-B cell; PB, pre-B cell; TPB, transitional pre-B; B, mature B cell. Antigens: DR, HLA-DR; TDT, terminal deoxynucleotidyltransferase; cIg μ, cytoplasmic immunoglobulin μ chains; sIg μ, surface immunoglobulin μ chains; sIg κ or λ, surface immunoglobulin κ or λ light chain expression.

by the Vpre-B and 5/14.1 genes and are only produced by B cells (77,467). The genes encoding for these proteins do not undergo rearrangements as do the genes encoding for λ light chains. TPB cells constitute less than 2% of the normal bone marrow cells. The function of the μ heavy chain/ψ LC complexes on the B cell is presently unknown.

With further maturation, the B cell produces either κ or λ light chains that complex with the μ heavy chains, and complete IgM complexes are transported to the surface of the cell (Fig. 8). Concordant with the expression of surface immunoglobulins, CD20 density increases and CD21 may be expressed. Subsequently, B lymphocytes migrate to the peripheral lymphoid organs. Further

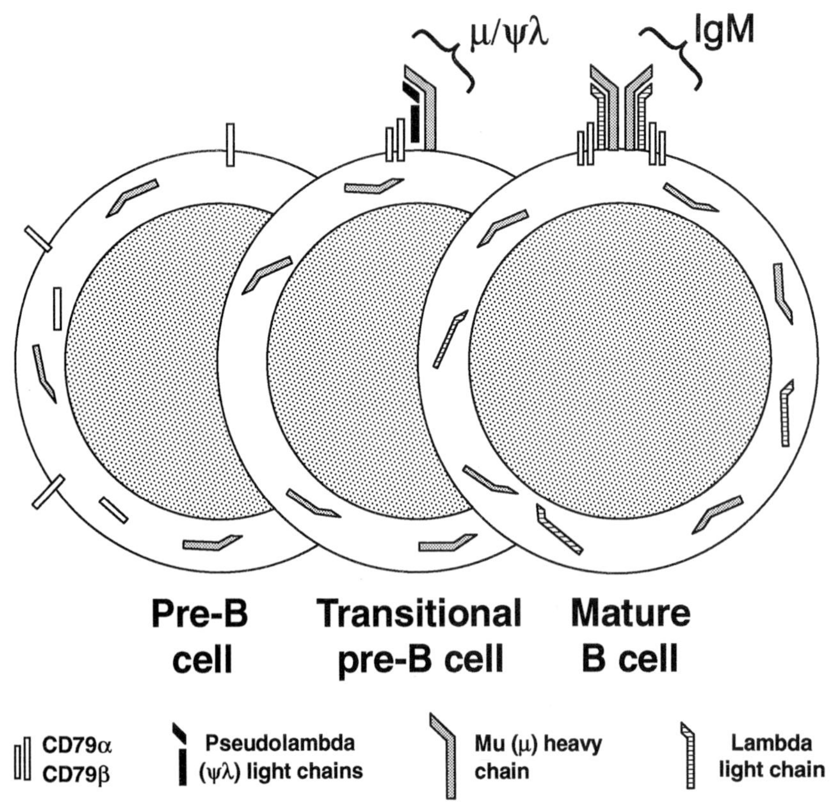

FIG. 8. Immunoglobulin heavy and light chain expression during B-cell maturation. Only μ chain immunoglobulins are produced by the pre-B cell. In the transition from pre-B to mature B cell, cells express cytoplasmic and surface μ chain immunoglobulins. During the transitional pre-B stage, μ chains complex with proteins that are known as pseudolambda light chains because of their resemblance to the constant and variable portions of the λ light chain. The CD79 molecules provide a bridge between the activities of surface immunoglobulins and the cytoplasmic signaling pathway.

immunoglobulin heavy gene rearrangements in the B cell result in the production of IgD in addition to IgM or complete switches to IgG or IgA production. Proliferating mature B cells located in the germinal centers of lymphoid tissues may reexpress CD10 but not TDT. A small number of mature B cells return to the bone marrow from peripheral lymphoid organs.

T-Cell Development and Antigen Expression

T lymphocytes are thought to be derived from multipotential bone marrow cells that express CD34, CD7, and TDT. Subsequent T-lineage commitment and maturation takes place in the thymus gland. The earliest T cell is found in the cortical areas of the thymic lobules. These early cells are identified by their expression of CD34, CD7, CD5, usually CD2, cytoplasmic CD3, and nuclear TDT (Fig. 9) (80,224,323,487). With further maturation, the cortical lymphocytes add CD4, CD8, and CD1 to their surface and move to the medullary portions of the thymic lobule. Molecules of CD3, carried by T-cell receptor (TCR) proteins α plus β or, less commonly, γ plus δ, make their appearance on the cell surface (110,305). The medullary thymocytes that weakly express surface CD3 are referred to as $CD3^{lo}$ cells. Variable numbers of medullary thymic lymphocytes also express CD10 and CD21. Finally, the mature thymic lymphocyte resembles peripheral blood T cells and brightly displays CD3 ($CD3^{hi}$) and either CD4 or CD8. TDT becomes undetectable by immunofluorescent assays in the final stage of T-cell maturation.

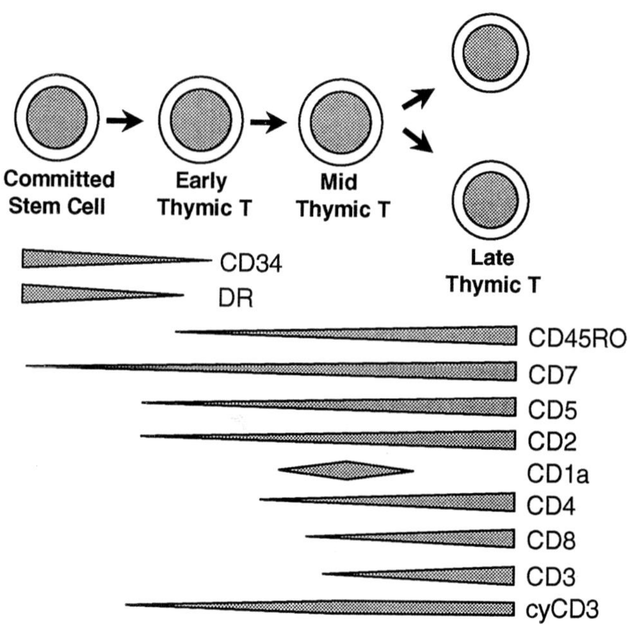

FIG. 9. T-cell development and expression of T-cell-associated antigens. Except for cyCD3 (cytoplasmic CD3), the listed antigens represent cell surface expression.

Myeloid and Monocytic Lineage Development and Antigen Expression

The changes in cell markers during myeloid and monocytic maturation are not as dramatic and are less clearly defined than those accompanying lymphocytic development. Unlike B and T cells, differences in marker expression between myeloid and monocytic lineage cells are largely due to differences in intensity rather than the presence of unique lineage-associated markers. The myeloid- and monocytic-associated antigens most commonly screened for in nonlymphoid leukemias include CD13, CD14, CD15, CD33, CD36, and CDw65 (82,106,168). Myeloblasts express CD13, CD33, CD34, and HLA-DR. With myeloid cell maturation, CD34 is lost, CD13 and CD33 antigen densities decrease, and CD15 and CD11b appear (Fig. 10) (106). Early marrow monocytes or promonocytes express CD33 and HLA-DR and with further development display CD14 (Fig. 11).

Megakaryocyte and Erythroid Lineage and Antigen Expression

Mature megakaryocytes express the platelet antigens CD36, CD41, CD42, and CD61, but little known about the surface antigen composition of early megakaryocytes and megakaryoblasts (400,580). Studies of megakaryocytic malignancies imply that as megakaryocytes mature there is an orderly and progressive appearance of platelet antigens (Fig. 12) (162). Antibodies that detect the glycoprotein IIb/IIIa complex (CD41a) or glycoprotein IIIa (CD61) are assumed to be the earliest markers of megakaryocytic development, whereas anti–factor VIII–related antigens are only detected in the later stages of megakaryocyte maturation.

Very few monoclonal antibodies have been developed for studies of erythroid precursors. Most descriptions of antigen expression by erythroid precursors are derived from studies of cultured erythroid cells and may not accurately reflect in vivo states (26,45,131,291,328). Early proerythroblasts express glycoprotein IV (CD36) and possibly glycoprotein IIa/IIIa (CD41a) but not hemoglobin or glycophorin A (Fig. 13). Further erythroblast development sees the appearance of glycophorin A and the production of hemoglobin (205).

Leukemic Cell DNA Content (DNA Index)

The flow cytometric study of cellular DNA content using compounds that fluoresce when bound to DNA, such as propidium iodide, is a rapid semiquantitative method of assessing leukemic blast chromosome content (ploidy). Approximately 40% of childhood ALLs have aneuploid peaks (235,331,537). In ALL, DNA indices

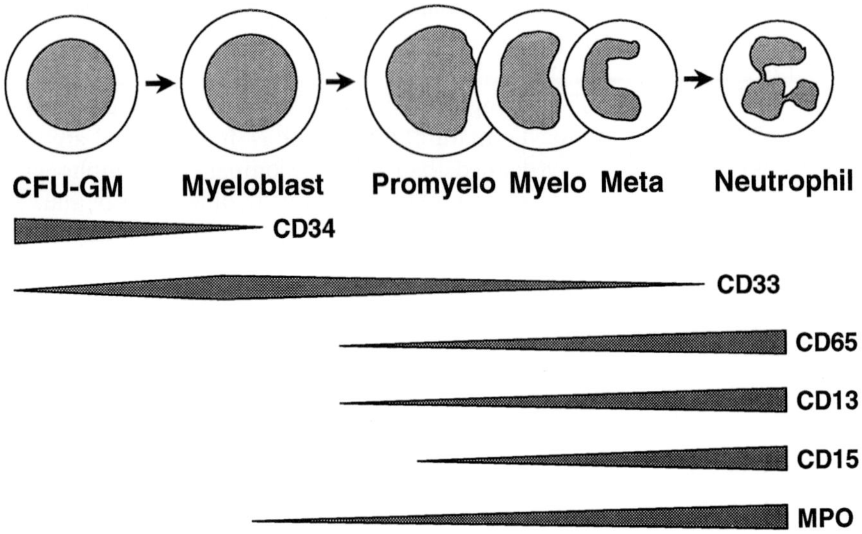

FIG. 10. Myelocytic cell development correlated with myeloid-associated antigen expression. Stages of myelocytic cell maturation: CFU-GM, colony-forming unit–granulocytic/monocytic; promyelo, promyelocyte; myelo, myelocyte; meta, metamyelocyte. MPO, myeloperoxidase enzyme.

(DIs) of ≥1.16 correspond to ≥53 chromosomes and are associated with a good clinical outcome (330). In contrast, only 25% of cases of AML display aneuploidy, and the degree of hyperdiploidy is usually less than 1.15 (10). In contrast to ALL, aneuploidy in AML does not appear to have any prognostic significance (10).

ACUTE LYMPHOBLASTIC LEUKEMIA (ALL)

EAB Classification of ALL

In 1976, the French–American–British (FAB) Cooperative Group proposed criteria for classifying ALL into three subtypes based on blast cytology as seen in Romanowsky's stained bone marrow smears (31). Assignment to one of three groups, L1, L2, or L3, depended on cell size, nuclear-to-cytoplasmic ratio, nuclear contours, presence of nucleoli and vacuoles, and presence of cytoplasmic basophilia (Table 4, Figs. 14–16; see figures in color plate section). Using FAB guidelines, the morphologic and cytochemical diagnosis of ALL is one of exclusion because no cytochemical marker is specific for this type of leukemia (Table 1). As such, MPO-negative acute nonlymphocytic leukemias, excluding the ANB-positive monocytic leukemias, would be included with ALL if no additional laboratory studies were performed.

The goal of the FAB classification of ALL was to identify its clinically relevant morphologic subtypes. Indeed, L3 cytology is associated with the B-cell type of ALL and the presence of chromosome translocation t(8;14), which in turn dictates a specific therapeutic approach. Although ALL-L1 is more common in childhood and ALL-L2 more common in adults (31,575), no unique

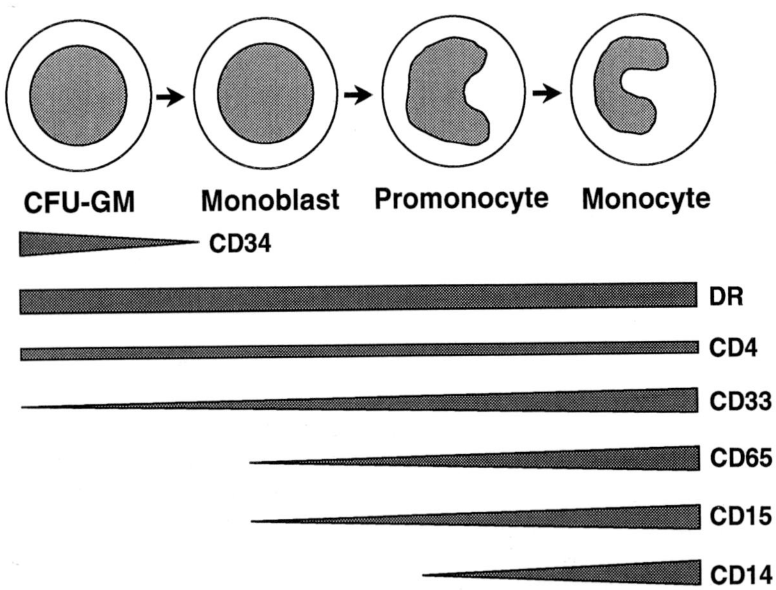

FIG. 11. Monocytic cell development correlated with myeloid/monocytic-associated antigen expression. CFU-GM, colony-forming unit–granulocytic/monocytic.

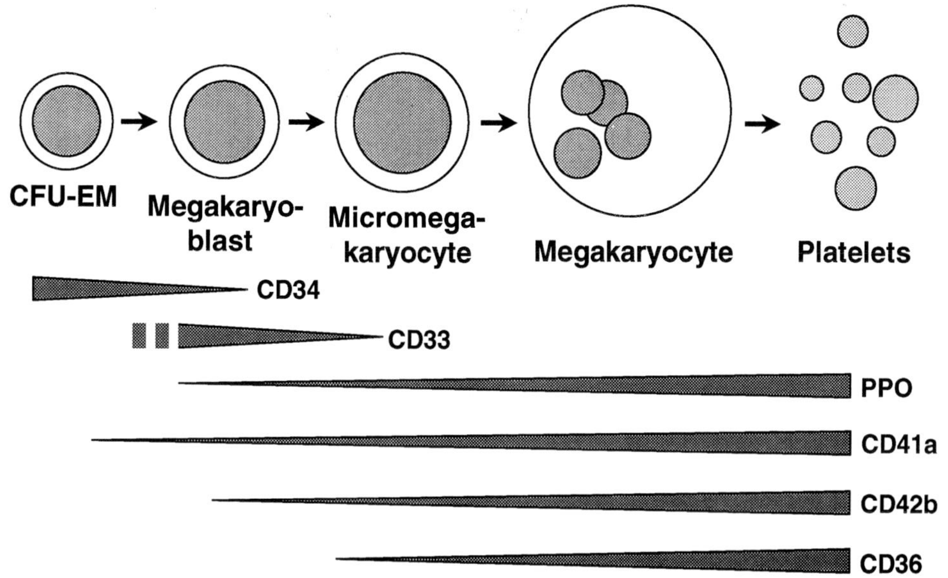

FIG. 12. Megakaryocytic development correlated with megakaryocyte-platelet antigen expression. CFU-EM, colony-forming unit–megakaryocytic/erythroid; PPO, platelet peroxidase.

immunophenotypic patterns or cytogenetic abnormalities are directly associated with these two morphologic variants (358,379). After adjusting for age, WBC count, and chromosomal abnormalities, the FAB classification of ALL contributes no additional prognostic information (265,574). Thus, the FAB classification has very little to offer the physician in confirming the diagnosis of ALL or identifying children at risk of poor treatment response.

Immunologic Classification of ALL

The development of antibodies reactive with lineage and differentiation-association cell antigens has provided reagents for the classification of leukemias. By the early 1980s, ALL could be classified as B-ALL, T-ALL, common ALL, and null ALL based on the reactivity of leukemic blasts with several immunologic reagents (204,258) (Table 5). Further subgrouping of ALL has become possible with the development of newer monoclonal antibodies (Table 6). In contrast to the FAB morphologic classification, the immunologic classification has been shown to be useful in predicting clinical outcome and is used along with other clinical features for treatment decisions (418).

Studies indicate that the expression of most known cell surface "differentiation" antigens lacks lineage specificity. This is even true for cytoplasmic expressions of CD3 and CD22, which were at one time thought to be lineage-specific. Therefore, current immunologic classifications of ALL are based on the patterns of reactivity of leukemic blasts with panels of monoclonal antibodies to lineage-associated antigens. With this immunophenotyping approach, childhood ALLs are classified as T-lineage (CD7+ plus surface or cytoplasmic CD3+) or

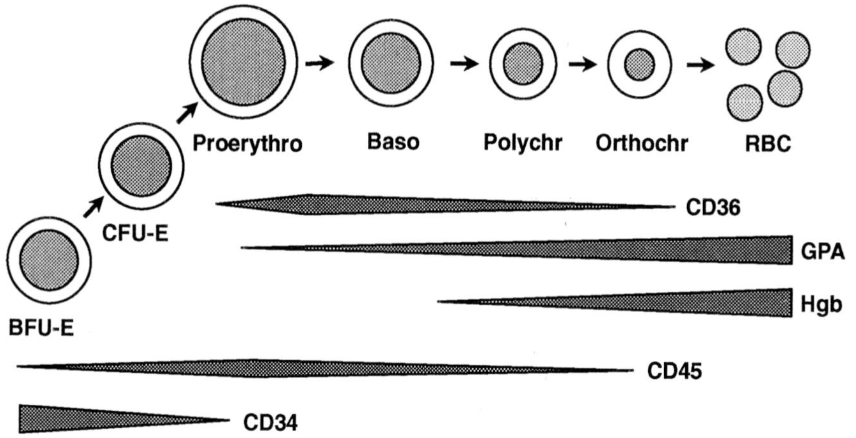

FIG. 13. Schematic of erythrocytic development correlated with erythroid antigen expression. BFU-E, burst-forming unit–erythroid; CFU-E, colony-forming unit–erythroid; proerythro, proerythroblast; baso, basophilic normoblast; polychr, polychromatic normoblast; orthochr, orthochromatic normoblast; RBC, red blood cells; GPA, glycophorin A; Hgb, hemoglobin.

TABLE 4. *French–American–British (FAB) Cooperative Group classification of acute lymphoblastic leukemia (ALL)*

Blast feature	L1	L2	L3
Cell size	Small (<15 μm)	Large (>15 μm)	Large (>15 μm)
Cytoplasm	Scant; ±vacuoles	Moderate to abundant; pale to moderately basophilic; ±vacuoles	Moderate to abundant; deeply basophilic; vacuoles often prominent
Nucleus	Regular contour; dense, homogeneous chromatin	Regular to irregular clefting; fine to coarse chromatin	Round to oval; homogeneously coarse chromatin
Nucleolus	None or vague	One or more; distinct; prominent	One or more; ill defined to prominent
FAB score[a]	0 to 2+	−1 to −4	Scoring not applicable
Frequency	~85%	~15%	~1%

Feature	Score
1. Blast size	
Small	0
Large (≥50% of cells)	−1
2. Nucleocytoplasmic ratio	
High (≥75% of cells)	+1
Low (≥25% of cells)	−1
3. Nucleoli	
0–1 small (≥75% of cells)	+1
>1 distinct (≥25% of cells)	−1
4. Nuclear contour	
Regular	0
Irregular (≥25% of cells)	−1

[a] The sum of scores for each blast feature as listed above (see ref. 31).

TABLE 5. *Early immunologic classification of acute lymphoblastic leukemia (ALL)*

Immunologic type:	sIg	E-rosette	CALLA	Frequency	Includes modern subgroups:
B-ALL	+	−	−	<3%	B-ALL
T-ALL	−	+	−	~12%	T-ALL
Common ALL	−	−	+	~75%	Early pre-B-ALL Pre-B ALL E-rosette-negative T-ALL
Non-B, non-T ALL	−	−	−	~10%	Early pre-B ALL Pre-B-ALL E-rosette-negative T-ALL MPO-negative AML Megakaryoblastic leukemia

Abbreviations: sIg, surface immunoglobulin; E-rosette, sheep red blood cell rosettes; CALLA, common ALL antigen (CD10); MPO, myeloperoxidase; AML, acute myeloid leukemia.

TABLE 6. *Immunologic classification of acute lymphoblastic leukemia*

Subgroup:	TDT	DR	CD34	CD10	CD19	CD22[a]	CD79[a]	CD7	CD5	CD3[a]	cIg μ	sIg μ	sIg κ or λ	Frequency (%)
EPB	++	+++	+	++	+++	+++	+++	(+)	−	−	−	−	−	60–65
PB	++	+++	+	++	+++	+++	+++	−	−	−	+++	−	−	20–25
TPB	+	+++	+	++	+++	+++	+++	−	−	−	+++	+++	−	1
B	−	+++	−	+	+++	+++	+++	−	−	−	+++	+++	+++	2
T	++	(+)	+	+	−	−	−	+++	+++	+	−	−	−	15–18

Abbreviations: EPB, early pre B; PB, pre-B; TPB, transitional pre-B; B, mature B (FAB-L3); T, T cell lineage; cIg μ, cytoplasmic immunoglobulin heavy chain μ; sIg μ, surface immunoglobulin heavy chain μ; sIg λ or κ, surface immunoglobulin λ or κ light chains; −, no expression of marker; (+), <5% of cases express marker; +, 40–60% of cases express marker; ++, >90% of cases express marker; +++, 100% of cases express marker.

[a] Cytoplasmic or surface expression of CD22, CD79, or CD3.

B-lineage (CD19+ plus CD22+ or CD79+) (Table 6). B-lineage ALL accounts for 80–85% of newly diagnosed childhood ALL. These leukemias are further subclassified as early pre-B, pre-B,, transitional pre-B-, and B-ALL based on their pattern of cytoplasmic and surface immunoglobulin expression (Table 6). T-lineage ALLs compose 15–20% of childhood ALL and are less readily subclassified than B-lineage leukemias.

The distribution of immunophenotypic subgroups of ALL is influenced by age, socioeconomic, and possibly hereditary factors. In infants there is a preponderance of CD10-negative early pre-B-ALL and a paucity of T-ALL. T-ALL is more common in the adolescent years and accounts for about 25% of cases. Black African children have a lower incidence of ALL, a higher proportion of T-ALL, and significantly fewer cases of CD10-positive B-lineage ALL. It appears that the incidence of CD10-expressing B-lineage ALL increases with improved socioecomonic situation and hygiene.

Early Pre-B ALL

Early pre-B ALL (EPB-ALL) resembles the normal marrow B-cell precursor that lacks immunoglobulin. Leukemic blasts of almost all EPB-ALLs express surface CD19, CD72, CD79, and HLA-DR. More than 85% of cases weakly display surface CD22, and almost all have cytoplasmic CD22. Although μ heavy chain genes are rearranged in most of these leukemias, immunoglobulins are not detectable. More than 90% of EPB ALLs have TDT and CD10, and about 83% of cases express CD34 (418). The CD20 antigen that normally appears with the production of μ heavy chains is present on a portion of blasts in 55% of cases. CD45 is weakly expressed and may be undetectable in up to 13% of these leukemias (24).

Pre-B-ALL

About 25% of newly diagnosed ALLs have a pre-B (PB) phenotype. Like the EPB ALL, CD19, CD22, CD72, CD79, and HLA-DR are expressed by almost all cases. By definition every PB-ALL will have cytoplasmic μ heavy chains without surface immunoglobulins (418,579). Although rearrangements of light chain genes is evident in many of these leukemias, κ and λ proteins are not detectable. More than 95% of these leukemias express CD10 and TDT, and 61% express CD34 (418,429,436). In contrast to normal marrow pre-B cells, only 40% of PB-ALLs have surface CD20.

Compared with EPB ALL, PB leukemias are more likely to have higher WBC counts, serum lactic acid levels, and Hgb levels. A DNA index less than 1.16, ploidy less than 50, and chromosomal translocations are more common in PB-ALL. About 25% of PB-ALLs have either the balanced form of t(1;19)(q23;p13) or its unbalanced form, der(19)t(1;19)(q23;p13). Initial clinical studies suggested that children with PB-ALL had poorer clinical outcomes than those with EPB ALL (117). However, subsequent clinical trials ascribed the poorer outcome to the presence of t(1;19), because patients with PB-ALL and no t(1;19) had outcomes similar to EPB ALL (120,449). With intensified chemotherapy, patients with the t(1;19) appear to have the same outcome as those without this rearrangement.

Transitional Pre-B-ALL (Late Pre-B-ALL)

Leukemic blasts that express cytoplasm plus surface μ heavy chains without κ or λ light chains have been called transitional pre-B-ALL (TPB ALL) on the assumption that these leukemias represent a transition between pre-B and B stages of differentiation (287,485,579). The μ heavy chains are thought to be transported to the surface of the immature B cell by pseudolambda light chains (77,467,485). Unlike B-ALL, the blasts of TPB ALL have L1 or L2 morphology and lack t(8;14), t(8;22), or t(2;8) translocations (287). Similar to PB-ALL, blasts of these cases usually present with CD10, TDT, and not infrequently CD34. The initial report of TPB ALL found this phenotype in only 1% of childhood ALLs. However, this study was performed by immunofluorescence microscopy, which lacks sensitivity for small amounts of cell surface immunoglobulin. Since the μ/pseudolambda complexes on the leukemic cell surface are relatively few, studies of B-lineage ALL using more sensitive flow cytometry methods may find that this immunophenotype is more common than thus far reported.

Patients with TPB-ALL compose less than 1% of childhood acute leukemias (287). These children do not usually present with bulky extramedullary masses or central nervous system leukemia. The leukocyte count and serum lactate dehydrogenase levels are usually low. Unlike PB-ALL with its associated t(1;19), no unique chromosomal abnormality is found in TPB ALL. Patients with TPB ALL have an excellent response to chemotherapy.

B-ALL

The blasts of approximately 3% of childhood ALLs express surface μ heavy chains together with κ or λ light chains. Childhood B-ALL consists of two clinically and phenotypically distinct leukemias (Table 7). The more common leukemic B-cell process is characterized by FAB-L3 morphology; extramedullary disease (abdominal and head/neck masses); chromosomal translocations t(8;14), t(8;22), or t(2;8); and blasts lacking PAS-reactive granules, TDT, and CD34. Most childhood L3 leukemias are the leukemic phase of Burkitt's lymphoma (130).

A lesser encountered type of B-ALL leukemia lacks extramedullary masses at presentation, translocations

somes 4, 6, 10, 14, 17, 18, 20, 21, and X. Up to 60% of these cases will have structural chromosomal abnormalities and 20% will have chromosomal translocations. Patients with hyperdiploid ALL have more favorable presenting features and higher cure rates than the other numeric groups (330,332,432,499,561). These favorable features include early pre-B immunophenotype, low leukocyte counts, low serum lactic dehydrogenase levels, white race, and age between 2 and 10 years. Leukemic cell hyperdiploidy is particularly uncommon in infants and patients with T-ALL. An association of hyperdiploidy with weak or absent expression of CD45 is seen in EPB and PB-ALL (24). Blast cells of patients with hyperdiploidy demonstrate increased accumulations of methotrexate and its active polyglutamate metabolites (590), higher drug sensitivities (543), and marked propensity for apoptosis (84). Hyperdiploid leukemias with additional chromosomes 4 and 10 appear to respond more favorably to treatment (217). Patients with hyperdiploid ALL and concurrent structural abnormalities of chromosomes, such as isochromosome 17q, tend to fare more poorly than those with only numeric abnormalities (425,432).

About 10–15% of cases of childhood ALL have hyperdiploidy 47–50 (549). The most commonly added chromosomes are 8, 10, and 21. A complement of 47–50 chromosomes confers a prognosis intermediate between pseudodiploid and hyperdiploid (449,454).

The pseudodiploid group comprises 40% of ALLs and includes patients whose leukemic blasts contain a net 46 chromosomes but with structural changes. This group contains the majority of leukemias having translocations t(9;22) and t(4;11) that are associated with poor clinical outcomes. As a group these patients have an unfavorable treatment response; however, when patients with t(9;22) and t(4;11) are excluded and intense multidrug therapy is instituted, the clinical outcome approaches that of the hyperdiploid group (465).

The diploid group includes cases of ALL that lack apparent cytogenetic abnormalities. The incidence of this chromosomal numeric group varies from 10% to 15% of ALLs and depends on the patient population studied, the sophistication of the cytogenetic laboratory performing the study, and the quality of the leukemic sample analyzed. Up to 30% of T-ALLs will have a normal 46-chromosome karyotype (448).

Hypodiploidy, or less than 46 chromosomes, is found in up to 8% of pediatric ALLs (231,424,440,549). Approximately 80% of these ALLs have a modal chromosome number of 45 resulting from loss of a whole chromosome, unbalanced translocations, or formation of dicentric chromosomes (440,447). Chromosome 20 is most frequently lost. Although this ploidy group is associated with low leukocyte counts and a median age of 5 years, these patients have a poorer treatment outcome than children with hyperdiploid leukemias (440). Less than 1% of pediatric ALLs have leukemic blasts that are near-haploid or contain fewer than 30 chromosomes (79,194,440). The main clone contains at least one copy of each chromosome and frequently a second chromosome 21. Although most of these patients obtain a complete remission, the median survival is only 10 months (194,440).

Triploid leukemias with 66–73 chromosomes are identified in fewer than 1% of childhood ALLs (423). Near-tetraploidy, 82–94 chromosomes, is found in fewer than 1% of pediatric ALLs (1,229,423). Almost any chromosome can be duplicated in the trisomy cases, but blasts with tetraploidy usually display extra chromosomes X, 8, 10, 11, 18, and 21. Leukemic blasts with more than 66 chromosomes frequently have large, and grooved or tightly folded nuclei, which may represent an attempt by the blasts to accommodate the extrachromosomal material. The outcome of patients with trisomy ALL does not appear to differ from that of ALL patients in general. Near-tetraploid ALL is associated with a slightly older patient age, FAB-L2 morphology, T-cell immunophenotype, a high frequency of atypical myeloid-associated antigen expression, and a poorer clinical outcome as compared with other ploidy groups (423).

The t(1;19)(q23;p13)

The t(1;19)(q23;p13) and its derivative form, der(19)t(1;19)(q23;p13), are the most common chromosomal translocations in childhood ALL, occurring in 5% of B-lineage ALL and 20–25% of PB-ALL (59,90, 120,433,449). The t(1;19)(q23;p13) is rarely found in EPB ALL (59,416,559). Rare examples of t(1;19) are also described in cases of acute myelomonocytic leukemia, T-ALL, chronic myelogenous leukemia, null cell leukemia, follicular lymphoma, and Burkitt's lymphoma (371,380,544,567,597).

The t(1;19) breakpoints in PB-ALL involve the *E2A* gene on chromosome 19 and the *PBX1* gene on chromosome 1 (267,390). The *E2A* gene encodes the ubiquitously expressed κ E2 immunoglobulin enhancer–binding proteins E12 and E47. Both of these proteins contain an N-terminal transactivation domain and C-terminal helix-loop-helix DNA binding and dimerization motifs. The *PBX1* gene is not normally expressed in hematopoietic and lymphoid cells. However, the t(1;19) results in the formation of a *E2A/PBX1* chimeric gene on the der(19) chromosome which in turn encodes a fusion product that contains the transactivation domain of E2A fused to the DNA binding homeobox domain of *PBX1*. It is postulated that leukemic blast transformation may result from the activity of the *E2A/PBX1* transcription factor on genes normally regulated by the PBX1 protein (132,266,572). Most cases of EPB ALL and other nonlymphoblastic malignancies with t(1;19)(q23;p13) have failed to show rearrangements of the *E2A* gene (416,597).

The presence of the t(1;19) correlates with several adverse prognostic factors: high leukocyte counts, elevated serum lactic dehydrogenase levels, nonwhite race, and DNA indices less than 1.16 (449). Early studies demonstrated an association with poor outcome (117); however, patients with this translocation who are treated with intensified chemotherapy fare similarly to other patients with PB-ALL (120,449). Patients with the der(19)t(1;19) may have a less favorable prognosis than those with the balanced translocation (498). EPB ALLs with t(1;19) frequently display chromosomal hyperdiploidy with >50 chromosomes and have a favorable prognosis (59,416,433).

Immunophenotyping studies recognize a cohort of patients likely to have the t(1;19) translocation (59,433). The antigen profile of CD19+, CD22+, CD20±, and CD34– identifies B-lineage ALLs likely to have the t(1;19), but it lacks specificity. Suspected cases of t(1;19) can now be confirmed by a rapid and specific reverse transcriptase–polymerase chain reaction (RT-PCR) assay that detects the E2A/PBX1 fusion transcript.

The *E2A* gene is also involved in the t(17;19)(q22;p13) translocation that is described in a few cases of EPB and PB-ALL (139,301,393,452). In the t(17;19), the transactivation domain of E2A is fused to the DNA binding and dimerization domains of the liver-specific transcription factor *HLF* (hepatic leukemic factor) (244,251). t(17;19)-positive B-lineage ALL is associated with early adolescence, hypercalcemia, disseminated intravascular coagulation, lytic bone lesions, and poor clinical response to conventional ALL therapy (139,393,452).

The t(9;22)(q34;q11)

The Philadelphia chromosome (Ph[1]) resulting from the t(9;22)(q34;q11) is identified in more than 95% of cases of chronic myelogenous leukemia (CML) and in up to 25% of adult and 3–5% of childhood cases of ALL (274,461,500,549). In the t(9;22), the c-*ABL* proto-oncogene from the distal q arm of chromosome 9 is translocated into the *BCR* gene on the q arm of chromosome 22, resulting in the formation of a *BCR/ABL* chimeric gene (Fig. 17). At the cytogenetic level, the t(9;22) of CML and ALL appear identical; however, two different fusion genes can be formed depending on the breakpoint location in *BCR* (Fig. 18). Breaks in the major breakpoint cluster region (M-BCR) are found in the majority of CML and one half of adult ALL cases. Chimeric transcripts of this translocation encode for a 210-kd hybrid protein. The majority of pediatric ALLs and one half of adult ALLs with t(9;22) produce a 190-kd BCR/ABL protein. This chimeric protein is the result of a break in a region 50 kb upstream of M-BCR that is termed m-BCR (107). The 190- and 210-kd chimeric proteins have enhanced tyrosine-specific protein kinase activity as compared with the wild type of c-abl protein (278,292,541). Both chimeric proteins are thought to play an important role in cell transformation and proliferation (123,232,278,336).

The clinical and laboratory features of children with Ph[1] ALL include older age, higher leukocyte counts, higher frequencies of FAB-L2 morphology, and DNA indices less than 1.16 (118,179,461,549). The lineage distribution is similar to cases without Ph[1]: early pre-B ALL, 75%; pre-B ALL, 16%; and T-ALL, 9% (118). Ph[1]

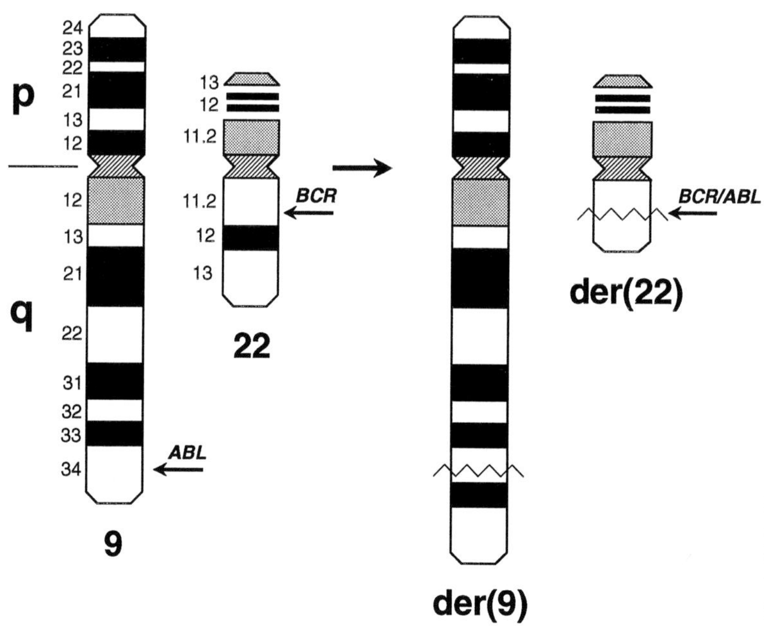

FIG. 17. Schematic representation of the t(9;22)(q34;q11). The *ABL* gene on chromosome 9 is translocated into the *BCR* gene on chromosome 22, resulting in the formation of a *BCR/ABL* chimeric gene on the derivative (der) chromosome 22.

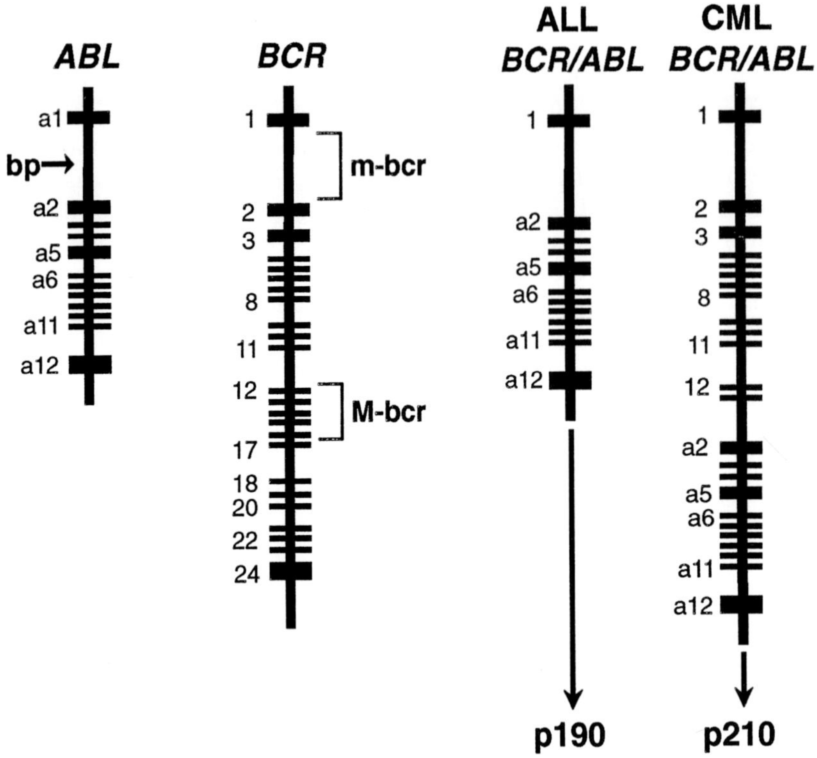

FIG. 18. The *ABL*, *BCR*, and chimeric *BCR/ABL* genes. The breakpoint (bp) in *ABL* is indicated by an arrow. The breakpoint regions in BCR are indicated by m-bcr (minor breakpoint region) and M-bcr (major breakpoint region). Possible recombinations of *BCR* and *ABL* in acute lymphoblastic leukemia (ALL *BCR/ABL*) and chronic myelocytic leukemia (CML *BCR/ABL*) are shown. The fusion protein products of the chimeric genes are represented by p190 and p210.

ALLs are usually pseudodiploid (58%) or hypodiploid (26%) (118). The t(9;22) is the sole chromosomal abnormality in one half of cases. A significantly lower proportion of patients with Ph[1] ALL enter a complete remission, and two thirds of Ph[1] ALL patients attaining a remission will relapse (118).

Fluorescence in situ hybridization (FISH) and RT-PCR assays for detection of t(9;22) have been established (240,276). Unlike conventional cytogenetics, these assays are independent of the ability to obtain mitotic cells and require small numbers of cells. Thus, FISH and PCR methods are more sensitive assays for the Ph[1] defect and are valuable for monitoring patient response to therapy.

The t(4;11) and Other Translocations Involving 11q23

Chromosome 11q23 abnormalities are identified in 4–7% of pediatric ALLs (427,428,435,451) and 13% of childhood AMLs (435). Chromosome band 11q23 is involved in translocations with several different partner chromosomes including 1p32, 4q21, 9p22, 19p13, and Xq13 in ALL and 1q21, 2q21, 6q27, 9p22, 10p11, 17q25, and 19p13 in AML (113,271,385,401,435,451).

The t(4;11)(q21;q23) is identified in 2% of pediatric ALLs (427). Infants account for only 2–3% of pediatric ALLs (117) but compose 60% of cases with t(4;11) (427). ALLs with t(4;11) have higher median leukocyte counts than most other karyotypic subgroups. More than 98% of cases with t(4;11) are either EPB ALL or PB-ALL. This translocation is rarely found in T-ALL or in B-ALL (170,326).

The blasts of B-lineage ALL with t(4;11) usually present with a characteristic antigen profile of $CD19^-$, $CD24^{\pm}$, $CD10^-$, and $CD15^+$ (427). The CD24 expression is usually weak or absent on blasts carrying the t(4;11) but is strongly expressed on cells of other B-lineage ALLs. Blasts of two thirds of cases atypically express the myeloid-associated antigens CD15 and CDw65 (417,427). The pan-T-cell antigen CD7 and the myeloid-associated antigens CD13 and CD33 may also be detected in some cases. A chondroitin sulfate proteoglycan molecule that is not produced by normal bone marrow hematopoietic cells is uniquely expressed by leukemic blasts with reciprocal translocations of 11q23 (25,508). When incubated with 12-*O*-tetradecanoylphorbol-13-acetate, lymphoblasts with the t(4;11) can switch to a monocytic phenotype (311,534,535). These myeloid/monocytic features may indicate the origin of t(4;11) leukemias from a primitive hematopoietic progenitor with multilineage differentiation potential. Alternatively, transcriptional factors produced by the t(4;11) may directly or indirectly induce the expression of myeloid and monocytic features. The t(4;11) is associated with an extremely poor prognosis. Only 10% of children under 1 year or more than 10 years of age are expected to survive long term (419,427,428). Children between 1 and 9 years of age may have a better outcome than infants or older adolescents.

The t(11;19)(q23;p13) is found in <1% of childhood ALLs and 1% of pediatric AMLs. In patients with ALL, this translocation is associated with age <1 year, hyperleukocytosis, myeloid-associated antigen expression, and chromosomal pseudodiploidy (243). The ALLs with t(11;19) may be of B or T lineage (243). Similar to B-lineage ALLs with the t(4;11), leukemic blasts usually do not express CD10. Infants less than 1 year old invariably fail induction therapy or relapse, whereas older children appear to fare better (243).

The *MLL* (mixed lineage leukemia) gene, also named *HRX, ALL1,* and *HTRX1,* is located in the chromosome 11q23 band and is disrupted in most reciprocal translocations involving this chromosomal region (144,145, 210,245,553,605). This gene encodes a 431-kd protein that contains two DNA binding regions, a cysteine-rich zinc finger region and an AT hook motif, which bind to DNA in the major and minor grooves, respectively. The zinc finger domains and C-terminal region share homology to the *Drosophila trithorax* gene (337). It is assumed that the *MLL* gene normally functions as a transcription factor and that this function is disrupted by translocations.

Several of the partner genes involved in 11q23 translocations have been cloned. The t(4;11) fuses *MLL* to the *AF4* or *FEL* gene on chromosome 4q21 (Fig. 19) (210,374). *AF4* encodes a 140-kd serine/proline-rich protein containing GTP-binding and nuclear localization sequences, suggesting a role in transcriptional regulation (145,374,385). *AF4* is widely expressed in normal tissues. The t(4;11) results in a chimeric gene on both the der(4) and der(11) chromosomes (Fig. 19). The der(11) chromosome encodes a fusion protein containing the N-terminal portion of *MLL* with its AT hook and methyltransferase domains fused to the C-terminal portion of *AF4* (210,553). The function of the fusion protein and its role in leukemogenesis is unknown. The *ENL, AF9,* and *AFX* genes involved in t(11;19)(q23;p13.3), t(9;11)(p22;q23), and t(X;11)(q13;q23), respectively, also encode for serine/proline-rich proteins and result in chimeric genes resembling the *MLL/AF4* fusion gene (113,385,553). Most if not all 11q23 translocations involving the *MLL* gene can be detected by Southern blotting with a single cDNA probe to sequences from exons 5 to 11 region of MLL (550). More rapid and sensitive detection of the t(4;11) and the t(11;19) is available with RT-PCR (148,553).

The t(8;14), t(2;8), and t(8;22)

Leukemic cells of B-ALL with L3 morphology contain translocations involving the c-*MYC* gene on chromosome 8, e.g., t(8;14)(q24;q32), t(8;22)(q24;q11), and t(2;8)(p12;q24). More than 90% of cases have the t(8;14), in which c-*MYC* is translocated onto the μ immunoglobulin chain gene on chromosome 14q32 (Fig. 20) (4,134). In the t(2;8) and the t(8;22), the κ or λ immunoglobulin light chain genes of chromosome 2 and 22, respectively, are joined 3′ of c-*MYC* on chromosome 8. As a result of these translocations, transcriptional regulatory sequences of the immunoglobulin genes are positioned next to c-*MYC* (Fig. 20), leading to its dysregulated transcription. The MYC protein belongs to the basic helix-loop-helix family of transcription factors and binds to DNA in a heterodimeric complex with a protein called MAX. Increased production of c-MYC protein leads to the formation of activated MYC/MAX protein complexes, which in turn are thought to result in changes in the expression of yet another unidentified target gene. The dysregulation of c-*MYC*, induced by introducing a t(8;14) into transgenic mice, leads to the formation of monoclonal B-cell malignancies (5).

Translocations of T-Cell Receptor Loci on 14q11, 7q34-36, and 7p15

Similar to B-lineage ALL, in which immunoglobulin genes are involved in translocations, cases of T-cell ALL frequently carry abnormalities of chromosomes 14q11, 7q34-36, and, rarely, 7p15 that are the location of genes encoding for T-cell receptor proteins α and δ, β, and γ, respectively. These loci are involved in about 35% of chromosomal abnormalities of T-ALL (447). Unlike B-lineage ALL, no unique relationships between particular translocations and the level of T-leukemic blast maturation have been identified (448).

The t(11;14)(p13;q11) is the most common abnormality in T-ALL, occurring in 7% of patients (302,448,463). The breakpoint on 14q11 is within the α/δ T-cell receptor locus (55,165,478). The breakpoint on 11p13 involves *RBTN2* (rhombotin), or *Ttg2* (T-cell translocation gene 2) (582). *RBTN2* encodes for a cysteine-rich protein with an LIM motif that is expressed in T-ALL but not in normal T cells (475). Although essential for normal mouse erythropoietic differentiation, *RBTN2* induces T-cell tumors in transgenic mice (582). The t(11;14)(p15;q11) also disrupts the TCR α/δ locus on 14q11 (56,582), but the break on chromosome 11p15 occurs in a gene called *RBTN1,* or *Ttg1.* The *RBTN1* also encodes for an LIM protein (57,357).

The t(10;14)(q24;q11) occurs in 5–10% of T-cell leukemias. The breakpoints include the TCRδ locus on 14q11 and the *HOX11* on 10q24 (156,262,611). The translocation results in the dysregulated expression of *HOX11* (155,219,334). *HOX11* is normally expressed during embryogenesis but not in normal T cells; how it contributes to T-ALL leukemogenesis is not known at present.

The t(1;14)(p32;q11) is detected in 3% of patients with T-ALL (89,174). The *TAL1* gene (also known as *TCL5* or *SCL*) is located on 1p32, and its product is markedly overexpressed with this translocation (74,260). In up to 25% of cases of childhood T-ALL, a cryptic cytogenetic interstitial mutation is present on the 5′ side of the *TAL1*

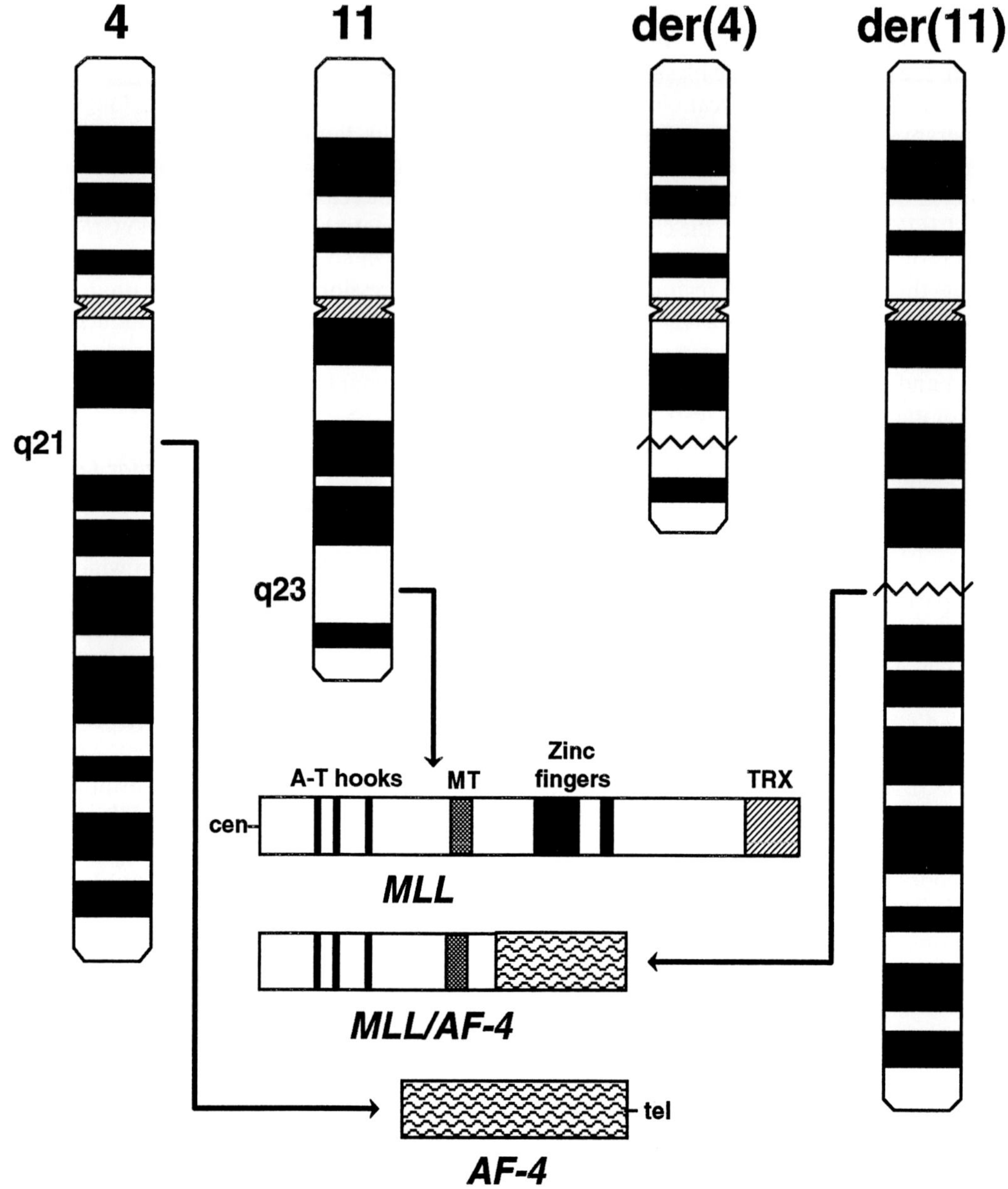

FIG. 19. The t(4;11)(q21;q23). The *AF-4* gene on chromosome 4 is fused with the *MLL* (*HRX, HTRX1, AML1*) gene on chromosome 11, resulting in the derivative (der) 11 chromosome. The centromeric (cen) and telomeric (tel) ends of the *MLL* and *AF-4* genes are respectively indicated. The *MLL* gene contains the a cysteine-rich zinc finger, an AT hook (AT), methyl-transferase (MT), and *Drosophila trithorax* homology (TRX) regions.

gene (11,41). The *TAL1* gene is a member of the helix-loop-helix family of transcriptional factors involved in the control of cell growth and differentiation (101). The chromosomal translocation and 5′ *TAL* deletions are thought to cause abnormal TAL1 production with subsequent activation of target genes that are normally quiescent in T cells.

The t(8;14)(q24;q11) is found in 1–2% of T-ALL but is also rarely found in B-lineage malignancies (154, 303,448). This translocation involves c-*MYC* on 8q24 and the TCRα locus on 14q11. In a manner analogous to the t(2;8) and t(8;22) of B-ALL, the constant regions of the TCRα are translocated distal to c-*MYC*, resulting in overproduction of c-*MYC* protein (40,517).

7q34 Abnormalities

Chromosome abnormalities involving the *TCR*β gene occur infrequently in T-ALL (269,453,512). Translocations involving this region include t(7;9)(q34;q34), t(7;19)(q34;p13), and t(1;7)(p34;q34). In all three trans-

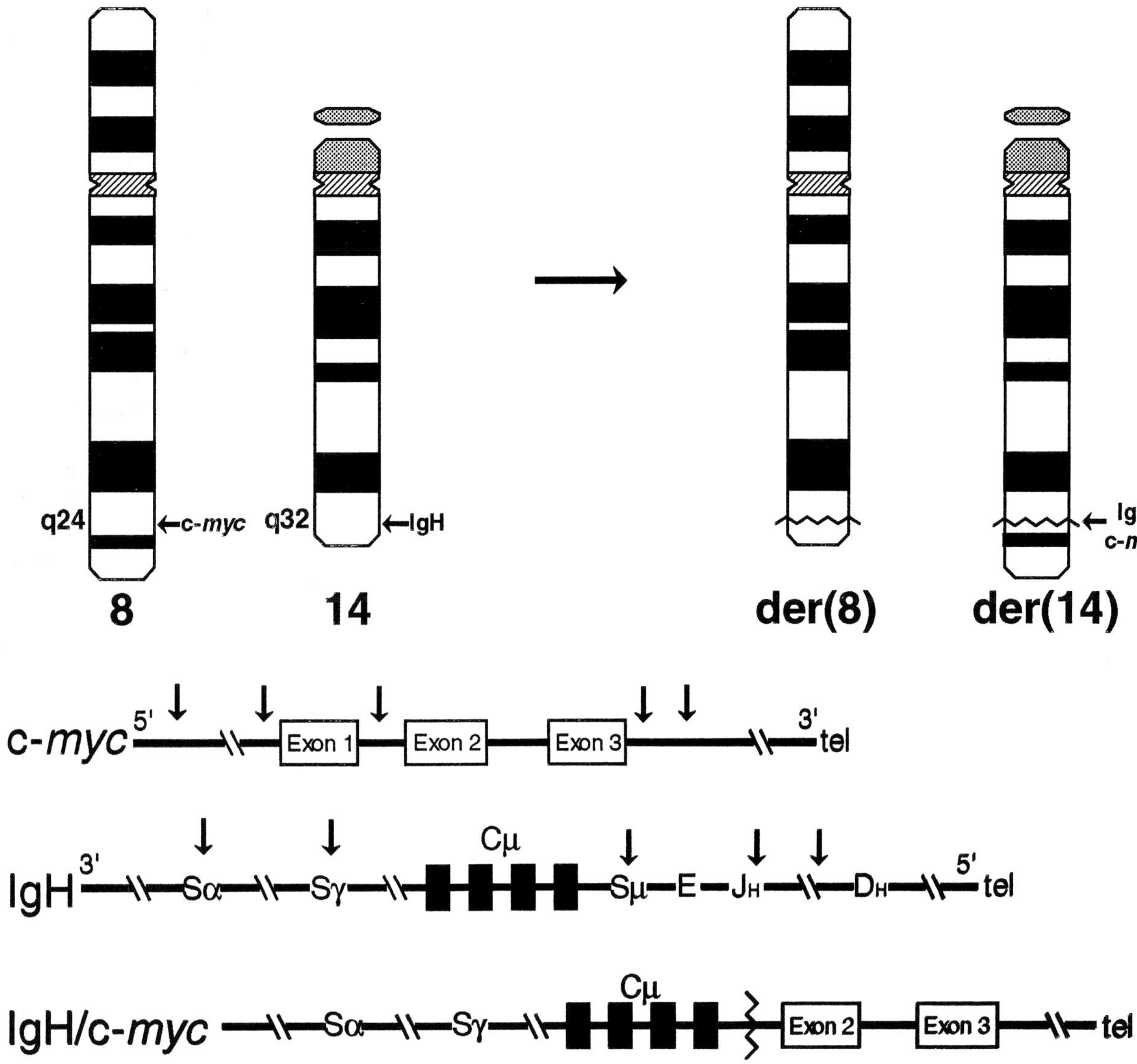

FIG. 20. The t(8;14)(q24;q32) and its chimeric gene derivatives. C-*myc* and immunoglobulin heavy chain (IgH) genes, respectively, located on chromosomes 8 and 14, are indicated. The t(8;14) results in a derivative (der) chromosome 14 that contains c-*myc* fused to IgH. Possible breakpoints in the c-*myc* and IgH gene are indicated by the vertical arrows. The breakpoints of most American and European B-ALLs with the t(8;14) involve $S\alpha$, $S\tau$, and $S\mu$ switch sequences of IgH and intronic regions telomeric to exon I of c-*myc*. The endemic or African-associated B-cell malignancies involve the J_H (joining) or D_H (diversity) regions of IgH.

locations the *TCRβ* locus is involved. In the t(7;9), the breakpoint on chromosome 9 does not alter the *ABL* oncogene but involves another gene, *TAN1* (460,588). The t(7;19)(q34;p13) results in a truncated *LYL1*, a gene with homology to the *TAL1* gene (12,109,362). The *TAL1* locus is placed near the *TCRβ* enhancer in the t(1;7)(q24;q11) (178).

Structural Abnormalities of Chromosomes 6q, 9p, and 12p

Deletions and balanced or unbalanced translocations of chromosomes 6q, 9p, and 12p constitute the most frequent structural abnormalities of newly diagnosed ALLs. Deletions and other structural alterations of the long arm of chromosome 6 (6q) are found in 4–13% of cases (222). Most breakpoints occur at 6q15 and 6q21 (273,415,444). No unique clinical, morphologic, or immunophenotypic features are associated with 6q abnormalities (222). The *MYB* gene is positioned on 6q but does not appear to be involved in alterations of this region in ALL (19,394).

Alterations of the short arm of chromosome 9 (9p) are observed in 7–12% of pediatric ALLs (87,105,381,511). Childhood ALLs with 9p abnormalities are associated with older age, lymphadenopathy, splenomegaly, medi-

been shown (253,351). The male-to-female ratio of the pre-ALL syndrome is the reverse of that for the usual presentation of childhood ALL, suggesting that inherent host factors may have a role in the initial hypoplastic presentation (585).

Benign Lymphocytosis Mimicking Leukemia

Lymphocytes constitute 10–15% of the marrow cellularity at birth and rapidly increase thereafter. By 1 month of age, 38–55% of the marrow cells are lymphocytes. This active lymphopoiesis persists through the first several years of life. During the first year of life the lymphoid population is a mixture of lymphoblasts and immature and mature lymphocytes. The immature lymphocytes are almost exclusively B-lineage cells that express CD19+, CD10+, CD20±, and TDT±, a phenotype characteristic of most B-lineage ALLs. Increased proportions of these nonneoplastic, immature B cells have been reported in a variety of clinical settings, including postchemotherapy for lymphoblastic leukemia (530, 568), post–bone marrow transplantation (286), immune thrombocytopenic purpura (112), neuroblastoma (237, 343,538), transient erythroblastopenia (182), and following viral infections. The marrow examination and immunophenotyping studies of a patient from one of these clinical settings can lead to an inappropriate diagnosis of lymphoblastic leukemia.

From 1 to 2 months after cessation of therapy for ALL, a "rebound" or "off-therapy" lymphocytosis begins and lasts for 12–18 months. The lymphoid population may account for more than 55% of the marrow cellularity, with a median of 31% at 1–2 months and decreasing thereafter (568). Most of the lymphocytes are normal mature lymphocytes, but others will have features of blasts such as increased cell size, fine nuclear chromatin, and scanty to moderate amounts of cytoplasm. These blasts resemble those present in normal, healthy infants and usually differ from the patient's original leukemic blast cytology. In contrast, the majority of relapses in patients with ALL occur from 4 months to 2 years after cessation of therapy. Concurrent with these relapses, the number of normal lymphocytes in the bone marrow usually decreases, and cytopenias develop in the peripheral blood.

Immunologic marker studies of regenerating marrow, if not appropriately chosen, may mislead more than clarify the nature of the lymphocytosis. In the first month of the "rebound" lymphocytosis, a high proportion of these cells express the CD10 (568). Increased numbers of mononuclear cells with nuclear TDT, sometimes two to three times normal, are common in regenerating marrows (524). However, well-devised panels that include antibodies to antigens appearing early and late in B-cell differentiation will distinguish between benign and leukemia lymphoid proliferations. Benign lymphoproliferations will consists of a mixture of early (CD19+, CD10+, TDT±), immature (CD19+, CD20+, CD10±, cytoplasmic μ+), and late (surface IgM+) lymphocytes, whereas a single stage of lymphocyte maturation is reflected by leukemic cells. Monoclonal or oligoclonal immunoglobulin gene rearrangements are not detected by Southern blotting methods in these marrows (312). Most of the problems connected with discerning the nature of the marrow lymphocytosis are avoided if the morphologist remains aware of the clinical diagnosis and treatment history.

Metastatic Small Cell Tumors Mimicking AML and ALL

Neuroblastoma, rhabdomyosarcoma, Ewing's sarcoma, medulloblastoma, and retinoblastoma, referred to as "small cell tumors" or "small round cell tumors," can pose diagnostic problems when initially detected in the bone marrow (2,9,226,411). These tumors are commonly mistaken for leukemia or lymphoma. Usually the cytologic features of metastatic tumor cells are not sufficient to distinguish among the different types of small cell tumors. Immunohistochemical or ultrastructural studies can be resorted to when the primary site is not evident from radiologic studies or when other laboratory studies, such as urinary catecholamines, are not sufficient for diagnosis. Bone marrow metastases of retinoblastoma and medulloblastoma are uncommon and generally occur only with extensive metastatic disease (retinoblastoma) or following cranial surgery (medulloblastoma) (403,414,602).

Most small cell tumors incite very little marrow fibrosis. Thus, the marrow involved by these tumors is fairly easily aspirated. In contrast, carcinomas usually provoke intense desmoplastic reactions resulting in difficult aspirates or "dry taps." A bone marrow needle biopsy should accompany all aspirates in metastatic workups because these two sampling techniques together offer the best odds of detecting metastases. Additionally, the histologic appearance of the tumor in the biopsy core is sometimes sufficient to distinguish among the small cell tumors. In biopsy material, metastatic alveolar rhabdomyosarcoma usually consists of alveolarlike collections of malignant cells surrounded by thin fibrous bands. Neuroblastoma cells frequently form rosettes and bands of neurofibrillary material. The biphasic cell pattern of Ewing's sarcoma is also often retained in marrow biopsies.

Most metastatic tumor cells are larger and have more cytoplasm than blasts of AML and ALL. Although metastatic small cell tumors tend to present with two- and three-dimensional clumps or cell aggregates in marrow aspirate smears, diffuse noncohesive cell spreads are not infrequent. The possibility of megakaryoblastic leukemia should always be included in the differential diagnosis of small cell tumors. Megakaryoblastic disease can have a tumorlike presentation with bony and sometimes extramedullary masses (15,140,506). Malignant megakaryoblasts often tend to be cohesive and can form small clumps in marrow aspirate smears (404,437). Megakaryoblastic disorders also tend to incite marrow reticulin fibrosis, resulting in dry taps that further mimic metastatic cancer.

Small cell tumors, lymphomas, and leukemias may all result in extensive necrosis in the marrow (115,280,388, 439). Thus, necrosis cannot be used as a feature to differentiate these malignancies. Indeed, necrosis of the marrow may be found in acute immunodeficiency syndrome (AIDS), disseminated intravascular coagulation, sickle cell disease, and infections (115). Smudge or basket cells on aspirate smears are not unique to any particular type of cancer and may be found in nonneoplastic conditions. Similarly, streaking of basophilic material derived from the DNA–histone complex, or the "Azzopardi phenomenon," in biopsy or aspirate material can be seen with metastatic small cell tumors as well as with leukemias and lymphomas (558). Malignant cells may engulf red blood cells, leukocytes, and platelets. Rhabdomyosarcomas most often demonstrate this activity. Phagocytosis by leukemic blasts is common in monoblastic leukemias but also occurs in other subtypes of myeloid and lymphoblastic leukemias (111,180,197, 200,430,589). Rhabdomyosarcoma and Ewing's sarcoma cells frequently have deposits of PAS-positive material resembling the "block" PAS reactivity of ALL and AML-M6. The ANA and ANB esterase reactions also may be positive in rhabdomyosarcoma leading to confusion with the monocytic leukemias.

Immunohistochemical and ultrastructural studies of bone marrow aspirates or biopsies can be used to distinguish metastatic tumor from leukemia. With the exception of some B-lineage lymphoblastic and megakaryocytic malignancies, leukemias are CD45-positive and small cell tumors are CD45-negative. Small cell tumors do not express TDT, CD3, CD5, or CD79 lymphoid-associated antigens. Useful markers for the identification of small cell tumors include muscle actin, desmin, chromogranin, neuron-specific enolase, and synaptophysin (see related chapters); a panel approach is recommended.

Remission and Relapse Bone Marrows

A patient treated for ALL is considered to be in complete remission when (a) no leukemic blasts are identifiable; (b) the bone marrow shows orderly maturation of erythroid, myeloid, and megakaryocytic lineages; and (c) the peripheral blood counts approach normal values. Because it may be difficult, if not impossible, to distinguish between normal marrow blasts and leukemic blasts when they are present in small numbers, some treatment protocols include criteria for remission that allow for the presence of up to 4% nonmyeloid, nonerythroid blasts in the bone marrow. Sometimes the cytology of the leukemic blasts may be so distinctive as to strongly suggest persistent or relapsed ALL, even when the blasts number only 1% or less. This situation is particularly true for L3 blasts, vacuolated blasts, blasts of G-ALL, and blasts containing large blocks of PAS-positive glycogen.

Lymphoblasts of recurrent ALL usually resemble those observed at diagnosis. On occasion the cytology of the leukemic cells differs at relapse. These transitions usually are in the direction of L1 to L2 cytology (304,318,586). An example of conversion of L1 to L3 cytology has also been described (3). Reverse changes, conversion from L3 or L2 to L1, have not been reported. Children treated for ALL are also at risk for developing myelocytic or monocytic leukemias later in their clinical course.

ACUTE MYELOID LEUKEMIA

In the strictest sense, the term "acute myeloid leukemia" (AML) indicates a malignancy of the myeloid or granulocytic lineage. However, most clinicians use the term to refer to all nonlymphoid leukemias including myelocytic, monocytic, erythroid, and megakaryocytic subtypes. These leukemias are also referred to as acute nonlymphocytic leukemia, but this designation has lost favor with many morphologists in recent years (103). In the following discussions, "AML" implies any nonlymphoid leukemia, and the specific cell lineage of AML is designated by the French–American–British (FAB) Cooperative Group's proposed nomenclature, e.g., AML-M3 represents acute promyelocytic leukemia (30,33, 34,35).

The FAB Cooperative Group classification is based on morphologic features and cytochemical studies (Table 1). In this classification, the diagnosis of AML requires 30% or more myeloid blasts in the bone marrow (34). In several types of AML the dominant leukemic cell may not be the myeloblast. Examples of this include acute promyelocytic leukemia, acute monocytic leukemia with differentiation, and acute myelocytic leukemia with differentiation. Two types of leukemia, AML with minimal differentiation and megakaryoblastic leukemia, require ultrastructural or immunologic marker studies for identification. Although the FAB classification identifies major subtypes of AML, several distinct subtypes of leukemia with potentially different responses to therapy and clinical outcomes are included in each FAB subgroup. Similarly, AML as defined by nonrandom chromosomal abnormalities may include leukemias from two or more FAB subgroups. Only a combined morphologic, immunologic, cytogenetic, and molecular approach to diagnosis will accurately identify these different leukemic entities.

Acute Myeloblastic Leukemia with Minimal Differentiation (AML-M1)

The blasts of this leukemia are predominantly type I and may be indistinguishable from ALL-L2 and, rarely, ALL-L1 lymphoblasts. Type I or II blasts constitute 90% or more of the marrow nonerythroid cells (Fig. 1). Auer rods may be present but are rarely numerous. Auer rods not readily evident in Wright- or Giemsa-stained smears are frequently observed in MPO- and SBB-stained smears. More than 3% of the myeloblasts are MPO/SBB positive, but the intensity of enzymatic activity and the percentage of positive blasts is less than in AML-M2 and AML-M3. The CAE stain is often weak or negative. Bone marrow biopsy material usually shows extensive replacement of normal marrow cells by myeloblasts and may resemble biopsies harboring ALL.

The pediatric patient with AML-M1 often presents with fatigue, fever, and malaise. Most patients are anemic and thrombocytopenic. The peripheral blood blast count may be high, but some children present with leukopenia. Hepatomegaly and splenomegaly are common.

The majority of pediatric cases of AML-M1 have myeloblasts that express CD13, CD33, CD34, CDw65, and HLA-DR (Table 9). The detection of CD15, CD11b, and nuclear TDT is variable, whereas the expression of CD4, CD14, and CD36 is uncommon.

A variety of chromosomal abnormalities have been described in AML-M1, including monosomy 7 (-7), 7q-, t(8;21), t(9;22), and t(6;9) (Table 10), suggesting the presence of multiple underlying oncogenic mechanisms. These cytogenetic defects also relay prognostic information. Patients with monosomy 7 and t(6;9) have a very poor response to chemotherapy, whereas patients with t(8;21) may be expected to have a more favorable clinical outcome (264,279,347).

Acute Myelocytic Leukemia with Differentiation (AML-M2)

The nonerythroid bone marrow population of patients with AML-M2 consists of 30–89% blasts, 10% or more maturing granulocytic elements (promyelocytes to segmented neutrophils), and less than 20% monocytic cells. AML-M2 composes up to 40% of childhood AML (247). The most common presenting symptoms include fatigue, fever, petechiae, and purpura. Many patients have hepatosplenomegaly and, less commonly, lymphadenopathy. Central nervous system leukemia may be present at diagnosis. Granulocytic sarcomas are particularly common in this type of leukemia. Almost all patients are anemic and thrombocytopenic. There may be overt or subclinical evidence of disseminated intravascular coagulation.

Morphologic, immunologic, and cytogenetic studies identify several different leukemic processes within AML-M2. One group with characteristic morphologic changes and the t(8;21)(q22;q22) composes 35–45% of childhood AML-M2 (50). These patients have a high incidence of central nervous system leukemia and granulocytic sarcoma (264,347). The bone marrow often shows a prominent component of differentiating granulocytic elements (promyelocytes to segmented neutrophils), with type II myeloblasts and type III blasts (promyelocytes with blastlike nuclei) outnumbering type I blasts (Fig. 2). The maturing granulocytic cells usually demonstrate marked nuclear atypia and nuclear/cytoplasmic maturation asynchrony. The peripheral rim of cytoplasm of myelocytes, metamyelocytes, and neutrophils may be basophilic and devoid of granules. Myeloid elements can show hypergranulation or hypogranulation. Abnormally large secondary granules are often present and are best observed in smears stained for MPO and CAE. Binucleated and pseudo–Pelger–Huet cells are common. Most blasts and maturing granulocytes are MPO/SBB and CAE-positive, but frequently a small number of myeloid precursors and neutrophils fail to re-

TABLE 9. *Immunophenotypes of acute myeloid leukemia*[a]

FAB subtype	CD34	DR	CD13	CD14	CD15	CD33	CD36	CD41	CD65	CD2	CD4	CD7	CD19	CD56
M0	++	++	++	0.	++	++	±	0	++	+	±	+	+	±
M1	++	++	++	0	++	+++	±	0	+++	+	±	+	+	±
M2	+++	+++	+++	0	++	+++	±	0	+++	+	±	+	+	+
M3	±	±	+++	0	++	+++	±	0	+++	+	±	±	±	±
M4	++	+++	++	++	++	++	++	0	+++	+	+++	+	±	+
M5	±	+++	++	+	++	+++	++	±	+++	±	+++	+	±	+
M7	+	+	+	0	+	++	++	+++	+	++	+	++	±	±

Abbreviations: FAB, French–American–British classification (33–35).

[a] Percentage of cases expressing CD antigen: 0 = none; ± = <10%; + = 10–49%; ++ = 50–80%; +++ = >80%.

TABLE 10. *Cytogenetic abnormalities in childhood AML and MDS*[a]

Chromosomal abnormality	Involved genes[b]	FAB group	Frequency
Normal			<10%
t(8;21)(q22;q22)	*ETO; AML1*	M2; M1; M4	20% overall (45% of M2)
t(15;17)(q22;q11)	*PML; RARα*	M3	4–7% overall (>99% of M3[c])
t(11;17)(q24;q11)	*PLZF; RARα*	M3-like	Rare
inv(16)(p13q22)	*MYH11; CBFβ*	M4 > M2	10%
t(16;16)(p13;q22)	*MYH11; CBFβ*	M4	Rare
del(16)(q22)	?deleted *CBFβ*	M4	2%
t(8;16)(p11;p13)	?; ?	M5	Rare
t(4;11)(p21;q23)	*AF4; MLL*	M4; M5	<1%
t(9;11)(q22;q23)	*AF9; MLL*	M4; M5	5–10% overall (25–35% of M5)
t(10;11)(q11-15;q23)	*AF10; MLL*	M5	Uncommon
t(11;19)(q23;p13.3)	*MLL; ENL*	M4; M5	<2%
t(11;19)(q23;p13.1)	*MLL; ELL*	M4; M5	<2%
t(11;17)(q23;q21)	*MLL; AF17*	M5	Uncommon
t(1;22)(p13;q13)	?; ?	M7	Rare
t(6;9)(p23;q34)	*DEK; CAN*	MDS; M4; M2; M1	Rare
t(3;21)(q26;q22)	*EAP; AML1*	MDS	Rare
−7		MDS; M2; M4; M6; M7	Common
del(7q)		MDS; M1; M2; M4	Common
del(5q)		MDS; M7	Rare
+8		MDS; M1-M4; M7	Common
+21		MDS; M1-M7	Common
i(17)		MDS; AML	Uncommon

Abbreviations: Gene names explained in text; MDS, myelodysplastic syndrome; AML, acute myeloid leukemia; FAB, French–American–British classification.
[a] See refs. 264, 279, and 347.
[b] See ref. 445.
[c] Rare cases of AML-M3 will have molecular but no cytogenetic evidence of t(15;17).

act with these cytochemical stains. Auer rods are found in most cases. Occasionally, Auer rods are observed in differentiating metamyelocytes and segmented neutrophils. Erythropoiesis and thrombopoiesis usually show little or no dysplastic changes. Bone marrow biopsy sections reflect the aspirate findings, but the blast percentage usually appears higher because of the difficulty in distinguishing between blasts and dysplastic granulocytic precursors.

AML-M2 cases with the t(8;21) usually have a distinct immunophenotype to complement the morphologic findings. The blasts are positive for HLA-DR, CD13, CD33, CD34, and CDw65. The expression of CD13 and CD33 is usually very weak and sometimes not detectable (282,562). Leukemic blasts commonly express B-cell-associated CD19 and, less commonly, the NK cell CD56 antigens (246,282,562). Unlike AML-M2 without the t(8;21), T-cell-associated CD2 and CD7 antigens are rarely expressed (246).

The chromosomal breakpoints of the t(8;21) involve the *AML1* on 21q22 and *ETO* on 8q22. The translocation results in the fusion of these genes on the der(8) chromosome, producing a novel chimeric *AML1/ETO* gene and transcript (Fig. 23) (164,191). The 8q22 and 21q22 breakpoints are restricted to the same introns of *AML1* and *ETO* (348). The AML1 protein binds to a DNA sequence belonging to a family of enhancer core binding motifs that include the myeloperoxidase gene, CD13 antigen, and the T-cell antigen receptors. In normal myeloid cells, AML1 complexes with core-binding factor–β (CBFβ) and binds as a heterodimeric complex to DNA. The aberrant AML1/ETO product retains the ability to complex with CBF and binds DNA through the *runt* homology domain of AML1 (364). The chimeric AML1/ETO product may induce cellular transformation and differentiation through its altered interaction with genes normally regulated by *AML1,* but its direct contribution to leukemogenesis is unclear.

Although the t(8;21) is most common to AML-M2, this translocation is occasionally found in AML-M1 and rarely in AML-M4 (Table 10) (450). Reports of a t(8;21) in de novo myelodysplastic syndromes most likely represent cases of AML-M2 with low type I and II blast percentages. Cases of AML with the t(8;21) are associated with an initial favorable response to chemotherapy, but long-term survival may be poor (264,279,347,542). Thus, in future treatment programs the identification of this chromosomal translocation may be more important than the FAB subgroup assignment.

The molecular characterization of the t(8;21)(q22;1q21) has provided information for the design of DNA probes for Southern blot analysis and oligonucleotide primers for RT-PCR assays. Although the t(8;21) is fairly easy to detect by cytogenetic techniques, Southern blot analysis for ETO breaks is useful in cases where this evaluation is not available or is unsatisfactory (164,349). The

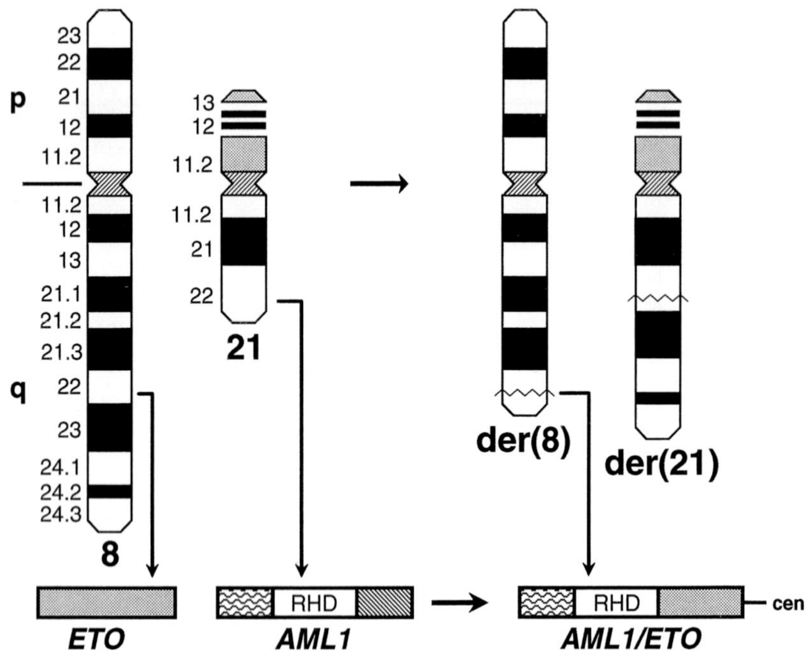

FIG. 23. The t(8;21)(q22;q22). The t(8;21) results in the translocation of *AML1* gene on chromosome 21 onto the *ETO* gene of chromosome 8, resulting in a derivative (der) chromosome 8 with a chimeric *AML1/ETO* gene. The sequence encoding for the *runt* homology domain (RHD) of *AML1* is retained in the chimeric gene.

more rapid and specific RT-PCR assay may be useful for diagnosis and monitoring response to therapy (147,348). Surprisingly, *AML1/ETO* transcripts are detected by RT-PCR in peripheral blood and bone marrow from most patients in long-term remission (300,348,391). Thus, the use of RT-PCR for detecting *AML1/ETO* transcripts may have limited value for documenting minimal residual disease and predicting impending relapse.

A subtype of AML-M2 occurs that is relatively uncommon in children, is common in adults, and shows dysplastic changes in erythropoiesis or megakaryopoiesis as well as granulopoiesis. Type I and II blasts usually dominate the marrow cellularity, with granulocytic differentiation being less exuberant than M2 leukemias with the t(8;21). Cytogenetic studies may disclose monosomy 7, 7q-, a normal karyotype, the rare t(6;9)(p23;q34), or a variety of other less well-characterized cytogenetic abnormalities (Table 10). A history of anemia, leukopenia, or thrombocytopenia sometimes precedes the diagnosis of AML. Patients with monosomy 7 or t(6;9) frequently have a preceding myelodysplastic syndrome. Frequently, marrow basophilia and sometimes eosinophilia is seen in association with the t(6;9) (321,402).

The leukemic myeloblasts in the non-t(8;21) AML-M2 group commonly express HLA-DR, CD13, CD33, CD34, and CDw65, but rarely CD19. The intensity of CD13 and CD33 antigen expression by leukemic blasts usually exceeds that of myeloblasts from AML-M2 cases with the t(8;21). Myeloblasts may express TDT and not infrequently the T-cell-associated antigens CD2 and CD7 (7,246).

The recognition of the t(6;9) is important because patients with this translocation respond poorly to chemotherapy. It is doubtful that the AML-M2 morphology can be attributed directly to the t(6;9) because this translocation is also found in the myelodysplastic syndrome, AML-M1, and AML-M4 (Table 10) (7,321,402). The 6;9 translocation results in the production of a fusion gene involving the *CAN* on 9q and the *DEK* on 6p. An altered fusion DEK/CAN protein (p165) is generated from the 6p-derivative chromosome, but the function of this protein as well as the normal DEK (p43) and CAN (p220) proteins is unknown (513).

Bone marrows of a third subtype of AML-M2 in children show a dimorphic leukemic cell population consisting of large myeloblasts and differentiating dysplastic granulocytic elements plus a significant component of small, lymphoidlike blasts with scant, agranular cytoplasm. The smaller blasts often have hand–mirror configurations (434). The myeloblasts may contain Auer rods and are MPO/SBB-positive. The small blasts do not contain Auer rods and produce no or only weak reactions with MPO and SBB stains. Both blast cell populations usually express HLA-DR, CD13, CD33, CD34, and CDw65, and sometimes the lymphoid-associated antigens CD2, CD7, or CD19. The smaller blasts usually express fewer myeloid antigens and one or more lymphoid-associated antigens. No unique cytogenetic abnormality characterizes this group of leukemias. These leukemias may respond more readily to induction chemotherapy for ALL than to drugs used in AML inductions (434).

All three of the preceding subtypes of AML-M2 may present with a significant marrow eosinophilia comprising immature and mature eosinophils. Cases of AML-M2 with eosinophilia and inv(16)(p13q22), a cytogenetic abnormality more commonly found in AML-M4, have also been reported (542). Granules may be increased or decreased or atypically large in the eosinophils, and they may produce atypical reactions with PAS and CAE stains (254,542). The eosinophilic proliferation may dominate the marrow cellularity and be confused with hypereosinophilic syndrome or with the rare case of ALL with associated hypereosinophilia (256,268).

Acute Promyelocytic Leukemia (AML-M3 and AML-M3v)

Acute promyelocytic leukemia, AML-M3, is a distinct subtype of myeloid leukemia with unique clinical, biologic, and molecular features. This subtype accounts for 4–7% of myeloid leukemias in North American children and 20–32% of those in South American, African, and Italian ones (91,136,195,207,247,471,592). Hepatosplenomegaly and lymphadenopathy are uncommon (91). Most patients are anemic and thrombocytopenic. The WBC count is frequently normal, but leukopenia and hyperleukocytosis are not uncommon (91). Among the myeloid leukemias, AML-M3 has the longest duration of complete remission and is the only leukemia to show a clinical remission response to the differentiation agent all-*trans*-retinoic acid (ATRA) (16,207).

Hemorrhagic complications are more common in AML-M3 than in any other type of childhood leukemia. Laboratory evidence of coagulopathy is present in most patients (91,195). Patients frequently have a hemorrhagic syndrome involving the skin, mucosal membranes, retina, urinary system, or gastrointestinal tract. The coagulopathy is presumably due to the release of procoagulant activity from the granules of leukemic cells. Although laboratory studies implicate diffuse intravascular coagulation as the cause of bleeding diatheses, fibrinogenolytic or proteolytic activity due to leukocyte proteases may be an important associated process (16,546). The initiation of chemotherapy may increase the risk of bleeding due to lysis of leukemic cells and further release of granules. The leukemic cells of AML-M3 resemble large promyelocytes with prominent azurophilic cytoplasmic granulation (Fig. 24; see figure in color plate section). However, unlike normal promyelocytes these cells have abundant cytoplasm and characteristic large-folded, monocytoid or bilobate nuclei (44). Type I and type II blasts usually constitute less than 30% of the marrow cellularity. Variable numbers of smaller leukemic cells with markedly basophilic cytoplasm, sparse granules, and oval to lobated nuclei may be present (359). In some cases, these basophilic cells are the dominate cell type. Auer rods are easily identified. Cells containing multiple rods, "faggot" cells, are present in almost all cases (Fig. 24; see figure in color plate section). With electron microscopy, Auer rods in AML-M3 consist of tubular arrays with a periodicity that differs from that of Auer rods of other leukemias (67,564). Leukemic cells may show maturation through the metamyelocyte stage and infrequently to segmented neutrophils but with persistence of prominent azurophilic granulation. Rare cases of M3 leukemia have a significant component of basophils in the marrow and show basophilic differentiation of the leukemic promyelocytes on ATRA therapy (545).

The leukemic cells are intensely MPO-, SBB-, and CAE-positive and may give weak reactions with ANB or ANA with partial NaF resistance (Table 1) (129,352, 495,555). The outer surface but usually not the core of Auer rods reacts with MPO, SBB, and CAE. In thin sections of paraffin-embedded bone marrow biopsies, the leukemic cells retain their monocytoid nuclear shapes and demonstrate eosinophilic granular cytoplasm. The CAE reaction is usually positive in formalin and B-5 fixed tissues. Auer rods may be discernible in very thin sections stained with hematoxylin and eosin.

A subset of AML-M3, AML-M3v, is composed of leukemic cells with fine pink granules or cells that appear void of granules (Fig. 25; see figure in color plate section). "Hypogranular" and "microgranular" are often used to describe this variant (199,359). Auer rods and faggot cells are usually present but often require a concerted search. The CAE reaction is useful in unmasking Auer rods (158). The presence of the characteristic folded or monocytoid nucleus of AML-M3 is a significant clue to the correct diagnosis. Despite the apparent diminution of granules, the leukemic cells are intensely MPO- and SBB-positive (483). Hyperleukocytosis is usually present at diagnosis as compared with the lower leukocyte count typically found in the hypergranular form (471). Severe coagulopathy and death from central nervous system and lung hemorrhages are more common in M3v than in classical M3 during the first 10 days after diagnosis (471).

The differential diagnosis of AML-M3 includes acute agranulocytosis with a marked left shift of marrow myeloid elements, monocytic (AML-M4 and M5) leukemias, and myelocytic leukemias showing cellular differentiation (AML-M2). During the recovery stage of acute agranulocytosis, the bone marrow may demonstrate a predominance of myeloblasts and promyelocytes that may be misinterpreted as AML-M3. Unlike M3 promyelocytes, the regenerating promyelocytes have prominent Golgi, lack marked nuclear folding, and lack Auer rods (252). Some cases of AML-M2 have a prominent component of type II blasts and promyelocytic forms and occasional blasts containing multiple Auer rods. With these leukemias the definitive diagnosis of AML-M3 often rests on the demonstration of the t(15;17) by cytogenetic or molecular studies. The prominent folded

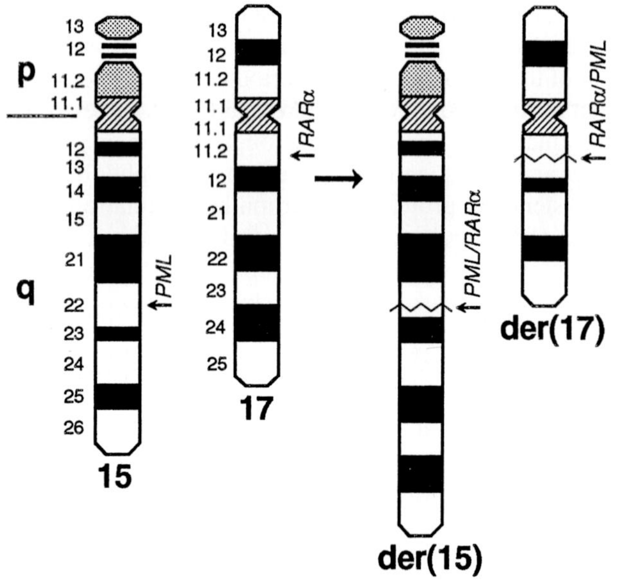

FIG. 26. The t(15;17)(q22;q21). A fusion gene, *PML/RARα*, results from the translocation of part of the *RARα* gene on chromosome 17 onto the *PML* gene on chromosome 15, the derivative (der) chromosome 15.

nuclei and fine azurophilic granulation of the leukemic cells of AML-M3v may be confused with cells of the monocytic leukemias (294). The confusion is compounded if the leukemic cells have ANB or ANA esterase activity (199,223,294,352,359,495,555). Perinuclear microfilaments, an ultrastructural finding in monocytic diseases, may be found in AML-M3 (359). In contrast to AML-M3, monocytic leukemias do not have faggot cells and show a weak MPO/SBB and an intense ANB reaction pattern.

Cells of AML-M3 and -M3v express a characteristic surface antigen pattern (Table 9). Leukemic cells strongly express CD9, CD13, CD33, and CDw65 but lack CD14, CD34, and HLA-DR (149,193,398). CD11b and CD15 are variable in their expression. The T-cell-associated CD2 antigen is atypically expressed in approximately 40–45% of cases (293). The expression of CD2 may occur more frequently in the M3v subtype (108,325,350,398,471). Other anomalous but infrequently expressed antigens include CD4 and CD56 (294,576).

Almost every patient with AML-M3 or its variant M3v has cytogenetic evidence of a translocation between the long arms of chromosomes 15 and 17, the t(15;17)(q22;q11) (Fig. 26) (306). As a consequence of the 15;17 translocation, recombinant 15q- and 17q-chromosomes are formed. Breakpoints of chromosome 17 are within the gene coding for the retinoic acid receptor–α (*RARα*) (62,138). RARα mediates the effect of its ligand retinoic acid, triggering myeloid cell differentiation by binding to DNA. The chromosome 15 break site falls within the *PML* (promyelocytic) gene. Although the presence of a zinc finger DNA binding sequence suggests that the protein coded by *PML* acts as a transcriptional factor, PML proteins also localize to electron dense regions of the nucleus known as nuclear bodies (289). The interplay of PML with nuclear bodies may regulate cell growth (289).

Two fusion genes are formed as a result of the 15;17 reciprocal translocation: the *PML/RARα* gene on the derivative 15q-chromosome and its reciprocal *RARα/PML* gene on the derivative 17q-chromosome (Fig. 27). The *PML/RARα* gene encodes for an aberrant PML protein that is found in every case of AML-M3, whereas the RARα/PML protein is expressed in only 70–80% of cases. This suggests that the derivative 15q- or *PML/RARα* transcript is involved in leukemogenesis (61, 63,207). The PML/RARα protein binds to nuclear bodies resulting in dispersal of other nuclear body–associated antigens, whereas retinoic acid reverses this dispersal (289). PML/RARα inhibits myeloid cell differentiation and promotes survival in the absence of

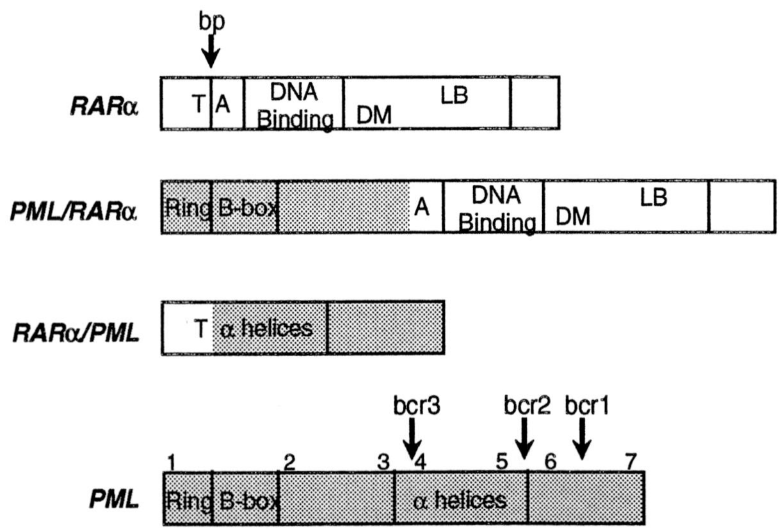

FIG. 27. The *RARα, PML,* and chimeric genes *PML/RARα* and *PML/RARα*. The common breakpoint of *RARα* is indicated by arrow labeled bp. The three breakpoint cluster regions of *PML* are indicated by arrows labeled bcr1, bcr2, and bcr3. The chimeric protein PML/RARα is thought to be involved in the leukemogenesis of AML-M3. The structure of *RARα* begins with an N-terminal transactivation (TA) domain. The N-terminal region of the *PML* contains zinc finger domains (ring and B-box) that are retained in all *PML/RARα* isoforms. Located C-terminal to the zinc finger region is an α-helices region with codes for DNA-binding and dimerization-coding sequences.

retinoic acid (207). Paradoxically, in the presence of high concentrations of retinoic acid, the PML/RARα protein induces terminal myeloid differentiation (207). Three breakpoint cluster regions (bcr 1, bcr 2, bcr 3) are present in the *PML* gene (Fig. 27). The bcr 1 and bcr 3 (introns 6 and 3) breaks are found in 90–95% of M3-leukemias, whereas bcr 2 (exon 6) breaks are detected in 5–10% of patients. The chromosome 17 break always occurs in intron 2 of the *RARα*. Thus the *RARα* component of *PML/RARα* gene is the same in all cases, whereas the *PML* portion differs because of chromosome 15 break site heterogeneity. Evidence suggesting an association of the location of *PML* breakpoints with patient age, WBC count, M3 type (M3 vs. M3v), coagulopathy, and atypical expression of CD2 is conflicting (108,142,325,350, 471). The clinical response to ATRA may be related to the specific type of 15;17 rearrangement (47,324,368).

AML-M3 must be accurately and rapidly diagnosed because of the high risk of fatal coagulopathy. Only M3 leukemias with t(15;17) will respond to ATRA, and long-term complete remissions may require specific combinations of chemotherapy that incorporate anthracyclins (207). The t(15;17) is rapidly detected by classic cytogenetic techniques in more than 95% of patients with AML-M3. Molecular diagnosis can be accomplished rapidly when cytogenetic testing is unavailable or is unsatisfactory. Two or three RARα genomic DNA probes will identify rearrangements by Southern blot analysis in 100% of cases (142,325). However, Southern blot techniques have the disadvantage of taking 5–10 days to complete. The confirmation of t(15;17) can also be performed by testing with RT-PCR for the PML/RARα transcript (368). RT-PCR analysis has the advantages of being specific for t(15;17) and requiring only 48–72 hours to perform.

Rare leukemias that morphologically resemble AML-M3 but lack the t(15;17) have molecular evidence of rearrangements of *RARα* and sometimes *PML* (63,102, 316,368). Cytogenetic abnormalities in AML-M3-like leukemias include t(11;17)(q24;q21), t(3;15)(q21;q22), and t(X;15)(p11;q22) (63,102,225,316,383). Because leukemias with the t(11;17) are not responsive to retinoic acid, it is important to separate these from AML-M3 with the t(15;17) (316). In the t(11;17), *RARα* is fused to *PLZF* (promyelocytic leukemia zinc finger), which resembles *PML* structurally. Like the t(15;17), the t(11;17) is detected by Southern blot analysis with DNA probes to *RARα* (102).

The *PML/RARα* transcript permits unambiguous diagnosis and monitoring of minimal residual disease. RT-PCR amplification of the *PML/RARα* transcript identifies one neoplastic cell in a background of 10^5 normal cells (47,143). *PML/RARα* transcripts are detected during remission induction, but these transcripts disappear after complete remission. The persistence of abnormal transcripts in patients in complete morphologic remission is predictive of clinical relapse (143,242, 327,368).

ATRA therapy may be the first choice of treatment because it has the advantage of not exacerbating hemorrhagic diatheses. However, hyperleukocytosis and thromboembolism may be serious complications. With ATRA therapy, leukemic promyelocytes undergo terminal differentiation and lose the capacity to proliferate. The thromboembolic events occurring during ATRA therapy may be due to hyperleukocytosis but may also occur with low leukocyte counts, possibly as a result of ATRA interacting with endothelium or interfering with fibrinolysis.

Acute Monocytic Leukemia (AML-M5a and AML-M5b)

In acute monoblastic leukemia, AML-M5, the marrow contains 80% or more monocytic cells that include monoblasts, promonocytes, and monocytes. AML-M5 may present as an extramedullary mass (or monocytic sarcoma) with few or no blasts in the bone marrow (127,407). It accounts for 15–25% of pediatric AML, and 50% of these patients are under 2 years of age (392). AML-M5 is associated with high white counts, lymphadenopathy, leukemia cutis, gingival hypertrophy, central nervous system leukemia, elevated serum muramidase, and disseminated intravascular coagulation (127, 247,259,264,554).

Leukemia with 80% or more monocytic cells resembling monoblasts is termed AML-M5a or acute monocytic leukemia, undifferentiated (34). Most childhood monocytic leukemias are the M5a subtype. Marrows with this disease contain large blasts with abundant cytoplasm and cell diameters of 30–45 μm (Fig. 28; see figure in color plate section). The cytoplasm can vary from pale to intensely basophilic and often contains a few azurophilic granules in the Golgi region. The nuclei are round to reniform with finely dispersed chromatin. Many blasts have a single, prominent, centrally located nucleolus, whereas other blasts show multiple, distinct nucleoli. The MPO reaction varies from negative to moderately strong. The SBB stain usually results in stronger reactions than MPO. A slight blush of CAE reactivity is frequently observed, but the strong reaction of myelocytic cells is uncommon (468). With rare exception, the ANB and ANA esterase stains produce a strong diffuse reaction pattern that is abolished by NaF treatment (Fig. 5) (223). The small number of monoblasts of some cases exhibit hemophagocytosis or leukophagocytosis. The majority of de novo AML-M5's show little if any erythroid or megakaryocytic dyspoiesis. Bone marrow biopsies usually show replacement of normal hematopoietic elements by large cells with ample eosinophilic to amphophilic cytoplasm and prominent, inclusionlike eosinophilic nucleoli.

The monocytic leukemias showing monocytic cell maturation or fewer than 80% monoblasts are termed AML-M5b and are uncommon in childhood. Promonocytes and incompletely differentiated monocytes usually dominate the marrow picture, with monoblasts composing less than 80% of the monocytic population. The leukemic cells contain a reniform to folded nucleus and usually fine to coarse azurophilic cytoplasmic granules. Auer rods are rarely observed and probably indicate a leukemic myeloid component. MPO is negative to weakly reactive, whereas the SBB stain usually shows a small number of positive granules. With rare exception, the ANB and ANA esterase reactions are positive and inhibited by NaF. Bone marrow biopsies show hypercellular marrows that are populated with medium to large cells with monocytoid nuclei and small vague or distinct nucleoli.

The monocytic leukemias have a characteristic pattern of surface antigen expression that in most cases distinguishes them from other subtypes of AML (496). With rare exception, monoblasts express HLA-DR, CD4, CD11b, CD11c, CD33, and CDw65, but not CD34 (Table 9). The majority of M5 leukemias also express CD13, CD15, CD14, and CD36. Most monocytic leukemias also express CD45RO, a glycoprotein often mistakenly thought by the inexperienced to be unique to T lymphocytes and T-cell lymphomas. CD56 is commonly expressed by leukemic monoblasts. Often, a subpopulation of leukemic cells demonstrates CD41a due to adherence of platelets or adsorbance of glycoprotein IIb/IIIa to the surface of the blasts (46,295). This misleading CD41a expression may result in the leukemic process being confused with a megakaryoblastic leukemia.

Structural abnormalities of chromosome 11q23 are present in 15–20% of AMLs and more than 50% of M5a types (184,264,474). These abnormalities in order of frequency include the t(9;11)(p22;q23), t(11;19)(q23;p13.1), t(10;11)(p11-15;q23), t(11;17)(q23;q21), t(4;11)(p21;q23), t(6;11)(q27;q23), t(1;11)(p32;q23), and del(11)(q23) (37,184,271,272,474). Although most common to AML-M5, translocations involving 11q23 can also be found in AML-M4 and AML-M1. The t(4;11) and t(11;19) translocations are also relatively common in ALL. All of these translocations result in breaks of the *MLL* (or *HRX*) gene at 11q23. Most of the partner genes for the 11q23 translocations have been identified (113,210,385,413,553) (Table 10). The functions of these partner genes are unknown, but all except *ELL* appear to encode for serine/proline rich proteins. The *ELL* gene on 19p13.1 has coding sequences for a lysine-rich protein (551). Rearrangement of the *MLL* gene is more frequent in pediatric AML than is indicated by classic cytogenetic studies. Up to 58% of infants with AML have breaks of the *MLL* gene demonstrable with Southern blot/hybridization techniques (516). Like the translocations involving 11q23 in ALL, it is thought that the product of the derivative 11q23 chromosome of these translocations is involved in leukemogenesis. Less commonly observed chromosome abnormalities in AML-M5 include t(10;11)(p14-21;q23), t(8;16)(p11;p13), and monosomy 7 (73,230).

The differential diagnosis of AML-M5 includes AML-M0, AML-M3v, AML-M7, ALL-M2, large cell lymphoma, and metastatic small cell tumor. The intense diffuse ANB esterase reaction of AML-M5 should differentiate this process from AML-M0, AML-M7, ALL-L2, and large cell lymphomas. The blasts of megakaryoblastic leukemias usually display a diffuse granular reaction with ANA esterase stains that is NaF-resistant. The blasts of the microgranular variant of promyelocytic leukemias, AML-M3v, may produce a positive reaction with ANB and ANA esterases, resulting in a mistaken diagnosis of AML-M5b. The presence of the t(15;17) and the immunophenotype pattern of HLA-DR–, CD33+, CD13+, and CD4– will correctly identify AML-M3.

Children under 2 years of age with monoblastic malignancy frequently present with masses of skin, gingiva, soft tissue, lacrimal gland, or bone but with little peripheral blood and marrow evidence of disease (407). Bone marrow biopsies can show patchy infiltrates of large cells with prominent nucleoli. The monoblasts in biopsies of these lesions share cytologic features with the immunoblasts of large cell lymphomas, i.e., large size with copious acidophilic cytoplasm, large nuclei, and prominent nucleoli. However, most monoblastic lesions also contain cells with monocytoid nuclei that should create a high degree of suspicion for a sarcomatous presentation of monoblastic disease. Appropriate immunologic marker studies will differentiate between most cases of lymphoma and monoblastic leukemia.

Acute Myelomonocytic Leukemia (AML-M4 and AML-M4Eo)

Acute myelomonocytic leukemia, AML-M4, is thought to have neoplastic myeloid and monocytic components. This implies a common malignant precursor cell of origin. The bone marrow contains 30% or more blasts, greater than 20% monocytic cells, and more than 20% myeloid elements (34). The monocytic component can consist of monoblasts, promonocytes, and monocytes (Fig. 29; see figure in color plate section). The monocytic component should be confirmed by cytochemical stains. The cytochemical pattern of blast reactivity varies among patients. MPO/SBB-positive blasts comprise 3% or more of the nonerythroid elements. In most cases more than 20% of the marrow cells react with ANA and ANB esterase stains. An elevated serum lysozyme level, three times normal, or a peripheral blood monocytic count more than 5×10^9/L qualifies a leukemia for AML-M4 status in the absence of a demonstrable monocytic component in the marrow (34). The granulocytic component often resembles AML-M2 with cells representing all stages of myelocytic development. Auer rods are present in some cases but are not numerous. Some cases will also present with dysplastic changes in erythropoiesis and megakaryopoiesis.

AML-M4 composes 15–22% of pediatric AMLs. Patients may present with fever, fatigue, bleeding diathesis, gingival hyperplasia, leukemia cutis, lymphadenopathy, hepatosplenomegaly, and central nervous system leukemia. Most patients have an increased leukocyte count, anemia, and thrombocytopenia.

An uncommon variant, AML-M4Eo, is associated with increased numbers of marrow eosinophils with or without peripheral blood eosinophilia (14,49). All stages of eosinophilic development are present (Fig. 30; see figure in color plate section). Promyelocytic stage eosinophils contain a mixture of eosinophilic and basophilic cytoplasmic granules. The basophilic granules often persist through maturation to the metamyelocyte stage, presenting as "monocytoid" eosinophils. Unlike the granules of basophils, the basophilic granules of the eosinophils are MPO-positive and nonmetachromatic. Often the eosinophilic granules react atypically with CAE and PAS (48,49). Ultrastructural studies of the abnormal eosinophils show a mixture of large electron-lucent and small electron-dense granules (125). Typical crystalloid-containing eosinophil granules are usually absent (75).

AML-M4Eo is associated with abnormalities of the q22 band of chromosome 16, including inv(16) (p13q22), del(16)(q22), and t(16;16)(p13;q22) (Table 10) (14,49, 50,307,308). The inv(16) and del(16) abnormalities are occasionally observed in AML-M4 without marrow eosinophilia and in other types of myeloid leukemias, including AML-M2, AML-M5, myelodysplastic syndrome, and chronic granulocytic leukemia (42,85). Bone marrows from cases of inv(16) contain the chromosomal abnormality in monocytes, eosinophils, and basophils (599). The inv(16) is associated with a more favorable prognosis, hyperleukocytosis, and an increased incidence of central nervous system leukemia relapse (6,14,38,308,347).

The inv(16)(p13q22) and t(16;16)(p13;q22) result in a new *CBFβ/MYHII* chimeric gene (322,503). This chimeric gene contains part of *CBFβ* (core-binding factor *β*) on 16q fused to a variable portion of *MYHII* (a smooth muscle myosin heavy chain gene) on 16p (Fig. 31). CBFβ is a ubiquitous protein that binds to the *runt* homology domain of AML1, a DNA-binding protein. The CBFβ/MYHII protein appears to retain its ability to interact with the AML1 protein, thus possibly altering the activity of target genes normally regulated by AML1 or acting as a functional inhibitor of the normal AML1/CBFβ complex through a dominant negative mechanism (364). It is important to note that the t(8;21) and inv(16), which account for 25–30% of chromosomal abnormalities in AML, appear to disrupt a single transcriptional factor complex, AML1/CBFβ.

Acute Erythroleukemia (AML-M6) and Acute Erythroblastic Leukemia

Leukemias composed primarily of erythroid precursors include erythroleukemia, erythremic myelosis, and acute erythroblastic leukemia. Erythroleukemia and

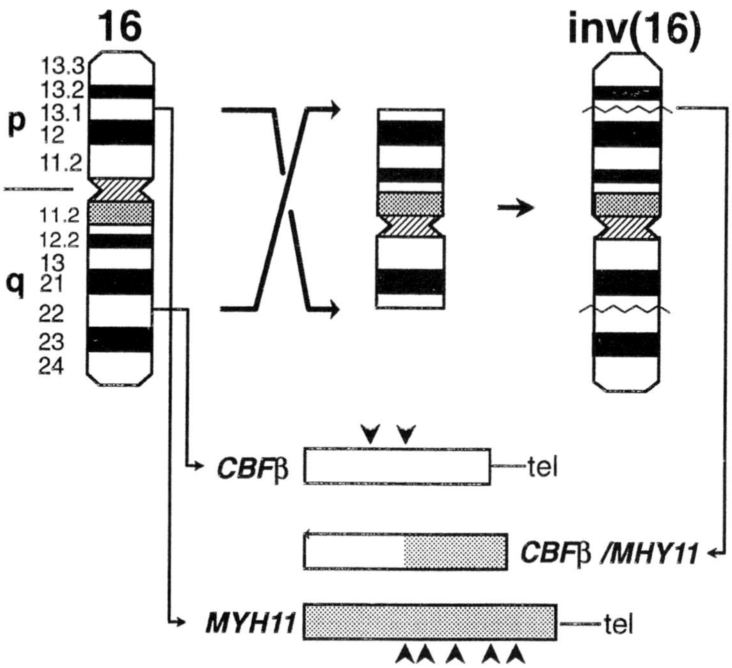

FIG. 31. The inv(16)(p13;q22). Chromosome 16 detaches in the *CBFβ* and *MYHII* gene loci and reassembles in an inverted orientation. The inversion causes fusion of parts of centromeric portion of *CBFβ* and telomeric portion of *MYHII*, resulting in the chimeric gene *CBF/MYHII*. Breakpoint regions of *CBFβ* and *MYHII* are indicated by arrowheads.

TABLE 11. *Diagnostic criteria for acute myeloid leukemia without differentiation (AML-M0)*

Criteria used at SJCRH[a]	Criteria according to FAB Cooperative Group[b] (35)
1. <3% of blasts positive with MPO or SBB	1. <3% of blasts positive for MPO or SBB
2. <3% of blasts positive with ANB esterase[c]	2. Blasts negative for all lymphoid antigens except CD2, CD4, or CD7
3. <3% of blasts express platelet antigens CD36, CD41a, CD42b, or CD61	**plus**
4. <3% of blasts express cytoplasmic CD3 and CD79	3. Ultrastructural evidence of MPO
plus	**or**
5. Ultrastructural evidence of MPO	4. Blasts react with anti-MPO antibody
or	**or**
6. >10% of blasts react with anti-MPO antibody	5. Blasts express one or more of the following antigens: CD11b, CD13, CD14, CD15, or CD33
or	
7. >10% of blasts express two or more of the following antigens: CD13, CD15, CD33, or CD65	

Abbreviations: SJCRH, St. Jude Children's Research Hospital; MPO, myeloperoxidase; SBB, Sudan black B; ANB, α-naphthylbutyrate.

[a] Blasts must meet all of first four criteria and one of last three.

[b] Blasts must meet both of first two criteria and one of last three.

[c] Monocyte pattern.

MYELODYSPLASTIC SYNDROME

Myelodysplastic syndrome (MDS) is a heterogeneous group of bone marrow disorders characterized by ineffective hematopoiesis of one or more cell lineages and a propensity for developing AML. The myelodysplastic disorders are uncommon in childhood and account for 1–3% of pediatric bone marrow malignancies (116,218). Boys are three to four times more likely to develop MDS than girls. The etiology of the majority of de novo pediatric cases is unknown, but several genetic disorders predispose to MDS, including Fanconi's anemia, neurofibromatosis, ataxia-telangiectasia, xeroderma pigmentosa, and constitutional trisomy 8 (17,270). Carcinogenic agents, irradiation, viral infections, and possibly immunodeficiency states also may have a causative role (159,341,531). Irradiation and alkylating-agent chemotherapy are associated with secondary MDS (see Chapter 12).

The initial clinical manifestations of MDS are usually due to cytopenias secondary to bone marrow failure. Some children will have a recent history of recurrent infections. Patients may present with malaise, weakness, pallor, or anorexia. Physical exam may show petechiae, ecchymosis, hepatosplenomegaly, and sometimes adenopathy. Some children will have a recent history of recurrent infections. Central nervous system disease at the time of diagnosis is uncommon.

Classification

The classification of MDS proposed by the FAB Cooperative Group has found widespread acceptance (32,34,64,218). Subtypes of MDS are defined by peripheral blood and bone marrow percentages of blasts, monocytes, and ringed sideroblasts (Table 12). Dysplastic changes in hematopoiesis are usually present in one

TABLE 12. *Classification of myelodysplastic syndromes*[a]

Subtype	Peripheral blood	Bone marrow
Refractory anemia (RA) or refractory cytopenia	Anemia, neutropenia, or thrombocytopenia, no blasts	<5% blasts
Refractory anemia with ringed sideroblasts (RARS)	Anemia, no blasts	<5% blasts; >15% ringed sideroblasts
Refractory anemia with excess blasts (RAEB)	<5% blasts	5–20% blasts
Refractory anemia with excess blasts in transformation (RAEB-IT)	≥5% but <15% blasts[b]; or presence of Auer rods	>20% but <30% blasts; or Auer rods present
Chronic myelomonocytic leukemia (CMMoL)	Peripheral blood monocytes $>1 \times 10^9$/L, and <5% blasts	≤20% blasts
Chronic myelomonocytic leukemia in transformation (CMMoL-IT)	Peripheral blood monocytes $>1 \times 10^9$/L and ≥5% but <15% blasts[b]	>20% but <30% blasts

[a] Based on a modification of the French–American–British (FAB) classification (32, 34).

[b] The disease process should be classified as acute myeloid leukemia when the peripheral blood blasts are ≥15%.

or more major cell lineages. Most childhood MDS diseases are classified as refractory anemia with excess blasts (RAEB), refractory anemia with excess blasts in transformation (RAEB-IT), or chronic myelomonocytic leukemia (CMMoL). Refractory anemia (RA) and refractory anemia with ringed sideroblasts (RARS) are uncommon in the pediatric age group.

Refractory Anemia and Refractory Anemia with Ringed Sideroblasts

Patients with RA and RARS usually present with a single cytopenia, anemia or neutropenia being the most common. Erythrocytes are usually normochromic and normocytic. Marrow and peripheral blood leukocytes may show very little evidence of dysplasia. The marrow may be normocellular or hypercellular. The marrow myeloid/erythroid ratio can be normal, increased, or decreased. In RARS, 15% or more of the nucleated erythroid precursors will have ringed sideroblastic changes.

Refractory Anemia with Excess Blasts and Refractory Anemia with Excess Blasts in Transformation

Patients with refractory anemia with excess blasts (RAEB) and refractory anemia with excess blasts in transformation (RAEB-IT) usually present with anemia, neutropenia, or thrombocytopenia. Red blood cells may be normochromic or include a macrocytic component. Anisopoikilocytosis is common. Nucleated red blood cells are often present. Neutrophils can display a range of changes including hypogranulation, abnormal nuclear lobulation, hypersegmentation, pseudo–Pelger–Heut changes, toxic granulation, and Chiediak–Higashi–like inclusions. Myeloid precursors including blasts are commonly present. Monocytes may have nuclear atypia and decreased granulation. Platelets can be overly large and lack the granular appearance of normal platelets.

The bone marrow is usually hypercellular, but hypocellularity is not uncommon in the pediatric patient. Erythropoiesis can be megaloblastic or megaloblastoid with accompanying atypical nuclear budding. Myelopoiesis is left-shifted with increased mitotic pool forms, easily identifiable myeloblasts, and nuclear/cytoplasmic maturation asynchrony. Metamyelocytes may display pseudo–Pelger–Huet changes. Dysplastic megakaryocytic changes include abnormal nuclear hyper- or hypolobulation, excessive cytoplasmic vacuolization, and retention of cytoplasmic basophilia. Increased reticulin fibrosis is uncommon and when present is usually accompanied by pooling of dysplastic megakaryocytes.

Chronic Myelomonocytic Leukemia

Childhood chronic myelomonocytic leukemia (CMMoL) more closely resembles the myeloproliferative disorder, chronic myelogenous leukemia, than MDS (94). In contrast to the adult form of CMMoL, most childhood cases of CMMoL show productive granulo- and monocytopoiesis with little evidence of dysplasia. The absolute peripheral blood monocyte count exceeds 1.0×10^9/L. In most cases only a few immature granulocytic and monocytic forms are found in the peripheral blood. The percentage of blasts in the marrow may be normal or slightly increased. Other cases of CMMoL show obvious dysplastic changes in one or more major cell lineages in addition to increased numbers of bone marrow blasts. If the marrow or peripheral blast count at diagnosis exceeds 20% or 5%, respectively, the process is referred to as CMMoL in transformation (CMMoL-IT).

Patients with CMMoL usually present with hepatosplenomegaly and frequently have lymphadenopathy and skin rashes (213). Fetal hemoglobin levels and serum immunoglobulins may be elevated. The course may progress rapidly to a myeloid blast crisis or follow a chronic course marked by progressive thrombocytopenia, anemia, and massive organomegaly.

By morphology alone, CMMoL is difficult to distinguish from CML or a congenital leukemoid reaction to Epstein–Barr virus or cytomegalovirus (Table 13). However, CMMoL differs from CML in not having the t(9;22) translocation and rearrangements of *BCR/ABL* (384). The LAP scores may be decreased, normal, or elevated and are not useful for confirming the diagnosis. Subclinical infections with Epstein–Barr virus or cytomegalovirus may mimic CMMoL with granulocytosis, monocytosis, and organomegaly (234,281,296,399,531). These infections can be identified by serologic and molecular techniques, but these tests do not always settle the question as to whether the infection is the cause or a symbiont of the proliferative process. The detection of a clonal chromosomal defect confirms the diagnosis of a malignant process but is found in less than 20% of cases (341).

Monosomy 7

Monosomy 7 is the most common cytogenetic abnormality in childhood MDS. The combination of MDS and monosomy 7 is sometimes considered to be a separate clinical entity because of its very poor clinical outcome (18,104,122,166,211,587). However, this cytogenetic abnormality may accompany all FAB morphologic subtypes of MDS. Some reports of childhood monosomy 7 have also included examples of de novo and secondary AML. As a result, no unifying set of morphologic changes characterizes this group of diseases.

Differential Diagnosis of MDS

The differential diagnosis of MDS includes early aplastic anemia, Fanconi's anemia, sideroblastic anemias,

TABLE 13. *Presenting features of chronic myelogenous leukemia (CML), chronic myelomonocytic leukemia (CMMoL), and leukemoid reactions*

Feature at diagnosis	CML	CMMoL	Leukemoid reaction[a]
Age	Usually >4 yr	Commonly >4 yr	Variable
Splenomegaly	Common	Common	Absent or slight
Hepatomegaly	Common	Common	Uncommon
WBC $>100 \times 10^9$/L	Common	Uncommon	Uncommon
Hemoglobin <12 g/dL	Variable	Common	Uncommon
Platelets	↑, normal, or ↓	Normal or ↓	Normal to ↑
Monocytes $<1 \times 10^9$/L	Uncommon	Always	Variable
Eosinophilia	Common	Occasional	Uncommon
Basophilia	Common	Occasional	Uncommon
LAP score	Low in 90% of cases	Variable	Normal to ↑
Marrow dysplasia	Mild	Mild to marked	Uncommon
Hemoglobin F levels	Normal	Commonly ↑	Normal
t(9;22)(q34;q11)	Present in >90%	Absent	Absent
BCL/ABL fusion gene[b]	Present in 100%	Absent	Absent

Abbreviations: CML, chronic myeloid leukemia; CMMoL, chronic myelomonocytic leukemia; ↑, increased; ↓, decreased; LAP, leukocyte alkaline phosphatase score (see text).

[a] Marked leukocytosis due to bacterial, parasitic, or viral infections; metastatic malignancy; or congenital heart disease.

[b] As detected by the polymerase chain reaction (see text).

congenital dyserythropoietic syndromes, megaloblastic anemia, transient myeloproliferative disorder of childhood, acute leukemia, and congenital viral infections. Comprehensive clinical history and laboratory studies will identify some of these disease processes. Some cases of de novo AML can present with less than 30% type 1 and type 2 blasts. If the t(8;21) or inv(16) chromosome anomalies of AML-M2 or AML-M4 are found, the patient should be classified as AML, as the clinical course of these AML patients with low blast percentages is more akin to AML than MDS.

Clinical Course

The clinical course in MDS is variable. Features associated with short survival include pancytopenia, greater than 5% blasts in the peripheral blood, abnormal localization of immature precursors in trephine biopsy, and cytogenetic abnormalities. The risk of progression to AML is greater for RAEB and RAEB-IT than RA with or without ringed sideroblasts. The preleukemic phase in children is usually short, i.e., 12–18 months, with rapid progression to AML. A rare case of MDS may transform into ALL (382). Prolonged aplasia with fatal infections or hemorrhages frequently complicates the posttherapy course. Abnormal colony forming unit (CFU-GM) in vitro growth features may be used as a clinical indicator of the disease course. Undetectable or low colony growth, increased numbers of clusters, and abnormal colony/cluster ratio in cultures of myeloid progenitors from bone marrow aspirates are related to leukemic transformation.

CHRONIC MYELOGENOUS LEUKEMIA

Chronic myelogenous leukemia (CML) is a clonal disorder of a multipotent hematopoietic stem cell (172,346). All cases of CML have the Ph[1] chromosome. Initially the disease presents with excessive numbers of neutrophils and their precursors in the peripheral blood and bone marrow. This indolent or chronic phase is invariably interrupted by transformation to an acute blastic process or blast crisis. The incidence of CML is less than 1 case per 100,000 for patients less than 20 years old. The male-to-female ratio is 1.8:1. Except for an association with the nuclear blasts in Japan (51), the cause of pediatric CML is unknown.

Pathogenesis

Cytogenetic, isoenzyme, and molecular studies have confirmed that myeloid, monocytic, eosinophilic, basophilic, erythroid, megakaryocytic, and lymphoid lineages are involved in CML. These cell lineages are the clonal progeny of a single early hematopoietic stem cell (167,171,172). In the patient with CML, nonhematopoietic cells such as the bone marrow fibroblast do not contain the Ph[1] chromosome (206). It is not understood as to why CML primarily presents as a granulocytic proliferation. The accumulation of granulocytes is in part due to more neutrophils being produced per myeloblast and to an increased life span of the mature neutrophil (533,536).

Classic cytogenetics detect the Ph[1] chromosome in more than 90% of cases of CML. All cases have evidence of this chromosome abnormality if molecular techniques are used (233). The Ph[1] is a result of a reciprocal translocation between chromosomes 9 and 22, the t(9;22)(q34;q11) (Fig. 17) (473). By cytogenetic studies, this translocation is indistinguishable from the t(9;22) found in ALL. In the t(9;22) translocation, the *ABL* gene on chromosome 9 is juxtaposed to the breakpoint cluster region (*BCR*) on chromosome 22 (Fig. 18). A new chimeric *BCR/ABL* gene results that encodes for a 210-kd protein, p210 (299,521). The normal *ABL* protooncogene codes for a tyrosine kinase that is located on the inner surface of the cell membrane and participates in signal transduction during cell differentiation (573). Compared with the normal ABL protein, the p210 protein has enhanced tyrosine kinase activity that may allow for unregulated cell growth (161). The cause of the t(9;22) translocation is unknown, and it is unclear as to whether the Ph[1] initiates the neoplastic transformation or is one of several events in a multistep process (173). The mechanism that underlies the transition of the chronic phase of CML to a blastic phase is unknown but is usually accompanied by the acquisition of additional chromosomal abnormalities.

Clinical Features

The most common presenting symptoms of patients with CML include malaise, fever, night sweats, weight loss, abdominal discomfort, a bleeding diathesis, and bone and joint pains (93). Splenomegaly is present in the majority of patients, whereas hepatomegaly and lymphadenopathy are less common. Skin nodules and extramedullary masses are uncommon. Leukostasis due to high WBC counts is uncommon in children but may give rise to papilledema, strokes, cerebellar signs, and priapism (93,472,540).

Laboratory Findings

The peripheral blood counts may fluctuate significantly during the course of CML (578). At diagnosis the WBC counts usually exceed 100×10^9/L (93,472). Platelet numbers are frequently increased above 400×10^9/L but may be normal or decreased. Anemia is variable and when present is usually normocytic and normochromic (93,510). At diagnosis, the granulocytic cells are predominantly banded and segmented neutrophils with fewer metamyelocytes and myelocytes. Myeloblasts and promyelocytes usually account for under 2% of the peripheral white cell differential. The myeloid elements are morphologically normal, whereas significant dysplastic change may herald an accelerated phase of the disease. Absolute eosinophilia and basophilia are common. The alkaline phosphatase activity of neutrophils, or leukocyte alkaline phosphatase score (LAP), is decreased in more than 90% of patients (470).

The bone marrow is always hypercellular due to a myeloid hyperplasia. Myelopoiesis is dominated by myelocytes, metamyelocytes, and neutrophils. Myeloblasts constitute less than 5% of the cellularity. Significantly increased percentages of myeloblasts and promyelocytes may be an indication of a more aggressive stage of disease or an impending blast crisis. Dysplastic cell changes are usually minimal. Megakaryocyte, eosinophil, and basophil numbers are commonly increased. Erythropoiesis is orderly, normoblastic, and occasionally increased. Pseudo-Gaucher cells or lipid-filled histiocytes are seen in many cases (146). Reticulin fibrosis, the increase of reticulin fibers without mature collagen fibrosis, is uncommon at diagnosis.

Clinical Course

Patients with CML may remain in a chronic phase of their disease for months to years. Control of hyperleukocytosis and thrombocytosis is maintained by treatment with busulfan or hydroxyurea. Therapy with α-interferon results in the return of normal blood counts in three quarters of patients and, unlike chemotherapy, often normalizes the bone marrow cytogenetics (547). However, these cytogenetically normal marrows will demonstrate *BCR/ABL* transcripts by PCR.

Inevitably, patients with CML develop a more aggressive form of the disease. A blast transformation intervenes at a median of 3 years (93). The blast crisis may be preceded by a transitional period or an accelerated phase, characterized by a shift in myelopoiesis to more immature forms and relative resistance to therapy (345). The presence of 30% or more blasts in the bone marrow or peripheral blood is considered evidence of blastic transformation (469). Extramedullary collections of blasts may be the initial presentation of blast transformation in some patients (375,469). The blast crisis of 40–50% of childhood cases is characterized by blasts with myelocytic morphology and immunophenotype. However, approximately 30–40% of patients develop a lymphoid blast crisis with early pre-B or, less commonly, pre-B immunophenotype. Blast transformations can also be megakaryoblastic, rarely T-lymphoblastic, or occasionally a mixture of two or more cell lineages. The blast phase is frequently accompanied by the appearance of additional Ph[1] chromosomes, trisomy 8, or isochromosome 17 (514). The LAP score may return to normal during the accelerated and blast phases (470).

Differential Diagnosis

In the pediatric age group the differential diagnosis of CML includes CMMoL and leukemoid reactions to bacterial or viral infections (Table 13). The myeloproliferative disorders, polycythemia vera and primary myelofibrosis, can also be confused with CML, but these are very rare malignancies in childhood. The correct diagnosis of CML is rapidly confirmed by cytogenetic or molecular studies. RT-PCR and FISH techniques can be performed with peripheral blood and have the advantage of being more sensitive than classic cytogenetics. The nonspecific LAP score should be abandoned for diagnostic purposes.

HUMAN LYMPHOTROPIC VIRUS-1–ASSOCIATED LEUKEMIA/LYMPHOMA

A mixed leukemia/lymphoma process with unique clinical, morphologic, and immunophenotypic features was first recognized in the southwestern part of Japan, particularly on the island of Kyushu (565,584). A retrovirus isolated from a Japanese case of this malignancy had the same DNA sequence of a retrovirus isolated from an American patient with mycosis fungoides (409,601). At a joint conference between Japanese and U.S. investigators, the names "adult T-cell leukemia" (ATL) and "human T-lymphotropic virus type 1" (HTLV-1) were proposed for the disease process and the virus, respectively (53). ATL was subsequently recognized in other HTLV-1 endemic areas, including western Africa, the Caribbean Islands, and parts of South America (96).

Cases of childhood HTLV-1-related malignancies are very uncommon in the United States and in endemic regions of the world (183,227). In the United States, most adult and the few recognized pediatric patients have been from southeastern states and Hawaii, i.e., regions receiving immigrants from endemic areas of the world. Most pediatric cases of ATL are the result of perinatal acquisition of HTLV-1. The incidence of ATL among HTLV-1-infected persons is low, and a long latent period exists between viral infection and development of ATL (395).

Clinical and Laboratory Features

The pediatric presentation of ATL is similar to that of adults. ATL is characterized by peripheral lymphadenopathy, skin involvement, hepatosplenomegaly, and absence of thymic enlargement. Increased serum lactic dehydrogenase and hypercalcemia are common at presentation.

In the leukemic phase, the peripheral blood will contain distinctly abnormal lymphoid cells that are slightly larger than normal. The nuclei of these cells display characteristic prominent lobulation and deep, wide indentations (Fig. 36). The chromatin is clumped and nucleoli are absent or vague. Cytoplasmic granules are uncommon. Initially, the bone marrow shows no or little leukemic disease even in the presence of high peripheral blood counts. Involvement of the central nervous system occurs in more than 50% of patients.

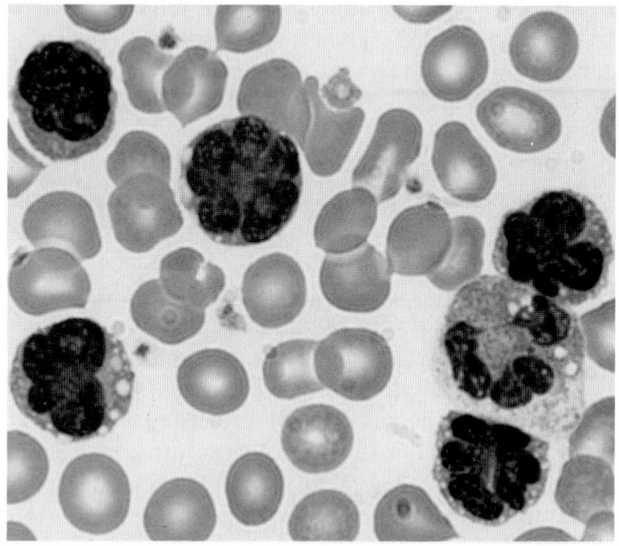

FIG. 36. HTLV-1 leukemia. Leukemic cells have multilobated nuclei with dense chromatin. (Wright's stain.)

The immunophenotype of ATL cells resembles that of activated T-helper cells and is thus characterized by expression of CD2, CD3, CD4, CD5, and CD25. Unlike blasts of T-ALL, cells of ATL lack CD7. The diagnosis of HTLV-1-associated ATL is confirmed by serologic evidence of antibodies to HTLV-1, demonstration of viral antigens in malignant cells, or the finding of HTLV-1 DNA by Southern blot hybridization or PCR.

CHRONIC LYMPHOCYTIC LEUKEMIA

Chronic lymphocytic leukemia (CLL) is the most common type of leukemia in elderly adults, who present with a marked peripheral blood lymphocytosis, lymphadenopathy, splenomegaly, and bone marrow lymphocytosis. In contrast, there are only a few well-documented cases of CLL in children (23,169,459, 515,600). Children with CLL may present with lymphadenopathy, splenomegaly, and, less commonly, hepatomegaly. They have a peripheral blood lymphocytosis, and their marrow is infiltrated by small mature-appearing lymphocytes. Similar to adult CLL, the lymphocytes express monoclonal IgM, sometimes with coexpression of IgD. Lymphocytes in one described case coexpressed CD19, CD20, and CD5, a pattern also characteristic of adult CLL (23). Unlike most lymphoblastic leukemias, lymphoid cells of CLL do not express CD34 or TDT. A t(2;14)(p13;q32) translocation has been found in several pediatric CLLs and is a very uncommon chromosomal anomaly in adult CLL (515,600).

DOWN SYNDROME AND TRANSIENT MYELOPROLIFERATIVE DISORDER AND LEUKEMIA

Children with Down syndrome have an estimated 10- to 15-fold increased risk of developing acute leukemias (181). These patients comprised about 2% of the children enrolled in two large ALL studies (431,446,466). In these reports, ALL patients with or without Down syndrome did not differ with regard to race, sex, organomegaly, central nervous system leukemia at diagnosis, initial leukocyte count, and FAB subtype (263). However, Down syndrome patients are less likely to have T-ALL or the t(9;22), t(4;11), or t(1;19) (431). Down syndrome patients experience more chemotherapy-related toxicities as a result of their inability to clear methotrexate and other drugs, putting them at increased risk for induction failure (52,192).

The proportion of AML cases among Down syndrome patients with acute leukemia is similar to that of other children. However, 75% of cases of AML in Down syndrome occur in patients less than 3 years of age, as compared with 25% of cases in other patients. A considerably larger proportion of AMLs in Down syndrome are acute megakaryoblastic leukemias (or AML-M7) (313,606, 607). A myelodysplastic syndrome precedes the megakaryoblastic leukemia in 50–85% of patients (221, 288,608). The ultrastructural characteristics and surface antigens of leukemic megakaryoblasts of Down patients do not differ from those of other childhood AML-M7 cases (608). Up to 35% of megakaryocytic leukemias associated with Down syndrome have trisomy 8 (608).

Infants with Down syndrome may present with a transient myeloproliferative process that may be morphologically indistinguishable from acute leukemia (607). The peripheral white cell count may be as high as 500×10^9 cells/L but is usually less than 60×10^9/L. Blasts may constitute 75% or more of the circulating leukocytes. The marrow blast percentage is often less than that of the peripheral blood. The blasts are usually MPO-, SBB-, and NSE-negative. With ultrastructural and immunologic studies, the blasts commonly show evidence of megakaryocytic, erythroid, and basophilic differentiation (114,607). The megakaryocytic elements may be monoclonal in origin (298). The proliferative process usually regresses within 2 months (607), but up to 30% of affected patients develop leukemia within the first 3 years of life (607).

ACUTE LEUKEMIA WITH ABERRANT LYMPHOID/MYELOID ANTIGEN EXPRESSION (Acute Mixed Lineage Leukemia, Biphenotypic Leukemia, Hybrid Leukemia)

The choice of therapy for an acute leukemia is based on whether the lineage of the leukemia is lymphoid or myeloid. According to earlier concepts, leukemias represent a clonal expansion of an original, transformed cell. Furthermore, a leukemia was considered a reflection of a frozen stage of hematopoietic cell differentiation. From this theorem it followed that these clonal expansions should mirror the differentiation or biologic features of their normal cellular counterparts (lineage fidelity). However, subsequent immunologic and molecular studies have shown that many leukemias simultaneously express characteristics of more than one lineage (lineage infidelity) (27,128,369,525).

Acute leukemias containing blasts that simultaneously demonstrate features of more than one lineage, e.g., lymphoid plus myeloid, have been given names that include acute mixed lineage, hybrid, chimeric, and biphenotypic leukemia (Table 14). Not to be confused with these terms, the names "biclonal," "bilineal," or "oligoclonal" are used to refer to leukemias that consist of two or more separate lineages. The terms "lineage switch" and "secondary" leukemia refer to sequential changes of lineage with time or changes of lineage during

TABLE 14. *Definitions of leukemias with features of more than one lineage*

Term	Definition
Acute mixed lineage, hybrid, or biphenotypic leukemia	A single blast population that simultaneously expresses antigens of two or more lineages
Biclonal, oligoclonal, or bilineal leukemia	Coexistence of two or more populations of blasts representing different lineages
Asynchronous maturation	A single lineage with leukemic cells that simultaneously expresses "differentiation" antigens of early and late stages of development
Lineage switch or metachronous leukemia	A complete cell lineage change (eg, ALL to AML or ALL to ALL) with time but with evidence that both leukemic processes are derived from the same clone
Secondary leukemia	A complete lineage change with time with no evidence that the first and subsequent leukemic processes are derived from the same malignant clone. This term implies but does not require an external influence (e.g., chemotherapy)

therapy or with relapse. The mixed lineage or hybrid types of leukemia have been defined by morphologic, cytochemical, immunologic, ultrastructural, and molecular studies. Most of these leukemias have been identified by immunologic studies.

Acute mixed lineage leukemia consists of two different categories of leukemia: ALL with myeloid-associated antigens (My$^+$ALL), and AML with lymphoid-associated antigen expression (Ly$^+$AML). Despite our ability to recognize these types of leukemia, we have been burdened with little agreement as to diagnostic criteria, nomenclature, and therapeutic or prognostic implications (152,153). This disharmony is not surprising, as reported investigations differ significantly as to patient population studied (pediatric, adult, or a mixture); stringency of initial definitions of lymphoblastic and myeloblastic lineages; methods of analysis (flow cytometry vs. fluorescence microscopy vs. immunohistochemistry); single- or two-color analysis (proof of coexpression of lineage-associated antigens); types and numbers of monoclonal antibody studies; consideration for epitopic heterogeneity among antibodies within a CD group; cutoff values for the discrimination of positive vs. negative tests; inclusion of antigens that are not lineage-specific (e.g., CD4, CD11b, CD14, TDT, CD10); and source of sample analyzed (marrow, blood, fresh vs. old vs. cryopreserved).

The general consensus among several large pediatric studies of ALL is that myeloid-associated antigen expression in childhood ALL has no independent prognostic significance (60,335,422,434,438), although several articles conclude otherwise (175,591). Similarly, studies of pediatric Ly$^+$AML suggest no effect of lymphoid antigen expression on clinical outcome (434,507). Until a clear consensus as to the importance of atypical antigen expression in acute leukemias is agreed on, Ly$^+$AML and My$^+$ALL should not be singled out for different therapeutic approaches.

The ongoing studies of acute leukemias at St. Jude Children's Research Hospital use the criteria in Table 15 to define My$^+$ALL, Ly$^+$AML, and true mixed lineage leukemia. Central to this classification is the establishment of criteria for classifying a leukemia as lymphoid or myeloid. When blasts of a leukemic process coexpress "lineage-specific" (CD3, CD79, and MPO) markers for more than one lineage, the leukemia may be an example of a true mixed lineage leukemia.

The recognition of My$^+$ALL and Ly$^+$AML may be useful for the screening of leukemic processes for cytogenetic abnormalities that may be associated with clinical outcome. Infants and possibly older adolescents with leukemias having the t(4;11)(q21;q23) have a increased risk of relapse and subsequent poor response to chemotherapy reinduction (419,427). The blasts from these patients usually are B-lineage (CD19+ and CD22+), usually lack CD10, and commonly express the myeloid-associated antigens CD15 and CDw65 (419,427). Since more than 90% of B-lineage ALLs express CD10 and less than 10% express CD15, the immunophenotype of CD19+, CD10–, and CD15+ or CDw65+ is highly predictive for the t(4;11).

Similarly, AML-M2 and uncommonly AML-M1 blasts with a t(8;21)(q22;q22) have a characteristic immunophenotype. The leukemic blasts of these cases weakly express CD13 and CD33 but commonly have detectable CD19 and sometimes CD56 (246). In contrast, the blasts of AML-M2 without the t(8;21) often strongly express CD13 and CD33, frequently demonstrate CD2

TABLE 15. *SJCRH criteria for My$^-$ALL, Ly$^-$AML, and true mixed-lineage leukemia*

B-lineage My^{+1}ALL[a]	Ly$^+$AML[a]
1. ≥90% of blasts are CD19$^+$ plus CD79$^+$	1. ≥3% blasts are MPO$^+$
2. Leukemic blasts are cytoplasmic CD3$^-$	2. Leukemic blasts are cytoplasmic CD3$^-$
3. Leukemic blasts are MPO$^-$[b,c]	3. Leukemic blasts are CD79$^-$
4. Leukemic blasts express ≥1 myeloid-associated antigens: CD13, CD15, CD33, CD36, or CD65	4. Leukemic blasts express ≥1 lymphoid-associated antigens: CD2, CD5, CD7, CD19, CD22, CD56
T-lineage My$^+$ALL[a,b]	**True mixed-lineage leukemia**
1. ≥90% of blasts are CD7$^+$ plus CD3$^-$	≥60% of blasts coexpress MPO[d] and CD79
2. Leukemic blasts are CD79$^-$	*or*
3. Leukemic blasts are MPO$^-$[c]	≥60% of blasts coexpress MPO[d] and CD3[e]
4. Leukemic blasts express ≥1 myeloid-associated antigens:	*or*
CD13, CD15, CD33, CD36, or CD	≥60% of blasts coexpress CD3[e] and CD79

Abbreviations: SJCRH, St. Jude Children's Research Hospital; My$^-$ALL, acute lymphoblastic leukemia (ALL); expressing myeloid-associated antigens; Ly$^-$AML, acute myeloid leukemia expressing lymphoid-associated antigens; MPO, myeloperoxidase.

[a] All four criteria must be met.
[b] MPO by cytochemical testing <3%.
[c] MPO-negative by anti-MPO antibody testing or ultrastructural analysis.
[d] MPO-positive by cytochemistry, anti-MPO antibody testing, or ultrastructural analysis.
[e] Surface or cytoplasmic CD3-positive.

or CD7, but rarely show CD19 and CD56 (246). There are exceptions to these atypical immunophenotypes but their presence should alert one to the possible presence or absence of a t(8;21), which may be associated with a better clinical outcome.

ACKNOWLEDGMENT

Supported in part by Cancer Center Support CORE grant P30 CA21765 and by American Lebanese Syrian Associated Charities (ALSAC).

REFERENCES

1. Abe R, Raza A, Preisler HD, Tebbi CK, Sandberg AA. Chromosomes and causation of human cancer and leukemia. LIV. Near tetraploidy in acute leukemia. *Cancer Genet Cytogenet* 1985;14:45–59.
2. Abildgaard CF. Unique features of metastatic neuroblastoma in the bone marrow. *Am J Clin Pathol* 1980;74:363–364.
3. Abromowitch M, Williams DL, Melvin SL, Stass S. Evidence for clonal evolution in pre B-cell leukemia. *Br J Haematol* 1984;56:409–416.
4. Adams JM, Gerondakis S, Webb E, Corcoran LM, Cory S. Cellular myc oncogene is altered by chromosome translocation to an immunoglobulin locus in murine plasmacytomas and is rearranged similarly in human Burkitt lymphomas. *Proc Natl Acad Sci USA* 1983;80:1982–1986.
5. Adams JM, Harris AW, Pinkert CA, et al. The c-myc oncogene driven by immunoglobulin enhancers induces lymphoid malignancy in transgenic mice. *Nature* 1985;318:533–538.
6. Adriaansen HJ, te Boekhorst PAW, Hagemeijer AM, van der Schoot CE, Delwel HR, van Dongen JJ. Acute myeloid leukemia M4 with bone marrow eosinophilia (M4E0) and inv(16)(p13q22) exhibits a specific immunophenotype with CD2 expression. *Blood* 1993;81:3043–3051.
7. Adriaansen HJ, van Dongen JJM, Hooijkaas H, van't Veer MB, Lo¨wenberg B, Hagemeijer A. Translocation (6;9) may be associated with a specific TdT-positive immunological phenotype in ANLL. *Leukemia* 1988;2:136–140.
8. Alexander E, Henkart P. The adherence of human Fc receptor-bearing lymphocytes to antigen–antibody complexes. *J Exp Med* 1976;143:329–347.
9. Almanaseer IY, Trujillo YP, Taxy JB, Okuno T. Systemic rhabdomyosarcoma with diffuse bone marrow involvement. *Am J Clin Pathol* 1984;82:349–353.
10. Andreff MM. Flow cytometry of leukemia. In: Melamed MR, Lindmo T, Mendelson ML, eds. *Flow Cytometry and Sorting.* New York: Wiley-Liss; 1990.
11. Aplan PD, Lombardi DP, Kirsh IR. Structural characterization of SCL, a gene frequently disrupted in T-cell acute lymphoblastic leukemia. *Mol Cell Biol* 1991;11:5462–5469.
12. Aplan PD, Lombardi DP, Reaman GH, Sather HN, Hammond D, Kirsch I. Involvement of the putative hematopoietic transcription factor SCL in T-cell acute lymphoblastic leukemia. *Blood* 1992;79:1327–1333.
13. Armata J, Grzeskowiak-Melanowska J, Balwierz W, Najbar-Pabiam A, Pawlik-Niesytto E. Prognosis in acute lymphoblastic leukemia (ALL) in children preceded by an aplastic phase. *Leuk Lymph* 1994;13:517–518.
14. Arthur DC, Bloomfield CD. Partial deletion of the long arm of chromosome 16 and bone marrow eosinophilia in acute nonlymphocytic leukemia: a new association. *Blood* 1983;61:994–998.
15. Ashfaq R, Weinberg AG, Argyle CA. Acute megakaryoblastic leukemia simulating carcinoma. *Am J Clin Pathol* 1992;98:55–60.
16. Avvisati G, ten Cate JW, Mandelli F. Acute promyelocytic leukemia. *Br J Haematol* 1992;81:315–320.
17. Bader JL, Miller RW. Neurofibromatosis and childhood leukemia. *J Pediatr* 1978;92:925–929.
18. Baranger L, Baruchel A, Leverger G, Schaison G, Berger R. Monosomy-7 in childhood hemopoietic disorders. *Leukemia* 1990;4:345–349.
19. Barletta C, Pelicci P-G, Kenyon LC, Smith SD, Dalla-Favera R. Relationship between the c-myb locus and the 6q-chromosomal aberration in leukemias and lymphomas. *Science* 1987;235:1064–1067.
20. Bates MN. Extremely low frequency electromagnetic fields and cancer. The epidemiologic evidence. *Environ Health Perspect* 1991;95:147–156.
21. Bearman RM, Winberg CD, Maslow WC, et al. Terminal deoxynucleotidyl transferase in neoplastic and non-neoplastic hematopoietic cells. *Am J Clin Pathol* 1981;75:794–802.
22. Behm FG, Head DR, Pui C-H, Rivera GR, Riberio RC, Raimondi SC. B-precursor ALL with unexpected expression of surface immunoglobulin (sIg) mu and lambda. *Mod Pathol* 1995;8:106.
23. Behm FG, McWilliams NB, Westin EH, et al. Chronic lymphocytic leukemia in a child. *Proc Am Pediatr Soc* 1985;19:258 (abstract).
24. Behm FG, Raimondi SC, Schell MJ, Look AT, Rivera GK, Pui C-H. Lack of CD45 antigen on blast cells in childhood acute lymphoblastic leukemia is associated with chromosome hyperdiploidy and other favorable prognostic features. *Blood* 1992;79:1011–1016.
25. Behm FG, Smith FO, Raimondi SC, Pui C-H, Bernstein ID. The human homologue of the rat chondrotin sulfate proteoglycan, NG2, detected by monoclonal antibody 7.1, identifies childhood acute lymphoblastic leukemias with t(4;11)(q21;q23) or t(11;19)(q23;p13) and MLL gene rearrangements. *Blood.* In press.
26. Bellucci S, Han ZC, Pidard D, Caen JP. Identification of a normal human bone marrow cell population co-expressing megakaryocytic and erythroid markers in culture. *Eur J Haematol* 1992;48:259–265.
27. Ben-Bassat I, Gale RP. Hybrid acute leukemia. *Leuk Res* 1986;8:929–936.
28. Ben-Ezra J, Sheibani K, Hwang DL, Lev-Ran A. Megakaryocyte synthesis is the source of epidermal growth factor in human platelets. *Am J Pathol* 1990;137:755–759.
29. Ben-Ezra J, Weinberg CD, Wu A, Rappaport H. Leu-9 (CD7) positivity in acute leukemias: a marker of T-cell lineage? *Hematol Pathol* 1987;1:147–156.
30. Bennett JM, Catovsky D, Daniel M-T, et al. Proposals for the classification of acute leukemia. *Br J Haematol* 1976;33:451–458.
31. Bennett JM, Catovsky D, Daniel M-T, et al. The morphologic classification of acute lymphoblastic leukemia: concordence among observers and clinical correlations. *Br J Haematol* 1981;47:553–561.
32. Bennett JM, Catovsky D, Daniel M-T, et al. Proposals for the classification of the myelodysplastic syndromes. *Br J Haematol* 1982;51:189–199.
33. Bennett JM, Catovsky D, Daniel M-T, et al. Criteria for the diagnosis of acute leukemia of megakaryocyte lineage (M7). A report of the French–American–British Cooperative Group. *Ann Intern Med* 1985;103:460–462.
34. Bennett JM, Catovsky D, Daniel M-T, et al. Proposed revised criteria for the classification of acute myeloid leukemia. A report of the French–American–British Cooperative Group. *Ann Intern Med* 1985;103:626–629.
35. Bennett JM, Catovsky D, Daniel M-T, et al. Proposal for the recognition of minimally differentiated acute myeloid leukemia (AML-M0). *Br J Haematol* 1991;78:325–329.
36. Beran A, Burns CF, Gray L, Cawley JC. Cytochemistry of human T cell subpopulations. *Scand J Immunol* 1980;11:223–233.
37. Berger R, Bernheim A, Sigaux F, Daniel M-T, Valensi F, Flandrin G. Acute monocytic leukemia chromosome studies. *Leuk Res* 1982;6:17–26.
38. Berger R, Flandrin G, Bernheim A, et al. Cytogenetic studies on 519 consecutive de novo acute nonlymphocytic leukemias. *Cancer Genet Cytogenet* 1987;29:9–21.

39. Bernard A, Boumsell L, Dausset J, Milstein C, Schlossman SF. Leucocyte typing. Human leucocyte differentiation antigens detected by monoclonal antibodies. New York: Springer-Verlag; 1984.
40. Bernard O, Larsen C-J, Hampe A, Mauchautte M, Berger R, Mathieu-Mahul D. Molecular mechanisms of a t(8;14)(q24;q11) translocation juxtaposing c-myc and TCR-α genes in a T-cell leukaemia: involvement of a Vα internal heptamer. *Oncogene* 1988;2:195–200.
41. Bernard O, Lecointe N, Jonveaux P, et al. Two site-specific deletions and t(1;14) translocation restricted to human T-cell acute leukemias disrupt the 5′ part of the tal-1 gene. *Oncogene* 1991;6: 1477–1488.
42. Bernard P, Dachary D, Reiffers J, et al. Acute nonlymphocytic leukemia with marrow eosinophilia and chromosome 16 abnormality: a report of 18 cases. *Leukemia* 1989;3:740–745.
43. Bernasconi C, Brusamolino E, Castelli G. Eosinophilia in T-cell acute lymphoblastic leukemia. *Abstracts of the XVII Congress of the International Society of Hematology.* Paris, 1978;760 (abstract).
44. Bessho F, Fujiu M, Kinumaki H. Acute non-lymphocytic leukemia showing abnormal nuclear lobulation. *Am J Clin Pathol* 1981;75:684–692.
45. Bettaieb A, Villeval JL, Kieffer N, Farace F, Edelman L, Cartron JP, Vainchenker W. Early erythroid markers as probes for normal and leukemic erythroid differentiation. *Ann Inst Pasteur Immunol* 1987;138:877–883.
46. Betz SA, Foucar K, Head DR, Chen I-M, Willman CL. False-positive flow cytometric platelet glycoprotein IIb/IIIa expression in myeloid leukemias secondary to platelet adherence to blasts. *Blood* 1992;79:2399–2403.
47. Biondi A, Rambaldi A, Pandolfi PP, et al. Molecular monitoring of the myl/retinoic acid receptor-α fusion gene in acute promyelocytic leukemia by polymerase chain reaction. *Blood* 1992;80: 492–497.
48. Bitter MA, Le Beau MM. Comparison of eosinophils in acute nonlymphocytic leukaemia associated with the t(8;21) and inv(16). *Br J Haematol* 1985;59:185–187.
49. Bitter MA, Le Beau MM, Larson RA, Rosner MC, Golomb HM, Rowley JD, Vardiman JW. A morphologic and cytochemical study of acute myelomonocytic leukemia with abnormal marrow eosinophils associated with inv(16)(p13q22). *Am J Clin Pathol* 1984;81:733–741.
50. Bitter MA, Le Beau MM, Rowley JD, Larson RA, Golomb HM, Vardiman JW. Associations between morphology, karyotype and clinical features in myeloid leukemias. *Hum Pathol* 1987;18: 211–225.
51. Bizzozero OJ, Jr, Johnson KG. Radiation-related leukemias in Hisroshima and Nagasaki, 1946–1964. II. Observations on type-specific leukemia, survivorship, and clinical behavior. *Ann Intern Med* 1967;66:522–526.
52. Blatt J, Albo V, Prin W, Orlando S, Wollman M. Excessive chemotherapy-related myelotoxicity in children with Down's syndrome and acute lymphoblastic leukemia. *Lancet* 1986;2: 914.
53. Blattner WA, Takatsuki Y, Steele PE, Tykocins M, Martin MA. Human T-cell leukemia/lymphoma virus and adult T-cell leukemia. *JAMA* 1981;250:1074–1080.
54. Boder E. Ataxia-telangiectasia: an overview. In: Gratti RA, Swift M, eds. *Ataxia Telangiectasia: Genetics, Neuropathology, and Immunology of a Degenerative Disease of Childhood.* New York: Alan R. Liss Inc; 1985:1–63.
55. Boehm T, Baer R, Lavenir I, Forster A, Waters JJ, Nacheva E, Rabbitts TH. The mechanism of chromosomal translocation t(11;14) involving the T-cell receptor of Cδ locus on human chromosome 14q11 and a transcribed region of chromosome 11q15. *EMBO J* 1988;7:385–394.
56. Boehm T, Buluwela L, Williams D, White L, Rabbitts TH. A cluster of chromosome 11p13 translocations found via distinct D-D and D-D-J rearrangements of the human T cell receptor δ chain gene. *EMBO J* 1988;7:2011–2017.
57. Boehm T, Foroni L, Kaneko Y, Perutz MF, Rabbitts TH. The rhombotin family of cysteine-rich LIM-domain oncogenes: distinct members are involved in T-cell translocations to human chromosomes 11p15 and 11p13. *Proc Natl Acad Sci USA* 1991;88:4367–4371.
58. Bollum FJ. Terminal deoxynucleotidyl transferase as a hematopoietic cell marker. *Blood* 1979;54:1203–1215.
59. Borowitz MJ, Hunger SP, Carroll AJ, Shuster JJ, Pullen DJ. Steuber CP, Cleary ML. Predictability of the t(1;19) (q23;p13) from surface antigen phenotype: implications for screening cases of childhood acute lymphoblastic leukemia for molecular analysis: a Pediatric Oncology Group study. *Blood* 1993;82:1086–1091.
60. Borowitz MJ, Shuster JJ, Land VJ, et al. Myeloid antigen expression in childhood acute lymphoblastic leukemia. *N Engl J Med* 1991;325:1379–1380.
61. Borrow J, Goddard AD, Gibbons B, et al. Diagnosis of acute promyelocytic leukemia by RT-PCR: detection of PML-RARα and RARα-PML fusion transcripts. *Br J Haematol* 1992;82:529–540.
62. Borrow J, Goddard AD, Sheer D, Soloman E. Molecular analysis of acute promyelocytic leukemia breakpoint cluster region on chromosome 17. *Science* 1990;249:1577–1579.
63. Borrow J, Shipley J, Howe K, et al. Molecular analysis of simple variant translocations in acute promyelocytic leukemia. *Genes Chrom Cancer* 1994;9:234–243.
64. Brandwein JM, Horsman DE, Eaves AC, et al. Childhood myelodysplasia: suggested classification of myelodysplastic syndromes based on laboratory and clinical findings. *Am J Pediatr Hematol Oncol* 1990;12:63–70.
65. Braziel RM, Keneklis T, Donlon JA, Hsu S-M, Cossman J, Bollum FJ, Jaffe ES. Terminal deoxynucleotidyl transferase in non-Hodgkin's lymphoma. *Am J Clin Pathol* 1983;80:655–659.
66. Breatnach F, Chessells JM, Greaves MF. The aplastic presentation of childhood leukemia: a feature of common-ALL. *Br J Haematol* 1981;49:387–393.
67. Breton-Gorius J, Houssay D. Auer rods in acute promyelocytic leukemia: demonstration of their structure and peroxidase localization. *Lab Invest* 1973;28:135–141.
68. Breton-Gorius J, Lewis JC, Guichard J, Kieffer N, Vainchenker W. Monoclonal antibodies specific for human platelet membrane glycoproteins bind to monocytes by focal absorption of platelet membrane fragments: an ultrastructural immunogold study. *Leukemia* 1987;1:131–141.
69. Breton-Gorius J, Reyes F, Duhamel G, Najman A, Gorin NC. Megakaryoblastic acute leukemia: identification by the ultrastructural demonstration of platelet peroxidase. *Blood* 1978;51: 45–60.
70. Breton-Gorius J, Vanhaeke D, Pryzwansky KB, Guichard J, Tabilio A, Vainchenker W, Carmel R. Simultaneous detection of membrane markers with monoclonal antibodies and peroxidatic activities in leukemia: ultrastructural analysis using a new method of fixation preserving the platelet peroxidase. *Br J Haematol* 1984;58:447–458.
71. Breton-Gorius J, Villeval JL, Mitjavila MT, et al. Ultrastructural and cytochemical characterization of blasts from early erythroblastic leukemias. *Leukemia* 1987;1:173–181.
72. Breton-Gorius J, Villeval JL, Kieffer R, Mitjavila MT, Guichard J, Vainchenker W. Limits of phenotypic markers for the diagnosis of megakaryoblastic leukemia. *Blood Cells* 1989;15:259–277.
73. Brizard A, Guilhot F, Huret JL, Benz-Lemoine E, Tanzer J. The 8p11 anomaly in "monoblastic" leukemia. *Leuk Res* 1988;12: 693–697.
74. Brown L, Cheng J-T, Chen Q, Siciliano MJ, Crist W, Buchanan G, Baer R. Site-specific recombination of the tal-1 gene is a common occurrence in human T cell leukemia. *EMBO J* 1990;9: 3343–3351.
75. Brunning RD, Parkin JL, Hanson CA. Hematopoietic and lymphoreticular neoplasms. In: Azar HA, ed. *Pathology of Human Neoplasms: An Atlas of Diagnostic Electron Microscopy and Immunohistochemistry.* New York: Raven Press; 1988:221–303.
76. Buccheri V, Shetty V, Yoshida N, Morilla R, Matutes E, Catovsky D. The role of an anti-myeloperoxidase antibody in the diagnosis and classification of acute leukaemia: a comparison with light and electron microscopy cytochemistry. *Br J Haematol* 1992;80:62–68.
77. Burrows PD, Cooper MD. B-cell development in man. *Curr Opin Immunol* 1993;5:201–206.

78. Caldwell CW, Patterson WP. Relationship of T200 antigen expression to stages of B-cell differentiation in marrow resurgent hyperplasia. *Blood* 1987;70:1165–1172.
79. Callen DF, Raphael K, Michael PM, Garson OM. Acute lymphoblastic leukemia with a hypodiploid karyotype with less than 40 chromosomes: the basis for division into two subgroups. *Leukemia* 1989;3:749–752.
80. Campana D. The developmental stages of the human T cell receptors. *Thymus* 1989;13:3–18.
81. Campana D, Coustan-Smith E, Behm FG. The definition of remission in acute leukemia with immunologic techniques. *Bone Marrow Transpl* 1991;8:429–437.
82. Campana D, Janossy G. Analysis of myeloid antigens on the cell surface and in the cytoplasm. In: McMichael AJ, ed. *Leucocyte Typing III. White Cell Differentiation Antigens.* New York: Oxford University Press; 1987:661–666.
83. Campana D, Janossy G, Bofill M, et al. Human B cell development. I. Phenotypic differences of B lymphocytes in the bone marrow and peripheral lymphoid tissues. *J Immunol* 1985;134:1524–1529.
84. Campana D, Kumagai M, Manabe A, Murti KG, Behm FG, Mahmoud H, Raimondi SC. Hyperdiploid acute lymphoblastic leukemia (ALL): a distinct biological entity with marked propensity to programmed cell death. *Blood* 1993;82:49a (abstract).
85. Campbell LJ, Challis J, Fox T, Garson DM. Chromosome 16 abnormalities associated with myeloid malignancies. *Genes Chrom Cancer* 1991;3:55–61.
86. Cantu`-Rajnoldi A, Invernizzi R, Biondi A, et al. Biological and clinical features of acute lymphoblastic leukemia with cytoplasmic granules or inclusions: description of eight cases. *Br J Haematol* 1989;73:309–314.
87. Carroll AJ, Castleberry RP, Crist WM. Lack of association between abnormalities of the chromosome 9 short arm and either "lymphomatous" features of T cell phenotype in childhood acute lymphocytic leukemia. *Blood* 1987;69:735–738.
88. Carroll A, Civin C, Schneider N, et al. The t(1;22)(p13;q23) is nonrandom and is restricted to infants with acute megakaryoblastic leukemia: a Pediatric Oncology Group study. *Blood* 1991;78:748–752.
89. Carroll AJ, Crist WM, Link MP, et al. The t(1;14)(p34;q11) is non-random and restricted to T-cell acute lymphoblastic leukemia. A Pediatric Oncology group study. *Blood* 1990;76:1220–1224.
90. Carroll AJ, Crist WM, Parmley RT, Roper M, Cooper MD, Finley WH: Pre-B cell leukemia associated with chromosome translocation 1;19. *Blood* 1984;63:721–724.
91. Carter M, Kalwinsky DK, Dahl GV, Santana VM, Mason CA, Schell MJ. Childhood acute promyelocytic leukemia: a rare variant of nonlymphoid leukemia with distinctive clinical and biological features. *Leukemia* 1989;3:298–302.
92. Castella A, Davey FR, Kurec AS, Nelson DA. Presence of Burkitt-like cells in non-Burkitt's neoplasms. *Cancer* 1982;50:1764–1770.
93. Castro-Malaspina H, Schaison G, Briere J, et al. Philadelphia chromosome-positive chronic myelocytic leukemia in children. Survival and prognostic factors. *Cancer* 1983;52;721–727.
94. Castro-Malaspina H, Schaison G, Passe S, et al. Subacute and chronic myelomonocytic leukemia in children (juvenile CML). Clinical and hematologic observations, and identification of prognostic factors. *Cancer* 1984;54:675–686.
95. Catovsky D, Bernasconi C, Verdonck PJ, et al. The association of eosinophilia with lymphoblastic leukemia or lymphoma: a study of seven patients. *Br J Haematol* 1980;45:523–534.
96. Catovsky D, Greaves MF, Rose M, et al. Adult T-cell lymphoma-leukemia in blacks from the West Indies. *Lancet* 1982;1:639–643.
97. Cerezo L, Head DR, Pullen J, Humphrey B. The prevalence of hand–mirror cells in acute myeloblastic and lymphoblastic leukemia. *Am J Clin Pathol* 1981;81:355–357.
98. Cerazo L, Shuster JJ, Pullen DJ, et al. Laboratory correlates and prognostic significance of granular acute lymphoblastic leukemia in children. *Am J Clin Pathol* 1991;95:526–531.
99. Chan WC, Brynes RK, Kim TH, Verras A, Schick C, Green RJ, Ragab AH. Acute megakaryoblastic leukemia in early childhood. *Blood* 1983;62:92–98.
100. Charak BS, Advani SH, Karandikar SM, et al. Sudan black B positivity in acute lymphoblastic leukemia. *Acta Haematol* 1988;80:199–202.
101. Chen Q, Cheng J-T, Tsai L-H, et al. The tal gene undergoes chromosome translocation in T cell leukemia and potentially encodes a helix-loop-helix protein. *EMBO J* 1990;9:415–424.
102. Chen S-J, Zelent A, Tong J-H, et al. Rearrangements of the retinoic acid receptor alpha and promyelocytic leukemia zinc finger genes resulting from t(11;17)(q23;q21) in a patient with acute promyelocytic leukemia. *J Clin Invest* 1993;91:2260–2267.
103. Cheson BD, Cassileth PA, Head DR, et al. Report of the National Cancer Institute–sponsored workshop on definitions of diagnosis and response in acute myeloid leukemia. *J Clin Oncol* 1990;8:813–819.
104. Chessels JM, Sieff CA, Harvey BAM, Pickthall JT, Lawler SD. Monosomy 7 in childhood: a preleukemic state. *Br J Haematol* 1981;49:129–130.
105. Chilcote RR, Brown E, Rowley JD. Lymphoblastic leukemia with lymphomatous features associated with abnormalities of the short arm of chromosome 9. *N Engl J Med* 1985;313:286–291.
106. Civin CI, Strauss LC, Brovall C, Fackler MJ, Schwartz JF, Shaper JH. Antigenic analysis of hematopoiesis. III. A hematopoietic progenitor cell surface antigen defined by a monoclonal antibody raised against KG-1a cells. *J Immunol* 1984;133:157–165.
107. Clark SS, McLaughlin J, Crist WM, Champlin R, Witte ON. Unique forms of the abl tyrosine kinase distinguish Ph[1]-positive CML from Ph[1]-positive ALL. *Science* 1987;235:85–88.
108. Claxton DF, Reading CL, Nagarajan L, et al. Correlation of CD2 expression with PML gene breakpoints in patients with acute promyelocytic leukemia. *Blood* 1992;80:582–586.
109. Cleary ML, Mellentin JD, Spies J, Smith SD. Chromosomal translocation involving the T cell receptor gene in acute leukemia. *J Exp Med* 1988;167:682–687.
110. Clevers H, Alacon B. Wileman T, Terhorst C. The T cell receptor/CD3 complex: a dynamic protein ensemble. *Annu Rev Immunol* 1988;6:629–662.
111. Colon-Otero G, Li C-Y, Dewald GW, et al. Erythrophagocytic acute lymphocytic leukemia with B-cell markers and with a 20q chromosome abnormality. *Mayo Clin Proc* 1984;59:678–681.
112. Cornelius AS, Campbell D, Schwartz E, Ponecz M. Elevated common acute lymphoblastic leukemia antigen expression in pediatric immune thrombocytopenic purpura. *Am J Pediatr Hematol Oncol* 1991;13:57–61.
113. Corral J, Forster A, Thompson S, et al. Acute leukemias of different lineages have a similar MLL gene fusions encoding related chimeric proteins resulting from chromosomal translocations. *Proc Natl Acad Sci USA* 1993;90:8538–8542.
114. Coulombel K, Derycke M, Villeval JL, et al. Characterization of the blast population in two neonates with Down's syndrome and transient myeloproliferative disorder. *Br J Haematol* 1987;66:69–76.
115. Cowan JD, Rubin RN, Kies MS, Cerezo L. Bone marrow necrosis. *Cancer* 1980;46:168–217.
116. Creutzig U, Cantu`-Rajnoldi A, Ritter J, et al. Myelodysplastic syndromes in childhood. Report of 21 patients from Italy and West Germany. *Am J Pediatr Hematol Oncol* 1987;9:324–330.
117. Crist W, Boyett J, Pullen J, Van Eys J, Viehi T. Clinical and biological features predict poor prognosis in acute lymphoid leukemias in children and adolescents: a Pediatric Oncology Group review. *Med Pediatr Oncol* 1986;14:135–139.
118. Crist W, Carroll A, Shuster J, et al. Philadelphia chromosome positive childhood acute lymphoblastic leukemia: clinical and cytogenetic characteristics and treatment outcome. A Pediatric Oncology Group study. *Blood* 1990;76:489–494.
119. Crist W, Pullen J, Boyett J, et al. Clinical and biologic features predict a poor prognosis in acute lymphoid leukemias in infants: a Pediatric Oncology Group study. *Blood* 1986;67:135–140.
120. Crist WM, Carroll AJ, Shuster JJ, et al. Poor prognosis of children with pre-B acute lymphoblastic leukemia is associated with the t(1;19)(q23;p13): a Pediatric Oncology Group study. *Blood* 1990;76:117–122.
121. Cuneo A, Nucucii C, Kevin S, et al. Multipotent stem cell involvement in megakaryoblastic leukemia: cytologic and cytogenetic evidence in 15 patients. *Blood* 1989;74:1781–1790.
122. Daghistani D, Toledano SR, Curless R. Monosomy 7 syndrome.

Clinical heterogeneity in children and adolescents. *Cancer Genet Cytogenet* 1990;44:263–269.
123. Daley GQ, McLaughlin J, Witte ON, Baltimore D. The CML-specific p210 bcr/abl protein, unlike v-abl, does not transform NIH/3T3 fibroblasts. *Science* 1987;237:532–535.
124. Dalton W, Stass SA. A morphologic and cytochemical approach to the diagnosis of acute leukemia. In: Stass SA, ed. *The Acute Leukemias.* New York: Marcel Dekker; 1987:27.
125. Dalton WT, Ahearn MJ, Cork A, et al. Acute myelomonocytic leukemia associated with abnormalities of chromosome 16: a light and electron microscopic study. *Hematol Pathol* 1987;1:105–112.
126. Darbyshire PJ, Lilleyman JS. Granular acute lymphoblastic leukemia of childhood: a morphological phenomenon. *J Clin Pathol* 1987;40:251–253.
127. Darbyshire PJ, Smith JHF, Oakhill A, Mott MG. Monocytic leukemia in infancy. A review of eight children. *Cancer* 1985;56:1584–1589.
128. Das Gupta A, Advani SH, Nair CN, et al. Acute leukemia and coexpression of lymphoid and myeloid phenotypes. *Hematol Oncol* 1987;5:189–196.
129. Davey FR, Davis RB, MacCullum JM, et al. Morphologic and cytochemical characteristics of acute promyelocytic leukemia. *Am J Hematol* 1989;30:221–227.
130. Dayton YD, Arthur DC, Gajl-Peczalska KJ, Brunning R. L3 acute lymphoblastic leukemia. Comparison with small non-cleaved cell lymphoma involving the bone marrow. *Am J Clin Pathol* 1994;101:130–139.
131. Debili N, Kieffer N, Mitjavila MT, et al. Expression of platelet glycoproteins by erythroid blasts in four cases of trisomy 21. *Leukemia* 1989;3:669–678.
132. Dedera DA, Waller EK, LeBrun DP, Sen-Majumdar, Stevens ME, Barsh GS, Cleary ML. Chimeric homeobox gene E2A-PBX1 induces proliferation, apoptosis, and malignant lymphomas in transgenic mice. *Cell* 1993;74:833–843.
133. DeKorte D, Haverkort WA, Behrendt H, Roos D, Van Gennip AH. Abnormal nucleotide pattern in the eosinophils of a patient with acute lymphoblastic leukemia associated with eosinophilia. *Leuk Res* 1986;10:1419–1424.
134. Della-Favera R, Bregni M, Erikson J, Patterson D, Gallo RC, Croce CM. Human c-myc oncogene is located on the region of chromosome 8 that is translocated in Burkitt lymphoma cells. *Proc Natl Acad Sci USA* 1982;79:7824–7827.
135. De Oliveira MSP, Gregory C, Matutes E, Parreira A, Catovsky D. Cytochemical profile of megakaryoblastic leukemia: a study with cytochemical methods, monoclonal antibodies, and ultrastructural cytochemistry. *J Clin Pathol* 1987;40:663–669.
136. De Salvo L, Weir-Medina J, Gomez-Sanchez O, et al. Leucemia promielocitica aguda en el occidente de Venezuela. *Sangre* 1989;34:329–331.
137. Desiderio SV, Yancopoulos GD, Paskin M, et al. Insertion of N regions into heavy-chain genes is correlated with expression of terminal deoxytransferase in B cells. *Nature* 1984;311:752–755.
138. de The´ H, Chomienne C, Lanotte M, Degos L, Dejean A. The t(15;17) translocation of acute promyelocytic leukemia fuses the retinoic acid receptor α gene to a novel transcriptional locus. *Nature* 1990;347:558–561.
139. Devaraj PE, Foroni L, Sekhar M, et al. E2A/HLF fusion cDNAs and the use of RT-PCR for detection of minimal residual disease in t(17;19)(q22;p13) acute lymphoblastic leukemia. *Leukemia* 1994;8:1131–1138.
140. Dharmasena F, Wickham N, McHugh PJ, Catovsky D, Galton DAG. Osteolytic tumors in acute megakaryoblastic leukemia. *Cancer* 1986;58:2273–2277.
141. Dijkstra K, Kluin-Nelemans HC. No difference between cytochemical and immunological detection of myeloperoxidase in AML. *Br J Haematol* 1990;75:630.
142. Diverio D, Lo Cocco F, D'Adamo F, et al. Identification of DNA rearrangements at the retinoic acid receptor (RAR-α) locus in all patients with acute promyelocytic leukemia (APL) and mapping of breakpoints within the RAR-α second intron. *Blood* 1992;79:3331–3336.
143. Diverio D, Pandolfi PP, Rossi V, Biondi A, Pelicci PG, Lo Coco F. Monitoring of treatment outcome in acute promyelocytic leukemia by RT-PCR. *Leukemia* 1994;8:1105–1107.
144. Djabali M, Sallen L, Parry P, Bower M, Young B, Evans GA. A trithorax-like gene is interrupted by chromosome 11q23 in acute leukemia. *Nat Genet* 1992;2:113–118.
145. Domer PH, Fakharzadeh SS, Chen C-S, et al. Acute mixed lineage leukemia t(4;11)(q21;q23) generates an MLL-AF4 fusion product. *Proc Natl Acad Sci USA* 1993;90:7884–7888.
146. Dosik H, Rosner F, Sawitshy A. Acquired lipidosis: Gaucher-like cells and "blue cells" in chronic myelogenous leukemia. *Semin Hematol* 1972;9:309–316.
147. Downing JR, Head DR, Curcio-Brint AM, et al. An AML1/ETO fusion transcript is consistently detected by RNA-based polymerase chain reaction in acute myelogenous leukemia containing the t(8;21)(q22;q22) translocation. *Blood* 1993;81:2860–2865.
148. Downing JR, Head DR, Raimondi SC, et al. The der(11)-encoded MLL/AF-4 fusion transcript is consistently detected in t(4;11)(q21;q23)-containing acute lymphoblastic leukemia. *Blood* 1993;83:330–335.
149. Drexler HG. Classification of acute myeloid leukemias: a comparison of FAB and immunophenotyping. *Leukemia* 1987;1:697–705.
150. Drexler HG, Messmore HL, Menon M, Monowada T. A case of Tdt-positive B-cell acute lymphoblastic leukemia. *Am J Clin Pathol* 1986;85:735–738.
151. Drexler HG, Sperling C, Ludwig W. Terminal deoxynucleotidyl transferase (TdT) expression in acute myeloid leukemia. *Leukemia* 1993;7:1142–1150.
152. Drexler HG, Theil E, Ludwig W-D. Review of the incidence and clinical relevance of myeloid antigen-positive acute lymphoblastic leukemia. *Leukemia* 1991;5:637–645.
153. Drexler HG, Theil E, Ludwig W-D. Acute myeloid leukemia expressing lymphoid-associated antigens: diagnostic incidence and prognostic significance. *Leukemia* 1993;7:489–498.
154. Dube´ ID, Greenberg ML. Phenotyic heterogeneity in three cases of lymphoid malignancy with chromosomal translocations in 14q11. *Cytogenet Cell Genet* 1986;41:215–218.
155. Dube´ ID, Kamel-Reid S, Yuan CC, et al. A novel human homeobox gene lies at the chromosome 10 breakpoint in lymphoid neoplasias with chromosomal translocation t(10;14). *Blood* 1991;78:2996–3003.
156. Dube´ ID, Raimondi SC, Pi D, Kalousek DK. A new translocation, t(10;14)(q24;q11), in T-cell neoplasia. *Blood* 1986;67:1181–1184.
157. Dvorak AM, Monahan RA, Dickersin GR. Diagnostic electron microscopy. I. Hematology: differential diagnosis of acute lymphoblastic and acute myeloblastic leukemia. Use of ultrastructural peroxidase cytochemistry and routine electron microscopic technology. *Pathol Annu* 1981;16:101–119.
158. Edelman BB, Groosman NJ. Microgranular acute promyelocytic leukemia: a case with multiple Auer rods demonstrable only after staining for chloroacetate esterase. *Am J Clin Pathol* 1983;79:621–625.
159. Editorial: Childhood leukaemia: An infectious disease? *Lancet* 1990;336:1477–1479.
160. Eguchi M, Ozawa T, Sakakibara H, Sugita K, Iwama Y, Furukawa T. Ultrastructural and ultracytochemical differences between megakaryoblastic leukemia in children and adults. *Cancer* 1992;70:451–458.
161. Epner DE, Koeffler HP. Molecular genetic advances in chronic myelogenous leukemia. *Ann Intern Med* 1990;113:3–5.
162. Erber WN, Breton-Gorius J, Villeval JL, Oscier DG, Bai Y, Mason DY. Detection of cells of megakaryocytic lineage in haematopoietic malignancies by immuno-alkaline phosphatase labelling of cell smears with a panel of monoclonal antibodies. *Br J Haematol* 1987;65:870–874.
163. Erber WN, Phil D, Mason DY. Immunoalkaline phosphatase labeling of terminal transferase in hematologic samples. *Am J Clin Pathol* 1987;88:43–50.
164. Erickson P, Gao J, Chang K-S, Look T, et al. Identification of breakpoints in t(8;21) acute myelogenous leukemia and isolation of a fusion transcript, AML1/ETO, with similarity to Drosophila segmentation gene, runt. *Blood* 1992;80:1825–1831.
165. Erikson J, Williams DL, Finan J, Nowell PC, Croce CM. Locus of the α-chain of the T-cell receptor is split by chromosome translocation in T-cell leukemias. *Science* 1985;229:784–786.
166. Evans JPM, Czepulkowski B, Gibbons B, Swansbury GJ, Ches-

sells JM. Childhood monosomy 7 revisited. *Br J Haematol* 1988; 69:41–45.
167. Fauser AA, Kanz L, Bross KJ, Lo¨hr GW. T cells and probably B cells arise from the malignant clone in chronic myelogenous leukemia. *J Clin Invest* 1985;75:1080–1082.
168. Favaloro EJ, Bradstock KF, Kabral A, Grimsley P, Zowtwj H, Zola H. Further characterization of human myeloid antigens (gp 160, 95; gp 150; gp 67): investigation of epitopic heterogeneity and non-hemopoietic distribution using panels of monoclonal antibodies belonging to CD-11b, CD-13, and CD-33. *Br J Haematol* 1988;69:163–171.
169. Fell HP, Smith RG, Tucker PW. Molecular analysis of the t(2;14) translocation of childhood chronic lymphocytic leukemia. *Science* 1986:232:491–494.
170. Ferro MT, San Roma´n C, Mun˜oz A, Madero L, Olmeda F, Ferna´ndez-Ran˜ada JM, Mecucci C. Translocation (4;11) in ALL: a new morphologic aspect? *Cancer Genet Cytogenet* 1986;23:145–149.
171. Fialkow PJ, Denman AM, Jacobsen RJ, Lowenthal MN. Chronic myelocytic leukemia. Origin of some lymphocytes from leukemic stem cells. *J Clin Invest* 1978;62;815–823.
172. Fialkow PJ, Jacobson RJ, Papayannopoulou T. Chronic myelocytic leukemia: clonal origin in a stem cell common to the granulocytic, erythrocytic, platelet and monocytic/macrophage. *Am J Med* 1977;63:125–130.
173. Fialkow PJ, Martin PJ, Najfeld V, Penfold GK, Jacobson RJ, Hansen JA. Evidence for a multistep pathogenesis of chronic myelogenous leukemia. *Blood* 1981;58:158–163.
174. Finger LR, Kagan J, Christopher G, Kurtzberg J, Hershfield MS, Nowell PC, Croce CM. Involvement of the Tcl5 gene on human chromosome 1 in T-cell leukemia and melanoma. *Proc Natl Acad Sci USA* 1989;86:5039–5043.
175. Fink FM, Ko¨ller U, Mayer H, et al. Prognostic significance of myeloid-associated antigen expression on blast cells in children with acute lymphoblastic leukemia. *Med Pediatr Oncol* 1993;21: 340–346.
176. Finlay JL, Borchevding W. Acute B-lymphocytic leukemia with L1 morphology: a report of two pediatric cases. *Leukemia* 1988;2:60–62.
177. Fioretos T, Heisterkamp N, Groffen J. No evidence for genomic imprinting of the human BCR gene. *Blood* 1994;83:3441–3444.
178. Fitzgerald TJ, Neale GAM, Raimondi SC, et al. c-tal, a helix-loop-helix protein, is juxtaposed to the T-cell receptor–chain gene by a reciprocal chromosomal translocation: t(1;17)(p32;q35). *Blood* 1991;78:2686–2695.
179. Fletcher JA, Lynch EA, Kimball VM, Donnelly M, Tantravahi R, Sallan SE. Translocation (9;22) is associated with extremely poor prognosis in intensively treated children with acute lymphoblastic leukemia. *Blood* 1991;77:435–439.
180. Foadi MD, Slater AM, Pegrum GD. Erythrophagocytosis by acute lymphoblastic leukemia cells. *Scand J Haematol* 1978;20: 85.
181. Fong C, Brodeur GM. Down's syndrome and leukemia: epidemiology, genetics, cytogenetics and mechanisms of leukemogenesis. *Cancer Genet Cytogenet* 1987;28:55–76.
182. Foot ABM, Potter MN, Ropner JE, Wallington TB, Oakhill A. Transient erythroblastopenia of childhood with CD10, TdT, and cytoplasmic lymphocyte positivity in bone marrow. *Br J Haematol* 1990;43:133–134.
183. Fort JA, Graham-Pole J, Mottshaw G. Adult-type T-cell lymphoma in an adolescent with human T-lymphotropic virus type 1 seropositivity. *Med Pediatr Oncol* 1989;17:236–238.
184. Fourth International Workshop on Chromosomes in Leukemia, 1982: Rearrangements of 11q. *Cancer Genet Cytogenet* 1984;11: 294–295.
185. Fradera J, Velez-Garcia E, White JG. Acute lymphoblastic leukemia with unusual cytoplasmic granulation: a morphologic, cytochemical, and ultrastructural study. *Blood* 1986;68:406–411.
186. Fraumeni Jr JF, Manning MD, Mitus WJ. Acute childhood leukemia: epidemiologic study by cell type of 1,263 cases at the Children's Cancer Research Foundation in Boston, 1947–1965. *J Natl Cancer Inst* 1971;46:461–470.
187. Freeman JA. Origins of Auer bodies. *Blood* 1966;27:499–510.
188. Freeman JA. The ultrastructure and genesis of Auer bodies. *Blood* 1960;15:449–465.
189. Fuchs CAR, Marin CA, Bezares RF, Carreras LO, Pinto MT. Granular acute leukemia not always of myeloid origin. *Lancet* 1984;1:636.
190. Ganick DJ, Finlay JL. Acute lymphoblastic leukemia with Burkitt cell morphology and cytoplasmic immunoglobulin. *Blood* 1980;56:311–314.
191. Gao J, Erickson P, Gardiner K, et al. Isolation of a yeast artificial chromosome spanning the 8;21 translocation breakpoint t(8;21)(q22;q22.3) in acute myelogenous leukemia. *Proc Natl Acad Sci USA* 1991;88:4882–4886.
192. Garre´ ML, Relling MV, Kalwinsky D, et al. Pharmocokinetics and toxicity of methotrexate in children with Down's syndrome and acute lymphocytic leukemia. *J Pediatr* 1987;111:606–612.
193. Geller RB, Zahurak M, Hurwitz CA, Burke PJ, Karp JE, Piantadosi S, Civin CI. Prognostic importance of immunophenotyping in adults with acute myelocytic leukemia: the significance of the stem-cell glycoprotein CD34 (My10). *Br J Haematol* 1990;76: 340–347.
194. Gibbons B, MacCallum P, Watts E, et al. Near haploid acute lymphoblastic leukemia: seven new cases and a review of the literature. *Leukemia* 1991;5:738–743.
195. Gilbert RD, Karabus CD, Mills AE. Acute promyelocytic leukemia. A childhood cluster. *Cancer* 1987;59:933–935.
196. Gilfillan S, Dierich A, Lemeur M, Benoist C, Mathis D. Mice lacking TDT: mature animals with an immature lymphocyte repertoire. *Science* 1993;261:1175–1178.
197. Glasser EF. Phagocytosis in acute leukemia. *Cancer* 1980;45: 1365–1369.
198. Glassy EF, Sun NCJ, Okun DB. Hand–mirror cell leukemia. Report of nine cases and a review of the literature. *Am J Clin Pathol* 1980;74:651–656.
199. Golomb HM, Rowley JD, Vardiman JW, Testa JR, Butler A. "Microgranular" acute promyelocytic leukemia: a distinct clinical, ultrastructural, and cytogenetic entity. *Blood* 1980;55:253–259.
200. Gori-Bergammi Z, Spremolla G. Erythrophagocytosis in acute myeloblastic leukemia: A morphological and ultrastructural study. *Haematologica* 1979;64:597–601.
201. Gramatzki M, Strong DM, Duval-Arnould B, Morstyne G, Schumacher HR. Hand mirror variant of acute lymphoblastic leukemia: evidence for early T-cell lineage in two cases by evaluation with monoclonal antibodies. *Cancer* 1985;55:77–83.
202. Greaves MF. Speculations on the cause of childhood acute lymphoblastic leukemia. *Leukemia* 1988;2:120–125.
203. Greaves MF, Alexander FE. An infectious etiology for common acute lymphoblastic leukemia in childhood? *Leukemia* 1993;7: 349–360.
204. Greaves MF, Janossy G, Peto J, et al. Immunologically defined subclasses of acute lymphoblastic leukemia in children: their relationship to presentation features and prognosis. *Br J Haematol* 1981;48:179–197.
205. Greaves MF, Sieff C, Edwards PAW. Monoclonal antiglycophorin as a probe for erythroleukemias. *Blood* 1983;61:645–651.
206. Greenberg BR, Wilson FD, Woo L, Jenks HM. Cytogenetics of fibroblastic colonies in Ph[1]-positive chronic myelogenous leukemia. *Blood* 1978;51:1039–1044.
207. Grignani F, Fagioli M, Alcalay M, et al. Acute promyelocytic leukemia: from genetics to treatment. *Blood* 1994;83:10–25.
208. Grimaldi JC, Meek TC. The t(5;14) chromosomal translocation in a case of acute lymphocytic leukemia joins the interleukin-3 gene to the immunoglobulin heavy chain gene. *Blood* 1989;73: 2081–2085.
209. Grogan TM, Insalaco SJ, Savage RA, Vail MC. Acute lymphocytic leukemia with prominent azurophilic granulation and punctate acidic nonspecific esterase and phosphatase activity. *Am J Clin Pathol* 1981;75:716–722.
210. Gu Y, Nakamura T, Alder H, et al. The t(4;11) chromosomal translocation of human acute leukemias fuses the ALL-1 gene, related to Drosophila trithorax, to the AF-4 gene. *Cell* 1992;71: 701–708.
211. Gyger M, Bonny Y, Forest L. Childhood monosomy 7 syndrome. *Am J Hematol* 1982;13:329–334.
212. Haas OA, Argyriou-Tirita A, Lion T. Parental origin of chromosome involved in the t(9;22). *Nature* 1992;359:414–416.
213. Haas OA, Zoubek A, Ko¨ller U, et al. Generalized lymphadenop-

athy in juvenile chronic myelomonocytic leukemia is due to lymph node infiltration with myelomonocytic cells and immature T-cells. In: Schmalzl F, Mufti GJ, eds. *Myelodysplastic Syndromes*. Berlin: Springer-Verlag; 1992:146–154.
214. Haider YS, Phillips TM, Schumacher HR. Acute myeloid leukemia with hand-mirror cells. *Arch Pathol Lab Med* 1982;106:271–274.
215. Hannon GJ, Beach D. p15^{INK4B} is a potential effector of TGF cell cycle arrest. *Nature* 1994;371:257–261.
216. Harnden DG. Inherited factors in leukaemia and lymphoma. *Leuk Res* 1985;9:705–707.
217. Harris MB, Shuster JJ, Carroll A, et al. Trisomy of leukemic cell chromosomes 4 and 10 identifies children with B-progenitor cell acute lymphoblastic leukemia with a very low risk of treatment failure. A Pediatric Oncology Group study. *Blood* 1992;79:3316–3324.
218. Hasle H. Myelodysplastic syndromes in childhood—classification, epidemiology and treatment. *Leuk Lymph* 1994;13:11–26.
219. Hatano M, Roberts CWM, Minden M, Crist WM, Korsmeyer SJ. Deregulation of a homeobox gene, HOX11, by the t(10;14) in T-cell leukemia. *Science* 1991;253:79–82.
220. Hay CRM, Barnett D, James V, Woodcock BW, Brown MJ, Lawrence ACK. Granular common acute lymphoblastic leukemia in adults: a morphologic study. *Eur J Haematol* 1987;39:299–305.
221. Hayashi Y, Eguchi M, Sugita K, et al. Cytogenetic findings and clinical features in acute leukemia and transient myeloproliferative disorder in Down's syndrome. *Blood* 1988;72:15–23.
222. Hayashi Y, Raimondi SC, Look AT, et al. Abnormalities of the long arm of chromosome 6 in childhood acute lymphoblastic leukemia. *Blood* 1990;76:1626–1630.
223. Hayhoe FGJ, Quaglino D. *Haematological Cytochemistry*. 3rd ed. Edinburgh: Churchill Livingstone; 1994.
224. Haynes BF, Denning SM, Singer KH, Kurtzberg J. Ontogeny of T-cell precursors: a model for the initial stages of human T cell development. *Immunol Today* 1989;10:87–90.
225. Head DR, Behm FG, Raimondi SC, et al. Genetic heterogeneity of acute myeloid leukemia (AML) with FAB-AML M3 morphology. *Mod Pathol* 1995;8:112A (abstract).
226. Head DR, Kennedy PS, Goyette RE. Metastatic neuroblastoma in bone marrow aspirate smears. *Am J Clin Pathol* 1979;72:1008–1011.
227. Head DR, Kjeldsberg CR, Kadin ME, Pick T, Bybee B, Longbotham J, Shumski E. Childhood T-cell malignancy resembling adult T-cell leukemia/lymphoma. *Hematopathology* 1987;1:15–25.
228. Hebert J, Cayuella JM, Berkeley J, Sigaux F. Candidate tumor-suppressor genes MTS1 (p16^{INK4A}) and MTS2 (p15^{INK4B}) display frequent homozygous deletions in primary cells from T- but not from B-cell lineage acute lymphoblastic leukemia. *Blood* 1994;84:4038–4044.
229. Heerema NA, Palmer CG, Baehner RL. Karyotypic and clinical findings in a consecutive series of children with acute lymphocytic leukemia. *Cancer Genet Cytogenet* 1985;17:165–179.
230. Heim S, Avanzi GC, Billströ¨m R, et al. A new specific chromosomal rearrangement, t(8;16)(p11;p13), in acute monocytic leukemia. *Br J Haematol* 1987;66:323–326.
231. Heim S, Bekassy AN, Garwicz S, et al. Bone marrow karyotypes in 94 children with acute leukemia. *Eur J Haematol* 1990;44:227–233.
232. Heisterkamp N, Jenster G, ten Hoeve J, et al. Acute leukaemia in bcr/abl transgenic mice. *Nature* 1990;344:251–253.
233. Heisterkamp N, Stephenson JR, Groffers J, Hansen PF, de Lein A, Bartram CR, Grosveld G. Localization of the c-abl oncogene adjacent to a translocation breakpoint in chronic myelocytic leukemia. *Nature* 1983;306:239–242.
234. Herrod HG, Dow LW, Sullivan JL. Persistent Epstein-Barr virus infection mimicking juvenile chronic myelogenous leukemia: immunologic and hematologic studies. *Blood* 1983;61:1098–1104.
235. Hiddemann W, Buchner T, Andreeff M, Wormann B, Melamed MR, Clarkson BD. Cell kinetics in acute leukemia. A critical reevaluation based on new data. *Cancer* 1982;50:250–258.
236. Hirt A, Luethy AR, Mueller B, Gugler E, Wagner HP. Acute megakaryoblastic leukemia in children identified by immunologic marker studies. *Am J Pediatr Hematol Oncol* 1990;12:27–33.
237. Hirt A, Morell A, Frei H, Imbach P, Wagner HP. Proliferation of lymphoid precursor cells in the bone marrow of patients with various disorders of the immune system. *Exp Hematol* 1988;16:38–41.
238. Ho FCS, Chan GTC, Todd D. Non-specificity of Sudan black B in the diagnosis of acute myeloid leukemia. *Br J Haematol* 1983;53:171–172.
239. Hogan TF, Koss W, Murgo AJ, Amato RS, Fontana JA, Van Scoy FL. Acute lymphoblastic leukemia with chromosomal 5;14 translocation and hypereosinophilia: case report and literature review. *J Clin Oncol* 1987;5:382–390.
240. Hooberman AL, Westbrook CA. Molecular diagnosis of the Philadelphia chromosome in acute lymphoblastic leukemia. *Leuk Lymph* 1990;1:3–10.
241. Hopton PA, McKinney PA, Cartwright RA, et al. X-rays in pregnancy and the risk of childhood cancer. *Lancet* 1985;ii:773.
242. Huang W, Sun G-L, Li X-S, et al. Acute promyelocytic leukemia: clinical relevance of two major PML-RARα isoforms and detection of minimal residual disease by retrotranscriptase polymerase chain reaction to predict relapse. *Blood* 1993;82:1264–1269.
243. Hudson MM, Raimondi SC, Behm FG, Pui C-H. Childhood acute leukemia with t(11;19)(q23;p13). *Leukemia* 1991;5:1064–1068.
244. Hunger SP, Ohyashiki K, Toyama K, Cleary ML. Hlf, a novel hepatic bZIP protein, shows altered DNA-binding properties following fusion to E2A in t(17;19) acute lymphoblastic leukemia. *Genes Dev* 1992;1608–1620.
245. Hunger SP, Tkachuk DC, Amylon MD, et al. HRX involvement in de novo and secondary leukemias with diverse chromosome 11q23 abnormalities. *Blood* 1993;81:3197–3203.
246. Hurwitz CA, Raimondi SC, Head D, et al. Distinctive immunophenotypic features of t(8;21)(q22;q22) acute myeloblastic leukemia in children. *Blood* 1992;80:3182–3188.
247. Hurwitz CA, Schell MJ, Pui C-H, Crist WM, Behm FG, Mirro J, Jr. Adverse prognostic features in 251 children treated for acute myeloid leukemia. *Med Pediatr Oncol* 1993;21:1–7.
248. Imamura N, Kuramoto A. Acute unclassifiable leukemias in adults, demonstrating myeloid antigens and myeloperoxidase protein. *Br J Haematol* 1988;69:427–428.
249. Immamura N, Kuramoto A. Analysis of peroxidase negative acute leukemias by monoclonal antibodies: III. Acute lymphoblastic leukemia. *J Clin Lab Anal* 1989;3:88–94.
250. Imamura N, Tanaka R, Kajihara H, Kuramoto A. Analysis of peroxidase-negative acute unclassifiable leukemias by monoclonal antibodies. I. Acute myelogenous leukemia and acute myelomonocytic leukemia. *Eur J Haematol* 1988;41:420–428.
251. Inaba T, Roberts WM, Shapiro LH, et al. Fusion of the leucine zipper gene HLF to the E2A gene in human acute B-lineage leukemia. *Science* 1992;257:531–534.
252. Innes DJ, Hess CE, Bertholf MF, Wade P. Differentiation of acute promyelocytic leukemia from benign myeloid proliferations. *Am J Clin Pathol* 1987;88:725–729.
253. Ireland R, Gillett D, Mieli-Vergani G, Mufti G. Pre-ALL and non-A, non-B hepatitis infection. *Leuk Res* 1988;12:795–797.
254. Ishibashi T, Kimura H, Abe R, Matsuda S, Uchida T, Kariyone S. Involvement of eosinophils in leukemia: cytogenetic study of eosinophilic colonies from acute myelogenous leukemia associated with translocation(8;21). *Cancer Genet Cytogenet* 1986;22:189–194.
255. Jablon S. Tachikawa K, Belsley JL, Steer A. Cancer in Japanese exposed as children to atomic bombs. *Lancet* 1971;i:927–932.
256. Jacobsen RJ, Temple MJ, Sacher RA. Acute myeloblastic leukaemia and t(8;21) translocation. *Br J Haematol* 1984;57:539–541.
257. Jaffe ES, Berard CW. Lymphoblastic lymphoma: a term rekindled with new precision. *Ann Intern Med* 1978;89:415–417.
258. Janossy G, Hoffbrand AV, Greaves MF, et al. Terminal transferase assay and immunological membrane markers in the diagnosis of leukaemia: a multiparameter analysis of 300 cases. *Br J Haematol* 1980;44:221–234.
259. Janvier M, Tobelem G, Daniel MT, Bernheim A, Marty M, Boiron M. Acute monoblastic leukemia. Clinical, biological data and survival in 45 cases. *Scand J Haematol* 1984;32:385–390.
260. Jonsson OG, Kitchens RL, Baer RJ, Buchanan GR, Smith RG. Rearrangements of the tal-1 locus as clonal markers for T cell acute lymphoblastic leukemia. *J Clin Invest* 1991;87:2029–2035.
261. Juneja HS, Rajaraman S, Alpern JB, Bainton DF. Auer rod-like

inclusions in prolymphocytic leukemia. *Acta Haematol* 1987;77: 115–119.

262. Kagan J, Finan J, Letofsky J, Besa EC, Nowell PC, Croce CM. α-chain locus of the T-cell antigen receptor is involved in the t(10;14) chromosome translocation of T-cell acute lymphoblastic leukemia. *Proc Natl Acad Sci USA* 1987;84:4543–4546.
263. Kalwinsky DK, Raimondi SC, Bunin NJ, et al. Clinical and biological characteristics of acute lymphoblastic leukemia in children with Down syndrome. *Am J Med Genet* 1990;7:267–271.
264. Kalwinsky DK, Raimondi SC, Schell MJ, et al. Prognostic importance of cytogenetic subgroups in de novo pediatric acute nonlymphocytic leukemia. *J Clin Oncol* 1990;8:75–83.
265. Kalwinsky DK, Roberson P, Dahl G, et al. Clinical relevance of lymphoblastic biological features in children with acute lymphoblastic leukemia. *J Clin Oncol* 1985;3:477–484.
266. Kamps MP, Baltimore D. E2A-Pbx1, the t(1;19) tranlocation protein of human pre-B-cell acute lymphocytic leukemia, causes acute myeloid leukmeia in mice. *Mol Cell Biol* 1993;13:351–357.
267. Kamps MP, Murre C, Sun X-H, Baltimore D. A new homeobox gene contributes the DNA binding domain of the t(1;19) translocation protein in pre-B ALL. *Cell* 1990;60:547–555.
268. Kaneko Y, Kimpara H, Kawai S, Fujimoto T. 8;21 chromosome translocation in eosinophilic leukemia. *Cancer Genet Cytogenet* 1983;9:181–183.
269. Kaneko Y, Maseki N, Homma C, et al. Chromosome translocations involving band 7q35 or 7p15 in childhood T-cell leukemia/lymphoma. *Blood* 1988;72:534–538.
270. Kaneko Y, Maseki N, Sakurai M, et al. Chromosome pattern in juvenile chronic myelogenous leukemia, myelodysplastic syndrome, and acute leukemia associated with neurofibromatosis. *Leukemia* 1989;3:36–41.
271. Kaneko Y, Maseki N, Takasaki N, et al. Clinical and hematologic characteristics in acute leukemia with 11q23 translocations. *Blood* 1986;67:484–491.
272. Kaneko Y, Rowley JD, Mauer HS, Variakojis D, Moohr JW. Chromosome pattern in childhood acute nonlymphocytic leukemia (ANLL). *Blood* 1982;60:389–399.
273. Kaneko Y, Rowley JD, Variakojis D, Chilcote RR, Check I, Sakurai M. Corrleation of karyotype with clinical features in acute lymphoblastic leukemia. *Cancer Res* 1982;42:2918–2929.
274. Kantarjian HM, Deisseroth A, Kurzrock R, Estrov Z, Talpaz M. Chronic myelogenous leukemia: a concise update. *Blood* 1993;82:691–703.
275. Kaplow LS. Leukocyte alkaline phosphatase. Applications and methods. *Ann NY Acad Sci* 1968;155:911–914.
276. Kawasaki ES, Clark SS, Coyne MY, Smith SD, Champlin R, Witte ON, McCormick FP. Diagnosis of chronic myeloid and acute lymphocytic leukemias by detection of leukemia-specific mRNA sequences amplified in vitro. *Proc Natl Acad Sci USA* 1988;85:5698–5702.
277. Keifer J, Abromowitch M, Stass SA. Chloroacetate esterase positivity in acute lymphoblastic leukemia. *Am J Clin Pathol* 1985;83:647–649.
278. Kelliher M, Knott A, McLaughlin J, Witte ON, Rosenberg N. Differences in oncogenic potency but not target cell specificity distinguish the two forms of the BCR/ABL oncogene. *Mol Cell Biol* 1991;11:4710–4716.
279. Keverger G, Bernheim A, Daniel M-T, Flandrin G, Schaison G, Berger R. Cytogenetic study of 130 childhood acute nonlymphocytic leukemias. *Med Pediatr Oncol* 1988;16:227–232.
280. Kinney TR, Kock PA, Gottlieb RP, et al. Bone marrow necrosis in children. Three instances. *Clin Pediatr* 1977;16:565–567.
281. Kirby MS, Weitzman S, Freedman MH. Juvenile chronic myelogenous leukemia: differentiation from infantile cytomegalovirus infection. *Am J Pediatr Hematol Oncol* 1990;12:292–296.
282. Kita K, Nakase K, Miwa H, et al. Phenotypical characteristics of acute myelocytic leukemia associated with the t(8;21)(q22;q22) chromosomal abnormality: frequent expression of immature B-cell antigen CD19 together with stem cell antigen CD34. *Blood* 1992;80:470–477.
283. Klitz W. Viruses, cancer and the MHC. *Nature* 1992;356:17–18.
284. Knapp W, Do¨rken B, Gilks WR, Rieber EP, Schmidt RE, Stein H, von dem Borne AEGR, eds. *Leucocyte Typing. vol IV. White Cell Differentiation Antigens.* New York: Oxford University Press; 1989.
285. Knox EG, Marshall T. Leukemia and childhood cancer in twins. *J Epidemiol Common Health* 1984;38:12–14.
286. Kobayashi SP, Seki K, Suwa N, et al. The transient appearance of small blastoid cells in the marrow after bone marrow transplantation. *Am J Clin Pathol 1991;*96:191–195.
287. Koehler M, Behm FG, Shuster J, et al. Transitional pre-B-cell acute lymphoblastic leukemia of childhood is associated with favorable prognostic clinical features and an excellent outcome: a Pediatric Oncology Group study. *Leukemia* 1993;7:2064–2068.
288. Kojima S, Matsuyama T, Sato T, et al. Down's syndrome and acute leukemia in children: an analysis of phenotype by use of monoclonal antibodies and electron microscopic platelet reaction. *Blood* 1990;76:2348–2353.
289. Koken MHM, Puvion-Dutilleul F, Guillemin MC, et al. The t(15;17) translocation alters a nuclear body in a retinoic acid-reversible fashoin. *EMBO J* 1994;13:1073–1083.
290. Komori T, Okada A, Stewart V, Alt FW. Lack of N regions in antigen receptor variable region genes of TDT-deficient lymphocytes. *Science* 1993;261:1171–1175.
291. Kondo K, Sakai M, Isobe H, Taniguchi N, Nishi S, Kawakami Y. Induction of carbonic anhydrase I isozyme precedes the globin synthesis during erythropoiesis in K562 cells. *Am J Hematol* 1991;38:201–206.
292. Konopka JB, Watanabe SM, Witte ON. An alteration of the human c-abl protein in K562 leukemia cells unmasks associated tyrosine kinase activity. *Cell* 1984;37:1035–1042.
293. Krause JR, Penchansky L, Contis L, Kaplan SS. Flow cytometry in the diagnosis of acute leukemia. *Am J Clin Pathol* 1988;89: 341–346.
294. Krause JR, Stolc V, Kaplan SS, Penchansky L. Microgranular promyelocytic leukemia: a multiparameter examination. *Am J Hematol* 1989;30:158–163.
295. Krissansen GW, Lucas CM, Stomski FC, et al. Blood leukocytes bind platelet glycoprotein (IIb-IIIa) but do not express the vitronectin receptor. *Int Immunol* 1990;267–277.
296. Kuis W, Roord JJ, Zegers BJM, et al. Heterogeneity of immune defects in three children with a chronic active Epstein-Barr virus infection. *J Clin Immunol* 1985;5:377–381.
297. Kung PC, Long JC, McCaffery RP, Ratliff RL, Harrison TA, Baltimore D. Terminal deoxynucleotidyl transferase in the diagnosis of leukemia and malignant lymphoma. *Am J Med* 1978;64:788–794.
298. Kuruhashi H, Junichi H, Keiko Y, et al. Monoclonal nature of transient abnormal myelopoiesis in Down's syndrome. *Blood* 1991;77:1161–1163.
299. Kurzrock R, Gutterman JU, Talpaz M. The molecular genetics of Philadelphia chromosome-positive leukemias. *N Engl J Med* 1988;319:990–998.
300. Kusec R, Laczika K, Kno¨bl P, et al. AML1/ETO fusion mRNA can be detected in remission blood samples of all patients with t(8;21) acute myeloid leukemia after chemotherapy of autologous bone marrow transplantation. *Leukemia* 1994;8:735–739.
301. Laı¨ JL, Fenaux MH, Estienne JJ, et al. Translocation t(1;19) (q23;p13) in acute lymphoblastic leukemia. A report on six new cases and an unusual t(17;19)(q11;913), with special reference to prognostic factors. *Cancer Genet Cytogenet* 1989;37:9–17.
302. Lambert F, Harbott J, Ritterbach J, et al. T-cell acute childhood lymphoblastic leukemia with chromosome 14q11 anomaly: a morphologic, immunologic, and cytogenetic analysis of 10 patients. *Blut* 1988;56,117–121.
303. Lange BJ, Raimondi SC, Heerema N, et al. Pediatric leukemia/lymphoma with t(8;14)(q24;q11). *Leukemia* 1992;6:613–618.
304. Lanham GR, Rivera G, Weiss K, Stass S. Comparison of morphology in ALL at presentation and relapse. *Med Pediatr Oncol* 1985;13:1–3.
305. Lanier LL, Allison JP, Phillips JH. Correlation of cell surface antigen expression of human thymocytes by multi-color flow cytometric analysis: implications for differentiation. *J Immunol* 1986;137:2501–2507.
306. Larson RA, Kondo K, Vardiman JW, Butler AE, Golomg HM, Rowley JD. Evidence for a 15;17 translocation in every patient with acute promyelocytic leukemia. *Am J Med* 1984;76:827–841.
307. Larson RA, Williams SF, Le Beau MM, Bitter MA, Vardiman JW, Rowley JP. Acute myelomonocytic leukemia with abnormal

eosinophils and inv(16) or t(16;16) has a favorable prognosis. *Blood* 1986;68:1242–1249.

308. Le Beau MM, Larson RA, Bitter MA, Vardiman JW, Golomb HM, Rowley JP. Association of an inversion of chromosome 16 with abnormal marrow eosinophils in acute myelomonocytic leukemia. A unique cytogenetic-clinicopathologic association. *N Engl J Med* 1983;309:630–636.
309. Leder L-D. Diagnostic experiences with the naphthol AS-D chloroacetate esterase reaction. *Blut* 1970;21:1–8.
310. Lee EJ, Pollack A, Leavitt RD, Testa JR, Sciffer CA. Minimally differentiated acute nonlymphocytic leukemia: a distinct entity. *Blood* 1987;70:1400–1406.
311. Le´glise M-C, Rivie`ve D, Le Calvez G, Le Bris M-J, Sensebe´ L, Brie`re J. In vitro study of translocation t(4;11) acute leukemia. Sequential range of phenotype. *Arch Pathol Lab Med* 1989;113: 164–168.
312. Leitenberg D, Rappeport JM, Smith BR. B-cell precursor bone marrow reconstitution after bone marrow transplantation. *Am J Clin Pathol* 1994;102:231–236.
313. Levitt GA, Stiller CA, Chessells JM. Prognosis of Down's syndrome with acute leukemia. *Arch Dis Child* 1990;64:212–216.
314. Li FP, Hecht F, Kaiser-McCaw B, Baranko PV, Potter NU. Ataxia-pancytopenia: syndrome of cerebellar ataxia, hypoplastic anemia, monosomy 7, and acute myelogenous leukemia. *Cancer Genet Cytogenet* 1981;4:189–196.
315. Liang R, Chan TK, Todd D. Childhood acute lymphoblastic leukemia and aplastic anemia. *Leuk Lymph* 1994;13:411–415.
316. Licht JD, Chomienne C, Goy A, et al. Clinical and molecular characterization of a rare syndrome of acute promyelocytic leukemia associated with translocation (11;17). *Blood* 1995;1083–1094.
317. Lilleyman JS, Britton JA, Anderson SM, Richards SM, Bailey CC, Chessels JM. Periodic acid Schiff reaction in childhood lymphoblastic leukaemia. *J Clin Pathol* 1994;47:689–692.
318. Lilleyman JS, Britton JA, Laycock BJ. Morphologic metamorphosis in relapsing lymphoblastic leukemia. *J Clin Pathol* 1981;34:60–62.
319. Lilleyman JS, Hann IM, Stevens RF, Richards SM, Eden OB. Blast cell vacuoles in childhood lymphoblastic leukemia. *Br J Haematol* 1988;70:183–186.
320. Lilleyman JS, Hann IM, Stevens RF, et al. Cytomorphology of childhood lymphoblastic leukaemia: a prospective study of 2000 patients. *Br J Haematol* 1992;81:52–57.
321. Lillington DM, MacCallum PK, Lister TA, Gibbons B. Tranlocation t(6;9)(p23;q34) in acute myeloid leukemia without myelodysplasia or basophilia: two cases and a review of the literature. *Leukemia* 1993;7:527–531.
322. Liu P, Tarle SA, Hajra A, et al. Fusion between transcription for CBF /PEBP2 and a myosin heavy chain in acute myeloid leukemia. *Science* 1993;261:1041–1044.
323. Lobach DF, Hensley LL, Ho W, Haynes B. Human T cell antigen expression during early stages of fetal thymic maturation. *J Immunol* 1985;135:1752–1759.
324. Lo Coco F, Avvisati G, Diverio D, et al. Molecular evaluation of response to all-trans-retinoic acid therapy in patients with acute promyelocytic leukemia. *Blood* 1991;77:1657–1659.
325. Lo Coco F, Avvisati G, Diverio D, et al. Rearrangements of the RAR-α gene in acute promyelocytic leukaemia: correlations with morphology and immunophenotype. *Br J Haematol* 1991;78: 494–499.
326. Lo Coco F, di Celle PF, Alimena G, et al. Acute lymphoblastic leukemia with the 4:11 translocation exhibiting early T cell features. *Leukemia* 1989;3:79–82.
327. Lo Coco F, Diverio D, Pandolfi PP, et al. Molecular evaluation of residual disease as a predictor of relapse in acute promyelocytic leukaemia. *Lancet* 1992;340:1437–1438.
328. Loken MR, Shah VO, Dattilo KL, Civin CI. Flow cytometric analysis of human bone marrow. I. Normal erythroid development. *Blood* 1987;69:255–263.
329. Loken MR, Shah VO, Dattilio KL, Civin CI. Flow cytometric analysis of human bone marrow. II. Normal B lymphocyte development. *Blood* 1987;70:1316–1324.
330. Look T. The emerging genetics of acute lymphoblastic leukemia: clinical and biologic implications. *Semin Oncol* 1985;12:92–104.
331. Look AT, Melvin SL, Williams DL, et al. Aneuploidy and percentage of S-phase cells determined by flow cytometry correlate with cell phenotype in childhood acute leukemia. *Blood* 1982;60: 959–967.
332. Look AT, Roberson PK, Williams DL, et al. Prognostic importance of blast cell DNA content in childhood acute lymphoblastic leukemia. *Blood* 1985;65:1079–1086.
333. Lu G, Altman AJ, Benn PA. Review of the cytogenetic changes in acute megakaryoblastic leukemia: one disease or several? *Cancer Genet Cytogenet* 1993;67:81–89.
334. Lu M, Gong Z, Shen W, Ho AD. The tcl-3 proto-oncogene altered by chromosomal translocation in T-cell leukemia codes for a homeobox protein. *EMBO J* 1991;10:2905–2910.
335. Ludwig W-D, Harbott J, Bartram CD, et al. Incidence and prognostic significance of immunophenotypic subgroups in childhood acute lymphoblastic leukemia: experience of BFM Study 86. In: Ludwig W-D, Thiel E, eds. *Recent Advances in Cell Biology of Acute Leukemia.* New York: Springer-Verlag; 1993:269–282.
336. Lugo TG, Pendergast A-M, Muller AJ, Witte ON. Tyrosine kinase activity and transformation potency of bcr-abl oncogene products. *Science* 1990;247:1079–1082.
337. Ma Q, Alder H, Nelson K, et al. Analysis of the murine All-1 gene reveals conserved domains with human ALL-1 and identifies a motif shared with DNA methyltransferases. *Proc Natl Acad Sci USA* 1993;90:6350–6354.
338. MacMahon B. Prenatal X-ray exposure and childhood cancer. *JNCI* 1962;28:1173–1191.
339. Mahmoud H, Carroll AJ, Behm FG, et al. The nonrandom dic(9;12) translocation in acute lymphoblastic leukemia is associated with B-progenitor phenotype and an excellent prognosis. *Leukemia* 1992;6:703–707.
340. Mahmoud HM, Ridge SA, Behm FG, Pui C-H, Ford AM, Raimondi SC, Greaves MF. Intrauterine monoclonal origin of neonatal concordant acute lymphoblastic leukemia in monozygotic twins. *Med Pediatr Oncol* 1995;24:77–81.
341. Mahoney DH, McClain KL, Hanson IC, Taylor LD, Steuber CP. Acquired immune deficiency, myelodysplasia, and acute nonlymphocytic leukemia associated with monosomy 7 and t(3;3)(q21;q26) in a child with Langerhans cell histiocytosis. *Am J Pediatr Hematol Oncol* 1989;11:153–157.
342. Malkin D, Freedman MH. Childhood erythroleukemia: review of clinical and biological features. *Am J Pediatr Hematol Oncol* 1989;11:348–359.
343. Mandel M, Rechavi MM, Neumann Y, et al. Bone marrow cell populations mimicing common acute lymphoblastic leukemia in infants with stage IV-S neuroblastoma. *Acta Haematol* 1991;86: 86–89.
344. Marks SM, Baltimore D, McCaffrey R. Terminal transferase as a predictor of initial responsiveness to vincristine and prednisone in blastic crisis chronic myelogenous leukemia. *N Engl J Med* 1978;298:812–814.
345. Marks SM, McCaffery R, Rosenthal DS, Moloney WC. Blastic transformation in chronic myelogenous leukemia: experience with 50 patients. *Med Pediatr Hematol Oncol* 1978;4:159–167.
346. Martin PJ, Najfeld V, Hansen JA, Penfold GK, Jacobson RJ, Fialkow PJ. Involvement of the B-lymphoid system in chronic myelogenous leukemia. *Nature* 1980;287;49–50.
347. Martinez-Climent JA, Lane NJ, Rubin CM, et al. Clinical and prognostic significance of chromosomal abnormalities in childhood acute myeloid leukemia de novo. *Leukemia* 1995;9:95–101.
348. Maruyama F, Stass SA, Estey EH, et al. Detection of AML1/ETO fusion transcript as a tool for diagnosing t(8;21) positive acute myelogenous leukemia. *Leukemia* 1994;8:40–45.
349. Maseki N, Miyoshi H, Shimizu K, Homma C, Ohki M, Sakurai M, Kaneko Y. The 8;21 chromosome translocation in acute myeloid leukemia is always detectable by molecular analysis using AML1. *Blood* 1993;81:1573–1573.
350. Maslak P, Miller WH, Heller G, Scheinberg DA, Dmitrovsky E, Warrell Jr RP. CD2 expression and PML/RAR-α transcripts in acute promyelocytic leukemia. *Blood* 1993;81:1666.
351. Matloub YH, Brunning RD, Arthur DC, Ramsey NKC. Severe aplastic anemia preceding acute lymphoblastic leukemia. *Cancer* 1993;71:264–268.

352. Matsuo T, Jain NC, Bennett JM. Nonspecific esterase of acute promyelocytic leukemia (M3). *Am J Hematol* 1988;29:148–151.
353. McCaffrey R, Harrison TA, Parkman P, Baltimore D. Terminal deoxynucleotidyl transferase in human leukemic cells and in normal thymocytes. *N Engl J Med* 1975;292:775–780.
354. McConnell TS, Foucar K, Hardy WR, Saiki J. Three-way reciprocal chromosome translocation in an acute lymphoblastic leukemia patient with hypereosinophilia syndrome. *J Clin Oncol* 1987;5:2042–2044.
355. McFarland W, Scheeter GP. The lymphocytes in immunological reactions in vitro: ultrastructural studies. *Blood* 1969;34:832.
356. McGrath IT, Ziegler JL. Bone marrow involvement in Burkitt's lymphoma and its relationship to acute B cell leukemia. *Leuk Res* 1979;4:33–39.
357. McGuire EA, Hockett RD, Pollock KM, Bartholdi MF, O'Brien SJ, Korsmeyer SJ. The t(11;14)(p15;q11) in a T-cell acute lymphoblastic leukemia cell line activates multiple transcripts, including Tlg-l, a gene encoding a potential zinc finger protein. *Mol Cell Biol* 1989;9:2124–2132.
358. McKenna RW, Brynes RK, Nesbit ME, et al. Cytochemical profiles in acute lymphoblastic leukemia. *Am J Pediatr Hematol Oncol* 1979;1:263–269.
359. McKenna RW, Parkin J, Bloomfield CD, Sundberg RD, Brunning RD. Acute promyelocytic leukemia: a study of 39 cases with identification of a hyperbasophilic microgranular variant. *Br J Haematol* 1982;50:201–204.
360. McMichael AJ. *Leucocyte Typing. vol III. White Cell Differentiation Antigens.* New York: Oxford University Press; 1987.
361. Meeker TC, Hardy D, Wilman C, Hogan T, Abrams J. Activation of the interleukin-3 gene by chromosome translocation in acute lymphoblastic leukemia with eosinophilia. *Blood* 1990;76:285–289.
362. Mellentin JD, Smith SD, Cleary ML. ly1-1, a novel gene altered by chromosomal translocation in T cell leukemia, codes for a protein with a helix-loop-helix DNA binding motif. *Cell* 1989;58:77–83.
363. Melo JV, Yan X-H, Diamond J, Goldman JM. Lack of imprinting of the ABL gene. *Nat Genet* 1994;8:318–319.
364. Meyers S, Downing JR, Hiebert SW. Identification of AML1 and the (8;21) translocation protein (AML1/ETO) as sequence specific DNA binding proteins: the runt homology domain is required for DNA binding and protein–protein interactions. *Mol Cell Biol* 1993;13:6336–6345.
365. Michiels JJ, Adraiaansen HJ, Hagemeijer A, Hooijkaas H, Van Dongen JTM, Abels J. Tdt positive B-cell acute lymphoblastic leukemia (B-ALL) without Burkitt characteristics. *Br J Haematol* 1988;68:423–426.
366. Miller DR, Leikin S, Albo V, et al. Prognostic factors and therapy in acute lymphoblastic leukemia of childhood: CCG-41. *Cancer* 1983;51:1041–1049.
367. Miller DR, Steinherz PG, Feurer D, et al. Prognostic significance of hand mirror cell variant of childhood acute lymphoblastic leukemia. *Proc Am Assoc Cancer Res* 1981;22:403 (abstract).
368. Miller Jr WH, Kakizuka A, Frankel SR, et al. Reverse transcription polymerase chain reaction for the rearranged retinoic acid receptor α clarifies diagnosis and detects minimal residual disease in acute promyelocytic leukemia. *Proc Natl Acad Sci USA* 1992;89:2694–2698.
369. Mirro J, Zipf TF, Pui C-H, et al. Acute mixed lineage leukemia: clinicopathologic correlations and prognostic significance. *Blood* 1985;66:1115–1123.
370. Miyazono K, Takaku F. Platelet-derived growth factors. *Blood Rev* 1989;3:269–276.
371. Miyamoto K, Tomita N, Ishii A, Nonaka H, Knodo T, Tanaka T, Kitajima K-i. Chromosome abnormalities of leukemic cells in adult patients with T-cell leukemia. *JNCI* 1984;73:353–362.
372. Morishita Y, Morishima Y, Ogura M, Nagai Y, Ohno R. Biochemical characterization of human peroxidase using three specific monoclonal antibodies. *Br J Haematol* 1986;63:435–444.
373. Morrell D, Cromartie E, Swift M. Mortality and cancer incidence in 263 patients with ataxia-telangiectasia. *JNCI* 1986;77:89–92.
374. Morrissey J, Tkachuk DC, Miltovich A, Franke U, Link M, Cleary ML. A serine/proline rich protein is fused to HRX in t(4;11) acute leukemia. *Blood* 1993;81:1124–1131.
375. Muehleck SD, McKenna RD, Arthur DC, Parkin JL, Brunning RD. Tranformation of chronic myelogenous leukemia: clinical, morphologic, and cytogenetic features. *Am J Clin Pathol* 1984;82:1–14.
376. Mufti GJ, Hamblin TJ, Oscier PG, Johnson S. Common ALL with pre-B-cell features showing (8;14) and (14;18) chromosomal translocations. *Blood* 1983;62:1142–1146.
377. Mulvihill JJ, Miller RW. *Genetics of Human Cancer.* New York: Raven Press; 1977.
378. Murphy S, Jaffe ES. Terminal transferase activity and lymphoblastic neoplasms. *N Engl J Med* 1984;311:1373–1374.
379. Murphy SB, Borrella L, Sen L, Mauer A. Lack of correlation of lymphoblastic cell size with presence of T-cell markers or with outcome in childhood lymphoblastic leukemia. *Br J Haematol* 1975;31:95–101.
380. Murphy SB, Harris A, Williams DL. Chromosomal translocations and timing of malignant transformation in Burkitt's lymphoma. *N Engl J Med* 1984;311:195–196.
381. Murphy SB, Raimondi SC, Rivera GK, et al. Nonrandom abnormalities of chromosome 9p in childhood acute lymphoblastic leukemia: association with high-risk clinical features. *Blood* 1989;74:409–415.
382. Nagler A, Brenner B, Tatarsky I. Secondary refractory anemia with excess blasts in transformation terminating as acute lymphoblastic leukemia. *Acta Haematol* 1986;76:164–165.
383. Najfeld V, Scalise A, Troy A. A new variant translocation 11;17 in a patient with acute promyelocytic leukemia together with t(7;12). *Cancer Genet Cytogenet* 1985;43:103–105.
384. Nakamura H, Sadamori N, Ichimaru M, et al. Juvenile chronic myeloid leukemia: no rearrangement of the breakpoint cluster region. *Cancer Genet Cytogenet* 1988;36:227–229.
385. Nakamura T, Alder H, Gu Y, et al. Genes on chromosomes 4, 9, and 19 involved in 11q23 abnormalities in acute leukemia share sequence homology and/or common motifs. *Proc Natl Acad Sci USA* 1993;90:4631–4635.
386. Narod SA. Radiation, genetics and childhood leukaemia. *Eur J Cancer* 1990;26:661–664.
387. Neglia JP, Robinson LL. Epidemiology of the childhood acute leukemias. *Pediatr Clin North Am* 1988;35:675–692.
388. Nelson DA. Cytomorphological diagnosis of the acute leukemias. *Semin Oncol* 1976;3:201–217.
389. Niebrugge DJ, Benjamin DR. Bone marrow necrosis preceding acute lymphoblastic leukemia in childhood. *Cancer* 1983;52:2162–2164.
390. Nourse J, Mellentin JD, Galili N, Wilkinson J, Stanbridge E, Smith SD, Cleary ML. Chromosomal translocation t(1;19) results in synthesis of a homeobox fusion mRNA that codes for a potential chimeric transcriptional factor. *Cell* 1990;60:535–545.
391. Nucifora G, Larson RA, Rowley JD. Persistence of the 8;21 translocation in patients with acute myeloid leukemia type M2 in long term remission. *Blood* 1993:82:712–715.
392. Odom LF, Lampkin BC, Tannous R, Buckley JD, Hammond GD. Acute monoblastic leukemia: a unique subtype—a review from the Childrens Cancer Study Group. *Leuk Res* 1990;14:1–10.
393. Ohyashiki K, Fujieda H, Miyauchi J, et al. Establishment of a novel heterotransplantable acute lymphoblastic leukemia cell line with a t(17;19) chromosomal translocation the growth of which is inhibited by interleukin-3. *Leukemia* 1991;5:322–331.
394. Ohyashiki K, Ohyashiki JH, Kinniburgh AJ, Toyama K, Ito H, Minowada J, Sandberg AA. myb Oncogene in human hematopoietic neoplasia with 6q- anomaly. *Cancer Genet Cytogenet* 1988;33:83–92.
395. Okamoto T, Ohno Y, Tsugane S, et al. Multi-step carcinogenesis model for adult T-cell leukemia. *Jap J Cancer Res* 1989;80:191–195.
396. Okuda T, Shurtleff SA, Valentine MB, et al. Frequent deletion of $p16^{INK4a}$/MTS1 and $p15^{INK4b}$/MTS2 in pediatric acute lymphoblastic leukemia. *Blood.* 1995;85:3416–3422.
397. Orazi A, Cotton J, Cattoretti G, Kotylo PK, John K, Manning JT, Neiman RS. Terminal deoxynucleotidyl transferase staining in acute leukemia and normal bone marrow in routinely processed paraffin sections. *Am J Clin Pathol* 1994;102:640–645.
398. Paietta E, Andersen J, Gallagher R, et al. The immunophenotype of acute promyelocytic leukemia (APL): an ECOG study. *Leukemia* 1994;8:1108–1112.

399. Palmer CG, Provisor AJ, Weaver DD, Hodes ME, Heerema N. Juvenile chronic granulocytic leukemia in a patient with trisomy 8, neurofibromatosis, and prolonged Epstein–Barr virus infection. *J Pediatr* 1983; 102:888–892.
400. Parravicini CL, Soligo D, Berti E, Cattoretti G, Gaiera G, Vago L. Immunohistochemical reactivity of anti-platelet mAb in normal human tissues and bone marrow. In: Knapp W, ed. *Leucocyte Typing. vol 4. White Cell Differentiation Antigens.* New York: Oxford University Press; 1989:981–985.
401. Parry P, Wei Y, Evans G. Cloning and characterization of the t(X;11) breakpoint from a leukemia cell line identifies a new member of the forkhead gene family. *Genes Chrom Cancer* 1994; 11:79–84.
402. Pearson MG, Vardiman JW, Le Beau MM, et al. Increased numbers of marrow basophils may be associated with a t(6;9) in ANLL. *Am J Hematol* 1985; 18:393–403.
403. Penchansky L. Bone marrow biopsy in the metastatic work-up of solid tumors in children. *Cancer* 1984; 1447–1448.
404. Penchansky L, Taylor SR, Krause JR. Three infants with acute megakaryoblastic leukemia simulating metastatic tumor. *Cancer* 1989;64:1366–1371.
405. Pendergrass TW. Epidemiology of acute lymphoblastic leukemia. *Semin Oncol* 1985; 12:80–91.
406. Pereira F, Moreno H, Crist W, Ermocilla R. Loffler's endomyocardial fibrosis, eosinophilia, and acute lymphoblastic leukemia. *Pediatrics* 1977;59:950–951.
407. Peterson L, Dehner LP, Brunning RD. Extramedullary masses as presenting features of acute monoblastic leukemia. *Am J Clin Pathol* 1981;75:140–148.
408. Pippard EC, Hall AH, Barker DJP, Bridges BA. Cancer in homozygotes and heterozygotes of ataxia telangiectasia and xeroderma pigmentosum in Britain. *Cancer Res* 1988;48:2929–2932.
409. Poiesz BJH, Ruscetti FW, Gazdar AF, Bunn PA, Minna JD, Galo RC. Detection and isolation of type C retrovirus particles from fresh and cultured lymphocytes of a patient with cutaneous T-cell lymphoma. *Proc Natl Acad Sci USA* 1980;77:7415–7419.
410. Pollack C, Hagemeijer A. Abnormalities of the short arm of chromosome 9 with partial loss of material in hematological disorders. *Leukemia* 1987; 1:541–548.
411. Pollack ER, Miller HJ, Vye MV. Medulloblastoma presenting as leukemia. *Am J Clin Pathol* 1981;76:98–100.
412. Potter VP, Sorell M, Baglivo JA, Sather H, Miller DR. Prognostic significance of vacuoles in L1 lymphoblasts in childhood acute lymphoblastic leukemia: a report from the Children's Cancer Study Group. *Br J Haematol* 1984;56:215–222.
413. Prasad R, Gu H, Alder T, et al. Cloning of the ALL-1 fusion partner, the AF-6 gene, involved in acute myeloid leukemias with the t(6;11) chromosome translocation. *Cancer Res* 1993;53:5624–5628.
414. Pratt CB, Meyer W, Chenaille D, Crom DB. The use of bone marow aspirations and lumbar punctures at the time of diagnosis of retinoblastoma. *J Clin Oncol* 1989;7:140–143.
415. Prigogina EL, Puchkova GP, Mayakova SA. Nonrandom chromosomal abnormalities in acute lymphoblastic leukemia of childhood. *Cancer Genet Cytogenet* 1988;32:183–302.
416. Privitera E, Kamps MP, Hayashi Y, et al. Different molecular consequences of the 1;19 chromosomal translocation in childhood B-cell precursor acute lymphoblastic leukemia. *Blood* 1992;79:1781–1788.
417. Pui C-H. Acute leukemias with the t(4;11)(q21;q23). *Leuk Lymph* 1991;7:173–179.
418. Pui C-H, Behm FG, Crist WM. Clinical and biological relevance of immunologic marker studies in childhood acute lymphoblastic leukemia. *Blood* 1993;82:343–362.
419. Pui C-H, Behm FG, Downing JR, et al. 11q23/MLL rearrangement confers a poor prognosis in infants with acute lymphoblastic leukemia. *J Clin Oncol* 1994; 12:909–915.
420. Pui C-H, Behm FG, Raimondi SC, et al. Risk and pathogenesis of secondary acute myeloid leukemia in childhood acute lymphoblastic leukemia. *N Engl J Med* 1989;321:136–142.
421. Pui C-H, Behm FG, Singh B, et al. Heterogeneity of presenting prognostic features and their relation to treatment outcome in 120 children with T-cell acute lymphoblastic leukemia. *Blood* 1990;75:174–179.
422. Pui C-H, Behm FG, Singh B, et al. Myeloid-associated antigen expression lacks prognostic value in childhood acute lymphoblastic leukemia treated with intensive multiagent chemotherapy. *Blood* 1990;75:198–202.
423. Pui C-H, Carroll AJ, Head D, et al. Near-triploid and near-tetraploid acute lymphoblastic leukemia of childhood. *Blood* 1990;76: 590–596.
424. Pui C-H, Carroll AJ, Raimondi SC, et al. Clinical presentation, karyotypic characterization, and treatment outcome of childhood acute lymphoblastic leukemia with a near-haploid or hypodiploid 45 line. *Blood* 1990;75:1170–1177.
425. Pui C-H, Carroll AJ, Raimondi SC, et al. Isochromosomes in childhood acute lymphoblastic leukemia: a collaborative study of 83 cases. *Blood* 1992;79:2384–2391.
426. Pui C-H, Crist WM. Cytogenetic abnormalities in childhood acute lymphoblastic leukemia correlates with clinical features and treatment outcome. *Leuk Lymph* 1992;7:259–274.
427. Pui C-H, Frankel LS, Carroll AJ, et al. Clinical characteristics and treatment outcome of childhood acute lymphoblastic leukemia with the t(4;11)(q21;q23): a collaborative study of 40 cases. *Blood* 1991;77:440–447.
428. Pui C-H, Hancock ML, Crist WM. Prognosis in children with the t(4;11)(q21;q23) acute leukemia. *Blood* 1991;78:2472–2473.
429. Pui C-H, Hancock ML, Head DR, Rivera GK, Look AT, Sandlund JT, Behm FG. Clinical significance of CD34 expression in childhood acute lymphoblastic leukemia. *Blood* 1993;82:889–894.
430. Pui C-H, Mirro J, Woodruff L, Motroni T, Stass S. Phagocytic activity and expression of myeloid-associated cell surface antigens by blast cells in acute lymphoblastic leukemia. *Med Pediatr Oncol* 1986;14:12–16.
431. Pui C-H, Raimondi SC, Borowitz MJ, et al. Immunophenotypes and karyotypes of leukemic cells in children with Down syndrome and acute lymphoblastic leukemia. *J Clin Oncol* 1993;11: 1361–1367.
432. Pui C-H, Raimondi SC, Dodge RK, et al. Prognostic importance of structural chromosomal abnormalities in children with hyperdiploidy (>50 chromosomes) acute lymphoblastic leukmeia. *Blood* 1989;73:1963–1967.
433. Pui C-H, Raimondi SC, Hancock ML, et al. Immunologic, cytogenetic, and clinical characterization of childhood acute lymphoblastic leukemia with the t(1;19)(q23;p13) or its derivative. *J Clin Oncol* 1994; 12:2601–2606.
434. Pui C-H, Raimondi SC, Head DR, et al. Characterization of childhood acute leukemia with multiple myeloid and lymphoid markers at diagnosis and at relapse. *Blood* 1991;78:1327–1337.
435. Pui C-H, Raimondi SC, Murphy SB, et al. An analysis of leukemic cell chromosome features in infants. *Blood* 1987;69:1289–1293.
436. Pui C-H, Rivera GK, Hancock ML, et al. Clinical significance of CD10 expression in childhood acute lymphoblastic leukemia. *Leukemia* 1993;7:35–40.
437. Pui C-H, Rivera G, Mirro J, Stass S, Peiper S, Murphy SB. Acute megakaryoblastic leukemia: blast cell aggregates simulating metastatic tumor. *Arch Pathol Lab Med* 1985; 109:1033–1035.
438. Pui C-H, Schell MJ, Raimondi SC, et al. Myeloid-antigen expression in childhood acute lymphoblastic leukemia. *N Engl J Med* 1991;325:1378–1379.
439. Pui C-H, Stass S, Green A. Bone marrow necrosis in children with malignant disease. *Cancer* 1985;56:1522–1525.
440. Pui C-H, Williams DL, Raimondi SC, et al. Hypodiploidy is associated with a poor prognosis in childhood acute lymphoblastic leukemia. *Blood* 1987;70:247–253.
441. Pui C-H, Williams DL, Roberson PK, et al. Correlation of karyotype and immunophenotype in childhood acute lymphoblastic leukemia. *J Clin Oncol* 1988;6:56–61.
442. Pui C-H, Williams DL, Scarborough V, Jackson CW, Price R, Murphy S. Acute megakaryoblastic leukaemia associated with intrinsic platelet dysfunction and constitutional ring 21 chromosome in a young boy. *Br J Haematol* 1982;50:191–200.
443. Quesnel B, Preudhomme C, Philippe N, et al. p16 gene homozygous deletions in acute lymphoblastic leukemia. *Blood* 1995;85: 657–663.
444. Rabbitts TH. Translocations, master genes and differences between the orgins of acute and chronic leukemias. *Cell* 1991;67: 641–644.

445. Rabbitts TH. Chromosomal translocations in human cancer. *Nature* 1994;372:143–149.
446. Ragab AH, Abdel-Mageed A, Shuster JJ, et al. Clinical characteristics and treatment outcome of children with acute leukemia and Down's syndrome. *Cancer* 1991;67:1057–1063.
447. Raimondi SC. Current status of cytogenetic research in childhood acute lymphoblastic leukemia. *Blood* 1993;81:2237–2251.
448. Raimondi SC, Behm FG, Roberson PK, Pui C-H, Rivera GK, Murphy SB, Williams DL. Cytogenetics of childhood T-cell leukemia. *Blood* 1988;72:1560–1566.
449. Raimondi SC, Behm FG, Roberson PK, et al. Cytogenetics on pre-B-cell acute lymphoblastic leukemia with emphasis on prognostic implications of the t(1;19). *J Clin Oncol* 1990;8:1380–1388.
450. Raimondi SC, Kalwinsky DK, Hayashi Y, Behm FG, Mirro Jr J, Williams DL. Cytogenetics of childhood acute nonlymphocytic leukemia. *Cancer Genet Cytogenet* 1989;40:13–27.
451. Raimondi SC, Peiper SC, Kitchingman GR, Behm FG, Williams DL, Hancock ML, Mirro J. Childhood acute lymphoblastic leukemia with chromosomal breakpoints at 11q23. *Blood* 1989;73:1627–1634.
452. Raimondi SC, Privetera E, Williams DL, et al. New recurring chromosomal translocations in childhood acute lymphoblastic leukemia. *Blood* 1991;77:2016–2022.
453. Raimondi SC, Pui C-H, Behm FG, Williams DL. 7q32-q36 translocation in childhood T cell leukemia: cytogenetic evidence for involvement of the T cell receptor β-chain gene. *Blood* 1987;69:131–134.
454. Raimondi SC, Roberson PR, Pui C-H, Behm FG, Rivera GK. Hyperdiploid (47–50) acute lymphoblastic leukemia in children. *Blood* 1992;79:3245–3252.
455. Raimondi SC, Williams DL, Callihan T, Peiper S, Rivera GK, Murphy SB. Nonrandom involvement of the 12p12 breakpoint in chromosome abnormalities of childhood acute lymphoblastic leukemia. *Blood* 1986;68:69–75.
456. Reid MM, Summerfield GP. Distinction between aleukemic prodrome of childhood acute lymphoblastic leukemia and aplastic anaemia. *J Clin Pathol* 1992;45:697–700.
457. Reilly JT, Barnett D, Dolan G, Forrest P, Eastham J, Smith A. Characterization of an acute micromegakaryocytic leukemia: evidence for the pathogenesis of myelofibrosis. *Br J Haematol* 1993;83:58–62.
458. Reinherz EL, Haynes BF, Nadler LM, Bernstein ID. *Leukocyte Typing*. vol II. New York: Springer-Verlag; 1985.
459. Rewald E, Estevez ME, Sen L. Monoclonal B cell lymphocytosis in early childhood: a case report. *Am J Pediatr Hematol Oncol* 1985;7:331–335.
460. Reynolds TC, Smith SD, Sklar J. Analysis of DNA surrounding the breakpoints of chromosomal translocations involving the T cell receptor gene in human lymphoblastic neoplasms. *Cell* 1987;50:107–117.
461. Ribeiro RC, Abromowitch M, Raimondi SC, Murphy SB, Behm FG, Williams DL. Clinical and biologic hallmarks of the Philadelphia chromosome in acute childhood acute lymphoblastic leukemia. *Blood* 1987;70:948–953.
462. Ribeiro RC, Oliveira MSP, Fairclough D, et al. Acute megakaryoblastic leukemia in children and adolescents: a retrospective analysis of 24 cases. *Leuk Lymph* 1993;10:299–306.
463. Ribeiro RC, Raimondi SC, Behm FG, Cherrie J, Crist WM, Pui C-H. Clinical and biological features of childhood T-cell leukemia with the t(11;14). *Blood* 1991;78:466–470.
464. Ritter J, Vormoor J, Creutzig U, Schellong G. Prognostic significance of Auer rods in childhood acute myelogenous leukemia: results of the studies AML-BFM-78 and -83. *Med Pediatr Oncol* 1989;17:202–209.
465. Rivera GK, Raimondi SC, Hancock ML, et al. Improved outcome in childhood acute lymphoblastic leukemia with reinforced early treatment and rotational combination chemotherapy. *Lancet* 1991;337:61–66.
466. Robinson LL, Nesbit ME, Sather HN, Level C, Shahidi N, Kennedy A, Hammond D. Down's syndrome and acute leukemia in children: a 10-year retrospective survey from Children's Cancer Study Group. *J Pediatr* 1984;105:235–242.
467. Rolink A, Melchers F. Generation and regeneration of cells of the B-lymphocyte lineage. *Curr Opin Immunol* 1993;5:207–217.
468. Rosenthal NS, Farhi DC. Acute monocytic leukemia with chloroacetate esterase positivity. FAB M4 or M5? *Am J Clin Pathol* 1992;98:41–45.
469. Rosenthal S, Canellos GP, DeVita VT, Galnick HR. Characteristics of blast crisis in chronic granulocytic leukemia. *Blood* 1977;49;705–714.
470. Rosner F, Schreiber ZR, Parise F. Leukocyte alkaline phosphatase: fluctuations with disease status in chronic granulocytic leukemia. *Arch Intern Med* 1972;130:892–894.
471. Rovelli A, Biondi A, Rajnoldi AC, et al. Microgranular variant of acute promyelocytic leukemia in children. *J Clin Oncol* 1992;10:413–1418.
472. Rowe JM, Lichtman MA. Hyperleukocytosis and leukostasis: common features of childhood chronic myelogenous leukemia. *Blood* 1984;63:1230–1234.
473. Rowley JD. A new consistent chromosomal abnormality in chronic myelogenous leukemia identified by quinacrine fluorescence and Giemsa staining. *Nature* 1973;243:290–295.
474. Rowley JD. Consistent chromosome abnormalities in human leukemia and lymphoma. *Cancer Invest* 1983;1267–1272.
475. Royer-Pokora B, Loos U, Ludwig W-D. TTG-2, a new gene encoding a cysteine-rich protein with the LIM motif, is overexpressed in acute T-cell leukemia with t(11;14)(p13;q11). *Oncogene* 1991;6:1887–1893.
476. Rubin CM, LeBeau MM, Mick R, et al. Impact of chromosomal translocations on prognosis in childhood acute lymphoblastic leukemia. *J Clin Oncol* 1991;9:2183–2192.
477. Saarinen UM, Wegelius R: Preleukemic syndrome in children. *Am J Pediatr Hematol Oncol* 1984;6:137–145.
478. Sanchez-Garcia I, Kaneko Y, Gonzalez-Samieto R, Campbell K, White L, Boehm T, Rabbitts TH. A study of chromosome 11p13 translocations involving TCR and TCRδ in human T cell leukemia. *Oncogene* 1991;6:577–582.
479. Sandler DP. Epidemiology and etiology of acute leukemia: an update. *Leukemia* 1992;6(suppl 4):3–5.
480. Sandler DP, Collman GW. Cytogenetic and environmental factors in the etiology of the acute leukemias in adults. *Am J Epidemiol* 1987;126:1017–1021.
481. Sariban E, Oliver C, Corash L, et al. Acute megakaryoblastic leukemia in childhood. *Cancer* 1984;54:1423–1428.
482. Savage RA, Hoffman GC. Sudan black B positivity in nonmyeloid leukemia. *Br J Haematol* 1983;54:494–495.
483. Savage RA, Hoffman GC, Lucas Jr FV. Morphology and cytochemistry of "microgranular" acute promyelocytic leukemia (FAB M3m). *Am J Clin Pathol* 1981;75:548–552.
484. Savitz D. Overview of epidemiologic research on electric and magnetic fields and cancer. *Am Ind Hyg Assoc J* 1993;54:197–204.
485. Schiff C, Milili M, Bossy D, et al. λ-like and V pre-B genes expression: an early B-lineage marker of human leukemias. *Blood* 1991;78:1516–1525.
486. Schlossman SF. *Leucocyte Typing*. vol 5. Oxford: Oxford University Press. 1995.
487. Schmitt C, Ktorza S, Sarun S, Blanc C, De Jong R, Debre P. CD34-expressing human thymocyte precursors proliferate in response to interleukin-7 but have lost myeloid differentiation potential. *Blood* 1993;82:3675–3685.
488. Schumacher HR, Champion JE, Thomas WJ, Pihs LL, Stass SA. Acute lymphoblastic leukemia hand mirror variant. An analysis of a large group of patients. *Am J Hematol* 1979;7:11–17.
489. Schumacher HR, Clapp WL, Thomas WJ, Mandavia SG, Pihs LL. Acute lymphoblastic leukemia. Hand mirror variant. *Arch Pathol Lab Med* 1980;104:134–136.
490. Schumacher HR, Desai SN, McClain KL, Domenico DR, Dizikes GJ, Bird ML. Acute lymphoblastic leukemia hand mirror variant. Analysis for endogenous retroviral antibodies in bone marrow plasma. *Am J Clin Pathol* 1989;91:410–416.
491. Schumacher HR, Perlin E, Klos JR, et al. Hand-mirror cell leukemia, a new clinical and morphological variant. *Am J Clin Pathol* 1977;68:531–534.
492. Schumacher HR, Rainey T, Davidson L, et al. American Burkitt's lymphoma: hand mirror variant. *Am J Clin Pathol* 1978;70:937–944.
493. Schumacher HR, Thomas WJ, Strong M, et al. Acute lymphoblastic leukemia hand mirror variant: viral immune interrelation-

ship as demonstrated by ultrastructural studies. *Am J Hematol* 1981;10:399–403.
494. Schwartz CL, Cohen HJ. Preleukemic syndromes and other syndromes predisposing to leukemia. *Pediatr Clin North Am* 1988; 35:853–871.
495. Scott CS, Patel D, Drexler HG, Master PS, Limbert HS, Roberts BE. Immunophenotypic and enzymatic studies do not support the concept of mixed monocytic-granulocytic differentiation in acute promyelocytic leukemia (M3): a study of 44 cases. *Br J Haematol* 1989;71:505–509.
496. Scott CS, Stark AN, Limbert HJ, Master PS, Head C, Roberts BE. Diagnostic and prognostic factors in acute monocytic leukemia: an analysis of 51 cases. *Br J Haematol* 1988;69:247–252.
497. Secker-Walker L, Stewart E, Norton E, Campana D, Thomas A, Hoffbrand V, Prentice G. Multiple chromosome abnormalities in a drug resistant Tdt positive B-cell leukemia. *Leuk Res* 1987;11: 155–161.
498. Secker-Walker LM, Berger R, Fenaux P, et al. Prognostic significance of the balanced t(1;19) and the unbalanced der(19)t(1;19) translocations in acute lymphoblastic leukemia. *Leukemia* 1992;6:363–369.
499. Secker-Walker LM, Chessells JM, Stewart EL, Swansburry GJ, Richards S, Lawler SD. Chromosomes and other prognostic factors in acute lymphoblastic leukemia: a long-term follow-up. *Br J Haematol* 1989;72:336–342.
500. Secker-Walker LM, Craig JM, Hawkins JM, Hoffbrand AV. Philadelphia positive acute lymphoblastic leukemia in adults: age distribution, bcr breakpoint and prognostic significance. *Leukemia* 1991;5:196–199.
501. Serrano M, Hannon GJ, Beach D. A new regulatory motif in cell-cycle control causing specific inhibition of cyclin D/CDK4. *Nature* 1993;366:704–707.
502. Shaw MT, Dwyer JM, Allaudeen HS, Weitzman HA. Terminal deoxyribonucleotidyl transferase activity in B-cell acute lymphocytic leukemia. *Blood* 1978;51:181–187.
503. Shurtleff SA, Meyers S, Hiebert SW, et al. Heterogeneity in CBF/MYH11 fusion messages encoded by the inv(16)(p13q22) and the t(16;16)(p13;q22) in acute myelogeneous leukemia. *Blood.* 1995;85:3695–3703.
504. Shuster JJ, Falletta JM, Pullen DJ, et al. Prognostic factors in childhood T-cell acute lymphoblastic leukemia: a Pediatric Oncology Group study. *Blood* 1990;75:166–173.
505. Silverstone AE, Cantor H, Goldstein G, Baltimore D. Terminal deoxynucleotidyl transferase is found in prothymocytes. *J Exp Med* 1976;144:543–548.
506. Slavc I, Urban C, Haas OA, Kroisel PM, Ko¨ller U. Acute megakaryocytic leukemia in children. *Cancer* 1991;68:2266–2272.
507. Smith FO, Lampkin B, Versteeg C, et al. Expression of lymphoid-associated cell surface antigens by childhood acute myeloid leukemia cells lacks prognostic significance. *Blood* 1992;79:2415–2422.
508. Smith FO, Rauch C, Williams DE, et al. The human homologue of rat NG2, a chondroitin sulfate proteoglycan, is not expressed on the cell surface of normal hematopoietic cells but is expressed by acute myeloid leukemia blasts from poor prognosis patients with abnormalities of chromosome band 11q23. *Blood.* 1996.
509. Smith H, Collins RJ, Sarnat HB, Trevenen CL. Pecular cytoplasmic inclusions in cells of acute lymphoblastic leukemia. *Am J Clin Pathol* 1986;86:261–263.
510. Smith KL, Johnson W. Classification of chronic myelocytic leukemia in children. *Cancer* 1974;34:670–679.
511. Smith SD, Link MP, Treia M, Amylon M, Sklar J, Morgan R, Hecht F. Chromosome 9 abnomalities in childhood T-cell leukemia. *N Engl J Med* 1986;315:195–196.
512. Smith SD, Morgan R, Gemmell R, et al. Clinical and biologic characterization of T-cell neoplasias with rearrangements of chromosome 7 band q34. *Blood* 1988;71:395–402.
513. Soekarman D, von Lindern M, van der Plas DC, et al. Dek-Can rearrangement in translocation (6;9)(p23;q34). *Leukemia* 1992;6:489–494.
514. Sokal JE, Gomez GA, Baccarani M, et al. Prognostic significance of additional cytogenetic abnormalities at diagnosis of Philadelphia chromosome–positive chronic granulocytic leukemia. *Blood* 1988;72:294–298.
515. Sonnier JA, Buchanan GR, Howard-Peebles PN, Rutledge J, Smith RG. Chromosomal translocation involving the immunoglobulin kappa-chain and heavy-chain loci in a child with chronic lymphocytic leukemia. *N Engl J Med* 1983;309:590–594.
516. Sorensen PHB, Chen C-S, Smith FO, et al. Molecular rearrangements of the MLL gene are present in most cases of infant acute myeloid leukemia and are strongly correlated with monocytic or myelomonocytic phenotypes. *J Clin Invest* 1994;93:429–437.
517. Soudon J, Bernard O, Mathieu-Mahul D, et al. c-myc gene expression in a leukemic T-cell bearing a t(8;14)(q24;q11) translocation. *Leukemia* 1991;5:60–65.
518. Spiers AS, Bain BJ, Turner JE. The peripheral blood in chronic granulocytic leukemia: Study of 50 untreated Philadelphia-positive cases. *Scand J Haematol* 1977;18:25–32.
519. Spitzer G, Garson OM. Lymphoblastic leukemia with marked eosinophilia: a report of two cases. *Blood* 1973;42:377–384.
520. Spry CJF. *Eosinophils: A Comprehensive Review and Guide to the Scientific and Medical Literature.* New York: Oxford University Press; 1988:150.
521. Stam K, Heisterkamp N, Grosveld G, et al. Evidence of a new chimeric bcr/c-abl mRNA in patients with chronic myelogenous leukemia and the Philadelphia chromosome. *N Engl J Med* 1985;313:1429–1433.
522. Stamberg J. Chromosome abnormalities in erythroleukemia. Cancer 1987;60:2649–2653.
523. Stass SA, Dean L, Peiper SC, Bollum FJ. Determination of terminal deoxynucleotidyl transferase on bone marrow smears by immunoperoxidase. *Am J Clin Pathol* 1982;77:174–176.
524. Stass SA, McGraw TP, Folds J, et al. Terminal transferase in acute lymphoblastic leukemia in remission. *Am J Clin Pathol* 1981;75:838–841.
525. Stass S, Mirro J. Unexpected heterogenity in acute leukemia: mixed lineages and lineage switch. *Hum Pathol* 1985;16:864–866.
526. Stass SA, Perlin E, Jaffe ES, et al. Acute lymphoblastic leukemia hand mirror cell variant: a detailed cytological and ultrastructural study with analysis of the immunological surface markers. *Am J Hematol* 1978;4:67–77.
527. Stass SA, Phillips TM, Weislow OS, Perlin E, Schumacher HR. Antigen–antibody complexes related to the baboon endogenous virus in humans with acute lymphoblastic leukemia hand mirror cell variant: (ALL-HMV). *Blood* 1980;56:661–666.
528. Stass SA, Pui H-C, Melvin S, et al. Sudan black B positive acute lymphoblastic leukemia. *Br J Haematol* 1984; 57:413–421.
529. Stein P, Peiper S, Butler D, Melvin S, Williams D, Stass S. Granular acute lymphoblastic leukemia. *Am J Clin Pathol* 1983;79: 426–430.
530. Stekhoven JHS, Langenhuysen CAM, Bakkeren JAJM, et al. Morphology and incidence of the "post-therapeutic lymphoid cell" in the bone marrow of children with acute lymphoblastic leukemia. *Am J Clin Pathol* 1986;124:46–52.
531. Stollmann B, Fonatsch C, Havers W. Persistent Epstein–Barr virus infection associated with monosomy 7 or chromosome 3 abnormality in childhood myeloproliferative disorders. *Br J Haematol* 1985;60:183-196.
532. Stoor J, Dolan G, Coustan-Smith E, Barnett D, Reilly JT. Value of monoclonal anti-myeloperoxidase (MPO7) for diagnosing acute leukaemia. *J Clin Pathol* 1990;43:847–849.
533. Strife A, Lambek C, Wisniewski D, et al. Discordant maturation as the primary biological defect in chronic myelogeneous leukemia. *Cancer Res* 1988;48:1035–1040.
534. Strong RC, Kersey JH. In vitro culture of leukemic cells in t(4;11)(q21;q23) acute leukemia. *Blood* 1985;66:439–443.
535. Strong RC, Korsmeyer SJ, Parkin JL, Arthur DC, Kersey JH. Human acute leukemia cell line with the t(4;11) chromosomal rearrangement exhibits B lineage and monocytic characteristics. *Blood* 1985;65:21–31.
536. Stryckmans PA, Debusscher L, Collard E. Cell kinetics in chronic myelogenous leukemia. *Clin Haematol* 1977;6:21–40.
537. Suarez C. DNA and RNA determinations in 111 cases of childhood acute lymphoblastic leukemia (ALL) by flow cytometry: correlation of FAB classification with DNA stemline and proliferation. *Br J Haematol* 1985;60:677–686.

538. Sugimoto T, Sawada T, Metsumura T, et al. Diagnosis of neuroblastoma metastasis in bone marrow with a panel of monoclonal antibodies. *Med Pediatr Oncol* 1988;16:190–196.
539. Sullivan MP, Crist W, Pullen J, et al. Childhood B-cell acute lymphoblastic leukemia (ALL) is unexpectedly clinically heterogeneous: a Pediatric Oncology Group (P.O.G.) study. *Proc Am Soc Clin Oncol* 1978;6:148 (abstract).
540. Suri R, Goldman JM, Catovsky D, Johnson A, Wiltshaw E, Galton DAG. Priapism complicating chronic granulocytic leukemia. *Am J Hematol* 1980;9:295–299.
541. Suryanarayan K, Hunger SP, Cleary ML, et al. Consistent involvement of the bcr gene by 9;22 breakpoints in pediatric acute leukemia. *Blood* 1991;77:324–330.
542. Swirsky DM, Li YS, Matthews JG, Flemans RJ, Rees JKH, Hayhoe FGJ. 8;21 translocation in acute granulocytic leukaemia: cytological, cytochemical and clinical features. *Br J Haematol* 1984;56:119–213.
543. Synold T, Relling M, Boyett J, et al. In vivo intracellular concentrations of methotrexate polyglutamates (MTX-PG) in acute lymphoblastic leukemia (ALL) blasts from children randomized to receive either high dose (HDMTX) or low dose (LDMTX) methotrexate. *Proc Am Soc Clin Oncol* 1993;12:131 (abstract).
544. Takimoto Y, Sakatani K, Kuramoto A, Tanaka K, Oguma N, Kamuda N. Isochromosome i(22q-) confirmed by in situ hybridization of v-alb gene in a case of CML in blast crisis. *Jap J Clin Haematol* 1986;27:2155–2161.
545. Tallman MS, Hakimian D, Snower D, Rubin CM, Reisel H, Variakojis D. Basophilic differentiation in acute promyelocytic leukemia. *Leukemia* 1993;7:521–526.
546. Tallman MS, Rowe JM. Acute promyelocytic leukemia: a paradigm for differentiation therapy with retinoic acid. *Blood Rev* 1994;3:70–78.
547. Talpaz M, Kantarjian H, Kurzock R, Trujillo JM, Gutterman JU. Interferon-alpha produces sustained cytogenetic responses in chronic myelogenous leukemia Philadelphia-positive patients. *Ann Intern Med* 1991;114:532–538.
548. Tauchi T, Ohyashiki K, Ohyashiki JH, et al. Acute lymphoblastic leukemia with azurophilic granules that contain ultrastructural myeloperoxidase activity. *Am J Hematol* 1991;36: 288–290.
549. Third International Workshop on Chromosomes in Leukemia, 1980: clinical significance of chromosomal abnormalities in acute lymphoblastic leukemia. *Cancer Genet Cytogenet* 1981;4:111–137.
550. Thirman MJ, Gill HJ, Burnett RC, et al. Rearrangement of the MLL gene in acute lymphoblastic and acute myeloid leukemias with 11q23 chromosomal translocations. *N Engl J Med* 1993; 329:909–914.
551. Thirman MJ, Levitan DA, Kobayashi H, Simon MC, Rowley JD. Cloning of ELL, a gene that fuses to MLL in a t(11;19)(q23;p13.1) in acute myeloid leukemia. *Proc Natl Acad Sci USA* 1994;91: 12110–12114.
552. Thomas WJ, Duval-Arnould B, Creegan WJ, Schumacher HR, Forman DS, Strong DM. Morphologic observations of contact-induced lysis of EBV-infected B lymphocytes by autologous hand mirror T cells. *Am J Hematol* 1982;12:109–119.
553. Tkachuk DC, Kohler S, Cleary ML. Involvement of a homolog of *Drosophila trithorax* by 11q23 chromosomal translocations in acute leukemias. *Cell* 1992;71:691–700.
554. Tobelem G, Jacquillat C, Chastang C, et al. Acute monoblastic leukemia: a clinical and biological study of 74 cases. *Blood* 1980;55:71–76.
555. Tomonaga M, Yoshida Y, Tagawa M, et al. Cytochemistry of acute promyelocytic leukemia (M3): leukemic promyelocytes exhibit heterogeneous patterns in cellular differentiation. *Blood* 1985;66:350–357.
556. Tono-oka T, Sato Y, Matsumoto T, Ueno N, Ohkawa M, Shikano T, Takeda T. Hypereosinophilic syndrome in acute lymphoblastic leukemia with a chromosome translocation [t(5q;14q)]. *Med Pediatr Oncol* 1984;12:33–37.
557. Tricot G, Orshoven ABV, Hoof AV, Verwilghen RL. Sudan black B positivity in acute lymphoblastic leukemia. *Br J Haematol* 1982;51:615–621.
558. Triche T, Askin FB, Kissane JM. Neuroblastoma, Ewing's sarcoma, and the differential diagnosis of small-, round-, blue cell tumors. In: Finegold M, ed. *Pathology of Neoplasia in Children and Adolescents*. Philadelphia: WB Saunders; 1986;145–195.
559. Troussard X, Valensi F, Salomon-Nguyen F, Debert C, Flandrin G, MacIntyre E. Correlation of cytoplasmic Ig μ ($C\mu$) and E2A-PBX1 fusion transcripts in t(1;19) B lineage ALL: discrepancy in $C\mu$ detection by slide immunofluorescence and flow cytometry. *Leukemia* 1995;9:518–519.
560. Troxell ML, Mills GM, Allen RC. The hypereosinophilic syndrome in acute lymphocytic leukemia. *Cancer* 1984;54:1058–1061.
561. Trueworthy R, Shuster J, Look T, et al. Ploidy of lymphoblasts is the strongest predictor of treatment outcome in B-progenitor cell acute lymphoblastic leukemia of childhood: a Pediatric Oncology Group study. *J Clin Oncol* 1992;10:606–613.
562. Tsuchiya H, ElSonbaty SS, Nagano K, et al. Acute myeloblastic leukemia (ANLL-M2) with t(8;21)(q22;q22) variant expressing lymphoid but not myeloid surface antigens with a high number G-CSF receptors. *Leuk Res* 1993;17:375–377.
563. Tucker MA, Meadows AT, Boice Jr JD, et al. Leukemia after therapy with alkylating agents for childhood cancer. *JNCI* 1987;87:459–464.
564. Tulliez M, Breton-Gorius J. Three types of Auer bodies in acute leukemia. Visualization of their protein by negative contrast after peroxidase cytochemistry. *Lab Invest* 1979;41:419–423.
565. Uchiyama T, Yodoi J, Sagawa K, Takatsuki K, Uchino H. Adult T-cell leukemia: clinical and hematologic features of 16 cases. *Blood* 1977;50:481–492.
566. Uckun FM, Gajl-Peczalska KJ, Provisor AJ, Heerema NA. Immunophenotype-karyotype associations in human acute lymphoblastic leukemia. *Blood* 1989;73:271–280.
567. Vagner-Capodano AM, Mozzionacci MJ, Zattara-Cannoni H, Guitard AM, Thuret I, Michel G. t(1;19) in a M4-ANLL. *Cancer Genet Cytogenet* 1994;73:86–88.
568. van den Doel LJ, Pieters R, Huisman DR, et al. Immunological phenotype of lymphoid cells in regenerating bone marrow of children after treatment for acute lymphoblastic leukemia. *Eur J Haematol* 1988;41:170–175.
569. van der Shoot CE, Daams GM, Pinkster J, Vet R, von dem Borne AEGK. Monoclonal antibodies against myeloperoxidase are valuable immunological reagents for the diagnosis of acute myeloid leukemia. *Br J Haematol* 1990;74:173–178.
570. van der Shoot CE, von dem Borne AEGK, Tettetoo PAT. Characterization of myeloid leukemia by monoclonal antibodies, with an emphasis on antibodies against myeloperoxidase. *Acta Haematol* 1987;78(suppl 1):32–40.
571. van der Valk P, Mullink H, Huijgens PC, Tadema TM, Vos W, Meijer CJLM. Immunohistochemistry in bone marrow diagnosis. Value of a panel of monoclonal antibodies on routinely processed bone marrow biopsies. *Am J Surg Pathol* 1989;13:97–106.
572. van Dijk MA, Voorhoeve M, Murre C. Pbx1 is converted into a transcriptional activator upon acquiring the N-terminal region of E2A in pre-B-cell acute lymphoblastoid leukemia. *Proc Natl Acad Sci USA* 1993;90:6061–6065.
573. Van Etten RA, Jackson P, Baltimore D. The mouse type IV c-abl gene product is a nuclear protein, and activation of transforming ability is associated with cytoplasmic localization. *Cell* 1989;58: 669–678.
574. van Eyes J, Pullen J, Head D, et al. The French–American–British (FAB) classification of leukemia: the Pediatric Oncology Group experience with lymphocytic leukemia. *Cancer* 1986;57: 1046–1051.
575. Viana MB, Maurer HS, Ferenc C. Subclassification of acute lymphoblastic leukemia in children: analysis of the reproducibility of morphological criteria and prognostic implications. *Br J Haematol* 1980;44:383–388.
576. Vidriales MB, Orfao A, Gonza´lez M, et al. Expression of NK and lymphoid-associated antigens in blasts of acute myeloblastic leukemia. *Leukemia* 1993;7:2026–2029.
577. Villeval JL, Cramer P, Lemoine F, et al. Phenotype of early erythroblastic leukemias. *Blood* 1986;68:1167–1174.
578. Vodopick H, Rupp EM, Edwards CL, Goswitz FA, Beauchamp JJ. Spontaneous cyclic leukocytosis and thrombocytosis in chronic granulocytic leukemia. *N Engl J Med* 1972;286:284–290.

579. Volger LB, Crist WM, Bockman DE, Pearl ER, Lawton AR, Cooper MD. Pre-B-cell leukemia. A new phenotype of childhood lymphoblastic leukemia. *N Engl J Med* 1978;298:872–878.
580. vom dem Borne AEGKR, Modderman PW, Admiraal LG, Nieuwenhuis HK. Platelet antibodies, the overall results. In: Knapp W, Do¨rken B, Gilks WR, Rieber EP, Schmidt RE, Stein H, von dem Borne AEGKR, eds. *Leucocyte Typing. vol 4. White Cell Differentiation Antigens.* New York: Oxford University Press; 1989:951–966.
581. Walle AJ, Al-Katib A, Wong GY, Jhanwar SC, Chaganti RSK, Koziner B. Multiparameter characterization of L3 leukemia cell populations. *Leuk Res* 1987; 11:73–83.
582. Warren AJ, Colledge WH, Carlton MBL, Evans MJ, Smith AJH, Rabbitts TH. The oncogenic cysteine-rich LIM domain protein Rbtn2 is essential for erythroid development. *Cell* 1994;78:45–57.
583. Washio S, Ido M, Azuma E, et al. Acute megakaryoblastic leukemia with translocation t(1;22)(p13;q13) in a 10-week-old infant. *Am J Hematol* 1992;39:56–60.
584. Watanabe S, Shimosato Y, Shimoyama M. Lymphoma and leukemia of T-lymphocytes. *Pathol Annu* 1981;16(2):155–203.
585. Wegelius R. Preleukemic states in children. *Scand J Haematol* 1986; 36(suppl 45):133–139.
586. Weinblatt ME, Ortega JA, Kaplan S. Morphologic changes in blast cells of children with acute lymphoblastic leukemia in relapse. *Med Pediatr Oncol* 1983;11:339–342.
587. Weiss K, Stass S, Williams D, et al. Childhood monosomy 7 syndrome: clinical and in vitro studies. *Leukemia* 1987;1:97–104.
588. Westbrook CA, Rubin CM, LeBeau MM, Kaminer LS, Smith SD, Rowley JD, Diaz MO. Molecular analysis of TCRB and ABL in a t(7;9)-containing cell line (SUP-T3) from a human T-cell leukemia. *Proc Natl Acad Sci USA* 1987;84:251–255.
589. Wheeler MS, Wilson EC, Stass SA. Erythroleukophagocytosis by leukemic cells: a nonspecific finding. *Am J Clin Pathol* 1981;75: 266–267.
590. Whitehead VM, Vuchich MJ, Lauer SJ, et al. Accumulation of high levels of methotrexate polyglutamates in lymphoblasts from children with hyperdiploid (>50 chromosomes) B-lineage acute lymphoblastic leukemia: a Pediatric Oncology Group study. *Blood* 1992;80:1316–1323.
591. Wiersma SR, Ortega J, Sobel E, Weinberg KI. Clinical importance of myeloid-antigen expression in acute lymphoblastic leukemia of childhood. *N Engl J Med* 1991;324:800–808.
592. Williams CKO, Folami AO, Saditan AAO, Ukaejiofo EO. Childhood acute leukemia in a tropical population. *Br J Cancer* 1982;46:89–94.
593. Williams DL, Harber J, Murphy SB, et al. Chromosomal translocations play a unique role in influencing prognosis in childhood acute lymphoblastic leukemia. *Blood* 1986;68:205–212.
594. Williams DL, Raimondi SC, Rivera G, George S, Berard CW, Murphy SB. Presence of clonal chromosome abnormalities in virtually all cases of acute lymphoblastic leukemia. *N Engl J Med* 1985;313:640–641.
595. Williams DL, Tsiatis A, Brodeur GM, et al. Prognostic importance of chromosome number in 136 untreated children with acute lymphoblastic leukemia. *Blood* 1982;60:864–871.
596. Windebank KP, Teffer A, Smithson WA, et al. Acute megakaryocytic leukemia (M7) in children. *Mayo Clin Proc* 1989;64: 1335–1351.
597. Wlodarska I, Stul M, Wolf-Peeters CD, Verhoef G, Mecucci C, Cassiman J-J, Van den Berghe H. t(1;19) without detectable E2A rearrangements in two t(14;18)-positive lymphoma/leukemia cases. *Genes Chrom Cancer* 1994;10:171–176.
598. Yanagihara ET, Naeim F, Gale RP, Austin G, Waisman J. Acute lymphoblastic leukemia with giant intracytoplasmic inclusions. *Am J Clin Pathol* 1980;74:345–349.
599. Yanagisawa K, Fukuska T, Fujita S. Evidence for the neoplastic involvement of monocytic, eosinophilic and basophilic lineages in acute myelomonocytic leukemia with eosinophilia. *Acta Haematol* 1990;83:145–148.
600. Yoffe G, Howard-Peebles PN, Smith RG, Tucker PW, Buchanan GR. Childhood chronic lymphocytic leukemia with t(2;14) translocation. *J Pediatr* 1990;116:114–117.
601. Yoshida M, Miyoshi I, Hinuma Y. Isolation and characterization of retrovirus from cell lines of human adult T cell leukemia and its implication in the disease. *Proc Natl Acad Sci USA* 1982;72: 2031–2035.
602. Youness E, Barlogie B, Ahearn M, Trujillo J. Tumor cell phagocytosis: its occurence in a patient with medulloblastoma. *Arch Pathol Lab Med* 1980;104:651–653.
603. Young Jr JL, Ries LG, Silverberg E, Horm JW, Miller RW. Cancer incidence, survival, and mortality for children younger than age 15 years. *Cancer* 1986;58:598–602.
604. Youro J. Burkart P, Lizzi F, Tartaglia A. Enzymologic classification of acute leukemias: nonspecific esterase markers distinguish myeloid and lymphoid varieties. *Blood* 1982;60:304–308.
605. Zieman-van der Poel S, Mccabe NR, Gill HJ, et al. Identification of a gene MLL that spans the breakpoint in 11q23 translocations associated with human leukemias. *Proc Natl Acad Sci USA* 1991;88:10735–10739.
606. Zipursky A, Peeters M, Poon A. Megakaryoblastic leukemia and Down's syndrome. A review. *Pediatr Hematol Oncol* 1987;4: 211–230.
607. Zipursky A. Poon A, Doyle J. Leukemia in Down's syndrome. A review. *Pediatr Hematol Oncol* 1992;9:139–149.
608. Zipursky A, Thorner P, De Harven E, Christensen H, Doyle J. Myelodysplasia and acute megakaryoblastic leukemia in Down's syndrome. *Leuk Res* 1994;18:163–171.
609. Zuelzer WW, Cox OE. Genetic aspects of leukemia. *Semin Hematol* 1969;6:228–249.
610. Zur Hausen H. Viruses in human cancers. *Science* 1991;254: 1167–1173.
611. Zutter M, Hockett RD, Roberts CWM, et al. The t(10;14) (q21;q11) of T-cell acute lymphoblastic leukemia juxtaposes the δ T-cell receptor with TCL-3, a conserved and activated locus at 10q24. *Proc Natl Acad Sci USA* 1990;87:3161–3165.

Pediatric Neoplasia: Morphology and Biology, edited by David M. Parham.
Lippincott-Raven Publishers, Philadelphia © 1996.

CHAPTER 16

Tumors of the Lymphoid Organs

Robert E. Hutchison and Aysegul H. Uner

INTRODUCTION

The lymphoid immune system comprises an extraordinarily complex though subtle mechanism for protecting the body against foreign organisms and substances. Although lymphoid tissue is easily recognizable at the microscopic level, it appears relatively monotonous compared to distinct structures of many other organ systems. It is only recently, since the development of immunologic and molecular genetic methods of investigation, that the wealth of diversity within lymphoid tissue has been fully appreciated. Not only are there distinct lineages of lymphoid cells (T cells, B cells, natural killer cells, antigen-presenting cells) that each show maturational sequences, but there is also genetic rearrangement and selection within at least the B cells and T cells that provide clones of lymphocytes to recognize and combat essentially any potential foreign antigen. There are therefore many thousands of distinct lymphoid cell populations in a person at any time, any one of which may also develop disease, such as through malignant transformation. Mistakes that occur during the normal processes of genetic rearrangement probably account for the majority of lymphoid malignancies that, as acute lymphoblastic leukemia and malignant lymphomas, constitute the first and third most common malignant tumors of children. It is fortunate, and a tribute to the vigor of children, that childhood lymphoid neoplasms are much less common (in absolute numbers), of more limited types, and generally more responsive to therapy than those of adults.

ORIGIN OF LYMPHOID CELLS

Lymphoid cells of each lineage derive initially from a pluripotential hematopoietic precursor cell that gives rise to bone marrow myeloid, erythroid, and some stromal cells as well as to lymphocytes and monocytes. These cells are present in the bone marrow and in small numbers in the peripheral blood throughout life. In fetal life they derive from the yolk sac, liver, and bone marrow. Lineage-specific differentiation of these stem cells is thought to be initially due to stochastic, or random, differential gene expression followed by selective events influenced by local microenvironmental factors, soluble factors (interleukins), and subsequent contact with antigens (196).

Lymphoid neoplasms are made up of expanded clones of cells that remain in an arrested state of development at any stage of maturation and usually have monotonous cytologic features corresponding to that level of maturation. In children, these are usually clones of precursor (blast) cells or cells in midlevels of differentiation. Neoplasms of mature or terminally differentiated lymphocytes, while common in adults, are rare in children.

Because of the correspondence of arrested maturational states in leukemias and lymphomas with stages of normal development, much of our understanding of the immunology of lymphocyte development in humans has come from study of malignancies. Animal-derived antibodies against human leukocyte products and membrane constituents have been used extensively to characterize and define lymphoid populations and compare them to data from animal experiments. Antibodies reacting with similar determinants have been organized into "clusters of differentiation" (CD groups) by a series of international workshops on human leukocyte differentiation (87) (see chapter 15 for additional information). Many of these are available as diagnostic reagents that, in conjunction with cytomorphology, are helpful in characterizing lymphomas and leukemias. Clinical features, such as sites of presentation, are often related to the normal sites of development of the corresponding cells.

The earliest recognizable B cells (early pre-B or pre-,

R. E. Hutchison and A. H. Uner: Department of Pathology, State University of New York Health Science Center, Syracuse, New York 13210.

pre-B-cells) have undergone immunoglobulin heavy chain (IgH) rearrangement and express HLA-DR, CD45, CD19, and CD10 (72). Subsequent maturation is accompanied by the presence of cytoplasmic mu heavy chain immunoglobulin, Ig light chain gene rearrangement, and CD20 expression (pre-B cells). Mature B cells express surface immunoglobulin, first IgM, then both IgM and IgD, and then, after heavy chain switching, IgG or IgM and either kappa or lambda light chains. Terminally differentiated B cells (plasma cells) produce (and secrete) cytoplasmic immunoglobulin and lack CD19. B-cell maturation, development, and expansion occur in the peripheral lymphoid system, principally the lymph nodes, spleen, and gastrointestinal and other mucosal-associated lymphoid tissue.

The thymus constitutes the primary organ for T-cell maturation and selection, including development of self-tolerance, and is active in young children (72). T-cell precursors migrate to the thymus in the first trimester of gestation and there undergo maturation, differentiation, and proliferation. The thymus is a bilobed organ in the anterior superior mediastinum that is arranged in lobules separated by connective tissue septae. Each lobule contains lymphoid cells referred to as thymocytes, which are arranged as an outer cortex and an inner medulla. The least mature proliferating thymocytes are present in the outer cortex with increasingly mature cells found in the inner cortex and mature thymocytes in the medulla. Throughout the lobules are epithelial cells of varying maturation, with islands of squamous epithelium, known as Hassall's corpuscles, present in the medulla. Dendritic cells and macrophages are found principally at the cortico-medullary junction.

The earliest T-cell precursors (T lymphoblasts) have undergone rearrangement of T-cell receptor complex genes (either alpha/beta or, less frequently, gamma/delta T-cell receptors), contain the nuclear enzyme terminal deoxynucleotidal transferase (TDT), and exhibit T-cell antigen CD7 and stem cell antigen CD34. With maturation in the thymic cortex, these cells lose CD34, acquire cytoplasmic CD3 (T-cell receptor complex), and express both CD4 and CD8, as well as CD1, CD2, and CD5. Selection occurs in conjunction with antigen presentation on the major histocompatibility complex (MHC) antigen of thymic epithelial cells, and subsequent maturing cells express either CD4 (helper cells) or CD8 (cytotoxic-suppressor cells), as well as surface CD3. Mature cells of the thymic medulla lack TDT and CD1, express either CD4 or CD8, and continue to express CD2, CD5, and CD7. They also express CD44, which is characteristic of trafficking T cells. Mature peripheral T cells proliferate in response to activation, giving rise to additional mature CD4 and CD8 lymphocytes (196).

Natural killer (NK) cells are an additional type of lymphoid cell that to some extent phenotypically resemble T-suppressor cells, frequently expressing CD2, CD7, CD8, and CD38, but usually lacking CD3. They generally express CD16, CD56, and CD57. These cytotoxic cells usually have the morphology of large granular lymphocytes. They are of obscure origin but likely derive from lymphoid precursors. NK cell–derived neoplasms are uncommon in adults and extremely rare in children (196).

Antigen-presenting cells include macrophages, Kupffer cells of the liver, Langerhan cells of the skin, follicular and interdigitating dendritic cells of the lymph nodes, and veiled cells of the spleen. All of these cells are considered to be derived from bone marrow monocyte precursors. Their functions are in part mediated by a diversity of adhesion molecules that facilitate cell-to-cell contact (72).

ORGANIZATION OF THE SECONDARY LYMPHOID ORGANS

The secondary, or peripheral, lymphoid organs are the sites at which antigens are processed and the immune response is mounted (102). They are anatomically positioned to provide comprehensive surveillance of the body. The spleen provides defense from bloodborne antigens, the mucosal-associated lymphoid tissue (MALT) provides defense from antigens penetrating the mucosa, and the lymph nodes process antigens draining with excess extracellular fluid in the lymph from visceral organs and from the skin. Chronic stimulation can lead to the additional formation of organized lymphoid tissue (lymphoid hyperplasia) at virtually any site in the body.

The spleen is composed of a red pulp, with vascular sinuses and cellular cords with marcophages that filter the blood to destroy senescent and damaged erythrocytes and platelets, and a white pulp made up of nodules of lymphocytes arranged around the arterioles that subsequently terminate in the red pulp sinuses. A periarteriolar lymphoid sheath (PALS) containing predominantly T cells is located immediately adjacent to the arteriole and the white pulp also contains B cell follicles that prior to stimulation lack germinal centers and are referred to as primary follicles. Following antigenic stimulation, secondary follicles form prominent germinal centers and distinct mantle zones. Around the entire PALS is a marginal zone that contains macrophages, T cells, and marginal zone B cells that have abundant cytoplasm and a somewhat monocytoid appearance. Hyperplasia of the marginal zone can result in a peculiar inverted follicle appearance. Malignant lymphomas originating in splenic lymphoid tissue (usually low-grade lymphomas) are rare in children, but the white pulp is frequently involved by spread of lymphomas, notably Hodgkin's disease, originating at other sites.

The mucosal-associated lymphoid tissue includes Waldeyer's ring (tonsils and adenoids), Peyer's patches of the gastrointestinal tract (so-called gut-associated lymphoid tissue, or GALT), and bronchial-associated lymphoid tissue (BALT), and it is also found in the genitourinary tract. In inflammatory circumstances it is associated with other mucosae, such as salivary glands. These unencapsulated lymphoid tissues are embedded in the lamina propria and submucosa of their respective organs. They generally show prominent germinal centers with mantle zones. Lamina propriae contain T lymphocytes and plasma cells, which often bear IgA.

The lymph nodes and lymphatic vessels compose a system for drainage and immune surveillance of extracellular fluids from throughout the body and terminate in the thoracic duct, which drains lymph into the left subclavian vein. The lymph nodes, located at lymphatic vessel junctions, are small kidney-shaped structures with an outer fibrous capsule and a system of supporting fibrous trabeculae. Underneath the capsule is an endothelial-lined subcapsular sinus that overlies the cellular cortex containing B-cell follicles. Unstimulated primary follicles in the cortex are made up predominantly of small lymphocytes, but most are stimulated secondary follicles containing germinal centers (GC). Within the GC are a variety of proliferating lymphoid cells, including small round lymphocytes, small cleaved cells and large cleaved cells (centrocytes), and small noncleaved cells and large noncleaved cells (centroblasts). Mitoses are frequent, and the majority of cells label with proliferating cell-specific antibodies such as Ki-67. Interspersed macrophages (tingible body macrophages) contain cell debris from dead cells, presumably resulting from apoptotic (programmed) cell death. The majority of germinal center lymphocytes are phenotypically mature B cells that exhibit surface immunoglobulin as well as pan-B and mature B-cell markers (CD19, CD20, CD22, and CD24). Scattered CD4−T cells are also present, as well as macrophages and dendritic cells. Germinal center cells in benign follicles often show "polarization," with darker cells and more macrophages to one side of the follicle.

Around the germinal center is a distinct mantle zone of small, dark-staining lymphocytes with condensed chromatin. These mantle zone mature B cells show low proliferative activity (Ki-67 negative) but express BCL-2 protein, which is an inhibitor of programmed cell death and indicates long-lived cells.

Underlying and between the cortical B-cell follicles is the paracortex, which is composed of small mature T cells with admixed large immunoblasts, interdigitating cells, plasma cells, histiocytes, and has a rich network of small vessels, including postcapillary "high endothelial" venules from which lymphocytes enter the lymph node.

The deeper portion of the lymph node, the medulla, contains cords of T cells, B cells, plasma cells, and converging medullary sinuses that terminate in the efferent lymphatic vessel at the hilum. Lymph travels centrally from here toward the thoracic duct.

Antigenic stimulation of the lymph node or other lymphoid organ results in enlargement (hyperplasia) of the normal cellular components. Excess lymphatic drainage from a diseased organ results in "sinus histiocytosis," T-cell stimulation causes paracortical expansion, and a humoral antibody response results in follicular hyperplasia. Hyperplasia generally affects the entire organ; however, in some circumstances it only affects one portion, resulting in an unbalanced hyperplasia that sometimes mimics lymphoma.

OVERVIEW OF PEDIATRIC LYMPHOMAS

Cancer in children is much less common than in adults and shows a different distribution of histologic types. While adults suffer most frequently from epithelial neoplasms (85%), these are rare in children. Children's cancers tend to be mesenchymal or hematopoietic and include, in descending order of frequency, acute leukemia, central nervous system tumors, lymphomas, neuroblastoma, Wilms' tumor, bone sarcomas (Ewing's and osteogenic), rhabdomyosarcoma, and retinoblastoma (24). Five to ten percent of pediatric neoplasms are lymphomas, of which 60% are non-Hodgkin's lymphoma (NHL) and 40% are Hodgkin's disease (Table 1). In children both tumor types occur in children, most frequently between the ages of 5 and 15 years. Although Hodgkin's disease has a second peak of incidence in early adulthood, it shows a relatively stable incidence throughout life, in contrast to many other malignancies, including leukemias, lymphomas, and carcinomas, that increase in incidence with age, particularly after 60 years. The lymphomas of later life include many low-grade types that occur only very rarely in childhood.

The most common histologic subtypes of Hodgkin's disease are mixed cellularity and nodular sclerosis types, and this is true in both children and adults. Lymphocyte-predominant Hodgkin's disease, often a disease of young to middle-aged men, and lymphocyte-depleted type,

TABLE 1. *Lymphoma types occurring in children*

1. Hodgkin's disease
   a. Lymphocyte-predominant
   b. Nodular sclerosis
   c. Mixed cellularity
   d. Lymphocyte-depleted
2. Non-Hodgkin's lymphoma
   a. Lymphoblastic
   b. Diffuse small noncleaved cell
      (1) Burkitt's
      (2) Non-Burkitt's
   c. Large cell
      (1) Immunoblastic
         a. Polymorphous
         b. Plasmacytoid
         c. Clear cell
      (2) Diffuse large cell
   d. Others (account for less than 3% of lymphomas in children)

most often occurring in older people, are proportionally even less common in children than in adults. The histologic and immunophenotypic features of Hodgkin's disease are essentially the same for all age groups.

Non-Hodgkin's lymphomas (NHL) of children, however, show a very different distribution of histologic types than occur in adults, with an almost exclusive predominance of diffuse aggressive types with rapidly progressive natural courses (24,86,119). These consist of nearly equivalent proportions of lymphoblastic, diffuse small noncleaved cell (Burkitt's and variants), and diffuse large cell lymphomas. There is a 2–3:1 male vs. female predominance in the incidence of childhood NHL. Fortunately, we now see high cure rates with both NHL and Hodgkin's disease in children with modern therapy (119).

Historically, accurate descriptions of the malignant lymphomas date at least back to Thomas Hodgkin's detailed 1832 observations of "tumours of the absorbent glands and spleen" (64,106). His necropsy studies with accompanying illustrations provided information on the gross pathology and natural course of disease that is valid to this day. He thought that he was describing a peculiar form of tuberculosis (TB), and in fact some of the patients he studied may have had TB. Samuel Wilks later restudied Hodgkin's material and concluded that the pathology represented neoplasms "separate from the tubercle" and named it "Hodgkin's disease" (207). Sternberg (186) and Reed (151) provided histologic descriptions of the malignant cells, but it is interesting that we still do not know the cause or even the cell of origin of Hodgkin's lymphoma.

The great German pathologist Rudolf Virchow provided the first detailed studies of non-Hodgkin's lymphoma in the 1850s and 1860s and coined the terms "lymphoma" and "lymphosarcoma" (199,200). These remained the names for essentially all NHLs, until Frederic Roulet referred to large cell or undifferentiated forms as "reticulum cell sarcoma" *(retothelsarkom)* in 1930 (163). This was also approximately the time that some follicular lymphoid proliferations were recognized as neoplastic (13,192).

Perhaps, it was irrelevant that a number of tumors of strikingly different clinical behaviors were lumped under just a few names until the potential for successful therapies existed. Some lymphomas, probably localized, were cured by radiation in the 1950s, but the advent of chemotherapy and combined modalities clearly called for better categorization of lymphomas.

In 1958, Denis Burkitt described a tumor in Ugandan children that was later recognized to be a malignant lymphoma with worldwide distribution in addition to endemic foci in equatorial Africa and New Guinea (16,17,130,132). In 1966, this was included in Rappaport's updated NHL classification (150); this schema was demonstrated to be clinically useful though lacking some relevance for childhood lymphoma because it included lymphoblastic types with "poorly differentiated lymphocytic" (PDL) types that are entirely different biologically and clinically. In the Rappaport Classification, Burkitt's tumor was included in "undifferentiated" lymphoma and large cell types were called "histiocytic." Today we recognize "histiocytic" lymphoma to be a misnomer, but it still includes most of the lymphomas that are considered together as large cell types for treatment purposes. Lukes and Butler concurrently described a classification of Hodgkin's disease that, with minor modifications by the Rye Conference, is still in use (98,101).

Classifications for NHL utilizing emerging knowledge of immunology were developed by Lukes and Collins (99) and by Lennert (92) in the 1970s, whereas Rappaport's purely morphologic approach was refined by Dorfman (33) and others. A system for translation between the various clinically relevant classifications, the Working Formulation (WF), was proposed in 1982 by the U.S. National Cancer Institute (211) after a major international comparative study and is still in use, although it utilizes only morphologic criteria. Karl Lennert's Kiel Classification, utilizing immunologic as well as morphologic data, has been updated and refined and is also in current widespread use (181). Both describe low- and high-grade lymphomas (also intermediate grade in the WF) and include both follicular and diffuse histology. Pediatric lymphomas are generally contained within the diffuse high-grade types (overlapping into diffuse intermediate grade in the WF). The updated Kiel Classification includes anaplastic large cell lymphoma, which has recently received a great deal of attention. Another recent proposal, the Revised European–American Classification, includes features of both the WF and the Kiel Classification as well as several entities (mostly occurring in adults) that are not addressed by either the WF or the Kiel. This system also includes lymphoproliferative disorders such as leukemias and myeloma that in the past have been categorized separately (58). Regardless of the classification utilized, additional information of immunologic, cytogenetic, and molecular features are now frequently used along with clinical information to qualify or augment a morphologic diagnosis.

NON-HODGKIN'S LYMPHOMA

Lymphoblastic Lymphoma

Approximately one third of childhood NHLs are lymphoblastic lymphomas (LBLs) (1,85) with estimates varying from 26% to 47% in some series (50,119). Despite the frequency of this disease, terminologic shifts in the 1960s led to neglect of the entity that had been previously referred to as "lymphoblastic lymphosarcoma" (74). It was known to present with supradiaphragmatic disease with frequent mediastinal mass formation and pleural effusion, consist of immature lymphoid cells, and often evolve into acute leukemia, and it had been postulated to be of thymic origin as early as 1948 (123). Following a period during which LBL was lumped with Rappaport's poorly differentiated lymphocytic lymphoma (PDL), Berard pointed out in 1972 the cytologic similarity between "PDL" of children and acute lymphoblastic leukemia (ALL) (9). Smith in 1973 reported a mediastinal lymphoid neoplasm of T-cell origin (179), and Barcos and Lukes in 1975 further described cases of convoluted cell mediastinal lymphoma of T-cell origin, reestablishing it as a distinct entity (2). It was subsequently recognized that the proper therapies for these tumors are those designed for high-risk T-cell ALL, and it is now known that most cases of LBL are essentially equivalent to nonleukemic T-cell ALL, with only subtle differences separating them from de novo T-cell ALL, and that leukemic progression ultimately occurs. B-lineage and other variants of LBL also exist, however (11,95,176,203) (see Chapter 15).

LBL in childhood presents at any age from early infancy throughout adolescence, with a male predominance that is accentuated in older children (70). The majority of patients present with advanced stage disease, and mediastinal involvement occurs in approximately one third of cases (50,70). About 20% of LBL patients have bone marrow or CNS disease, although marrow involvement with >25% blasts is generally classified as ALL. Abdominal disease is uncommon and pleural effusion common.

Histology

LBL shows diffuse infiltration of lymph nodes and other organs. When involvement is partial, there may be selective involvement of the paracortical T zone with relative sparing of the cortex and with residual germinal centers (Fig. 1). The capsule and surrounding tissue are often infiltrated with blastic cells appearing in single files between connective tissue cells as in leukemic infiltrates. When involvement is extensive, architectural effacement may be complete.

On hematoxylin and eosin–stained paraffin sections, the blasts appear as discohesive cells with nuclei that are usually smaller than those of the intermingled macrophages, which are often interspersed as in Burkitt's lymphoma to give a "starry sky" appearance. Nuclear membranes are frequently, though not uniformly, convoluted. The chromatin is finely dispersed and appears dusty, imparting a homogeneous light blue–gray color when viewed at low power. Nucleoli are variable in number but usually inconspicuous. Cytoplasm is scant and lightly basophilic. These features, particularly the small nuclear size, fine chromatin, and inconspicuous nucleoli, set LBL apart from diffuse small noncleaved cell (SNC) lymphoma (Fig. 2).

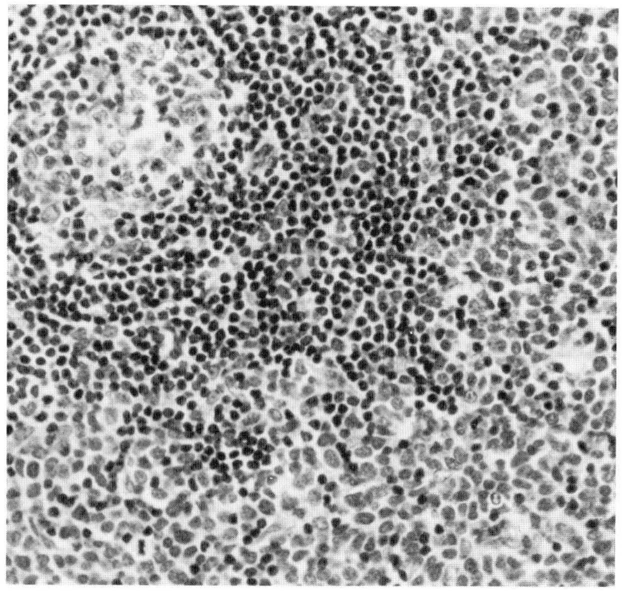

FIG. 1. Lymphoblastic lymphoma may show focal involvement with T-zone infiltration and sparing of follicles. (Hematoxylin and eosin slide courtesy of Dr. C. W. Berard, Memphis, TN.)

Some cases of LBL (approximately 10%) show larger cells and/or more prominent nucleoli than usual and have been referred to as the large cell variant of LBL (50). This is not surprising, given a similar heterogeneity in ALL. These large cell variants may be analogous to the L2 type of ALL described in French–American–British Cooperative Group (FAB) criteria (6) (see Chapter 15). On a practical histologic level, large cell variants of LBL may mimic small noncleaved cell (SNC) NHL, particularly when fixation artefacts are present. Cytologic examination of Wright–Giemsa– or other Romanowsky–stained touch imprints are helpful in identifying blast morphology in these difficult cases and should be examined whenever possible (88).

Cytologically, typical lymphoblasts in LBL are small cells with high nuclear/cytoplasmic (N/C) ratios; diffuse chromatin; irregular, convoluted, or sometimes smooth nuclear membranes; and inconspicuous nucleoli (Fig. 3; see figure in color plate section). Even when cytoplasm is more abundant and nucleoli prominent, as in L2 ALL, the chromatin pattern is usually more diffuse than SNC.

Immunophenotypic (and molecular) data are also helpful in diagnosing LBL because the vast majority of cases are of T-cell derivation, contrasting with the B-cell lineage of small noncleaved cell NHL. LBL has been shown to have an immunophenotype similar to that of T-cell ALL, except that there is a tendency toward more advanced thymocyte maturity (10,25,203). Although most T-ALLs have an early (TDT+/CD7+/CD1+/CD3+/CD4+/CD8+) or mid- (TDT+/CD7+/CD1+/

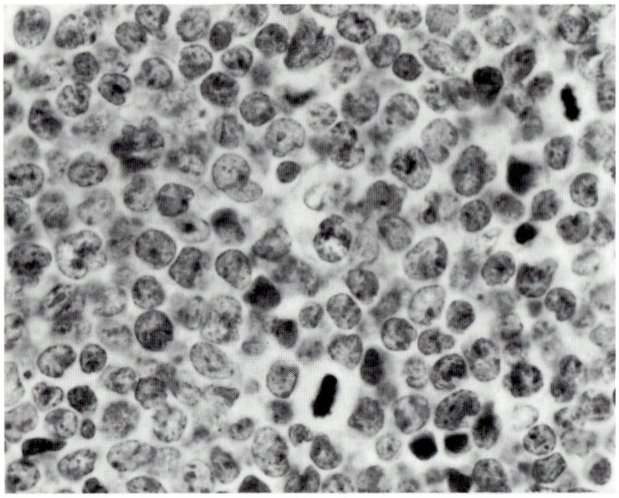

FIG. 2. Lymphoblastic lymphoma shows small cells with diffuse chromatin, usually inconspicuous nucleoli, scant cytoplasm and often irregular nuclear membranes. (Hematoxylin and eosin slide courtesy of Dr. C. W. Berard, Memphis, TN.)

CD3+/CD4+/CD8+) cortical thymocyte phenotype, most LBLs have a mid- or late (TDT+/CD7+/CD3+/CD4 or CD8+/CD1+) cortical thymocyte phenotype.

Complete immunophenotyping is best performed by flow cytometric immunofluorescent examination of viable cells or by immunohistochemical examination of frozen tissue or cytologic specimens. Partial immunophenotyping can also be performed on paraffin-embedded tissue, which will generally answer the question of T-cell vs. B-cell lineage, but the results provide less detailed information and are more technically variable than flow cytometric results. LBL are variably reactive with one or more T-cell markers (CD3/CD43/CD45RO) in paraffin-based studies, though these may be absent in immature phenotypes. These tumors show a high proliferative rate by Ki-67 immunohistochemical antibody labeling (205).

Most LBL show rearrangement of the alpha/beta T-cell receptor genes, and Southern blot assays for clonal rearrangement of the beta chain gene are commonly used. This technique and newer polymerase chain reaction (PCR)-based assays augment a complete phenotypic evaluation. Monoclonality is usually not a question, however, in an extensive blastic infiltrate.

Infrequent cases of LBL are of early B-lineage and are analogous to B-lineage or common ALL. These have been described with lymph node, skin, bone, and even mediastinal presentations (10,11,78,95,166,188,203). LBL of NK phenotype has also been reported (176), as have mixed lineage T-cell/myeloid and lineage shift from T-cell to myeloid phenotypes (31,129).

Characteristic cytogenetic abnormalities are not described in LBL, though this may be due to a lack of systematic studies, and those abnormalities that have been noted overlap with those of T-ALL. Structural abnormalities with breakpoints 9q32-34, 7q35, and 7p15 have been reported as have translocations involving 14q11 and 14q12, and t(9;17)(p34;q23) (79,171,177). The latter translocation may be specific for LBL (79). Abnormalities involving chromosome band 11q23, which are associated with poor prognosis in acute lymphoid and myeloid leukemias, have also been noted in LBL (194).

Diffuse Small Noncleaved Cell (SNC) (Burkitt's) Lymphoma

As noted above, the British surgeon Denis Burkitt in 1958 described a rapidly growing tumor usually arising in the jaw in children in Uganda (16). Subsequently recognized to be a malignant lymphoma (17,130,131), Burkitt's tumor has been the subject of intense epidemiologic and biologic investigation.

Because of a geographic distribution coinciding with certain mosquito populations and appearing to be temperature- and humidity-related, arboviruses were initially suspected to be etiologic, and a relationship with holoendemic falciparum malaria was finally concluded (210). Subsequently, a herpesvirus was isolated from tumor material by Epstein and associates and found to be characteristically associated with the disease (38,128). However, the Epstein–Barr virus (EBV) was also found to be nearly ubiquitous in those without neoplasia. It has generally been considered that immune suppression associated with malarial infection and malnutrition predispose to Burkitt's lymphoma (BL) associated with EBV. The more recent phenomenon of EBV-associated BL in immunosuppressed patients with human immunodeficiency virus (HIV) (124) supports the concept of an interplay between immune dysfunction, EBV, and Burkitt's tumor.

In addition to the endemic incidence of BL, predominant in tropical Africa and Papua New Guinea, a nonendemic or sporadic form was identified (132). The sporadic form is histologically and cytogenetically identical to the endemic form but is not associated with EBV. Subtle clinical differences also occur, with tendencies to abdominal presentation and bone marrow involvement but less tendency to present in the head and neck or with central nervous system involvement (167). Each form may involve the kidneys, adrenals, thyroid, other endocrine organs, ovaries, or breasts, often with bilateral involvement. Serum lactic dehydrogenase (LDH) is typically elevated.

To standardize the diagnostic criteria of BL, a histopathologic definition of BL was published by the World Health Organization in 1969 (8). This definition required adherence to a relatively strict histologic uniformity, with atypical cases fitting some but not all criteria excluded from the category of BL. These atypical cases have been referred to as undifferentiated non-Burkitt's lymphoma, diffuse small noncleaved cell lymphoma (211), or "Burkitt-like" lymphomas (58).

SNC NHL is a diffusely infiltrating tumor, sometimes with pushing borders and a tendency to surround organs. Occasionally, follicle formation or lymph node germinal center replacement is seen. The cells contain medium-size nuclei that are approximately the same size as those of the frequently interspersed macrophages that give a "starry sky" appearance. The nuclei of the Burkitt's type are uniformly round to oval (sometimes slightly indented) with distinct membranes. They contain coarsely reticulated chromatin and two to five moderately prominent nucleoli in a relatively clear parachromatin (8) (Fig. 4). Cytoplasm is moderate in amount and basophilic or amphophilic, with a characteristic "squared-off" appearance of acute angles between adjacent cells. The cytoplasm contains abundant RNA that stains red with methyl green pyronine (MGP).

Romanowsky-stained touch imprints and other cytologic preparations show greater nuclear heterogeneity than do paraffin sections. Nuclei in Burkitt's type vary from 12 to 25 μm in diameter with round to oval outlines, moderately clumped chromatin, and 2–5 nucleoli. Cytospin preparations may show irregular nuclei due to spin artefact. The cytoplasm is moderate in amount, deeply basophilic, and characteristically contains lipid vacuoles (Fig. 5; see figure in color plate section).

Non-Burkitt's (NB) SNC NHL is similar but with greater heterogeneity of nuclear size and outline. Both small and large cells may be present, and nucleoli tend to be fewer and more prominent, including cells with single prominent nucleoli (Fig. 6). If more than 25% of the cells in such cases have large nuclei, however, a diagnosis of large cell lymphoma may be more appropriate.

Cytologic specimens of non-Burkitt's SNC NHL show

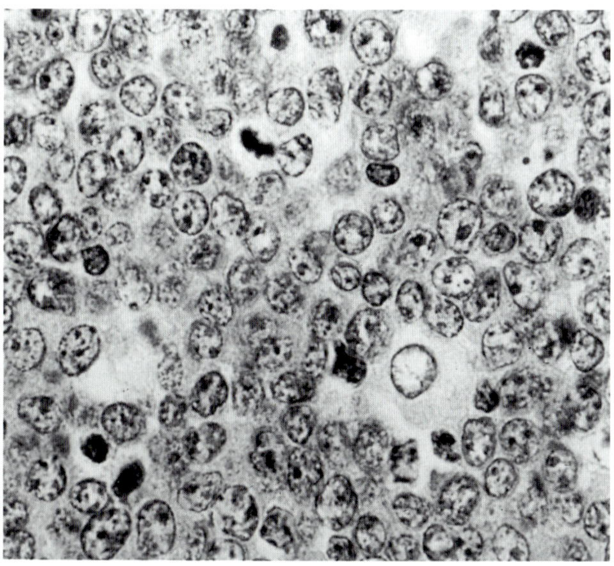

FIG. 4. Burkitt's lymphoma (diffuse small noncleaved cell) shows diffuse infiltrates of cells with homogeneously round to oval medium-size nuclei with multiple nucleoli, clumped chromatin in a clear parachromatin, and a high mitotic index.

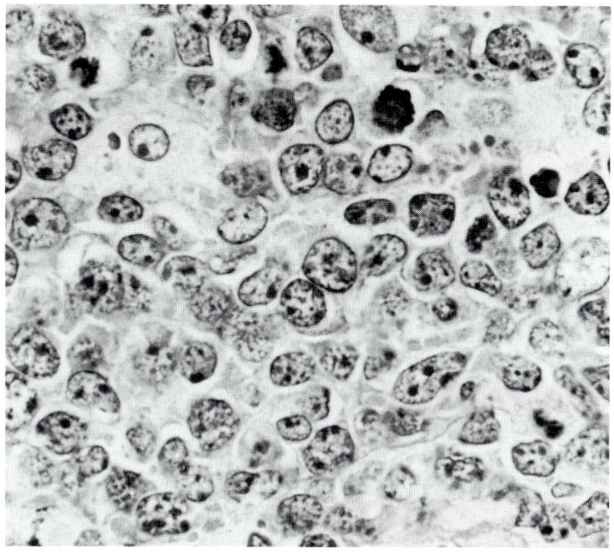

FIG. 6. Diffuse small noncleaved cell, non-Burkitt's lymphoma (Burkitt-like lymphoma). This lymphoma resembles Burkitt's tumor but shows greater nuclear size and shape heterogeneity, often with fewer, more prominent nucleoli.

nuclei from 15 to 35 μm in diameter, sometimes with giant or bizarre cells (211). Chromatin is often more dispersed and nuclear membranes less distinct than Burkitt's type. There is often a single nucleolus and moderate to scant pale cytoplasm that may not be vacuolated. These features may overlap with LBL or large cell lymphomas.

The immunophenotype of BL and most NB is that of mature B cells and is consistent with derivation from follicular center cells. The majority of cases express CD19, CD20, CD10, and monoclonal surface immunoglobulin. There is clonal rearrangement of the immunoglobulin heavy chain gene and one light chain gene.

Paraffin section immunochemistry shows positivity for antibodies against CD45 and B-cell-associated antigens, including CD20, CD45RA, and the antigen recognized by MB2 as well as others (LN1, LN2, etc.). Clonal surface immunoglobulin (Ig) can be detected in paraffin sections in some but not all cases (for technical reasons), but CD20 (L26) is usually strongly expressed.

Rare cases of NB show other immunophenotypes, including early B-lineage, pre-B-, and T-cell phenotypes (133). This bespeaks the heterogeneity of NB and its overlap with other entities.

Studies that have compared the clinical features of BL vs. NB histologic subtypes of sporadic SNC NHL have found no conclusive differences (52,68,82,93,113,140). This may be in part due to the fact that histologic discrimination between BL and NB is difficult to reproduce (208). Cytogenetic study has noted that the NB types less frequently show the characteristic abnormalities of BL, but more often show the presence of a rearranged *BCL-2* region due to the t(14;18), which is associated with follicular lymphomas and diffuse large cell lymphoma of B-cell immunophenotype (212). This, again, indicates that NB overlaps with other entities.

The characteristic cytogenetic and molecular abnormalities of BL consist of translocation of the c-*myc* proto-oncogene on chromosome 8 to transcriptionally active sites encoding immunoglobulin heavy chain on chromosome 14, kappa light chain on chromosome 2, or lambda light chain on chromosome 22, with resulting t(8;14), t(2;8), or t(8;22). Production of myc protein, associated with proliferation, is deregulated. In endemic BL, the breakpoints involve the immunoglobulin switch regions and the c-*myc* gene is not rearranged, whereas in the sporadic form, the breakpoints occur within the Ig joining regions and the c-*myc* is rearranged (truncated) (167).

The Epstein–Barr virus is characteristically associated with both the endemic form of BL and with BL occurring in immunosuppressed patients who are HIV-infected or have transplanted organs. It is not associated with SNC NHL in other children in Western countries. In immunosuppressed patients, clonal involvement of EBV in tumor cells can be detected by Southern blot analysis of EBV termini, which are of uniform number in clonal circumstances resulting in discreet bands on Southern blot analysis.

Large Cell Lymphoma

Large cell lymphoma (LCL) of childhood is a clinically and biologically heterogeneous group of neoplasms of large lymphoid cells. It is the least characterized of the childhood lymphomas, even though it occurs with an incidence similar to that of both lymphoblastic and SNC lymphomas. Until very recently it was assumed to share biologic features with large cell lymphoma of adults, but recent information shows a different spectrum of disease, with a greater frequency of high-grade immunoblastic histologies and T-cell immunophenotypic features (66).

In contrast to the relatively predictable presentations of lymphoblastic and small noncleaved cell NHL, LCL presents in a heterogeneous fashion with thoracic, abdominal, nodal, bone, or skin involvement (169). There is also a somewhat variable response to therapy, with good outcome in limited stage disease but disappointing results in advanced stage, particularly with bone marrow involvement. Age less than 5 years is also a poor prognostic feature (69,169). Recent data suggest that immunophenotype plays a prognostic role and that T-cell LCL is less favorable than its B-cell counterpart (118). T-cell phenotype is also associated with advanced stage disease (66).

The histology of LCL is quite variable and includes a number of distinct but overlapping subtypes. Hematopathologists commonly utilize terminology from several lymphoma classifications to describe cases. In the WF, LCLs are included in two groups: diffuse large cell and immunoblastic (211).

The term "diffuse large cell lymphoma" (DLCL) is primarily used to describe those lymphomas with a diffuse growth pattern derived from or resembling large follicular center B cells, but it is also used as a "wastebasket" category for those LCLs that don't fit clearly into a distinct subtype. Thus, although many of these are of B lineage, T-cell and other phenotypes also occur in this morphologic category. It is important to stress that immunophenotype cannot be accurately predicted from morphology alone.

In Luke's camera lucida drawings of germinal centers, he illustrated small lymphocytes with cleaved nuclei (small cleaved cells) and large cells with cleaved (large cleaved cells) or round (large noncleaved cells) as well as medium sized cells with round nuclei (so-called small noncleaved cells). Large cleaved cells have indented or cleaved nuclei larger than those of benign histiocytes or usual reactive endothelial cells, with minimal cytoplasm and inconspicuous nucleoli. Large noncleaved cells have oval vesicular nuclei with one or more distinct nucleoli that are often situated at the nuclear membrane and, and they contain a narrow rim of basophilic/amphophilic cytoplasm (99). Lennert called both small and large cleaved cells "centrocytes" and large noncleaved cells "centroblasts" (92).

One or both type(s) of these cells predominate in DLCL, and small cleaved lymphocytes are frequently admixed as a minority population (Fig. 7). Sclerosis may be present. DLCL includes the Lukes and Collins categories of follicular center cell, diffuse large cleaved cell and diffuse large noncleaved cell. It also encompasses Kiel Classification categories of centroblastic/centrocytic–diffuse, and centroblastic–diffuse.

Malignant lymphoma, large cell, immunoblastic (IBL) is the other main category of LCL in the WF and is even more heterogeneous than DLCL. It includes the variants designated plasmacytoid, clear cell, and polymorphous (with or without an epithelioid cell component). Immunophenotype (T cell or B cell) is not specified in the WF as it is in the Kiel and Lukes-Collins classifications and cannot be predicted from histology alone. Immunoblasts in IBL generally have uniform round or oval vesicular nuclei with one or more prominent central nucleoli.

In addition, the *plasmacytoid* variant has abundant basophilic/amphophilic (and pyroninophilic) cytoplasm with an eccentrically placed nucleus producing a resemblance to large plasma cells (Fig. 8A). The erroneous assumption that these are all "B-immunoblastic" lymphomas may have contributed in the past to overestimations of B-cell IBL in children, as some T-cell lymphomas also have this morphology.

The *polymorphous* variant contains large clear, pleomorphic, multinucleated or hyperlobated cells mixed

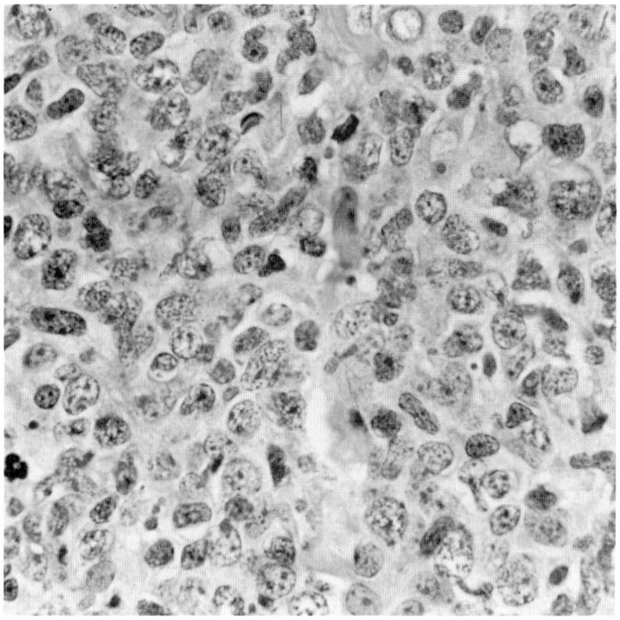

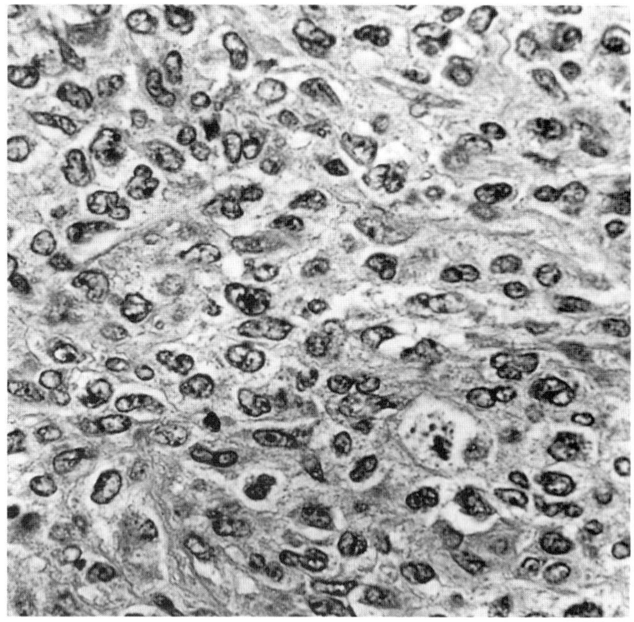

A B

FIG. 7. A. This diffuse large cell lymphoma is composed predominately of large noncleaved cells. **B.** This diffuse large cell lymphoma is composed predominately of large cleaved cells and contains sclerosis.

with atypical small cells with twisted nuclei and sometimes with variable numbers of plasma cells and/or epithelioid histiocytes. The large cells sometimes resemble Reed–Sternberg cells of Hodgkin's disease, with which this variant is often confused (Fig. 8B). The category was included in the WF partially in response to cases submitted from Japan and likely encompasses many of the pleomorphic lymphomas associated with HTLV-1 virus. It also encompasses many cases of anaplastic large cell lymphoma of the Kiel Classification (see below), a tumor that is much more common in children.

The *clear cell* variant has abundant optically clear cytoplasm with a distinct border surrounding a nucleus with fine, evenly dispersed chromatin and one or more distinct small nucleoli (Fig. 8C). These tumors were referred to as "T-immunoblastic sarcoma" by Lukes and Collins (99). They may be most often of T-cell origin, particularly when arising as clusters of clear cells in angioimmunoblastic lymphadenopathy, but are very uncommon as de novo lymphomas. Cases having this morphology but exhibiting a B-cell phenotype also exist. Clear cytoplasm may be occasionally seen as a focal fixation artefact in other immunoblastic lymphomas.

Anaplastic large cell lymphoma (ALCL) has sparked a great deal of interest and excitement since its description by Stein et al. in 1985 (185). It seems to provide a bridge linking the enigmatic disorders of Hodgkin's disease and malignant histiocytosis with large cell NHL. Furthermore, it appears to be a somewhat common childhood lymphoma, representing as many as 40% of childhood LCLs and approximately 10% of childhood NHLs overall (118).

ALCL was detected immunologically by tumor cell reactivity with an antibody (Ki-1; anti-CD30) raised against a Hodgkin's disease–derived cell line (172). This antibody labels T- and B-lymphoid cells activated in vitro by EBV, HTLV-1, and some mitogens. It labels Reed–Sternberg cells in HD and tumor cells in cases of T-cell and less commonly B-cell NHL, including cases previously designated as malignant histiocytosis (21,29,48,57,81,112, 137,138,144,146,198). CD30 ligand is a member of a family of cytokines having homology to tumor necrosis factor (178).

ALCL was described in the spectrum of T-cell lymphomas by Suchi et al. in 1987 (189) and incorporated into an updated version of the Kiel Classification in 1988 (181). It is characterized histologically by diffuse infiltration with large cells with indented nuclei and abundant cytoplasm. Multinucleated cells and cells with horseshoe or multilobated wreathlike nuclei are often seen (Fig. 9A; see figure in color plate section). There is frequently a T-zone distribution with infiltration of lymph node sinuses by cohesive sheets of tumor cells that mimic metastatic carcinoma or melanoma. Phagocytic, reactive histiocytes and sinus involvement have led to a frequent pathologic diagnosis of malignant histiocytosis. Morphologic variants of ALCL that have smaller cells and a relatively monomorphic appearance have been described.

Reactivity with anti-CD30 antibodies results in membrane and/or Golgi zone cytoplasmic staining (Fig. 9B; see figure in color plate section) (159). Tumor cells most often show a peripheral T-cell immunophenotype, often with an incomplete T-cell antigen profile when analyzed

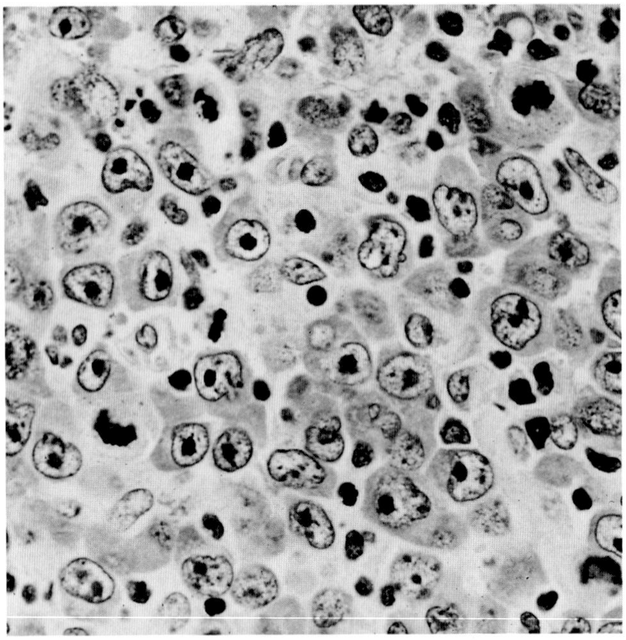

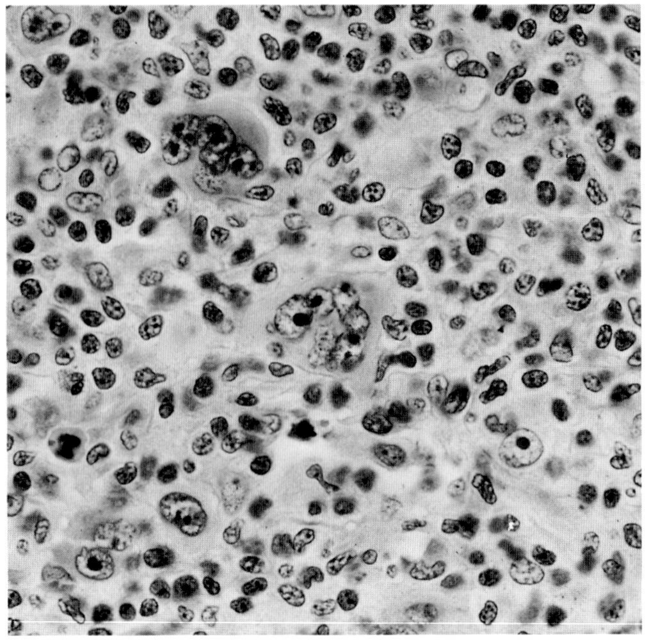

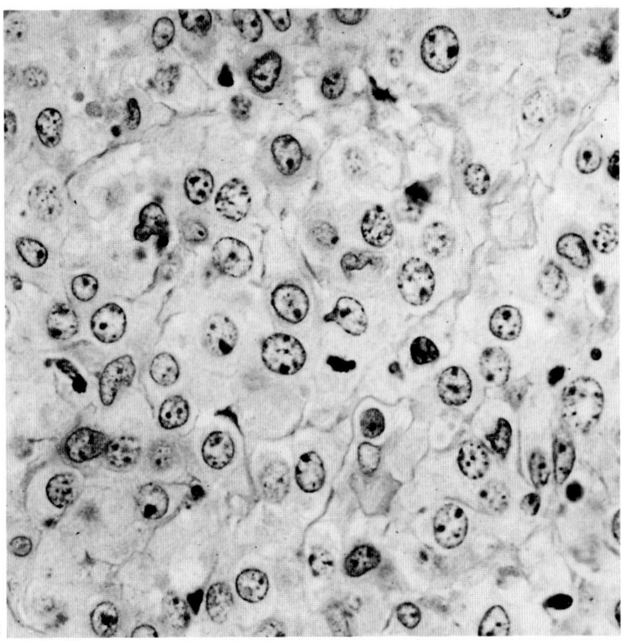

FIG. 8. A. The plasmacytoid subtype of immunoblastic (IB) lymphoma show cells resembling large plasma cells with prominent nucleoli. **B.** The polymorphous subtype of IB lymphoma contains pleomorphic cells, often resembling those of Hodgkin's disease, in a background of reactive cells. **C.** Clear cell IB lymphoma shows large cells with medium size nuclei and abundant clear cytoplasm with distinct cytoplasmic membranes.

by frozen section immunochemistry. Paraffin section immunochemistry usually shows labeling for CD45RO, CD43, and/or CD3. CD25 (interleukin-2 receptor) is characteristically present, as is epithelial membrane antigen (EMA) and BNH-9. T-cell receptor β-chain gene rearrangement is also often seen, though some cases are B-cell (most of which are in adults) and a greater number show no evidence of T- or B-cell lineage. Occasional cases with monocyte/macrophage markers such as CD68 occur, variably accompanied by T-cell markers and gene rearrangements.

ALCL is associated with a nonrandom chromosome abnormality, t(2;5)(p23;q35) (155). Recent cloning and characterization of this abnormality shows that a protein kinase gene *(ALK)* on chromosome 2 is fused with the region on chromosome 5 of the nucleophosmin gene *(NPM)*, which is associated with transport of ribosome components from the cell nucleus (115).

The clinical presentation of ALCL usually includes peripheral lymphadenopathy with frequent involvement of the skin and other extranodal sites including bone, soft tissue, gastrointestinal tract, lung, and pleura. Bone marrow involvement appears infrequently (77,153,168). Lymph node involvement typically includes sinusoidal and T-zone infiltration, frequently with cohesive sheets of tumor cells and areas in which tumor cells become admixed with reactive cells to produce a Hodgkin's-like appearance. There is also a characteristic "homing" to areas surrounding secondary B-cell follicles (182).

Both HD and ALCL cells express CD30, but ALCL usually lacks the CD15 expression that is characteristically present in HD. Whereas HD cells characteristically lack CD45, ALCL may or may not express it. Both share frequent association with EBV as detected by RNA in situ hybridization (EBER) and immunologic staining for EBV latent membrane protein (LMP) (60,61).

Results of treatment of ALCL indicate that, as with other NHLs of childhood, the majority of cases have a favorable outcome, but treatment failures occur. Results of the Pediatric Oncology Group (POG) suggest that the outcome of ALCL is similar to that of other T-cell and null cell LCLs (118). Advanced stage ALCL may have a better outcome than other advanced stage LCLs, and skin involvement has been reported to be associated with variably better or worse prognosis (153,168).

The category of ALCL now encompasses most cases previously designated malignant histiocytosis (MH) (see below). MH is characterized by lymph node sinus involvement and extranodal disease similar to ALCL and frequently exhibits hemophagocytosis by tumor cells or reactive histiocytes. Furthermore, the presence of enzymes and/or antigens suggesting derivation from monocytes or macrophages is generally described. Recently, however, cases previously designated MH have been reexamined and classified as T-cell lymphomas, often with CD30 expression (134,209). Controversy arises with cases that express myeloid/monocyte-associated antigens, including CD14, CD15, CD11c, CD68, and Mac387, and monocyte-associated enzymes such as α-naphthyl acetate esterase (nonspecific esterase), lysozyme, acid phosphatase, and α_1-antitrypsin. Coexpression of T-cell-associated antigens in these tumors is frequent. It is possible that these represent a lymphoma counterpart of mixed lineage phenotype in acute leukemia, but systematic studies are limited.

Some authors prefer to retain the category of MH (125). Hsu et al. described tumors with monocyte-associated enzymes and separated them into malignant histiocytosis (with CD11b, CD11c, CD14, and CD45 expression) and histiocytic lymphoma (with CD30 and lack of the above) (65). None of their cases showed T- or B-cell gene rearrangements. In studies of consecutively accrued large cell lymphomas, those with monocytic/histiocytic differentiation appear to be rare (66). In the future these entities may be better defined, but currently most investigators include MH with other types of LCL.

Uncommon NHL Histologies in Childhood

While the vast majority of childhood NHLs are lymphoblastic, small noncleaved cell, or diffuse large cell types, a very small proportion have other histologies more commonly seen in adults. A recent multi-institutional study identified 2.7% having unusual histologies in 1,336 childhood NHLs (154). These included 1 case of low-grade small lymphocytic, 6 cases of low-grade follicular mixed small and large cell, 9 of intermediate grade follicular large cell, 18 of intermediate grade diffuse mixed small and large cell, and 2 of high-grade small noncleaved cell with a follicular component. Most of those cases with follicular histology also showed variably extensive areas of diffuse involvement, but cases of purely follicular lymphoma (small cleaved cell, mixed, and large cell) have also been reported (46,145). SNC NHL with a focal follicular pattern is well described and behaves as aggressively as typical SNC. The other follicular lymphomas reported in children and adolescents have shown a remarkably favorable outcome.

Follicular lymphomas in adults have a strong tendency toward recurrence and/or slow progression with a frequently intractable course. In reports of follicular lymphoma in children, however, most cases have achieved remission with sustained long-term disease-free survival using a variety of therapies (46,145,154). This suggests that follicular lymphomas in children may be biologically different from those in adults.

Diffuse mixed small and large cell lymphomas have shown behaviors similar to those of diffuse large cell lymphomas in children. This category includes both B-cell and T-cell lymphomas and shows considerable morphologic overlap with diffuse large cell lymphomas. Polymorphous immunoblastic lymphomas, for example, contain pleomorphic immunoblasts admixed with small neoplastic cells and inflammatory cells. Lacking recognition of pleomorphism and Reed–Sternberg–like cells due to sample variation or artefacts, many of these could be categorized as mixed lymphomas. An entity often referred to as "Lennert's lymphoma," diffuse T-cell NHL with abundant epithelioid histiocytes, is heterogeneous and includes cases of diffuse mixed lymphoma in the WF as well as polymorphous immunoblastic with epithelioid histiocytes (and some cases of HD) (83,84). Furthermore, Nathwani et al. have argued that mixed lymphomas of T-cell phenotype should be categorized with immunoblastic lymphomas due to their aggressive behavior (122). The presence of inflammatory T lymphocytes in otherwise typical diffuse large cell lymphoma, so-called T-cell-rich large B-cell lymphoma, also results in morphologic overlap between large cell and mixed histologies (89,103,105,158). Due to the rarity of mixed small and large cell lymphomas in children as well as both clinical and histologic overlap, they may best be treated as diffuse large cell types.

Additionally, rare cases of mycosis fungoides (MF) have been described in pediatric patients (143). MF must be distinguished from skin involvement by other T-cell lymphomas such as ALCL as well as from inflammatory disorders. MF shows a typical clinical presentation with erythema and pruritis or with multiple macules or papules. The histologic feature is that of a bandlike or sometimes patchy dermal infiltrate that includes perivascular and periadnexal involvement by a lymphoid infiltrate containing small to medium-size abnormal cells with fine "cerebriform" nuclear convolutions. Histiocytes, small lymphocytes, and eosinophils are also frequently present. The upper dermis is relatively spared, but there is lymphocytic involvement and disruption of the epidermal basal layer and exocytosis of lymphocytes into the epidermis. Characteristically, there is no spongiosis (edema) associated with the exocytosis as one sees in inflammatory processes, but up to one third of cases of MF in adults will show this feature (174). Small collections of abnormal lymphocytes (Pautier's microabscesses) are present in cleared spaces in the epithelium, which may be atrophic or hyperplastic and which often shows hyperkeratosis.

The immunophenotype of MF, best assayed on frozen sections, consists of CD4+ peripheral T cells that frequently lack the pan-T-cell antigen CD7. There is characteristically clonal rearrangement of the T-cell receptor β-chain gene, but due to dilution with epithelial DNA it is difficult to obtain sufficient material from small skin specimens for Southern analysis. Polymerase chain reaction (PCR) techniques for T-cell receptor clonality may prove more helpful in this regard.

Other lymphomas occur in the skin and include rare lymphoblastic NHL (214), which may be B- or T-lineage, and, more frequently, large cell types including ALCL. Granulocytic sarcoma (tissue involvement by acute myeloblastic leukemia) also occurs in the skin and often shows monocytic differentiation (see Chapter 15). Secondary ALCL may also arise in MF (at least in adults).

Acute T-cell leukemia/lymphoma (ATLL) associated with HTLV-1, or precursor lesions, may rarely also arise in children (see Chapter 15) (56). The disease in adults is classically characterized by an aggressive course with leukemia, skin involvement, lymphadenopathy, and hypercalcemia. Tumor cells are typically medium-size with polylobated nuclei and a CD4+, CD25+ peripheral T-cell phenotype. However, virtually any histology associated with T-cell lymphomas has been seen in HTLV-1 disease in adults, including T-cell CLL, MF, lymphoblastic, mixed, and large cell types (26). The histologic features usually best fit in the polymorphous immunoblastic category in the WF (or pleomorphic in the Kiel).

HODGKIN'S DISEASE

Hodgkin's disease (HD), although most common in young adults (15–34 years), also occurs in childhood (0–14 years) and in older adults (55+ years) (53). The incidence in the United States is approximately 1 per 1 million in children under 15 years (85). Children tend to have more localized disease and an overall better prognosis when compared with adults, with both young age and limited stage being favorable prognostic factors (32). The majority of patients present with supradiaphragmatic disease, and spread of disease is usually contiguous (32), as was originally described by Hodgkin (64). Therapy consists of radiation, chemotherapy (usually MOPP and/or ABVD), or a combination modality (32,195). Long-term survival is as high as 90% in some series (195).

Generally, the initial diagnosis of HD is made on lymph node biopsies. Rarely, lung, liver, spleen, or bone marrow samples may be examined for initial diagnosis. HD may involve the lymph nodes totally or partially, and involved lymph nodes may be interspersed with normal lymph nodes. Focal involvement may also create a sampling problem in other sites, such as liver or bone marrow.

The histologic features of HD are well described (15,51). The diagnosis depends on the identification of diagnostic Reed–Sternberg (RS) cells in a background of reactive cells. The RS cell is a large cell with abundant eosinophilic cytoplasm, a polylobated nucleus, and a prominent, usually eosinophilic inclusionlike nucleolus in each lobe (Fig. 10; see figure in color plate section). There is usually parachromatin clearing around the nucleolus and a thick nuclear envelope. Mononuclear variants with similar nuclear features are also seen in most cases. RS-like cells can be found in other conditions such as infectious mononucleosis, peripheral T-cell lymphoma, and immunoblastic polymorphous type of non-Hodgkin's lymphoma. Thus, the demonstration of the reactive cell component in the background is essential for the correct diagnosis.

Another type of cell typically seen in nodular sclerosis HD is the lacunar cell. This is a large cell with a hyperlobated nucleus and abundant pale cytoplasm that retracts in formalin-fixed sections, leaving a clear space or "lacuna" around the cell. Eosinophilic nucleoli may be present in lacunar cells, although they tend to be inconspicuous. Clusters of lacunar cells are seen in the nodules in nodular sclerosing HD. Degenerated forms of "Hodgkin's cells" with pyknotic nuclei, dark eosinophilic smudged cells, or "mummified" cells are frequently encountered in tissue sections. A type-specific cell seen in lymphocyte/histiocyte (L/H) predominance HD is the "L/H variant," or "popcorn cell," which is a large cell with a convoluted or polylobated nucleus containing a moderately prominent (though smaller than that of an RS cell) nucleolus.

The reactive background component of HD is composed of variable proportions of lymphocytes, histiocytes, eosinophils, neutrophils, and plasma cells. Lymphocytes are generally small with round nuclei. Occasionally, irregular angulated forms and activated lymphoid cells may also be present. Immunohistochemical studies have demonstrated that the majority of these reactive elements are T cells of helper cell phenotype (51). A histiocytic response may also be quite prominent in some biopsies, with formation of granulomas or with scattered individual histiocytes. The host response, as judged by the reactive background elements, may provide prognostic information. For example, the presence of granulomas in lymph nodes involved by HD may be associated with a better prognosis (18), whereas a prominent polymorphonuclear cell infiltrate and necrosis correlate with B symptoms and worse prognosis (41).

Classification of Hodgkin's Disease

In 1947, Jackson and Parker proposed a classification scheme for Hodgkin's disease that involved three types; paragranuloma, granuloma, and sarcoma (73). Then, in 1966, Lukes and Butler proposed a histopathologic classification based on the relative proportions of RS cells and the accompanying lymphocytic proliferation and sclerosis observed in pretherapy lymph node biopsies (98). This classification had four major categories, which are shown in Table 1. The original Lukes and Butler classification was modified at an international meeting in Rye, New York, resulting in the scheme widely accepted today (101). The Rye Classification divides HD into four types: lymphocyte predominance (LP); nodular sclerosis (NS); mixed cellularity (MC); and lymphocyte depletion (LD).

The Ann Arbor staging classification was put forward in 1971 to assess the extent and pattern of Hodgkin's disease involvement at presentation (18). Currently, this scheme is widely used and divides Hodgkin's disease into four stages, depending on the extent of nodal and/or extranodal disease and whether or not systemic symptoms such as fever, sweats, and/or weight loss is present.

Lymphocyte Predominance HD

LP HD comprises between 5% and 10% of childhood Hodgkin's disease (193). Cervical lymph nodes (LNs), followed by inguinal LNs, are most commonly involved. This type encompasses nodular and diffuse subtypes, with the diffuse subtype being the more common of the two (Fig. 11). The histopathologic features of both subtypes include prominence of mature lymphocytes and histiocytes. Lymphocytic and histiocytic RS cell variants (L/H cells) are also frequent, but definitive diagnosis relies on the identification of classical RS cells, which are rare in this type of HD. Multiple sections may be necessary to identify a single diagnostic RS cell, and this scarcity itself provides an important feature in differentiating LP HD from other types, especially MC type. L/H cells characteristically have folded, complex vesicular nuclei with inconspicuous nucleoli. Abnormal mitotic figures,

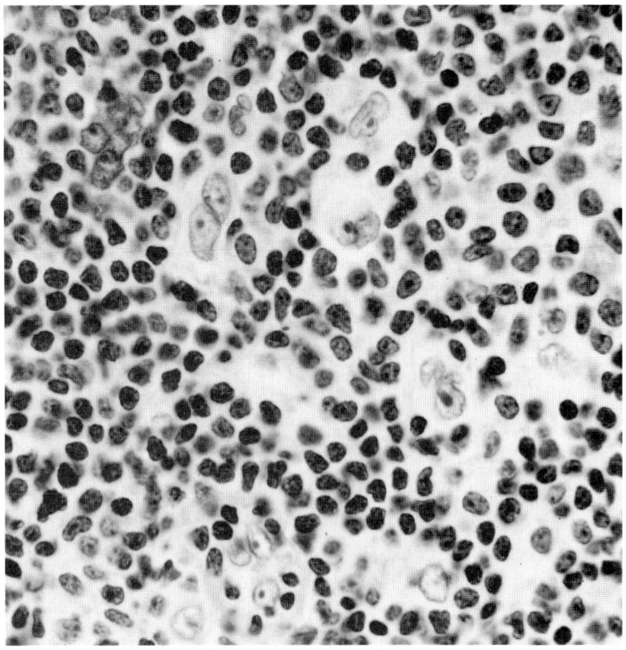

FIG. 11. Lymphocyte-predominant Hodgkin's disease shows "L/H" cells in a background of small lymphocytes. The pattern may be nodular or diffuse.

mummified cells, and mononuclear Hodgkin's cells may also be encountered. Infrequently, scattered eosinophils, plasma cells, and polymorphonuclear cells may be identified in lymph nodes involved by LP HD. The absolute requirement for typical (though rare) RS cells in LP HD has been challenged (51,126), and it may be that in many cases L/H cells with lobated nuclei stand in for true RS cells.

The diffuse subtype of LP HD generally shows complete effacement of the lymph node by a lymphohistiocytic infiltrate with scattered L/H cells. In the nodular subtype, the lymph nodes show a nodularity that may be vague or prominent. The L/H cells are concentrated within the nodules, which often compress the paracortex. Fibrosis is not present, although increased reticulum fibers may be demonstrated with special stains.

Immunophenotyping studies have demonstrated that in LP HD, especially the nodular variant, the L/H cells express B-cell markers, including paraffin-reactive CD20 (23,51,76,183). This has lead to the proposal that the nodular subtype of LP HD is actually a low-grade B-cell lymphoma or premalignant B-cell proliferation originating from the follicular center (76,147). In 2–10% of cases, transformation to large cell lymphoma with B-cell immunophenotype has been observed (76). Diffuse-type LP HD, on the other hand, may show histologic progression to MC and eventually LD HD.

The differential diagnosis of LP HD includes reactive hyperplasias, other types of HD, and non-Hodgkin's lymphomas. In this context, an entity that deserves a special comment is progressive transformation of germinal centers (PTGC). This is a form of follicular hyperplasia in which the follicles are expanded and disrupted due to infiltration by small lymphocytes. Usually, reactive follicular hyperplasia is observed in the rest of the lymph node with foci of PTGC and there is an absence of RS cells. However, an association between PTGC and LP-HD has been reported (147).

Nodular Sclerosis Hodgkin's Disease

NS is the most common type of HD, both in children and adults, accounting for approximately 60% of cases (15,148). This type is characterized by a triad of sclerosis, lacunar cells, and classical RS cells (Fig. 12; see figure in color plate section). The most commonly involved sites include mediastinal, cervical, and supraclavicular lymph nodes. The sclerosis is defined as "orderly bands of dense interconnecting collagenous tissue that circumscribe nodules of abnormal lymphoid tissue" (97). The collagen bands have a birefringent character in polarized light. The amount of sclerosis present in LN biopsies may be highly variable and, while it may be limited to focal capsular thickening in some specimens, total sclerosis of the lymph node may be present in others. The former variant, having sparse sclerosis and abundant lacunar cells, is referred to as the cellular phase of NS. In general, lacunar cells are concentrated within the nodules, sometimes forming cohesive sheets, and central necrosis may be present.

The cellular makeup within the nodules of NS HD is quite variable. Depending on the relative proportions of lymphocytes, other reactive cells, RS cells, and lacunar cells present, subtypes, or phases, of NS HD have been described. These include lymphocyte predominance, mixed cellularity, and lymphocyte depletion phases. The lymphocyte depletion phase has also been referred to as the syncytial variant (187). In these cases, sheets of lacunar and RS cells within nodules resemble a syncytium, often with areas of central necrosis. With recurrences, progression from LP to MC and LD phases may be observed within the nodules. The clinical relevance of subtyping NS HD is not well established, but it is important to recognize the variation that occurs.

Immunophenotyping studies have demonstrated that RS cells in NS HD, MC, and LD types have a unique phenotype (76). They are positive for Leu M1 (CD15) and Ki-1 (CD30), and negative for CD45 and, usually, for T- and B-cell markers. An occasional case may exhibit T- or B-cell marker positivity, adding difficulty in defining the boundary between NS HD and NHL.

The differential diagnosis of NS HD includes metastatic carcinoma, melanoma, sarcomas, and NHL with sclerosis. Especially in the mediastinum, the distinction between large cell NHL with sclerosis and NS HD may be difficult. However, the absence of lacunar cells and the results of immunophenotyping studies usually help in establishing the correct diagnosis. It has recently been pointed out that there are regional differences in criteria for diagnosing cases of the syncytial variant of NS HD, which in Europe is often referred to as Hodgkin's-like ALCL with sclerosis (58).

Mixed Cellularity HD

Mixed cellularity is the second most common type of HD, accounting for approximately 26% of cases in children. The histologic picture and prognosis is intermediate between LP and LD HD. Generally, nodal architecture is completely effaced; however, interfollicular and focal involvement may be seen in some cases. As the name indicates, the cellular infiltrate is composed of a heterogeneous population with readily apparent admixed RS cells and mononuclear variants (Fig. 13). Variable amounts of plasma cells, eosinophils, lymphocytes, histiocytes, and neutrophils may be present. Fibrosis can be observed in some cases, although in contrast to the sclerosis in NS HD, the fibers are disorderly and birefringence is not typical. Most cases of interfollicular HD, which show partial nodal involvement and lack typical features of other types of HD, are placed in the category of MC.

The differential diagnosis of MC HD includes various NHL, peripheral T-cell lymphomas, and reactive lymphadenopathies. A distinct type of peripheral T-cell lymphoma with abundant epithelioid histiocytes, also known as Lennert's lymphoma (see above), may occasionally create a diagnostic problem. Immunohistochemistry and the subsequent clinical course are usually helpful.

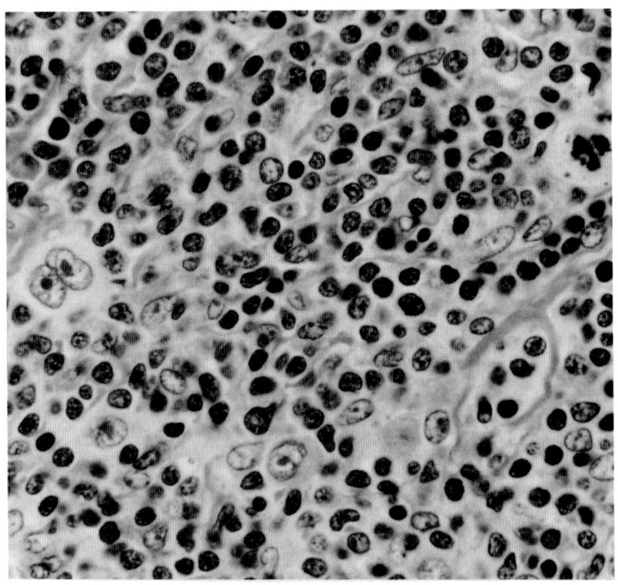

FIG. 13. In mixed-cellularity Hodgkin's disease, Reed–Sternberg cells are readily identified in a reactive background.

Lymphocyte Depletion HD

Lymphocyte depletion is the least common type of HD in both children and adults. It is characterized by a predominance of RS cells, depletion of reactive lymphocytes, and fibrosis. Clinically, it is an aggressive, rapidly fatal disease. Some studies have shown that subdiaphragmatic lymph nodes are more commonly involved (3). In the Lukes and Butler classification, reticular and diffuse fibrosis subtypes were recognized (98). In the Rye modification these subtypes were unified under the lymphocyte depletion category (101).

The lymph node architecture is generally totally effaced by a mononuclear cell infiltrate composed primarily of RS cells with highly pleomorphic and bizarre shapes. Lymphocytes and other reactive cells, including eosinophils, plasma cells, and histiocytes, are depleted (Fig. 14; see figure in color plate section). Fibrosis and necrosis of varying degrees are characteristically present. In contrast to the orderly sclerosis seen in NS HD, the fibrosis is disorderly and nonbirefringent. Fibrosis may range from acellular to a sarcomatoid fibroblastic proliferation, with scattered RS cells usually readily seen.

The differential diagnosis of LD HD includes sarcomas, other types of Hodgkin's disease, and non-Hodgkin's lymphomas (especially immunoblastic or ALCL). In addition, fibrosis secondary to previous chemotherapy or radiotherapy should be differentiated from the diffuse fibrosis of active LD HD.

Hodgkin's Disease and the Epstein–Barr Virus

Abundant recent data have supported the hypothesis that HD is etiologically related to infection with EBV. In situ hybridization and immunohistochemical studies reveal EBV in the neoplastic cells of many cases (approximately 50%), particularly of MC and NS types (60, 63,184,202,204). Herbst et al. postulate that HD results from activation of an immature lymphoid cell, such as by EBV, resulting in malignant transformation and that HD is closely related to ALCL (62). However, the precise pathogenesis of this most enigmatic neoplasm remains to be elucidated.

HISTIOCYTIC PROLIFERATIONS

Histiocytoses comprise a broad group of disorders that share a proliferation of elements from the diverse group of macrophages and antigen-presenting cells. These cells are probably all derived from bone marrow monocyte precursors. Their putative neoplasms, like Hodgkin's disease, are enigmatic disorders partly because of a lack of full understanding of the basic biology of the cells of origin as well as the diversity of clinical behavior of morphologically similar lesions. This group includes reactive processes, aggressive malignant diseases, and those of unpredictable nature such as Langerhans cell histiocytosis.

To facilitate research, diagnosis, and patient management, the Histiocyte Society proposed in 1987 a general classification of the histiocytoses (22). Langerhans cell histiocytosis (LCH; class I) has distinctive pathologic features, including principally the presence of the Langerhans cell. LCH may be diagnosed with certainty from adequate samples of tissue, but its clinical behavior is highly variable. Histiocytoses of mononuclear phagocytes other than Langerhans cells (class II) are generally considered reactive conditions, although some have adverse outcomes. These include hemophagocytic lymphohistiocytosis and infection-associated hemophagocytic syndrome, sinus histiocytosis with massive lymphadenopathy, xanthogranuloma, reticulohistiocytoma, and other unclassified proliferations of active histiocytes and lymphocytes. Malignant histiocytic disorders (class III) include acute monocytic leukemia, malignant histiocytosis, and true histiocytic lymphomas.

Langerhans Cell Histiocytosis

Langerhans cells (LCs) are epidermal antigen-presenting cells that are mobile and have been found in most tissues. They are dendritic cells that express CD1 antigen, HLA-DR, and S-100 protein. They have moderately abundant cytoplasm and a medium-size, usually oblong nucleus with vesicular chromatin and an elongate central groove resembling a zipper. Their cytoplasm contains characteristic structures known as "Birbeck granules." These cells bind antigen at their surface and migrate through dermal lymphatics to the regional lymph nodes, where presentation of antigens to T cells occurs in the paracortex.

Langerhans cell histiocytosis (LCH), previously known as histiocytosis X, is a disease with various clinical manifestations that were previously called eosinophilic granuloma (localized), Hand–Schuller–Christian disease (multiple lesions), and Letterer–Siwe disease (multiorgan progressive disease) (40,75). These were grouped together as one entity by Lichtenstein in 1953 (94).

The clinical presentation and course of LCH are extremely variable and somewhat unpredictable (75). LC4 usually presents in children, from newborns to 15 years of age (median = 2–3 years). Eighty percent of patients have lytic (radiologically punched out) bone lesions in active hematopoietic sites such as the skull and femur, often with associated bone pain. Jaw lesions frequently are associated with soft tissue involvement and loose teeth. Skin lesions occur frequently in the scalp, axilla, postauricular areas, hands, and feet, have vesiculopustular hemorrhagic features, but are usually not contiguous with bone lesions. External otitis is common. Lymph node involvement is usually associated with regional skin or bone disease, but it may be the solitary site of involvement and is sometimes seen as an incidental finding in lymph nodes removed for other reasons. Spleen, bone marrow, thymus, lung, liver, gastrointestinal tract, and nervous system involvement may be present. With hepatic involvement, there may be elevated liver enzymes, hypoproteinemia, edema, ascites, and/or hyperbilirubinemia. LCH may be discovered at any age, but young age and organ dysfunction at presentation indicate a poor prognosis (22).

The diagnosis of LCH depends on finding proliferations of LC with characteristic abundant cytoplasm and medium-size, usually bland-appearing, oval or oblong nuclei with a central groove. The typical nucleus resembles a coffee bean and is often also found in syncytial multinucleated giant cells within a lesion of predominantly solitary cells (Fig. 15). LC morphology should be substantiated by immunochemistry and/or electron microscopy to differentiate them from reactive histiocytes.

In bone lesions (see Chapter 9), there is destruction of the bone with marrow replacement by variable numbers of LC, lymphocytes, eosinophils, foamy non-LC macrophages (sometimes with phagocytic debris), neutrophils, and stromal cells. Skin lesions typically involve the papillary dermis and epidermis with similar cellularity. In the lung (see Chapter 14) LCH may be solitary or multiple. Small perivascular, peribronchial, and parenchymal lesions are usually interstitial, whereas large lesions may fill the alveolar spaces as well. LC must be differentiated from alveolar macrophages.

Lymph node involvement usually consists of variably extensive aggregates or sheets of LC centered in the sinuses or occasionally in the paracortex. The node may be replaced by the process. The thymus sometimes shows similar involvement by LC, often with involution of the normal architecture, resulting in a "dysplastic" or abnormal architecture in which there is a lack of cortical-medullary demarcation and Hassall's corpuscles as well as lymphocyte depletion, or it may show these architectural changes without evidence of LC infiltration (55). This phenomenon has been cited as evidence that LCH is an immune dysfunction rather than a neoplasm. Other evidence of immune dysfunction includes altered CD4/CD8 ratios, but these ratios have been variable.

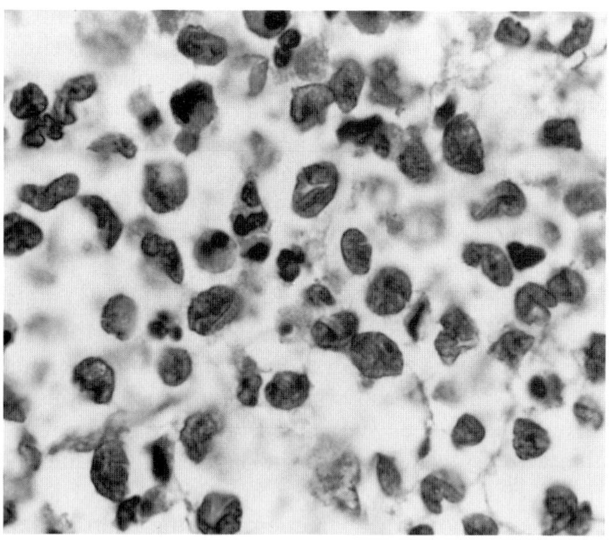

FIG. 15. Langerhans cell histiocytosis with histiocytelike cells having folded bean-shaped nuclei.

When the spleen is involved, there is usually diffuse sinusoidal or nodular red pulp involvement. When patients suffer from extensive multiorgan disease with organ failure, extensive activation of non-LC histiocytes may obscure the true nature of LCH at autopsy.

Electron microscopy (EM) provides the most definitive confirmation of the presence of LCs. However, because LCs are present in normal skin and EM is highly selective and sample-dependent, it is important that the microscopist be confident that any LC identified is representative of lesional material. The characteristic feature of the LC is the Birbeck granule, a membrane-bound racquet-shaped structure with a vesicular bulb and a tail of opposed membranes forming a pentalaminar rod, 180–360 nm in length, with a central striation showing a regular 10-nm periodicity. The appearance resembles a zipper (111) (Fig. 16).

Immunochemical studies of LCH in frozen sections or touch imprints reveal expression of CD1 (OKT-6), HLA-DR, and often CD4, CD11c, CDw32, and CD68 (59,116,117,135). The cells are characteristically CD14-negative. In paraffin section immunochemistry, S-100 protein and peanut agglutinin (PNA) distinguish LC from typical macrophages (213) (Fig. 17). Adhesion molecules described on LCs in LCH include ICAM-1, β-1 integrins α-4 and α-5, and β-2 integrins LFA-1, MAC-1, and p150,95 (164).

Many patients, even with multifocal disease without organ dysfunction, have a good outlook for long-term survival. A variety of therapies have been utilized, including conservative surgical therapy, radiation, and single-agent chemotherapy (etoposide). Refractory disease has been treated on occasion with bone marrow transplantation (190).

Malignant Histiocytosis

Malignant histiocytosis (MH) is also discussed with large cell non-Hodgkin's lymphomas (see above). It is now generally felt that many if not most cases of MH are either T-cell lymphomas or other phenotypic variants of NHL, including ALCL (Fig. 18). The authors are convinced that many examples of tumors that would have at one time been classified as MH are now included in

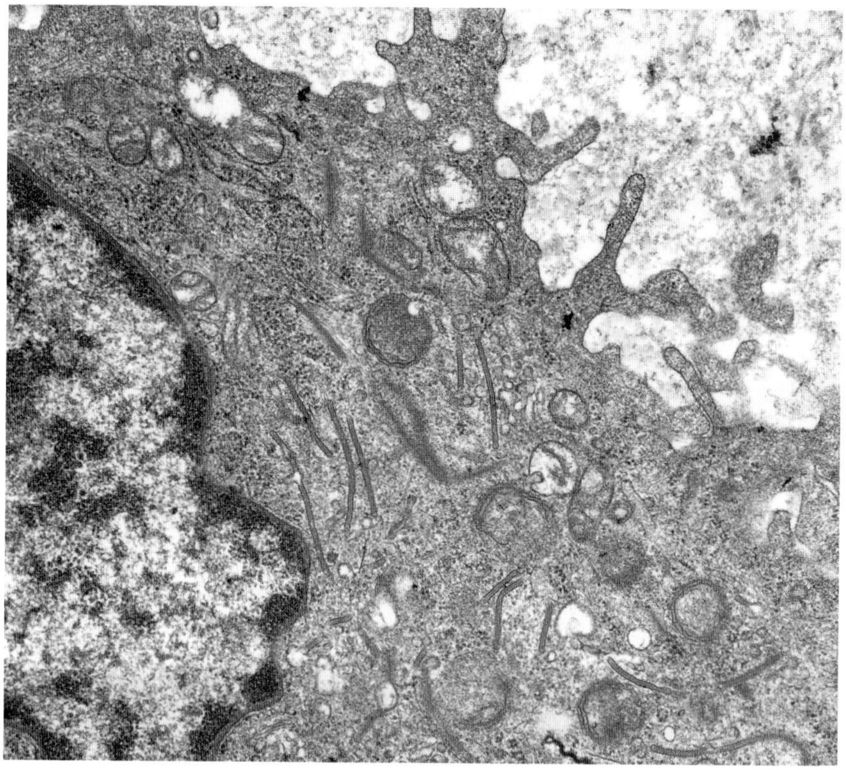

FIG. 16. Langerhans cell containing numerous Birbeck granules, membrane-bound racquet-shaped pentalaminar structures with striations showing 10 nm periodicity. (Photograph courtesy of Dr. Noel Florendo. Duckworth Pathology Group. Memphis, TN)

therapeutic protocols for large cell NHL, with results comparable to those for T-cell NHL (or ALCL), so that these cases are not clinically obvious as unique tumors. Thus, it is more practical to consider them as LCL for treatment purposes. It is also likely, however, that some LCLs are derived from precursors of the antigen-presenting cells that occur in smaller numbers in lymphoid tissue than do T or B cells. Therefore, remembering the lesson of lymphoblastic lymphoma, we should not forget that these tumors have been previously described as unique entities, even though their descriptions suffer from imprecision. As therapies for lymphoid malignancies in children continue to evolve, we may again need to segregate these unusual lesions.

"Histiocytic medullary reticulosis" (HMR) was the

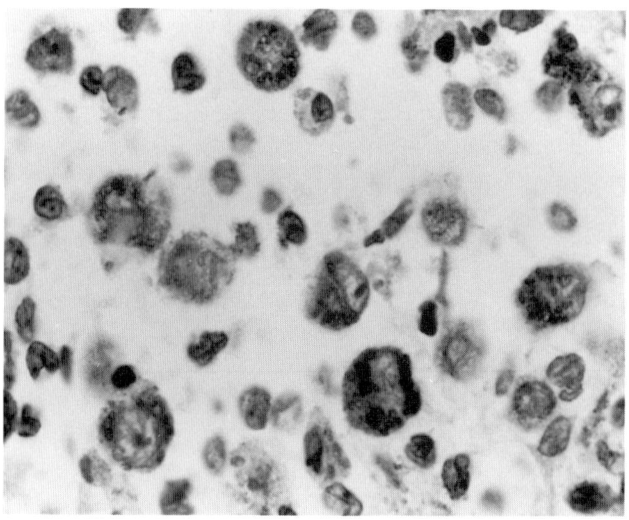

FIG. 17. Langerhans cell histiocytosis. Cells in paraffin sections characteristically exhibit reactivity with peanut agglutinin (PNA), as in this photomicrograph, and contain S-100 protein.

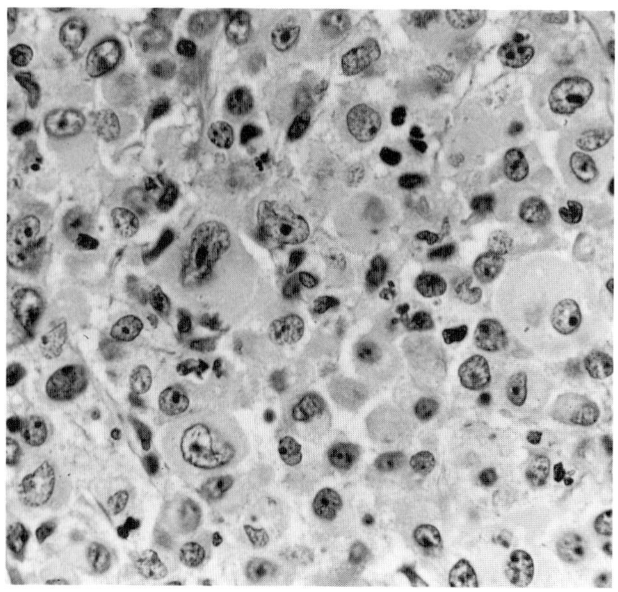

FIG. 18. This "histiocytic" tumor showed a morphology consistent with anaplastic large cell lymphoma, exhibited histiocyte-associated antigens CD68 and lysozyme, and lacked lymphoid antigens.

term used by Scott and Robb-Smith to describe what has generally been called malignant histiocytosis (173). This was a progressive cellular hyperplasia of the hematopoietic system leading uniformly to a fatal outcome and affecting all age groups. It was characterized by a wasting syndrome variably including hemolytic anemia, fever, weakness, weight loss, lymphadenopathy, hepatosplenomegaly, and soft tissue and skin lesions (100). Anemia and sometimes thrombocytopenia and neutropenia were associated with erythrophagocytosis by histiocytes. Cytologic features of cells involving lymph node sinuses, bone marrow, and/or splenic red pulp varied from mitotically active immunoblasts to benign-appearing histiocytes. MH is thus likely to be a heterogeneous group of lesions.

Hemophagocytic Syndromes

Familial erythrophagocytic lymphohistiocytosis (FEL) is a disorder of early infancy with a familial pattern suggesting autosomal recessive transmission (190). It is characterized by fever, failure to thrive, hepatosplenomegaly, and anemia. Involvement may include lymphoid, pulmonary, central nervous system, pericardial, bone, soft tissue, and gastrointestinal infiltration. There may be coagulopathy and neutropenia, and liver dysfunction is common. There is organ infiltration by benign-appearing histiocytes, some of which may contain phagocytosed red blood cells, with associated lymphocyte depletion (Fig. 19). This is histologically similar to both HMR (which overlaps with NHL) and viral-associated hemophagocytic syndrome. The diagnosis is thus dependent on the early age of onset (usually less than 3 months) and the familial association. There is currently no accepted successful therapy. Large cell lymphoma, should be considered in the differential diagnosis.

Virus-associated hemophagocytic syndrome (VAHS), described by Risdall et al. (157), is a disorder consisting of proliferation of benign-appearing histiocytes that appears in response to an infection. It often occurs in patients with immunosuppression due to chemotherapy for other malignancies, following transplantation, or on steroid therapy for autoimmune diseases. It has been associated with numerous infectious processes, notably viral (EBV, cytomegalovirus, herpes simplex, varicella, adenovirus, and parvovirus B19) as well as bacterial, fungal, mycobacterial, rickettsial, and parasitic infections and has also been seen with malignancies (12,109,152,156,157,190). The benign appearance of the histiocytes belies the high mortality rate associated with the syndrome.

VAHS is characterized by fever and generalized constitutional symptoms. Hepatosplenomegaly, lymphadenopathy, pancytopenia, liver function abnormalities, and frequently severe coagulopathy are present. Early in the course of the disease, lymph nodes show immunoblastic proliferation and the bone marrow is hypercellular. Subsequently, the lymph nodes show lymphoid depletion, and the bone marrow is hypocellular with histiocytic infiltration. The liver shows portal and sinusoidal infiltration by lymphocytes, immunoblasts, and histiocytes with frequent erythrophagocytosis.

VAHS associated with acute viral infection (usually EBV) may respond to antiviral therapy (acyclovir), but immunosuppressive therapy is deleterious (190). Therefore, a diagnosis of VAHS should be considered prior to therapy for a supposed malignancy.

Sinus histiocytosis with massive lymphadenopathy (SHML), described by Rosai and Dorfman (161), is a benign massive enlargement of cervical lymph nodes of unknown etiology. There is often associated fever, leukocytosis, and polyclonal hyperglobulinemia. It usually presents as painless bilateral enlargement of cervical nodes in patients under 10 years of age. Extranodal in-

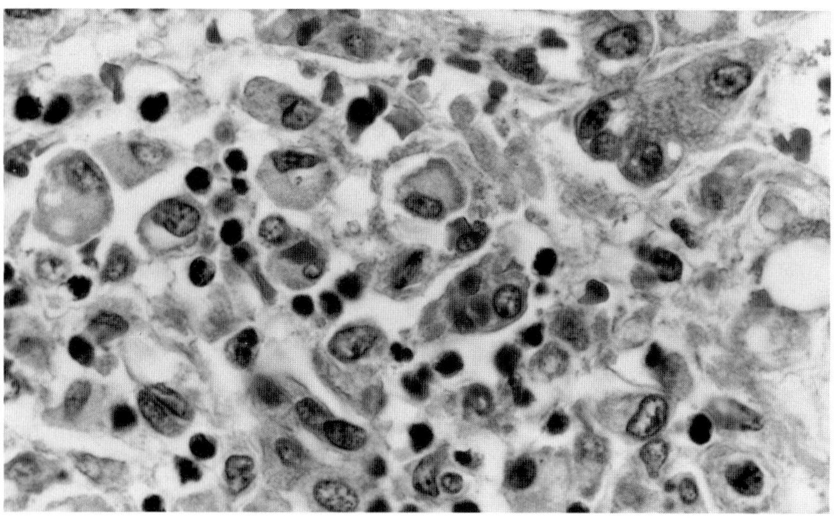

FIG. 19. Hepatic infiltrates of histiocytes in familial erythrophagocytic lymphohistocytosis showing the presence of engulfed erythrocytes.

volvement occurs in 40% of cases and sometimes occurs without nodal disease. It may involve the orbit, eyelid, or cranium.

Histologically, the lymph node sinuses or extranodal tissues in SHML are infiltrated by benign-appearing histiocytes that distend the sinuses, enlarge the node, and may obliterate the normal architecture (43,107,139, 162,175). Although the histiocytes appear normal, they bear an immunohistochemical marker, protein S-100 (37). They are CD1-negative, differentiating the disease from LCH. Typically, there is emperipolesis or leukocytophagocytosis (including the presence of viable-appearing lymphocytes in histiocytes), and erythrophagocytosis may be present as well (Fig. 20; see figure in color section). EBV and measles virus antibody titers are frequently elevated. The course is benign with resolution in 3–6 months or occasionally longer (up to 5 years). Therapy is not required.

NODAL PRESENTATION OF LEUKEMIC DISEASE

Lymph node involvement is a common occurrence in acute leukemias in children, particularly in acute lymphoblastic leukemia (ALL) (Chapter 15). It occurs on presentation in 30–40% of newly diagnosed ALL, as do hepatic and splenic involvement. Mediastinal (thymic) involvement occurs in approximately 10% of ALL and is characteristically (95%) associated with a thymic T-cell phenotype (127). When lymph node or other soft tissue is involved by a lymphoblastic process, the distinction between ALL and LBL is based on the percentage of blasts in the bone marrow. POG protocols define cases with more than 25% marrow blasts to be leukemia and those with less than 25% to be lymphoblastic lymphoma. Most cases of ALL of B-lineage phenotype present with much higher blast counts, so that this distinction is most often important with T-cell disease, particularly because T-cell LBL frequently evolves to T-cell ALL. The histopathology and cytology are essentially identical in nodal involvement by ALL or LBL. Leukemic disease in general, and also LBL, frequently shows an infiltrative pattern of nodal involvement in the sinus, paracortex, and adjacent extranodal soft tissue. Files of blasts often separate muscle or collagen fibers and surround fat cells. The diagnosis of ALL is best made from a bone marrow examination (6).

Nodal involvement is less often a feature of acute myeloblastic leukemia (AML), myeloproliferative, or myelodysplastic syndromes. It occurs in approximately 25% of AML, most often with monocytic differentiation (49). Diagnosis is, again, best made from a bone marrow examination (6,7).

Myeloid leukemias may also present in extramedullary tissue in the absence of diagnosable bone marrow disease; these cases are referred to as granulocytic sarcoma (GS) or chloroma (67). They most often occur in the orbit, bones including the cranium, sternum, ribs and vertebrae, skin, lymph nodes, and dura. Children and young adults show a proportionately greater frequency of GS than older adults relative to the incidence of AML. Monoblastic leukemia is the most common type, but virtually any myeloid malignancy may present as GS. In the absence of therapeutic intervention the vast majority of cases evolve to AML (with marrow involvement) within a year of diagnosis.

Morphologically, GS in the lymph nodes often resembles both lymphoblastic and large cell lymphomas (Fig. 21). Typically, there is a diffuse infiltrate of large blastic cells, often with starry sky macrophages and a high mitotic rate. The presence of eosinophils and eosinophilic myelocytes has been considered characteristic of GS, but these may not be present. They are certainly not specific for GS because T-cell lymphomas also exhibit them. A clue to the presence of GS is a high-grade neoplasm suggestive of lymphoma but not easily subclassifiable. Touch imprints are extremely helpful to demonstrate blasts and/or differentiating myeloid cells as well as to possibly identify Auer rods. Bone marrow and peripheral blood should always be examined when malignancies involve the lymph nodes, for diagnosis of difficult and unusual cases as well as for staging purposes.

The diagnostic features of GS have been previously reviewed (67). Cytochemistry, immunologic markers and cytogenetics are best studied from fresh cell suspensions and are identical to those of myeloid leukemias. Some studies may be performed in paraffin sections as well. Chloroacetate esterase (Leder stain) may be helpful to

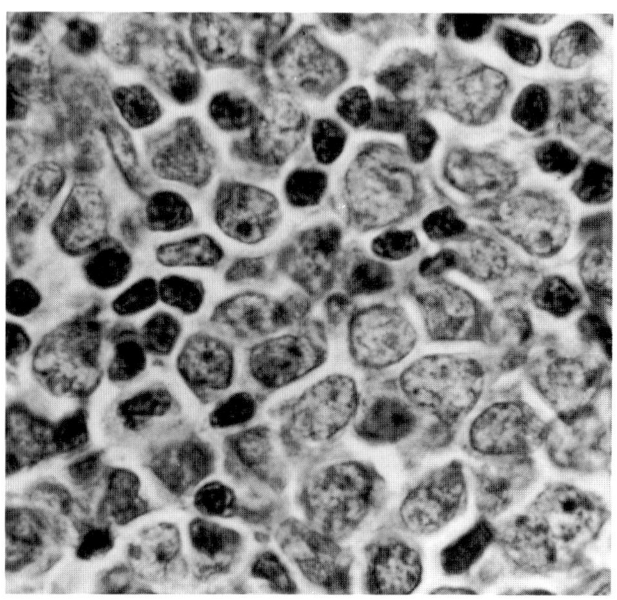

FIG. 21. Granulocytic sarcoma often shows large blastlike cells resembling lymphoma but not fitting usual classifications.

identify GS but is not present in primitive granulocytic or virtually any monocytic blasts. Antibodies against myeloid determinants (including Mac387, CD68/KP1, antielastase, antilactoferrin, antilysozyme, and antiglycophorin C) (90) help differentiate myeloid from lymphoid neoplasms. CD45RO and CD43, frequently used to identify T-cell lineage, also cross-react with myeloid cells. The difficulties of differentiating myeloid from lymphoid malignancies are compounded in mixed lineage leukemias or those with features borderline between monocytic leukemia and histiocytic/T-cell lymphoma.

THYMOMA

Thymoma is a mediastinal neoplasm relatively common in adults but rare in children. Fewer than 50 pediatric cases have been described in the literature (149). More commonly, mediastinal tumors in children represent lymphomas or involvement by acute leukemia. Thymic hyperplasia and thymic cyst are also in the differential diagnosis, as are carcinoids and germ cell tumors.

Thymomas most often occur in the anterior-superior mediastinum, are lobulated with the presence of fibrous septae, are usually encapsulated, and may be calcified. They are composed of a variable mixture of neoplastic epithelial cells and benign thymic lymphocytes (Fig. 22; see figure in color section). Hassall's corpuscles and/or epithelial rosettes are sometimes present. Histologic types may be defined by the predominant cell type and the patterns of growth, i.e., lymphocyte-rich, epithelial, and spindle cell types, but variation occurs within individual thymomas (160,201). Thymomas may also be categorized by the predominance of thymic cortical vs. medullary histology. Whereas thymomas may show areas of both cortical and medullary differentiation, thus mimicking thymic hyperplasia, organoid cortical areas are generally irregularly lobated in thymoma and predominate over medullary areas (142).

Cases with marked epithelial atypia are referred to as thymic carcinomas and include squamous cell, lymphoepitheliomalike, sarcomatoid, small cell, and undifferentiated histologies (149,160). A recent study of childhood thymoma suggests that histologic features may correlate with clinical behavior (149). Cases of lymphocyte-rich thymoma without atypia fare well, those with spindle cell atypia show multiple recurrences and metastases but prolonged survival, and those with frank carcinoma have a short survival. In general, however, clinical outcome has been difficult to predict, (80). DNA ploidy studies have not provided prognostic assistance (170).

As in adults (114), encapsulated thymomas in children are frequently cured by complete surgical resection (142). Patients with incompletely resectable disease due to infiltrative growth often succumb to the disease (180). Aggressive surgery for infiltrative cases may lead to prolonged survival (120).

The immunophenotype of the T lymphocytes in thymoma corresponds to the stages of thymocyte differentiation in cortical and medullary areas and similar to histology may be heterogeneous in a given tumor (71,136). This limits the role of immunophenotyping in the diagnosis of thymoma vs. other mediastinal tumors, as lymphoblastic malignancies of the mediastinum also commonly show thymocyte differentiation. Cells that are morphologically blastic may also be present among the thymocytes in a thymoma, leading to further confusion between thymoma and lymphoblastic leukemia or lymphoma. Concurrent lymphoblastic malignancies and T-cell proliferations have been described with thymoma in adults, and etiologic associations have been postulated (30,44,104,110).

Only recognition of the epithelial cell component (morphologically, immunophenotypically, or electron microscopically) can result in the accurate diagnosis of thymoma. Immunocytochemistry shows reactivity of epithelial cells with antibodies against cytokeratins, whereas electron microscopy shows the presence of desmosomes and bundles of tonofilaments. With this in mind, extreme caution should be utilized in the interpretation of cytologic preparations from mediastinal tumors. This caution extends to the fact that other neoplasms involving the mediastinum, such as Hodgkin's disease, large cell lymphomas, or germ cell tumors, may be misdiagnosed as lymphoblastic neoplasms if cytologic or flow cytometric material includes thymic cells.

Thymomas have been associated with paraneoplastic syndromes, including myasthenia gravis, hypogammaglobulinemia, pure red cell aplasia, and a variety of other immune-mediated disorders in approximately 40% of adult patients (114). Myasthenia gravis associated with thymoma is most often seen in patients over the age of 50 but has rarely also been noted in children (160). Other immune disorders may also occur in children with thymoma but are not prominent in the literature, likely due to the rarity of this tumor in pediatric patients.

SPINDLE CELL AND STROMAL PROLIFERATIONS

Benign and malignant spindle cell neoplasms involving lymph nodes are very rare. They may originate from blood vessels or from mesenchymal cells present in the lymph nodes such as fibroblasts, myofibroblasts, smooth muscle cells, or dendritic cells. Lymph nodes may also be secondarily involved by tumors originating elsewhere, through direct extension from the adjacent soft tissue.

Inflammatory pseudotumor of the lymph nodes was first described in 1988 (141). This is a proliferative pro-

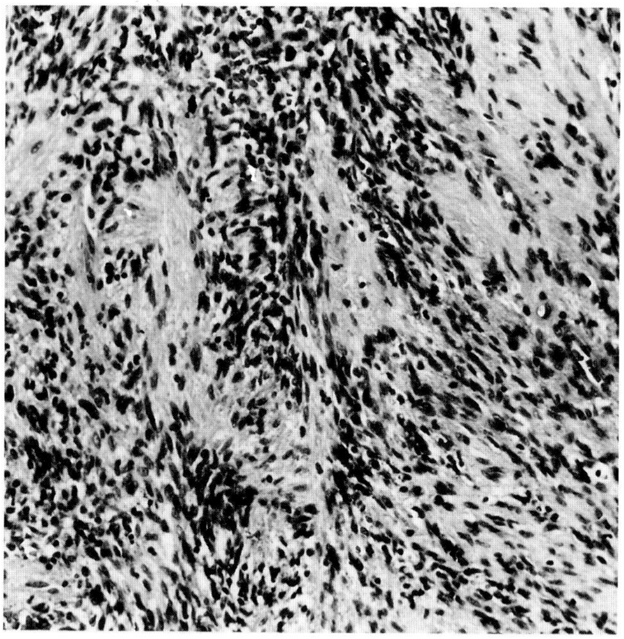

FIG. 23. Intranodal myofibroblastoma is a benign spindle cell tumor that displaces normal lymph node tissue. Nuclei are bland and sometimes form palisades. (Hematoxylin and eosin slide courtesy of Dr. Michelle Rooney, Syracuse, NY.)

cess with an apparent inflammatory etiology that primarily involves the connective tissue framework of lymph nodes (27,39,141). A similar process is described in a number of other locations (see Chapters 8, 11, and 14). The patients reported to date show a wide age range and include individuals in the second decade. Constitutional symptoms including fever and night sweats and laboratory abnormalities such as hypergammaglobulinemia, elevated erythrocyte sedimentation rate, and anemia are present in most patients. Microscopically, the process mainly involves the connective tissue framework. The hilum, trabeculae, and capsule may be expanded to variable degrees, compressing the lymphoid parenchyma and usually with extension of the process into the perinodal fat. It is characterized by a proliferation of spindle cells, inflammatory cells, and small blood vessels, often giving rise to a storiform pattern (141). Edematous and fibrotic areas may be intermixed with more densely cellular areas. The spindle cell component is composed mainly of fibroblasts and myofibroblasts. Vascular proliferation, focally accentuated by a cuff of inflammatory cells and fibrosis, and vasculitis are frequently present. The inflammatory cell component is composed of histiocytes, numerous polyclonal plasma cells, small lymphocytes, and occasional immunoblasts. Although moderate numbers of mitotic figures may be present, necrosis and cytologic atypia are absent.

The differential diagnosis includes malignant fibrous histiocytoma, "histiocytic" and peripheral T-cell lymphomas, Hodgkin's disease, Castleman's disease, atypical reactive hyperplasias, and drug lymphadenopathies. The prognosis is generally very good. Spontaneous resolutions and remissions after chemotherapy, surgical excision, and/or anti-inflammatory therapy have been reported (141).

Intranodal myofibroblastoma is another rare benign mesenchymal tumor of lymph nodes. The vast majority of cases reported involve the inguinal lymph nodes; however, two cases involving other sites have also been reported (42,91,191,206). Grossly, involved lymph nodes are well circumscribed and show focal hemorrhages. At the microscopic level, the tumor is surrounded by an area of compressed normal lymphoid tissue. It is composed of slender spindle cells with ill-defined pale eosinophilic cytoplasm, vesicular nuclear chromatin, and occasional nucleoli (Fig. 23). Nuclear atypia and hyperchromasia are absent, and mitotic activity is generally very low. The cells tend to arrange themselves in short, intersecting fascicles with focal prominent nuclear palisades often simulating the pattern of neurilemmoma (so-called palisading myofibroblastoma). Immunohistochemical studies have demonstrated that the proliferating spindle cells are positive for muscle-specific actin and are negative for *Ulex*, factor VIII–related antigen, cytokeratin, epithelial membrane antigen, S-100, and desmon. These findings suggest that the cells are related to myofibroblasts or a specialized smooth muscle cell.

Various vascular proliferations involving lymph nodes have also been described. Striking vascular proliferation can occur in response to a wide variety of stimuli and in association with diverse conditions including Castleman's disease, angioimmunoblastic lymphadenopathy, and peripheral T-cell lymphomas. Primary vascular lesions comprise entities such as vascular transformation of lymph node sinuses (54), hemangiomatoid lesions (96), nodal angiomatosis (5), and bacillary angiomatosis (197), all of which probably represent reactive processes. True neoplastic proliferations, including hemangioma, lymphangiomas, angiomatous hamartomas, epithelioid vascular tumors, polymorphous hemangioendotheliomas, Kaposi's sarcoma, and angiosarcoma, can also occur in lymph nodes (4,19). These neoplastic lesions are exceedingly rare in children, with only a few cases reported (19).

TABLE 2. *Reactive lymphadenopathies*

1. Infectious
   a. Viral
   b. Toxoplasmosis
   c. Cat-scratch disease
   d. Kichuchi's necrotizing lymphadenitis
   e. Kawasaki's disease
2. Other
   a. Sinus histiocytosis with massive lymphadenopathy (Rosai–Dorfman disease)
   b. Giant lymph node hyperplasia (Castleman's disease)

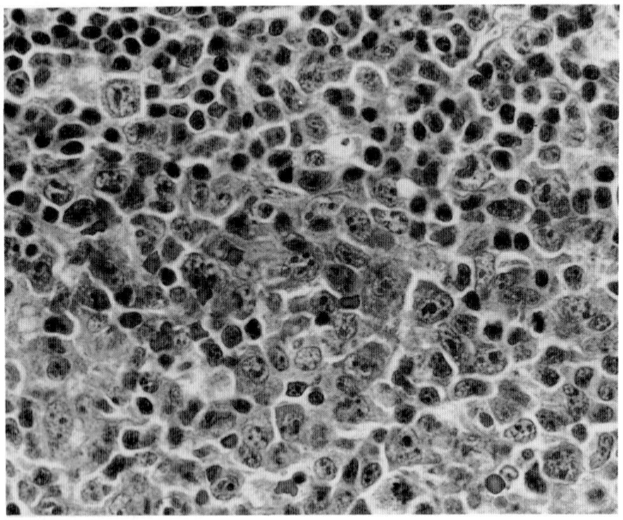

FIG. 25. Infectious mononucleosis results in a polyclonal immunoblastic infiltration mimicking immunoblastic lymphoma. (Hematoxylin and eosin slide courtesy of Dr. Celeste Powers, Syracuse, NY.)

REACTIVE LYMPHADENOPATHIES

A majority of the lymphadenopathies encountered in daily practice are due to reactive processes rather than neoplastic conditions (Table 2). However, the reactive hyperplasias can closely mimic the morphologic features of lymphomas, so that pathologists should be familiar with different patterns of nonneoplastic lymphadenopathies. Four architectural patterns are recognized: follicular, diffuse, sinus, and mixed (14).

Reactive follicular hyperplasia is commonly seen in childhood. It is characterized by an increase in the size and number of follicles, with overall preservation of the lymph node architecture (Fig. 24; see figure in color plate section). The follicles are variable in size, and the expanded germinal centers contain a mixture of lymphocytes, moderate to high numbers of mitoses, and variable numbers of macrophages containing cellular debris ("tingible-body macrophages"). Polarization of transformed lymphocytes within the germinal centers may be seen in some follicles. The mantle zones around the germinal centers are generally present and separated from the germinal center by a sharp border. In some cases, however, the mantle zones may be absent due to extensive enlargement of the germinal centers. In most cases, this may represent a nonspecific response and the etiology is unknown. An exuberant follicular hyperplasia may be seen in HIV-positive individuals.

The sinus pattern of hyperplasia is characterized by expansion of the lymph node sinuses with accumulation of various types of cells. Sinus histiocytosis is the most commonly encountered form and is associated with increased numbers of histiocytes in dilated sinuses. It is a nonspecific finding and may be associated with follicular hyperplasia.

Lymphadenopathies with diffuse pattern are most commonly associated with viral infections. They are also seen with other infections and in noninfectious inflammatory states, and they may contain large numbers of immunoblasts, mimicking large cell lymphomas (121). In infectious mononucleosis the lymph node architecture is generally effaced by a diffuse infiltrate of lymphocytes, plasma cells, and scattered immunoblasts (Fig. 25). Occasionally, clusters and singly dispersed binucleated immunoblasts resembling RS cells may be present. The reticulin structure of the lymph node is preserved, however, and immunohistochemical staining may be helpful in the differential diagnosis because these cells are negative for CD15 (20).

Some of the lymphadenopathies seen in children show predominantly a mixed architectural pattern of hyper-

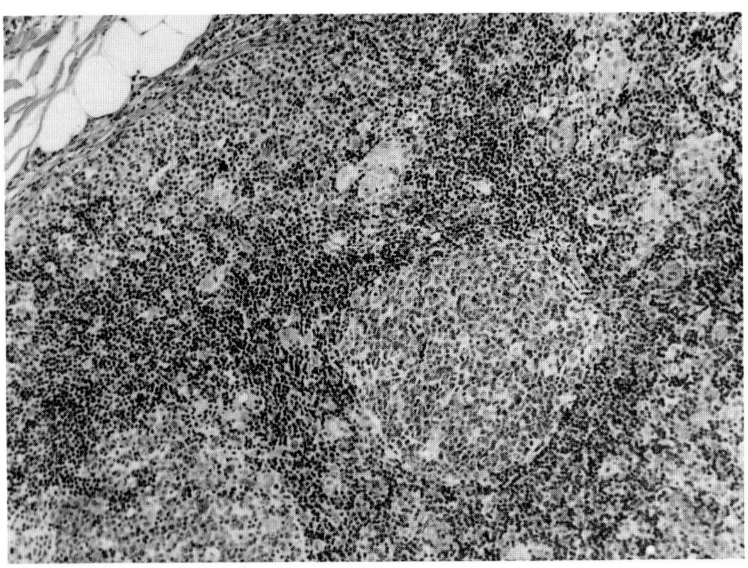

FIG. 26. Toxoplasmosis shows increased numbers of epithelioid histiocytes that, singly or in clusters, impinge on germinal centers. Monocytoid B cells are present in the sinuses. (Hematoxylin and eosin slide courtesy of Dr. Michelle Rooney, Syracuse, NY.)

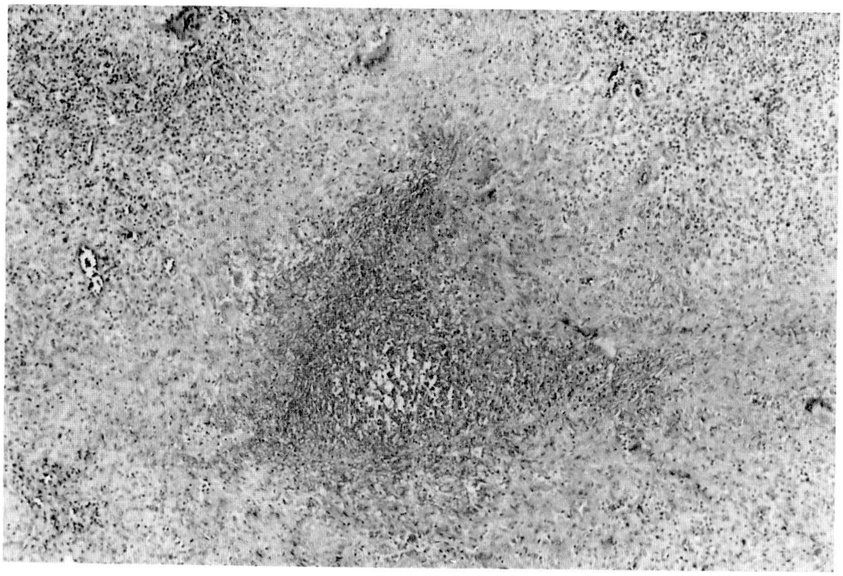

FIG. 27. Cat-scratch disease results in stellate necrosis of the lymph node. (Hematoxylin and eosin slide courtesy of Dr. Celeste Powers, Syracuse, NY.)

plasia. These include toxoplasmosis, necrotizing granulomatous inflammation (e.g., cat-scratch), Kikuchi's disease, and Kawasaki's disease. Some features that are characteristic of these entities enable the pathologist to determine the etiology of the lymphadenopathy.

Toxoplasmic lymphadenitis is characterized by a mixed pattern of hyperplasia including florid follicular hyperplasia and distension of sinuses by monocytoid B cells. Proliferation of epithelioid histiocytes that blur the border between germinal centers and mantle zones are characteristic (108) (Fig. 26).

Cat-scratch disease is characterized by the presence of stellate abscesses containing polymorphonuclear cells mainly located in the cortical areas (Fig. 27). Necrotizing granulomas and distension of sinuses with monocytoid B cells can also be seen in some cases (28).

Kikuchi's disease also shows patchy necrosis mainly located in the paracortical areas; however, polymorphonuclear leukocytes are absent or very rare (34–36). The necrotic areas show prominent karyorrhexis and are surrounded by foamy histiocytes. A reactive cellular component includes irregular lymphocytes and immunoblasts (Fig. 28).

Lymph nodes from patients with Kawasaki's disease may show features similar to those seen in Kikuchi's disease (36,47). Patchy necrosis is, however, associated with the presence of polymorphonuclear cells, and small vessel thrombi are often found. In all of these cases pertinent clinical information aids greatly in establishing the correct diagnosis.

Angiofollicular (giant) lymph node hyperplasia, or Castleman's disease, is a benign lymphadenopathy of unknown etiology (45). It may occur in children and has been described as in patients as young as 8 years (165). This disease usually presents as localized lymphadenopathy. Histologically, it causes altered follicles with enlarged or compact germinal centers showing pale eosinophilic backgrounds containing vesicular nuclei and decreased follicular center cells surrounded by concentric rings of mantle zone lymphocytes, imparting an "onion skin" appearance (Fig. 29; see figure in color plate section). Vessels are increased and often hyalinized in the follicles, and there is increased paracortical vasculature. This most common form is referred to as the hyaline-vascular type. Variable numbers of plasma cells are present in the paracortex. When these form sheets encasing reactive germinal centers, often without the follicular changes of the hyaline-vascular type, it is referred to as the plasma cell type. Mixed patterns also occur.

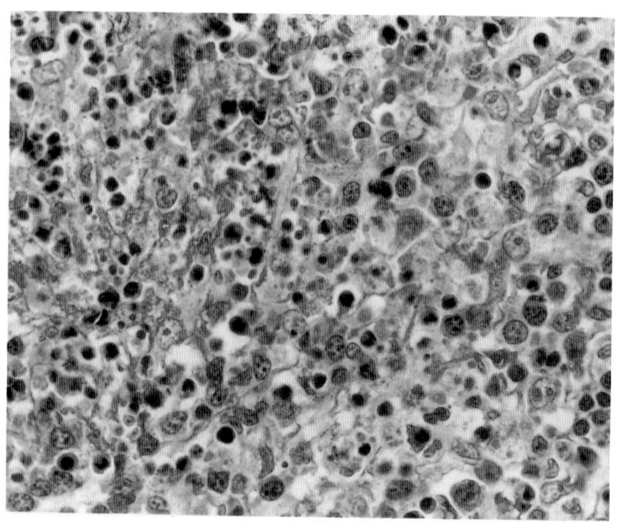

FIG. 28. Kikuchi's necrotizing lymphadenitis shows focal necrosis with karyorrhectic debris but without neutrophils and with adjacent immunoblastic proliferation. Abundant benign histiocytes are usually present. (Hematoxylin and eosin slide courtesy of Dr. Celeste Powers, Syracuse, NY.)

Multicentric Castleman's disease, probably a distinct entity, is associated with an aggressive course.

By nature of their immune surveillance function, lymph nodes are common sites of metastases from tumors arising in other organs. They may be involved by virtually any metastasizing neoplasm, with typically an interstitial sinus involvement that may spread to involve the entire node and surrounding tissue following establishment of the metastasis. Diagnostic criteria are those of the original tumor.

SUMMARY

The lymphoid immune system is essential for protection from invasive microorganisms, foreign substances, and even endogenous threats such as neoplasia. However, it is also the site of origin of neoplasias that are among the most common malignancies of children.

Because of recent improvements in the outcome of children with lymphoid malignancies, it is imperative that thorough evaluation of lymphoid disorders be performed to lead to accurate diagnoses. Thus, appropriate therapies can offer potential cure for the majority of these children. Conversely, it is imperative to exclude a nonmalignant, reactive process, which may closely mimic neoplasia clinically and even morphologically.

REFERENCES

1. Anderson JR, Wilson JF, Jenkin DT, et al. Childhood non-Hodgkin's lymphoma: the results of a randomized therapeutic trial comparing a 4-drug regimen (COMP) with a 10-drug regimen (LSA2-L2). *N Engl J Med* 1983;308:559–565.
2. Barcos MP, Lukes RJ. Malignant lymphoma of convoluted lymphocytes: a new entity of possible T-cell type. In: Sinks LF, Godden JO, eds. *Conflicts in Childhood Cancer: An Evaluation of Current Management. Proceedings.* New York: Alan R Liss; 1975: 147–177.
3. Bearman RM, Pangalis GA, Rappaport H. Hodgkin's disease, lymphocyte depletion type: a clinicopathologic study of 39 patients. *Cancer* 1978;41:293–302.
4. Beckstead JH, Wood GS, Fletcher V. Evidence for the origin of Kaposi's sarcoma from lymphatic endothelium. *Am J Pathol* 1985;119:294–300.
5. Bedrosian SA, Goldman RL. Nodal angiomatosis: relationship to vascular transformation of lymph nodes. *Arch Pathol Lab Med* 1984;108:864–865.
6. Bennett JM, Catovsky D, Daniel MT, et al. Proposals for the classification of the acute leukaemias. French-American-British (FAB) co-operative group. *Br J Haematol* 1976;33:451–458.
7. Bennett JM, Catovsky D, Daniel MT, et al. Proposed revised criteria for the classification of acute myeloid leukemia. A report of the French-American-British Cooperative Group. *Ann Intern Med* 1985;103:620–629.
8. Berard C, O'Conor GT, Thomas LB, Torloni H. Histopathological definition of Burkitt's tumour. *Bull WHO* 1969;40:601–607.
9. Berard CW. Histopathology of the lymphomas. In: Williams WJ, Beutler E, Erslev AJ, Rundles RW, eds. *Hematology.* New York: McGraw-Hill; 1972:901–912.
10. Bernard A, Boumsell L, Reinherz EL, et al. Cell surface characterization of malignant T cells from lymphoblastic lymphoma using monoclonal antibodies: evidence for phenotypic differences between malignant T cells from patients with acute lymphoblastic leukemia and lymphoblastic lymphoma. *Blood* 1981;57: 1105–1110.
11. Borowitz MJ, Croker BP, Metzgar RS. Lymphoblastic lymphoma with the phenotype of common acute lymphoblastic leukemia. *Am J Clin Pathol* 1983;79:387–391.
12. Boruchoff SE, Woda BA, Pihan GA, Durbin WA, Burstein D, Blacklow NR. Parvovirus B19-associated hemophagocytic syndrome. *Arch Intern Med* 1990;150:897–899.
13. Brill NE, Baehr G, Rosenthal N. Generalized giant lymph follicle hyperplasia of lymph nodes and spleen: a hitherto undescribed type. *JAMA* 1925;84:668–671.
14. Burke JS. Reactive lymphadenopathies. *Semin Diag Pathol* 1988;5:312–316.
15. Burke JS. Hodgkin's disease: histopathology and differential diagnosis. In: Knowles DM, ed. *Neoplastic Hematopathology.* Baltimore: Williams and Wilkins; 1992:497–533.
16. Burkitt D. A sarcoma involving the jaws in African children. *Br J Surg* 1958;46:218–223.
17. Burkitt D, O'Conor GT. Malignant lymphoma in African children. I. A clinical syndrome. *Cancer* 1961;14:258–269.
18. Carbone PP, Kaplan HS, Musshoff K, Smithers DW, Tubiana M. Report of the committee on Hodgkin's disease staging classification. *Cancer Res* 1971;31:1860–1861.
19. Chan JK, Frizzera G, Fletcher CD, Rosai J. Primary vascular tumors of lymph nodes other than Kaposi's sarcoma. Analysis of 39 cases and delineation of two new entities. *Am J Surg Pathol* 1992;16:335–350.
20. Childs CC, Parham DM, Berard CW. Infectious mononucleosis. The spectrum of morphologic changes simulating lymphoma in lymph nodes and tonsils. *Am J Surg Pathol* 1987;11:122–132.
21. Chott A, Kaserer K, Augustin I, et al. Ki-1-positive large cell lymphoma. A clinicopathologic study of 41 cases. *Am J Surg Pathol* 1990;14:439–448.
22. Chu T, D'Angio GJ, Favara BE, Ladisch S, Nesbit M, Pritchard J. Histiocytosis syndromes in children. *Lancet* 1987;2:41–42.
23. Coles FB, Cartun RW, Pastuszak WT. Hodgkin's disease, lymphocyte-predominant type: immunoreactivity with B-cell antibodies. *Mod Pathol* 1988;1:274–278.
24. Cossman J, Berard CW. Histopathology of childhood non-Hodgkin's lymphomas. In: Graham-Pole J, ed. *Masson Monographs in Pediatric Hematology/Oncology: Non-Hodgkin's Lymphomas in Children.* New York: Masson; 1980:13–36.
25. Crist WM, Shuster JJ, Faletta J, et al. Clinical features and outcome in childhood T-cell leukemia-lymphoma according to stage of thymocyte differentiation. *Blood* 1988;72:1891–1897.
26. Davey FR, Hutchison RE. Pathology and immunology of adult T-cell leukemia/lymphoma. *Curr Opin Oncol* 1991;3:13–20.
27. Davis RE, Warnke RA, Dorfman RF. Inflammatory pseudotumor of lymph nodes. Additional observations and evidence for an inflammatory etiology. *Am J Surg Pathol* 1991;15:744–756.
28. De Almeida PC, Harris NL, Bhan AK. Characterization of immature sinus histiocytes (monocytoid cells) in reactive lymph nodes by use of monoclonal antibodies. *Hum Pathol* 1984;15: 330–335.
29. de Mascarel I, Trojani M, Eghbali H, Coindre JM, Bonichon F. Prognostic value of phenotyping by Ber-H2, Leu-M1, EMA in Hodgkin's disease. *Arch Pathol Lab Med* 1990;114:953–955.
30. Delannoy A, Philippe M, Hamels J, Beauduin M. Clonal rearrangement of the T-cell receptor beta-chain gene in the pleural fluid of a patient with thymoma. *Nouv Rev Fr Hematol* 1993;35: 121–124.
31. Delia D, Polli N, Borrello MG, et al. Mixed-lineage leukemias and phenotypic shifts occurring in relapsed cases of acute T lymphoblastic lymphomas. *Leukemia* 1988;2:192S–197S.
32. Donaldson SS. Hodgkin's disease in children. [Review]. *Semin Oncol* 1990;17:736–748.
33. Dorfman RF. Classification of non-Hodgkin's lymphomas. *Lancet* 1974;2:961–962.
34. Dorfman RF. Necrotising lymphadenitis without granulocytic infiltration (Kikuchi's disease). *J Clin Pathol* 1986;39:811–812.
35. Dorfman RF. Histiocytic necrotizing lymphadenitis of Kikuchi and Fujimoto. *Arch Pathol Lab Med* 1987;111:1026–1029.
36. Dorfman RF, Berry GJ. Kikuchi's histiocytic necrotizing lymphadenitis: an analysis of 108 cases with emphasis on differential diagnosis. *Semin Diag Pathol* 1988;5:329–345.

37. Eisen RN, Buckley PJ, Rosai J. Immunophenotypic characterization of sinus histiocytosis with massive lymphadenopathy (Rosai-Dorfman disease). *Semin Diag Pathol* 1990;7:74–82.
38. Epstein MA, Achang BG, Barr YM. Virus particles in cultured lymphoblasts from Burkitt's lymphoma. *Lancet* 1964;702–703.
39. Facchetti F, De Wolf Peeters C, De Wever I, Frizzera G. Inflammatory pseudotumor of lymph nodes. Immunohistochemical evidence for its fibrohistiocytic nature. *Am J Pathol* 1990;137:281–289.
40. Favara BE, McCarthy RC, Mierau GW. Histiocytosis X. In: Finegold M, Bennington JL, eds. *Pathology of Neoplasia in Children and Adolescents.* Philadelphia: WB Saunders; 1986:126–144.
41. Ferry JA, Linggood RM, Convery KM, Efird JT, Eliseo R, Harris NL. Hodgkin disease, nodular sclerosis type. Implications of histologic subclassification. *Cancer* 1993;71:457–463.
42. Fletcher CD, Stirling RW. Intranodal myofibroblastoma presenting in the submandibular region: evidence of a broader clinical and histological spectrum. *Histopathology* 1990;16:287–293.
43. Foucar E, Rosai J, Dorfman R. Sinus histiocytosis with massive lymphadenopathy (Rosai–Dorfman disease): review of the entity. *Semin Diag Pathol* 1990;7:19–73.
44. Friedman HD, Inman DA, Hutchison RE, Poiesz BJ. Concurrent invasive thymoma and T-cell lymphoblastic leukemia and lymphoma. A case report with necropsy findings and literature review of thymoma and associated hematologic neoplasm. *Am J Clin Pathol* 1994;101:432–437.
45. Frizzera G. Castleman's disease and related disorders. *Semin Diag Pathol* 1988;5:346–364.
46. Frizzera G, Murphy SB. Follicular (nodular) lymphoma in childhood: a rare clinical-pathological entity. Report of eight cases from four cancer centers. *Cancer* 1979;44:2218–2235.
47. Giesker DW, Pastuszak WT, Farquar FA, et al. Lymph node biopsy for early diagnosis in Kawasaki disease. *Am J Surg Pathol* 1982;6:493–501.
48. Gordon BG, Weisenburger DD, Warkentin PI, et al. Peripheral T-cell lymphoma in childhood and adolescence. A clinicopathologic study of 22 patients. *Cancer* 1993;71:257–263.
49. Grier HE, Civin CI. Acute and chronic myeloproliferative disorders and myelodysplasia. In: Nathan DG, Oski FA, eds. *Hematology of Infancy and Childhood.* Philadelphia: WB Saunders; 1992:1288–1317.
50. Griffith RC, Kelly DR, Nathwani BN, et al. A morphologic study of childhood lymphoma of the lymphoblastic type. The Pediatric Oncology Group experience. *Cancer* 1987;59:1126–1131.
51. Grogan TM. Hodgkin's disease. In: Jaffe ES, ed. *Surgical Pathology of the Lymph Nodes and Related Organs.* Philadelphia: WB Saunders; 1995:133–192.
52. Grogan TM, Warnke RA, Kaplan HS. A comparative study of Burkitt's and non-Burkitt's "undifferentiated" malignant lymphoma: immunologic, cytochemical, ultrastructural, cytologic, histopathologic, clinical and cell culture features. *Cancer* 1982;49:1817–1828.
53. Grufferman S, Delzell E. Epidemiology of Hodgkin's disease. *Epidemiol Rev* 1984;6:76–106.
54. Haferkamp O, Rosenau W, Lennert K. Vascular transformation of lymph node sinuses due to venous obstruction. *Arch Pathol* 1971;92:81–83.
55. Hamoudi AB, Newton WA Jr, Mancer K, Penn GM. Thymic changes in histiocytosis. *Am J Clin Pathol* 1982;77:169–173.
56. Hanchard B, LaGrenade L, Carberry C, et al. Childhood infective dermatitis evolving into adult T-cell leukaemia after 17 years. *Lancet* 1991;338:1593–1594.
57. Hansen H, Lemke H, Bredfeldt G, Konnecke I, Havsteen B. The Hodgkin-associated Ki-1 antigen exists in an intracellular and a membrane-bound form. *Biol Chem Hoppe Seyler* 1989;370:409–416.
58. Harris NL, Jaffe ES, Stein H, et al. A revised European–American classification of lymphoid neoplasms: A proposal from the international lymphoma study group. *Blood* 1994;84:1361–1392.
59. Harrist TJ, Bhan AK, Murphy GF, et al. Histiocytosis-X: in situ characterization of cutaneous infiltrates with monoclonal antibodies. *Am J Clin Pathol* 1983;79:294–300.
60. Herbst H, Pallesen G, Weiss LM, et al. Hodgkin's disease and Epstein–Barr virus. *Ann Oncol* 1992;3 (Suppl 4):27–30.
61. Herbst H, Stein H. Tumor viruses in CD30-positive anaplastic large cell lymphomas. *Leuk Lymphoma* 1993;9:321–328.
62. Herbst H, Stein H, Niedobitek G. Epstein–Barr virus and CD30-malignant lymphomas. *Crit Rev Oncog* 1993;4:191–239.
63. Herbst H, Steinbrecher E, Niedobitek G, et al. Distribution and phenotype of Epstein–Barr virus-harboring cells in Hodgkin's disease. *Blood* 1992;80:484–491.
64. Hodgkin T. On some morbid appearances of the absorbent glands and spleen. *Trans Med Chir Soc Lond* 1832;17:68.
65. Hsu SM, Ho YS, Hsu PL. Lymphomas of true histiocytic origin. Expression of different phenotypes in so-called true histiocytic lymphoma and malignant histiocytosis. *Am J Pathol* 1991;138:1389–1404.
66. Hutchison RE, Fairclough DL, Holt H, Pui CH, Sandlund JT, Berard CW. Clinical significance of histology and immunophenotype in childhood diffuse large cell lymphoma. *Am J Clin Pathol* 1991;95:787–793.
67. Hutchison RE, Kurec AS, Davey FR. Granulocytic sarcoma. *Clin Lab Med* 1990;10:889–901.
68. Hutchison RE, Murphy SB, Fairclough DL, et al. Diffuse small noncleaved cell lymphoma in children, Burkitt's versus non-Burkitt's types. Results from the Pediatric Oncology Group and St. Jude Children's Research Hospital. *Cancer* 1989;64:23–28.
69. Hutchison RE, Pui CH, Murphy SB, Berard CW. Non-Hodgkin's lymphoma in children younger than 3 years. *Cancer* 1988;62:1371–1373.
70. Hvizdala EV, Berard C, Callihan T, et al. Lymphoblastic lymphoma in children—a randomized trial comparing LSA2-L2 with the A-COP- therapeutic regimen: a Pediatric Oncology Group Study. *J Clin Oncol* 1988;6:26–33.
71. Ichikawa Y, Shimizu H, Yoshida M, Arimori S. Two-color flow cytometric analysis of thymic lymphocytes from patients with myasthenia gravis and/or thymoma. *Clin Immunol Immunopathol* 1992;62:91–96.
72. Inghirami G, Knowles DM. The immune system: structure and function. In: Knowles D, ed. *Neoplastic Hematopathology.* Baltimore: Williams and Wilkins; 1993:27–72.
73. Jackson H Jr, Parker F Jr. *Hodgkin's Disease and Allied Disorders.* New York: Oxford University Press; 1947.
74. Jaffe ES, Berard CW. Lymphoblastic lymphoma, a term rekindled with new precision. *Ann Intern Med* 1978;89:415–417.
75. Jaffe R. Pathology of histiocytosis X. *Perspect Ped Pathol* 1987;9:4–47.
76. Kadin ME. Hodgkin's disease: immunobiology and pathogenesis. In: Knowles D, ed. *Neoplastic Hematopathology.* Baltimore: Williams and Wilkins; 1991:535–553.
77. Kadin ME. Ki-1/CD30- (anaplastic) large-cell lymphoma: maturation of a clinicopathologic entity with prospects of effective therapy. *J Clin Oncol* 1994;12:884–887.
78. Kamps WA, Poppema S. Pre-B-cell non-Hodgkin's lymphoma in childhood. Report of a case and review of the literature. *Am J Clin Pathol* 1988;90:103–107.
79. Kaneko Y, Frizzera G, Shikano T, Kobayashi H, Maseki N, Sakurai M. Chromosomal and immunophenotypic patterns in T cell acute lymphoblastic leukemia (T ALL) and lymphoblastic lymphoma (LBL). *Leukemia* 1989;3:886–892.
80. Kaplinsky C, Mor C, Cohen IJ, et al. Childhood malignant thymoma: clinical, therapeutic, and immunohistochemical considerations. *Pediatr Hematol Oncol* 1992;9:261–268.
81. Kaudewitz P, Stein H, Dallenbach F, et al. Primary and secondary cutaneous Ki-1(CD30)-anaplastic large cell lymphomas. Morphologic, immunohistologic, and clinical-characteristics. *Am J Pathol* 1989;135:359–367.
82. Kelly DR, Nathwani BN, Griffith RC, et al. A morphologic study of childhood lymphoma of the undifferentiated type. The Pediatric Oncology Group experience. *Cancer* 1987;59:1132–1137.
83. Kim H, Jacobs C, Warnke RA, Dorfman RF. Malignant lymphoma with a high content of epithelioid histiocytes: a distinct clinicopathologic entity and a form of so-called "Lennert's lymphoma." *Cancer* 1978;41:620–635.
84. Kim H, Nathwani BN, Rappaport H. So-called "Lennert's lymphoma": is it a clinicopathologic entity? *Cancer* 1980;45:1379–1399.
85. Kjeldsberg CR, Wilson JF. Malignant lymphoma in children. In:

Finegold M, Bennington JL, eds. *Pathology of Neoplasia in Children and Adolescents.* Philadelphia: WB Saunders; 1986;87–108.
86. Kjeldsberg CR, Wilson JF, Berard CW. Non-Hodgkin's lymphoma in children. *Hum Pathol* 1983;14:612–627.
87. Knapp W, Dorken B, Gilks WR, et al. *Leukocyte Typing. vol 4. White Cell Differentiation Antigens.* Oxford: Oxford University Press; 1994.
88. Koo CH, Rappaport H, Sheibani K, Pangalis GA, Nathwani BN, Winberg C. Imprint cytology of non-Hodgkin's lymphomas based on a study of 212 immunologically characterized cases: correlation of touch imprints with tissue sections. *Hum Pathol* 1989;20:1–137.
89. Krishnan J, Wallberg K, Frizzera G. T-cell-rich large B-cell lymphoma. A study of 30 cases, supporting its histologic heterogeneity and lack of clinical distinctiveness. *Am J Surg Pathol* 1994;18: 455–465.
90. Kurec AS, Cruz VE, Barrett D, Mason DY, Davey FR. Immunophenotyping of acute leukemias using paraffin-embedded tissue sections. *Am J Clin Pathol* 1990;93:502–509.
91. Lee JY, Abell E, Shevechik GJ. Solitary spindle cell tumor with myoid differentiation of the lymph node. *Arch Pathol Lab Med* 1989;113:547–550.
92. Lennert K, Mohri N, Stein H, Kaiserling E. The histopathology of malignant lymphoma. *Br J Haematol* 1975;31(suppl):193–203.
93. Levine AM, Pavlova Z, Pockros AW, et al. Small noncleaved follicular center cell (FCC) lymphoma: Burkitt and non-Burkitt variants in the United States. I. Clinical features. *Cancer* 1983;52: 1073–1079.
94. Lichtenstein L. Histiocytosis X, integration of eosinophilic granuloma of bone, Letterer–Siwe disease and Schuller–Christian disease as related manifestations of a single nosologic entity. *Arch Pathol* 1953;56:84–102.
95. Link MP, Roper M, Dorfman RF, Crist WM, Cooper MD, Levy R. Cutaneous lymphoblastic lymphoma with pre-B markers. *Blood* 1983;61:838–841.
96. Lott MF, Davies JD. Lymph node hypervascularity: haemangiomatoid lesions and pan-nodal vasodilatation. *J Pathol* 1983;140: 209–219.
97. Lukes R, Butler JJ, Hicks EB. Natural history of Hodgkin's disease as related to its pathologic picture. *Cancer* 1966;19:317–344.
98. Lukes RJ, Butler JJ. The pathology and nomenclature of Hodgkin's disease. *Cancer Res* 1966;26:1063–1081.
99. Lukes RJ, Collins RD. Immunological characterization of human malignant lymphomas. *Cancer* 1974;34:1488–1503.
100. Lukes RJ, Collins RD. *Atlas of Tumor Pathology. Second series. Tumors of the Hematopoietic System.* Washington, D.C.: Armed Forces Institute of Pathology; 1992.
101. Lukes RJ, Craver LF, Hall TC, Rappaport H, Ruben P. Report of the nomenclature committee. *Cancer Res* 1966;26:1311.
102. Lydyard P, Grossi C. The lymphoid system. In: Roitt IM, Brostoff J, Male DK, eds. *Immunology.* London: CV Mosby; 1993:3.1–3.11.
103. Macon WR, Cousar JB, Waldron JA Jr, Hsu SM. Interleukin-4 may contribute to the abundant T-cell reaction and paucity of neoplastic B cells in T-cell-rich B-cell lymphomas. *Am J Pathol* 1992;141:1031–1036.
104. Macon WR, Rynalski TH, Swerdlow SH, Cousar JB. T-cell lymphoblastic leukemia/lymphoma presenting in a recurrent thymoma. *Mod Pathol* 1991;4:524–528.
105. Macon WR, Williams ME, Greer JP, Stein RS, Collins RD, Cousar JB. T-cell-rich B-cell lymphomas. A clinicopathologic study of 19 cases. *Am J Surg Pathol* 1992;16:351–363.
106. Magrath I. Historical perspective: the origins of modern concepts of biology and management. In: Magrath I, ed. *The non-Hodgkin's lymphomas.* Baltimore: Williams and Wilkins; 1990: 15–28.
107. McAlister WH, Herman T, Dehner LP. Sinus histiocytosis with massive lymphadenopathy (Rosai–Dorfman disease). *Pediatr Radiol* 1990;20:425–432.
108. McCabe RE, Brooks RG, Dorfman RF, Remington JS. Clinical spectrum in 107 cases of toxoplasmic lymphadenopathy. *Rev Infect Dis* 1987;9:754–774.
109. McKenna RW, Risdall RJ, Brunning RD. Virus associated hemophagocytic syndrome. *Hum Pathol* 1981;12:395–398.
110. Medeiros LJ, Bhagat SK, Naylor P, Fowler D, Jaffe ES. Malignant thymoma associated with T-cell lymphocytosis. A case report with immunophenotypic and gene rearrangement analysis. *Arch Pathol Lab Med* 1993;117:279–283.
111. Mierau GW, Favara BE, Brenman JM. Electron microscopy in histiocytosis X. *Ultrastruct Pathol* 1982;3:137–142.
112. Miettinen M. CD30 distribution. Immunohistochemical study on formaldehyde-fixed, paraffin-embedded Hodgkin's and non-Hodgkin's lymphomas. *Arch Pathol Lab Med* 1992;116:1197–1201.
113. Miliauskas JR, Berard CW, Young RC, Garvin AJ, Edwards BK, DeVita VTJ. Undifferentiated non-Hodgkin's lymphomas (Burkitt's and non-Burkitt's types). The relevance of making this histologic distinction. *Cancer* 1982;50:2115–2121.
114. Morgenthaler TI, Brown LR, Colby TV, Harper CM Jr, Coles DT. Thymoma. *Mayo Clin Proc* 1993;68:1110–1123.
115. Morris SW, Kirstein MN, Valentine MB, et al. Fusion of a kinase gene, ALK, to a nucleolar protein gene, NPM, in non-Hodgkin's lymphoma. *Science* 1994;263:1281–1284.
116. Murphy GF, Bhan AK, Sato S, Harrist TJ, Mihm MC Jr. Characterization of Langerhans cells by the use of monoclonal antibodies. *Lab Invest* 1981;45:465–468.
117. Murphy GF, Harrist TJ, Bhan AK, Mihm MC Jr. Distribution of cell surface antigens in histiocytosis X cells. Quantitative immunoelectron microscopy using monoclonal antibodies. *Lab Invest* 1983;48:90–97.
118. Murphy SB. Pediatric lymphomas: recent advances and commentary on Ki-1- positive anaplastic large-cell lymphomas of childhood. *Ann Oncol* 1994;5 (Suppl 1):S31–S33.
119. Murphy SB, Fairclough DL, Hutchison RE, Berard CW. Non-Hodgkin's lymphomas of childhood: an analysis of the histology, staging, and response to treatment of 338 cases at a single institution. *J Clin Oncol* 1989;7:186–193.
120. Nakahashi H, Maeo S, Osaki T, Dobashi K, Horiuchi Y, Miyazaki Y. Complete excision and panpleuropneumonectomy resulting in long-term survival for a teenager with invasive thymoma: report of a case. *Surg Today–Jap J Surg* 1992;22:558–560.
121. Nathwani BN, Brynes RK. Reactive immunoblastic proliferations. *Semin Diag Pathol* 1988;5:317–328.
122. Nathwani BN, Metter GE, Gams RA, et al. Malignant lymphoma, mixed cell type, diffuse. *Blood* 1983;62:200–208.
123. Neale AE, Menten ML. Tumors of the thymus in children. *Am J Dis Child* 1948;76:102.
124. Neri A, Barriga F, Inghirami G, et al. Epstein–Barr virus infection precedes clonal expansion in Burkitt's and acquired immunodeficiency syndrome–associated lymphoma. *Blood* 1991;77:1092–1095.
125. Nezelof C, Barbey S, Gogusev J, Terrier Lacombe MJ. Malignant histiocytosis in childhood: a distinctive CD30-positive clinicopathological entity associated with a chromosomal translocation involving 5q35. *Semin Diag Pathol* 1992;9:75–89.
126. Nicholas DS, Harris S, Wright DH. Lymphocyte predominance Hodgkin's disease—an immunohistochemical study. *Histopathology* 1990;16:157–165.
127. Niemeyer CM, Sallan SE. Acute lymphoblastic leukemia. In: Nathan DG, Oski FA, eds. *Hematology of Infancy and Childhood.* Philadelphia: WB Saunders; 1992:1249–1287.
128. Nonoyama M, Huang CH, Pagano JS, Klein G, Singh S. DNA of Epstein–Barr virus detected in tissue of Burkitt's lymphoma and nasopharyngeal carcinoma. *Proc Natl Acad Sci USA* 1973;70: 3265–3268.
129. Nosaka T, Ohno H, Doi S, et al. Phenotypic conversion of T lymphoblastic lymphoma to acute biphenotypic leukemia composed of lymphoblasts and myeloblasts. Molecular genetic evidence of the same clonal origin. *J Clin Invest* 1988;81:1824–1828.
130. O'Conor GT. Malignant lymphoma in African children. II. A pathological entity. *Cancer* 1961;14:270–283.
131. O'Conor GT, Davies JNP. Malignant tumors in African children. *J Pediatr* 1960;56:526.
132. O'Conor GT, Rappaport H, Smith EB. Childhood lymphoma resembling "Burkitt tumor" in the United States. *Cancer* 1965;18: 411–417.
133. Oliver JD, Grogan TM, Payne CM, Spier C, Richter LC, Rangel

CS. Burkitt's-like lymphoma of T-cell type. *Mod Pathol* 1988;1: 15–22.

134. Ornvold K, Carstensen H, Junge J, Gyhrs A, Ralfkiaer E. Tumours classified as "malignant histiocytosis" in children are T-cell neoplasms. *APMIS* 1992;100:558–566.

135. Ornvold K, Ralfkiaer E, Carstensen H. Immunohistochemical study of the abnormal cells in Langerhans cell histiocytosis (histiocytosis x). *Virchows Arch A Histopathol Anat* 1990;416:403–410.

136. Palestro G, Geuna M, Novero D, Godio L, Ciccone G, Azzoni L. Immunophenotype of thymoma-associated lymphoid cell component of T-cell type. A new analytic procedure in keeping with structural heterogeneities. *Virchows Arch B Cell Pathol* 1990;59: 297–304.

137. Pallesen G. The diagnostic significance of the CD30 (Ki-1) antigen. *Histopathology* 1990;16:409–413.

138. Paloczi K, Pocsik E, Kotlan B, Ujhelyi E, Timar L, Petranyi GG. The pattern of activation antigen expression on T-lymphocyte subpopulation in infectious mononucleosis. *Haematologia (Budap)* 1991;24:83–90.

139. Paulli M, Locatelli F, Kindl S, et al. Sinus histiocytosis with massive lymphoadenopathy (Rosai–Dorfman disease). Clinicopathological analysis of a paediatric case. *Eur J Pediatr* 1992;151: 672–675.

140. Pavlova Z, Parker JW, Taylor CR, Levine AM, Feinstein DI, Lukes RJ. Small noncleaved follicular center cell lymphoma: Burkitt's and non-Burkitt's variants in the US. II. Pathologic and immunologic features. *Cancer* 1987;59:1892–1902.

141. Perrone T, De Wolf-Peeters C, Frizzera G. Inflammatory pseudotumor of lymph nodes. A distinctive pattern of nodal reaction. *Am J Surg Pathol* 1988;12:351–361.

142. Pescarmona E, Giardini R, Brisigotti M, Callea F, Pisacane A, Baroni CD. Thymoma in childhood: a clinicopathological study of five cases. *Histopathology* 1992;21:65–68.

143. Peters MS, Thibodeau SN, White JW Jr, Winkelmann RK. Mycosis fungoides in children and adolescents. *J Am Acad Dermatol* 1990;22:1011–1018.

144. Pfreundschuh M, Pohl C, Berenbeck C, et al. Detection of a soluble form of the CD30 antigen in sera of patients with lymphoma, adult T-cell leukemia and infectious mononucleosis. *Int J Cancer* 1990;45:869–874.

145. Pinto A, Hutchison RE, Grant LH, Trevenen CL, Berard CW. Follicular lymphomas in pediatric patients. *Mod Pathol* 1990;3: 308–313.

146. Piris M, Brown DC, Gatter KC, Mason DY. CD30 expression in non-Hodgkin's lymphoma. *Histopathology* 1990;17:211–218.

147. Poppema S, Kaiserling E, Lennert K. Hodgkin's disease with lymphocytic predominance, nodular type (nodular paragranuloma) and progressively transformed germinal centres—a cytohistological study. *Histopathology* 1979;3:295–308.

148. Poppema S, Lennert K. Hodgkin's disease in childhood: histopathologic classification in relation to age and sex. *Cancer* 1980;45:1443–1447.

149. Ramon, Suster S. Primary thymic epithelial neoplasms in children. *Am J Surg Pathol* 1991;15:466–474.

150. Rappaport H. *Tumors of the Hematopoietic System.* Washington, D.C.: Armed Forces Institute of Pathology; 1966.

151. Reed DM. On the pathological changes in Hodgkin's disease with especial reference to its relation to tuberculosis. *Johns Hopkins Hosp Rep* 1902;10:133–196.

152. Reisman RP, Greco MA. Virus-associated hemophagocytic syndrome due to Epstein–Barr virus. *Hum Pathol* 1984;15:290–293.

153. Reiter A, Schrappe M, Tiemann M, et al. Successful treatment strategy for Ki-1 anaplastic large-cell lymphoma of childhood: a prospective analysis of 62 patients enrolled in three consecutive Berlin–Frankfurt–Munster group studies. *J Clin Oncol* 1994;12: 899–908.

154. Ribeiro RC, Pui CH, Murphy SB, et al. Childhood malignant non-Hodgkin lymphomas of uncommon histology. *Leukemia* 1992;6:761–765.

155. Rimokh R, Magaud JP, Berger F, et al. A translocation involving a specific breakpoint (q35) on chromosome 5 is characteristic of anaplastic large cell lymphoma ('Ki-1 lymphoma'). *Br J Haematol* 1989;71:31–36.

156. Risdall RJ, Brunning RD, Hernandez JI, Gordon DH. Bacteria-associated hemophagocytic syndrome. *Cancer* 1984;54:2968–2972.

157. Risdall RJ, McKenna RW, Nesbit ME, et al. Virus-associated hemophagocytic syndrome: a benign histiocytic proliferation distinct from malignant histiocytosis. *Cancer* 1979;44:993–1002.

158. Rodriguez J, Pugh WC, Cabanillas F. T-cell-rich B-cell lymphoma. *Blood* 1993;82:1586–1589.

159. Rohde D, Hansen H, Hafner M, et al. Cellular localizations and processing of the two molecular forms of the Hodgkin-associated Ki-1 (CD30) antigen. The protein kinase Ki-1/57 occurs in the nucleus. *Am J Pathol* 1992;140:473–482.

160. Rosai J. Mediastinum. In: Rosai J, ed. *Surgical Pathology.* St. Louis: CV Mosby; 1989:348–365.

161. Rosai J, Dorfman RF. Sinus histiocytosis with massive lymphadenopathy. A newly recognized benign clinicopathological entity. *Arch Pathol* 1969;87:63–70.

162. Rosai J, Dorfman RF. Sinus histiocytosis with massive lymphadenopathy: a pseudolymphomatous benign disorder. Analysis of 34 cases. *Cancer* 1972;30:1174–1188.

163. Roulet F. Das primare retothelsarkom der lymphknoten. *Virchows Arch* 1930;277:15.

164. Ruco LP, Stoppacciaro A, Vitolo D, Uccini S, Baroni CD. Expression of adhesion molecules in Langerhans' cell histiocytosis. *Histopathology* 1993;23:29–37.

165. Salisbury JR. Castleman's disease in childhood and adolescence: report of a case and review of literature. *Pediatr Pathol* 1995;10(4):609–615.

166. Sander CA, Jaffe ES, Gebhardt FC, Yano T, Medeiros LJ. Mediastinal lymphoblastic lymphoma with an immature B-cell immunophenotype. *Am J Surg Pathol* 1992;16:300–305.

167. Sandlund JT, Hutchison RE, Crist WM. Non-Hodgkin's Lymphoma. In: Fernbach DJ, Vietti TJ, eds. *Clinical Pediatric Oncology.* 1991;337–354.

168. Sandlund JT, Pui C-H, Santana VM, et al. Clinical features and treatment outcome for children with CD30+ large-cell non-Hodgkin's lymphoma. *J Clin Oncol* 1994;12:895–898.

169. Sandlund JT, Santana V, Abromowitch M, et al. Large cell non-Hodgkin lymphoma of childhood: clinical characteristics and outcome. *Leukemia* 1994;8:30–34.

170. Sauter ER, Sardi A, Hollier LH, Cooper ES, Bolton JS. Prognostic value of DNA flow cytometry in thymomas and thymic carcinomas. *South Med J* 1990;83:656–659.

171. Schouten HC, Sanger WG, Weisenburger DD, Armitage JO. Chromosomal abnormalities in patients with non-cutaneous T-cell non-Hodgkin's lymphoma. The Nebraska Lymphoma Study Group. *Eur J Cancer* 1990;26:618–622.

172. Schwob C, Stein H, Gerdes J, et al. Production of a monoclonal antibody specific for Hodgkin and Sternberg–Reed cells of Hodgkin's disease and a subset of normal lymphoid cells. *Nature* 1982;299:65–67.

173. Scott RB, Robb-Smith AHT. Histiocytic medullary reticulosis. *Lancet* 1939;2:194–198.

174. Shapiro PE, Pinto FJ. The histologic spectrum of mycosis fungoides/Sezary syndrome (cutaneous T-cell lymphoma). A review of 222 biopsies, including newly described patterns and the earliest pathologic changes. *Am J Surg Pathol* 1994;18:645–667.

175. Shaver EG, Rebsamen SL, Yachnis AT, Sutton LN. Isolated extranodal intracranial sinus histiocytosis in a 5-year- old boy. Case report. *J Neurosurg* 1993;79:769–773.

176. Sheibani K, Nathwani BN, Winberg CD, et al. Antigenically defined subgroups of lymphoblastic lymphoma. Relationship to clinical presentation and biologic behavior. *Cancer* 1987;60:183–190.

177. Shikano T, Ishikawa Y, Naito H, Kobayashi R, Nakadate H, Hatae Y. Cytogenetic characteristics of childhood non-Hodgkin lymphoma. *Cancer* 1992;70:714–719.

178. Smith CA, Gruss HJ, Davis T, et al. CD30 antigen, a marker for Hodgkin's lymphoma, is a receptor whose ligand defines an emerging family of cytokines with homology to TNF. *Cell* 1993;73:1349–1360.

179. Smith JL, Barker CR, Clein GP, Collins RD. Characterisation of malignant mediastinal lymphoid neoplasm (Sternberg sarcoma) as thymic in origin. *Lancet* 1973;1:74–77.

180. Spigland N, Di Lorenzo M, Youssef S, Russo P, Brandt M. Malignant thymoma in children: a 20-year review. *J Pediatr Surg* 1990;25:1143–1146.
181. Stansfeld AG, Diebold J, Noel H, et al. Updated Kiel classification for lymphomas. *Lancet* 1988;1:292–293.
182. Stein H, Dallenbach F. Diffuse large cell lymphomas of B and T cell type. In: Knowles DM, ed. *Neoplastic Hematopathology.* Baltimore: Williams and Wilkins; 1992:675–714.
183. Stein H, Handsman ML, Lennert K, Brandtzaeg P, Gatter KC, Mason DY. Reed-Sternberg and Hodgkin cells in lymphocyte-predominant Hodgkin's disease of nodular subtype contain J chain. *Am J Clin Pathol* 1986;86:292–297.
184. Stein H, Herbst H, Anagnostopoulos I, Niedobitek G, Dallenbach F, Kratzsch HC. The nature of Hodgkin and Reed–Sternberg cells, their association with EBV, and their relationship to anaplastic large-cell lymphoma. *Ann Oncol* 1991;2 (Suppl 2): 33–38.
185. Stein H, Mason DY, Gerdes J, et al. The expression of the Hodgkin's disease associated antigen Ki-1 in reactive and neoplastic lymphoid tissue: evidence that Reed–Sternberg cells and histiocytic malignancies are derived from activated lymphoid cells. *Blood* 1985;66:848–858.
186. Sternberg C. Uber eine eigenartige unter dem Bilde der Pseudoleukamie verlaufende Tuberculose des lymphatischen Apparates. *Ztschr Heilk* 1898;19:21–90.
187. Strickler JG, Michie SA, Warnke RA, Dorfman RF. The "syncytial variant" of nodular sclerosing Hodgkin's disease. *Am J Surg Pathol* 1986;10:470–477.
188. Stroup R, Sheibani K, Misset JL, Szekely AM, Tremblay G, Rappaport H. Surface immunoglobulin-positive lymphoblastic lymphoma. A report of three cases. *Cancer* 1990;65:2559–2563.
189. Suchi T, Lennert K, Tu LY, et al. Histopathology and immunohistochemistry of peripheral T cell lymphomas: a proposal for their classification. *J Clin Pathol* 1987;40:995–1015.
190. Sullivan JL, Woda BA. Lymphohistiocytic disorders. In: Nathan DG, Oski FR, eds. *Hematology of Infancy and Childhood.* Philadelphia: WB Saunders; 1992:1354–1374.
191. Suster S, Rosai J. Intranodal hemorrhagic spindle-cell tumor with "amianthoid" fibers. Report of six cases of a distinctive mesenchymal neoplasm of the inguinal region that simulates Kaposi's sarcoma. *Am J Surg Pathol* 1989;13:347–357.
192. Symmers D. Follicular lymphadenopathy with splenomegaly: A newly recognized disease of the lymphatic system. *Arch Pathol* 1927;3:816.
193. Tan CTC. Hodgkin's disease in children and adolescents: experiences from the Memorial Sloan-Kettering Cancer Center, New York. In: Kamps WA, Humphrey GB, Poppema S, eds. *Hodgkin's Disease in Children: Controversies and Current Experience.* Boston: Kluwer Academic; 1989:291–302.
194. Thirman MJ, Gill HJ, Burnett RC, et al. Rearrangement of the MLL gene in acute lymphoblastic and acute myeloid leukemias with 11q23 chromosomal translocations. *N Engl J Med* 1993; 329:909–914.
195. Thompson EI. Hodgkin's disease. In: Fernbach DJ, Vietti TJ, eds. *Clinical Pediatric Oncology.* St. Louis: Mosby Year Book; 1991;1:355–375.
196. Trinchieri G. The hematopoietic system and hematopoiesis. In: Knowles D, ed. *Neoplastic Hematopathology.* Baltimore: Williams and Wilkins; 1993:1–25.
197. Tsang WY, Chan JK. Bacillary angiomatosis. A "new" disease with a broadening clinicopathologic spectrum. *Histol Histopathol* 1992;7:143–152.
198. Tsuji M, Kobashi A, Hashimoto K, et al. A case of adult T-cell leukemia/lymphoma, histologically presenting CD30-positive large cell lymphoma. *Acta Pathol Jpn* 1992;42:512–517.
199. Virchow RLK. *Die krankhaftern geschwue.* Berlin: Hirschwald; 1863.
200. Virchow RLK. *Die cellularpathologie in irher begrueudung auf physiologische und pathologische gewebelehre.* Berlin: Hirschwald; 1868.
201. Walker AN, Mills SE, Fechner RE. Thymomas and thymic carcinomas. *Semin Diag Pathol* 1990;7:250–265.
202. Weinreb M, Day PJ, Murray PG, et al. Epstein-Barr virus (EBV) and Hodgkin's disease in children: incidence of EBV latent membrane protein in malignant cells. *J Pathol* 1992;168:365–369.
203. Weiss LM, Bindl JM, Picozzi VJ, Link MP, Warnke RA. Lymphoblastic lymphoma: an immunophenotype study of 26 cases with comparison to T cell acute lymphoblastic leukemia. *Blood* 1986;67:474–478.
204. Weiss LM, Chen Y-Y, Liu XF, Shibata D. Epstein–Barr virus and Hodgkin's disease: a correlative in situ hybridization and polymerase chain reaction study. *Am J Pathol* 1991;139:1259–1265.
205. Weiss LM, Strickler JG, Medeiros LJ, Gerdes J, Stein H, Warnke RA. Proliferative rates of non-Hodgkin's lymphomas as assessed by Ki-67 antibody. *Hum Pathol* 1987;18:1155–1159.
206. Weiss SW, Gnepp DR, Bratthauer GL. Palisaded myofibroblastoma. A benign mesenchymal tumor of lymph node. *Am J Surg Pathol* 1989;13:341–346.
207. Wilks S. Cases of enlargement of the lymphatic glands and spleen, (or, Hodgkin's disease), with remarks. *Guys Hosp Rep* 1865;11: 56–67.
208. Wilson JF, Kjeldsberg CR, Sposto R, et al. The pathology of non-Hodgkin's lymphoma of childhood: II. Reproducibility and relevance of the histologic classification of "undifferentiated" lymphomas (Burkitt's versus non-Burkitt's). *Hum Pathol* 1987;18: 1008–1014.
209. Wilson MS, Weiss LM, Gatter KC, Mason DY, Dorfman RF, Warnke RA. Malignant histiocytosis. A reassessment of cases previously reported in 1975 based on paraffin section immunophenotyping studies. *Cancer* 1990;66:530–536.
210. Wright DH. Pathogenesis of non-Hodgkin's lymphoma: clues from geography. In: Magrath IT, ed. *The Non-Hodgkin's Lymphomas.* Baltimore: Williams and Wilkins; 1990:122–134.
211. Writing committee. National Cancer Institute sponsored study of classifications of non-Hodgkin's lymphomas; summary and description of a working formulation for clinical usage. *Cancer* 1982;49:2112–2135.
212. Yano T, van Krieken JH, Magrath IT, Longo DL, Jaffe ES, Raffeld M. Histogenetic correlations between subcategories of small noncleaved cell lymphomas. *Blood* 1992;79:1282–1290.
213. Ye F, Huang SW, Dong HJ. Histiocytosis X. S-100 protein, peanut agglutinin, and transmission electron microscopy study. *Am J Clin Pathol* 1990;94:627–631.
214. Zaatari GS, Chan WC, Kim TH, Williams DL, Kletzel M. Malignant lymphoma of the skin in children. *Cancer* 1987;59:1040–1045.

Subject Index

Subject Index

K

L

ISBN 0-7817-0273-9